AF616524

Ultrasonography in Vascular Diagnosis

Wilhelm Schäberle

Ultrasonography in Vascular Diagnosis

A Therapy-Oriented Textbook and Atlas

Third Edition

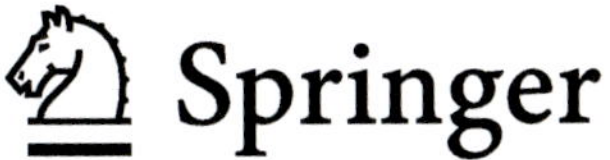

Wilhelm Schäberle
Department of Visceral, Vascular, Thoracic, and Pediatric Surgery
Alb Fils Kliniken
Göppingen, Germany

Translated by Bettina Herwig
Berlin, Germany

The Work was first pulished in 2016 by Springer-Verlag GmbH with the following title: Ultraschall in der Gefäßdiagnostik, 4. Auflage. © Springer-Verlag Berlin Heidelberg 2016

ISBN 978-3-319-64996-2 ISBN 978-3-319-64997-9 (eBook)
https://doi.org/10.1007/978-3-319-64997-9

Library of Congress Control Number: 2018954360

Printed on acid-free paper

This Springer imprint is published by the registered company Springer International Publishing AG part of Springer Nature
The registered company address is: Gewerbestrasse 11, 6330 Cham, Switzerland

To my wife Solange and my children Jan and Philip

Preface to the Third English and Fourth German Edition

The third English edition of this textbook continues to promote the ultrasound philosophy already advocated by its successful predecessors. A brief outline is provided in the earlier prefaces, particularly that of the second English edition (third German edition). This new edition discusses the latest scientific insights, and the Atlas part has been supplemented by new instructive teaching cases. As before, the author attaches great importance to the therapeutic consequences that derive from abnormal ultrasound findings. The basic principle behind this approach is that the patient's clinical findings, in conjunction with the available therapeutic options, should guide the ultrasound examination. This principle also underlies the diagnostic algorithms proposed in this book and aims at providing detailed, highly resolved information on vascular pathology in a time-efficient examination. Individual treatment can thus be planned on the basis of the sonographic findings, and many patients do not need additional imaging tests. Such algorithms are presented for the sonographic evaluation of patients with a hemodialysis access fistula, the diagnosis of PAOD, the ultrasound examination of the carotid arteries, sonographic follow-up after stenting, and the diagnostic assessment and measurement of abdominal aortic aneurysm. Supplementary sonographic options such as contrast-enhanced ultrasound are discussed in greater detail and illustrated with figures to show their potential but also their limitations.

A patient's clinical symptoms are not only due to morphologic vascular changes but are primarily the consequence of pathological and in part intricate hemodynamic changes, which are best captured in the Doppler waveform. New case examples and drawings have been added to teach readers how to interpret Doppler waveforms and make the most of what they can tell us about the underlying vascular disease.

Recent scientific study results are discussed paying special attention to their value for the clinician and discussing differences among the various imaging modalities used for vascular diagnosis and discrepancies between the results of published ultrasound studies. In his critical appraisal, the author points out the strengths and weaknesses of the different methods, explaining discrepancies in terms of different study designs, underlying physical principles, and the laws of hemodynamics.

The author wishes to thank Dr. Rupp-Heim and Dr. Knödler, who provided radiological images for comparison with ultrasound findings, and Dr. Meinrenken for editorial assistance and other support throughout this project. Many thanks are also due to Ms. Herwig for her expert translation and tremendous support in preparing the new English version. Last but not least, I would like to express my thanks to the publishers, Springer-Verlag, and in particular to Mr. Quinones, Dr. Heilmann, Mr. Bachem, and Ms. Beisel, for their cooperation in preparing the new German and English editions of this textbook.

A final word belongs to my family. A project of this kind means less time spent as a family, and I therefore dedicate this edition to my wife and children.

Wilhelm Schäberle
Göppingen, Germany
November 2017

Preface to the Second English and Third German Edition

The longer and the more intensively one has been working with medical imaging, the more questions of a broader, more general kind one is confronted with: How well does the image represent the truth? Can our interpretation of the imaging findings explain the patient's disease? Which imaging appearances mean that the patient requires treatment, and if so, which treatment? When does imaging (including incidental findings) lead to unnecessary interventions – due to users not being aware of the intrinsic problems of a diagnostic method or failing to take its inherent limitations into account? These issues are relevant for all diagnostic modalities, including the traditional gold standard of angiography and more recent developments such as magnetic resonance and computed tomography angiography. Applied to diagnostic ultrasonography, the more specific question that arises is how we misinterpret echo patterns or ultrasound features and consequently make erroneous treatment decisions. These problems become particularly manifest when dealing with the morphology of internal carotid artery plaque, where the sonographic appearance of the plaque may be used as a criterion for making treatment recommendations. In the name of scientific rigor investigators sometimes end up focusing too heavily on a single aspect of a complex problem, in turn giving rise to specific assumptions and hypotheses that affect the study design and ultimately lead to wrong, contradictory, and biased results, as well as to the wrong therapeutic conclusions. Despite these cautionary remarks, however, there is good scientific evidence that vascular duplex ultrasonography – as long as both the morphologic appearance and hemodynamic findings are taken into account and as long as the examiner remains critically aware of the methodological basis – comes very close to depicting the true clinical situation in patients with vascular disease. Although somewhat neglected by some "schools of ultrasound," where color flow images (which are more angiography-like) are preferred, spectral Doppler analysis can provide some very valuable information. In particular it can depict the hemodynamic situation (in both normal and diseased vessels) with excellent sensitivity, making it highly useful in the diagnostic assessment of vascular disease and in solving problems of differential diagnosis.

In terms of method and didactic approach this second English edition continues in the tradition of the earlier German editions and of the first English edition and emphasizes the therapeutic relevance of the diagnostic measures being taken. For details on this approach please refer to the earlier prefaces. Staying in the same pedagogical vein but seeking to advance this method further, this extensively revised edition incorporates even more diagrams and tables. The hope is that this will help make examination protocols and complex diagnostic procedures even easier to visualize and understand. This new edition presents the most recent scientific insights as well as new developments in ultrasound technology, which are discussed with regard to their role in providing therapeutically relevant diagnostic information for treating patients with vascular disease. On points where there is no clear consensus regarding the diagnostic status of certain ultrasound features and findings, these controversies are discussed. The atlas sections of the individual chapters have also been expanded to include even more examples of ultrasound findings obtained in the routine clinical setting, along with examples of less common vascular diseases. A focus here is on showing the reader how to interpret Doppler waveforms and how to use the hemodynamic information to help make a diagnosis. As a little cultural aside, color flow ultrasound can also be counted on to produce images with highly artistic color compositions. My 4-year-old son's comment, upon seeing the proofs of the book, was, "Your new art book is really beautiful."

The author would like to thank Ms Zorn, Ms Rieker, Ms Mehlbeer, and Ms Lietz for secretarial assistance. My thanks are also due to Ms Mütschele for her support in preparing the diagrams and figures. Thank you also to Ms Herwig for the translation and excellent support through all stages of preparing this English edition. Further, I would like to thank the staff of Springer-Verlag for their excellent support in preparing this new edition, particularly Ms Heilmann and Mr Bachem. Most of all, however, I would like to thank my family for their patience and understanding and for the humor that is necessary and makes it easier to pull off a project like this.

Wilhelm Schäberle
Göppingen, Germany
November 2010

Preface to the First English Edition

Vascular ultrasonography becomes increasingly valuable the more the diagnostic query to be answered is based on the clinical findings and the more the examination is performed with regard to its therapeutic consequences. As with other specialties that make use of ultrasound findings, the diagnostic yield of vascular ultrasound relies crucially on the close integration of the examination into the routine of the clinician or physician treating the patient. That is why in the German-speaking countries, vascular ultrasound is chiefly performed by angiologists and vascular surgeons. Duplex ultrasound can indeed be regarded as an integral component of the angiologic examination or an extension of the clinical examination by fairly simple technical means. Thus the sonographic findings do not simply supplement other imaging modalities but, together with the clinical findings, provide the basis for deciding whether medical therapy, a radiologic intervention, or surgical reconstruction is the most suitable therapy for an individual patient. This means that in a patient with atherosclerotic occlusive disease of the leg arteries, the patient's clinical presentation determines whether or not surgical repair is necessary, while the duplex sonographic findings serve to plan the kind of repair required and to confirm the localization and extent of the vascular pathology suspected on clinical grounds. Up to this point, no invasive diagnostic tests are needed. Angiography continues to have a role in planning the details of the surgical procedure, i.e., identification of a suitable recipient vessel for a bypass graft. Some surgical procedures such as thromboendarterectomy of the carotid arteries or femoral bifurcation can be performed without prior angiography, which does not provide any additional information that would affect the surgical strategy. Duplex sonography has evolved into the gold standard for answering most queries pertaining to venous conditions (therapeutic decision-making in thrombosis, planning of the surgical intervention for varicosis, chronic venous insufficiency).

Special emphasis is placed on the therapy-oriented presentation of indications for vascular ultrasonography, including the sonographic differentiation of rare vascular pathology and the role of the ultrasound examination in conjunction with the patient's clinical findings. The abundant images provided are intended to facilitate morphologic and hemodynamic vascular evaluation and put the reader in a position to become more confident in identifying rare conditions as well, which often have a characteristic appearance and are thus recognizable at a glance. The high acceptance of the diagnostic concept advocated here as reflected in the success of the first two editions of the book in the German-speaking countries led to the decision to have an English edition. I would like to thank Springer-Verlag, in particular Dr. Heilmann, for making this English edition possible.

Wilhelm Schäberle
Göppingen, Germany
August 2005

Preface to the Second German Edition

Vascular duplex sonography is the continuation of the clinical examination of vascular disease by fairly simple technical means. A sonographic examination relies on interaction with the patient and is guided by the clinical findings, therapeutic relevance, and treatment options available. It is highly examiner-dependent and does not easily lend itself to full documentation of the results, which are thus difficult to communicate and verify. For these reasons, sonographers require thorough training, both to avoid inaccurate findings with disastrous consequences for patients and in order not to discredit the method.

The format of the first edition with a text section and an atlas for each vascular territory has been retained as has the subdivision of the individual chapters into sections on sonoanatomy, examination technique, normal findings, abnormal ultrasound findings, and diagnostic role of the sonographic findings. Given the special focus of this textbook on clinically and therapeutically relevant aspects of vascular ultrasonography, each of the main chapters (peripheral arteries and veins, extracranial arteries supplying the brain, hemodialysis shunts, and abdominal and retroperitoneal vessels) has been supplemented with a section on the clinical significance of ultrasound examinations in the respective vascular territory. This addition was considered necessary in order to do justice to the expanding and changing role of diagnostic ultrasound since the first German edition 6 years ago. While until only a few years ago vascular ultrasound was used for orientation or served as a supplementary diagnostic test only, it has since evolved into a key modality in this field. It has since even become a kind of gold standard in the diagnostic evaluation of veins, in particular in patients with thrombosis and varicosis. In this setting, venography has lost its significance and its use is now restricted to exceptional cases where it serves to obtain supplementary information to answer specific questions.

In patients with arterial disease, duplex ultrasound is an integral part of the step-by-step diagnostic workup. The sonographic findings provide the key to adequate therapeutic management (medical therapy, radiologic intervention, or vascular surgical repair). Together with the patient's clinical status, duplex sonography is thus decisive for establishing the indication for medical therapy or invasive vascular reconstruction. Duplex sonography has replaced angiography in the localization of a vascular obstruction and the evaluation of its significance. The invasive radiologic modality is used only to identify a suitable recipient segment in patients scheduled for a bypass procedure or in combination with a catheter-based intervention (PTA and stenting). The morphologic information provided on the vessel lumen and wall as well as on perivascular structures makes nonatherosclerotic vascular disorders a domain of ultrasound.

Ultrasonography is the method of first choice in evaluating carotid artery stenoses for stroke prevention by identifying those patients who would benefit from surgical repair on the basis of hemodynamic parameters but also taking into account morphologic information. Ultrasound can retain its central role in therapeutic decision-making only if its advantages are fully exploited, which means that the examination should be performed by the angiologist or vascular surgeon who is also treating the patient. This is why this second edition is again intended mainly for angiologists and vascular surgeons.

The revised edition also describes recent developments such as the use of ultrasound contrast media, or echo enhancers, in angiology and the B-flow mode although their role in the routine clinical setting is small from the angiologist's and vascular surgeon's perspective. The use of ultrasound contrast media in differentiating liver tumors is not dealt with in detail since it is mainly of interest to gastroenterologists and visceral surgeons and would therefore go beyond the scope of this textbook.

As in the first edition, great care was taken in selecting illustrative ultrasound scans of high quality for the atlas, following the motto "an ultrasound image must speak for itself". The sonomorphologic context is important for didactic purposes; that is why the pathology of interest is not shown in a magnified view (zoom) but presented in the constellation in which it appears in the course of a routine examination. In those settings where the sonication conditions are poor but an ultrasound examination nevertheless appears to be indicated from a clinical perspective as in postoperative patients, the examples shown were not selected specifically but are such as illustrate this fact. Angiograms, and in individual cases graphic representations, are intended to clarify the situation.

The abundant images contained in the atlas sections reflect the intention not only to present abnormal finding as such but to illustrate more clearly situations that are relevant from a therapeutic perspective and to also show the development of vascular pathology. Adhering to the ultrasound convention of depicting cranial on the left side of the image and caudal on the right, the blood flow direction is color coded in accordance with the defaults settings of the ultrasound equipment. This means, for instance, that the internal carotid artery is coded in blue, indicating arterial blood flow away from the transducer. Following this convention, it is thus not necessary to first have to look for the color key, and orientation is facilitated when complex vascular territories such as the abdominal and retroperitoneal vessels are examined.

The detailed introduction to the fundamental physical principles of diagnostic ultrasound and basic hemodynamics under normal and abnormal conditions as well as the detailed description of vascular anatomy, examination protocols, and of the interpretation of the findings aim at providing the beginner with an introduction to vascular ultrasound. It is hoped that the richly illustrated atlas sections will facilitate the first steps for the beginner. For experienced sonographers, the detailed illustrations also of rare vascular pathology are expected to broaden their knowledge and help them diagnose rare disorders with greater confidence. To this end the role of ultrasound examinations is compared with that of other diagnostic modalities and tips and tricks are described that facilitate the examination and provide a basis for tackling more difficult diagnostic tasks. That is why all diseases in which ultrasonography is indicated and that are of relevance for angiologists and vascular surgeons are represented by images in the atlas. Rare vascular conditions can often be identified sonographically at a glance. Where appropriate, additional angiograms illustrate the role of the respective modality in comparison, and occasionally the situation is further clarified by an intraoperative photograph.

The constant support I received from Professor R. Eisele is gratefully acknowledged. My special thanks are due to the co-workers of Springer-Verlag for their excellent cooperation in preparing the second edition and to Ms. R. Mütschele for her assistance in preparing the graphics.

Wilhelm Schäberle
Göppingen, Germany
February 2004

Preface to the First German Edition

Conventional and color duplex ultrasonography has evolved into an indispensable tool for the diagnostic evaluation of vascular pathology. As a non-invasive test that can be repeated any time, sonography is increasingly replacing conventional diagnostic modalities that cause more discomfort to the patient. The combination of gray-scale sonographic information for evaluating topographic relationships and morphologic features of vessels with the qualitative and quantitative data obtained with the Doppler technique enables fine diagnostic differentiation of vascular disorders. In particular, the hemodynamic Doppler information is a useful supplement to the findings obtained with radiologic modalities. Being noninvasive and easy to perform any time, duplex sonography precedes more invasive, stressful, and expensive diagnostic tests in the step-by-step diagnostic workup of patients with vascular disease. It provides crucial information for optimal therapy and will replace invasive modalities such as angiography and venography as examiners gain skills and experience and ultrasound equipment becomes more sophisticated.

The significance duplex ultrasonography has gained in the hands of angiologists and vascular surgeons is also reflected in the further education programs for these specialties. This book therefore aims at providing a detailed description of the diagnostic information that can be obtained by (color) duplex sonography in those vascular territories that are relevant to angiologists and vascular surgeons. Each of the main chapters introduces beginners to the relevant vascular anatomy and scanning technique while at the same time offering detailed discussions of the parameters involved and a thorough review of the pertinent scientific literature to help experienced sonographers become more confident in establishing their diagnoses.

The first chapter presents the basic hemodynamic concepts that are relevant to vascular sonography and the fundamental physical and technical principles of vascular ultrasonography. This introductory chapter is intended to help readers grasp the potential and limitations of the method.

The situation in Germany is different from that in many other countries in that duplex sonography is performed primarily by angiologists, internists, and increasingly by vascular surgeons rather than by radiologists. On the basis of a patient's clinical findings, it is thus possible to specifically address therapeutically relevant questions in performing the sonographic examination. Besides general assessment of the vascular status, ultrasound can thus serve to acquire additional diagnostic information important for therapeutic decision-making in general and for planning the surgical procedure in particular. Duplex sonography in the hands of the clinician who is also treating the patient is seen as the continuation of the clinical examination by technical means. That is why the emphasis in this book is on the clinical and therapeutic role of ultrasound findings, and the individual chapters are organized according to such pragmatic aspects.

Each of the six main chapters deals with a specific vascular territory and consists of a text section as well as an atlas section with ample illustrations and detailed descriptions of normal findings, variants, and abnormal findings. Whenever considered appropriate for better illustration of complex pathology, the sonographic images have been supplemented with angiograms or CT scans. The comparison also illustrates the advantages and disadvantages of the respective radiologic modalities. As many rare vascular disorders are diagnosed at a glance by an experienced sonographer, their appearance is shown in numerous figures. Series of ultrasound scans document the course of the examination and complex hemodynamic changes in vascular disorders as well as their clinical significance and changes under therapy. The legends provide detailed descriptions allowing the reader to use the atlas sections independently for reference when looking for information on specific vascular conditions.

Different ultrasound modes are described in detail and their respective merits and shortcomings are discussed for the benefit of readers using different equipment. Gray-scale sonography alone (compression ultrasound) is quite sufficient for the diagnostic assessment of thrombosis while conventional duplex ultrasonography is a valid modality for diagnosing therapeutically relevant abnormal changes of the femoropopliteal territory. In most instances, color flow images are shown together with the Doppler waveform but occasionally "only" the conventional duplex scan is presented to illustrate the fact that many abnormalities can be identified by conventional duplex ultrasound alone. Despite the additional diagnostic information obtained with the color-coded technique, quantitative evaluation relies on the Doppler frequency spectrum. The color duplex mode can facilitate the examination procedure (identification of small vessels, recanalization, differential diagnosis) but the sonographer needs some basic knowledge of the conventional Doppler technique for the proper interpretation of color flow images.

My special thanks are due to Professor R. Eisele for promoting the use of diagnostic ultrasound in the department of vascular surgery at our hospital and for his valuable advice. I thank Ms. G. Rieker and Ms. E. Stieger and Mrs. B. Sihler for typing the manuscript and Ms. R. Uhlig for the photographic work in preparing the figures.

Finally I would like to express my thanks to the publishers, Springer-Verlag, and in particular to Ms. Zeck and Dr. Heilmann, for their excellent cooperation and constructive support.

Wilhelm Schäberle
Göppingen, Germany
December 1997

Contents

Contents

Fundamental Principles

W. Schäberle, *Ultrasonography in Vascular Diagnosis*, https://doi.org/10.1007/978-3-319-64997-9_1

1.1 Technical Principles of Diagnostic Ultrasound

1.1.1 Gray-Scale Ultrasonography (B-Mode)

1.1.1.1 Historical Milestones

The potential for using the reflection of ultrasound in the visualization of the internal organs of the human body was recognized about 80 years ago. The first attempts at using ultrasound in medical diagnosis were made in the late 1930s by the Austrian neurologist K.T. Dussik. He developed what he referred to as hyperphonography, a sonographic transmission technique for the visualization of the cerebral ventricles. Also in the 1940s, American scientists began experimenting with ultrasound reflection to examine biological objects. Among the early pioneers were Ludwig and Struthers, who used this new technique for detecting gallstones. Other important milestones in the history of diagnostic ultrasound were the development of B-mode imaging by Howry and Bliss and the introduction of the echo pulse method by Leksell in Sweden, which he used to determine the position of midline brain structures in the intact skull, thus marking the start of echoencephalography. In 1954, Edler and Herz presented the first description of M-mode echocardiography.

The Japanese physicist Satomura is credited with implementing the first medical applications of the Doppler principle. He and his colleagues investigated the use of Doppler frequency shifts to evaluate moving cardiac structures and to measure the velocity of red blood cells. The advent of the first real-time scanner, developed by Krause and Soldner, completely changed the practice of medical ultrasound scanning and marks yet another important step in the success story of diagnostic ultrasound.

Modern ultrasound offers excellent image quality and diagnostic capabilities, with its outstanding position among radiologic imaging techniques being due to its versatility, low cost, flexibility, and safety.

This chapter introduces the physical and technical fundamentals of medical ultrasound and outlines the range of techniques available today, which will help readers to make optimal use of the diagnostic capabilities of ultrasound and choose the best technique for the intended application.

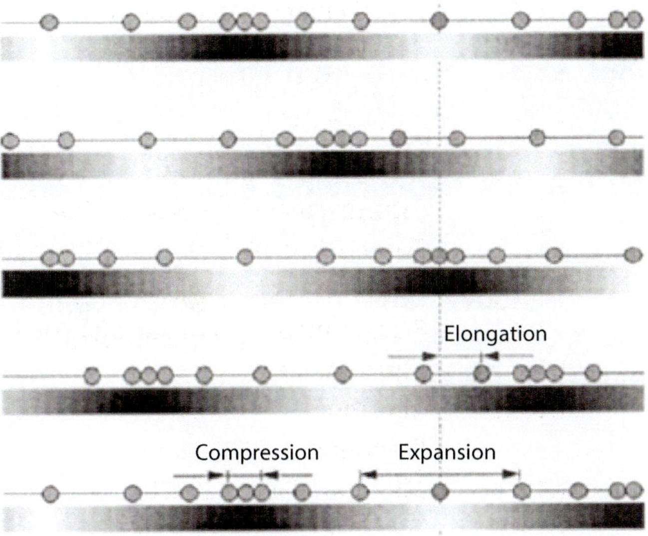

Fig. 1.1 Diagram of the propagation of a longitudinal wave illustrating cyclic compression and expansion (Courtesy of Hitachi Ltd., which also provided the historical material presented in ▶ Sect. 1.1.1.1)

Table 1.1 Typical sound velocities, densities, and attenuation values in some important biological tissues and other media in the body

Medium	Sound velocity (m/s)	Density (g/cm^2)	Attenuation (dB/MHz cm)
Fat	1470	0.97	0.5
Bone marrow	1700	0.97	–
Muscle	1568	1.04	2
Liver	1540	1.055	0.7
Brain	1530	1.02	1
Bone (compact)	3600	1.7	4–10
Water (20°C)	1492	0.9982	0.002
Air	331	0.0013	–

1.1.1.2 Sound Waves

When a molecule is activated to vibrate around its equilibrium position, the vibration is transmitted to a neighbor in the medium and from there to the next molecule and so on. In this way, kinetic energy is propagated from one molecule to the next, spreading through the medium in a sine wave pattern. This pattern of the spreading of kinetic energy is known as a continuous wave or an acoustic wave (sound wave). A sound wave alternately compresses (positive pressure) and expands (negative pressure) the medium it travels through (Fig. 1.1). Particles can vibrate parallel or perpendicular to the direction of energy propagation, giving rise to longitudinal waves (along the direction of travel) and transverse waves (perpendicular to the direction of travel). Particles excited in the ultrasound range vibrate around their resting positions at a rate of 20,000 to one billion times per second.

In gases and liquids, only longitudinal wave propagation is possible, as the shear forces necessary for the spread of transverse vibration are absent. In physical terms, biological tissues can be viewed as viscous fluids, which is why the effect of transverse waves is negligible. In such a medium the speed of sound increases with density, which in turn is defined by the force of molecular cohesion (Table 1.1). The average speed of sound in biological tissues is approx. 1540 m/s.

Waves can be described with reference to several properties. Wavelength λ is the distance between two consecutive

1

Table 1.2 Commonly used transmit frequencies and resulting properties of the ultrasound beam

Transmit frequency (MHz)	Wavelength (mm)	Penetration depth (cm)	Lateral resolution (mm)	Axial resolution (mm)
2	0.78	25	3	0.8
3.5	0.44	14	1.7	0.5
5	0.31	10	1.2	0.35
7.5	0.21	6.7	0.8	0.25
10	0.16	5	0.6	0.2
15	0.1	3.3	0.4	0.15

The following relationships exist between these parameters: the higher the transmit frequency (and therefore the shorter the wavelength), the higher the resolution – but the lower the penetration depth

Table 1.3 Parameters defining a sound wave

Property	Definition
Period	Duration of a complete vibration
Wavelength	Spatial extension of a period
Frequency	Number of periods per second
Amplitude	Measure of sound energy

points of maximum compression, and frequency f is the number of vibrations of a molecule per unit time, given in hertz (Hz). One hertz corresponds to one cycle per second, or 1 Hz = 1/s. The frequency range of diagnostic ultrasound is 2–30 MHz. The speed of a sound wave, C, is the product of wavelength and frequency:

$$C = \lambda \cdot f$$

The wavelengths occurring in diagnostic ultrasound are determined by the frequency emitted by the transducer (carrier frequency) and range from 0.78 to 0.15 mm over the 2–10 MHz frequency range typically used in vascular imaging (Table 1.2). The properties defining a sound wave are summarized in Table 1.3.

1.1.1.3 Generating Ultrasound Waves

In most ultrasonic transducers for medical imaging, the **piezoelectric effect** discovered by Pierre and Jacques Curie in 1880 is used to generate ultrasound waves. When mechanical stress is applied to piezoelectric materials such as ionic crystals, they experience an elastic deformation which results in a shift in internal charge distribution. In this way, electric voltages are generated at the surfaces – which are negative on one side and positive on the other. As the degree of stress increases, so does the voltage. Conversely, when a positive or negative voltage is applied to the surface of a piezoelectric crystal, the material expands or contracts, depending on the direction of the current. When an alternating current is applied, the piezoelectric crystal is activated and begins to vibrate. Materials possessing strong piezoelectric properties are quartz and tourmaline. State-of-the-art transducers use semicrystalline polymers such as polyvinylidene fluoride (PVDF).

1.1.1.4 Physical Factors Affecting the Ultrasound Scan

An ultrasound image is created by processing the echoes returning to the transducer from various depths of the body upon emission of an ultrasound pulse of a specific frequency (Fig. 1.2a). A two-dimensional (2D) image is generated from adjacent ultrasound lines. Two-dimensional morphologic images are acquired by applying short pulses of energy using only a small number of wavelengths to optimize spatial resolution. The round trip time is the time delay between the emission of an ultrasound pulse and the return of the reflected echo and is a function of the distance between the transducer and reflector. Reflection occurs at the boundaries between media that differ in their sound propagation properties, or acoustic impedance. Hence, an ultrasound image does not represent tissue structures directly but rather interfaces between tissues of different acoustic impedance. **Acoustic impedance** describes the frequency-dependent resistance that an ultrasound beam encounters as it passes through a tissue. It is equal to the speed of sound propagation multiplied by the density of the tissue. The greater the difference in impedance, the greater the reflection of the ultrasound wave (and therefore the greater the strength of the echo or signal) and the smaller its transmission into deeper tissue (Fig. 1.2a). Other physical processes besides reflection and scattering that affect the ultrasound scan are refraction, interference, diffraction, attenuation, and absorption.

1.1.1.4.1 Reflection and Refraction

The propagation of sound waves in biological tissues is governed by the laws of wave optics. Tissues vary in density and hence differ in acoustic impedance. Impedance Z is the product of the density of a medium and the speed of sound in it. At an acoustic interface in the body, an incident ultrasound beam is partially reflected and partially refracted. Refraction means that the wave passes through the interface, changing its direction of travel (Fig. 1.2b). The difference in acoustic impedance between the two tissues forming the interface determines how much of the beam is reflected and how much is transmitted: the greater the difference, the greater the amount of energy that is reflected back; the smaller the difference, the greater the amount of energy that is transmitted. Medical ultrasound thus functions like a sonar, exploiting differences in acoustic impedance between two adjacent tissues rather than absolute acoustic properties.

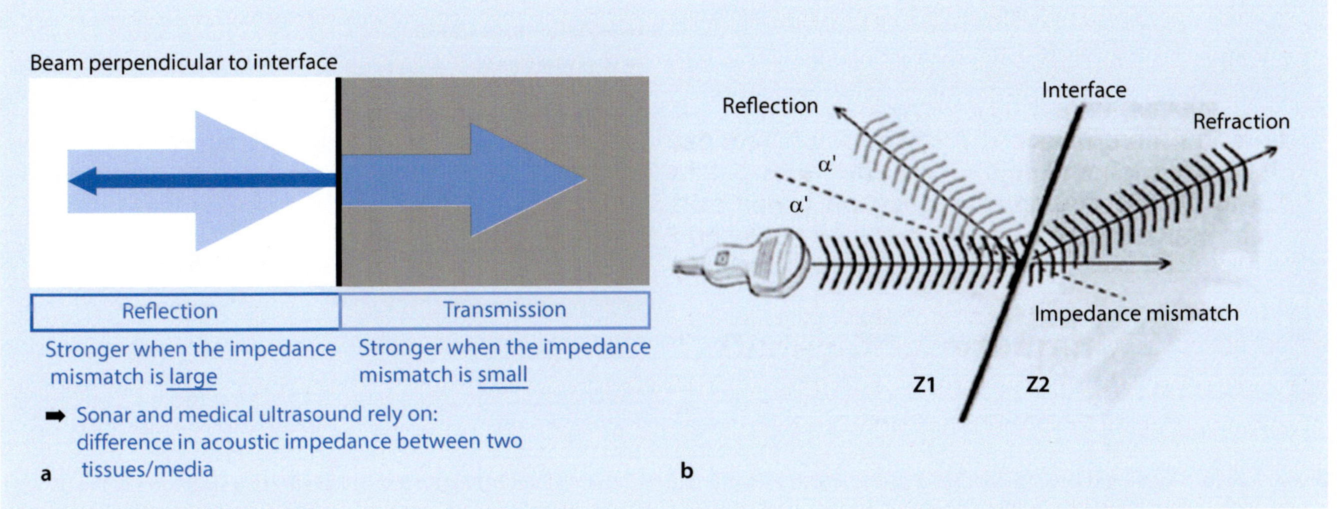

Fig. 1.2 **a** Generation of an ultrasound image: reflection – transmission. **b** Interaction of ultrasound with interfaces in the body according to the laws of wave optics (for details see text) (Courtesy of Hitachi Ltd.)

The reflection gradient, *R*, is given by the following equation for incident angles perpendicular to an interface:

$$R = \left(\frac{Z1 - Z2}{Z1 + Z2}\right)^2$$

For an ultrasound beam striking the interface between liver tissue ($Z1 = 1.66 \times 10^5$) and renal tissue ($Z2 = 1.63 \times 10^5$), the equation yields a reflection gradient of $R = 0.000008$, meaning that this boundary reflects less than one hundred thousandth of the incident energy. In contrast, nearly all of the incident energy (over 99%) is reflected from the interface between fatty tissue and air ($Z1 = 1.42 \times 10^5$, $Z2 = 43$, $R = 0.9987$), leaving virtually no ultrasound energy to travel deeper into the tissue. This is why the lungs or bowel loops containing air cannot be examined by ultrasonography and also why it is necessary to eliminate air intervening between the ultrasound probe and the skin surface by applying ultrasound gel.

The echoes reflected back from an interface between media of different acoustic impedance are available for image generation only if the interface is relatively perpendicular to the ultrasound beam (angles of incident and reflected beam). For this reason, structures such as vessel walls perpendicular to the beam appear fairly bright compared to vessel walls tangential to the beam since most echo pulses are reflected back to the transducer by the former. Reflection occurs at the surfaces of particles that are larger than the wavelength, while scattering predominates when they are smaller.

1.1.1.4.2 Scattering and Attenuation

The interface between tissues of different acoustic impedance is typically not smooth but rough. A sound wave interacting with a rough surface will be scattered in all directions in the form of a spherical wave rather than along one path (Fig. 1.3a). An incident ultrasound wave is also mostly scattered when it strikes an object that is much smaller than its wavelength, and it is reflected when it strikes an object much larger than its wavelength. Scattering gives rise to the characteristic echotexture of parenchymal organs in ultrasound images.

Since structures perpendicular to the beam are rare in clinical ultrasound examinations, an ultrasound image is chiefly generated from a mixture of reflected and scattered echoes. Aggregations of tissue cells scatter the beam diffusely in all directions. Therefore, a structure appears bright and is clearly defined when it is perpendicular to the ultrasound beam because the image information is mainly derived from reflected echoes; its visualization is weaker and less bright when the ultrasound beam strikes tangentially and only diffusely reflected echoes are available to generate the image, although impedance is identical in both cases.

Scattering contributes to the attenuation (loss of energy) of the ultrasound beam as it travels through the body and in turn depends on the transmitted frequency. A higher transmit frequency results in greater attenuation and limits the penetration depth of the ultrasound pulse. The emitted intensity decreases exponentially with distance and is influenced by an attenuation coefficient that varies with the type of tissue through which the beam travels in the human body (fat, muscle, blood). In the human body, it ranges from 0.3 to 0.6 dB/MHz cm. The energy is converted into absorption heat.

Higher carrier frequencies result in a lower penetration depth because attenuation loss is greater. The increasing attenuation can be compensated for to some extent by adjusting amplification (depth-dependent gain) (Fig. 1.3b). Using transducers with a wide frequency range results in the predominance of lower frequencies with greater penetration depths because attenuation of higher frequencies is more pronounced.

In addition to scattering and reflection, there is refraction at the interface between different media. Refraction in the

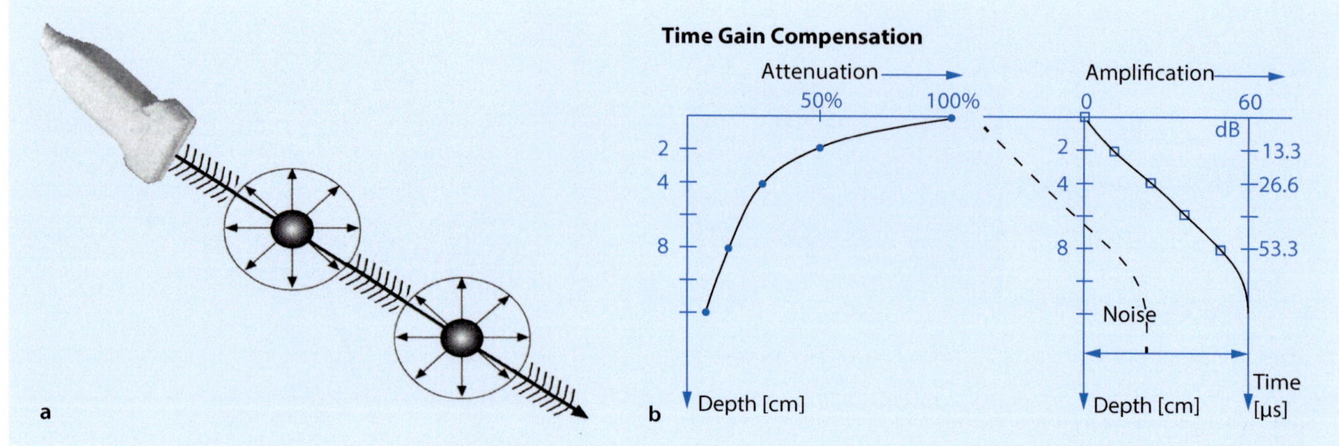

Fig. 1.3a, b Scattering and attenuation of sound waves. **a** Scattering: Most ultrasound beams do not strike reflecting structures in the body at a right angle, which is why the incident beam is scattered in all directions. As a result, only a small proportion of the emitted energy is backscattered to the transducer and available for generating the ultrasound image. An ultrasound beam reflected from an interface between two tissues with the same difference in acoustic impedance will yield much stronger echoes than a beam scattered at that interface (resulting in poorer visualization) (Modified from Widder and Görtler 2004). **b** Attenuation reduces the amplitude of the reflected ultrasound beam with echoes returning from structures deeper in the body being attenuated more strongly. To create a uniform image from all signals despite their different amplitudes, time gain compensation (TGC) is used, which changes the receive gain over time, applying greater amplification to echoes returing from deeper in the body (using a set of sliding knobs or paddles)

direction of the normal to the interface occurs when there is an increase in sound velocity in the next medium, and refraction away from the normal occurs when the velocity decreases. Refraction may lead to misinterpretation of the location and size of the structure visualized.

1.1.1.4.3 Interference

When two or more sound waves superimpose, they can be out of phase (i.e., one wave's compression phase coincides with the other's expansion phase), thus cancelling each other out (destructive interference), or they can be in phase (i.e., the compression and expansion phases line up), thus reinforcing each other (constructive interference). The spatial distribution of areas of constructive and destructive interference is known as the interference pattern. Such interference patterns are largely responsible for the visual appearance of an ultrasound image.

Interferences of sound waves can change the amplitude and thus the brightness of an image despite an identical acoustic impedance in the boundary zone. Depending on the momentary phase of the wave, the amplitude is either amplified or diminished.

1.1.1.4.4 Diffraction

Diffraction is the ability of a sound wave to bend around the corners of an obstacle in its path and to spread into the shadow region behind the obstacle.

1.1.1.4.5 Attenuation and Absorption

The intensity of an ultrasound wave diminishes as it propagates through the body. This loss of energy is known as attenuation and is caused by different processes, one of which is absorption – the conversion of ultrasound energy into heat. Body tissues roughly attenuate ultrasound energy at a rate of 1 dB/mHz cm. The attenuation values for a selection of biological tissues are given in Table 1.1. The rate of absorption depends not only on the tissue type but also on the emitted ultrasound frequency, with higher frequencies attenuating more quickly. Lower ultrasound frequencies, with long wavelengths, thus allow the examination of deeper structures, while high ultrasound frequencies are desirable for the better spatial resolution they afford. For an ultrasound frequency of 10 MHz, for instance, the attenuation is 10 dB/cm as opposed to only 3 dB/cm for 3 MHz. Assuming an output of 100 dB, the penetration depth would be 5 cm for 10 MHz and 17 cm for 3 MHz (corresponding to a total path length of 10 and 34 cm, respectively).

1.1.1.5 Generating an Ultrasound Image

1.1.1.5.1 Pulse-Echo Technique

Nearly all diagnostic ultrasound techniques rely on pulsed excitation signals. An ultrasound beam is generated by applying short electrical pulses of about 1 s to the piezoelectric crystal in the transducer, which converts the electrical energy into mechanical vibrations. The transducer is then switched to receive mode. The ultrasound wave passes into the body, is reflected from tissue interfaces, and returns to the transducer in the form of an echo. The incoming echoes are then converted back into electrical signals. The time, t, between transmission and reception of the pulse is measured in order to calculate the length of the path traveled, which is the product of ultrasound velocity, c, along the path and t. Dividing the product by the factor 2 yields z, the distance of the reflecting structure from the ultrasound probe.

$$z = ct/2$$

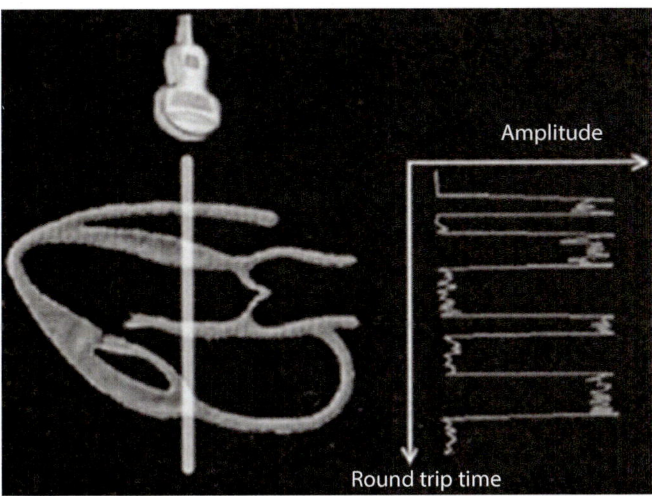

Fig. 1.4 In A-mode scanning, the amplitudes of the reflected echoes are displayed unidimensionally, representing the distances of the reflecting boundaries in the tissue from the transducer (Courtesy of Hitachi Ltd.)

If the time difference is 0.13 ms, for instance, the reflecting structure in the body is 10 cm from the ultrasound probe. Current ultrasound systems generate and transmit 3000–5000 ultrasound pulses per second and simultaneously receive and process returning echoes to generate an image.

1.1.1.5.2 Time Gain Compensation

Echoes returning from deeper within the body are weaker than those arising from structures closer to the transducer. Since the distance they have to travel is longer, they experience greater attenuation. To compensate for these differences and to display the signals returning from equally reflective boundaries with a similar brightness – regardless of the distance traveled – the incoming echoes are amplified in a depth-dependent manner. This method of variable amplification of echoes as a function of their round trip time is known as time gain compensation (TGC), depth-gain compensation, or swept gain (Fig. 1.3b). The user can set the gains for signals returning from different depths.

1.1.1.5.3 A-Mode

A-mode or amplitude mode is the simplest and oldest technique of diagnostic ultrasound. The amplitudes of the pulses returning to the transducer are displayed as spikes along a vertical baseline on a cathode ray oscilloscope with the position of a spike representing the distance between the reflecting boundary and the transducer (Fig. 1.4). This technique provides one-dimensional information and can be used to make precise length and depth measurements. Its use is now restricted to specialized applications including the measurement of corneal thickness in ophthalmology and the noninvasive evaluation of the paranasal sinuses in othorhinolaryngology.

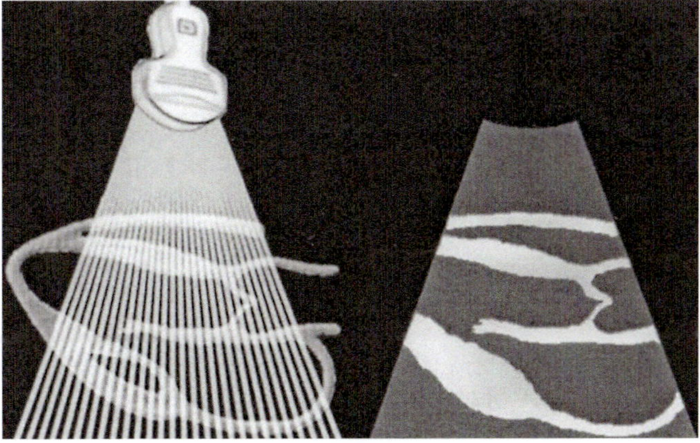

Fig. 1.5 In B-mode scanning, the echoes reflected from boundaries between tissues of different acoustic impedance are displayed two-dimensionally as bright/dark spots with brightness levels representing the intensity of the reflected echoes (Courtesy of Hitachi Ltd.)

1.1.1.5.4 B-Mode

B-mode or brightness mode scans differ from A-mode displays in that the amplitudes of the returning echoes are displayed on a monitor as dots of varying brightness rather than as spikes (Fig. 1.5). The brightness of the dots represents the strength of the echoes. Most modern ultrasound systems can display 256 levels of brightness (gray scales). The human eye in comparison can distinguish only about 20 gray levels in an image. The dots representing the echoes returning to the transducer after emission of a pulse are arranged along a straight line (beam line or scan line). After all echoes from preceding pulses have returned, pulses to generate successive scan lines are transmitted. Once all echoes have been detected and processed, the complete 2D B-mode image is displayed.

Suppose that we wish to generate a complete B-mode image with a penetration depth of 15 cm, a width of the scan area, x, of 5 cm, and a line spacing, Δx, of 1 mm. Using the pulse-echo technique, generation of one scan line takes about 0.2 ms. With the known ultrasound speed of 1540 ms in living tissue, the total scan time, T, can be calculated as:

$$T = (2zx)/(c\Delta x)$$

In our example, the total scan time is 10 ms, corresponding to a frame rate of 100 Hz. This means that 100 complete images can be generated per second, which is fast enough to allow real-time imaging.

1.1.1.5.5 M-Mode

M-mode or motion mode (also known as time-motion or TM-mode) differs from B-mode imaging in that the ultrasound beam is stationary and emitted repeatedly to obtain echoes from moving reflectors in the beam path at different times. The M-mode information is displayed along a time axis with the resulting tracing depicting the movement of a structure such as a cardiac valve in a wavelike manner (Fig. 1.6). As with B-mode imaging, using the pulse-echo

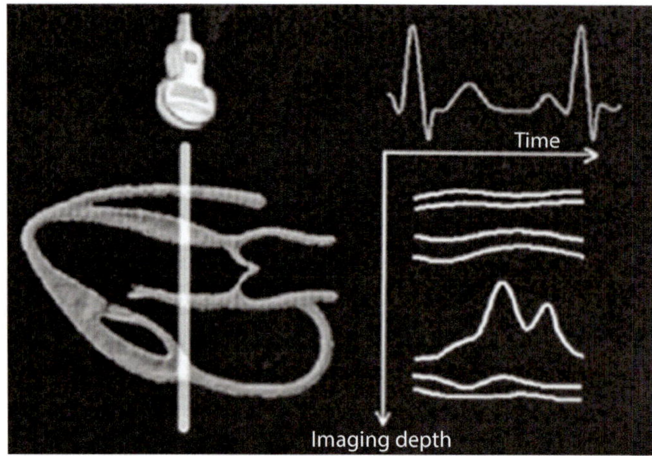

Fig. 1.6 In M-mode scanning, the temporal changes in returning echoes are displayed, representing the motion of reflecting interfaces toward and away from the transducer over time (Courtesy of Hitachi Ltd.)

technique, it takes 0.2 ms to generate a scan line with a penetration depth of 15 cm. This results in a high frame rate (up to about 5000 frames per second), affording a high temporal resolution, which is useful in evaluating rapidly moving structures such as cardiac valves or vessel walls. M-mode is used for echocardiography, allowing very precise measurement of the cardiac chambers and walls and quantitative evaluation of cardiac motion.

1.1.1.6 Resolution

Image resolution, which is given in millimeters, is defined as the smallest distance between two structures that is necessary to represent them as separate entities on a monitor. When applied to ultrasound scans, resolution describes the spatial discrimination between two structures differing in acoustic impedance. A distinction is made between axial resolution (resolution in the direction of sound propagation) and lateral resolution.

Axial resolution is determined by the length of the excitation pulse and is typically one or a few wavelengths. A higher-frequency transducer emits shorter wavelengths, resulting in better axial resolution. Attenuation, however, also increases with frequency, limiting the maximum depth from which echoes can be received. Hence, relatively low transmit frequencies are indispensible for imaging structures deeper in the body. The examiner must therefore strike a balance between spatial resolution and imaging depth (Fig. 1.7a). Axial resolution depends on wavelength alone and improves as the wavelength decreases (or the frequency increases), ranging from 0.2 to 1 mm (Table 1.2).

Lateral resolution is the ability to separate two closely spaced echoes that lie in a plane perpendicular to the direction of the sound wave. It is also influenced by the transmit frequency, and hence wavelength, but is mainly determined

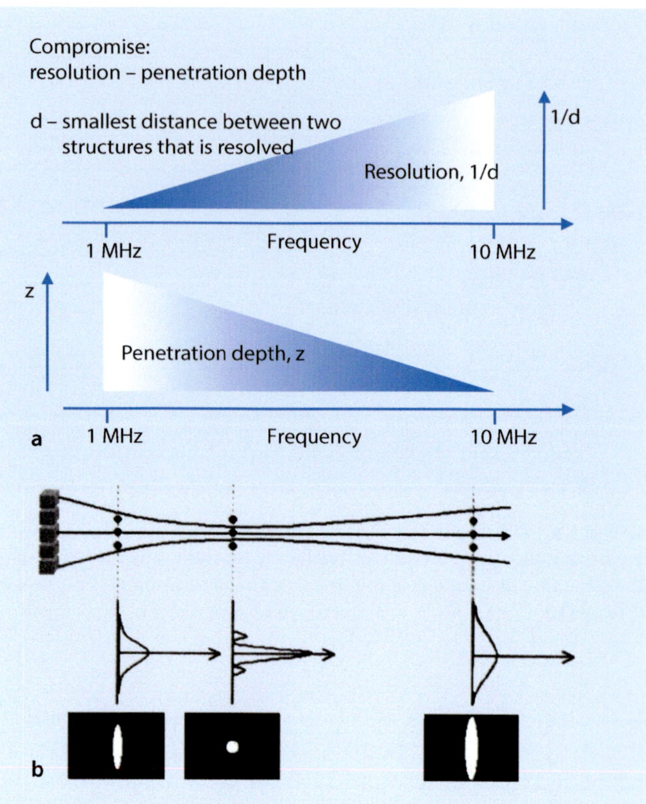

Fig. 1.7a, b Parameters affecting axial and lateral resolution. **a** Relationship between axial resolution and transmit frequency (wavelength): axial resolution increases with transmit frequency (but at the cost of penetration depth). **b** Effect of beam width on lateral resolution (Courtesy of Hitachi Ltd.)

by the focusing capabilities of the ultrasound system and the resulting beam properties.

Lateral resolution is determined by the width of the ultrasound beam and is best when the beam is narrow (Fig. 1.7b). The beam profile changes along the beam path, consisting of a well-focused, narrow near field and a divergent far field. The ultrasound beam can be focused to improve image quality. In this way, optimal resolution can be accomplished in a small target zone, while resolution outside this zone is much poorer. The slow speed of sound in human tissue (1540 m/s) and the aim of achieving a high frame rate (real-time imaging) limit the number of scan lines per image. In order to relate the echoes to a specific depth, it is necessary to wait for the arrival of the returning echo from the respective depth of the preceding pulse before emission of the next ultrasound pulse. The transmitted or received pulse is focused in a longitudinal direction relative to the transducer, and focusing of the returning pulse in the scan plane is optimized in smaller steps (dynamically, almost continuously with the arrival time of the pulse).

The achievable resolution is determined by the wavelength of the ultrasound beam. It is ½ λ (wavelength) for axial resolution and much poorer for lateral resolution with a value of 4 λ. Consequently, a high transmit frequency is desirable to achieve good axial and lateral resolution (Table 1.2). On the other hand, due to attenuation, lower transmit frequencies are necessary to achieve greater penetration depth. When deeper vessels are scanned, a compromise must be found at the expense of spatial discrimination of the vessel structures of interest (poorer spatial resolution resulting from a lower transmit frequency) (Fig. 1.7a).

The depth of a reflector in the body (encoded in the B-mode image) is calculated from the round trip time, which increases with depth, as does attenuation. Therefore, echo signals arriving from deeper within the body are progressively more strongly amplified in order to visualize them with the same intensity in the resulting image (see ▶ Sect. 1.1.1.5.2). Overall gain and depth gain are adjusted according to the distance of the vessel of interest from the body surface. The gain is crucial for the amplitude or intensity of the signal, and along with output energy and signal-to-noise limit, it must be set properly when assessing vascular structures.

1.1.1.7 Beam Focusing

There are several techniques for focusing an ultrasound beam. The simplest option is to use an acoustic lens, which has the same effect as a glass lens for visible light. A concave acoustic lens placed in front of the transducer provides weak focusing at a fixed depth. The site of maximum focusing is referred to as the focal point or focal zone. Alternatively, the crystal in the transducer can be made concave, providing internal focusing. This technique is used in single-element mechanical sector scanners.

More flexible beam forming, with a variable depth of the focal point, is accomplished using electronic beam focusing. Array transducers consist of multiple crystal elements placed side by side. Depending on the scanner type, the number of individual elements ranges from 60 to 256. Variable numbers of elements can be activated simultaneously to form an ultrasound beam. If the elements forming the beam are excited at slightly different times, a concave wavefront is generated, causing the beam to converge at the focal point. The site of the focal point can be manipulated by varying the number of active elements and the pattern of excitation of individual elements. The user can thus adjust the beam to achieve maximum lateral resolution at the anatomic site of interest. Modern scanners use multiple zone focusing, which reduces the frame rate, as several consecutive beams with different focal points are transmitted to generate a scan line. A technique known as dynamic focusing allows the focus of the beam to be altered during reception by imposing variable delays on signals from different depths. With this technique, the reception focus can be optimized without compromising the frame rate. Groups of 8–128 elements are used for focusing the beam (Fig. 1.8).

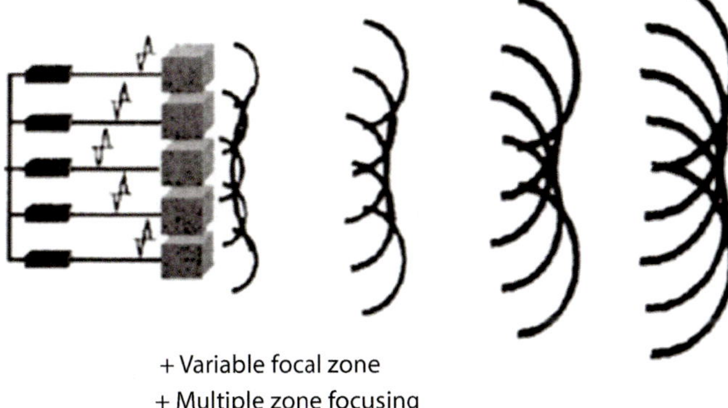

Fig. 1.8 Beam focusing in modern array probes. By delaying the firing of the central element after the firing of the outer elements a curved wavefront is produced, resulting in a focused beam (Courtesy of Hitachi Ltd.)

Lateral resolution is limited by the proximity of the transducer elements activated to emit an ultrasound pulse. Resolution along the longitudinal axis can be improved by exciting only a limited number of elements at a time and not the whole array. A more focused beam is achieved by later excitation of the transducer elements in the center. Dynamic focusing is accomplished by applying small time delays to the excitation pulses driving the individual transducer elements. Resolution in the third direction, or slice thickness, depends on the position in the image.

1.1.1.8 Types of Transducers

1.1.1.8.1 Principle of Operation

Most electronic ultrasound transducers used today contain a number of individual piezoelectric elements for transmitting and receiving ultrasonic waves. To create a complete image, the ultrasound beam has to pass through adjacent areas of tissue. Parallel ultrasound beams are generated by varying the groups of elements within the array that are simultaneously active. A group of elements is excited to generate the first scan line. The next adjacent scan line is formed by shifting the group of active elements along the transducer array, one element position from the first group – for example, elements 1–5 produce the first beam, 2–6 the second, 3–7 the third, and so on (Fig. 1.9). The second ultrasound beam generated in this way is said to be shifted by the width of one element. The number of scan lines used to generate an image can be increased by varying the number of elements activated simultaneously to generate each beam. For instance, if the second beam is generated using the same group of elements as for the first beam plus one additional element on the left side (and no element on the right side is switched off), then the axis of the second beam is shifted by half an element width relative to the first beam. The third beam is generated by removing one element on the right side without

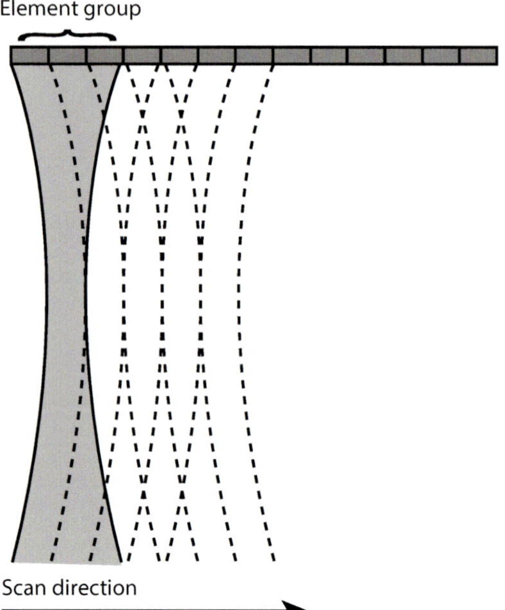

Fig. 1.9 Emission and reception of a series of parallel ultrasound beams by successive excitation of groups of transducer elements for generation of an ultrasound image (Courtesy of Hitachi Ltd.)

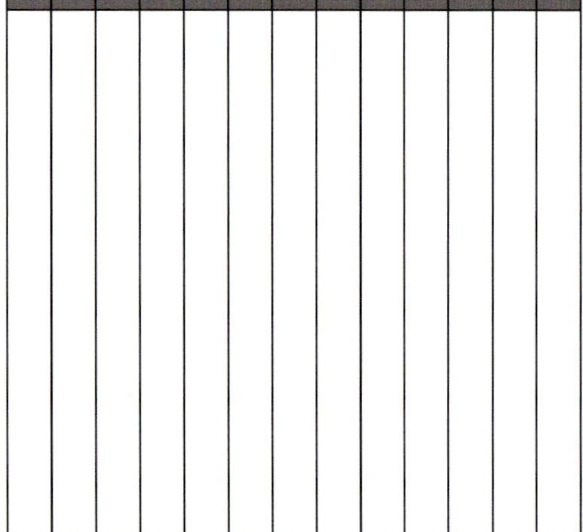

Fig. 1.10 Diagram of a linear array with the crystal elements arranged in a straight row (Courtesy of Hitachi Ltd.)

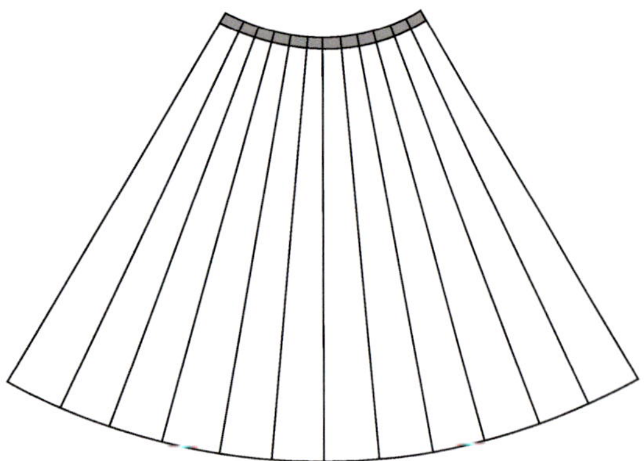

Fig. 1.11 Diagram of a curved array with the crystal elements arranged along a curved line (Courtesy of Hitachi Ltd.)

adding an element to the left side. In this way, the number of lines scanned to produce an image is doubled. A higher line density is desirable for improving image quality; however, it also reduces frame rate.

1.1.1.8.2 Linear Arrays

In a linear array transducer, the individual crystal elements are arranged in a straight row (Fig. 1.10) and can be pulsed to generate adjacent parallel ultrasonic beams, producing a rectangular image with nearly constant resolution over the entire scan depth. A linear array is made up of 60–196 elements, with an element width of 1–4 λ, and operates at a frequency of 5–13 MHz. An acoustic lens can be used for focusing perpendicular to the direction of beam propagation.

1.1.1.8.3 Curved or Convex Arrays

A curved or convex array transducer is a linear array, with the individual elements arranged along a curved line, to produce a sector image (Fig. 1.11). As the lines fan out with increasing distance from the transducer, lateral resolution decreases with depth. A typical curvilinear array consists of at least 96 elements and has a radius of 25–80 mm and a frequency range of 3–7 MHz. Most curvilinear scanners produce sector images ranging in size from 60° to 90°.

1.1.1.8.4 Sector Scanners

Sector scanners have a smaller radius (<25 mm) than curved arrays and also have a small footprint, resulting in a narrow near field. With a beam-steering angle >90°, these probes are especially useful where access is difficult, such as in the imaging of the heart through the intercostal spaces (echocardiography), or for endoluminal applications such as transvaginal ultrasound.

1.1.1.8.5 Phased Arrays

In a phased-array transducer, the elements are also arranged in a linear array. The difference is that all elements are excited to generate a scan line. However, time delays are introduced between pulsing consecutive elements to produce a wavefront that is no longer perpendicular to the transducer face (Fig. 1.12). By choosing appropriate delays between the excitation of individual elements, it is possible to direct the beam at a desired angle. Using this method, the beam can be steered through a range of angles to produce a sector image. Phased-array transducers use a smaller array of elements (64–128), resulting in a small footprint of 12–20 mm. The beam covers a sector of 80–90° with frequency ranging from 2 to 7 MHz. Since they require complex electronic circuitry, phased-array devices are expensive and are used mainly for cardiac and transcranial imaging.

1.1.1.8.6 Mechanical Sector Scanners

Compared with electronic phased arrays, mechanical systems are fairly simple regarding the control of transducer elements and signal processing. There are basically two designs of mechanical devices: the rotating wheel transducer and the wobbler transducer.

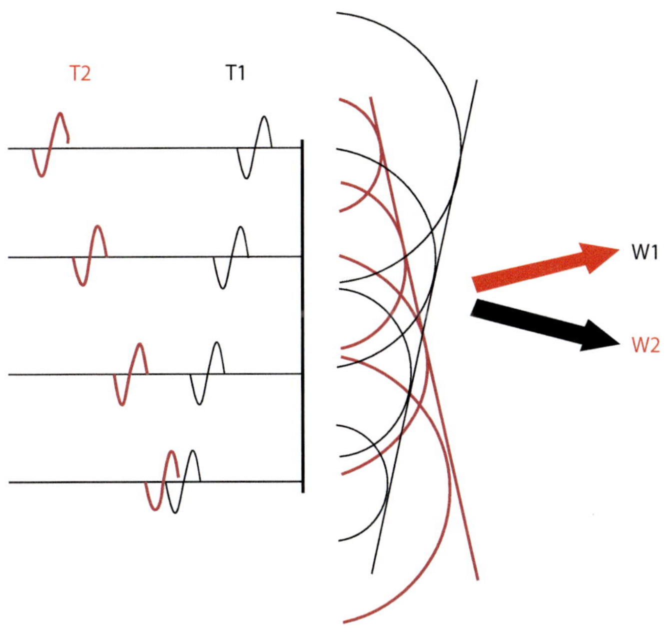

Fig. 1.12 Generation of a pie-shaped image by the successive excitation of groups of elements in a phased-array probe (Courtesy of Hitachi Ltd.)

- **Rotating wheel transducer.** This type usually comprises three to five transducer elements mounted 120–72° apart on a wheel. A motor housed in the handle turns the wheel at a constant rate in one direction. One of the crystal elements at a time is activated as it rotates past an acoustically transparent window. The active element scans a sector-shaped region. Then the next crystal rotates past the window, generating a second image.
- **Wobbler transducer.** In this type of mechanical sector scanner, a single crystal oscillates about a pivotal point, producing a beam that covers a sector of 60–100°. Since the wobbler transducer consists of a single crystal element, no complex adjustment is required. Another advantage it has over the rotating wheel transducer is that the sector angle is variable. Both mechanical devices are limited, however, by the fact that only a single element is used to produce the ultrasound beam and thus only fixed beam focusing is possible.

1.1.1.8.7 Annular Phased Arrays

An annular phased array is an oscillating transducer combining features of mechanical and electronic devices. Instead of a single element, the transducer consists of several concentric rings (annuli). Each ring can be excited separately, allowing variable focusing in two dimensions.

1.1.1.8.8 Disadvantages of Mechanical Transducers

Regardless of their design, mechanical probes are subject to wear and require maintenance. Moreover, they are relatively slow, not allowing rapid switching between different scan modes (B-mode, M-mode, Doppler). Real-time display of B-mode/M-mode or B-mode/Doppler information is generally not possible.

Table 1.4 Overview of ultrasound artifacts

Underlying mechanism	Type of artifact
Nonuniform ultrasound propagation in the human body	Structures with misregistered location Refraction artifact Reverberation artifact Mirror artifact
Nonuniform ultrasound attenuation	Acoustic shadowing Edge artifact Acoustic enhancement
Ultrasound beam characteristics	Side lobe artifact Line distortion Falsely perceived sediment
Structural artifacts	Speckles

1.1.1.9 Ultrasound Artifacts

Artifacts play a much greater role in diagnostic ultrasound compared with other imaging modalities such as computed tomography (CT) or magnetic resonance imaging (MRI). One fundamental issue is that several simplifying assumptions are made, namely that parameters such as the speed of sound in tissues, the propagation of ultrasound, and the attenuation are constant. Another important source of artifacts in the ultrasound image is the use of inadequate instrument settings. At the same time, however, some common artifacts can be exploited to advantage because they may provide additional diagnostic information on tissue composition. Often, artifacts can be identified by moving the transducer: artifacs will change position or disappear while actual tissue structures will not.

Table 1.4 provides an overview of ultrasound artifacts and their underlying causes. The artifacts that are most relevant to vascular applications are described in more detail in the following sections.

1.1.1.9.1 Posterior Shadowing

Acoustic shadowing is the occurrence of hypoechoic areas behind certain objects due to loss of energy; it is one of the most commonly encountered ultrasound artifacts. These artifacts can occur deep to a strong reflector such as air, which is difficult to penetrate by the ultrasound beam because of a strong acoustic mismatch, or behind highly attenuating structures such as bone or calculi, which absorb much of the ultrasound energy (Fig. 1.13).

1.1.1.9.2 Acoustic Enhancement

Acoustic enhancement is an increase in brightness behind a low-attenuating area, in particular fluid-filled spaces such as cysts. An ultrasound beam passing through fluid is nearly unchanged because fluid reflects and attenuates only little of the ultrasound energy. Time gain compensation therefore amplifies echoes returning from behind a low-attenuation region more than necessary. Acoustic enhancement can be exploited diagnostically in distinguishing a fluid-filled lesion such as a cyst from a solid mass (◘ Fig. 1.14).

1.1.1.9.3 Edge Effect

The edge effect is a form of acoustic shadowing that is observed at the margins of curved, fluid-filled spaces such as cysts and is assumed to be caused by a combination of refraction and reflection. When a parallel ultrasound beam passes through the lateral border of such a space, sound is diverted into the surrounding tissue. As a result, no ultrasound signal penetrates beyond the diverting structure, and hence no diagnostic information is obtained from that area. This phenomenon also explains the incomplete display of the margins of certain structures such as the fetal head or a blood vessel depicted in cross-section (◘ Fig. 1.15).

1.1.1.9.4 Side Lobes

A transducer transmits not only the main beam (also called the main lobe) but also some weaker beams, or side lobes, on either side of the primary beam in the near field. When a side lobe strikes a strong reflector, the obliquely deflected echoes are misrepresented in the resulting image because they are processed as if they had originated from the main beam (◘ Fig. 1.16). Modern ultrasound systems use various techniques, such as delay time calculation or suppression of echoes not returning along a path perpendicular to the transducer face, to minimize side lobe effects.

1.1.1.9.5 Reverberation Artifact

This type of artifact is also known as multiple reflection artifact and occurs when ultrasound is reflected back to the transducer from a strongly reflective surface in the near field. Part of the returning echo is properly processed by the transducer, while another part is reflected back into the body. Sound can thus bounce back and forth between the reflector and the transducer face (ping-pong effect). The resulting

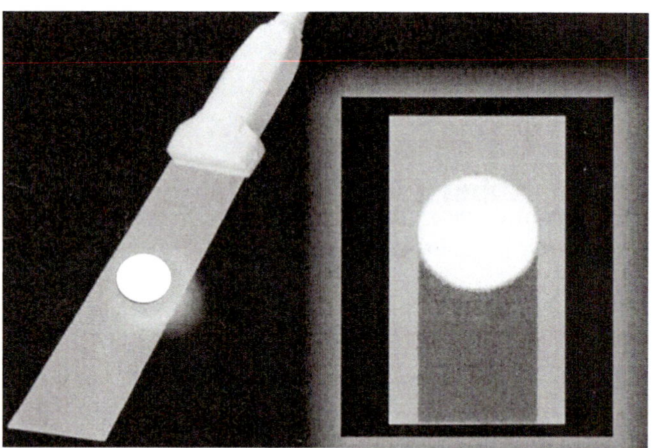

◘ **Fig. 1.13** Posterior shadowing occurs when a large impedance mismatch or object with high sound absorption is encountered (Courtesy of Hitachi Ltd.)

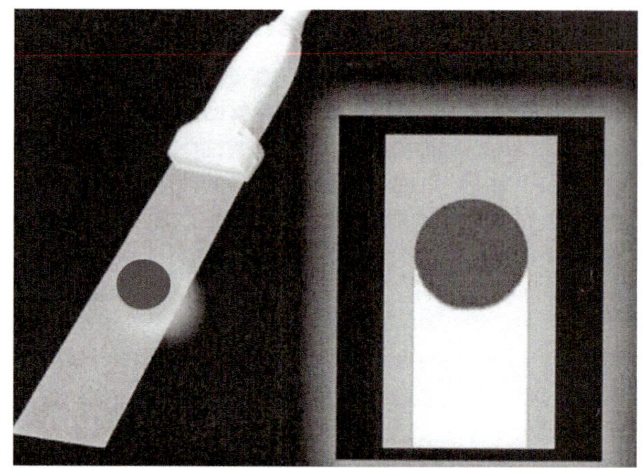

◘ **Fig. 1.14** Acoustic enhancement occurs behind low-attenuating areas (Courtesy of Hitachi Ltd.)

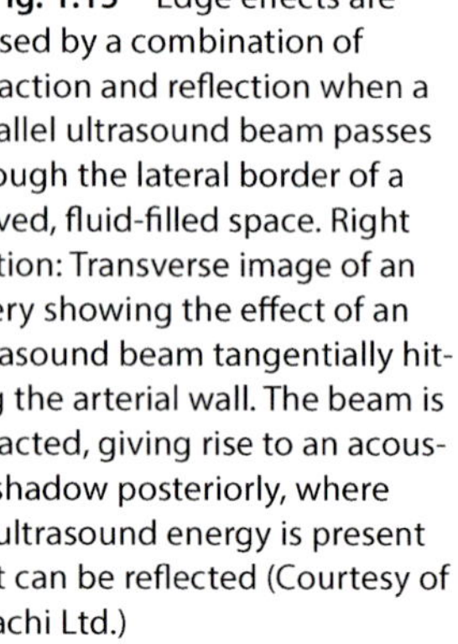

◘ **Fig. 1.15** Edge effects are caused by a combination of refraction and reflection when a parallel ultrasound beam passes through the lateral border of a curved, fluid-filled space. Right section: Transverse image of an artery showing the effect of an ultrasound beam tangentially hitting the arterial wall. The beam is refracted, giving rise to an acoustic shadow posteriorly, where no ultrasound energy is present that can be reflected (Courtesy of Hitachi Ltd.)

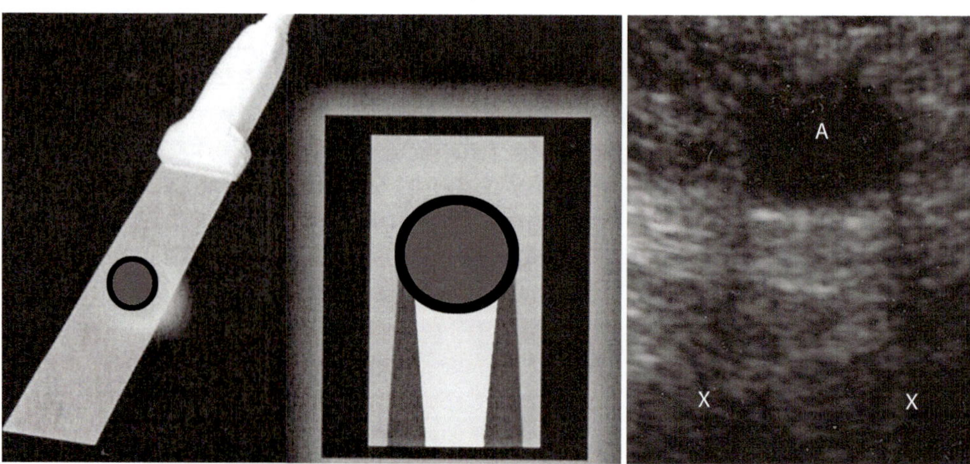

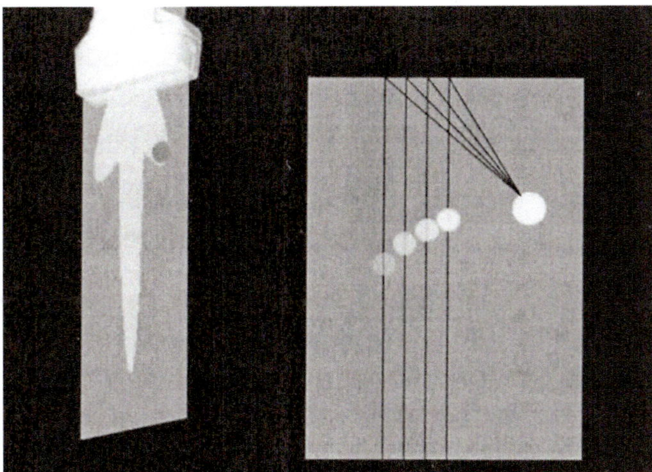

Fig. 1.16 Diagram of side lobe artifact (Courtesy of Hitachi Ltd.)

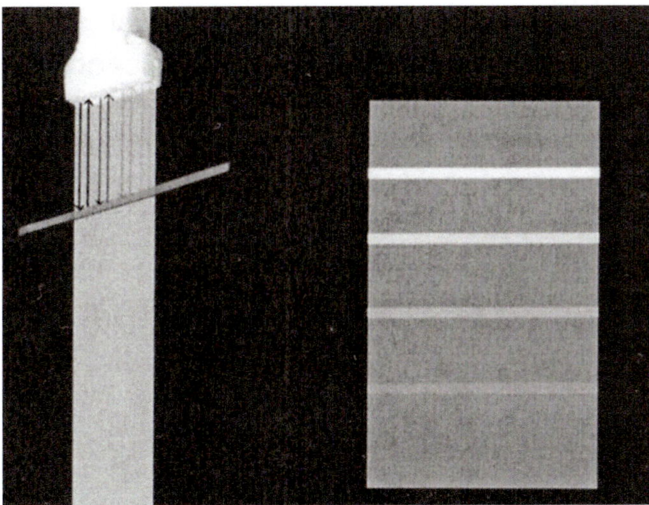

Fig. 1.17 Diagram of reverberation artifact. This is the repeat reflection of an ultrasound beam hitting a strong reflector near the transducer. In this situation, sound will bounce back and forth between the reflector and the transducer. Echoes from multiple reflections return to the transducer later than the direct echoes and are misrepresented in the image as a copy of the original object at a greater depth (Courtesy of Hitachi Ltd.)

reverberation artifact is seen in the display as several equidistant echoes decreasing in brightness with depth. This artifact typically arises when there is a large acoustic impedance mismatch near the transducer (soft tissue/air interface) (Fig. 1.17).

1.1.1.9.6 Geometric Distortion

In processing returning echoes and creating an image, the ultrasound system relies on certain assumptions, for example, that ultrasound travels in a straight line or at a constant speed in the body. In fact, however, an ultrasound beam can be deflected from its straight path, and the speed of sound varies slightly with the tissue. As a result, the ultrasound image may not reflect the exact anatomic location of a feature.

1.1.2 Basic Physics of Doppler Ultrasound

In 1842, the Austrian physicist and mathematician Christian Johann Doppler described what is now called the Doppler effect or Doppler shift. This phenomenon refers to the change in frequency of a wave resulting from relative movement between the source of the wave and an observer. A familiar example is an ambulance siren: although the emitted frequency remains the same, the siren has a higher pitch when the ambulance is approaching and a lower pitch when the vehicle is receding. The pitch changes abruptly at the moment the ambulance passes the observer. Thus, the pitch of the siren perceived by the human ear depends on the direction of motion relative to the observer and remains consistently high while the vehicle is approaching and consistently low while it is receding. This is different from the intensity of the sound, or the loudness of the siren, which increases gradually as the vehicle approaches and then decreases gradually after the vehicle has passed the observer. The Doppler effect occurs when the source or the observer is moving toward or away from the other or when both are moving relative to each other. For a vehicle traveling at a speed of 100 km/h, the difference in pitch due to the Doppler effect is almost two whole tones.

Compared to the emitted frequency, the received frequency is higher when the source and receiver approach each other and lower during the recession (Fig. 1.18a).

This difference in frequency, occurring when the source and/or receiver of a sound wave move relative to each other, is known as the Doppler effect or Doppler shift.

In diagnostic ultrasound, the Doppler effect is used to calculate blood flow velocity from the difference in frequency between the emitted and reflected waves; this was first reported by Satomura in 1959. The signals reflected by moving red blood cells have a different frequency than the emitted beam. In this case, the transducer transmitting and receiving the signals is stationary and the frequency shift is caused by the motion of the reflector (red blood cells). In this situation, the Doppler shift occurs twice – when the ultrasound beam emitting from the stationary transducer strikes the red blood cells and when the blood cells backscatter the signal, now acting as a moving source with the transducer becoming a stationary receiver. The Doppler shift frequency depends on the frequency of the transmitted ultrasound waves, the velocity of the moving red blood cells, and the angle at which the Doppler beam intersects the vessel. This angle is known as the Doppler angle.

The Doppler effect can be used to calculate blood flow velocity because the Doppler shift frequency depends on the direction of blood flow and is proportional to the speed of the moving red blood cells. The shift is detected by the Doppler probe. The direction of blood flow relative to the transducer determines whether the returning echoes have a higher or lower frequency, and the flow velocity determines the magnitude of the frequency shift (Fig. 1.18b). This relationship is expressed in the Doppler equation:

$$F_d = F_r - F_0 = \frac{2F_0 \cdot v \cdot \cos\alpha}{c}$$

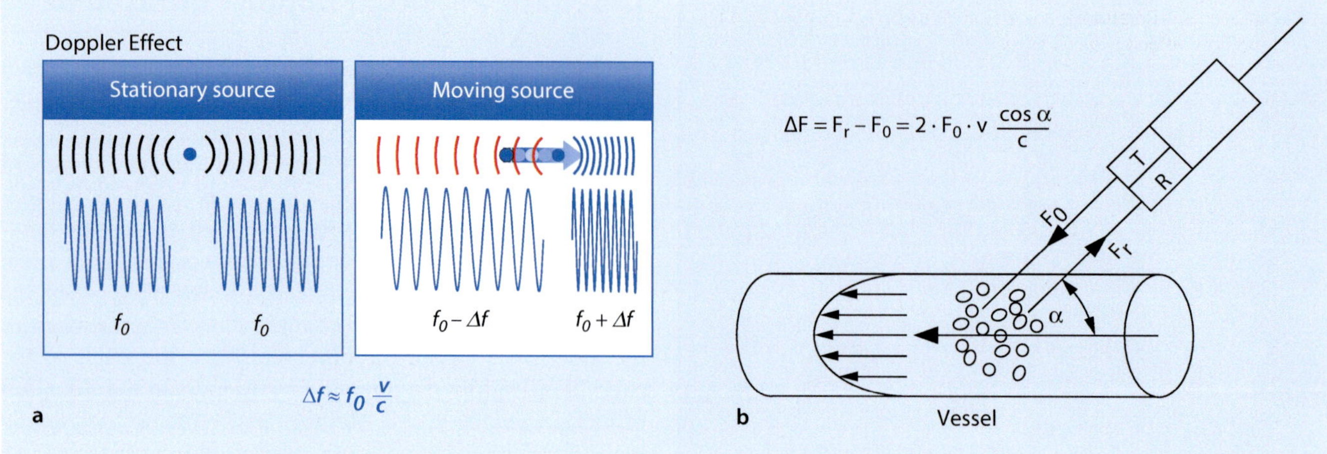

Fig. 1.18a, b Doppler effect. **a** Dependence of the Doppler shift (change in frequency between source and receiver) on the velocity of the moving source and its direction of motion relative to the reflector. **b** Diagram of Doppler interrogation of a vessel with laminar blood flow. The arrows in the vessel are vectors representing different flow velocities. Blood flow is fastest in the center and decreases toward the wall. The drawing illustrates the effect of the angle of incidence on the Doppler measurement. In the equation for calculating the Doppler shift, this angle is represented by the cosine function. The Doppler shift increases with the acuity of the angle (cosine of 90° = 0) (T, transmitter; R, receiver; F_0, emitted frequency; F_r, reflected frequency)

F_d Doppler frequency shift
F_0 emitted frequency
F_r reflected frequency
v mean flow velocity of the reflecting red blood cells
c speed of sound in soft tissue (about 1540 m/s)
α angle between ultrasound beam and direction of blood flow

In the transcutaneous measurement of blood flow by Doppler ultrasound, angle correction is necessary to calculate the flow velocity because the Doppler beam cannot be aligned parallel to the direction of flow. The transformation with representation of the different velocity vectors is expressed mathematically as a cosine function of the angle between the sound beam and the blood vessel (cos α).

F_d (or Δf) is proportional to the velocity of blood flow, cos α, and the carrier frequency of the ultrasound beam.

For angles of about 90°, the cosine function yields values around 0, at which there is no Doppler frequency shift, and the Doppler shift increases as the angle decreases (with a maximum cosα of 1 at $\alpha = 0°$).

The blood flow velocity is calculated by solving the Doppler shift equation for V:

$$V = \left(F_r - F_0\right) \cdot \frac{c}{\cos\alpha \cdot 2F_0}$$

This formula allows calculation of the blood flow velocity from the measured Doppler frequency shift at a given transmit frequency and angle of incidence. The accuracy of the calculation increases with the acuity of the angle. Ideally, the Doppler angle should be kept at or below 60° to minimize errors in the calculation of flow velocity. At angles above 60°, even minor errors in determining the Doppler angle (which are unavoidable in the clinical setting, especially when curved vessels are interrogated) unduly distort the velocity calculation. At angles around 90°, a Doppler shift is no longer detectable and the flow direction cannot be determined. This is reflected in the color duplex scan by the absence of color-coded flow signals although flow is present.

Table 1.5 Dependence of the Doppler shift frequency (Df) on the angle of insonation

Parameter	Values				
Angle α	0°	30°	45°	60°	90°
Cos α	1	0.866	0.707	0.5	0
Df (MHz)	7.79	6.75	5.51	3.90	0
Percentage error	0	13	29	50	100

Table 1.5 lists the Doppler shift frequencies for different angles of incidence, illustrating how the percentage error in calculating blood flow velocity increases with the Doppler angle. The values were calculated for a transmitted frequency of 6 MHz and a blood flow velocity of 1 ms/1.

It is apparent from the examples listed in Table 1.5 that no Doppler shift is detectable at a 90° angle of incidence. The reason is that when the ultrasound beam is perpendicular to the direction of blood flow, there is no relative movement between the Doppler probe and red blood cells. Velocity measurement is most accurate when the Doppler beam is aligned parallel to the blood flow. If this is not possible, accurate velocity estimates can only be made if the Doppler angle is measured using angle correction. The Doppler angle is measured by placing the angle correction cursor parallel to the direction of flow in the B-mode image. For precise calculation, a correction factor of 1/cosα is used. Table 1.6 lists the correction factors for different Doppler angles and the overestimation or underestimation of blood flow velocities

Table 1.6 Relationship between Doppler angle and error in blood flow velocity calculation

Angle α	Correction factor 1/cos α	Error in calculated blood flow velocity
30°	1.15	±3%
45°	1.41	±6%
60°	2.00	±9%
70°	2.92	±14%
75°	3.86	±21%
80°	5.76	±30%

resulting from cursor misplacement. The data in Table 1.6 illustrate how the error in calculating blood flow velocities increases with the Doppler angle. The examiner must therefore try to minimize the insonation angle for Doppler interrogation.

Doppler shift frequencies are extracted by the demodulator of the ultrasound system based on a comparison of the returning Doppler-shifted signal and the transmitted frequency. The Doppler shift frequencies occurring in medical imaging are in the audible range and can be output to a loudspeaker. Information about the direction of flow relative to the transducer can also be extracted from the Doppler signal; this, however, requires more sophisticated demodulation techniques. Blood flow toward the transducer produces a positive frequency shift, and blood flow away from the transducer a negative shift.

Blood flow velocity varies across the vessel lumen. Blood cells move faster in the center and slower near the wall due to friction, giving rise to a laminar flow profile. Other factors affecting the flow profile include the pulsatility of blood flow and the elasticity of the vessel wall or changes in flow resulting from bends in the vessel, branching, and narrowing. The Doppler signal derived from flowing blood thus contains a range of frequencies, which can be extracted using a mathematical algorithm called fast Fourier transform (FFT). This spectral analysis enables changes in blood flow velocity to be displayed over time. In the resulting Doppler spectrum or waveform, the magnitudes of positive and negative shifts are displayed above and below the baseline, respectively. The distribution of frequency shifts or velocities at any given point in time is encoded in the brightness of the pixels.

1.1.2.1 Continuous Wave Doppler Ultrasound

Continuous wave (CW) Doppler (Fig. 1.19) uses two transducer elements – one continuously transmitting and the other continuously receiving ultrasound. Blood flow velocity is calculated from the frequency shift of the signal reflected by the moving red blood cells.

CW Doppler systems may be directional or nondirectional. Nondirectional systems cannot discriminate between

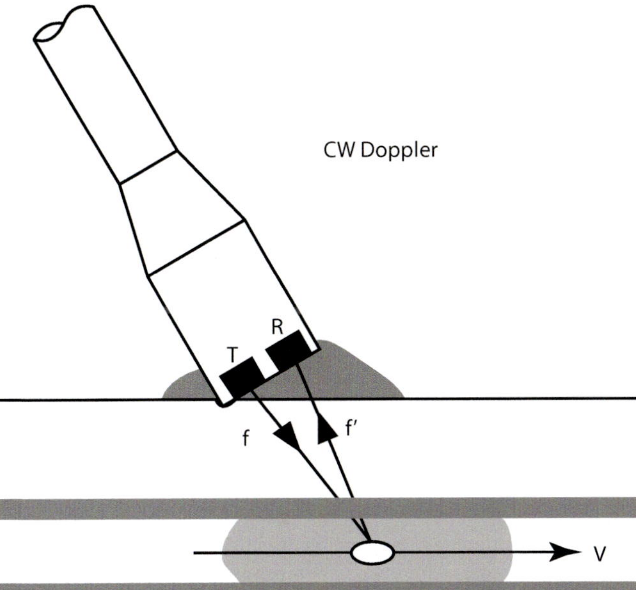

Fig. 1.19 Diagram of continuous wave (CW) Doppler ultrasound. Ultrasound pulses are continuously emitted by the transmitter (T), and frequency-shifted signals reflected by red blood cells moving at different velocities (V) are picked up by the receiver (R)

positive and negative flow directions. In a directional system, information on the flow direction is extracted from the phase shift. As ultrasound is continuously transmitted and received, CW Doppler cannot assign the returning Doppler signal to a specific depth. Hence, the returning signal contains flow information from all vessels along the beam path. With arteries and veins often lying close together, the CW Doppler signal simultaneously represents arterial and venous flow. When performed with a high transmit frequency, CW Doppler allows sensitive examination of superficial vessels.

The advantage of CW Doppler lies in the detection of high flow velocities without aliasing, which is accomplished by the use of separate transmit and receive crystals for the simultaneous emission and reception of ultrasound signals.

1.1.2.2 Pulsed Wave Doppler Ultrasound/Duplex Ultrasound

Pulsed wave (PW) Doppler (Fig. 1.20) is similar to conventional B-mode scanning in that the same piezoelectric elements alternately emit ultrasound pulses and receive the incoming echoes.

The depth from which a returning signal originates can be determined by calculating the round trip time (based on knowledge of the speed of sound in tissue) as follows: a short pulse is emitted, and the system is switched off for some time before the receive mode is switched on. In this way, only echoes arriving at the transducer face with the system in the receive mode are processed, ignoring echoes arriving during the off-mode. The time during which the transducer is in the receive mode is the range gate. By changing the range gate, the operator can define the sample volume or Doppler window. A typical sample volume encompasses the entire

1

diameter of the target vessel. The number of pulses emitted per second is the pulse repetition frequency (PRF). The maximum PRF that can be used decreases with the depth of the vessel interrogated, as it then takes longer for the echoes to return to the transducer.

Sound waves travel through the human body at a fairly constant speed of approx. 1540 m/s. Hence, the round trip time varies with the distance between the reflector and the transmitter, and the operator can define a scan depth using a time filter. An electronic gate then opens briefly, allowing only signals from this site to pass, while discarding all echoes coming in earlier or later. It is thus possible to selectively record Doppler signals from the specified depth. The combination of PW Doppler with real-time gray-scale imaging is the basis for duplex ultrasonography. PW Doppler has the advantage of providing axial resolution (discrimination of vessels along the ultrasound beam), but is limited by the fact that it fails to adequately record high-velocity signals (depending on the transmit frequency and penetration depth). Using a single crystal for transmitting and receiving signals requires a delay between pulses for the processing of returning echoes. The longer the pulse delay, the lower the peak flow velocity that can be detected.

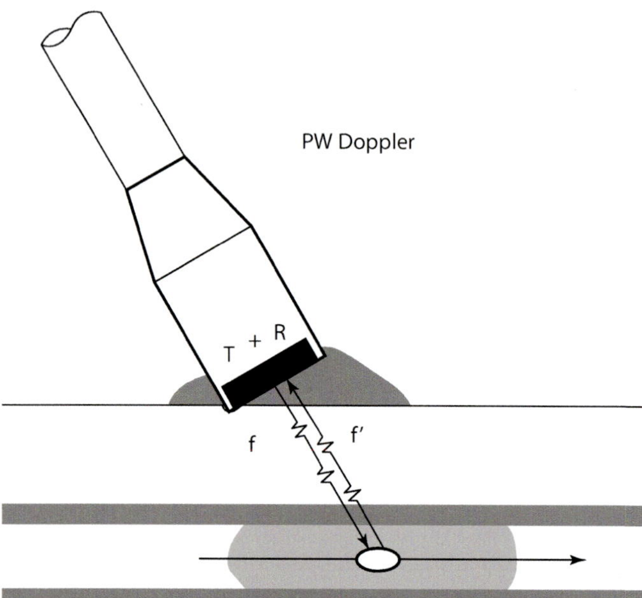

Fig. 1.20 Diagram of pulsed wave (PW) Doppler ultrasound. The transducer alternately emits short ultrasound pulses (T, transmitter) and records the reflected echoes at defined intervals (R, receiver)

Duplex ultrasound combines 2D real-time imaging with pulsed Doppler and thus provides flow information from a sample volume at a defined depth. Duplex scanning enables calculation of blood flow velocity from the Doppler frequency shift as the angle of incidence between the ultrasound beam and the vessel axis can be measured in the B-mode image.

1.1.2.3 Frequency Processing

In a blood vessel, blood components move with different velocities, which are represented in the Doppler spectrum by a range of frequencies with different amplitudes reflecting the distribution of flow velocities in the vessel. The spectrum is analyzed using fast Fourier transform (FFT), which breaks down the waveform into a series of sinusoidal waveforms. For the individual frequency values, the corresponding amplitudes are calculated and displayed in different shades of gray (Fig. 1.21).

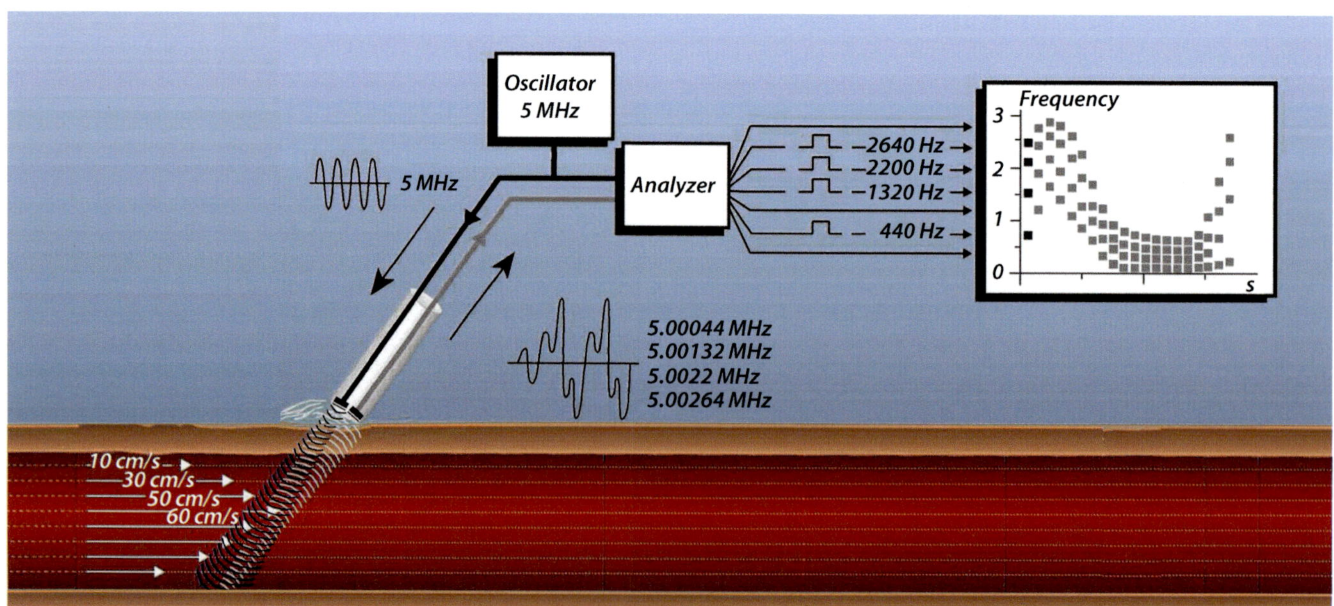

Fig. 1.21 Function of a Doppler transducer. Ultrasound waves are emitted by an oscillator and reflected by red blood cells moving through the vessel at different velocities. The signal is reflected with a shifted frequency, or Doppler shift, which depends on the speed and relative direction of the moving reflectors. The received Doppler signal is composed of a range of frequencies, which have to be sorted by fast Fourier transform (FFT) before they can be displayed over time in the form of a Doppler frequency spectrum or waveform (Diagram courtesy of GE Healthcare)

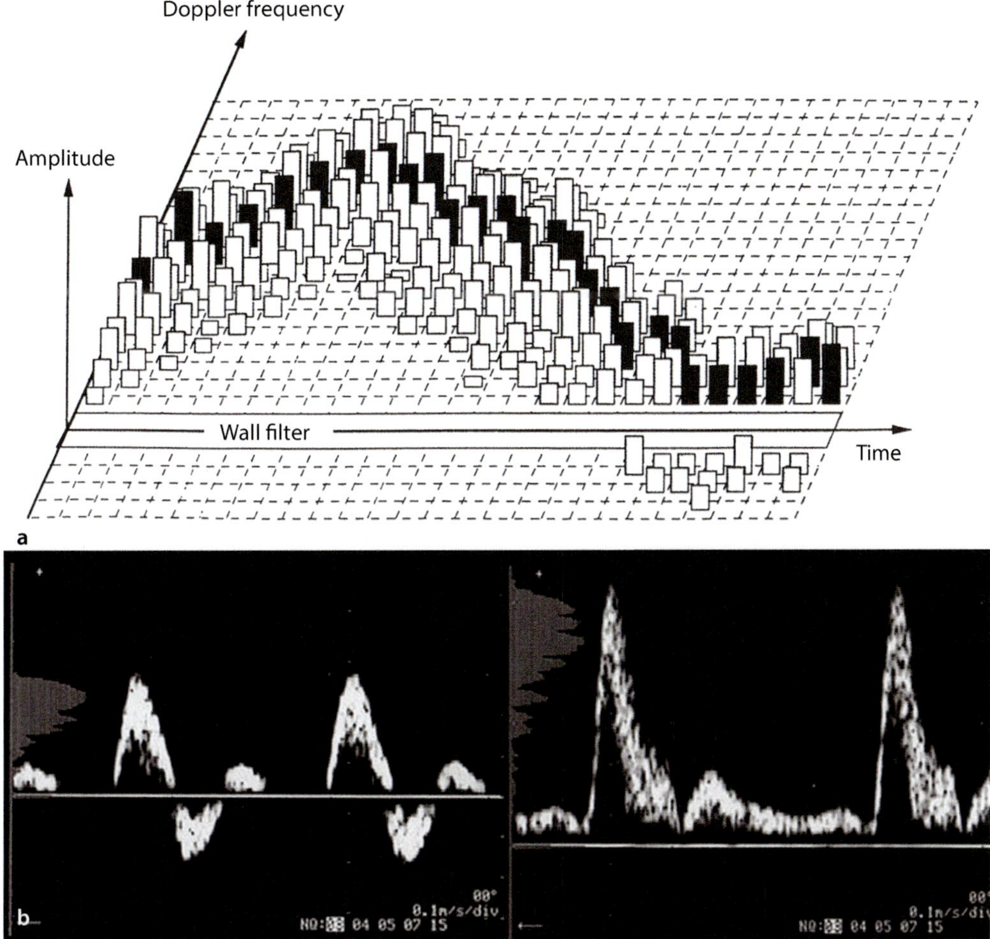

■ **Fig. 1.22** **a** Three-dimensional Doppler frequency spectrum showing the distribution of individual Doppler shifts (amplitudes), flow directions (above and below the time axis), and flow velocities (computed from Doppler frequency shifts). The heights of the boxes correspond to the amplitudes of the respective Doppler frequencies. A Doppler frequency spectrum represents amplitudes by different levels of brightness. In color-coded duplex ultrasound, the averaged flow velocity at a given point in time (black boxes) is displayed in color according to the flow direction and superimposed on the two-dimensional gray-scale image in real time (According to P.M. Klews, in Wolf and Fobbe 1993). **b** Doppler frequency spectrum of the superficial femoral artery (left section). The histogram plotted on the vertical axis on the left represents the distribution of the different Doppler frequency shifts during systole. In the Doppler waveform, this distribution is represented by different levels of brightness (laminar flow). The right section shows the corresponding distribution during systole in the common carotid artery, which has less pulsatile flow

According to Fourier's theorem, any periodic waveform can be reconstructed from its component waveforms. Conversely, in spectral analysis, a complex waveform of a given frequency (Doppler shift frequency) is decomposed into its frequency components. In this case, the FFT yields the amplitudes of the individual frequencies of the respective sine and cosine functions, which together make up the waveform. The individual frequencies thus separated are continuously displayed over time in the Doppler frequency spectrum (spectral waveform). The Doppler spectrum contains the following information on blood flow (■ Fig. 1.22a):

- The vertical axis representing different flow velocities as Doppler frequency shifts
- The horizontal axis representing the time course of the frequency shifts
- Density of points, or color intensity, on the vertical axis representing the number of red blood cells moving at a certain velocity (may also be plotted in the form of a histogram)

Flow toward and away from the transducer is processed simultaneously and respectively represented above and below the baseline (zero flow velocity line).

Alternatively, some ultrasound devices display the magnitudes of the different velocity components in a separate power spectrum. This is done by measuring the signal intensities of the individual Doppler frequencies at a specific time in the cardiac cycle and displaying the spectral distribution in a histogram (■ Fig. 1.22b; ■ Table 1.7).

1.1.2.4 Blood Flow Measurement

The most important parameters for evaluating and quantifying blood flow that can be derived from the Doppler frequency spectrum are:

- Peak systolic frequency (mainly relevant for quantifying stenosis)
- Peak end-diastolic frequency (stenosis, flow character)
- Averaged blood flow velocity

1

Table 1.7 Spectral displays

Type of spectrum	Information displayed
Power spectrum	Display of the power, or strength, of individual frequencies
Frequency spectrum	Display of shifted frequencies or blood flow velocities over time
Usual mode of display	Frequency spectrum
Levels of brightness or color represent the density of a given frequency in the frequency band	

- Intensity-weighted mean blood flow velocity (which is the basis for calculation of the volume flow rate)
- Variance (spectral broadening due to flow disturbances)

Based on these parameters, the following quantities can be calculated:

- Angle-corrected peak systolic velocity (PSV) and end-diastolic velocity (EDV) can be calculated from the Doppler waveform. Mean flow velocity is calculated on the basis of the signal intensities.
- The volume flow rate is calculated from the intensity-weighted mean blood flow velocity and the vascular cross-sectional area using the following equation:

$$Q(mL/min) = 60 \cdot mean\ flow\ velocity\ (cm/s) \cdot cross\text{-}sectional\ area\ (cm^2)$$

Quantitative evaluation of blood flow requires estimation of the Doppler angle to calculate angle-corrected blood flow velocity. The Doppler shift alone does not provide this information. To minimize errors in the calculation of blood flow velocity and other parameters, the angle should be as small as possible and not exceed 60°.

At a Doppler angle of 60°, an error of ±5° in the estimated angle of insonation will lead to a 20% error in the calculated velocity. The magnitude of the error increases disproportionately with the angle of insonation (Fig. 1.23).

Various measures are available to optimize the angle of insonation for spectral Doppler interrogation and measurement of blood flow velocity:

- Use of a unilateral waterpath (linear-array transducer).
- Electronic beam steering: Successive firing of the elements in a linear-array transducer produces an ultrasound wave that is emitted from the transducer at a specific angle (to steer the color box and make the insonation angle as small as possible).
- Manual manipulation of the transducer (sector and curved-array transducers): A curved-array transducer with a small footprint enables a wide range of motion including angulation for optimization of the Doppler angle. However, the examiner must be aware that the color coding may change as a result of a change in the flow direction relative to the sector-shaped ultrasound beam. In this case, the area of transition between red and blue is black (while it is yellow in aliasing). Black indicates that no Doppler frequency shift information is obtained because the ultrasound beam is at a 90° angle to the vessel axis.

In vitro waterbath experiments in which two precision pumps generated different flow profiles demonstrated good correlation ($r = 0.98$) between the volume flow rates measured by duplex ultrasound and volumetry (Schäberle and Seitz 1991; Fig. 1.24).

Even in deeper vessels, highly reproducible measurements can be obtained by performing Doppler interrogations at angles as close to 0° as possible to minimize the effects of errors in angle setting. Repeated ultrasound measurement of flow in the superior mesenteric artery performed in 28 fasting subjects in the morning revealed a day-to-day variation of 11% in peak systolic velocity (PSV) and of 9.7% in end-diastolic velocity (EDV) (Fig. 1.25). Repeated diameter measurement using the leading-edge method showed a day-to-day variation of 2.2% (Schäberle and Seitz 1991).

Another source of error that can lead to over- or underestimation of average flow velocity is to use inadequate transmit or receive gain settings (Fig. 1.26).

The main uncertainty in determining the volume flow rate, however, arises from the measurement of the vessel diameter and the resulting inaccuracy in calculating the cross-sectional area (Fig. 1.27). In B-mode images, vessel walls appear thicker than their true anatomic size. This is due to the so-called blooming effect resulting from the strong reflection of the ultrasound beam at the interface between blood and the vessel wall (Fig. 1.28b).

In summary, sonographic determination of volume flow rates is prone to the following pitfalls:

- Determination of average flow velocity
- Doppler angle error
- Uncertainty in the calculation of the vessel cross-sectional area
  - Inaccuracy in vessel diameter measurement (blooming effect)
  - Assumption of a circular vessel cross-section.
  - Variation in the cross-sectional area during the cardiac cycle
  - Respiratory variation in vascular cross-sectional area (veins)

The uncertainty in sonographic vessel diameter measurement can be minimized and systematized by using the leading-to-leading-edge (LTL) method and low gain settings. With the LTL method, the diameter is measured from the reflection of the nearest outer wall to that of the opposite inner wall (Fig. 1.28a). In vitro experiments found a greater accuracy for diameters below 13 mm and showed the overestimation

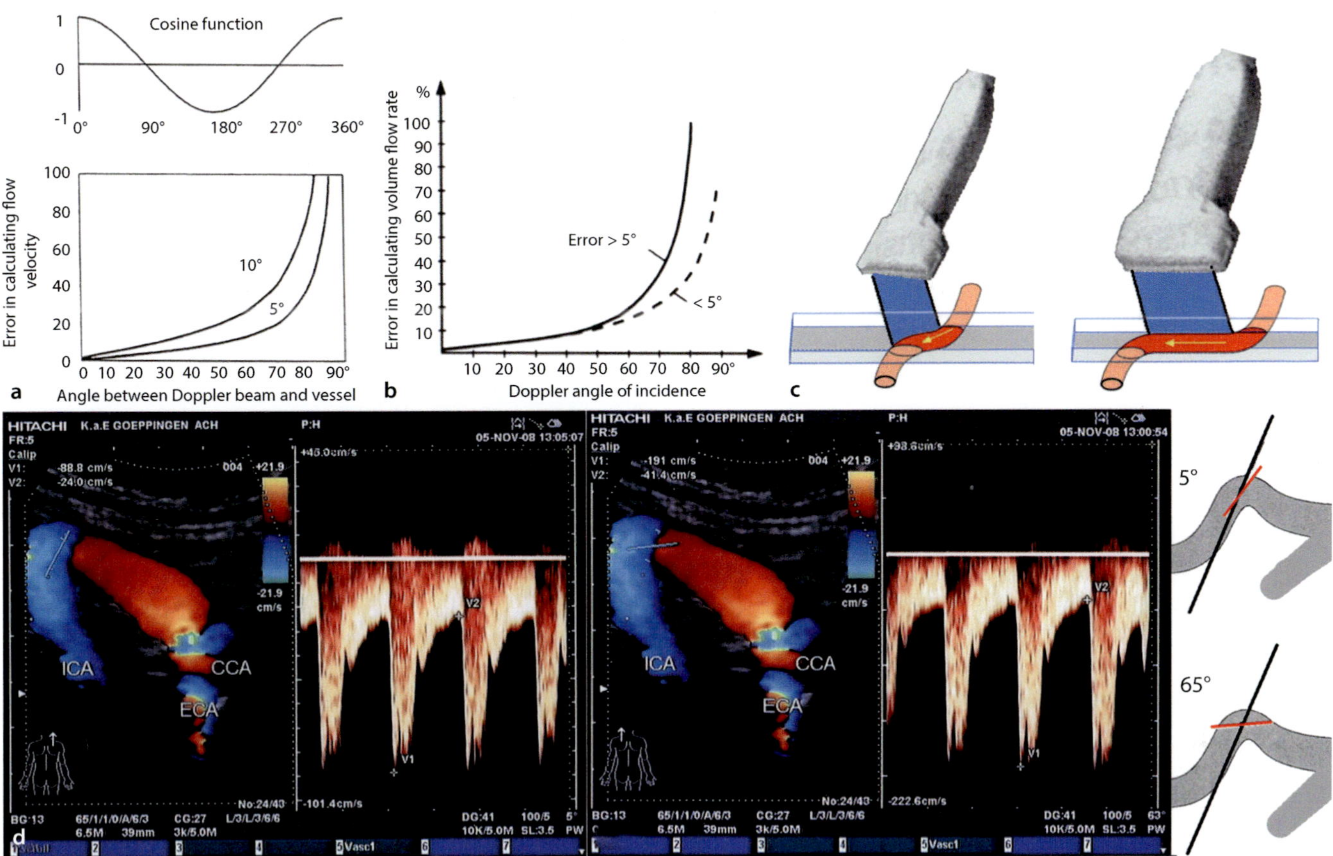

Fig. 1.23 **a** The Doppler equation incorporates the angle between the ultrasound beam and the flowing blood in the form of the cosine function (cosα), with the shift being highest when the beam strikes the vessel tangentially (cosine of 0° = 1) and lowest when the beam is perpendicular to the direction of blood flow (cosine of 90° = 0). The larger the Doppler angle, the greater the resulting error in the velocity calculation in case of inaccurate placement of the angle correction cursor (graphically shown for errors of 5° and 10°). Such errors are unavoidable, particularly when aligning the cursor with the vessel wall in curved vessel segments. **b** The graph illustrates the angle-dependent error in flow measurement for a misalignment of ±5°. Overestimation of the Doppler angle results in greater error in the velocity calculation than underestimation. **c** Error in blood flow velocity calculation resulting from misalignment of the angle correction cursor in vessels running obliquely through the scan plane. Alignment of the angle correction cursor is more difficult if a blood vessel passes obliquely through the scan plane in the B-mode image (left drawing). An oblique course is suggested if only a short segment of a long straight vessel is depicted. In such a case, the transducer should be turned to obtain a B-mode scan visualizing a long straight vessel segment (right drawing) for optimal positioning of the angle correction cursor. **d** Uncertainty concerning the Doppler angle of insonation in a tortuous vessel. In a curved vessel segment, the angle of insonation varies through a range of 5°–65° over a short stretch, making it difficult to accurately determine the Doppler angle for calculating flow velocity. Left color flow image and corresponding Doppler waveform: Velocity measurement in a very tortuous internal carotid artery (ICA). With the sample volume positioned in the curved segment (to confirm or rule out clinically suspected kinking stenosis), a maximum peak systolic velocity (PSV) of 88 cm/s and a peak end-diastolic velocity (EDV) of 24 cm/s were calculated with a Doppler angle of 5° (top drawing). Right color flow image and waveform: With an assumed Doppler angle of 65°, a PSV of 191 cm/s and an EDV of 41 cm/s were calculated in the curvature of the vessel (bottom drawing)

of diameters to be less severe than the underestimation reported for the inner-to-inner-edge method (ITI) (Smith 1984). Moreover, use of the LTL method systematizes the unavoidable measurement error, thereby improving the reproducibility of measurements.

Diameter variations during the cardiac cycle can be taken into account by measuring both systolic and diastolic diameters (in the time-motion mode) and considering them in the flow volume calculation with different weightings (1/3 systole +2/3 diastole).

Other parameters that characterize blood flow are the pulsatility index (PI) and the resistive index (RI) according to Pourcelot. These indices have the advantage that they are not dependent on the Doppler angle of insonation. The resistive indices, in particular the Pourcelot index, reflect wall elasticity as well as the peripheral resistance of the organ supplied (Fig. 1.28c, d).

The Pourcelot index increases with peripheral resistance, while end-diastolic velocity (EDV) decreases. Stenosis or occlusion in peripheral arteries with triphasic flow alters the Doppler waveform and hence the Pourcelot index. It can thus serve as a semiquantitative parameter for estimating the degree of stenosis. In an artery supplying a parenchymal organ, a relevant decrease in the Pourcelot index between the prestenotic and the poststenotic segment can be interpreted as indicating hemodynamically significant stenosis, for instance, when examining a patient with suspected renal artery stenosis.

1

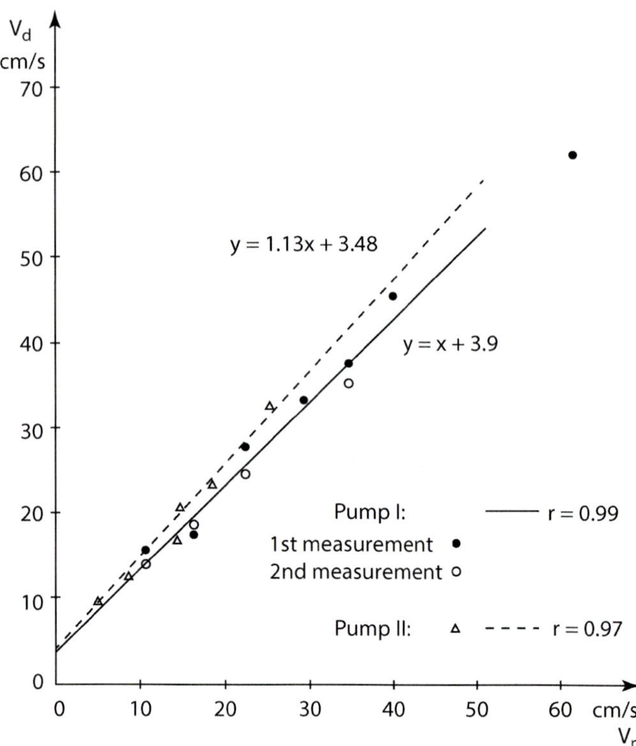

Fig. 1.24 In vitro flow measurement by duplex ultrasound. Comparison of mean flow velocity determined by duplex ultrasound (V_d) and volumetry (V_p). Different flow profiles were generated by two precision pumps (I and II). The mean axis shift of 3.75 cm/s with shift of the zero line was due to a software error and was corrected by the manufacturer following these experiments. V_p = mean actual flow velocity calculated from volumetrically determined flow rate/cross-sectional area of the tube; V_d = mean flow velocity determined by duplex ultrasound (mean of five individual measurements) (Schäberle and Seitz 1991)

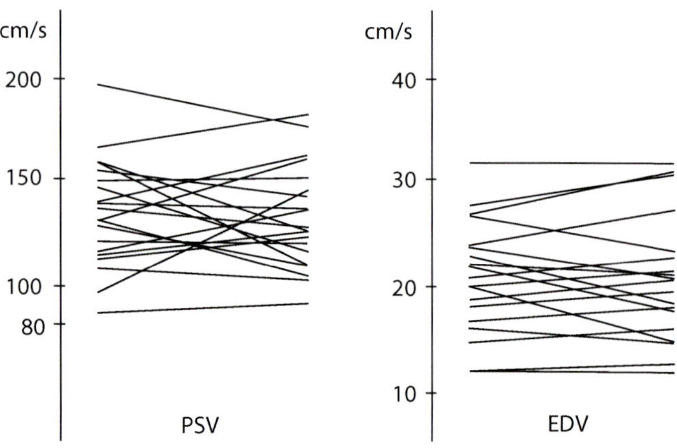

Fig. 1.25 Peak systolic velocities (PSV) and end-diastolic velocities (EDV) measured in the superior mesenteric artery of fasting subjects on two successive days (*n* = 28)

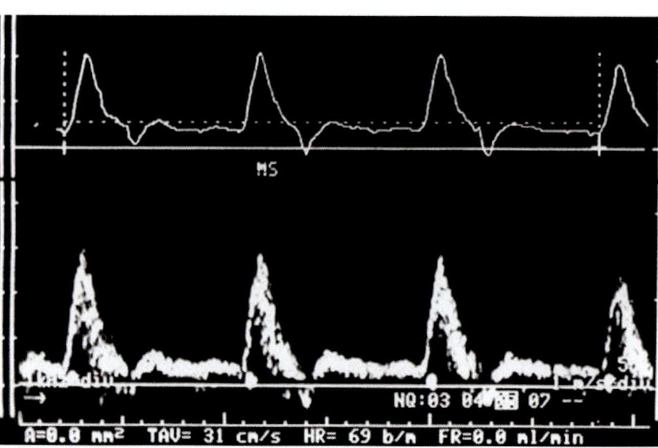

Fig. 1.26 Spectral Doppler waveform from the superior mesenteric artery (bottom) obtained with adequate settings and the corresponding curve of mean flow velocities over time automatically computed by the ultrasound machine (top). The blood flow velocity averaged over three cardiac cycles is 31 cm/s

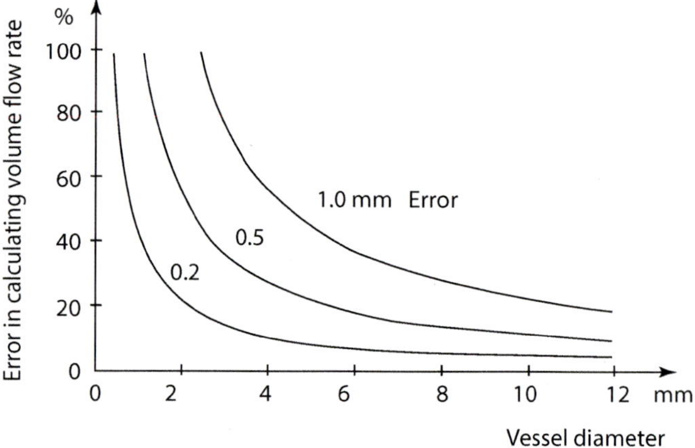

Fig. 1.27 Errors in volume flow rate calculation resulting from different measurement accuracies in determining vessel diameter (for errors ranging from 0.2 to 1.0 mm)

1.1.3 Physical Principles of Color-Coded Duplex Ultrasound

1.1.3.1 Velocity Mode

Color duplex ultrasound combines the presentation of two-dimensional (2D) morphologic information with superimposed flow data of a defined area displayed in color. The frame rate is much lower for the color-coded 2D display of flow information than for the conventional (black-and-white) display because it takes much longer to compute the 2D distribution of flow.

In conventional duplex ultrasound, a small gate (sample volume) is defined in the real-time gray-scale image for

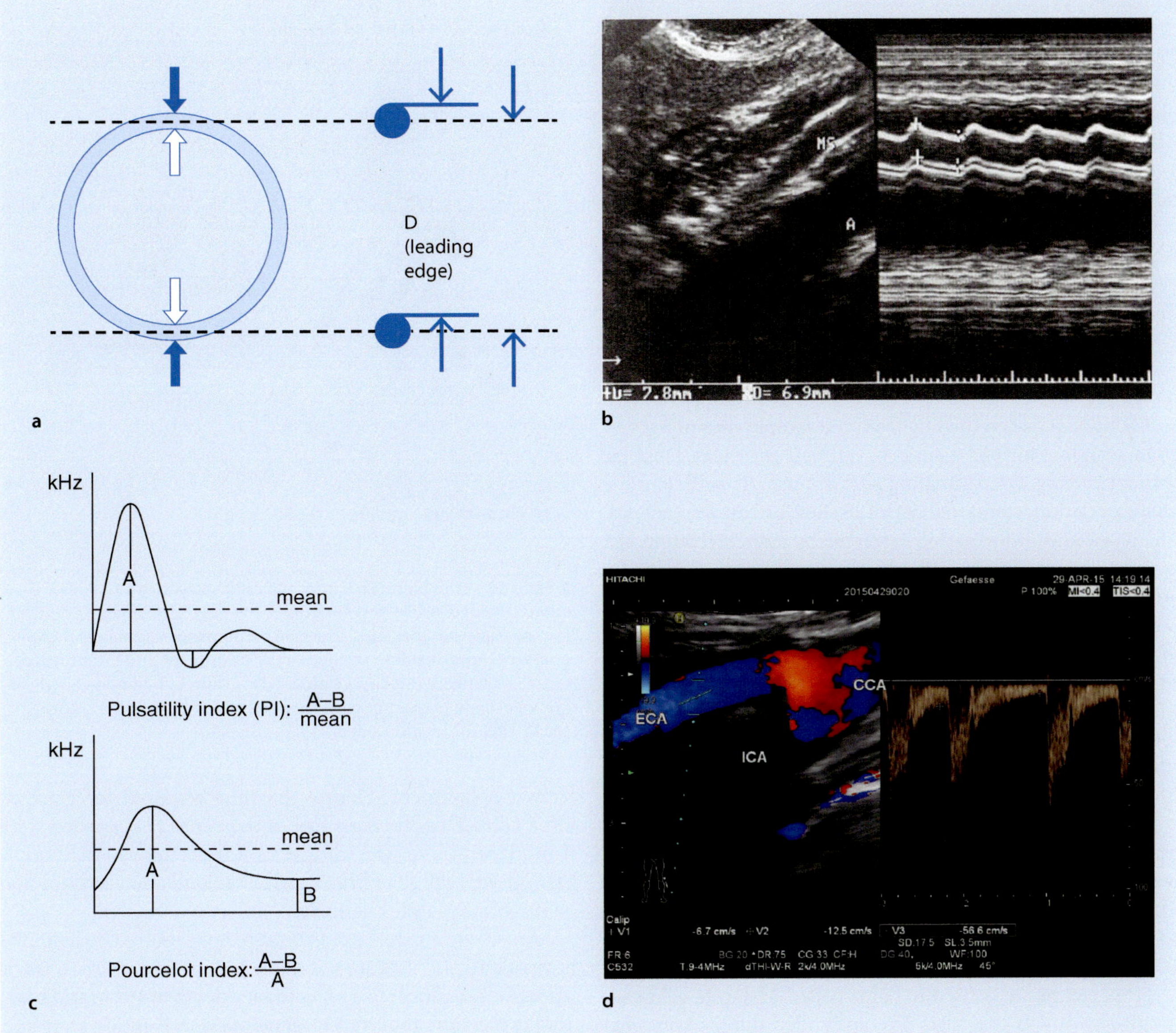

Fig. 1.28a–d Vessel diameter measurement and resistive indices. **a** Diagram illustrating the three main methods of sonographic vessel diameter measurement (left part of drawing): The diameter can be measured from the outer wall to the outer wall (outer-to-outer-edge method, OTO, blue arrows), from the inner wall to the inner wall (inner-to-inner-edge method, ITI, white arrows), or from the outer wall reflection closest to the transducer to the reflection from the opposite inner wall (leading-edge-to-leading-edge method, LTL, downward arrows). The LTL method minimizes and standardizes overestimation of vessel diameters due to blooming. **b** Measurement of the diameter of the superior mesenteric artery (MS) using the leading-edge method: The images illustrate how the vessel wall is overemphasized as a result of the blooming effect. Systolic-diastolic variation in diameter: the gray-scale scan on the left coincidentally depicts the maximum systolic extension of 7.8 mm, while the time-motion display shows the variation in diameter from 7.8 mm in systole to 6.9 mm in diastole. **c** Diagrams of resistive indices. The Pourcelot index is calculated from peak systolic (PSV) and end-diastolic velocities (EDVs), while the pulsatility index (PI) can only be calculated when the system's software allows calculation of time-averaged velocity (TAV). **d** The Pourcelot index, which is typically used in the spectral Doppler evaluation of parenchymal organ blood flow, is dependent on the patient's heart rate. In subjects with tachycardia, EDVs are cut off, resulting in a lower Pourcelot index than in patients with bradycardia and the same peripheral resistance. The variation in heart rate and the resulting effect on the Pourcelot index is illustrated here by the waveform from the external carotid artery (ECA) obtained in a patient with occlusion of the internal carotid artery (ICA) and absolute arrhythmia: EDV decreases with the length of diastole. In this patient, arrhythmia results in Pourcelot indices that differ by more than 10% (0.89 and 0.79, calculated from EDVs of 6.7 cm/s and 12.5 cm/s) (see Fig. 5.25)

which Doppler frequency shift data are obtained by analyzing separate scan lines. This information is displayed in the form of a Doppler waveform. To simultaneously measure flow velocities at different sites, several sample volumes are placed along adjacent beam paths. The distribution of sites defines a region of interest (ROI) for which flow velocity data are sampled. The Doppler signals from multiple sites cannot be analyzed using fast Fourier transform (FFT) because it would take too much time and also because it is not possible to simultaneously display all Doppler spectra generated using this approach. Consider that if we have 20 active scan lines, each with 50 sampling sites, this would mean data from 1000 sample volumes!

To cope with this amount of data, most systems use a technique known as autocorrelation, which compares two consecutive pulses returning from the sample sites of a given color scan line for phase shifts to estimate the mean Doppler shift frequency. Four sampling sites are usually sufficient for autocorrelation, compared with 128 sites for Fourier analysis. The phase shift information extracted by autocorrelation is a direct measure of the mean velocity distribution in a sample volume. The flow information is superimposed on a B-mode scan using red and blue to encode blood flow toward and away from the transducer, respectively. Different degrees of brightness encode blood flow velocity, with brighter colors indicating faster flow. As with PW Doppler, color Doppler ultrasound is also limited by angle dependence and aliasing. Aliasing is indicated by a color reversal in the color flow image.

Hence multigate pulsed Doppler uses several sample volumes, from which Doppler information is received and analyzed simultaneously using several independent channels. The flow information can thus be analyzed and displayed without delay compared with the conventional duplex scan (◘ Fig. 1.29).

This technique is used in color-coded M-mode echocardiography and is the basis of color-coded duplex sonography. An ultrasound line with several sample gates is swept over the B-mode scan or a defined region of the scan from which velocity information is extracted in 50–150 ms. The number of scan lines is limited by the geometric arrangement of the crystals in the transducer, and the available lines must be divided into those for generation of the gray-scale image (B-mode image lines) and those for blood flow velocity measurement (Doppler lines). Most scan lines are reserved for generation of the B-mode image with only every other to every fourth line being available for acquiring Doppler information. Due to the lower number of Doppler lines, the missing information between two Doppler lines must be interpolated. Using the multigate technique with placement of several sample volumes along the Doppler beam path, a 2D display of blood flow distribution is generated. About ten pulse packets are necessary for each color Doppler line to obtain precise information (as opposed to only one pulse packet for each B-mode scan line). Before emission of each new pulse packet, all echoes from the preceding pulse must have returned from the maximum scan depth to ensure correct assignment. Hence, the time required for generating a color Doppler scan line is ten times that needed for a B-mode scan line. The information from the 50–250 sample gates along each scan line is processed and analyzed simultaneously by separate channels.

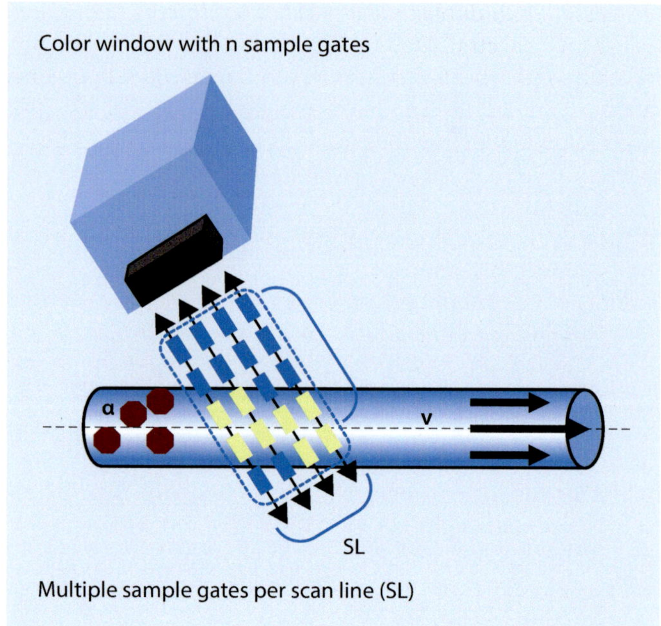

◘ **Fig. 1.29** The blood flow information displayed in a region of interest (color window or color box) of the gray-scale image is derived from multiple sample gates arranged along parallel scan lines. Color represents flow direction relative to the transducer, and brightness represents mean flow velocity. Laminar flow results in higher mean blood flow velocity in the center of a vessel, indicated by brighter colors (see ◘ Figs. 1.22a and 1.43)

Assuming a mean ultrasound propagation velocity in the human body of 1540 m/s, it takes 130 μs for a pulse to travel from the transducer to a reflector at a depth of 10 cm and back. This is the time required to generate one B-mode scan line. It takes ten times longer, that is, 1.3 ms, to generate a color Doppler scan line. If 50 color Doppler scan lines are used to generate a color Doppler image, the overall time required is about 65 ms, resulting in a frame rate of 15 images per second. The frame rate decreases when more color Doppler scan lines are required, which in turn depends on the width of the color box. A frame rate of at least 20/s is necessary for a smooth display with good temporal resolution.

When deeper structures in the body are imaged, as in abdominal ultrasound, the longer delay of the echo pulses makes it necessary to use a lower pulse repetition frequency (PRF) for precise spatial resolution of the echo pulses, which likewise decreases the frame rate.

In triplex ultrasound, the gray-scale morphologic information and Doppler-derived blood flow information in a defined portion of the image is supplemented by detailed spectral Doppler analysis of flow including velocity measurement at specific sites of the target vessel. The simultaneous use of these three modes reduces the performance of each. Specifically, the maximum PRF available is even lower compared with duplex ultrasound. Therefore, at higher flow velocities, spectral Doppler interrogation should be performed while the B-mode/color flow image is frozen once an abnormal vessel region requiring closer investigation has been identified in the color mode and the sample volume has been placed using the B-mode image.

A slightly better performance in the triplex mode can be achieved by processing a Doppler pulse echo cycle after each other to fourth B-mode scan line. This interleave technique improves the sampling rate compared with the analysis of one Doppler scan line after each B-mode line and thus generates images at an acceptable frame rate even at a low PRF, for example, when scanning deep body structures.

Conventional color flow imaging is based on spectral analysis of the frequency-shifted ultrasound echoes backscattered by moving red blood cells. The frequency shift information can be derived from blood flow velocity (velocity mode) or from the ultrasound energy (power mode).

In contrast, **color velocity imaging**, which is a so-called time-domain technique, derives blood flow velocity information from the round trip times of the emitted ultrasound pulses. This is done by comparing changes in the patterns of the reflected echoes between two successive B-mode scan line pulses and deriving blood flow information from changes in the echo pattern over time.

Quantitatively, the direction and velocity of flow can be determined using a cross-correlation technique. However, this procedure makes high demands on computing capacity and has not established itself although it is superior to shift-based techniques because there is no aliasing and angle dependence and it enables higher frame rates. The cross-correlation technique does not determine the Doppler frequency or phase shift of an echo compared to the transmitted pulse but compares two successive pulse echo cycles in a defined space and at a predetermined time delay. In other words, the positional change of two pulse echo cycles is determined in relation to time. The velocity of the moving medium with its characteristic echo pattern is then calculated from the temporal shift. This technique relies on the recognition of the echo pattern, which requires an excellent signal-to-noise ratio. The only factor that limits the PRF is the scanning depth.

The **autocorrelation technique** compares demodulated Doppler signals. The accuracy of determining the mean Doppler shift is higher when blood flow is constant and decreases when flow becomes more turbulent. The bandwidth of the different flow components is given by the variance, which can be displayed in color by adding a green shade. Analysis of several pulse cycles will yield a more accurate value of mean flow velocity.

The amount of Doppler information collected from the large number of sample volumes along the scan line (in contrast to a single, circumscribed gate in conventional duplex scanning) is too large to be processed by spectral analysis using the FFT with decomposition of the spectrum into its component parts and display of the proportions of different flow velocities at a given location. Instead, the faster autocorrelation technique is used to calculate the mean frequency shift and the corresponding mean velocity. Averaging of the frequencies reduces the spectral information to a color pixel that represents an intensity-weighted mean Doppler frequency shift in a direction-dependent manner (see ◘ Fig. 1.22a; average flow velocities at a given point in time (represented by black boxes in the 3D Doppler spectrum) are represented by levels of brightness in color flow images). Blood flow toward the transducer is displayed in red, and flow away from the transducer in blue. Brighter colors indicate faster flow. The system displays the gray-scale information, superimposing the color flow information in the selected color window whenever echoes reflected by moving structures are obtained.

In the inverse color mode, veins can be displayed in blue and arteries in red regardless of the true flow directions relative to the transducer. The use of this mode will cause problems when there is abnormal reversal of flow or when scanning abdominal regions with a complex vascular anatomy. The ultrasound convention of displaying cranial portions of the vascular anatomy on the left side of the monitor and peripheral segments on the right allows direct identification of the flow direction (toward the heart or toward the periphery) from the color coding when the transducer position is known (without first having to look for the information that indicates the inverse color display and varies from one manufacturer to the next).

1.1.3.2 Power Doppler Mode

Power Doppler uses the amplitude of the Doppler signal to detect flowing blood. The principle was first reported in the literature in 1994, and the technique is commercially available under a variety of names including color flow angio (CFA), power Doppler angio, color power Doppler, color angio, color Doppler energy (CDE), and color perfusion imaging.

While Doppler techniques processing frequency or phase information use a high-pass filter (HPF) to extract the blood signal and to distinguish it from tissue echoes, an amplitude-based flow technique additionally processes the intensity or amplitude of the received echoes to differentiate signals from stationary and moving reflectors. Tissue echoes typically have 1000 times higher intensity than echoes backscattered by moving blood cells, allowing much better separation of the two signal types. While conventional color Doppler requires a frequency analysis to process blood flow information, an amplitude-based technique assigns colors directly from the echo intensities, similar to the assignment of gray-scale values in B-mode ultrasound.

Blood flow is represented by different shades of a single color reflecting the strength of the returned Doppler signal, which is determined by the number of moving reflectors (◘ Fig. 1.30). Therefore, power Doppler is more sensitive to slow flow and flow with only a few reflectors than conventional frequency-based Doppler imaging. The signal-to-noise ratio improves with the number of gates placed along each color Doppler line. While power Doppler is similar to other

1

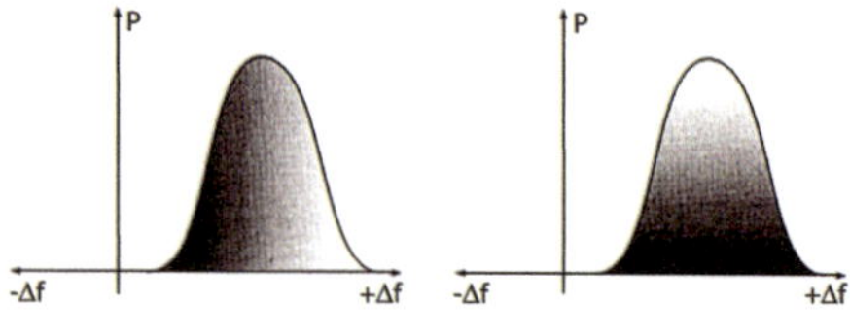

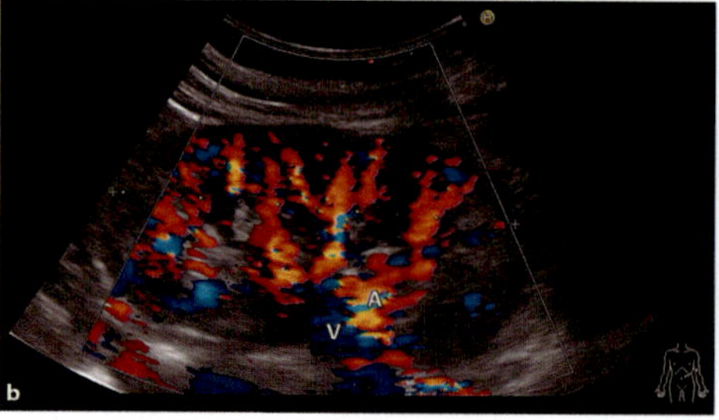

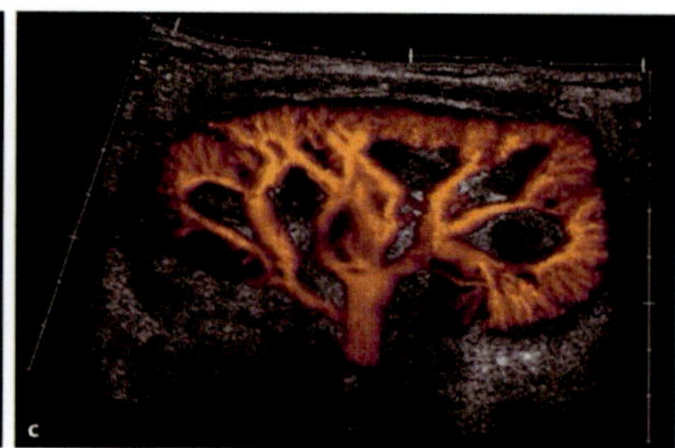

Fig. 1.30 **a** Illustration of the difference in display between frequency-based color flow imaging (velocity mode) and power Doppler: in the velocity mode (left), increasing levels of brightness of the colors used to encode flow direction (red and blue) represent increasing blood flow velocity. In a power Doppler image (right), increasing levels of brightness represent the amplitude or strength of the flow signal irrespective of its frequency or blood flow direction. **b** Color duplex image of the kidney: in the velocity mode, the color coding of the vessels indicates the blood flow direction. In this example, veins are shown in blue (flow away from the transducer) and arteries in red (toward the transducer). The renal vessels are visualized down to the interlobar level. Due to the angle dependence of this mode, depiction of flowing blood is difficult in the upper and lower kidney poles, where the beam is perpendicular to the direction of flow. **c** Power Doppler image of the kidney: the display provides no information on the direction of blood flow but enables evaluation of slow flow and is less angle-dependent, which is why this mode is superior in depicting renal parenchymal blood flow, even in small vessels

Table 1.8 Advantages and disadvantages of frequency-based color flow imaging (velocity mode) and power Doppler imaging (angio mode)

Ultrasound mode	Advantages	Disadvantages
Velocity mode	Display of flow velocity and direction, high temporal resolution	Accuracy depends on angle of insonation (which in turn affects color filling of lumen), aliasing
Power Doppler (angio mode)	Little angle dependence (resulting in good color filling), depiction of slow flow, sensitivity to low flow, few artifacts, better delineation of flowing blood	No information on flow velocity and direction, more difficult differentiation of arteries and veins, no hemodynamic information

techniques in that it only registers returning echoes within a certain range of Doppler frequency shifts, it is largely independent of the angle between the ultrasound beam and flowing blood. Since blood does not flow strictly in one direction, some echoes will always return to the transducer even at an unfavorable angle; however, color intensity is reduced at an angle around 90°. Power Doppler is particularly suitable for detecting slow flow in small vessels and can thus be used to assess peripheral perfusion as well as perfusion in small tumor vessels or in parenchymal organs (Table 1.8) or to identify sites from which spectral Doppler flow information should be obtained.

Power Doppler imaging is limited by the fact that it does not provide qualitative or semiquantitative information on blood flow velocity. Moreover, it is more susceptible to artifacts induced by organ movement and has a poorer temporal resolution. On the other hand, there is no aliasing because power Doppler is independent of the magnitude of the Doppler frequency shift. The main advantage of the power mode lies in the fact that it uses very low PRFs (in the range of some 100 Hz), which in turn enables the resolution of very small Doppler frequency shifts (slow flow). In summary, **power Doppler** is characterized by the **following features** (see Table 1.8):

- No information on blood flow direction (only presence vs absence of flow is encoded)
- No information on flow velocity
- Virtually independent of Doppler angle of insonation
- No aliasing
- Display of all flow components with color intensity representing the number of moving reflectors
- Dynamic gain:
  - Sensitive to low flow/perfusion
  - Susceptible to motion artifacts.

Conventional power Doppler images thus represent the sum of the signals returned from moving particles in terms of different levels of brightness, ignoring flow velocity and direction (Fig. 1.30). Bidirectional power Doppler allows color coding of flow direction (blue and red). Ultrasound systems with this capability employ some extra Doppler lines solely to sample and process flow direction information using the autocorrelation technique.

1.1.3.3 B-Flow Mode (Brightness Flow)

The B-flow mode is not a Doppler technique based on the processing of Doppler shift frequencies but a B-mode scanning technique that compares gray-scale scans over time to identify changes in the spatial positions of reflectors (blood cells) by the successive emission of coded pulse packets. If the echoes returning along the same scan line upon transmission of two successive ultrasound beams give an identical gray-scale pattern, the echoes have been reflected by stationary tissue. Conversely, if the echoes are reflected by stationary tissue and moving red blood cells, a slight difference in the pattern can be seen (Fig. 1.31). The echo signals are subtracted from one another, and the brightness is determined by the number of reflectors and partly also by their velocity.

Reflection (B-mode)

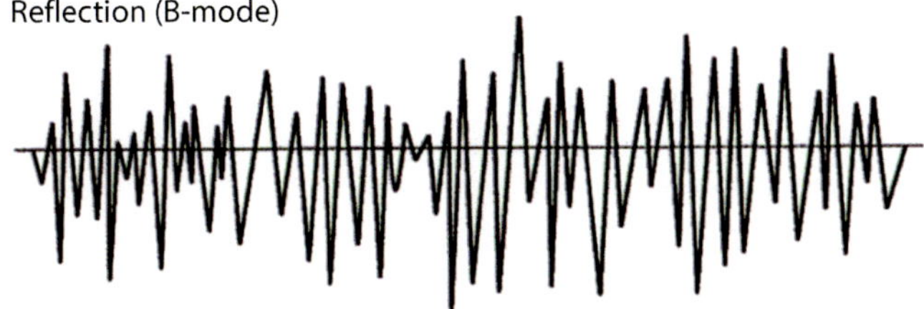

Reflection (B-mode) plus reflection from flowing blood (red)

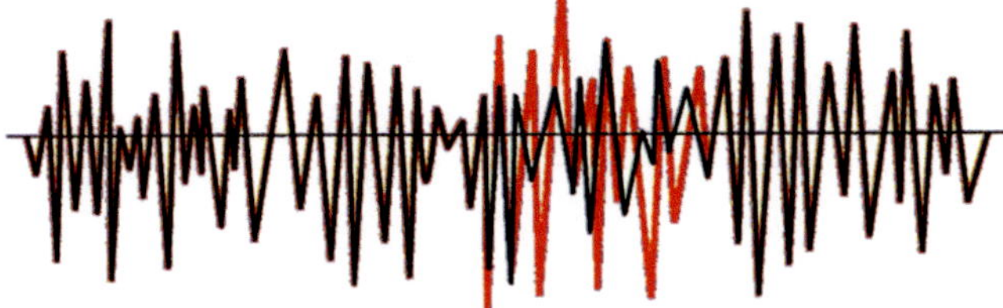

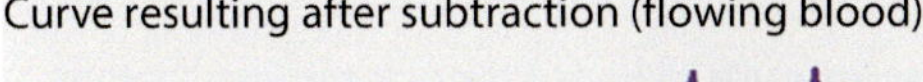

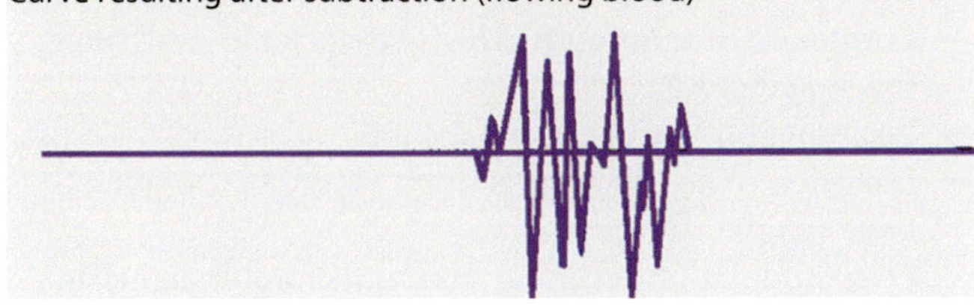

Fig. 1.31 Signal generation in B-flow ultrasound. Two reflections, I and II, produced by two successive ultrasound beams emitted along the same scan line give identical signals if the echoes are returning from stationary objects. Conversely, if signals are reflected from moving targets (red blood cells), there will be a circumscribed change in the signal pattern (seen when the two are superimposed). A subtraction image representing flowing blood can be generated by subtracting the echoes from stationary tissue, improving the differentiation between blood and surrounding stationary tissue (see Fig. 5.86 (Atlas))

The conventional B-mode image generated from the stationary echoes is displayed around the flow information. Since the successive pulses are emitted at defined intervals and in digitally encoded form, it is possible to eliminate interfering echoes and use only the encoded echoes in the subtraction procedure. Hence, only the amplitude signal reflected by moving particles is processed in the interval between two pulses. As the signal strength increases not only with the number of reflecting particles (volume flow) but also with flow velocity, a jet within a stenosis is depicted with higher signal intensity.

B-flow images depict blood flow with high spatial resolution and allow good delineation of flowing blood from the vessel wall. Echoes from stationary tissue are either suppressed or displayed with reduced gain to provide anatomic orientation. The advantage of this technique lies in the simultaneous display in a single image of blood flow information (comparable to angiography) and morphologic details of the vessel wall with high resolution and a high frame rate, while showing no or little angle dependence and no aliasing. B-flow ultrasound thus allows good differentiation of flowing blood from the vessel wall but provides no hemodynamic information. Disadvantages of B-flow imaging include the occurrence of artifacts in highly pulsatile, atherosclerotic vessels, susceptibility to wall motion artifacts, and the still limited scanning depth.

With further technical advancement, B-flow imaging could, in principle, enable morphologic quantification of stenosis and differentiation of the vessel wall from the patent lumen even if only slow flow is present (e.g., in ulceration). The B-mode provides a high-resolution display of the vessel wall contour with separate representation of blood flow in the B-flow mode. This is an advantage over the color duplex mode, which superimposes flow information onto an anatomic gray-scale image (see Figs. 5.18 and 5.86 (Atlas)).

1.1.3.4 Intravascular Ultrasound

Miniaturized ultrasound probes permit examination of a vascular region of interest (ROI) from within the vessel. Intravascular ultrasound (IVUS) is performed with a percutaneously inserted intravascular probe, which is advanced to the target site using a very small catheter system and thin guidewire under radiologic guidance. IVUS is used to assess atherosclerotic lesions, other vessel wall conditions such as dissection, and perivascular structures close to the vessel wall including tumor infiltration. The technique is highly suitable for evaluating catheter-based interventions of both coronary and peripheral arteries. In this setting, the ultrasound probe can be inserted through the introducer sheath already placed for the interventional procedure, providing high spatial resolution for identification of wall changes and postinterventional complications.

Various mechanical and electronic high-frequency **phased-array systems** are available for single use. A higher transmit frequency improves axial resolution but limits penetration depth. On a 360° IVUS image, the normal arterial wall has a three-layer appearance resulting from the reflection of the ultrasound beam at the boundaries between layers differing in acoustic impedance. The sonographic layers do not correspond to the histologic wall layers. The histologic thickness of the normal intima is below the axial resolution of IVUS. The bright inner ring thus represents the interface between blood and intima. The **intima** is seen only when it is **thickened by atherosclerosis**. The outer hyperechoic ring is the reflection of the interface between the adventitia and periadventitial tissue and is clearly distinct from the darker middle layer. This layer corresponds to the muscularis and results in the characteristic three-layer appearance of arteries of the muscular type. With its high resolution, IVUS is superior to percutaneous ultrasound in terms of demonstrating intimal thickening and plaques; it also improves plaque characterization as it allows better differentiation of plaque types such as fibrotic or necrotic plaques (Fig. 1.32).

Examination Procedure

With the patient positioned supine, the femoral artery is punctured and a 6F to 8F introducer sheath is placed using the Seldinger technique. A guidewire serves to advance the ultrasound probe to the target region under fluoroscopic guidance.

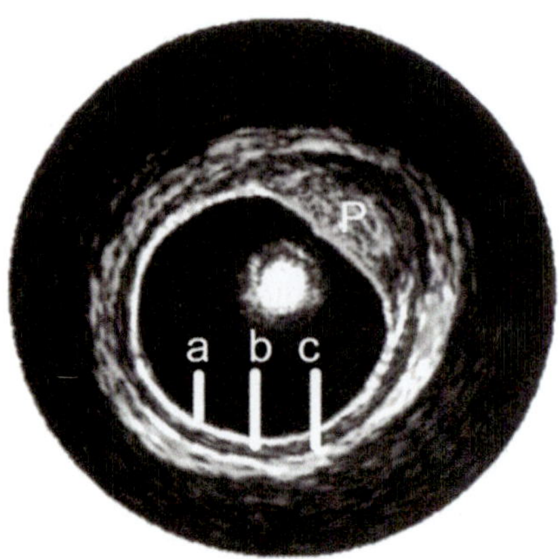

Fig. 1.32 Three-layer appearance of the arterial wall in intravascular ultrasound (IVUS). The layers distinguished by ultrasound do not represent the tissue layers that make up the arterial wall. The bright inner ring (a) is the interface between blood and the intima (which gives a high signal because of the large acoustic mismatch). The second, darker ring (b) roughly corresponds to the intima-media complex, and the third ring, which is also bright (c), is the transition from the adventitia to the perivascular connective tissue. The normal intima is not visualized by IVUS either - only a thickened intima due to atherosclerosis or plaque (P) is detectable

IVUS is used to identify and characterize atherosclerotic and other wall lesions and to evaluate perivascular changes, for instance, in patients with suspected tumor infiltration. Following an interventional procedure, IVUS can be performed to identify residual stenosis or complications such as an intimal flap or dissection. IVUS is an invasive and technically demanding procedure, and the single-use probes are expensive, which is why only specialized centers perform IVUS, typically in conjunction with a vascular intervention or as part of a study.

1.1.3.5 Three-Dimensional/Four-Dimensional Ultrasound

A three-dimensional (3D) ultrasound display is reconstructed from a series of 2D images acquired by manually or automatically moving the ultrasound probe across the body surface perpendicular to the transducer plane. There are several options for displaying the 3D information: either as a composite, as a transparent volume block, or as a display in which the observer can select a point, for which the information will then be presented in all three dimensions. These techniques enable a 3D display of wall lesions or plaques as well as their relationship to perivascular tissue.

However, these rendering techniques are most useful for the documentation and demonstration of sonographic findings. During scanning, the examiner is able to grasp spatial relationships more rapidly, making use of the flexibility of the ultrasound probe and switching to different scan planes. Compared with the fixed planes available in a 3D rendering, this flexibility is superior when it comes to evaluating challenging anatomy. It also provides more freedom in circumventing artifacts. Three-dimensional vascular ultrasound is degraded by vascular pulsation. With the computational capacity afforded by state-of-the-art ultrasound systems, complete volumes can be displayed in fractions of seconds. If the frame rate for volume generation is high enough to track motion, this is known as four-dimensional (4D) ultrasound (with the time course of the changes observed representing the fourth dimension).

1.1.4 Factors Affecting (Color) Duplex Imaging – Pitfalls

Duplex ultrasound is subject to a number of pitfalls (modified according to Seitz and Kubale 1988; Wolf and Fobbe 1993):

- Errors in estimating the Doppler angle (primarily with angles >60°), chiefly in curved vessels and branchings
- Errors in determining vessel diameter (blooming, diameter variation during cardiac cycle)
- Limitation of maximum velocity detectable (Nyquist limit)
- Limitation of minimum velocity detectable (wall filter, inadequate PRF)
- Position and size of sample volume
- Inclusion of nearby vessels (high PRF, CW Doppler, large sample volume)
- Overmodulation resulting from unfavorable signal-to-noise ratio (gain)
- Impairment by scattering structures (plaque, intestinal gas, edema)

1.1.4.1 Scattering and Acoustic Shadowing

Air (in the intestine and lungs) and calcified structures (bones, calcified plaque) produce scattering and acoustic shadowing. These structures are not penetrated by the ultrasound beam and thus prevent collection of morphologic and Doppler flow information from body regions behind them. Bowel gas can be pushed out of the way by pressing the transducer against the bowel, thereby enabling evaluation of retroperitoneal structures and blood flow. In all other cases, the examiner must try and circumvent such structures by changing the transducer position.

1.1.4.2 Mirror Artifact

Mirror artifacts occur at strongly reflecting surfaces (interfaces between structures with large differences in acoustic impedance), mimicking structures behind the reflector (e.g., liver behind diaphragm) in gray-scale imaging or patent vessels in color duplex ultrasound (e.g., subclavian artery behind pleura). The artifact will disappear when the reflector is scanned in oblique orientation (Fig. 1.33).

1.1.4.3 Maximum Flow Velocity Detectable – Pulse Repetition Frequency

Pulsed Doppler, unlike continuous wave (CW) Doppler, does not sample the Doppler signal continuously but at discrete points in time. The sampling rate is determined by the spacing of the emitted pulses and is inversely proportional to the **pulse repetition frequency (PRF)**. The maximum frequency that can be correctly measured is less than half the PRF. In other words, the PRF must be at least twice the maximum Doppler frequency that is being measured.

Let us consider an example. ◘ Fig. 1.34 shows a wave with frequency *f*. If we assume that the time interval between T1 and T3 is 1 s, *f* is 2 Hz. The signal is sampled at times T1, T2, and T3, that is, three times per second, corresponding to a sampling rate of 3 Hz. This sampling rate yields a frequency of <1 Hz, underestimating the true frequency. In this example, a sampling rate of at least 4 Hz is needed to measure the frequency correctly. The maximum frequency that can be accurately reproduced by means of sampling is known as the Nyquist frequency. Violation of the Nyquist limit or sampling theorem leads to aliasing (Lat. for "at another time", "in another place"). A form of aliasing seen in Western movies is the wagon-wheel effect or reverse rotation effect, which is an optical illusion in which a spoke wheel appears to rotate in the opposite direction from the true rotation. In a Doppler spectrum, aliasing leads to an underestimation of the high frequencies within the signal, as the peaks are cut off and displayed on the opposite side of the baseline (◘ Figs. 1.35 and 1.36).

Therefore, the PRF limits the maximum Doppler shift frequency for which reliable determination of blood flow direction and velocity is possible. The PRF is the rate at which ultrasound pulses are emitted from the transducer. In pulsed Doppler (conventional and color duplex), only

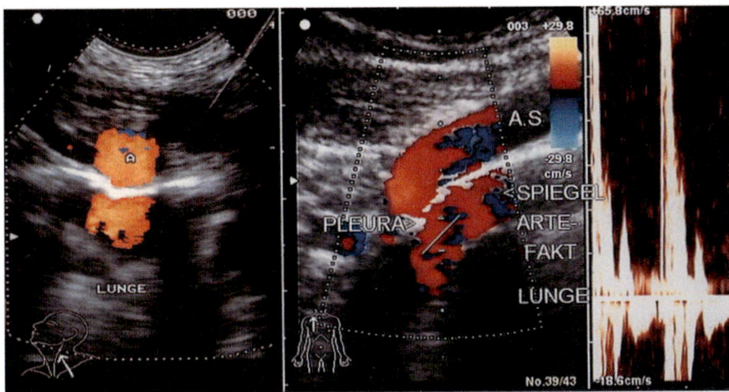

◘ **Fig. 1.33** Mirror artifact (subclavian artery scanned from supraclavicular approach). Here the strongly reflecting pleura (bright reflection) mirrors the subclavian artery (A), producing the impression of a second artery ("ghost") posterior to the true artery. The mirror artifact can be eliminated by changing the transducer position (transverse (left) and longitudinal (right) views of the subclavian artery). Mirroring can occur in all sonographic imaging modes. Spectral Doppler recording obtained over the duplicated subclavian artery with the sample volume placed in lung tissue behind the pleura

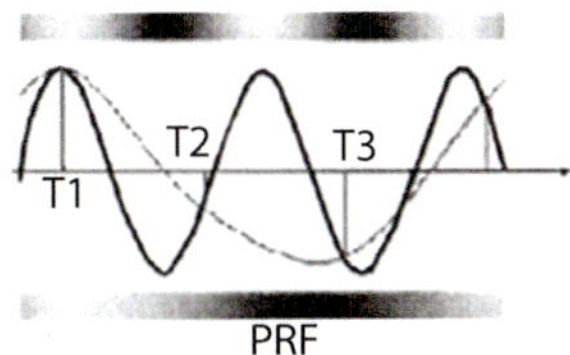

◘ **Fig. 1.34** Sampling of the Doppler signal. Temporal resolution is determined by pulse spacing, which is the inverse of the pulse repetition frequency (PRF)

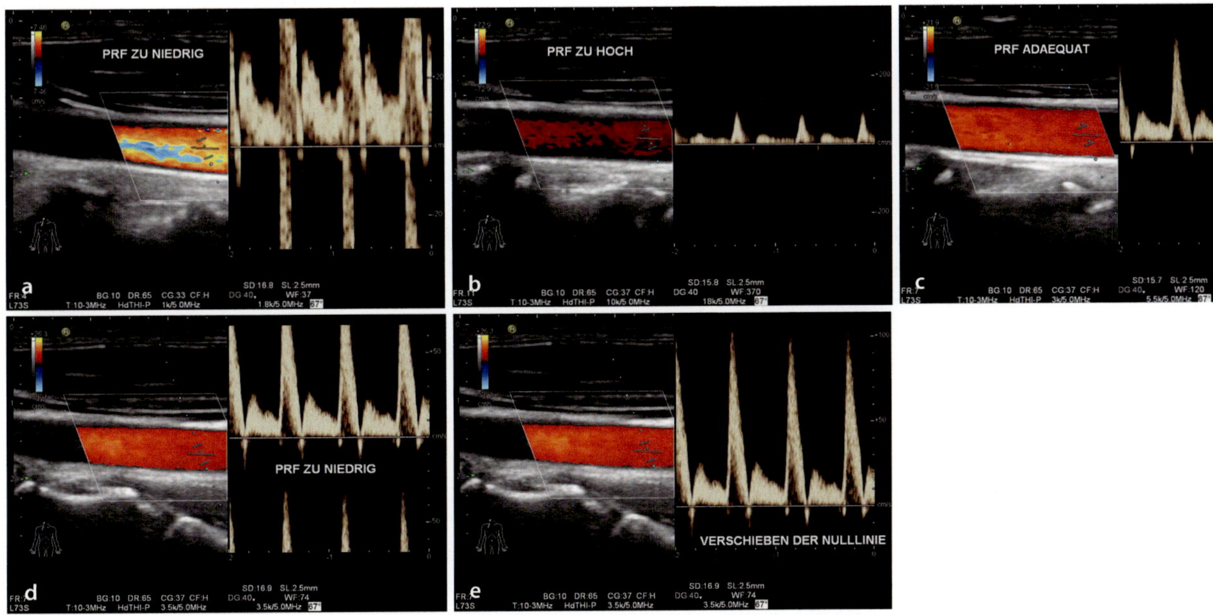

◘ **Fig. 1.35** Effects of different pulse repetition frequencies (PRF). Shown are identical views of the common carotid artery (CCA) obtained with different PRFs. **a** Examination with the PRF set too low. There is aliasing because the Doppler shift frequencies are above the Nyquist limit. In the color image, aliasing is seen as a color change from light red to yellow to blue. In the Doppler waveform, the peak velocity is cut off, wrapped around, and displayed on the opposide side of the baseline. **b** Examination with the PRF set too high. Slower flow is missed, resulting in poor color filling of the CCA (especially near the wall, where flow is slower). In the Doppler waveform, smaller amplitudes impair spectral analysis and give rise to measuring errors (see scale). **c** Color duplex image and waveform obtained with an adequate PRF: there is good color filling of the CCA lumen, and the waveform can be analyzed adequately. **d, e** When the PRF is only slightly lower than required for adequate sampling (**d**), a complete and adequate spectral Doppler display is obtained by shifting the baseline (**e**)

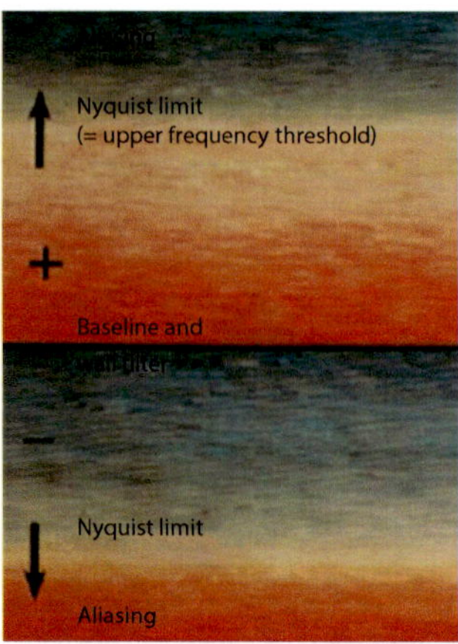

Fig. 1.36 In color duplex imaging, a positive Doppler shift is displayed in red and a negative shift in blue, and faster velocities are indicated by increasingly brigher shades of these colors. When true blood flow velocities are outside the range specified by the color velocity scale, aliasing will occur, with the flow peaks above the threshold being displayed in the color of the opposite flow direction. In aliasing, the color change from red to blue or vice versa progresses through a brighter shade (faster flow) and a yellow to white zone of transition (see Fig. 1.35a). In contrast, true flow reversal is characterized by a dark transition zone. Absence of color (black) may be due to a short cessation of flow or a change in flow direction relative to the transducer (curved-array transducer) with failure to depict flow signals at the site of transition, where the Doppler angle is 90°

echoes reflected from a predefined depth are accepted and processed (for determination of averaged flow velocity or FFT analysis) in the interval between transmissions. In color duplex ultrasound, this is accomplished by using multiple gates to which the returning Doppler shift frequency packets are assigned. The relatively low Doppler shift frequencies (some kilohertz with a period of approx. 1 ms) are extracted from short, successive ultrasound pulses less than 1 µs in duration. A minimum number of ultrasound pulses is necessary for correct frequency determination. The **Nyquist limit** states that only Doppler shifts below half the PRF can be unambiguously processed in terms of direction and flow velocity. Doppler shifts exceeding the Nyquist limit lead to **aliasing**. When aliasing occurs, portions of the spectral display representing the highest-frequency shifts wrap around and appear on the opposite side of the baseline. Aliased signals may thus misrepresent blood flow direction and flow velocity. In color flow images, aliased flow is displayed in the color of the opposite direction. In aliasing, the transition to the opposite color progresses from increasingly lighter shades to yellow, followed by a light shade of the opposite color (e.g., from light red to yellow to light blue). In contrast, true flow reversal is characterized by a color change from a dark shade of the initial color (or black for a transient period during which no flow information is obtained) to the opposite color. Various methods are available **to resolve aliasing**:

- Use of a higher PRF
- Shifting of the baseline
- Use of a lower transmit frequency
- Interrogation of the target vessel at a larger angle

The lower the transmit frequency, the lower the Doppler shift frequency. The latter can thus be reduced to below half the PRF by lowering the transmit frequency. Larger angles between the ultrasound beam and the blood vessel will also **decrease the Doppler shift frequency**; however, the extent to which this can be done is limited by the fact that errors in velocity measurement will increase unacceptably at angles above 70°. Shifting the zero baseline increases the velocity scale in one direction, allowing a higher flow velocity in that direction to be displayed without aliasing. In this way, the examiner can double the Doppler frequencies that can be displayed above or below the line, depending on the direction of the shift. Enlarging the positive frequency range in this way automatically reduces the negative frequency range by the same amount and vice versa.

Another parameter is the **scanning depth**, but this is difficult to manipulate. The greater the penetration depth, the longer the pulse delay. As the round trip time increases, the PRF must be reduced as successive pulses can only be emitted after all reflected echoes of the preceding pulse have been received.

Mathematically, the Nyquist limit is expressed in the following equation:

$$\delta F_{\max} = \frac{1}{2} PRF$$

It follows from this equation that the PRF must be at least twice the Doppler shift frequency (dF) expected to occur in the target vessel. With a PRF of 10 kHz, for example, a maximum Doppler shift of 5 kHz can be detected unambiguously. Let us consider two examples for illustration:

- 5 cm scanning depth:
  - Spacing of transmit pulses ≅ 0.06 ms
  - Maximum PRF of approx. 16.6 kHz (dF < 8.4 Hz)
  - High PRF is required to capture high Doppler shift frequencies (dF) and hence high flow velocities
- 15 cm scanning depth:
  - Spacing of transmit pulses ≅ 0.2 ms
  - Maximum PRF of approx. 5 kHZ (dF < 2.5 kHz)
  - Higher Doppler shift frequencies (dF) result in aliasing

The maximum flow velocity that can be measured without aliasing is given as:

$$V_{\max} = \frac{c}{4 \cdot T \cdot F_0 \cdot \cos\alpha}$$

It follows that this velocity is inversely proportional to the round trip time, T, or to the scan depth and the transmit frequency, F_0 (Figs. 1.35, 1.36, and 1.37).

The options available to overcome these limitations can be summarized as follows:

- Use of a higher PRF to register higher Doppler shift frequencies, but this will reduce the scan depth (longer pulse delays with greater depth; Fig. 1.38).
- Use of a lower transmit frequency, but this will reduce the spatial resolution of the gray-scale scan.

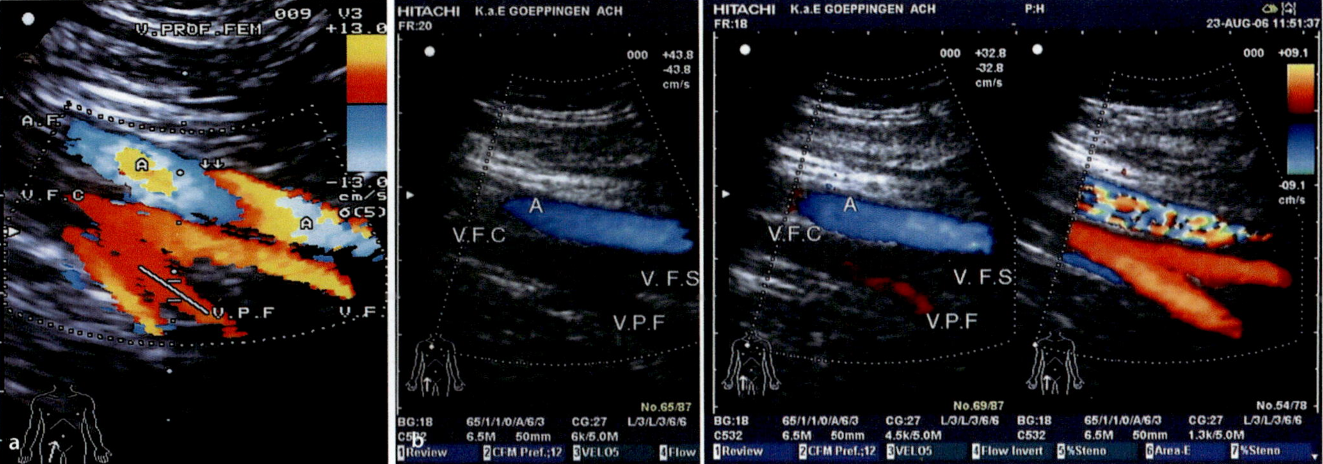

Fig. 1.37 **a** The pulse repetition frequency (PRF) is adequately set for evaluating venous flow (confirmed here in the deep femoral vein). The figure illustrates potential pitfalls of color duplex ultrasound in the superficial femoral artery. There is good color filling of the lumen of the deep femoral vein (duplicated in the example shown, V.P.F.) and in the superficial femoral vein. Flow is toward the transducer (red). Flow in the superficial femoral artery (A.F) is in the opposite direction (blue). The PRF is too low for arterial blood flow, resulting in aliasing indicated by brightening and a color change (through yellow). As a result of the low frame rate (proportional to the PRF), the color map also shows the change in flow direction from systole to early diastole (indicated by arrows in the center of the image). Unlike aliasing, this true flow reversal is indicated by a color change from dark blue to dark red. In the further course of the artery, there is a second region of aliased flow with color changing from red to yellow to blue. The increasingly smaller Doppler angle also contributes to these phenomena and is also responsible for the lighter color in the superficial femoral vein running posteriorly. **b** Adjustment of the PRF to the expected flow velocities in the (arterial/venous) vessels of interest. A lower PRF is required to detect slower venous flow. The leftmost image depicts the artery with good color filling (blue), while no flow signals are registered from the vein, which may be misinterpreted as thrombosis. With increasingly lower PRFs (from left to right), aliasing in the artery increases despite normal blood flow, which must not be misinterpreted to indicate stenosis. In the vein, on the other hand, more flow signals are displayed (from left to right) with increasing PRF. In the middle section, flow is only seen in the deep femoral vein (which is insonated at a smaller angle). The rightmost image shows good color filling (red, flow toward transducer) of the entire venous lumen, ruling out thrombosis

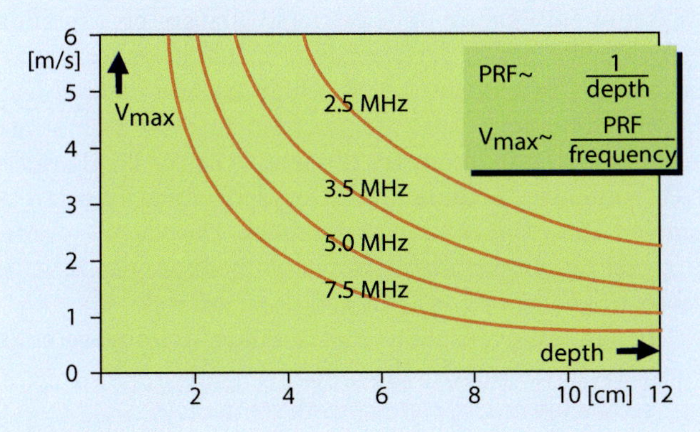

Fig. 1.38 The extent to which the pulse repetition frequency (PRF) can be increased to resolve aliasing is limited by the distance of the target vasculature from the transducer. The round trip time of a pulse increases with the depth of the target vessel, which means that the PRF has to be lower to ensure that all echoes from the previous pulse have been received before the next pulse is emitted – otherwise the range ambiguity problem may occur. Therefore, the maximum blood flow velocity (V_{max}) that can be recorded without aliasing is lower when a deeper vessel is examined. The relationships are illustrated in the graph. When an artery 6 cm from the skin surface is interrogated with a 5-MHz transducer, aliasing will occur at a peak systolic velocity (PSV) of 2 m/s. When the same artery is examined with a transmit frequency of 3.5 MHz, aliasing does not occur unless flow velocity increases to 3 m/s. This is because the Doppler shift frequency is lower when a smaller transmit frequency is used, enabling higher flow velocities to be measured without aliasing (Courtesy of GE Healthcare)

- Use of a larger Doppler angle (resulting in smaller cosα values), but this will degrade the signal and lead to larger measurement errrors.
- Shifting of the baseline, both in the spectral display and on the color bar. The PRF cannot be increased indefinitely as this would introduce range ambiguity. Alternatively, aliasing can be overcome by manipulating the measurement range as defined by the positive and negative Nyquist limits. The baseline is normally midway between these two limits, allowing equal forward and backward flow velocities to be detected. By shifting the baseline in either direction, the measurement range for one direction is expanded at the expense of the other (Fig. 1.35). The total range over which nonaliased flow can be displayed remains constant.
- Some ultrasound machines have a high PRF option for the detection of faster flow. The higher frequency is achieved by emitting ultrasound pulses before the preceding signals have been processed. Processing is done using additional Doppler lines. However, this approach introduces some unreliability in terms of spatial resolution as Doppler information from a larger number of gates must be processed to generate the spectral display.
- Continuous wave (CW) Doppler, using separate crystals for continuously transmitting and receiving signals, is not limited by an upper Doppler shift threshold. This technique, however, does not allow local differentiation of the returning signals since all frequencies reflected

back from along the beam path are processed to generate the Doppler waveform.

1.1.4.4 Minimum Flow Velocity Detectable – Wall Filter, Frame Rate

Doppler-shifted echoes return from flowing blood but also from the moving vessel wall. Shifts due to wall motion typically have a high amplitude but low frequency and affect the velocity spectrum. In contrast, the Doppler shifts caused by the flowing blood are of higher frequency and lower amplitude. To eliminate the interfering signals from the Doppler spectrum, a wall filter is used. The **wall filter** serves to eliminate low-frequency noise artifacts and vascular wall motion from the frequency spectrum. It is a high-pass filter, meaning that high frequencies pass the filter while low-frequency noise artifacts and vascular wall motion are filtered out and discarded. The user can select a filter cutoff to define the minimum frequency range to be displayed. Most filters have a cutoff range of 100–400 Hz, while a few ultrasound systems use cutoffs of up to 1600 Hz. The filter eliminates all frequencies below the selected cutoff, including Doppler shift frequencies caused by slow flow (◘ Fig. 1.39). When the cutoff is too high, the filter may inadvertently remove signals from slow-flowing venous blood, which can be misinterpreted to suggest absence of flow. Also, the mean flow velocity may be overestimated if slow flow components with low Doppler shifts are filtered out. More refined filters eliminate only low frequencies with high amplitudes (typical of wall motion) or identify and eliminate typical patterns of tissue motion.

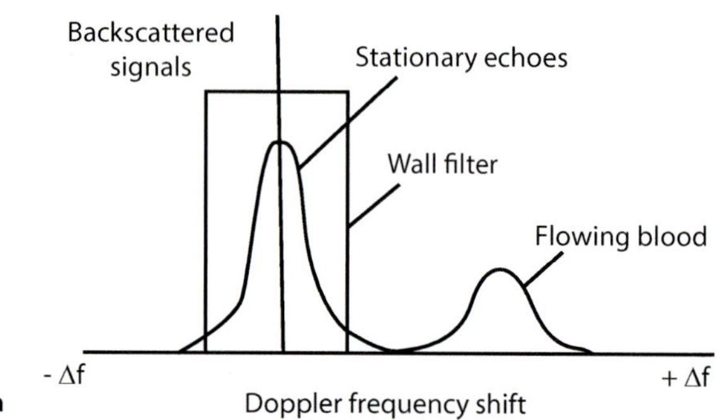

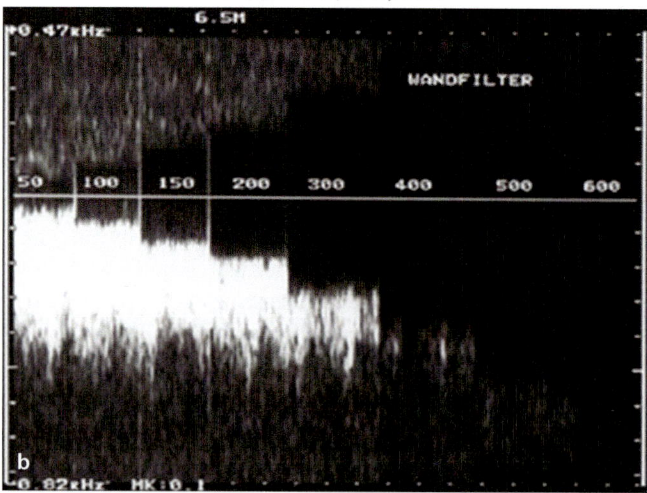

◘ **Fig. 1.39** **a** A wall filter is used to eliminate the low-frequency signals caused by motion of the vessel wall. The cutoff should be selected so as not to inadvertently remove flow-related low-frequency signals, for instance, when evaluating slow venous flow. **b** When the cutoff is gradually increased, at first only the low Doppler shift frequencies are eliminated, while further increments will eliminate venous flow signals as well. A wall filter of 500 Hz eliminates venous flow signals up to 450 Hz, while slower flow is already eliminated at lower values

◘ **Table 1.9** Factors affecting the frame rate in color Doppler imaging

Parameter	Frame rate	
	Higher	Lower
Size of color box	Smaller	Larger
Number of scan lines	Fewer	More
Scan depth	Smaller	Greater
Lower frequency limit	Higher	Lower

The **color Doppler frame rate** is the number of new color images created per second and is one of the factors determining the slowest flow velocity detectable. It is mainly dependent on the width of the color box and the scan depth selected by the examiner. A larger color box requires more color Doppler lines to be processed for generation of each image. Moreover, image generation is slower when deeper structures are scanned due to the longer round trip time (◘ Table 1.9). A lower frame rate means poorer temporal resolution with failure to detect rapid changes or short flow phenomena. Cardiac perfusion and flow in peripheral arteries can only be examined with a high frame rate of at least 20 color Doppler images per second. A lower frame rate, on the other hand, improves the sensitivity for low Doppler shift frequencies because more Doppler information can be sampled from the color Doppler lines. Despite the poorer temporal resolution, a low frame rate therefore yields better results when examining veins and small arteries.

The options available to the examiner to **improve color filling** can be summarized as follows:

- Use of a lower Doppler transmit frequency
- Use of a lower pulse repetition frequency (PRF)
- Use of a lower wall filter setting
- Optimization of the Doppler angle of insonation
- Use of higher color gain

1.1.4.5 Transmit and Receive Gain

The receive gain is another user-adjustable parameter and should be set to ensure that all information from the reflected echo pulses is displayed, while at the same time preventing artifacts due to overmodulation (◘ Fig. 1.40). The gain can be set separately for B-mode scanning, color flow imaging, and spectral Doppler. Readjustment during the examination may be required, for instance, when measuring intima-media thickness. Correct measurement requires careful tuning of

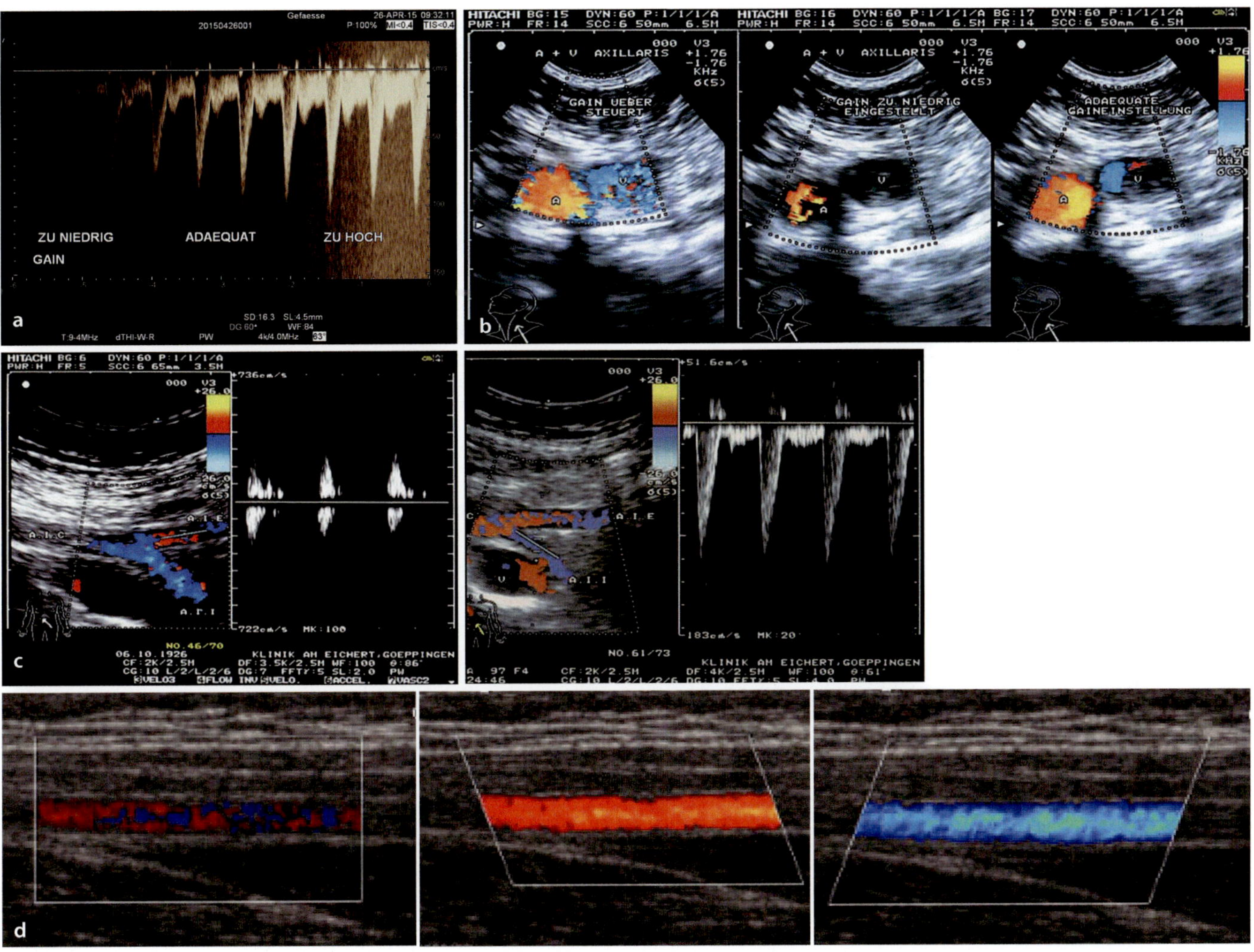

Fig. 1.40a–d Effects of gain and Doppler angle of insonation. **a** Doppler waveform obtained with continuously higher gain (from left to right): when receive gain is too low, there is hardly any spectral information and peak systolic velocity (PSV) is underestimated. In the middle portion of the display, obtained with adequate gain, there is a clear systolic window typical of laminar flow. The right portion was obtained with excessive gain. **b** Effects of different gain settings on the visualization of mural thrombosis in the axillary vein (V), as illustrated by a series of color flow images obtained with the same pulse repetition frequency (PRF). The left image, obtained with excessive gain, shows the mural thrombus to be largely obscured by artifacts extending beyond the patent lumen (blue). The next image depicts no flow signals along the thrombus in the axillary vein because the gain is too low. In addition, there is incomplete color filling of the axillary artery (red) cranial to the vein. The rightmost image illustrates adequate gain setting. There is proper color coding of the artery (red), and blue-coded flow is displayed in the vein along the thrombus. **c** An optimal gray-scale image is obtained with a beam perpendicular to an interface between tissues of different acoustic impedance. In contrast, angles of 80°–90° yield the lowest frequency shifts according to the Doppler equation and thus provide poor (color) duplex information. Therefore, interrogation of the iliac bifurcation at the preferred site of stenosis of the external iliac artery (A.I.E) poses a problem as adequate Doppler angles can be achieved only by tilting the transducer and moving it up or down (see Fig. 2.2b). In the color flow image, the change between red and blue at the origin of the external iliac artery illustrates the problem of determining the flow direction. The Doppler waveform is not helpful either, showing flow in both directions. As a result of the poor Doppler angle, an iliac artery stenosis with a peak systolic velocity (PSV) of 250 cm/s is suggested. **d** The posterior origin of the internal iliac artery (A.I.I), on the other hand, can be interrogated with a Doppler angle of less than 60° from the same transducer position, yielding a diagnostic Doppler waveform, from which a correct PSV of 120 cm/s is calculated. **e** When a linear-array transducer is used, electronic beam steering can help the examiner to obtain a better angle for Doppler interrogation. The leftmost color flow image was obtained with the beam path perpendicular to the transducer face, resulting in a large Doppler angle, at which only small Doppler shift frequencies are obtained. The poor Doppler angle results in a mix of red and blue color. With beam steering, the examiner can steer the beam through a small range of angles away from the perpendicular beam path. The smallest angle achieved with beam steering is 70° in the direction of flow or away from the direction of flow (red/blue)

the receive gain so that boundary lines are visible and overestimation resulting from the blooming effect is avoided.

Receive gain setting for spectral Doppler interrogation must ensure that, in the presence of laminar flow, the clear systolic window in the display of the Doppler spectrum contains no artifacts while not eliminating signals from slow flow. Conversely, some overmodulation of the receive gain may be necessary to calculate the correct peak systolic velocity (PSV) in subtotal occlusion (high-frequency Doppler shifts with low amplitudes due to the small number of reflecting red blood cells in stenosis jet), even if this results in more artifacts. In the color duplex mode, excessive gain will lead to color overflow and may obscure atherosclerotic lesions in arteries or thrombus in a partially occluded vein (◘ Fig. 1.40b). This phenomenon contributes to the unreliability of planimetric stenosis grading, which is based on the cross-sectional vessel area depicted in color duplex scans.

1.1.4.6 Doppler Angle

The evaluation of an artery or vein in the B-mode image combined with the spectral Doppler information obtained with a defined ultrasound beam and known angle of insonation enables reliable calculation of blood flow velocity from the Doppler shift. To ensure reliable Doppler angle correction for accurate measurement, **a long stretch of the vessel of interest should be displayed in** the longitudinal plane (parallel vessel walls along the width of the monitor). The smaller the angle between the Doppler beam and the direction of the flowing blood, the higher the Doppler frequency shift of the reflected echo and the higher the sensitivity for flow detection. At angles of 60–90°, the Doppler frequency shift decreases and flow velocity measurement becomes progressively more unreliable, and no flow signals are depicted when the Doppler beam is perpendicular to the vessel wall (◘ Fig. 1.40c–e). Conversely, **perpendicular insonation of a reflecting surface provides optimal B-mode information.** With a linear-array transducer, the examiner can use beam steering (lateral beam deflection) for electronically changing the direction of the beam to achieve a good Doppler angle relative to the direction of blood flow. Technically, the beam can only be steered either right or left by a maximum of 20°, resulting in a Doppler angle of ≥70°. Therefore, beam steering can improve the angle, but does not achieve the best Doppler angle of <60° (for minimizing measurement errors) when interrogating a vessel segment running parallel to the skin surface (◘ Fig. 1.40e).

In the clinical setting, the examiner must find a **compromise between optimal B-mode imaging and optimal flow evaluation**. The usual procedure is to first try and achieve a perpendicular beam angle for morphologic evaluation of the vessel wall and to then optimize the angle for spectral Doppler interrogation using either electronic beam steering or manual manipulation of the transducer (curved-array or sector probe). Another measure is to place the Doppler gate at the edge of the scan field.

In the color flow image of a vessel coursing parallel to the skin surface (e.g., carotid or femoral artery) examined with a curved-array transducer held perpendicular to the body surface, the colors representing the blood flow information may change in brightness (luminosity) without this reflecting different flow velocities. Under these conditions, flow near the margin of the image is displayed in brighter colors due to higher Doppler shifts and in increasingly darker colors toward the center, where the frequency shift decreases as the insonation angle increases (and no color as the angle approaches 90°). This phenomenon is relevant only in the velocity mode and not in the power mode, as the latter is virtually independent of the Doppler angle.

1.1.4.7 Physical Limitations of Color Duplex Ultrasound

As a result of the vast amount of information to be processed, color duplex scanning has a much poorer spatial and temporal resolution than pure B-mode imaging. Axial resolution is proportional to the wavelength in B-mode imaging, while it is dependent on the **number of sample volumes** placed along the color Doppler scan line in the color duplex mode. The use of smaller sample volumes improves axial resolution but at the expense of sensitivity and accuracy in Doppler shift evaluation as the signal-to-noise ratio deteriorates. Lateral resolution in color duplex imaging is determined by the number of color Doppler lines processed per centimeter. The frame rate decreases as the number of Doppler lines increases, compromising temporal resolution, in particular at greater scan depths.

As a result of these limitations, the axial resolution of color duplex ultrasound is on the order of 0.4–1.0 mm with a lateral resolution of only 1.0–2.0 mm, which is four to ten times lower than the B-mode scan resolution (Widder 1999).

In duplex ultrasound, it takes roughly 50–200 ms to create one color image, depending on the depth of the target vessel and size of the color box. This corresponds to a **frame rate** or sampling rate of 5 Hz. When a low PRF is selected, the speed at which the color Doppler lines sweep the sector is similar to or slightly below the mean flow velocity in arteries. Therefore, a single color flow frame may simultaneously depict systolic flow and early diastolic flow (e.g., displayed in red and blue, respectively, see ◘ Fig. 1.37). Due to the low temporal resolution, however, the color coding does not fully reflect the pulsatile character of flow.

Slow flow produces smaller Doppler frequency shifts, which have to be extracted from short echo pulse packets for each scan line consisting of a number of individual pulses. The scan lines must be processed successively.

Though the insonation angle should ideally be as small as possible for optimal velocity measurement, this is not always practical because there will be a **longer delay when the color box is tilted** (beam steering). This is why one must find a compromise, in particular when examining vessels deeper in the body. Tilting the color box by 20° and 30° prolongs the round trip time by 13% and 31%, respectively.

Color duplex imaging, like all diagnostic ultrasound techniques, is impaired by **scattering** and **acoustic shadowing** caused by bowel gas or calcified structures (bone or calcified plaques in the lumen). The examiner can circumvent such interfering structures by moving the transducer, but this often increases the distance between the transducer and the target anatomy, and hence the round trip time.

A strong reflector in the beam path can act like a mirror and generate a phantom image in another area of the scan. Such mirror images can be identified by angling the transducer, which will make the mirror artifacts disappear or appear in a different location. When the ultrasound beam strikes interfaces of high acoustic impedance at a right angle, reverberations (repeat echoes) may occur with the ultrasound pulses being reflected to and fro, resulting in a kind of ping-pong effect. Slight angulation of the transducer prevents reverberations but will also reduce reflection from the interface and thus degrade image quality.

1.1.5 Ultrasound Contrast Agents

Color duplex imaging with a high-resolution transducer usually allows adequate visualization of the peripheral arteries in the gray-scale mode; the evaluation of blood flow, however, may be impaired, either by the presence of sclerotic vascular lesions or by scattering due to edema or other localized soft tissue changes. In these situations, a microbubble contrast agent, or echo enhancer, can be used to improve blood flow imaging. For vascular ultrasound examinations in the clinical setting, however, a contrast agent is rarely needed as there are only a few situations (e.g., identification of a suitable recipient vessel for crural bypass grafting) in which color duplex and spectral Doppler imaging are degraded by poor imaging conditions and do not provide the information required for treatment planning.

Ultrasound contrast agents are gas-filled microbubbles and enhance the contrast between blood and surrounding tissue by **producing strong reflections in the vascular compartment** during their lifetime of 3–5 min after intravenous administration. Microbubbles can thus enable or improve the identification and evaluation of vessels with slow or low blood flow, which may be difficult to identify with conventional ultrasound techniques. While this is an advantage for vascular applications, ultrasound contrast agents are mainly used to evaluate organ and lesion perfusion, to characterize focal liver lesions for example. Contrast-enhanced ultrasound (CEUS) plays virtually no role in the routine clinical examination of patients with angiologic or vascular surgical conditions. Notable exceptions are CEUS examinations of small peripheral vessels and below-the-knee arteries with slow, postocclusive flow, transcranial duplex scanning, the search for endoleaks after stenting of the aorta, demonstration of intraplaque neovascularization in the assessment of plaque vulnerability, and evaluation of inflammatory activity in patients with vasculitis. With the use of contrast agents, ultrasound to some extent gives up the crucial advantages it normally has over other imaging modalities – low cost, short examination time, and noninvasiveness. Moreover, in those body regions where diagnostic improvement is achieved through the administration of an echo enhancer, competing imaging modalities are used because they provide high accuracy and often enable better documentation of the findings.

Ultrasound contrast agents with different compositions and properties are commercially available from various manufacturers. Basically, the contrast agents consist of microbubbles composed of a gas core encapsulated by a thin shell or stabilized by a carrier medium.

These two factors – the shell and the gas core – determine the **stability of ultrasound microbubbles**:

- The microbubble gas core is stabilized by a shell that contains surface stabilizers (palmitic acid, phospholipids) or substances that form a capsule on the molecular level (albumins, polymers).
- The stability of the core can be improved by using a heavier gas instead of air (sulfur hexafluoride, perfluoropropane). Such gases have lower diffusivity, higher physical density, and a lower saturation constant, reducing the solubility of the microbubbles.

The more stable microbubbles used in newer ultrasound contrast agent preparations have certain advantages, such as a longer blood half-life due to lower spontaneous solubility. Bubbles containing a high-molecular-weight gas can pass the pulmonary circulation because they are more resistant to destruction when exposed to changing pressures.

1.1.5.1 Approved Ultrasound Contrast Agents and Uses

While a variety of microbubble contrast agents differing in core and shell composition were investigated around the turn of the century, only a few microbubble preparations were ultimately approved for clinical use.

Levovist was the first ultrasound contrast agent approved in Europe but has since been taken off the European market. The preparation consists of a suspension of galactose-based air bubbles coated with a stabilizing palmitic acid layer.

SonoVue is approved in Europe as an echo enhancer for vascular applications. The microbubbles have a mean diameter of 5–10 μm, contain sulfur hexafluoride, and are stabilized by phospholipids. Being eliminated from the body by exhalation, SonoVue is not nephrotoxic.

The microbubbles are injected as a single bolus of 1–2.4 mL (at a rate of 1 mL/s) or as a smaller bolus of 0.5–1.0 mL followed by continuous infusion of 1 mL/min over a few minutes. After bolus injection, enhancement of the arterial lumen begins after 10–30 s and peaks after 30–60 s, followed by a gradual decrease in intensity over 3–8 min (imaging window). The imaging window can be extended by infusion of the microbubble preparation. Depending on the infusion rate, a 15–20 dB increase in intensity is observed after 1 min. Excessive enhancement with appearance of flow signals outside the vascular space (color blooming) immediately after bolus administration can be counteracted by adjusting transmit gain. The slow linear decrease in intensity following the initial peak after bolus injection ensures adequate enhancement for several minutes, which is long enough for most vascular applications. Dynamic contrast-enhanced ultrasound (CEUS) with generation of time-intensive curves (TIC) allows estimation of blood volume and regional blood flow in the target vasculature or a vascular segment of interest (Dietrich et al. 2012).

The intravascular half-life of the microbubbles primarily depends on their inherent stability and the acoustic energy applied, which in turn is determined by the ultrasound system's output and attenuation of the ultrasound beam while passing through the tissue.

Clinical CEUS examinations can be performed using conventional ultrasound techniques; however, the acoustic energy will rapidly destroy the microbubbles. The life span of the bubbles is longer when contrast-specific ultrasound modes such as low-mechanical (MI) index imaging are employed. This means that the examination is performed with a lower output power or decreased MI. With this technique, dynamic real-time imaging can be performed over several minutes after administration of the microbubbles. For most indications in vascular ultrasound, it is usually sufficient to inject an echo enhancer bolus of 1.2–2.4 mL, followed by a 10-mL saline flush (0.9%).

Ultrasound microbubbles do not diffuse from the blood into surrounding tissues. They do not leave the vascular system unless blood escapes through a hole in the vessel wall (e.g., an endoleak). Hence, they have no nephrotoxic effects and a low overall rate of adverse events. Life-threatening anaphylactic reactions have been reported to occur in less than 0.002% of cases.

There are several contraindications to the use of **SonoVue** as an echo enhancer:

- Severe pulmonary hypertension, uncontrolled arterial hypertension, acute lung failure
- Acute coronary syndrome, severe cardiac insufficiency, malignant arrhythmia
- Acute respiratory distress syndrome, e.g., bronchial asthma
- Pregnancy and breastfeeding (safety remains to be proven during pregnancy and lactation)
- Patient age below 18
- Known intolerance of sulfur hexafluoride

The preparation of a patient for an ultrasound examination with use of an echo enhancer includes obtaining written informed consent and placing a venous line.

1.1.5.2 Mechanisms of Action

Ultrasound contrast agents act by increasing the proportion of scattered and reflected ultrasound pulses from the blood, thereby improving both the Doppler signal and the signal-to-noise ratio (SNR). How strongly the microbubbles enhance reflection depends on their diameter (factor of 6), the transmit frequency used (factor of 4), and their compressibility. Most microbubbles used as echoenhancers contain gas and enhance backscatter because of the **acoustic mismatch between their gas cores and the liquid component of blood**. The intensity of backscatter is determined by the microbubble concentration in the blood and the reflection capacity of the individual bubbles, which is a function of their scatter cross-section. However, the maximum bubble size is limited by the fact that they must pass the lungs (bubble size <8 μm). It has been shown that backscatter enhances the echo signal intensity of blood by 15–25 dB (Kaps and Seidel 1999). Low ultrasound beam power induces linear oscillation of the microbubbles, transforming the bubbles into small "ultrasound transmitters." This is another mechanism by which microbubbles enhance the ultrasound signal. The resonance frequency is inversely proportional to the bubble diameter.

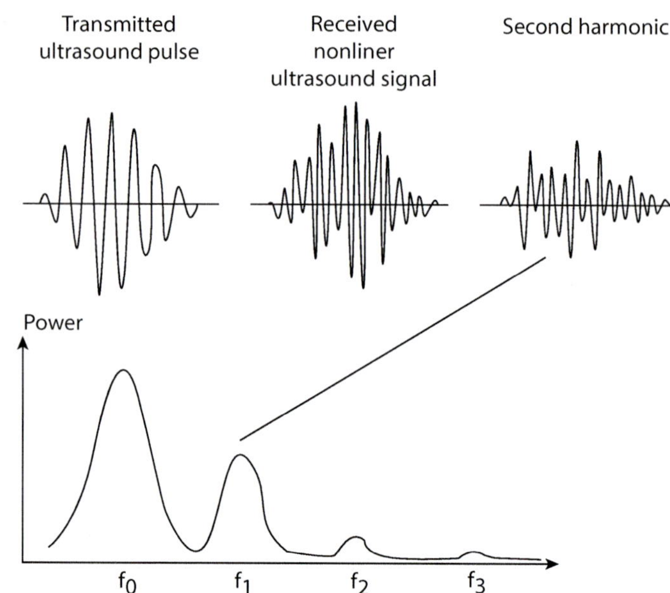

Fig. 1.41 The Doppler-shifted signal returning to the transducer contains both the fundamental and harmonics, which can be extracted by comparison with the emitted pulse

At higher power, the microbubbles oscillate in a nonlinear fashion, producing strong signals at fundamental and nonfundamental frequencies. The nonfundamental or **harmonic frequencies** are multiples of the transmitted frequency. The second harmonic has the highest energy and is therefore most relevant for diagnostic ultrasound (Fig. 1.41). Because the resonance frequencies of the 2–7-μm gas bubbles are within the range of the transmitted frequencies of 2.5–10 MHz typically used in diagnostic ultrasound, the bubble vibrations produce an additional signal amplification. The corresponding frequencies are received and processed along with the Doppler-shifted frequencies. This **resonance behavior of the microbubbles** improves the SNR by a further 30–35 dB, provided that the bandwidth of the ultrasound system extends over a sufficient range of frequencies to enable the generated harmonics to be detected (Correas et al. 1997).

Short pulses of high energy can be applied to make the microbubbles burst, producing ultrasound signals that are detected with high sensitivity. In contrast to the enhancing mechanisms outlined in the preceding sections, bursting is independent of blood flow and the resulting signals merely show the distribution of the collapsed microbubbles at the time of imaging.

Both SonoVue and Levovist are taken up and eliminated by the reticuloendothelial system of the liver. In the liver, the microbubbles can be made to burst by exposing them to a high-energy beam. In this way, they can contribute to the sonoscintigraphic identification of liver metastases, which do not have a reticuloendothelial system. Alternatively, focal liver lesions may be differentiated on the basis of their blood supply (predominantly portal venous versus arterial) and differences in contrast agent arrival times after bolus injection. Because of their selective uptake, the microbubbles also have the potential to be used as vehicles for the targeted local delivery of chemotherapy. Other echo enhancer preparations consist of suspensions (some of which contain human albumin) and bubbles stabilized for specific needs.

1.1.5.3 Ultrasound Techniques Using Contrast Agents

1.1.5.3.1 Contrast-Enhanced Duplex Ultrasound

The reflection of ultrasound by microbubbles present in the blood selectively enhances the vascular system, thus improving the delineation of arteries and veins from surrounding tissue (in color duplex and power Doppler). Blood flow velocity is not affected by the microbubbles, and therefore spectral Doppler analysis can be performed for quantification of blood flow velocity (CW/PW Doppler) in the same way as without contrast medium but with lower gain. When a frequency-based Dopppler technique is used, however, the effect of contrast enhancement can only be exploited in large and medium-sized vessels as the signals returning from slow microcirculatory flow in small vessels cannot be adequately separated from the echoes produced by moving tissue.

Microbubble contrast agents have been used to evaluate slow flow in peripheral vessels, including postocclusive flow, and carotid artery stenosis, and studies have shown that echo enhancers improve the accuracy of color duplex ultrasound in identifying pseudo-occlusion (Fürst et al. 1999; Ferrer et al. 2000). In the vertebral territory, ultrasound contrast agents can improve evaluation in patients with poor scanning conditions or with a hypoplastic vertebral artery.

Echo enhancers have also been advocated to improve the SNR in the examination of deep vessels such as the pelvic or renal arteries. Using state-of-the-art ultrasound equipment, however, these vascular areas rarely pose diagnostic problems. A study of duplex ultrasound with echo enhancer administration in renal artery stenosis found an increase in diagnostic yield from 64% to 84%, while the improvement in the sensitivity and specificity for identifying high-grade stenosis was negligible (Claudon et al. 2000).

1.1.5.3.2 Contrast Harmonic Imaging

This ultrasound technique can improve vascular imaging by selectively displaying the harmonics specific to microbubbles. A broadband transducer is used to detect the harmonics generated by the contrast microbubbles, especially the second harmonic. The backscatter from microbubbles allows better separation of the echoes from stationary tissues, thus offering advantages in the sonographic evaluation of slow flow.

1.1.5.3.3 Stimulated Acoustic Emission Imaging

Contrast agent microbubbles are destroyed when exposed to high ultrasound energy (high mechanical index) (◘ Fig. 1.42). The bursting bubbles emit transient ultrasound signals, which can be detected with a broadband transducer. The system registers the variation in signals from pulse to pulse. This information is displayed along with the spatial information of the B-mode image to show the contrast agent distribution in the macro- and microcirculation at a given point in time.

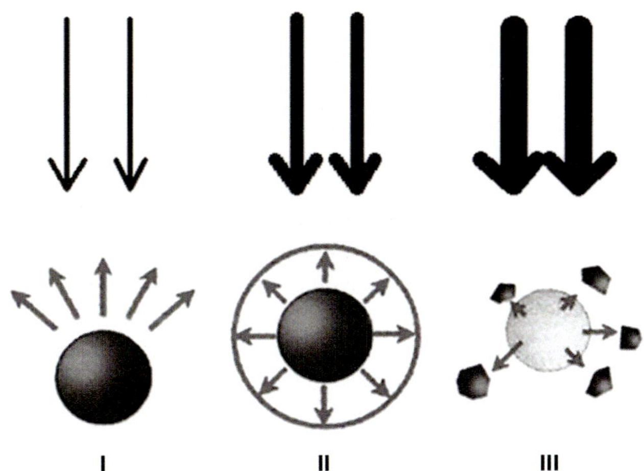

◘ **Fig. 1.42** Ultrasound techniques using contrast agents. The amount of ultrasound energy applied determines how the microbubbles interact with the ultrasound beam, giving rise to different techniques of image generation. Exposure of microbubbles to low energy (I) causes an increase in reflection and backscatter. Intermediate ultrasound energy levels (II) induce nonlinear oscillation of the microbubbles, resulting in the emission of second harmonics, which selectively enhance the blood signal (contrast harmonic imaging). High ultrasound energy (III) destroys the microbubbles, releasing frequencies that provide information on the distribution of the contrast bubbles in the circulation (stimulated acoustic emission)

1.1.5.4 Summary of Technical Aspects and Clinical Indications

In color duplex ultrasound, the administration of echo enhancers can lead to excessive enhancement of the color Doppler signal with color overflow obscuring perivascular structures and parts of the vessel wall, in particular when larger vessels are examined. This effect can be remedied by lowering the receive gain. On the other hand, the strong reflection produced by the contrast bubbles can attenuate structures farther away from the transducer than the enhanced vessel.

A Doppler waveform obtained after echo enhancer administration will show spectral broadening with almost complete filling-in of the systolic window. Again, the effect can be counteracted by lowering the receive gain.

Basically, all sonographic techniques exploiting the different effects of ultrasound contrast agents in the vascular compartment aim at improving sensitivity to blood flow phenomena. However, with the sophisticated ultrasound technology available today, most vascular applications do not require use of a contrast agent. Moreover, in those rare cases where an adequate diagnostic evaluation with color duplex imaging is not possible, the use of a microbubble contrast agent is often limited as well and offers no benefits. Despite these cautionary remarks, there are a few situations in which contrast microbubbles improve diagnostic yield. The most important **indications for vascular CEUS** are:

- Transcranial duplex imaging
- Evaluation for renovascular disease
- Vein mapping for identification of a suitable recipient segment before crural bypass graft surgery
- Search for endoleaks in patients with an aortic stent.

It is expected, however, that ultrasound contrast agents will be used increasingly in the evaluation of microcirculation, e.g., for identifying plaque neovascularization (Seidel et al. 2006; Claudon et al. 2008).

1.1.6 Safety of Diagnostic Ultrasound

Ever since the early 1960s, when this technique was first used for diagnostic imaging, the potential biological hazards of medical ultrasound have been discussed. Ultrasound traveling through the human body can have two effects known to cause changes in biological systems. Firstly there are the thermal effects resulting from the conversion of ultrasound energy into heat and secondly there are the mechanical effects arising from pressure changes associated with the propagation of sound waves in a medium.

1.1.6.1 Thermal Effects

Exposure to diagnostic ultrasound can increase tissue temperature because sound energy is absorbed and converted to heat. The ability to absorb energy varies with the tissue; it is low in body fluids (amniotic fluid, blood, urine) and high in bones. Adult bones absorb 60–80% of the incident ultrasound energy. In addition, absorption in the body is also affected by technical parameters, most notably the output frequency of the transducer. Higher frequencies are absorbed more rapidly. A temperature increase of 2.5°C can severely damage biological tissues, while an increase of 1°C is generally considered harmless. Experimental evidence suggests that the thermal effects of diagnostic ultrasound procedures pose no health hazard.

1.1.6.2 Mechanical Effects

Most of the mechanical effects of ultrasound that are potentially harmful to living tissues are related to the formation, growth, and possible collapse of tiny gas bubbles in the ultrasound field, a process known as **cavitation**. Recall that ultrasound propagates through tissue in waves of alternating high and low pressure. Bubble formation or the expansion of existing bubbles occurs when the negative pressure is large enough. The occurrence of cavitation and its effects depend on the frequency and intensity of the transmitted ultrasound waves as well as on the focus of the acoustic field. Two types of cavitation are commonly described: stable and inertial (or transient).

Stable cavitation refers to the continuous oscillation of gas-filled bodies in response to the alternating positive and negative pressures to which they are exposed in an ultrasound field. Such cyclic expansions and contractions result in an increased flow in the fluid-like medium surrounding the vibrating bubbles. This phenomenon is known as microstreaming and can generate very high pressures with disruption of cell membranes. In the other form of cavitation, **inertial cavitation**, existing bubbles or cavitation nuclei expand during the low-pressure phase and then collapse violently. Microbubble collapse is a highly localized process occurring on the order of microseconds. Collapsing bubbles can produce extremely high temperatures and pressures but these dissipate rapidly. Bursting bubbles therefore have the potential to destroy cells and tissues. There is scientific evidence to suggest that inertial cavitation is a threshold phenomenon and will only occur if microbubbles already present in the acoustic field are exposed to excessive acoustic pressures and frequencies. Pressure below the cavitation threshold will never by itself lead to cavitation, not even during extremely long exposure to ultrasound. Inertial cavitation induced by diagnostic ultrasound procedures therefore remains a mere theoretical possibility and has never been reported in vivo.

However, one must also be aware that in vivo evidence of potential bioeffects of ultrasound is very difficult, if not impossible, to obtain: cavitation can occur anywhere in the body, and the damage it produces may be very local, involving only a few cells. Modern ultrasound equipment incorporates safety mechanisms allowing the user to limit the average acoustic output, thus avoiding peak pressures that could theoretically lead to cavitation or other mechanical bioeffects.

1.1.6.3 Specific Risks of Individual Ultrasound Techniques

1.1.6.3.1 B-Mode

B-mode imaging is generally performed at very low acoustic output, resulting in intensities below 10 mW/cm^2. The individual pulses are very short (<1 ms) and are emitted at a PRF of less than 5 kHz to achieve high resolution. As the energy transmitted into the body is dissipated over a large volume, the resulting rise in tissue temperature is so small that it remains below the limit of detection. Diagnostic B-mode ultrasound is considered absolutely safe in terms of potential hazards to patients.

1.1.6.3.2 M-Mode

This technique uses higher energies and may theoretically cause tissue heating. In this mode, a stationary beam is emitted repeatedly to evaluate moving structures. The scan volume is smaller than in B-mode imaging, but the PRF is much lower (only approx. 1 kHz). M-mode sonography is also considered safe.

1.1.6.3.3 CW Doppler

As with M-mode techniques, the scan volume is small and there is continuous exposure. The power output can reach up to 100 mW, and some procedures have the potential to produce biologically significant temperature rises. Possible mechanical effects are much less of a concern than in B-mode or M-mode scanning, despite the higher acoustic output. The transmit power depends on the depth of the target anatomy. It is the operator's responsibility to keep the overall examination time as short as is consistent with achieving diagnostically useful results.

1.1.6.3.4 PW Doppler

Again, the exposed volume is relatively small and the PRF is high. The individual pulses are often twice as long as with B-mode or M-mode techniques. Taken together, the machine settings used in PW Doppler applications can result in considerable exposure, and the risk of tissue heating is far greater. Conversely, mechanical effects are negligible because the intensity of the emitted pulses is the same as in B-mode and M-mode imaging.

1.1.6.3.5 Color Doppler

The acoustic output in color Doppler imaging is intermediate between that of B-mode and PW Doppler. Mechanical effects are negligible. The emitted ultrasound pulses are distributed over a relatively large tissue volume. Temperature rises are higher than with B-mode imaging but lower than with PW Doppler techniques.

1.1.6.4 Conclusion

Current uses of diagnostic ultrasound expose the body to intensities that do not exceed 100 mW/cm². There is no evidence that these intensities damage living tissues.

Nevertheless, the examiner should always seek to minimize exposure by limiting both the power output and the duration of scanning to what is absolutely necessary to obtain the desired diagnostic information. This approach is known as the ALARA principle (as low as reasonably achievable) and applies to all diagnostic imaging modalities. Doppler ultrasound, which uses higher intensities, should not be employed during the first three months of pregnancy.

1.2 Hemodynamic Principles

1.2.1 Laminar Flow

Although blood flow is subject to specific conditions due to the solid components in plasma and the elasticity of the vessel wall, it basically follows the laws of flow dynamics. These laws govern the flow of a fluid in tubes and apply to watery or oily solutions of a constant viscosity (Newtonian fluid) and assume that flow velocity under these conditions is primarily a function of the pressure difference that exists between the two ends of the tube. These ideal conditions for continuous laminar flow are typically not met in a living organism because various factors such as elasticity of the vessel wall, pulsatility resulting from cardiac activity, curving of vessels, and branching affect blood flow, resulting in changing velocity distributions in the moving layers of the blood.

Moreover, **blood** is not a watery or oily solution of constant viscosity but a **suspension** of solid blood cells in plasma. Blood viscosity is primarily dependent on the hematocrit level and is only constant when hematocrit is below 10, increasing exponentially at higher levels. Other factors affecting blood viscosity are plasma viscosity and vessel diameter. In the terminal capillary bed, viscosity is additionally influenced by the deformation of red blood cells. Despite these specific features of blood flow, some basic hemodynamic terms and laws are useful and will make it easier to understand normal and abnormal flow in arteries and veins. In addition, in vitro experiments and in vivo blood flow measurements using duplex scanning have provided new insights into the flow behavior in specific vessels under normal and abnormal conditions as well as under the influence of pharmacologic agents.

Laminar flow is characterized by a constant velocity over time. Flow in a tube is brought about by a pressure difference between the two ends of the tube. The pressure difference ($P_1 - P_2$) is proportional to the volume flow rate. The volume flow rate (I) is proportional to the tube diameter (r) and inversely proportional to its length (l) and the viscosity of the fluid (η). Mathematically, this relationship is expressed in the **Hagen–Poiseuille law**:

$$I = \frac{(P_1 - P_2) \cdot \pi \cdot r^4}{8 \cdot l \cdot \eta} = \frac{(P_1 - P_2)}{R}$$

By analogy with Ohm's law, flow resistance can be calculated from the Hagen–Poiseuille equation:

$$R = \frac{8 \cdot l \cdot \eta}{\pi \cdot r^4}$$

It follows that resistance is proportional to the length of the tube (l) and the viscosity of the liquid (η). Overall resistance is most strongly affected by the radius (r) of the tube, which appears in the equation raised to the fourth power. This means that decreasing the vessel radius by one half, for example, increases flow resistance by a factor of 16. Peripheral resistance in the vascular system is regulated according to demand, primarily by the tone of the arterioles, and affects the pulsatility of blood flow in the large arteries supplying these territories. Therefore, it is also reflected in spectral Doppler tracings from these arteries.

The flow profile of **continuous flow** is determined by **inertial** and **frictional forces**. Friction produces a laminar or, in the 3D model, parabolic flow profile. Flow is fastest in the center of a vessel and decreases toward the wall, where it approximates zero.

In color duplex images, this decrease in blood flow velocity from midstream to the vessel wall is indicated by brighter colors in the center and darker colors near the wall (◘ Fig. 1.43a). The following factors determine the shape of the flow profile of blood:

- Velocity
- Viscosity (internal friction)
- Adhesion of the blood to the vessel wall (external friction)
- Cohesion (forces that occur between adjacent molecules of like composition).

1

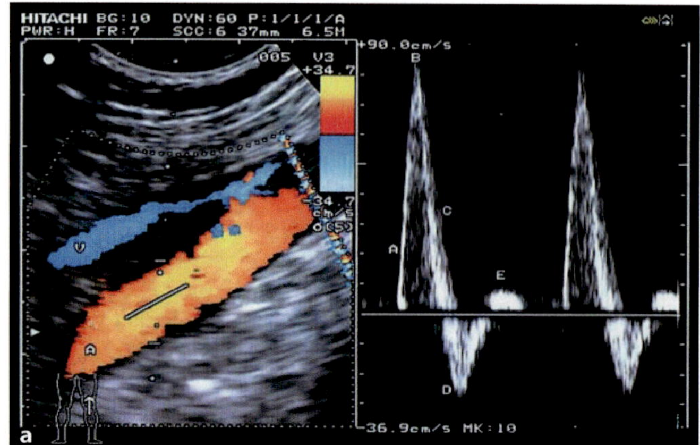

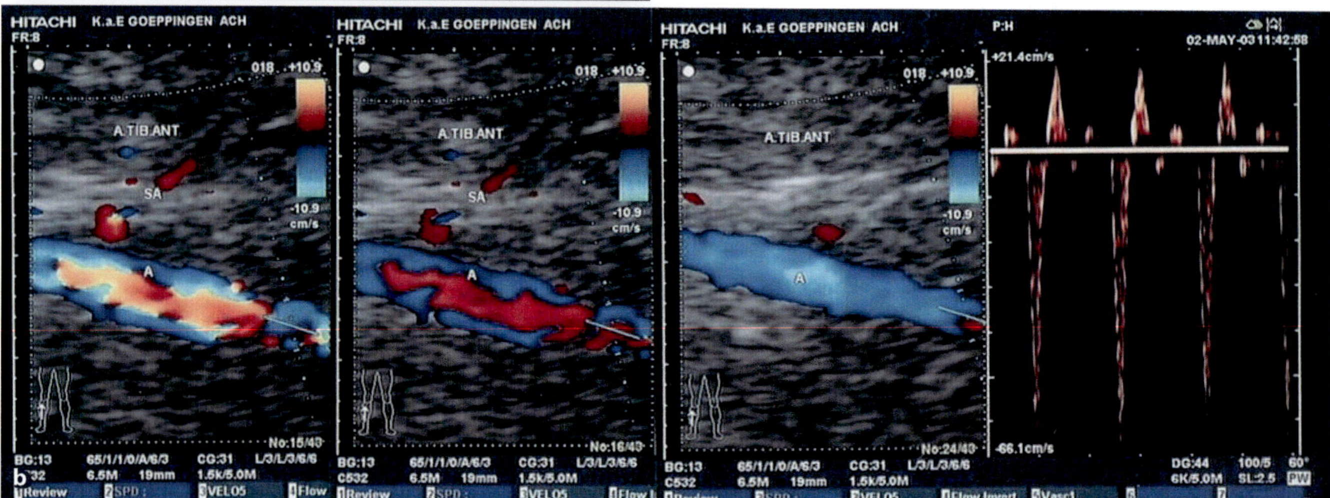

Fig. 1.43 **a** Typical triphasic Doppler waveform of the popliteal artery. In the color flow image, laminar flow is characterized by brighter coloring in the center with darker colors representing slow flow near the wall. Red indicates blood flow toward the transducer. A vein closer to the transducer is displayed in blue, indicating blood flow away from the transducer. The triphasic waveform consists of a steep upslope (A) to peak systolic velocity (PSV) (B), a deceleration phase (C), a short phase of early diastolic backward flow (D), and forward flow from the middle to the end of diastole (E). The magnitude and duration of diastolic forward flow (E) depend on peripheral resistance (sympathetic tone) and the thrust generated by the compliant aorta (windkessel effect). Blood flow toward the transducer is displayed above the baseline, and flow away from it below the line. The Doppler angle of insonation is 59°, and PSV is 85 cm/s. The different intensities of the individual pixels in the Doppler waveform reflect the number of red blood cells moving at a given velocity. The amplitude can also be represented in the form of a histogram. **b** Use of a low pulse repetition frequency (PRF) to ensure good color filling of arteries with slow flow below the knee. In the first color image (left), the anterior tibial artery (blue, flow toward the periphery, away from the transducer) is depicted with central aliasing (color change from blue to yellow to red). This example illustrates a laminar flow profile with fast flow in the center of the artery and lower flow velocities near the wall due to friction. The second color image depicts early diastolic blood flow at the same site, which is due to the fast image generation. In the center, arterial reflux due to high peripheral resistance is seen as a superimposed wave (red, toward transducer) while flow toward the periphery predominates nearer the walls (blue, away from transducer). The view illustrates true flow reversal relative to the ultrasound beam rather than aliasing. True flow reversal is characterized by a color change from blue to black to red. The third color flow image depicts blood flow (blue, away from transducer) toward the periphery without aliasing in mid-diastole. While each of the three color flow images depicts peripheral arterial blood flow at a specific time during the cardiac cycle, the corresponding Doppler waveform (right) displays the flow changes over time

Blood differs from Newtonian fluid in that its viscosity is not an inherent property that only varies with temperature but is mainly determined by the hematocrit level and other factors such as plasma viscosity (which in turn is predominantly dependent on the fibrinogen concentration), red blood cell deformability, and the degree of shearing. In an artery or vein with laminar flow, shear stress, like thrust, is weakest in the center and strongest near the wall (Fig. 1.43b).

According to the continuity law, a **decrease in the cross-sectional area** in the course of a vessel segment leads to an **increase in mean flow velocity**. Blood flow through a vessel segment with an abrupt change in caliber becomes flattened (plug flow) upon entering the narrower vessel segment. In plug flow, inertial forces are stronger than frictional forces, resulting in the same flow velocity of all fluid layers in the vessel except for a thin layer near the wall. So-called turbulent flow results when the inertial forces become even stronger than the frictional forces, which bring order to the course of flow. Turbulent flow is characterized by an irregular flow pattern with flow in different directions. The typical parabolic flow pattern develops after a certain stretch along which

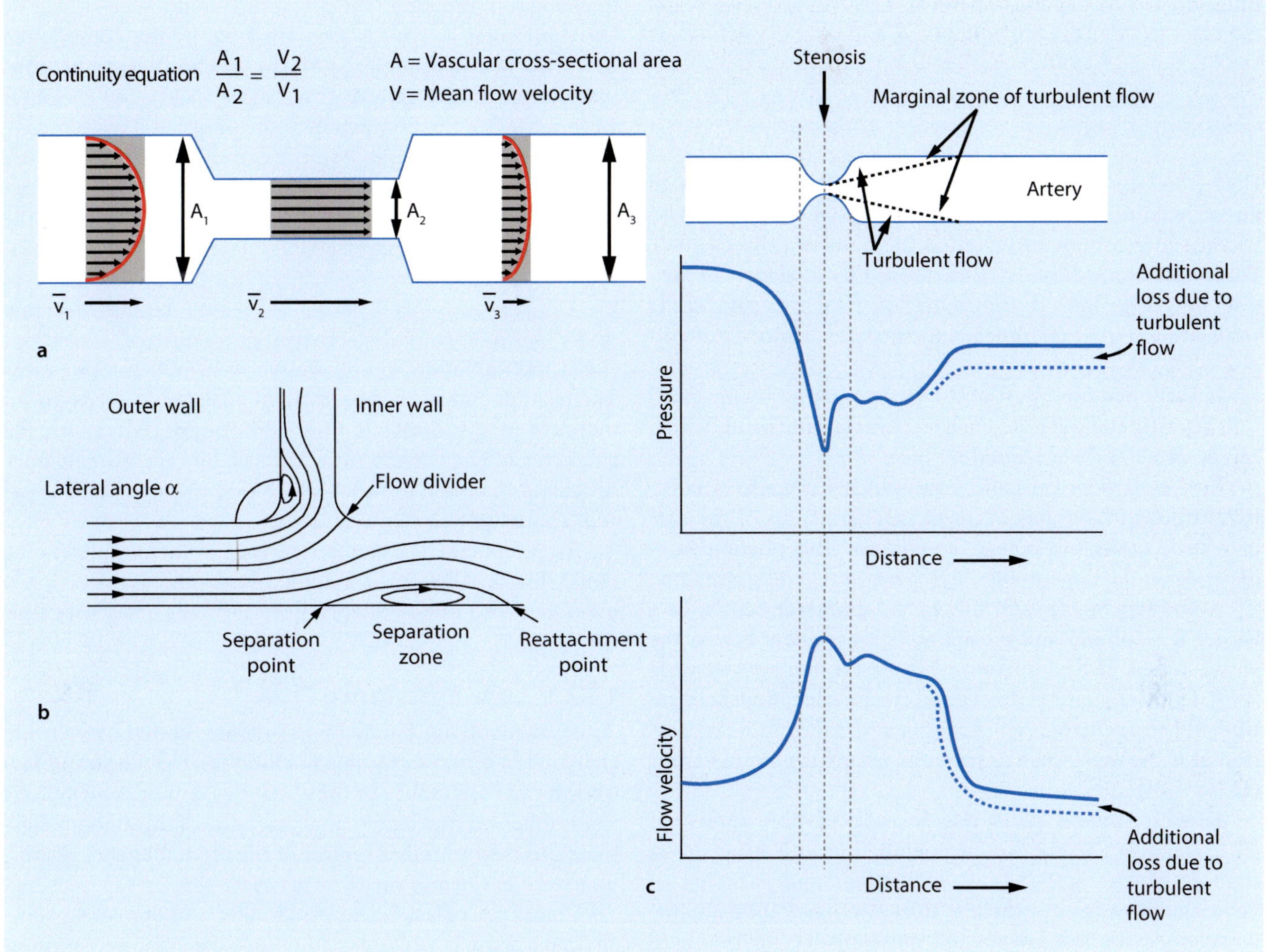

Fig. 1.44 **a** When a fluid such as blood enters a narrower lumen, parabolic flow changes into plug flow and returns to its original profile only after having traveled some distance under the influence of shear stress. According to the continuity equation, flow velocity increases in proportion to the decrease in diameter. **b** Flow in a vessel branching. Thrust and shearing are highest at the inner wall of the branching. Separation occurs at the outer wall, where thrust is rather low. Physiologic flow separation occurs in the carotid bulb (see Fig. 5.49 (Atlas)). **c** Diagram of flow in a vessel segment with higher-grade stenosis and corresponding curves (solid blue lines) representing the effects of the stenosis on pressure (top) and flow velocity (bottom) in the stenotic and poststenotic segment. The law of conservation of energy predicts that static energy (blood pressure) is converted to kinetic energy (flow velocity) (Bernoulli equation). It thus follows that the intrastenotic increase in flow velocity results in a proportional drop in pressure (neglecting other factors such as blood viscosity and systolic-diastolic flow variation). The actual pressure and flow velocity measured in a poststenotic vessel segment (dotted lines) are lower than theoretically predicted because the equation does not consider losses resulting from turbulence and friction

frictional forces predominate. Physiologically, this occurs when blood leaves the left ventricle and enters the ascending aorta. The sharp velocity gradient between flow in the center and the thin boundary layer near the wall in plug flow is associated with strong shear stress.

The law of conservation of energy states that the **total amount of energy** in a closed system remains constant. Applied to blood flow, this means that the total energy in a stenotic vessel is the same before and after the stenosis (unless there is loss of energy from the system) and that there is an inversely proportional relationship between static and dynamic components (Fig. 1.44):

$$E_{\text{total}} = E_{\text{static}} + E_{\text{kinetic}}$$

It follows from this law that increasing flow velocity within a stenosis (E_{kinetic}) is associated with decreasing tangential intravascular pressure (E_{static}). The reverse applies to the poststenotic segment: increasing pressure results in turbulent flow with slow flow components near the wall and can promote intramural hematoma formation.

An abrupt decrease in the cross-sectional area in a stenotic vessel segment and the resulting increase in flow velocity are associated with progressive disturbance of laminar flow, which will finally become turbulent. Turbulent flow above a critical velocity is characterized on color duplex ultrasound by a mosaic of colors reflecting the different flow directions. The transition from laminar to turbulent flow can be calculated by means of the dimensionless **Reynolds**

1

number, which depends on mean flow velocity (v), vessel diameter (d), density of the fluid (p), and viscosity (η):

$$Re = \frac{v \cdot d \cdot p}{\eta}$$

Data from in vitro model experiments show blood flow to be fairly laminar for Reynolds numbers up to 2000 and to become increasingly turbulent as the number exceeds 2000. **Turbulent blood flow** is characterized by a pattern of random flow directions, seen in color flow images as color shifts (indicating retrograde flow components) or a mosaic of colors.

In turbulent flow, part of the kinetic energy is converted into acoustic energy, producing a **characteristic bruit**, which can be detected by auscultation.

In vessels with pulsatile flow, which normally is laminar, turbulent flow may occur at specific phases of the cardiac cycle under physiologic conditions. This phenomenon depends on the flow profile (high pulsatility) and pulse rate.

A **sudden increase in the vessel diameter** results in a longer flow profile and greater velocity gradient across the vessel lumen. If the difference between a narrow and wide (poststenotic) segment exceeds a certain value, **flow separation** and eddy currents will occur near the wall. Flow separation near the wall is also observed in branching blood vessels (◘ Fig. 1.44).

Flow separation gives rise to **recirculation zones,** in which relative stasis of flow, in conjunction with shear stress, induces platelet aggregation with release and adhesion of procoagulative agents, which in turn can trigger local atherogenic processes. This is a possible mechanism contributing to the preferred occurrence of atherosclerotic lesions in dividing and branching vessel segments.

The most notable example of flow separation can be encountered when imaging the origin of the internal carotid artery (ICA), where it occurs as a result of both widening in the bulb area and branching (see ◘ Fig. 5.49 (Atlas)). The high wall pressure in this area, in conjunction with slow flow in separation zones, contributes to the preferred development of carotid bulb plaque on the wall opposite the external carotid artery origin (◘ Figs. 1.44b, 5.49 (Atlas), and 5.56 (Atlas)). Flow separation can also occur downstream of a stenosis, where the vascular cross-sectional area increases again (see ◘ Fig. 1.46a, b), and increased wall pressure can cause poststenotic dilatation.

Poststenotic vascular dilatation or even aneurysm is rare in atherosclerotic stenosis; it is more common in patients with other vascular conditions not causing wall sclerosis such as compression syndromes (see ◘ Figs. 3.101, 2.105, and 2.106 (all Atlas)) or fibromuscular dysplasia.

1.2.2 Flow Profiles and Perfusion Regulation

Unlike laminar flow, **pulsatile flow** changes periodically over time. Phases of acceleration and deceleration vary in relation to changes in pressure. The pressure amplitude generated by left ventricular activity is smoothed out by the **compliance of the aorta and other large elastic, or conducting, arteries** (windkessel effect), resulting in a more steady flow. Another factor affecting the flow profile is the peripheral resistance.

Flow is highly pulsatile in the extremity arteries because peripheral resistance is high at rest, giving rise to the characteristic triphasic Doppler waveform. An increase in the peripheral blood demand leads to dilatation of the arterioles, and the resulting decrease in peripheral resistance changes the Doppler waveform. Peripheral resistance may decrease under normal (muscle activity) or abnormal conditions (local inflammation, postocclusive ischemia, tumor perfusion). A **decrease in pheripheral resistance** leads to an **increase in the diastolic flow component**. Moreover, the character of the waveform is affected by central regulatory processes (increase in heart rate, blood pressure) and vessel wall elasticity (diabetes mellitus).

As peripheral resistance is a crucial factor influencing blood flow and hence the Doppler waveform, a distinction is made between low-resistance flow and high-resistance flow (◘ Fig. 1.45).

1.2.2.1 Low-Resistance Flow

Arteries supplying parenchymal organs and the brain are characterized by a fairly steady blood flow as a result of **low peripheral resistance**. In these arteries, a moderate systolic rise is followed by a steady flow that persists throughout diastole. This flow profile is typical of the renal, hepatic, splenic, internal carotid, and vertebral arteries.

Continuous diastolic flow in the arteries supplying parenchymal organs is necessary to ensure constant perfusion of these organs. This is accomplished by the lower peripheral resistance of these vascular beds and the windkessel function of the large conducting arteries including the aorta, which jointly produce a more continuous flow than would result from the action of the left ventricle and aortic valve alone (◘ Fig. 1.45).

1.2.2.2 High-Resistance Flow

High peripheral resistance results in a more pulsatile flow with a steep systolic upslope during the acceleration phase, followed by deceleration and a significant reflux in early diastole, short backward flow in mid-diastole, and typically zero flow in late diastole. This pattern is referred to as **triphasic flow**.

The systolic pulse wave is in part reflected by the high peripheral resistance and thus moves backward through the arterial system until the flow is again redirected toward the periphery by the influx of blood during the next cardiac cycle. This flow component is small due to the high peripheral resistance.

As a result of the high pressure in the arterioles supplied by the limb arteries, significant blood flow in these vessels occurs only during systole when systemic pressure is higher than peripheral pressure. The pressure during diastole is too low to produce blood flow toward the periphery.

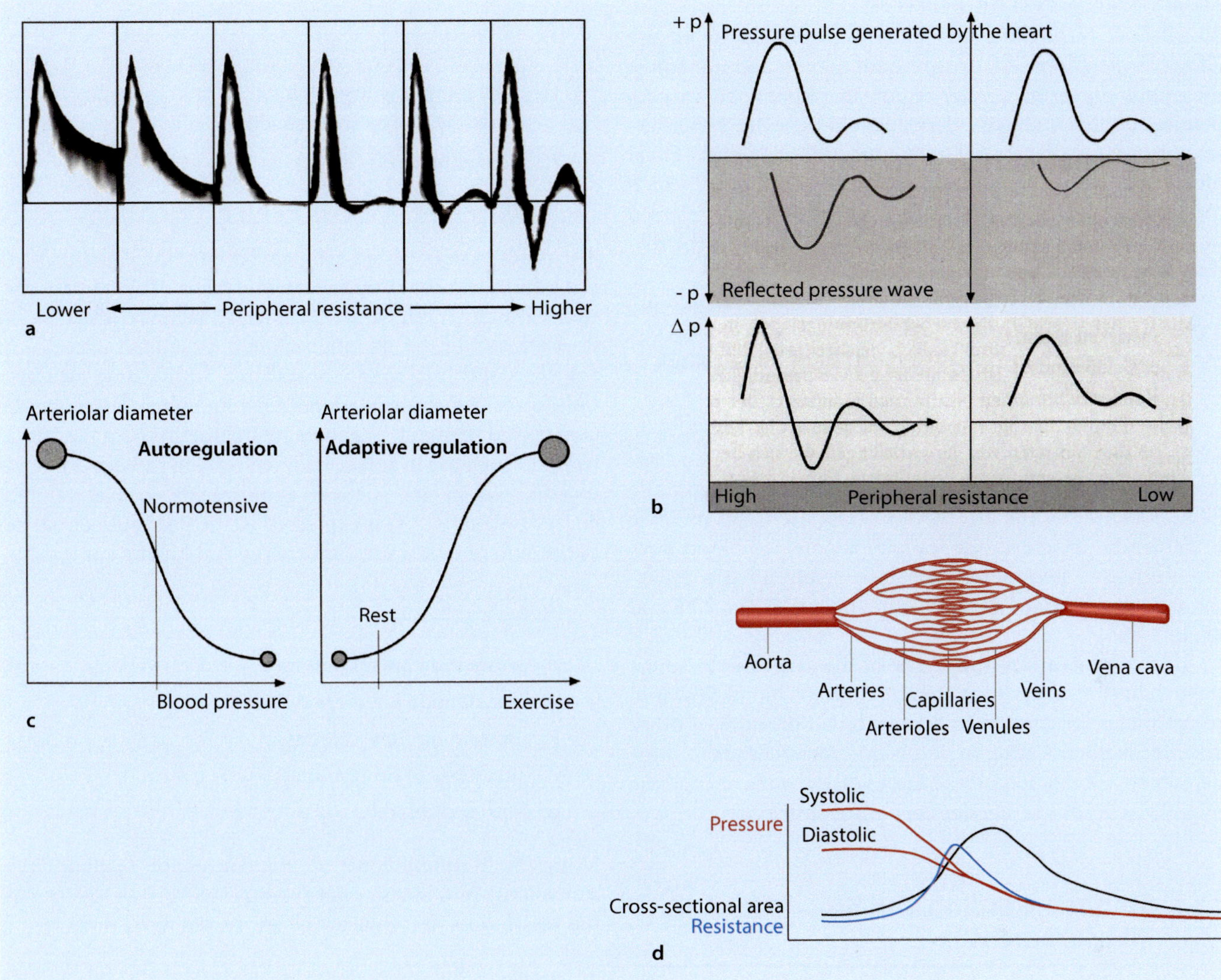

Fig. 1.45 **a** Effect of peripheral resistance on the Doppler waveform. Pulsatility increases with peripheral resistance. **b** Flow pulse curves resulting from superimposition of the pressure pulse generated by the heart and the pressure waves reflected by the distal vascular bed in arteries with high peripheral resistance (left) and low peripheral resistance (right). For an identical pressure pulse generated by the heart (above the baseline), the pulse curve resulting from interaction with the reflected pulse (below the baseline) is highly pulsatile when peripheral resistance is high and less pulsatile when peripheral resistance is low. The pressure gradient (Δp) calculated by subtracting the reflected pulse wave from the pulse wave emitted by the heart is directly proportional to blood flow velocity (according to the Hagen–Poiseuille law). **c** Changes in arteriolar diameter in response to blood pressure changes (autoregulation, left) and in response to exercise (adaptive regulation, right). **d** Simplified schematic illustration of changes in blood pressure (with flow velocity changing in proportion), peripheral resistance, and total area of the vascular bed through the circulatory system (arteries, capillaries, veins)

High-resistance flow occurs in the arteries supplying the muscles and the skin, such as the arteries of the arms and legs, and the external carotid artery. The ratio of skin to muscle supply determines the amount of diastolic forward flow. When peripheral demand increases (muscle activity, inflammation), the arterioles dilate to reduce local vascular resistance, and forward flow, primarily during diastole, increases.

Transitions between these two flow patterns may occur under normal and abnormal conditions. Besides, there are vessels with mixed patterns. An example is the superior mesenteric artery, which has pulsatile flow like a limb artery but also has a significant end-diastolic flow component. The amount of end-diastolic flow is regulated adaptively and increases with demand after ingestion of food. Adaptive adjustment of diastolic flow through arteriolar vasodilation occurs in all arteries with high-resistance flow. Other factors influencing late diastolic flow include systemic factors such as sympathetic tone and the windkessel function of the aorta. This is why loss of aortic compliance and of vascular elasticity results in more pulsatile flow.

An arteriovenous (AV) fistula turns high-resistance flow into low-resistance flow. A change from low-resistance to high-resistance flow in a transplant renal artery is an important diagnostic criterion in the diagnosis of graft rejection.

1.2.2.3 Perfusion Regulation

Blood flow throughout the body is regulated to ensure adequate perfusion of organs and tissues and to adjust the blood supply to a body region in response to varying demand (which is activity-dependent in the extremity arteries or increases after a meal in the mesenteric arteries). Local blood flow is regulated by arterioles and capillaries, which can dilate or constrict selectively and are therefore referred to as resistance vessels. Two types of regulation can be distinguished:

- autoregulation to maintain constant perfusion (cerebral perfusion, renal arteries) and
- adaptive regulation to adjust blood supply to varying demand (◻ Fig. 1.45c).

Normal **resting perfusion** is maintained by constricted arterioles, resulting in high peripheral resistance and pulsatile flow. Widening of the arterioles in response to an increase in demand during exercise leads to augmented blood flow. The decreased peripheral resistance results in less pulsatile flow and a larger diastolic component (◻ Fig. 2.15 and ◻ Fig. 1.45).

In **autoregulation**, the ability of the arterioles to adjust their diameter serves to maintain constant blood flow and compensates for changes in arterial blood pressure or other systemic factors. A drop in perfusion pressure leads to compensatory vasodilation of resistance vessels, while an increase in pressure leads to compensatory vasoconstriction.

1.2.3 Stenosis Grading and Blood Flow Measurement

Volumetric blood flow measurement plays no role in daily clinical practice, except for assessing flow in hemodialysis access fistulas. This topic is treated in a separate chapter and details of flow volume measurement are provided in ► Sect. 4.4.

Blood flow volume can be calculated from the vascular cross-sectional area and mean flow velocity; however, this method is prone to errors unless great care is taken in determining these two parameters (see ► Sect. 1.1.2.4). Therefore, it is not recommended to calculate flow volume using inbuilt software tools.

The **continuity equation** states that the volume flow rate (cross-sectional area multiplied by average flow velocity) remains constant throughout a vessel. Therefore, an abrupt decrease in arterial diameter in a stenotic vessel segment is associated with an increase in blood flow velocity (a 50% decrease in diameter, corresponding to a 75% decrease in cross-sectional area, will result in a four times higher flow velocity). The flow profile flattens out (plug flow) when the blood enters a narrower segment. If the increase in flow velocity is known, it is possible to estimate the degree of stenosis using the continuity equation (◻ Fig. 1.44a):

$$X = 100 \cdot \left(1 - \frac{V_1}{V_2}\right)$$

X percentage stenosis degree (cross-sectional area reduction)
V_1 prestenotic velocity
V_2 intrastenotic velocity

The result is an idealized estimate because the equation does not take into account other systemic factors (blood pressure, wall elasticity, peripheral resistance) that may affect blood flow velocity in the stenotic segment. A sudden decrease in the cross-sectional area is associated with strong acceleration forces, which turn laminar flow into plug flow along the constricted segment. The increase in kinetic energy resulting from the increase in average flow velocity in the stenosis leads to a decrease in static (lateral) pressure. This conservation of energy (► Sect. 1.2.1) is expressed in the **Bernoulli equation** as the sum of lateral pressure energy and kinetic energy:

$$P_1 + \frac{1}{2} \cdot \rho \cdot V_1^2 = P_2 + \frac{1}{2} \cdot \rho \cdot V_2^2$$

P_1 prestenotic lateral pressure
P_2 intrastenotic lateral pressure
V_1 prestenotic flow velocity
V_2 intrastenotic flow velocity
ρ density of blood

Using the Bernoulli equation, the conversion of static pressure energy into kinetic energy resulting from a reduction in the vessel cross-sectional area is expressed as follows:

$$P_1 - P_2 = \frac{1}{2} \cdot \rho \cdot \left(V_2^2 - V_1^2\right)$$

The **poststenotic increase in the cross-sectional flow area** leads to **turbulent flow**, **flow separation**, and vortexing. The pronounced turbulence occurring in the presence of high-grade stenosis is associated with eddy currents and backward flow, resulting in the irreversible loss of most of the kinetic energy, while the loss due to inertial and frictional forces is negligible (Weber et al. 1992). The pressure drop across a stenosis (substantial portion of the Doppler-derived blood pressure) thus predominantly **reflects the lost kinetic energy** in the stenosis. Therefore, the kinetic energy expressed as peak systolic velocity (PSV) in the stenosis can serve as a measure of the pressure drop across the stenosis (according to the simplified Bernoulli equation: $P_1 - P_2 = 4 \times V_2^2$; neglecting prestenotic velocity V_1 in favor of intrastenotic velocity V_2) and the degree of stenosis (see ► Sect. 2.1.6.1.1).

Blood flow resumes its laminar profile only farther downstream of the stenosis as a result of decreasing turbulence and the influence of mural friction. The conversion of much of the remaining kinetic energy into static pressure energy promotes dilatation of the atherosclerotic wall in the poststenotic arterial segment.

An examiner using the Doppler-derived PSV to grade stenosis should be aware, though, that, due to friction losses inside the stenosis, this method is subject to some inaccuracy. In high-grade stenosis with a reduced volume flow rate, flow velocity is already decreased in the prestenotic segment, resulting in an intrastenotic increase in velocity that is lower than expected from the diameter reduction. The maximum intrastenotic velocity may thus be lower in high-grade stenosis with a reduced volume flow rate than in moderate stenosis causing less pronounced flow reduction.

Stenosis grading based on absolute intrastenotic PSV thresholds is also unreliable in patients with multilevel steno-occlusive disease because the poststenotic pressure drop downstream of a more proximal stenosis results in a lower PSV upstream of the next (second or third) stenosis. To overcome this limitation, most examiners prefer to identify and grade stenosis by determining the increase in PSV in the stenosis in relation to the PSV in the prestenotic segment (known as the PSV ratio). In general, a PSV ratio greater than 2, indicating doubling of PSV inside the stenosis, is taken as the cutoff for hemodynamically significant stenosis (>50%). Calculation of PSV ratios is less straightforward for stenoses occurring immediately downstream of a vessel division, which is a common site of stenosis (origins of profunda femoris or renal arteries, carotid bifurcation). For these vessel segments, empirical threshold velocities (reference value, angiography) must be determined to identify hemodynamically significant stenosis. Such thresholds are affected by systemic factors (hypercirculation, hypertension).

Careful adjustment of the Doppler angle of insonation is crucial in measuring blood flow velocity for stenosis grading. Ideally, the Doppler angle should be 60° or less to minimize the effect of Doppler angle misreading on flow calculation; this effect becomes much larger when the Doppler angle is 70° or greater. Alignment of the angle correction cursor may be technically challenging in curved or branching vessels.

The maximum velocity, or PSV, is measured in the stenosis or the jet seen in the color duplex image. The intrastenotic increase in flow velocity in high-grade stenosis results in a higher Reynolds number and is associated with turbulent flow. Turbulence is characterized on color duplex images by a typical mosaic pattern around the central stenosis jet with backward flow near the wall. Depending on the increase in flow velocity, eddy currents may be seen over a length of several centimeters downstream of the stenosis (◘ Fig. 1.46).

The jet tapers off distal to the stenosis, while the zone of turbulent flow widens until it occupies the entire lumen. Further downstream, flow becomes laminar again. The pressure drop across a stenosis is determined by its length and degree. These two parameters, along with poststenotic turbulence, govern the loss of kinetic energy. The magnitude of the intrastenotic pressure drop correlates with the kinetic pressure energy present in the stenosis jet. Based on measurement of the stenosis jet, the pressure drop across the stenosis can be estimated using the simplified Bernoulli equation (neglecting prestenotic flow velocity) as

$$P_1 - P_2 = 4 \cdot V_2^{\,2} \left(jet\ velocity \right)$$

The jet axis is typically not parallel to the vessel wall, especially when the stenosis is eccentric. Depiction of the stenosis jet in the B-mode image can help the examiner in aligning the angle correction cursor with the direction of flow for reliable measurement of blood flow velocity in the jet (◘ Figs. 1.47 and 5.21).

A study comparing the invasively measured mean catheter pressure gradient across stenotic vessel segments with the pressure gradient determined from the stenosis jet using duplex ultrasound (Strauss et al. 1993) found a correlation of $R = 0.77$ for iliac artery stenoses. This investigation was based on preceding model calculations and neglected viscous friction losses and energy losses due to poststenotic turbulence.

In vitro measurements in a model of pulsatile flow in peripheral arteries demonstrated good agreement for the pressure decrease across a stenosis measured invasively and that determined by Doppler ultrasound. The correlation found for different degrees of stenosis was $R = 0.98$ (Strauss et al. 1990; Weber et al. 1992). Still, quantitative evaluation of stenosis using only the absolute values of maximum intrastenotic frequency shifts or peak velocities is discouraged, as the magnitude of intrastenotic flow velocity is also affected by various other factors including central regulatory mechanisms (blood pressure), collateral pathways, and peripheral resistance.

Empirical data show that a stenosis becomes hemodynamically relevant and **causes clinical symptoms** when the vessel diameter is reduced by at least 30–50% (corresponding to a cross-sectional area reduction of 50–75%). The pressure drop across a stenosis increases with its degree and length and is reflected in a decrease in the Doppler-derived peripheral blood pressure.

Because PSV measured in a stenosis is influenced by systemic factors (blood pressure during the examination, vessel wall elasticity), stenosis grading based on absolute PSV cutoffs for different degrees of stenosis identified by ROC analysis is limited. To overcome these limitations, the use of a ratio relating intrastenotic to prestenotic PSV (known as systolic velocity ratio (SVR) or PSV ratio) was proposed as an alternative velocity parameter for stenosis grading and explored in different vascular territories. Overall, the results come close to the theoretical predictions of the continuity equation (see ◘ Fig. 2.17), confirming that a ratio > 2 indicates hemodynamically significant stenosis (>50%) and a ratio > 4 high-grade stenosis (>75%).

While stenosis grading based on PSV ratios yields the most reliable results, there are some potential sources of error the examiner should be aware of (◘ Table 1.10):

- Measurements using in vitro flow models yielded slightly lower PSV ratios than theoretically predicted (loss due to intrastenotic friction)
- Cutoffs for diameter reduction only apply to concentric stenoses: an eccentric stenosis with the same diameter reduction as a concentric stenosis produces a smaller

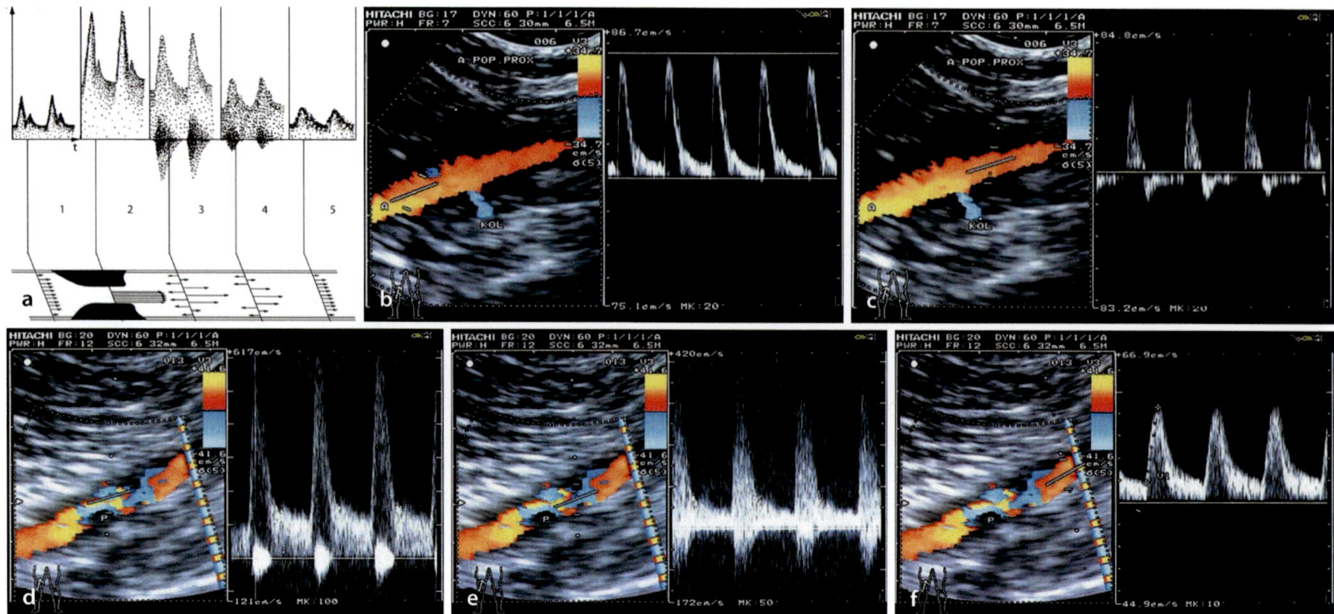

◘ Fig. 1.46 **a** Blood flow patterns and effects on Doppler waveforms from different sites within and around a stenosis of the internal carotid artery (ICA): 1 = prestenotic flow (laminar, pulsatile); 2 = intrastenotic flow (plug profile, maximum increase in peak systolic velocity (PSV), increase varies with diameter reduction); 3 = immediately poststenotic flow (marked turbulence, increased PSV); 4 = poststenotic flow (return to lower flow velocity, residual turbulence); 5 = poststenotic flow further downstream (return to laminar flow but decreased pulsatility, flattened waveform with larger diastolic component). **b-f** The waveform shapes in **a** illustrate stenosis-related flow changes in the carotid artery, but basically the same patterns occur in a stenotic peripheral artery (see direct and indirect stenosis criteria in ► Sect. 2.1.6.1.4), except that flow is more pulsatile (triphasic waveform). In this territory, loss of pulsatility in the poststenotic segment (with transition to a monophasic waveform) can serve as an indirect stenosis criterion. **b** Popliteal artery stenosis: Proximal to the origin of hemodynamically significant collaterals, the normal triphasic prestenotic waveform may show reduced pulsatility. The extent to which pulsatility is decreased depends on the amount of collateral flow and compensatory ischemic widening of arteries and arterioles in the periphery. When the sample volume is placed upstream of the origin of a collateral (KOL), there is only a subtle incisure in the Doppler waveform in early diastole and continuous blood flow throughout diastole. Farther away from the transducer, a collateral arising from the popliteal artery is seen, which provides significant compensatory circulation. The hemodynamic effects of collateralization are rarely depicted in such an impressive manner. In this situation, two different prestenotic PSV values are obtained (due to flow division): 75 cm/s proximal to the origin of the collateral versus 50 cm/s distal to it (see **c**). Hence, the continuity equation will yield two different results for the intrastenotic-to-prestenotic PSV ratio, depending on which of the two prestenotic PSVs is used (see ◘ Fig. 2.16). The PSV ratio calculated with the higher prestenotic PSV, measured proximal to the collateral origin, underestimates the degree of stenosis. **c** Distal to the collateral, the increased pulsatility reflects the flow resistance in the popliteal artery immediately before the stenosis. The abnormal diastolic flow is not only a function of the stenosis-related peripheral resistance but also of vessel elasticity. Proximal to the sample volume, the hemodynamically significant collateral (KOL) arising from the popliteal artery is displayed in blue. The stenotic popliteal artery segment is not depicted but is likely to be located to the right of the view presented. **d** The high-grade stenosis caused by a hypoechoic plaque produces aliasing in the color duplex image. The Doppler spectrum shows the flow velocity to be increased to over 600 cm/s (see waveform 2 in **a**). In the segment depicted in the B-mode scan, the popliteal artery stenosis appears to be less severe because the plaque predominantly involves the lateral vessel wall as compared with the spectral display, which reflects the hemodynamic significance of the stenosis (see ◘ Fig. 5.14). Like angiography, the B-mode scan reduces the three-dimensional lumen to a two-dimensional, longitudinal plane. Depending on the plane of the gray-scale image, the severity of the stenosis caused by plaque may be underestimated and may differ from the hemodynamic degree of stenosis based on PSV (see ◘ Fig. 5.27). **e** In the immediate poststenotic segment, turbulent flow is predominant both in the color duplex image and in the Doppler waveform. PSV is still increased (300 cm/s) (see waveform 3 in **a**). **f** Three centimeters downstream of the stenosis, flow is monophasic with a delayed systolic rise and reduced PSV (see waveform 5 in **a**)

reduction of the vascular cross-sectional area. Hence, the eccentric stenosis has a less marked hemodynamic effect and the resulting increase in PSV is smaller (see ◘ Fig. 2.17). This is important to keep in mind and explains some of the discrepancies between a morphologic stenosis grading technique such as angiography and a hemodynamic technique such as duplex ultrasound.

- When selecting the site of prestenotic PSV measurement it is important to be aware of the effect of collaterals: pre- and intrastenotic PSVs are higher in the absence of collateralization, and prestenotic PSV is higher upstream of the origin of a collateral than downstream of it (see ◘ Table 2.9 and ◘ Figs. 2.16b and 1.46).
- Ratios of intrastenotic to prestenotic PSV cannot be used to grade stenosis at sites of vessel branching (femoral and carotid bifurcation; see ► Sects. 2.1.6.1.9 and 5.6.1.2) due to differences in diameter and hemodynamics between stenotic and prestenotic segments and other influencing factors, e.g., steno-occlusive lesions in the other branch, that are difficult to control. Empirical cutoffs defined for the carotid bifurcation (see ◘ Table 5.9) can be used as secondary criteria but are only approximations.

Because stenosis most commonly develops at vessel origins (renal arteries) and in bifurcations (carotid, femoral, and iliac arteries), where the ratio of intrastenotic to prestenotic

PSV is of limited value, empirical data and graphic interpolations were used to establish nomograms and derive thresholds for stenosis grading on the basis of intrastenotic PSV in relation to PSV proximal or distal to the stenotic segment (Ranke et al. 1995). However, measuring the reference velocity distal to the stenosis may introduce new sources of error (hemodynamic effects of collaterals). Nomograms were originally developed for the peripheral arteries but have since been used to grade stenoses of the cerebral arteries as well. The use of nomograms for stenosis grading is based on the assumption that the nonstenotic vascular diameter in the stenotic segment is identical to the diameter of the prestenotic or poststenotic segment in which the reference velocity is measured (◘ Fig. 1.48). It follows that the intrastenotic to

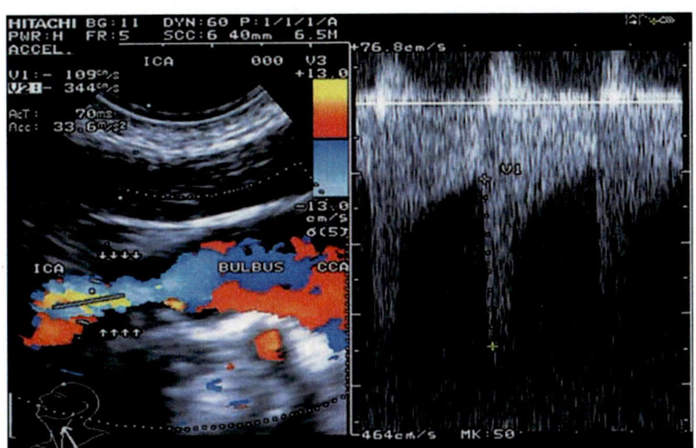

◘ **Fig. 1.47** In the eccentric high-grade stenosis of the internal carotid artery (ICA) shown, the Doppler angle adjusted relative to the vessel wall differs by approx. 10° from the angle relative to the stenosis jet. Flow in the ICA is shown in blue (away from transducer) with aliasing indicating the stenosis jet. Distal to the hypoechoic plaque, blood flow is red, indicating flow reversal resulting from flow separations and eddy currents. The color change in the common carotid artery and the bulb (red to blue) is due to a change in flow direction relative to the ultrasound beam (flow toward and away from transducer) and flow separation in the bulb (blue). Proper alignment of the Doppler angle with the stenosis jet would have yielded a higher flow acceleration. The turbulent flow components are reflected more adequately in the Doppler waveform (see ◘ Fig. 5.21)

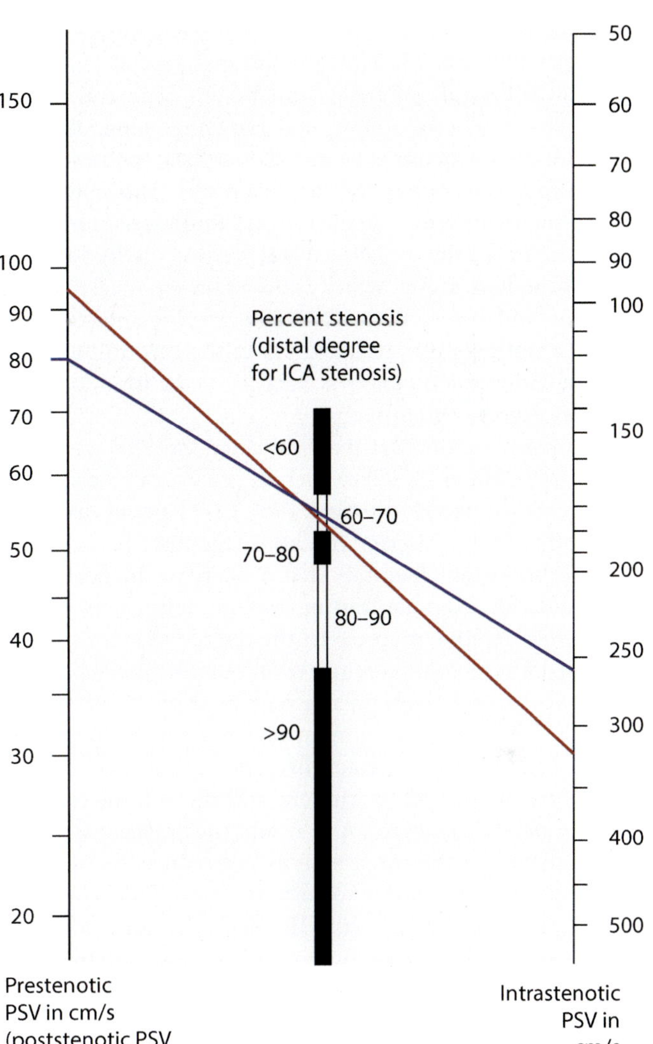

◘ **Fig. 1.48** Nomogram for grading stenosis (Modified from Ranke et al. 1995). Based on graphic interpolation, the degree of stenosis is determined from the ratio of intrastenotic peak systolic velocity (PSV) to the proximal or distal PSV. Example 1: 60–70% stenosis of the superficial femoral artery (red line) with a PSV of 320 cm/s in the stenosis and a prestenotic PSV of 95 cm/s. Example 2: Internal carotid artery (ICA) stenosis (blue line) with a PSV of 260 cm/s in the stenosis and a poststenotic PSV of 80 cm/s, yielding a distal stenosis degree of 60–70%. This can be converted to a local stenosis degree of 70–80% (▶ Sect. 5.5.1.1)

◘ **Table 1.10** Duplex ultrasound stenosis grading based on the continuity equation. Differences between theoretically predicted PSV ratios (intrastenotic PSV divided by prestenotic PSV) and PSV ratios measured in vitro are due to frictional losses within the stenosis. The thresholds apply to stenosis caused by concentric plaque occurring in straight vessel segments

Degree of stenosis		PSV ratio	
Vascular cross-sectional area reduction (%)	Diameter reduction(%)	Theoretically predicted PSV ratio	PSV ratio measured in vitro
> 50	> 30	> 2	> approx. 1.8
> 75	> 50	> 4	> approx. 3.6
> 85	> approx. 60	> 6.66	> approx. 6.2
> 95	> approx. 80	> 20	> approx. 15

poststenotic PSV ratio is used to grade a bifurcation stenosis, at the origin of the ICA, for instance (see ◘ Fig. 5.9b). Here, no collaterals enter the poststenotic segment, and in accordance with the continuity principle, identical flow velocities can be assumed proximal and distal to the stenosis (except for losses due to the stenosis itself). This is why the North American Symptomatic Carotid Endarterectomy Trial (NASCET) used the so-called distal grading method for stenosis at the ICA origin, which is based on the measurement of intra- and poststenotic PSV and graphic interpolation but does not take plaque thickness in the carotid bulb into account. Conversion tables (► Sect. 5.2.1) are used to derive the local degree of stenosis.

The main factors that may influence the PSV and must be considered in order not to over- or underestimate stenosis severity are discussed in ► Sect. 5.6.1.2.1 ("Critical Appraisal of PSV: The Main Criterion of Carotid Stenosis").

One important factor is that a decrease in peripheral resistance, for example, during muscle activity, is associated with a relative increase in the degree of stenosis. The increased blood volume required in the periphery per unit time leads to a relatively greater reduction of the blood flow through the narrowed segment above a certain degree of stenosis, resulting in a greater discrepancy between the flow volume required in the periphery and the volume that can pass the stenotic segment. As a result, the peripheral dilatation associated with muscle activity can reduce the stenosis-related perfusion pressure to such an extent that relative or absolute ischemia may occur. The hemodynamic effects of an **exercise-induced, hemodynamically significant perfusion reduction** in the presence of a stenosis that is not hemodynamically significant at rest are also reflected in the Doppler waveform: there is a more pronounced increase in the diastolic component during exercise but, above all, a longer rest after exercise is required before the postocclusive Doppler waveform returns to its normal triphasic pattern (as compared with the contralateral side). In addition to the local degree of stenosis, the severity of peripheral perfusion reduction is also affected by other occlusive processes and above all by cardiac function (in particular systolic pressure) and the extent of collateralization.

The decrease in pulsatility is primarily due to the high pressure gradient associated with luminal narrowing. The changes in the spectral waveform proximal to a vessel obstruction vary with collateral perfusion and the distance between the site of sampling and the vessel lesion. Close to the lesion, pulsatility increases as a result of the high resistance. When the Doppler information is sampled proximal to the origin of relevant collateral vessels, peripheral resistance causes a less pulsatile flow profile (◘ Fig. 1.46). The hemodynamic changes resulting from widening of the arterioles, which decrease their tone as the blood supply drops, affect the flow pattern in the prestenotic vessel segment through the collateral pathways.

Grading of stenosis at arterial origins (ICA, profunda femoris, and renal arteries) relies on empirical data as the continuity equation does not apply to vessel divisions. In the clinical setting, it is not generally necessary to determine an exact percentage as the therapeutic management of a hemodynamically significant stenosis is guided by the patient's clinical symptoms and the vessel segment affected.

On color duplex images acquired with adequate settings, aliasing will already suggest a stenosis. Nevertheless, quantitative evaluation must be performed by analysis of the Doppler waveform with angle-corrected velocity measurement using the criteria outlined above.

Again and again it has been proposed to measure the degree of a stenosis **planimetrically** by determining the **residual patent lumen**, visualized in the color flow mode, in relation to the vessel lumen (wall). However, this approach is often impaired or yields unsatisfactory results due to inaccuracies resulting from color overflow (few color scan lines with interpolation) and scattering or acoustic shadowing due to intrastenotic structures such as calcified plaques. Under ideal conditions with complete direct visualization of the stenotic segment, absence of aliasing, and localization of the stenosis outside a bifurcation, determination of the residual lumen by color duplex ultrasound was found to have a satisfactory diagnostic accuracy of 85% compared with angiography (Steinke et al. 1990). Planimetric measurement appears to be most suitable for estimating the degree of mild to moderate stenosis (see ◘ Figs. 5.53 (Atlas), 5.69 (Atlas), and 5.14) but should not be used unless plaque echogenicity enables reliable definition of the patent lumen on B-mode images. Planimetric stenosis grading on the basis of the cross-sectional area reduction is justified only because these stenoses have no hemodynamically relevant effect and therefore will not be detected by spectral Doppler. The more complex plaque configurations typically encountered when higher-grade stenosis is present may not allow adequate identification of the residual lumen, precluding grading on the basis of B-mode imaging.

The use of color duplex images for defining the patent lumen for stenosis grading has inherent methodological limitations and is discouraged.

With the angle of incidence perpendicular to the vessel (i.e., $\alpha = 90°$) in the transverse plane, the Doppler equation predicts Doppler-shifted frequencies approximating zero, resulting in poor or very inadequate visualization of blood flow. These limitations can be overcome to some extent, but the remedies are likewise subject to error:

- Slightly tilting the transducer to obtain a Doppler angle <90° will improve the Doppler signal, but this comes at the expense of introducing errors into the measurement of the vascular diameter and cross-sectional area, which becomes an oblique plane not showing the exact cross-section but rather an ellipsoid vessel section.
- The second remedy is to increase the color gain to make up for the inadequate color display of the patent lumen, but, as described above, this may result in color spillover obscuring the vessel wall and plaque edge.

1.2.3.1 Poststenotic Parameters

1.2.3.1.1 Acceleration Time – Resistive Index

Another important Doppler parameter is the systolic acceleration time (also known as the systolic rise time) or acceleration index. Normal arterial blood flow is characterized by a rapid systolic upstroke with a short rise time of a few hundredth of a second before peak systolic velocity (PSV) is reached. Distal to a high-grade stenosis or occlusion, the upstroke is delayed, resulting in a longer acceleration time and a reduced acceleration index ($\delta V/\delta T$) – mainly because flow through collaterals is slower.

Acceleration time measurement is mainly used in the sonographic evaluation of the renal arteries, where a prolonged acceleration time measured at the hilum is considered a sign of a severe proximal stenosis (◘ Figs. 1.49 and 6.8).

The delayed systolic upstroke in the poststenotic Doppler waveform is also due to the slower systolic pressure build-up in the poststenotic segment. A longer acceleration time in the poststenotic waveform is an indirect sign of a hemodynamically significant stenosis. Behind high-grade stenosis, the delayed equalization of central and peripheral (prestenotic and poststenotic) pressure during the cardiac cycle also contributes to the persistent diastolic flow. This postocclusive increase in diastolic pressure is due to the decreased peripheral resistance resulting from arteriolar widening in response to reduced perfusion (◘ Fig. 1.45). A stenosis may be identified faster by obtaining Doppler spectra at selected sites and evaluating them for prestenotic and poststenotic criteria. If a stenosis is suspected in a vessel segment that is difficult to interrogate directly, the so-called damping factor can be calculated from the resistive indices (pulsatility indices) proximal and distal to the suspected stenosis in order to estimate the significance of the flow obstruction.

$$Damping\ factor = \frac{Proximal\ pulsatility\ index}{Distal\ pulsatility\ index}$$

Stenosis of less than 60% has little effect on the poststenotic Doppler waveform. Only higher-grade stenoses are associated with an increasing reduction in poststenotic PSV, a less steep systolic upslope, and delayed diastolic decrease with persistent flow to the periphery. The decreased PSV and delayed systolic rise are primarily due to the proximal flow obstruction, while the monophasic flow profile results from peripheral vasodilatation secondary to a mismatch of blood supply and demand. The latter can thus also influence the prestenotic waveform via the collateral vessels.

1.3 Machine Settings

Proper selection of scanning parameters is of utmost importance for vascular examinations using color-coded duplex ultrasound (◘ Tables 1.11 and 1.12). Adjustment is done

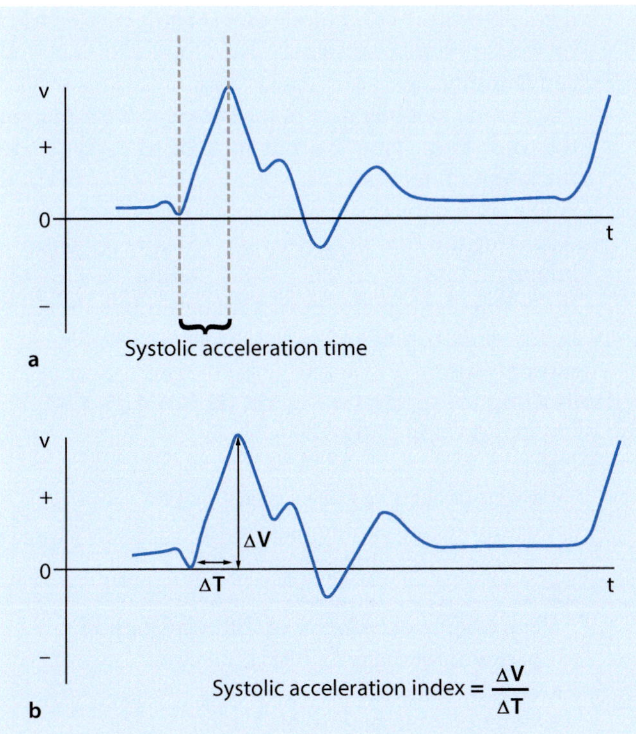

◘ **Fig. 1.49a, b** A longer systolic acceleration time and a reduced acceleration index in a postobstructive vessel segment indicate higher-grade stenosis and can be used as indirect stenosis criteria. The increase in acceleration time is proportional to the degree of stenosis (see ◘ Fig. 6.8)

◘ **Table 1.11** Optimal machine settings for specific diagnostic tasks: Color-coded duplex ultrasound

Parameter	Evaluation of flow pattern Evaluation for stenosis	Evaluation of small vessels Measurement of slow flow
PRF	As high as possible	Low
Color box	Small	Fairly large
Doppler angle	Intermediate (50°–60°)	As small as possible
Wall filter	Intermediate	Low
Color gain	Intermediate	High

◘ **Table 1.12** Optimal machine settings for specific diagnostic tasks: Pulsed Doppler ultrasound

Parameter	Evaluation of fast flow	Evaluation of slow flow
PRF	As high as possible	As low as possible
Wall filter	Intermediate	Low
Doppler angle	70°–90°	As small as possible
Transducer	Low frequency	Higher frequency

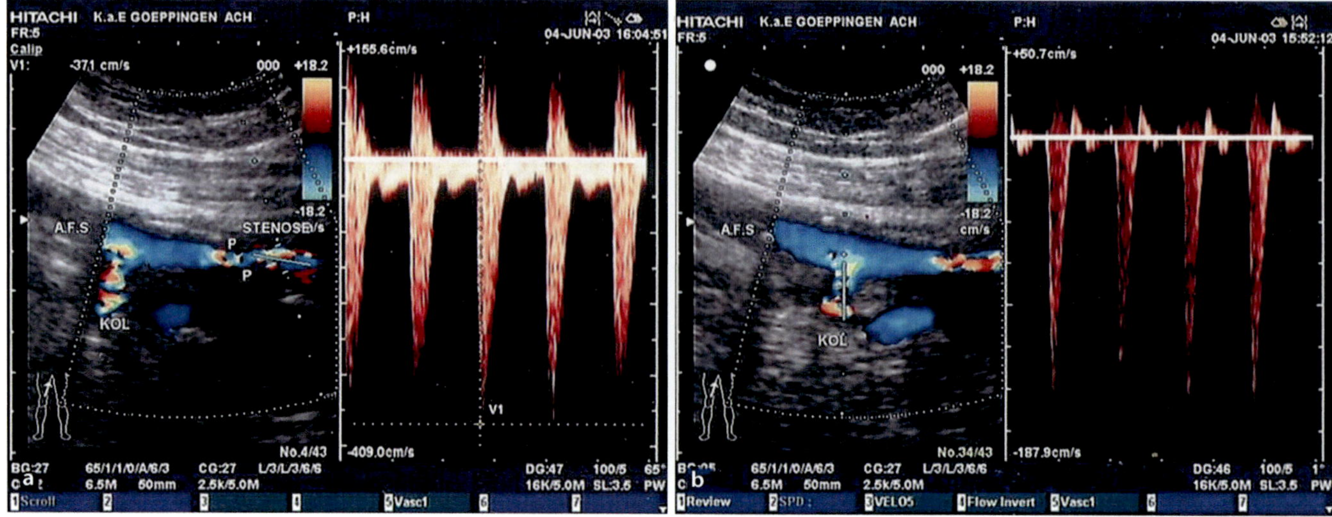

Fig. 1.50a, b An acute angle of insonation is a prerequisite for reliable Doppler-based stenosis grading including hemodynamic parameters. When the target vessel is insonated at a larger angle of say 70°, a small angle error of 5°, which is unavoidable, results in a disproportionate error in the measured fow velocity. Selection of a proper transducer can make it easier for the examiner to obtain an adequate Doppler angle. **a** A linear transducer, with a beam steering range of 20°, does not allow interrogation of an artery or vein coursing parallel to the skin surface with an angle of less than 70°. **b** A curved array transducer with a small footprint can be titlted and, with the sample volume placed at the edge of the scan sector, a Doppler waveform can be obtained with a small angle of insonation. In this way, vessels running parallel to the skin surface can be interrogated with a Doppler angle of 50–60° (57° in the example shown). For the higher-grade stenosis in **a** and **b**, a peak systolic velocity (PSV) of 380 cm/s was measured

individually for the respective vessel to be interrogated, in particular when spectral Doppler information is collected. The most important aspects are summarized below.

- **Transducer**
  - Selection of a suitable frequency
  - Adequate presetting (magnification, gain, focusing, PRF, wall filter, etc.)
- **Adjustment** of B-mode scanning parameters
  - Identification of the target vessel in the transverse plane
  - 90° clockwise rotation of the transducer to depict the vessel in the longitudinal plane
  - Focusing of the target vessel
  - Optimization of the image size
  - Optimization of gain and TGC: black vessel lumen, walls sharply delineated
- **Color Doppler**
  - Angling of the transducer to interrogate the vessel in the longitudinal plane (to improve angle of incidence)
  - Positioning of the color box, possibly tilting it (parallel transducer), to ensure the smallest angle possible in relation to the vessel axis
  - Selecting the size of the color box in such a way as to ensure a high enough frame rate
  - Optimizing gain
  - Adjusting PRF (Fig. 1.50):
    - Higher PRF when aliasing occurs
    - Lower PRF when no flow is detected but slow flow is expected
  - Adjusting high-pass filter (HPF) (rarely necessary as mostly coupled to PRF)
    - Lower cutoff to detect very slow flow
    - Higher cutoff when motion artifacts occur
  - If color filling of the vessel is insufficient, a lower-frequency transducer should be selected to improve penetration depth. The poorer spatial resolution is negligible in the color mode as it is compensated for by the superior color signal.
- **Pulsed Doppler**
  - Placing the Doppler gate in the center of the lumen in the color-mode viewfinder at an angle <70° relative to the longitudinal vessel axis
  - Angle correction
  - Adjusting the Doppler gate width to cover the entire lumen
  - If the Doppler signal is poor, the color mode should be frozen in triplex scanning to improve Doppler resolution
- **Optimizing** the spectral waveform (Figs. 1.35, 1.36, 1.37, 1.38, 1.39, and 1.40)
  - Gain:
    - Absent or sketchy curve: gain ↑
    - Overmodulation (complete filling-in of systolic window, mirror image): gain ↓
  - PRF:
    - Peak frequency/velocity cut off (aliasing): PRF ↑
    - Spectrum too "small": PRF ↓
  - Filter:
    - Depiction of slow flow: HPF ↓
    - Elimination of interfering low frequencies: HPF ↑

An optimal waveform can be sampled from the site interrogated by minimally changing the transducer position using for orientation the Doppler tracing but above all the acoustic

Doppler signal. An abnormal signal is often heard before the transducer provides the corresponding graphic information (in particular when there is scattering due to plaque).

It is important to note that, in vessel segments with high-grade stenosis and very turbulent flow, high-energy frequencies from slow flow are predominant. For stenosis grading, however, it is important to register the fast flow that often has a low energy and is concentrated in a thin jet. The following measures are recommended **to determine peak flow velocity in high-grade stenosis**:

- Selection of a high PRF
- Overmodulation of the spectrum by a higher gain to also depict the low-energy, high Doppler frequencies
- Localization of the jet by minimally and carefully changing the transducer position under acoustic and visual guidance.

Extremity Arteries

W. Schäberle, *Ultrasonography in Vascular Diagnosis*, https://doi.org/10.1007/978-3-319-64997-9_2

As the population ages, more people develop atherosclerotic occlusive disease. Atherosclerosis affects not only the coronary arteries and the arteries supplying the brain but also the arteries of the extremities. The prevalence of **symptomatic peripheral arterial occlusive disease** (PAOD) in men and women aged 55–75 is over 5% and, when asymptomatic disease is included, over 20%. Atherosclerosis impairs an individual's quality of life, causing immobility and disability. Life expectancy is reduced by about 10 years in male PAOD patients. The main causes of death are coronary heart disease (55% of patients with PAOD vs. 36% without PAOD) and cerebral conditions (11% vs. 4%). While PAOD is the manifestation of generalized atherosclerosis and affects all vascular territories, there is a high rate of concomitant involvement of the coronary and extracranial cerebral vessels, in particular in PAOD of the pelvic arteries. Patients in whom PAOD has been diagnosed require individual therapeutic management based on the stage of the disease and the suitability of their vascular system for surgical repair as well as further prophylactic diagnostic and therapeutic measures (coronary heart disease, carotid stenosis). The wider range of therapeutic options available today, percutaneous interventions in particular, can prevent the loss of a limb by reconstruction or recanalization of occluded arteries. Timely interventions restore perfusion and improve quality of life in patients with steno-occlusive disease. Early diagnosis is thus essential for the initiation of proper treatment, and duplex ultrasonography is a well-suited noninvasive modality for an efficient and low-risk primary diagnostic workup and treatment planning.

2.1 Pelvic and Leg Arteries

2.1.1 Vascular Anatomy

2.1.1.1 Pelvic Arteries

At the level of the L4–L5 vertebrae, or the umbilical level when scanning from the anterior approach, the abdominal aorta divides into the two common iliac arteries. They descend into the true pelvis taking an arched course along which they bifurcate at about the most posterior point (**iliac artery bifurcation**). The common and external iliac veins course behind the respective arteries. The internal iliac artery arises at the level of the sacroiliac joint, coursing in a posterior direction to supply the pelvic organs, pelvic wall, and buttocks. The external iliac artery is the continuation of the common iliac artery and arches into the lacuna vasorum under the inguinal ligament. It runs medial to the iliopsoas muscle and gives off the inferior epigastric and deep circumflex iliac arteries shortly before it reaches the inguinal ligament. These two arteries can **function as collaterals** in pelvic artery occlusion.

Diameters range from 0.6 to 1.4 cm in the common iliac artery, 0.5 to 1.0 cm in the external iliac artery, and 0.4 to 0.8 cm in the internal iliac artery.

2.1.1.2 Leg Arteries

The common femoral artery is about 2–4 cm long and, below the inguinal ligament, divides into the profunda femoris artery, which typically arises from the posterolateral aspect, and the superficial femoral artery (◘ Fig. 2.1a).

The **origin of the profunda femoris artery is variable**, and several branches may arise directly from the common femoral artery. Typically, one branch arises posteriorly, while the main branch arises posterolaterally or, in rare cases, posteromedially. Branches of the medial and lateral circumflex arteries arise from the femoral bifurcation or proximal profunda femoris artery and form important collateral pathways in patients with steno-occlusive disease of the distal pelvic segment and common femoral artery. The profunda femoris artery is the main collateral channel in femoropopliteal occlusion. Somewhat distal to the femoral bifurcation, the deep femoral veins converge and unite with the superficial femoral vein. The deep veins cross the bifurcation. The superficial femoral vein runs behind the artery on its course to the distal thigh. The plexus passes posteriorly through the vasoadductor membrane at the level of the adductor canal (Hunter canal), and the superficial femoral artery continues as the popliteal artery.

Interventional radiologists and vascular surgeons subdivide the **popliteal artery into three segments** with the P1 segment in angiography extending from the origin to the upper edge of the patella and the P2 segment to the knee joint cleft. The P3 segment extends to the origin of the anterior tibial artery, which passes anteriorly through the interosseous membrane at the lower edge of the popliteal muscle. It continues through the extensor compartment anterior to the interosseous membrane to the upper edge of the ankle joint with its proximal segment coursing relatively close to the fibula. The popliteal artery continues as the highly variable tibiofibular trunk with a length of about 1–5 cm (◘ Fig. 2.1b), branching into the posterior tibial and fibular arteries. The posterior tibial artery is the main artery of the lower leg and passes through the deep crural fascia between the superficial and deep flexors. It continues posterior to the medial ankle to the sole of the foot, where it divides into the larger lateral plantar artery and the smaller medial plantar artery. The lateral plantar artery extends to the deep plantar arch, which completes the arch of foot via its collaterals to the dorsalis pedis artery, establishing a connection to anterior tibial branches. The fibular artery courses posteromedial to the fibula, also at the level of the deep crural fascia. It ends in the distal lower leg and gives off several arteries supplying the muscles and serving as collaterals when other calf arteries become occluded.

The **arteries below the knee** vary widely in caliber. In cases of hypoplasia or, very rarely, aplasia, the other arteries act as collaterals. The anterior tibial artery is absent or shorter in 2% of the population, the posterior tibial artery in about 5%. In about 7% of individuals, the fibular artery is the main calf artery, communicating with the distal posterior tibial artery or dorsalis pedis artery via large collaterals arising at

2

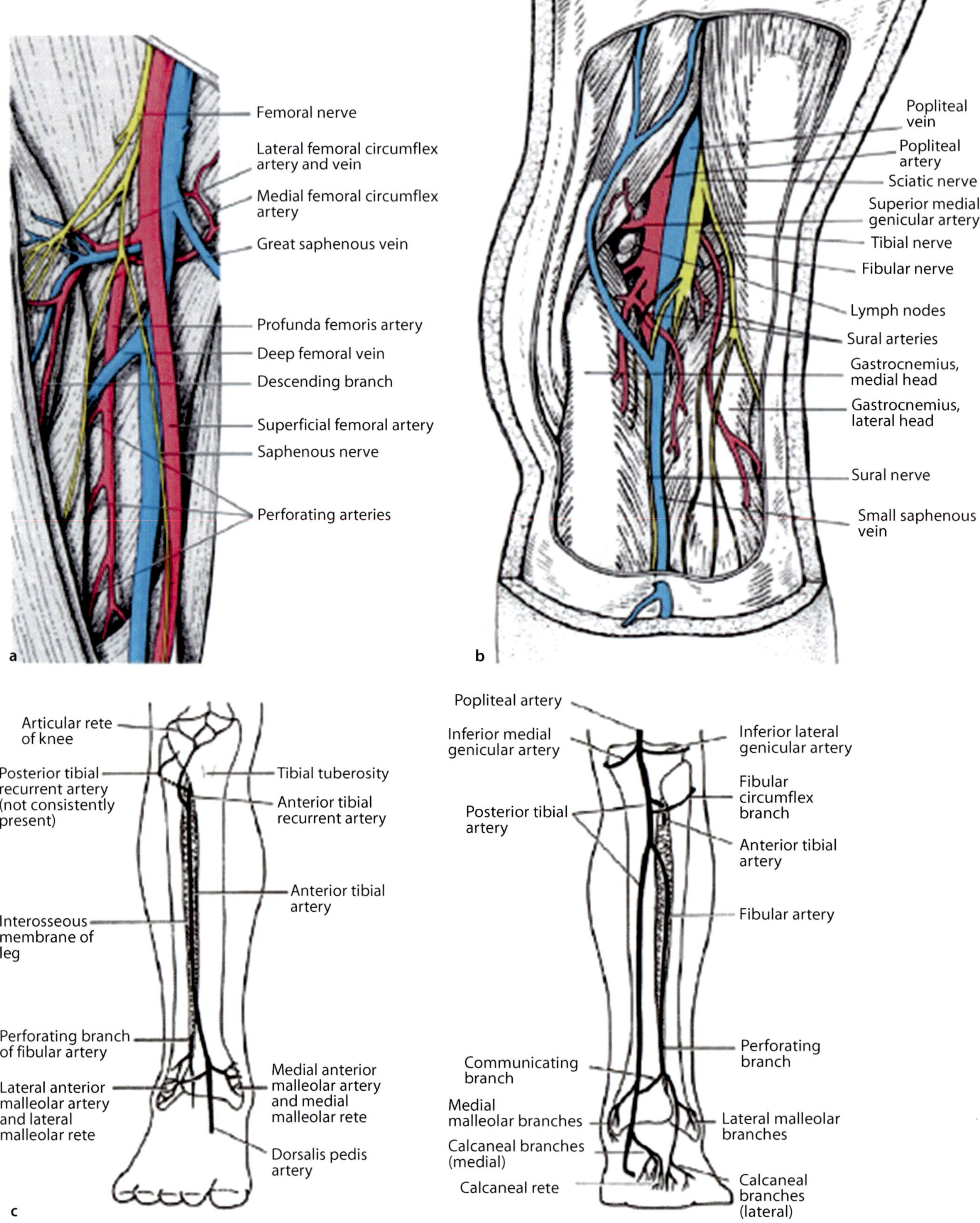

Fig. 2.1 **a** Arteries and veins in the groin (From Heberer and van Dongen 1993). **b** Arteries and veins in the popliteal fossa (From Heberer and van Dongen 1993). **c** Anterior and posterior views of the lower leg arteries

the level of the ankle joint. Collateralization through the malleolar network at the ankle joint plays an important role in atherosclerotic occlusion or hypoplasia.

2.1.2 Examination Protocol and Technique

2.1.2.1 Pelvic Arteries

The scanning depth required for an examination of the pelvic arteries makes it necessary to use a convex transducer with a frequency of 3.5–5 MHz. The proper pulse repetition frequency (PRF) (no aliasing) and gain are selected in a nondiseased arterial segment. The examination is performed with the patient in the supine position and after an adequate period of rest to prevent false-positive results due to reactive hyperemia. Exercise-induced hyperemia takes longer to return to normal in patients with atherosclerotic occlusive lesions.

Hemodynamically significant **stenosis** above the inguinal ligament can be identified quickly by spectral Doppler interrogation of the common femoral artery. A triphasic waveform with a peak systolic velocity (PSV) of at least 70 cm/s (comparison with contralateral side) rules out higher-grade stenosis at the pelvic level with a high degree of confidence.

For a closer evaluation, the **aortic bifurcation** is identified in the transverse plane at the umbilicus, and the **common and external iliac arteries** are scanned for **stenotic lesions** in longitudinal orientation (◘ Fig. 2.2a). Bowel loops, in particular when filled with air, produce marked scattering and attenuation, impairing continuous evaluation of the arteries at the pelvic level. The examiner can move the transducer around to avoid interfering bowel gas or exert pressure with the transducer to displace overlying gas-filled bowel loops.

The presence of **calcified plaques** impairs sonographic evaluation in all vascular territories. Calcification causes acoustic shadowing, obscuring both vascular structures and posterior anatomy in B-mode imaging. When long segments of a vessel are affected by calcified lesions, even higher gain settings may not allow the examiner to obtain an adequate Doppler signal for detecting stenosis. In this situation, indirect evidence must be obtained by taking spectral Doppler measurements upstream and downstream of the suspected stenotic lesion. If these waveforms show a constant PSV and unchanged triphasic pattern, the plaque in the nondiagnostic segment between the two sites of Doppler interrogation does not cause higher-grade stenosis (see ◘ Fig. 2.64 (Atlas)).

The arched course of the **iliac arteries** through the true pelvis makes it more difficult to achieve a small angle of incidence, especially at the deepest point, the iliac bifurcation (◘ Fig. 2.2b), where the origin of the external iliac artery is particularly prone to the development of stenosis. Therefore, it is important to optimize the Doppler angle by moving the transducer along the course of the artery in either direction and angling it (see ◘ Figs. 1.40b, c and 2.2b). However, aliasing cannot always be avoided, especially when the course of a deep artery such as the internal iliac artery at its origin results in a small angle relative to the Doppler beam. Aliasing means that higher velocity peaks wrap around and appear on the other side of the baseline (see ► Sect. 1.1.4.3 and ◘ Fig. 1.35).

If the examination is technically challenging and an abnormal Doppler waveform has been obtained in the groin, an attempt should be made to at least evaluate the preferred sites of stenotic disease at the pelvic level, namely the origin of the common iliac artery from the aorta and the external iliac artery close to the bifurcation and just proximal to the inguinal ligament. The spectral Doppler waveforms from these sites are analyzed for direct evidence of stenosis and compared for indirect evidence of steno-occlusive lesions between these sites.

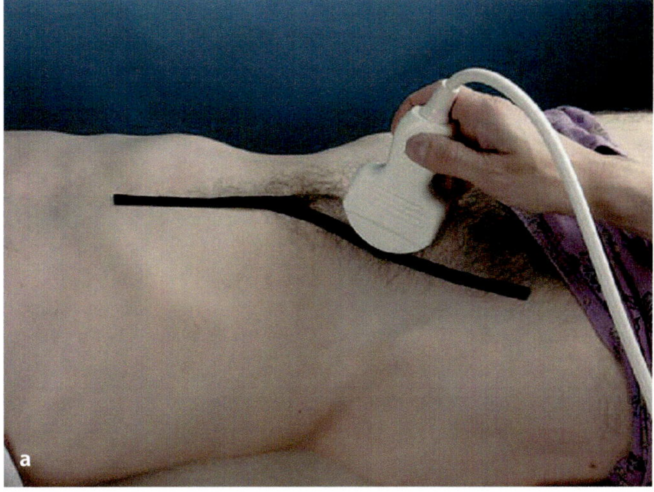

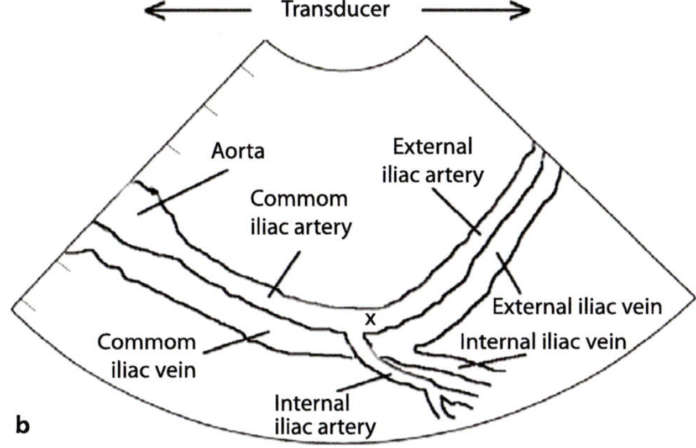

◘ **Fig. 2.2** **a** Transducer positioning for examination of the pelvic segment (aortic bifurcation at the umbilical level). **b** Diagram of the arched course of the iliac vessels through the true pelvis. The iliac bifurcation is situated at the most posterior point, where the common iliac artery gives off the internal iliac artery. The common and external iliac veins run posterior to the arteries of the same name. The origin of the external iliac artery is a common site of atherosclerotic stenosis (x). From the normal anterior transducer position, however, stenosis cannot be graded due to an extremely poor Doppler angle of approx. 90°. To obtain a better Doppler angle, the transducer must be moved upward or downward (arrows) and tilted (see ◘ Fig. 1.40c, d)

2

2.1.2.2 Leg Arteries

Because of their superficial course, the leg arteries can be examined with a higher-frequency transducer of 5–7.5 MHz, depending on the thickness of the intervening soft tissue layer.

There are **some useful rules** to follow when performing a vascular ultrasound examination (from identification of the target vessel to characterization of pathology) (◘ Fig. 2.4, ◘ Table 2.1):

- The examination begins with identification of the target artery and its course (arteries arising in bifurcations) in transverse **B-mode**. Next, the artery is followed in the longitudinal plane to evaluate the wall and differentiate the patent lumen from wall abnormalities such as plaque (atherosclerotic intimal lesions), medial thickening due to inflammatory vascular disease, or perivascular structures that might compress the vessel.
- The **color mode** is optional but helpful in obtaining an overview and rapidly identifying sites of stenosis (aliasing) and occlusion as well as collaterals arising from the main artery.
- **Waveform analysis using pulsed wave (PW) Doppler** is then performed for exact stenosis localization and grading. The length of an occluded segment is estimated by spectral analysis supplemented by color flow information. For an efficient, levelwise examination, it is essential to obtain Doppler waveforms from representative sites (common femoral artery and popliteal artery; anterior and posterior tibial arteries in patients with clinically relevant obstruction below the knee). Analysis of the waveforms from these sites using indirect stenosis criteria provides a fairly comprehensive overview, allowing the examiner to identify hemodynamically relevant stenosis or occlusion proximal to the respective sites. The segment is then mapped for confirmation of the suspected stenosis or occlusion including precise localization and grading. If a pulsatile, triphasic waveform with normal PSV (compared to the contralateral side) is obtained (whipping sound), an obstruction of the upstream segment is unlikely and mapping is not required.

The use of a **linear-array transducer** requires the activation of beam steering and careful alignment with the course of the vessel to achieve an adequate Doppler angle. A **curved-array transducer** with a small radius yields B-mode scans with somewhat poorer detail resolution but has the advantage of enabling fast Doppler angle correction (<60°) by tilting the transducer and placing the sample volume at the lateral edge of the imaging field. In contrast, beam steering in most ultrasound devices enables a maximum deflection of the emitted

◘ **Table 2.1** Duplex ultrasound examination of the pelvic and leg arteries (stepwise, segmental approach; ◘ Figs. 2.2, 2.3, 2.4, and 2.12)

Segment (level)	Ultrasound technique/steps	Purpose, diagnostic information, criteria of pathology
I Groin	**B-mode**: transverse	Overview of vascular anatomy including profunda femoris origin, evaluation of vessel walls
	B-mode: longitudinal (rotate transducer over the common femoral artery from transverse to longitudinal plane)	(Plaque?), femoral bifurcation
	Color duplex: (a) Longitudinal: curved array transducer tilted cranially or linear transducer with beam steered cranially; sample volume in distal external iliac artery/common femoral artery junction	Interpretation Spectral Doppler waveform Comparison with contralateral side Exclusion or signs of pelvic artery stenosis (triphasic/monophasic) Indirect criteria
	(b) Longitudinal: curved array transducer tilted caudally or linear transducer with beam steered caudally Doppler waveforms from profunda femoris and superficial femoral artery origins	Localization and grading of stenosis in femoral bifurcation (◘ Fig. 2.19) Stenosis of profunda femoris origin? PSV >180 cm/s
	(c) Longitudinal (suspected common femoral artery stenosis): possibly continuous examination of the common femoral artery with continuous spectral Doppler measurement (sliding the caudally tilted transducer toward the inguinal ligament)	Evaluation for stenosis/occlusion Localization of stenosis Grading of stenosis Demonstration of common femoral artery stenosis: PSV > 180 cm/s or PSV ratio (◘ Fig. 2.17)
Depending on findings: **Continuous evaluation of iliac arteries**	In case of abnormal common femoral artery Doppler waveform (monophasic or reduced pulsatility, reduced PSV compared with contralateral side): continuous color mapping of iliac artery in longitudinal plane (3.5–5 MHz transducer)	Evaluation for stenosis/occlusion Localization of stenosis Grading of stenosis Color duplex and spectral Doppler: Stenosis criterion: PSV ratio > 2/>4 In bifurcation: PSV >180 cm/s (◘ Fig. 2.12)

Table 2.1 (continued)

Segment (level)	Ultrasound technique/steps	Purpose, diagnostic information, criteria of pathology
II Popliteal fossa (popliteal artery)	**B-mode**: transverse	Identification of popliteal artery to evaluate wall and perivascular structures: nonatherosclerotic vascular disease/aneurysm?
	B-mode: longitudinal	Course of the artery, perivascular structures, evaluation of wall (nonatherosclerotic disease/aneurysm?)
	(Color) duplex (a) Longitudinal: curved array transducer tilted cranially linear transducer with beam steered cranially	Interpretation of Doppler waveform: indirect criteria for stenosis/occlusion of superficial femoral artery (triphasic/monophasic) Comparison of Doppler waveforms from proximal superficial femoral artery and proximal popliteal artery
	(b) Longitudinal: curved array transducer tilted caudally linear transducer with beam steered caudally	Popliteal artery stenosis? Evaluation of Doppler waveform: monophasic, reduced PSV compared with contralateral side
	(c) Mapping of popliteal artery if waveform from distal segment is abnormal	Evaluation for stenosis/occlusion Popliteal artery stenosis: PSV ratio > 2: 50% stenosis PSV ratio > 4: 75% stenosis
Depending on findings: **Continuous evaluation of femoral artery**	If popliteal artery exhibits monophasic flow or unilaterally reduced PSV: continuous longitudinal examination of superficial femoral artery with the tilted transducer (or beam steering) (color duplex as needed) and continuous spectral Doppler recording	Stenosis criteria (► Sect. 1.2.3): PSV ratio > 2: 50% stenosis PSV ratio > 4: 75% stenosis (◘ Figs. 2.14 and 2.20) Possibly measurement of occlusion length (color duplex) (◘ Fig. 2.25)
III Below the knee	**B-mode:** transverse	Identification of arteries
If therapeutically relevant (patients with stage III/IV PAOD): **Anterior and posterior tibial arteries at the ankle**	**Duplex:** longitudinal Distal anterior and posterior tibial arteries	Spectral Doppler sampling, indirect criteria Doppler waveform: postocclusive
If clinically relevant: **Mapping of calf arteries**	**(Color) duplex:** In case of abnormal Doppler waveform and clinical relevance: continuous examination of calf arteries Transverse: localization of arteries Longitudinal: color duplex and Doppler waveform to detect stenosis	Evaluation for stenosis/occlusion Localization of stenosis Grading of stenosis Stenosis criteria: PSV ratio > 2/>4, along the vessel (◘ Fig. 2.22) Search for target vessel for crural bypass graft

PSV peak systolic velocity

beam of only 20° either to the right or to the left of the perpendicular beam axis. Thus, the smallest Doppler angle achievable with beam steering is 70° when interrogating vessels running parallel to the skin surface. The evaluation of spectral tracings for indirect signs of occlusive lesions in the vicinity of the sample volume requires an angle of less than 60°.

The femoral (◘ Fig. 2.3a) and anterior tibial arteries are examined in the supine position, all other arteries below the knee and the popliteal artery in the prone position with slight elevation of the distal calf by a support placed under the ankles.

In general, vascular evaluation is performed **in two planes**. First, the artery is identified in the transverse plane. For a first overview, the transducer must be angled distally or cranially to achieve a small angle of insonation relative to the vessel cross section (◘ Fig. 2.4, ◘ Tables 2.1 and 2.2). Initial evaluation in the transverse plane has the advantage of enabling rapid identification of aneurysmal dilation, high-grade stenosis (aliasing), and occlusions (including origins of collaterals) once settings have been optimized. Abnormal findings need to be confirmed and quantified in the longitudinal plane. The pulse repetition frequency (PRF) and gain are set to allow complete color filling of the patent lumen without aliasing. An adequate angle of insonation and Doppler angle correction in the B-mode are prerequisites for accurate stenosis grading. As with gray-scale sonography, the monitor display of vascular images in the longitudinal plane depicts the cranial vessel segment on the left and the distal segment on the right.

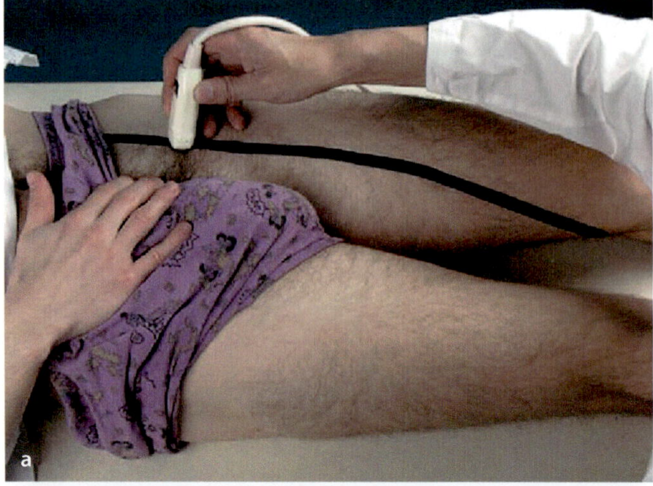

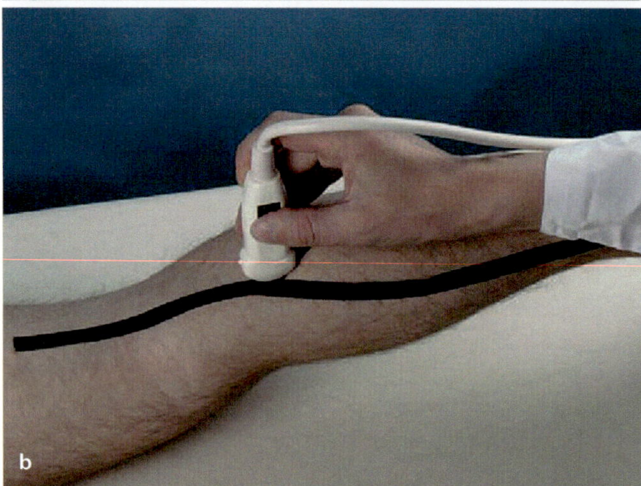

Fig. 2.3 **a** Transducer positioning for examination of the femoral arteries (transverse plane for identification of the target vessel, longitudinal plane for measuring blood flow velocity). **b** Transducer positioning for examination of the distal popliteal artery (at the junction of the P3 segment and tibiofibular trunk)

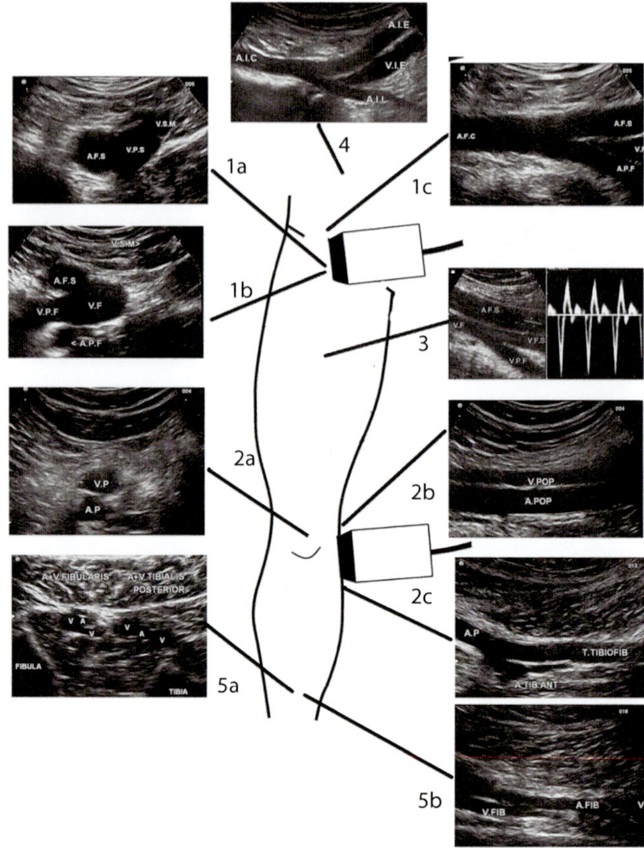

Fig. 2.4 Sonoanatomy of the leg arteries at representative sites (transverse views on the left for identification of the target arteries; longitudinal views on the right for evaluation and detection/characterization of stenosis with spectral Doppler measurement). Shown are images of vascular anatomy at the following sites:
1a and **1b** – transverse views of femoral bifurcation in the groin;
1c – longitudinal view of femoral bifurcation. **2a** – transverse view of popliteal fossa; **2b** – longitudinal view of popliteal artery; **2c** – longitudinal view of tibiofibular trunk. **3** – longitudinal view of superficial femoral artery.
4 – longitudinal view of iliac bifurcation. **5a** – transverse view of fibular and posterior tibial arteries from posterior approach; **5b** – longitudinal view of fibular artery and vein from posterior approach

With the patient in the supine position and after an adequate period of rest (>5 min), the **common femoral artery** is identified in the transverse plane and followed along its length to the bifurcation. The transducer is positioned (on the inner thigh in most patients) to view the bifurcation in such a way that the profunda femoris artery, which typically arises from the posterolateral aspect, comes to lie exactly behind the superficial femoral artery. The transducer is then turned longitudinally. In this view, the bifurcation appears as a tuning fork, which facilitates identification of vascular anatomy in this area and Doppler angle correction for evaluation of profunda femoris origin stenosis. Especially when occlusions have been identified in the femoropopliteal segment, the profunda femoris artery should be followed to the level of second-order branches to check for the presence of more distal stenosis. A step-by-step description of the examination is given in Table 2.1. The superficial femoral artery is scanned in longitudinal orientation down the inner thigh. When the leg arteries (or other vessels that run parallel to the body surface) are examined, **continuous mapping is most efficiently accomplished by moving the longitudinally oriented transducer along the artery of interest.** In this way, long arterial segments can be evaluated in the B-mode with simultaneous Doppler interrogation (optimal PRF and gain) at an angle of <60°. At the level of the adductor canal, scattering and attenuation due to connective tissue structures may require adjustment of receive gain for both B-mode and spectral Doppler imaging.

In the **adductor canal**, the artery is easier to follow with the leg turned outward and the knee slightly bent. The **popliteal artery** and **vein** are best examined with the patient lying prone. The vein runs posterior to the artery. Alternatively, the

Table 2.2 Diagnostic algorithm in peripheral arterial occlusive disease (PAOD) (key points)

	Question	Criteria
I	Is something to be done?	Clinical presentation! Duplex ultrasonography? Angiogram unnecessary (obsolete)
II	What is to be done?	(Color) duplex ultrasound (physical therapy, e.g., walking exercises, PTA, or bypass graft surgery) Angiogram unnecessary (obsolete)
III	How is it to be done?	Angiography with PTA MRA/CTA or duplex ultrasound (possibly with echo enhancer) to select a target segment for crural bypass procedure Supplementary invasive diagnostic tests (angiogram)

Ad I: Is the patient's pain even caused by PAOD? Consider clinical presentation, pulses, ankle-brachial index (ABI) (highly valid screening test for PAOD). The therapeutic strategy in PAOD is solely guided by clinical necessity (i.e., the patient's symptoms)
Ad II: Color duplex to identify the level of obstruction (pelvis, thigh, calf). Individual treatment approach based on clinical necessity as well as on therapeutic measures possible in a patient and their prognosis. Length of occlusion determines whether percutaneous transluminal angioplasty (PTA) can be attempted or bypass graft surgery is necessary. In occlusion of a pelvic or thigh artery, the decision for bypass graft surgery and the selection of a target segment can be made on the basis of duplex ultrasound
Ad III: Selective angiography with PTA without prior diagnostic angiogram. Selection of the crural target segment in multilevel obstruction or in combined popliteal/crural obstruction using angiography or magnetic resonance angiography (MRA). A pedal target artery is identified using color duplex ultrasound combined with angiography or MRA. The stepwise diagnostic approach demands that no additional diagnostic tests (e.g., more invasive and more expensive) be performed unless the results may affect the therapeutic decision

popliteal artery can be scanned with the patient supine, the knee at a 30°–60°angle of flexion, and the transducer placed in the popliteal fossa. As the anterior tibial artery arises from the anterolateral aspect of the popliteal artery, its origin appears farther away from the transducer (Figs. 2.3b and 2.2). The origin may be relatively high in individuals with a short P3 segment or very low when P3 is long. In about 4% of the population, all three lower leg arteries jointly arise in a trifurcation (Lippert and Pabst 1985). After having pierced the interosseous membrane, the anterior tibial artery is traced distally along its anterolateral course in longitudinal orientation.

The tibiofibular trunk varies in length from 1 to 6 cm, depending on the level of origin of the anterior tibial artery. Its division into the posterior tibial and fibular arteries is identified in the transverse plane. In the longitudinal view, the vessels are continuously scanned for stenosis or occlusion by following their courses distally (Fig. 2.5). If an artery disappears from the scanning plane, it can easily be identified again by rotating the probe into a transverse plane. The tibia and fibia, with their characteristic acoustic shadowing, can be used as landmarks. Further orientation is provided by the hyperechoic band of the deep crural fascia. Under good insonation conditions, the arteries below the knee can be visualized down to the ankle region. Time can be saved by recording two Doppler waveforms, one in the proximal and the other in the distal segment of the respective artery, which in general rules out a hemodynamically significant obstruction between the two sampling sites when both show the same flow profile and normal peak systolic velocity (PSV).

When there is poor color flow, the examiner should first try and adjust machine settings. Selection of a venous preset may improve detection of slow arterial flow below the knee. If the artery of interest is still difficult to identify, due to calcification, stenosis, or occlusion, the following measures may be helpful:

- Look for the accompanying veins, which may be easier to visualize. When the veins are not readily detected in the color duplex image, flow can be augmented by distal compression (sole of foot or ankle).
- Use the bright reflection of the tibia and fibula as an anatomic landmark in localizing the arteries below the knee; additional landmarks are the interosseous membrane and the deep crural fascia (Figs. 2.5 and 2.6).

The dorsalis pedis artery and the posterior tibial artery behind the medial ankle (Fig. 2.6) are examined in the supine position using a high-frequency transducer (7.5–10 MHz). These arteries are identified in the transverse plane to then perform spectral Doppler interrogation in the longitudinal plane. From there, the plantar artery can be scanned in the transverse plane to the level of the interdigital arteries.

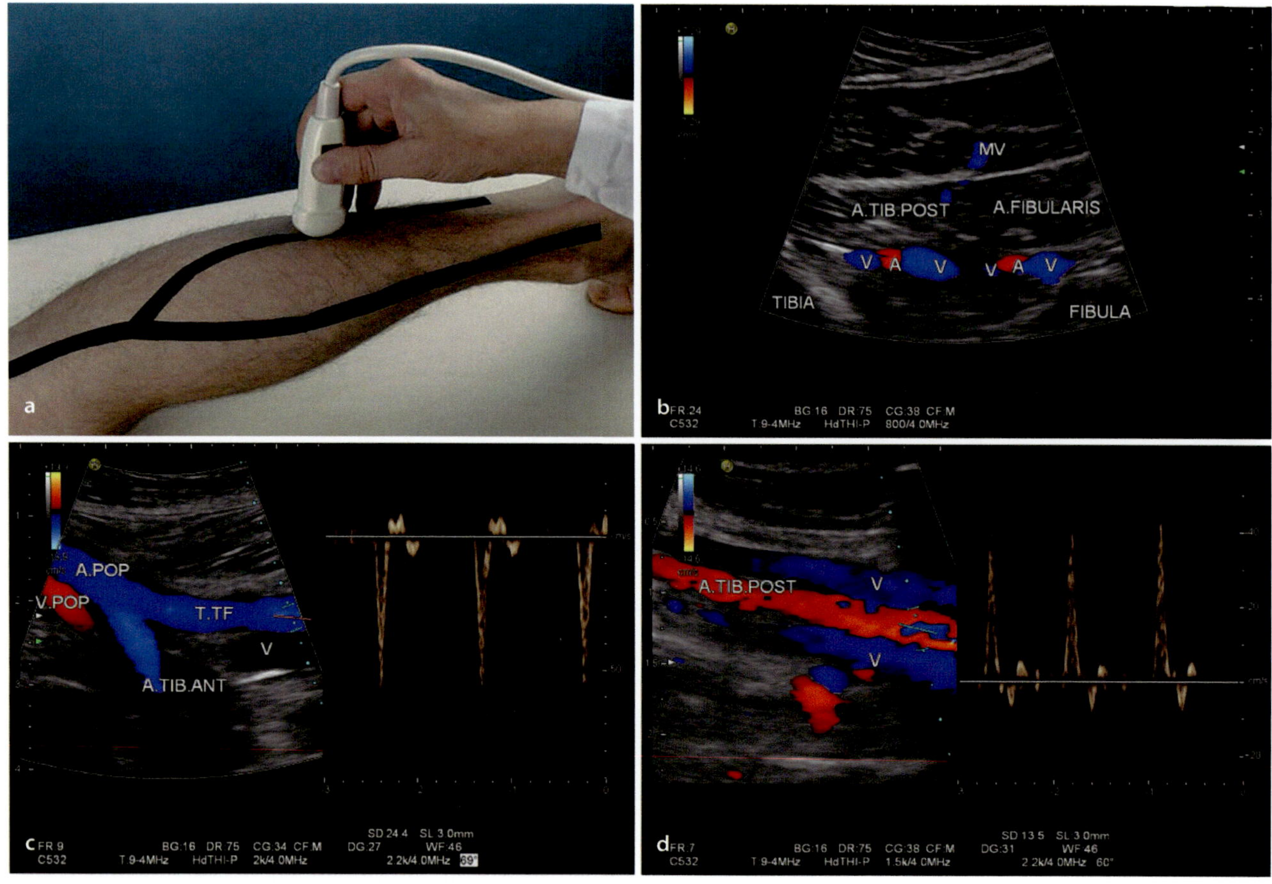

Fig. 2.5 **a** Transducer position for examination of fibular and posterior tibial arteries (courses indicated by thick black line). **b** Sonoanatomy of the posterior tibial artery (A.TIB POST) and fibular artery (A.FIBULARIS) scanned from a posterior approach. The arteries (A) are displayed in red between their paired accompanying veins (V, with flow displayed in blue). The posterior tibial artery courses posterior to the tibia, while the fibular artery courses medial to the fibula. Both arteries course in a thin, band-like structure of slightly higher echogenicity, the deep crural fascia, anterior to the soleus muscle. **c** Origins of the anterior tibial artery (A.TIB ANT) and tibiofibular trunk (T.TF) from the popliteal artery (A.POP); posterior approach with transducer placed in popliteal fossa. **d** Posterior tibial artery (A.TIB.POST) and its accompanying paired veins (V) at the mid-calf level

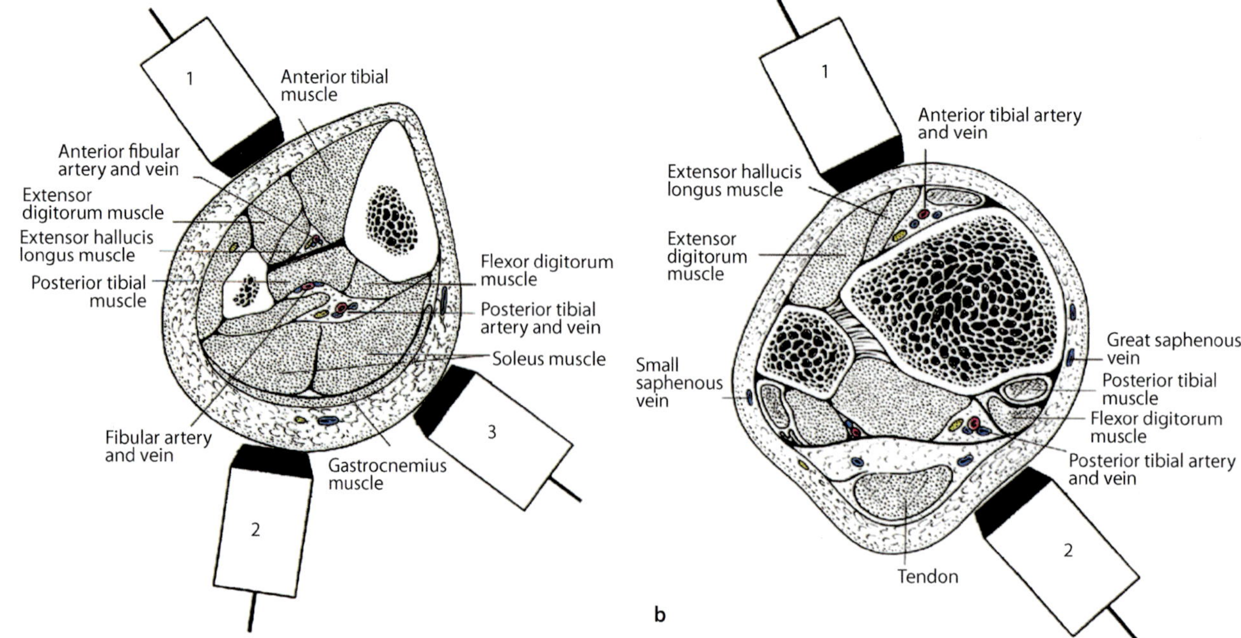

Fig. 2.6a, b Anatomy of the anterior and posterior tibial arteries at the mid-calf level (**a**) and at the ankle joint (**b**). At the mid-calf level, the arteries can be scanned from an anterior (1), posterior (2), or posteromedial transducer position (3). At the ankle, the transducer positions for scanning the anterior tibial artery (1) and posterior tibial artery (2) are shown

Table 2.3 Diagnostic and therapeutic management of patients with vascular disease in different territories

Vascular disease	Purpose of therapeutic management and diagnostic procedure
PAOD	Symptom-oriented
Nonatherosclerotic peripheral vascular disease	Prevention-oriented
Carotid artery stenosis	Prevention-oriented
Aneurysm	Prevention-oriented
Diagnostic procedure prior to:	
Symptom-oriented treatment	Levelwise duplex ultrasound examination informed by therapeutic options contemplated/stepwise diagnostic workup
Prevention-oriented treatment	Duplex sonographic vessel mapping of predilection sites based on clinical suspicion or in high-risk patients

PAOD peripheral arterial occlusive disease

2.1.3 Specific Aspects of the Examination from the Perspective of the Angiologist and Vascular Surgeon

Ultrasound examinations of the lower extremity arteries are performed for three purposes:
- Screening
- Diagnostic workup and treatment planning
- Follow-up after surgical and interventional procedures or medical treatment

Screening ultrasound is performed to identify individuals in need of treatment either in a group of the population or among patients presenting with suspected vascular disease. Vascular screening ultrasound is primarily performed in vascular territories where the findings serve to select patients for preventive interventions (Table 2.3). Screening tests should be inexpensive and not put patients at risk. In addition, they must have high sensitivity and a low false-negative rate. A false-positive diagnosis can be corrected by the subsequent (invasive) vascular examination.

The German Epidemiological Trial on Ankle-Brachial Index (GetABI; Lange et al. 2007) confirms earlier investigations (Neuerburg-Heusler 1984), showing that a simple Doppler examination combined with determination of the ankle-brachial index (ABI) is an ideal screening test for peripheral arterial occlusive disease (PAOD). This test has an accuracy of over 90% in differentiating patients with pain caused by PAOD from patients with pain of other etiologies when the clinical examination and pulse measurement are inconclusive (except for pelvic artery obstruction with good collateral circulation).

As the therapeutic management of patients with PAOD is symptom-oriented (vs. prevention-oriented management of patients with carotid artery disease), the clinical presentation determines the extent of the ultrasound examination, and no comprehensive vascular mapping is done in all cases (Table 2.3). A **stepwise algorithm** is proposed to ensure an efficient ultrasound examination of the lower extremity (Fig. 2.7). Noninvasive duplex ultrasound is performed if PAOD is suggested by the patient's history, clinical examination with full evaluation of peripheral pulses, and ABI measurement. Sonography provides information on the severity and localization of obstructive vascular lesions as well as on their cause (embolism, atherosclerosis, vascular compression syndrome) and is the basis for deciding about the therapeutic strategy (medical, interventional, surgical). Angiography is performed only as part of a therapeutic intervention (diagnostic angiogram plus angiographically guided percutaneous intervention) or to plan surgery (evaluation of outflow tract for bypass grafting and identification of the most suitable vessel segment for distal anastomosis). Alternatively, the distal leg arteries can be examined by magnetic resonance angiography (MRA) or computed tomography angiography (CTA) as well as color duplex or contrast-enhanced ultrasound (CEUS).

Further diagnostic tests, especially invasive ones such as angiography, are only done if the findings are expected to have therapeutic consequences. Hence, angiography has been abandoned as a routine modality for diagnosing PAOD or evaluating the vascular status in patients with definitive or inconclusive symptoms of claudication.

Adequate therapeutic measures in relation to the stage of disease are initiated on the basis of the clinical presentation in conjunction with the duplex ultrasound findings (Table 2.6, Fig. 2.8). The sonographically diagnosed site of obstruction and clinical stage allow interventional or surgical procedures to be performed without prior angiography.

Because ultrasound is not a prevention-oriented examination in PAOD, its extent can be restricted – based on clinical manifestations and disease stage. Patients with stage II PAOD, for instance, do not normally require a full duplex evaluation of the calf arteries below the tibiofibular trunk since vascular reconstruction for stenosis or occlusion in this territory is not indicated at this disease stage.

Steno-occlusive disease of the pelvic arteries, femoral bifurcation, and superficial femoral and popliteal arteries can be diagnosed and characterized by duplex ultrasound in a short amount of time and with a high degree of accuracy (>90–95% in the recent literature). Sonographic assessment allows reliable planning of bypass surgery with graft patency rates comparable to those in patients undergoing preoperative invasive angiography. Since the aim of surgical bypass grafting in patients with multilevel occlusive disease is to improve inflow, in stage III and IV PAOD as well, candidates for surgical recanalization above the popliteal artery do not require preoperative angiography or duplex mapping of the infrapopliteal arteries as long as the sonographic examination demonstrates a patent and nonstenotic popliteal segment. Comprehensive preoperative evaluation of the calf

2

Stepwise Diagonostic Management

- History (PAOD II-IV)
- Clinical examination (pulses)
- ABI/Oscillography
- Color/Duplex ultrasound
  Flow obstruction:
  - Pelvic arteries
  - Common femoral artery and bifurcation
  - Superficial femoral artery
  - Popliteal artery
  - Lower leg arteries
- Angiography (optional, depending on duplex findings)
- CT, MRI (optional)

a

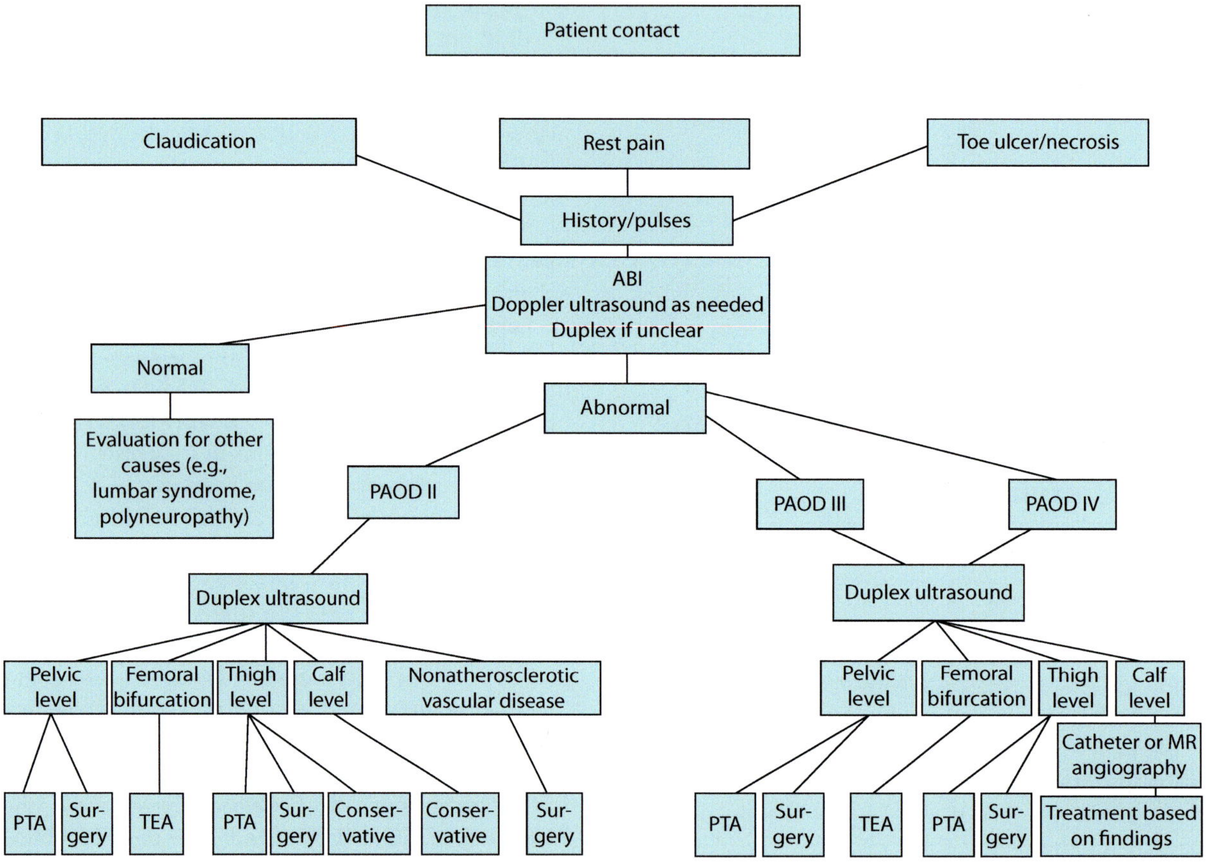

Patient contact

Claudication

Rest pain

Toe ulcer/necrosis

History/pulses

ABI
Doppler ultrasound as needed
Duplex if unclear

Normal

Evaluation for other causes (e.g., lumbar syndrome, polyneuropathy)

Abnormal

PAOD II

PAOD III

PAOD IV

Duplex ultrasound

Pelvic level

Femoral bifurcation

Thigh level

Calf level

Nonatherosclerotic vascular disease

PTA

Sur-gery

TEA

PTA

Sur-gery

Conser-vative

Conser-vative

Sur-gery

Duplex ultrasound

Pelvic level

Femoral bifurcation

Thigh level

Calf level

Catheter or MR angiography

PTA

Sur-gery

TEA

PTA

Sur-gery

Treatment based on findings

b

Fig. 2.7 **a** Stepwise diagnostic procedure and algorithm for diagnostic and therapeutic management based on the clinical presentation and localization of flow obstruction demonstrated by duplex ultrasonography. Symptom-oriented therapy → symptom-oriented diagnostic procedure. The key idea of this approach is that no subsequent diagnostic test is performed unless it is therapeutically relevant. **b** Diagnostic algorithm in peripheral arterial occlusive disease (PAOD). The examiner can deviate from the proposed algorithm in the following situations:

1. Crural reconstruction is not indicated in stage II PAOD: diagnostic evaluation of iliacofemoropopliteal arteries by color duplex alone is possible with therapeutic decision based on color duplex findings (plus clinical presentation and ABI)
2. Normal ankle-brachial index (ABI): patient may have pelvic level occlusion/stenosis with good collateralization; duplex scan if steno-occlusive disease is suggested by clinical symptoms
3. Multilevel occlusion and suboptimal duplex scan: supplementary angiography may be contemplated and should be used more liberally
4. Sonographic demonstration of popliteal aneurysm with occlusion: treatment (surgical repair) according to clinical symptoms; same diagnostic steps as for PAOD III/calf. If flow is detected in popliteal aneurysm: prophylactic surgical repair with bypass; same diagnostic steps as for PAOD III/calf
5. Diabetics with severe macroangiopathy and medial sclerosis precluding adequate evaluation (acoustic shadowing): more liberal use of diagnostic angiography
6. Patients with PAOD III or IV and multilevel occlusion: patent popliteal artery without hemodynamically relevant stenosis: surgery or intervention above the popliteal artery to improve inflow based on duplex findings (diagnostic angiography not required); additional obstruction of lower leg arteries does not affect the initial treatment strategy (e.g., bypass graft onto P1 segment). Steno-occlusive disease of popliteal segment: search for a suitable recipient artery for crural bypass using angiography (usually DSA), magnetic resonance angiography with dedicated coil, or color duplex (time-consuming), possibly contrast-enhanced ultrasound (CEUS)

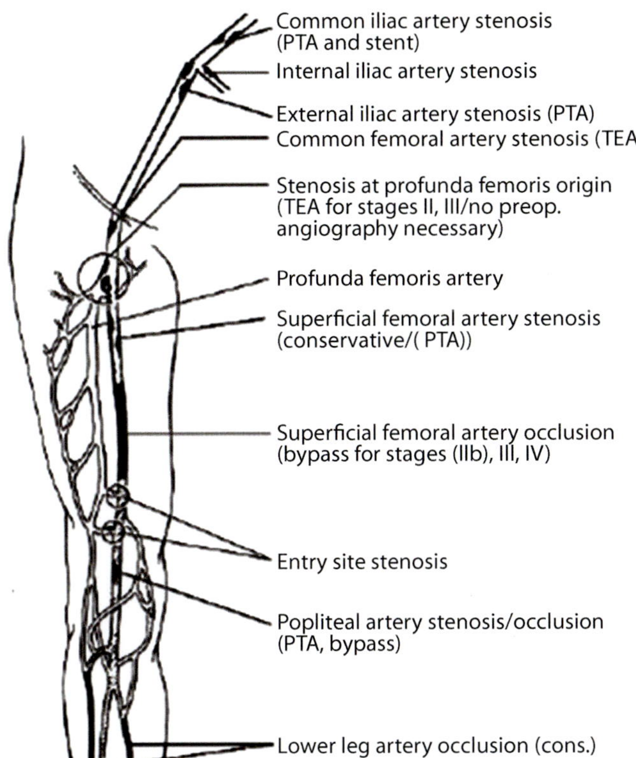

Fig. 2.8 Diagram of atherosclerotic stenotic lesions that can be diagnosed by duplex imaging and initial treatment based on duplex findings (different therapeutic management may be required based on the clinical stage or in patients with multilevel involvement)

arteries is not necessary in these cases as the primary surgical approach is not affected by occlusions distal to the popliteal artery or trifurcation. Outflow to the foot may be evaluated along with intraoperative completion angiography if this information is deemed necessary for patients who are likely to require additional surgical or interventional measures.

In the following two settings, the **decision to perform thromboendarterectomy (TEA)** can also be made without additional imaging tests: (1) if duplex ultrasound demonstrates stenosis of the common femoral artery or profunda femoris origin – with occlusion of the superficial femoral artery – and if the examination also rules out occlusion in the pelvic territory, or (2) if, in case of occlusion of the superficial femoral artery, the duplex examination confirms resupply of the P1 popliteal segment without major popliteal artery narrowing. In these cases, TEA at the inguinal level is the first therapeutic step, with further measures depending on the clinical outcome. This therapeutic approach is independent of the status of the arteries below the knee, and the benefit of using preoperative anteroposterior angiography to evaluate collateral circulation in the thigh in cases of superficial femoral artery occlusion is disputed.

Only the main branch of the profunda femoris artery provides relevant collateral flow in patients with an occluded superficial femoral artery. This branch runs almost parallel to the latter and is the only artery that needs to be evaluated with sonography as it is only here that a stenosis compromising collateral function would require surgical repair (see Fig. 2.60 (Atlas)).

The author's experience in 180 patients confirms that duplex sonography is a reliable preoperative imaging modality both for identifying patients with stenosis of the femoral bifurcation or arterial occlusion above the knee who require surgery and for planning the surgical procedure. In this patient population, the sonographic examination allowed adequate evaluation of the pelvic arteries in 95% of the patients; in these cases, ultrasound correctly diagnosed 96% of all pelvic artery stenoses and occlusions, and the therapeutic approach was modified accordingly (e.g., pelvic artery PTA). Overall, the sonographic findings led to a correct therapeutic decision in 94% of the patients with clinically indicated vascular reconstruction of the iliacofemoropopliteal segment (PTA, TEA, bypass with preoperative planning) (see Table 2.19).

A duplex ultrasound examination of the infrapopliteal arteries is time-consuming. Acoustic shadowing produced by calcified plaques or edema can impair detection and grading of stenosis in small arteries. This is especially problematic if indirect stenosis criteria (flow profile) do not apply because the patient has multilevel occlusive disease with proximal obstruction.

Several studies (Grassbaugh et al. 2003; Karacagil et al. 1996; Boström et al. 2002; Mazzariol et al. 2000) show duplex ultrasound to be highly accurate in localizing and grading steno-occlusive disease of the calf arteries and to enable reliable planning of the surgical approach and **identification of a potential bypass target below the knee**, with bypass patency rates similar to those in patients examined by preoperative angiography. The choice of the preoperative imaging modality in patients with popliteal occlusion and involvement of the calf arteries in stage III and IV PAOD depends not only on the expected diagnostic information but also, and importantly, on the examiner's skills and experience with duplex ultrasound, the time available (see ► Sect. 2.1.8), and the organization and workflow in the department (in Germany, most duplex ultrasound examinations are performed by clinicians, in particular angiologists and vascular surgeons).

An exception to the restrictive use of diagnostic angiography is the examination of patients with long-standing diabetes mellitus and secondary macro- and microangiopathy. Medial sclerosis in diabetics may preclude complete sonographic evaluation of the calf arteries, and serial stenoses may thus be overlooked. Nevertheless, the identification of all macro- and microangiopathic lesions is still necessary for initiation of appropriate therapeutic measures.

The **hemodynamic effect** of arterial stenosis is evaluated using hemodynamic parameters. Flow models and in vivo studies indicate that a reduction in arterial diameter of 50% or more becomes hemodynamically significant and will cause an increase in peak systolic velocity (PSV). In higher-grade stenosis, peak end-diastolic velocity (EDV) is increased as well. The increase in PSV correlates with the degree of stenosis (see Fig. 5.20).

In contrast to the carotid artery territory, B-mode evaluation of plaque morphology for estimating the risk of embolism has no role in the examination of the leg arteries. This is obvious given the difficulties one faces in assessing the risk of embolism associated with carotid artery stenoses in B-mode sonography and the rare occurrence of interdigital artery embolism (blue toe). Nevertheless, one must be aware that, as in the carotid territory, the risk of embolism increases with the degree of stenosis and plaque thickness.

Determining the degree of stenosis from the vessel diameter and the residual perfused lumen using transverse color flow images is less reliable than hemodynamic grading based on spectral Doppler velocity measurement. The former is done only for preliminary orientation and is susceptible to artifacts caused by calcified plaques. Moreover, physical and technical limitations necessitate the wider spacing of color scan lines, and the interpolation which then becomes necessary often overestimates the patent lumen and underestimates the stenosis.

The hemodynamic degree of stenosis determined by duplex ultrasound correlates better with its ischemic effects and with the patient's clinical symptoms than the morphologic degree determined by imaging modalities such as angiography or MRI. Morphologic methods have inherent limitations resulting from the fact that the apparent luminal narrowing caused by an eccentric plaque changes with the imaging plane. These limitations can only be minimized by evaluating all normal and diseased arterial segments in two or three planes. Another drawback of morphologic stenosis grading is the failure to adequately account for plaque configuration and how it affects the hemodynamic relevance of a stenosis. A concentric plaque causing the same diameter reduction as an eccentric plaque has more marked hemodynamic effects because the decrease in cross-sectional area is greater (see ◘ Fig. 2.17d).

2.1.4 Interpretation and Documentation

Minimum documentation of a duplex ultrasound examination of the legs consists of longitudinal B-mode images and angle-corrected spectral Doppler waveforms from the representative sites, which are the common femoral artery, the origins of the deep and superficial femoral arteries, and the popliteal artery (P1 and P3 segments). In patients in whom the arterial status below the knee is clinically relevant, the documentation is supplemented by B-mode images and Doppler waveforms from the anterior and posterior tibial arteries proximally and at the level of the ankle. If the findings at these sites are inconclusive or if a specific clinical question has to be answered, additional images and Doppler waveforms from the common and external iliac arteries, possibly the below-knee arteries as well, are documented. In addition, steno-occlusive lesions are documented with longitudinal images and waveforms. Intra- and peristenotic spectral Doppler waveforms are analyzed (◘ Table 2.9) to estimate the degree of stenosis based on pre- and intrastenotic peak systolic velocity (PSV) and the poststenotic flow pattern (from preserved triphasic profile to monophasic waveform). An aneurysm must be documented in two planes and its diameter measured in the transverse plane. Partial thrombosis, if present, should be reported as well. Documentation of additional color flow images (transverse view of aneurysm, longitudinal view of stenosis) may be helpful but is optional.

The report should describe the morphologic changes and Doppler results on which the diagnosis is based (◘ Table 2.4).

◘ **Table 2.4** Duplex ultrasound criteria for arterial evaluation

Technique	Criteria
B-mode	Assessability
	Anatomy (course, variants)
	Vessel contour (aneurysm, stenosis)
	Vessel wall changes (calcification, plaque, cysts)
	Pulsation (axial, longitudinal)
	Perivascular structures (hematoma, abscess, tumor, other compressing structures)
Doppler	Demonstration of flow
	Flow direction
	Flow pattern (laminar, turbulent)
	Flow profile (monophasic/triphasic)
	Flow velocity

2.1.5 Normal Duplex Ultrasound of Pelvic and Leg Arteries

Flow in the limb arteries is pulsatile and nearly laminar, due to the high peripheral resistance, which is reflected in the Doppler waveform by a narrow bandwidth with a clear systolic window. The typical triphasic waveform is characterized by a steep systolic upslope and rapid return to baseline, followed by a short early diastolic reversal of flow and subsequent diastolic forward flow varying in magnitude and duration with the body region supplied (◘ Fig. 1.43). The brief diastolic flow reversal is due to high peripheral resistance (► Sect. 1.2.2).

The **character of the Doppler waveform** varies with the elasticity of the vessel wall and peripheral resistance and is influenced by systemic and local hypercirculatory effects (fever, hyperthyroidism, phlegmon). The amount of flow persisting during diastole is subject to physiologic factors and pathologic changes including sympathetic tone, wall elasticity, compliance of the aorta, and heart rate. In addition, the waveform shape is influenced by the ratio of skin to muscle supply, which is why diastolic flow is higher in the profunda femoris than in the superficial femoral artery (◘ Fig. 2.9).

The main factors influencing the **flow profile** (Doppler waveform) can be summarized as follows:

- Wall elasticity (atherosclerosis, medial sclerosis)
- Peripheral resistance:
  - Physiologic:
    - Muscle activity
  - Abnormal:
    - Inflammation, phlegmon (stage IV PAOD) (◘ Fig. 2.9c)
    - Hypercirculation
    - Medications
    - Postocclusive vasodilatation

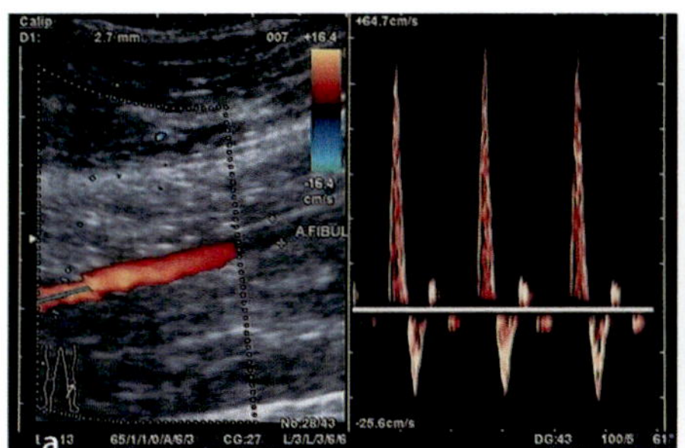

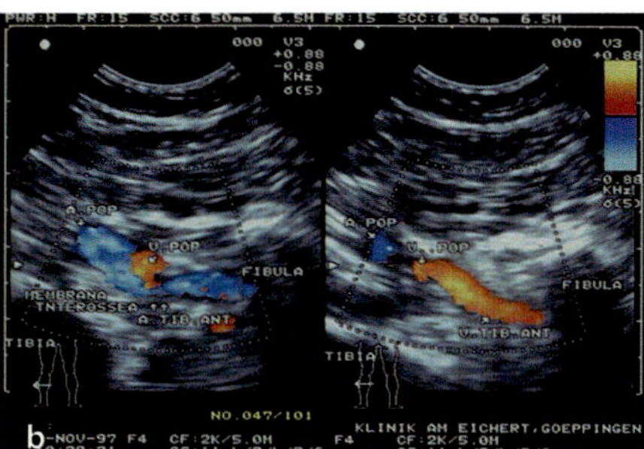

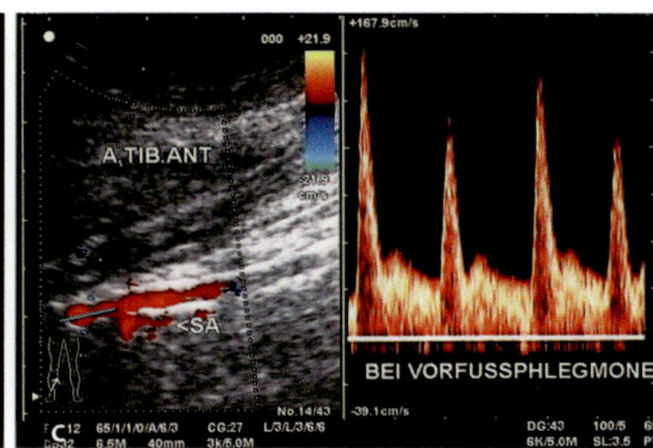

Fig. 2.9 **a** Peak systolic velocity (PSV) in the leg arteries decreases toward the periphery, but the triphasic flow pattern persists. The example shows normal blood flow in the fibular artery with the corresponding triphasic waveform. The artery has a diameter of 2.7 mm. **b** Sonoanatomy of the anterior tibial artery origin. The popliteal artery gives off the anterior tibial artery, which courses anteriorly to pierce the interosseous membrane, in front of which it descends, initially taking a course close to the fibula. The image shows the anterior tibial artery scanned from a posterior approach (transducer in popliteal fossa), with flow displayed in blue (flow away from transducer), below its origin from the popliteal artery (A.POP) as it pierces the interosseous membrane (hyperechoic structure between tibia and fibula). With the transducer slightly tilted, the anterior tibial vein comes into view (blue, flow toward transducer) along its course parallel to the artery and as it enters the popliteal vein. **c** Hyperemia. Peripheral inflammation is another factor that can alter the Doppler waveform besides an increased flow resulting from exercise-induced hyperemia or when an artery is recruited as a collateral. In the example, a phlegmon of the foot results in a monophasic waveform with reduced pulsatility and a rather high end-diastolic velocity (EDV) of 22 cm/s. An upstream stenosis is ruled out here as the steep systolic upslope is preserved and a PSV of 130 cm/s is measured (which is relatively high for an artery below the knee, see **a**). The variation in PSV in this patient is attributable to absolute arrhythmia. A mirror artifact is present (<SA)

Table 2.5 Normal diameters (D) and peak systolic velocities (PSV) with standard deviations determined in the lower extremity arteries of 30 healthy subjects

Artery	D (cm)	PSV (cm/s)
External iliac artery	0.85 ± 0.11	116 ± 29.7
Common femoral artery	0.81 ± 0.17	112.2 ± 22.7
Proximal superficial femoral artery	0.65 ± 0.14	93.95 ± 15.9
Profunda femoris artery	0.55 ± 0.14	95.1 ± 21.5
Popliteal artery	0.58 ± 0.12	71.6 ± 12.4

Arterial diameters and PSV are subject to wide interindividual variation and decrease toward the periphery (Table 2.5), while the triphasic flow profile is preserved.

Investigations of **normal flow velocity in the pelvic and leg arteries** (Jäger et al. 1985; Kohler 1990; Karasch et al. 1990; Polak et al. 1992) have revealed wide variations between different study populations and individual subjects within a study population. It is therefore somewhat more difficult to define an absolute systolic velocity threshold above which a hemodynamically effective stenosis should be assumed, as is the case for the diagnosis of carotid and renal artery stenosis. Given the wide variation in blood flow velocities in the peripheral arteries, the normal velocities measured by our group (Table 2.5) are comparable to those reported by others (Jäger et al. 1985; Kohler 1990).

In addition to PSV and changes in the normal triphasic flow profile, the **acceleration index** has become an established parameter for describing occlusive and postocclusive changes in blood flow. Higher-grade stenosis or occlusion is associated with a postocclusive decrease in PSV and delayed systolic upstroke (see Figs. 6.8 and 1.49). The acceleration index is the quotient of PSV and the pulse rise time from the onset of systole to the first peak.

The pulsatility index (PI) can be used to describe the pulsatility of flow (see formula in Fig. 1.29). As the poststenotic decrease in PSV (Fig. 2.10) and increase in EDV become more pronounced through dilatation of the arterioles and the resulting decrease in peripheral resistance, triphasic flow becomes monophasic, and the magnitude of this change correlates with the decrease in PI (see Figs. 1.29, 2.9, and 2.52 (Atlas)).

2.1.6 Abnormal Findings

The following subsections describe the therapy-oriented sonographic workup of vascular conditions affecting the leg arteries, including relevant sonographic findings and parameters, and discuss the role of ultrasound in the diagnostic management of the respective disease entities.

2.1.6.1 Atherosclerotic Occlusive Disease

Most atherosclerotic lesions occur in the thigh vessels (approx. 40%), followed by the pelvic and calf vessels, each accounting for approx. 20–30% (Schoop 1988). More than 20% of patients already have occlusive lesions of more than one level at the time of diagnosis. Since vascular sclerosis is a generalized process, it typically involves both legs, but often, one side will be affected more severely.

Vascular duplex ultrasound of the leg arteries is predominantly used for the stepwise diagnostic workup of patients presenting with typical symptoms of peripheral arterial occlusive disease (PAOD) (Fig. 2.7), treatment planning, and differentiation of atherosclerosis from other vascular conditions (Table 2.6).

The duplex ultrasound findings, in conjunction with the clinical disease stage, guide the further diagnostic and thera-

2

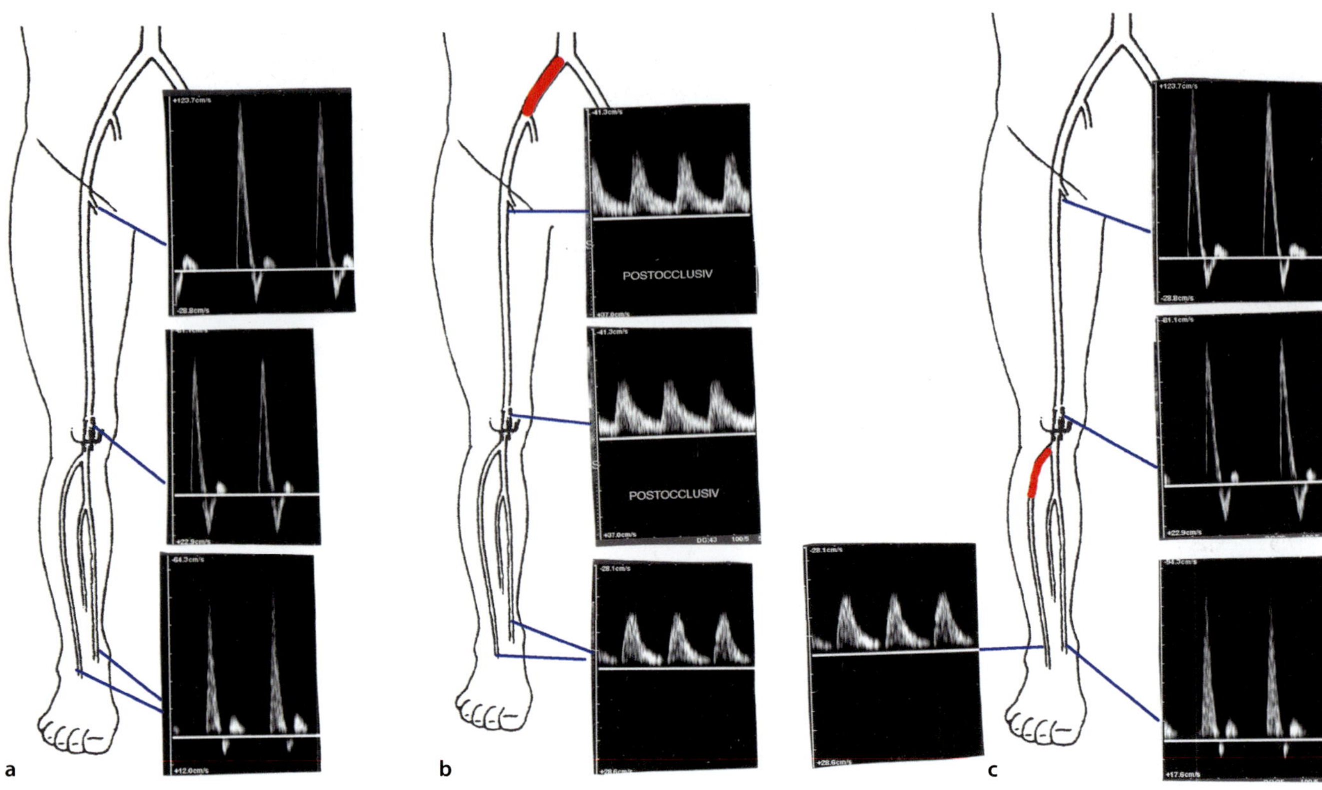

Fig. 2.10a–c Segmental duplex ultrasound of the lower extremity arterial tree based on spectral Doppler analysis and identification of postocclusive waveform changes to localize occlusive disease. **a** Normal triphasic Doppler waveforms (no hemodynamically relevant stenosis or occlusion) from the common femoral artery, popliteal artery, and anterior and posterior tibial arteries. **b** Pelvic artery occlusion is indicated by postocclusive monophasic waveforms from the common femoral, popliteal, and anterior and posterior tibial arteries. The postocclusive flow pattern is seen in all arteries distal to the occlusion. **c** In isolated occlusion of the proximal anterior tibial artery, flow is triphasic in the common femoral, popliteal, and posterior tibial arteries, while a postocclusive waveform is obtained from the anterior tibial/dorsalis pedis artery

Table 2.6 Indications for (color) duplex ultrasound of the leg arteries

Indication	Diagnostic tasks
Stepwise diagnostic workup of PAOD	Localization of flow obstruction (above the knee, below the knee, pelvic level, vessel origin) Identification of type of flow obstruction (stenosis, occlusion) Length of flow obstruction (length of occlusion, sequential stenoses) Stenosis grading (high-grade versus low-grade) Cause of occlusion (embolism, atherosclerosis, trauma, compression, dissection) Evaluation of postocclusive outflow tract Therapeutic decision making: medical treatment, radiologic intervention, surgery
Diagnostic evaluation of aneurysm	Localization Characterization (saccular, spindle-shaped, false) Extent (infrarenal, aortoiliac, popliteal) Thrombosis (partial, complete) Treatment: compression therapy of pseudoaneurysm, thrombin injection
Arterial compression	Entrapment syndrome Adventitial cystic disease Thoracic outlet syndrome Compression by tumor
AV fistula	Localization Flow volume in fistula
Follow-up of surgical or interventional procedures	Bypass grafting (anastomotic stenosis, suture aneurysm, infection, occlusion, flow velocity inside bypass graft: prognosis) PTA (residual stenosis, restenosis, puncture aneurysm, hematoma) Endovascular stenting (patency, stenosis)

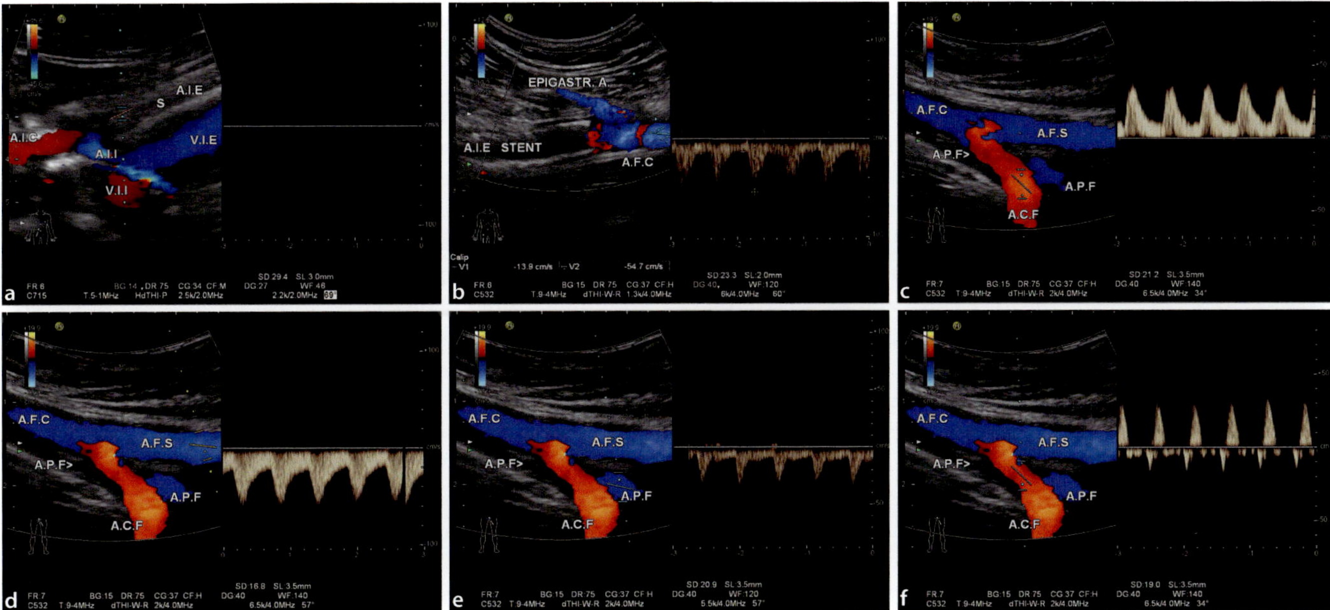

Fig. 2.11a–f Collateral circulation in pelvic artery occlusion. **a** Occlusion of the external iliac artery (A.I.E) after PTA and stent (S) implantation. The common iliac artery (A.I.C) is displayed in red. The internal iliac artery (A.I.I) is also patent with flow coded in blue. Flow in the external iliac vein (V.I.E) posterior to the artery is toward the center (blue); flow in the internal iliac vein (V.I.I) as it ascends from the true pelvis and enters the common iliac vein is displayed in red (toward transducer). **b** The common femoral artery (A.F.C) with flow toward the periphery (blue, postocclusive flow signal) is filled via the epigastric artery (EPIGASTR A), where flow is retrograde (blue). The stented external iliac artery (A.I.E) is occluded. **c** The femoral circumflex artery (A.C.F) with retrograde flow displayed in red fills the proximal profunda femoris artery (A.P.F), resulting in retrograde flow (red, toward transducer) in a short segment of the profunda femoris directly at the site of entry of the femoral circumflex. **d** In the superficial femoral artery (A.F.S), flow is orthograde with a postocclusive Doppler waveform (monophasic, delayed systolic rise). **e** Distal to the site of entry of the femoral circumflex artery (A.C.F), there is orthograde flow in the profunda femoris artery as well (A.P.F, blue, flow toward the periphery). **f** Doppler waveforms (flow volume, flow direction) reflect the changing intravascular pressure at the site of sampling (compare waveforms obtained at the sampling sites in **d** and **e**). While the color duplex image shows retrograde systolic flow toward the center (toward transducer) in the profunda femoris artery (A.P.F>) close to its origin from the common femoral artery (A.F.C), Doppler interrogation demonstrates to-and-fro flow in this segment. In contrast, the waveform in **c** shows high retrograde flow because part of the blood flows toward the periphery through the profunda femoris downstream of the sampling site (seen in **c** to the right of the A.C.F). The to-and-fro flow at the profunda femoris origin is due to the fact that this artery contributes to refilling of the common femoral artery, which receives only insufficient collateral flow from epigastric arteries. The Doppler waveform very accurately reflects the hemodynamic situation as a function of local pressure and pressure variation through the cardiac cycle (see Fig. 2.58 (Atlas)). In the absence of collateral flow through the femoral circumflex artery, the waveform sampled here would be the same as in **c**

peutic strategy (Fig. 2.7). The overall **motto** is: No further (invasive) diagnostic test without therapeutic consequences. This means that additional diagnostic tests, especially invasive ones, should not be ordered unless they are expected to provide relevant supplementary information for adequate treatment planning.

2.1.6.1.1 Pelvic Arteries

Lower extremity steno-occlusive disease affects the pelvic arteries in 11% of cases. Isolated occlusions at this level occur in the common iliac artery in approx. 54% of cases, in the external iliac in 21%, and in the internal iliac in 13% (Schoop 1988). The clinical presentation of pelvic artery occlusion varies with the presence of collateral pathways and concomitant involvement of distal arteries (40–50% incidence of combined femoropopliteal obstruction). Reconstruction of the occluded pelvic artery to improve inflow of blood is particularly important in patients with additional superficial femoral artery occlusion. Moreover, pelvic artery repair has a good long-term prognosis and patency rate. Important non-atherosclerotic conditions affecting the arteries at the pelvic level include aneurysmal disease (especially in patients with distal aortic anaeurysm), dissection (see ▸ Sect. 2.1.6.4.7), and stenosis due to fibromuscular dysplasia.

In patients with occlusion at the pelvic level, collateral flow mainly occurs through the internal iliac artery systems. Additional collateral pathways include the inferior mesenteric artery and internal iliac artery in common iliac artery occlusion and the epigastric arteries (entering just above the groin) in external iliac artery occlusion (Fig. 2.11a–f). In addition to the typical claudication symptoms of the lower leg, occlusion in this territory is associated with specific claudication pain of the gluteal, hip, and thigh muscles.

When the external iliac artery is occluded and the lateral circumflex artery provides collateral flow, backward flow occurs in the proximal profunda femoris and common femoral arteries. This is seen in the Doppler examination as reversed flow with a monophasic character. Additionally, collateral flow through the lateral circumflex artery fills the superficial femoral artery, while the common femoral artery often receives collateral flow from epigastric arteries entering just above the inguinal ligament (see Fig. 2.53i (Atlas)).

If direct evidence in the form of increased blood flow velocity in the stenotic segment cannot be obtained, especially when evaluation is impaired due to overlying bowel gas or obesity, spectral Doppler imaging of the proximal common femoral or distal external iliac artery can provide indirect evidence of upstream obstruction.

A stenosis of less than 50–60% has no relevant effect on the poststenotic Doppler waveform. Only higher-grade stenoses produce flow changes including a decrease in PSV, a less steep systolic rise, and a delayed diastolic drop with persistent flow toward the periphery in the poststenotic segment (see ◘ Fig. 2.52 (Atlas)). The lower PSV and the delayed systolic rise are primarily due to the upstream flow obstruction while monophasicity indicates peripheral vasodilatation in response to a mismatch of blood supply and demand. This peripheral situation in turn also influences the prestenotic waveform via the collaterals.

The ankle-brachial index (ABI) decreases after exercise, and flow becomes less pulsatile, which may result in a monophasic waveform. In the absence of vascular disease, the ABI and Doppler waveform will return to normal after a short rest. This is why a short **waiting period** following positioning of the patient on the couch (>3 min) is necessary to obtain accurate quantitative measurements and spectral Doppler information. On the other hand, an additional spectral Doppler measurement during the recovery phase can help in differentiating absence of stenosis from high-grade proximal stenosis with good collateralization. The latter is characterized by a relatively normal Doppler waveform at rest (◘ Fig. 2.53 (Atlas)) but a markedly delayed return to normal after activity (◘ Fig. 2.12).

2.1.6.1.2 Time-Efficient Examination Based on Waveform Analysis

Therapeutically relevant stenosis in the pelvis and thigh can be reliably and efficiently ruled out by segmental spectral Doppler evaluation of blood flow in the common femoral and popliteal arteries and comparison with the contralateral leg. Relevant stenosis is unlikely proximally if the waveform shows normal, triphasic flow. Compared with angiography, this method has 88–95% sensitivity and 81–98% specificity in identifying hemodynamically relevant stenosis at the pelvic level (Eiberg et al. 2001; De Morais Filho et al. 2004; Fontcuberta et al. 2005; Sensier et al. 2000; Cossman et al. 1989; Skaalan et al. 2003). Spronk et al. (2005) report poor sensitivity of only 56% but good specificity using the criterion of a sharp monophasic waveform for diagnosing aortoiliac obstructive disease. However, this study is limited by the use of MR angiography as the standard of reference.

Another parameter used to rule out hemodynamically significant, higher-grade stenosis is the **pulsatility index** (◘ Fig. 1.28c). A significant stenosis of the aortoiliac segment is unlikely if the pulsatility index is greater than 5.5 (Johnson et al. 1983; Neuerburg et al. 1991). The following pulsatility indices have been determined: 8.5 ± 3.5 in a normal population, 2.8 ± 1.6 in isolated stenosis at the pelvic level, 2.3 ± 1.0 in concomitant pelvic and thigh occlusion, and 6.3 ± 2.6 in isolated femoral artery occlusion. Note, though, that effective collateralization results in a higher pulsatility index (◘ Figs. 2.52 and 2.53 (both Atlas)), giving rise to false-negative results. A pulsatility index with a cutoff of 4 was found to have 94% sensitivity and 82% specificity for identifying isolated aortoiliac obstruction (Thiele et al. 1983). Indirect stenosis criteria can be used when the insonation conditions in the true pelvis are poor. Whenever abnormal findings are encountered, however, an attempt should also be made to identify the stenosis directly. Under normal scanning conditions, state-of-the-art (color) duplex ultrasound equipment often allows faster direct localization of stenosis or occlusion than is possible with use of indirect criteria.

While waveform analysis alone is used in many studies with a standardized design, one should be aware of potential pitfalls. Another important parameter, which is especially relevant in order not to miss moderate stenosis or steno-occlusive disease with very good collateralization, is measurement of **peak systolic velocity (PSV)** in comparison with the opposite side (>30% difference). Audible analysis of the Doppler signal is another option. Upstream stenosis is suggested when the systolic whipping sound is weaker compared with the contralateral side. However, to use this criterion, it is pivotal to perform the Doppler interrogation with a small (<50°) and identical angle on both sides (Schäberle et al. 2013). For an experienced examiner, the acoustic signal is the best criterion for ruling out pelvic artery stenosis. While this acoustic criterion does not lend itself to standardization, the change in the acoustic signal in the presence of upstream stenosis at the pelvic level is visually reflected in the waveform (damping and less steep systolic rise).

The potential pitfalls discussed above show that waveform phasicity alone is not a reliable criterion (e.g., stenosis of femoral artery bifurcation, ◘ Fig. 2.12f) and this may also explain the discrepancy of results reported by investigators using this parameter. To be on the safe side, the examiner should combine evaluation of **waveform phasicity, PSV, and acceleration time** on the affected side in comparison to the contralateral side to make allowance for the fact that the pelvis is rich in arteries that can be recruited as collaterals. This is how the author's group achieved 95% sensitivity and 98% specificity in the detection of >60% stenoses in 85 patients with suspected pelvic artery stenosis (intermittent claudication, pulses, ABI) (Schäberle et al. 1998). Stenosis was confirmed by angiography in 32 of the patients.

As noted, a triphasic waveform merely indictes that there is adequate peripheral perfusion at rest. To avoid misinterpretation, it is helpful to compare spectral Doppler findings obtained after activity (i.e., immediately after positioning of the patient on the couch) with the findings after the usual rest of approx. 3–4 min. Muscle activity induces physiological peripheral vasodilation, reflected in the waveform as a larger diastolic flow component (◘ Fig. 2.9). In individuals without vascular pathology, blood flow quickly returns to normal (within 1 min), and identical triphasic Doppler waveforms are obtained from both sides. In patients with moderate stenosis, well collateralized high-grade stenosis (◘ Figs. 2.12 and 2.53 (Atlas)), or with very well collateralized occlusion, the waveform will also return to normal but it takes longer. Therefore, spectral

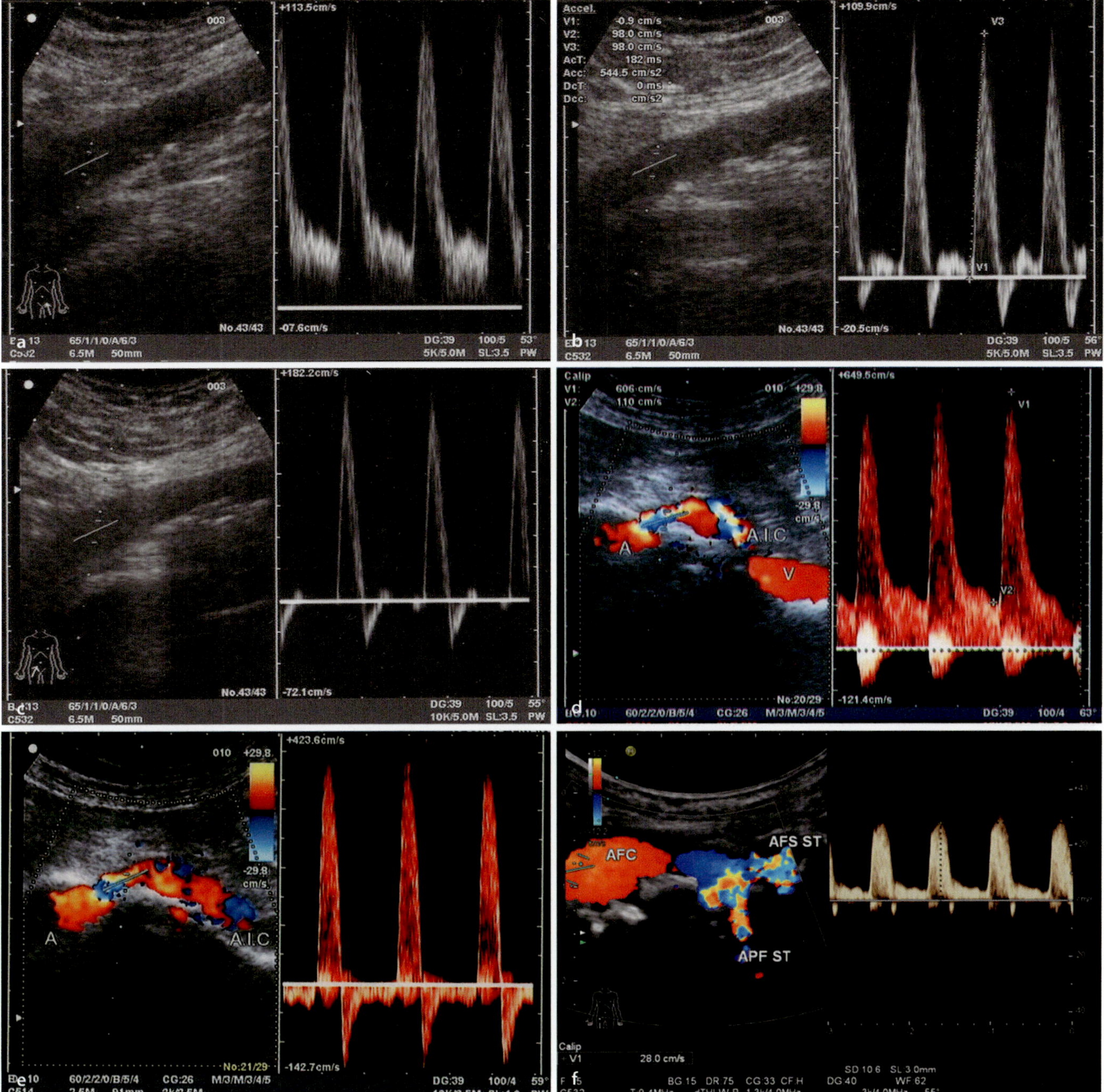

Fig. 2.12a–e Pitfalls in grading common iliac artery stenosis. **a** The Doppler waveform obtained in the left groin (common femoral artery) shows monophasic flow, consistent with upstream stenosis. The waveform was obtained immediately after positioning of the patient, who had walked from the waiting room to the examination room. **b** After 5 min of rest, the waveform shows normal triphasic flow with a slightly delayed systolic upstroke (acceleration time of 182 ms, peak systolic velocity (PSV) of 96 cm/s). However, the PSV here is markedly different from the PSV measured on the contralateral side (PSV of 170 cm/s), which should prompt continuous duplex imaging of the pelvic segment despite the triphasic waveform. **c** The Doppler spectrum from the contralateral common femoral artery is triphasic with a PSV of 170 cm/s. **d** Monophasic flow with delayed return to normal and reduced PSV in this patient was found to be caused by a stenosis of the common iliac artery at its origin from the aorta. The waveform recorded immediately after positioning of the patient for the examination shows criteria of high-grade stenosis (>90%; PSV > 6 m/s and end-diastolic velocity (EDV) > 1 m/s, monophasic flow). **e** The correct degree of stenosis can be estimated from the Doppler waveform obtained in the stenotic segment after 5 min of rest and is approx. 70% (PSV of 380 cm/s, triphasic flow). This example illustrates the importance of performing spectral Doppler analysis at rest to ensure accurate stenosis grading by spectral analysis (PSV, indirect criteria). **f** Another pitfall that must be borne in mind is that high-grade obstruction downstream of the spectral Doppler sampling site can mimic steno-occlusive disease at the pelvic level because it presents with the same changes in the waveform (monophasic flow, reduced PSV). In the example shown, the waveform from the external iliac artery/common femoral artery (AFC) junction is consistent with upstream obstruction (PSV of 30 cm/s, monophasic flow). However, this patient has no iliac artery stenosis and the abnormal waveform is due to high grade-stenosis at the origins of the superficial and profunda femoris arteries (PSV > 300 cm/s, not shown), as indicated by aliasing in the color flow image

Doppler analysis 1 min after activity allows differentiation of transient physiologic changes from vascular pathology.

In conclusion, segmental spectral Doppler analysis requires combined bilateral determination of **PSV and evaluation of waveform phasicity** in order not to overlook hemodynamically relevant stenosis. Any abnormality should prompt continuous mapping of the proximal territory to search for steno-occlusive lesions. A triphasic Doppler waveform alone is not sufficient to rule out upstream stenosis.

Another pitfall to be aware of is that high-grade obstruction downstream of the spectral Doppler sampling site can mimic iliac steno-occlusive disease, because it causes similar changes in the waveform (reduced pulsatility and lower PSV) (◘ Fig. 2.12f). For instance, a patient with profunda femoris stenosis and superficial femoral artery occlusion or high-grade stenosis at the superficial femoral artery origin will have a similar waveform as a patient with iliac artery obstruction (except that the steep systolic rise is preserved). In this situation, the examiner must rule out iliac artery stenosis by direct evaluation (see direct and indirect criteria in ► Sect. 2.1.6.1.4).

2.1.6.1.3 Stenosis Grading

An intrastenotic peak systolic velocity (PSV) of over 180–200 cm/s and focal doubling of PSV have emerged as criteria for hemodynamically relevant stenosis in flow models and in vivo. Using these thresholds, investigators reported sensitivities of 71–100% with specificities of 92–100% (Whyman et al. 1993; Moneta et al. 1992; Aly et al. 1998; Katsamouris et al. 2001). On the other hand, receiver operating characteristic (ROC) curve analysis identified markedly lower velocity thresholds of 120 cm/s for 50% stenosis and 160 cm/s for 70% stenosis (Sacks et al. 1990), but these turned out to be unsuitable in the routine clinical setting. The threshold velocities identified by ROC analysis vary greatly, depending on the study population investigated (e.g., proportion of patients with hypertension or diabetes mellitus).

Conventional angiography is limited in the grading of stenosis at the pelvic level, especially in patients with stenosis at the common iliac artery origin caused by eccentric posterior wall plaque. Strict lateral views are required for reliable grading of this type of stenosis. For more distally located pelvic artery stenoses, the standard anteroposterior projection (often the only projection available) should ideally be supplemented by left and right anterior oblique views (which are perpendicular to each other). Lateral projections are required for exact grading because most stenoses in this territory, especially in the external iliac artery, are caused by eccentric plaque on the posterior wall. CT angiography using thin slices (1 mm) is an alternative option, while MR angiography tends to overestimate stenosis severity.

Hemodynamic stenosis grading by **spectral Doppler imaging** is based on the identification of a focal increase in peak systolic velocity (PSV) compared to the blood flow velocity in the normal arterial segment upstream of the stenosis. The intrastenotic PSV increase is typically calculated as the ratio of intrastenotic PSV to prestenotic PSV, or PSV ratio for short. In general, a PSV ratio > 2 is interpreted to indicate >50% stenosis and a ratio > 4 to indicate >75% stenosis. PSV ratios cannot be used when a stenosis is located in a bifurcation or at the origin of an artery (iliac artery or profunda femoris origin). At these sites, threshold velocities determined by ROC analysis with angiography as the gold standard can be used instead. Several studies investigated a PSV cutoff of 180 cm/s, which was originally proposed for identification of hemodynamically relevant profunda femoris artery stenosis (Strauss et al. 1991), and found 71–96% sensitivities and 92–95% specificities (Moneta et al. 1992; Aly et al. 1998; Katsamouris et al. 2001). A drawback is that absolute PSV is influenced by systemic factors, as underlined by the results of a study using a PSV threshold of 200 cm/s, for which the authors found a high sensitivity of 95%, while specificity was only 55% (de Smet et al. 1996).

The increase in blood flow velocity in a stenotic segment is associated with a pressure drop. The pressure gradient across a hemodynamically relevant stenosis results in a decrease in peripheral systolic blood pressure and can be measured by determining the ankle-brachial index (ABI). A decrease in ABI suggests arterial disease. Strauss et al. (1995) used the PSV measured by duplex ultrasound in stenotic segments at the pelvic level to calculate the pressure gradient across the stenosis using the simplified Bernoulli equation and compared the results with direct intra-arterial pressure measurement. In this study, the following correlations were found between angiographic parameters and duplex ultrasound:

- Cross-sectional area reduction determined densitometrically and the hemodynamic degree of stenosis based on the PSV ratio: R = 0.64
- PSV and densitometrically determined cross-sectional area reduction: R = 0.56
- Pressure gradient calculated from the flow velocity determined by color duplex ultrasound using the Bernoulli equation (◘ Fig. 2.13) and the pressure gradient measured by intra-arterial catheter: R = 0.86

While this study found the best agreement between invasive angiography and noninvasive duplex ultrasound for the pressure gradient across the stenosis (◘ Fig. 2.13), the author's experience suggests that the pressure gradient calculated from PSV using the simplified Bernoulli equation can be misleading, especially when higher-grade stenosis is present. The pressure drop expressed in the ABI reflects the degree of stenosis but ignores the effects of collateralization. For a given degree of stenosis, the ABI is lower in the absence of collateralization and increases with the magnitude of collateralization. Better collateralization also results in less damping of the poststenotic waveform.

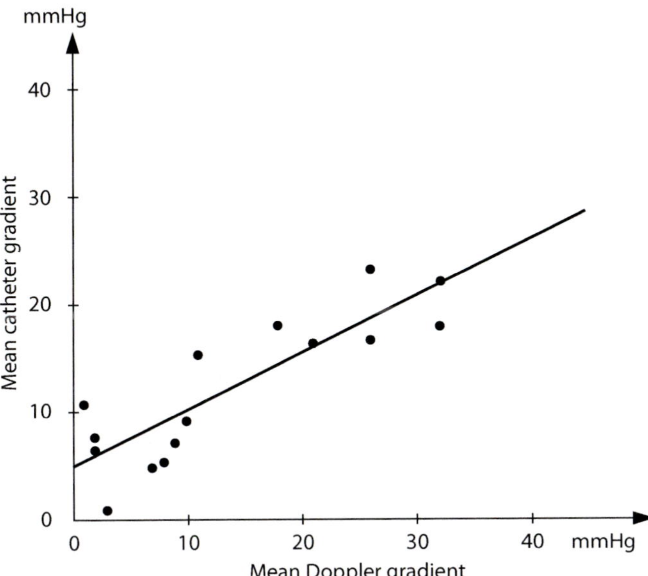

Fig. 2.13 Correlation (R = 0.86) of the mean pressure gradient across a pelvic artery stenosis calculated from color duplex ultrasound using the simplified Bernoulli equation ($p = 4 \times PSV^2$) and the pressure gradient measured by intra-arterial catheter (Strauss et al. 1995)

Theoretically, one would expect the magnitude of the pressure gradient across an iliac artery stenosis to also reflect collateralization, meaning that good collateralization should result in a smaller increase in PSV across the stenotic segment and hence a less steep pressure gradient compared with a stenosis of the same degree but poorer collateralization (comparable to the situation in superficial femoral artery stenosis; Fig. 2.16b). In steno-occlusive disease of more central arteries, however, the intrastenotic increase in PSV is less dependent on collateralization.

Another issue to be borne in mind is that **eccentric plaque**, which is frequent in the iliac and common femoral arteries, causes less severe stenosis in terms of hemodynamic relevance than **circumferential plaque** with the same degree of angiographic diameter reduction. This is due to the fact that a 50% diameter reduction reduces the vascular cross-sectional area by 75% when caused by circumferential stenosis as opposed to only 50% when caused by eccentric stenosis (Fig. 2.17d). Circumferential stenosis thus has more marked hemodynamic effects, resulting in a greater increase in intrastenotic PSV and more severe peripheral ischemia. This explains the discrepancies between morphologic and hemodynamic methods of stenosis grading and why a hemodynamic method such as duplex ultrasound is often a better indicator of the patient's clinical situation than radiologic methods based on morphology alone.

2.1.6.1.4 Leg Arteries

Preferred sites of atherosclerotic femoral artery stenosis are the **bifurcation** (superficial and profunda femoris origins) and the **adductor canal**.

Isolated stenosis or occlusion of the common femoral artery is rare (approx. 4%); most patients with common femoral artery stenosis have concomitant obstructions of the superficial femoral and below-knee arteries. Occlusion of the common femoral artery or femoral bifurcation is of considerable clinical significance and, whenever possible, should be treated by surgical repair (TEA); collateralization here is poor, as all collateral pathways (via the iliac and profunda femoris arteries) comprise the femoral bifurcation, and auxiliary collaterals have a low capacity. The **profunda femoris artery** supplies the thigh muscles and is the most important collateral in all arterial obstructions distal to the femoral bifurcation. As a phylogenetically old vessel, the profunda femoris artery is rarely affected by sclerotic changes distal to its origin. All isolated obstructions of the profunda femoris are due to embolism or occur in patients with diabetes mellitus. Stenosis at the origin of the profunda femoris artery is more common in patients with atherosclerosis of the femoral bifurcation and is clinically relevant due to the key role of the profunda femoris as a collateral in obstruction of the femoropopliteal circulation. Surgical repair of the profunda femoris artery is the treatment of choice.

The **superficial femoral artery** is the preferred site of atherosclerotic lesions and is the most common site of isolated occlusions, which have an incidence of 27%. Occlusion of both the femoral and popliteal arteries occurs in 40–45% of cases. In all cases of isolated popliteal artery occlusion, thrombosed popliteal aneurysm and nonatherosclerotic vascular disorders (which preferably affect the popliteal artery) must be ruled out in the differential diagnosis.

The **treatment** of femoropopliteal artery occlusion depends on the clinical presentation, cause, site, and length of the occluded segments. These frequently affected and hence clinically significant vessels are easily accessible to duplex scanning as they lie close to the surface and there are no intervening scatterers. Many studies have confirmed the diagnostic accuracy of duplex ultrasound in evaluating femoropopliteal occlusive disease (Table 2.7). The precise information on the site and length of an occlusion provided by duplex ultrasound is necessary for therapeutic decision making; however, treatment is ultimately dictated by what is required clinically (Fig. 2.8).

B-mode imaging will show atherosclerotic wall lesions as irregularities of the wall contour, intimal thickening, or plaques (Table 2.8). In larger arteries, the B-mode image already allows a rough estimate of the degree of luminal narrowing when caused by echogenic, noncalcified plaques; however, the hemodynamic degree of luminal narrowing is always derived from the Doppler waveform.

An atherosclerotic occlusion is suggested if extensive intraluminal plaques are depicted and the arterial wall is no longer visible. The B-mode examination thus allows differentiation of stenotic lesions caused by atherosclerosis from luminal narrowing caused by external structures.

Table 2.7 Sensitivity, specificity, and diagnostic accuracy of duplex ultrasonography compared with angiography in the diagnosis of hemodynamically relevant stenosis (>50%), occlusion, and aneurysm of the pelvic and leg arteries (see Table 2.20)

Author	Vascular territory	Duplex technique	Reference method	Sensitivity (%)	Specificity (%)	Accuracy (%)
Kohler et al. (1987)	Femoropopliteal	Conventional	Conventional angio	82	92	–
Legemate et al. (1991)	Aortoiliac	Conventional	IA DSA	89	92	91
Allard et al. (1994)	Aortoiliac Femoropopliteal	Conventional	Conventional angio	83 87	96 93	92 90
Cossman et al. (1989)	Iliac Common femoral Superficial femoral Profunda femoris Popliteal	Color	Conventional angio	81 70 87 71 85	98 97 85 95 97	92 93 87 93 93
Mulligan et al. (1991)	Femoropopliteal	Color	Conventional angio	89	91	
Moneta et al. (1992)	Iliac Common femoral Superficial femoral Profunda femoris Popliteal	Color	Conventional angio or IA DSA	89 76 87 83 67	99 99 98 97 99	
Strauss (2001)	Iliac Common femoral Superficial femoral Profunda femoris Popliteal	Color	Conventional angio or IA DSA	87 75 94 79 94	73 91 72 96 92	83 86 88 86 93
Schäberle (1998)	Femoropopliteal, iliac, proximal segments of crural arteries	Color	Conventional angio or IA DSA; intraoperative	97	98	97
Polak et al. (1990)	Femoropopliteal	Color	Angiography or IA DSA	88	95	93
Landwehr et al. (1990)	Femoropopliteal	Color	Angiography or IA DSA	92	99	96
Koennecke et al. (1989)	Femoropopliteal	Color	Angiography or IA DSA	97	97	97
Legemate et al. (1991)		Color	Angiography	84	96	
Ranke et al. (1992)		Color	Angiography	87	94	
Katsamouris et al. (2001)	Aortoiliac Femoropopliteal Tibial	Color	Angiography	86 99 80	90 94 91	88 96 83
Aly et al. (1998)	Aortoiliac Femoropopliteal Crural	Color	Angiography	89 100 82	99 99 99	
Khan et al. (2011)	Femoropopliteal	Color	Angiography	94.5	99	

IA DSA intra-arterial digital subtraction angiography

Table 2.8 Sonographic differentiation of vascular abnormalities in B-mode imaging

Diagnostic information provided by B-mode imaging	Suggested diagnosis	Measurement performed with duplex imaging (optimized settings)	Further diagnostic testing to resolve inconclusive duplex findings (if therapeutically relevant)
Circumscribed wall thickening (intima), low/high echogenicity, acoustic shadowing?	Atherosclerotic plaque	Stenosis grading: waveform (adjust PRF and gain settings)	CEUS, MRA, IA DSA (depending on treatment options contemplated)
Concentric wall thickening of long segment (Fig. 2.33)	Arteritis	Measurement of wall thickness and length of involved segment, stenosis grading, occlusion? (higher-frequeny transducer)	Inflammatory parameters, ESR, MRA
Dilated appearance (Fig. 2.27)	Aneurysm, dilated angiopathy	Measurement of aneurysm diameter, intravascular thrombus?	Color duplex, CT, IA DSA if surgery is indicated (periphery)
Anechoic cystic wall lesions (Fig. 2.29)	Adventitial cystic disease	Degree of stenosis, which may vary with cyst size (repeat examination)	CT, MRA
Abnormal arterial course, possibly with external compression (Fig. 2.31)	Vascular compression syndrome, stenosis or occlusion? (entrapment syndrome)	Functional assessment: increasing stenosis (or even occlusion) with increasing plantar flexion/vascular compression by muscle	CT for documentation of abnormal arterial course
Vascular lumen not anechoic	Embolic or thrombotic occlusion, artifact, inadequate machine settings (consider clinical presentation: symptoms of critical ischemia?)	Color duplex to determine length of occlusion (very low PRF, higher gain)	Angiography, MRA
Intraluminal echogenic structures, flap-like	Dissection	Color duplex to confirm diagnosis by identification of true and false lumen	Angiography, CTA

CEUS contrast-enhanced ultrasound, *CT* computed tomography, *CTA* computed tomography angiography, *ESR* erythrocyte sedimentation rate, *IA DSA* intra-arterial digital subtraction angiography, *MRA* magnetic resonance angiography, *PRF* pulse repetition frequency

Medial sclerosis in diabetics is characterized by diffuse calcification of the middle layer of the arterial wall. The calcifications produce irregular and inhomogeneous wall thickening with scattering and acoustic shadowing, impairing both B-mode and color flow imaging.

In the limb arteries, the high peripheral resistance gives rise to pulsatile, nearly laminar flow. The normal **Doppler waveform** is triphasic with a narrow bandwidth and a clear systolic window. A triphasic waveform is characterized by a steep systolic rise and subsequent decrease, followed by a short early diastolic reflux and forward flow, with the magnitude and duration depending on the vascular territory supplied. Physiologic changes in the laminar flow profile can occur at vessel origins and in curved segments.

An obstruction caused by stenosis or external compression leads to flow acceleration in proportion to the cross-sectional area reduction (see Fig. 1.44) and flow becomes turbulent (see Fig. 1.46). A slight increase in flow velocity can already be observed with 30–50% luminal narrowing, but a relevant drop in peripheral arterial blood pressure (ABI) is unlikely at rest. Low-grade stenosis (<50%) has only little effect on the flow profile. With increasing luminal narrowing, however, flow becomes less pulsatile with turbulence and eddy currents downstream of the stenosis. A reduction of the cross-sectional area exceeding 75% (>50% diameter reduction) is associated with a marked intrastenotic increase in PSV of more than 100% compared with the prestenotic arterial segment (Jäger et al. 1985; Moneta et al. 1992). Flow becomes less and less pulsatile, ultimately resulting in a **monophasic waveform** (Fig. 2.14), which characterizes blood flow both within and downstream of a **high-grade stenosis** (Cossman et al. 1989; Polak et al. 1991; Kohler 1990).

2

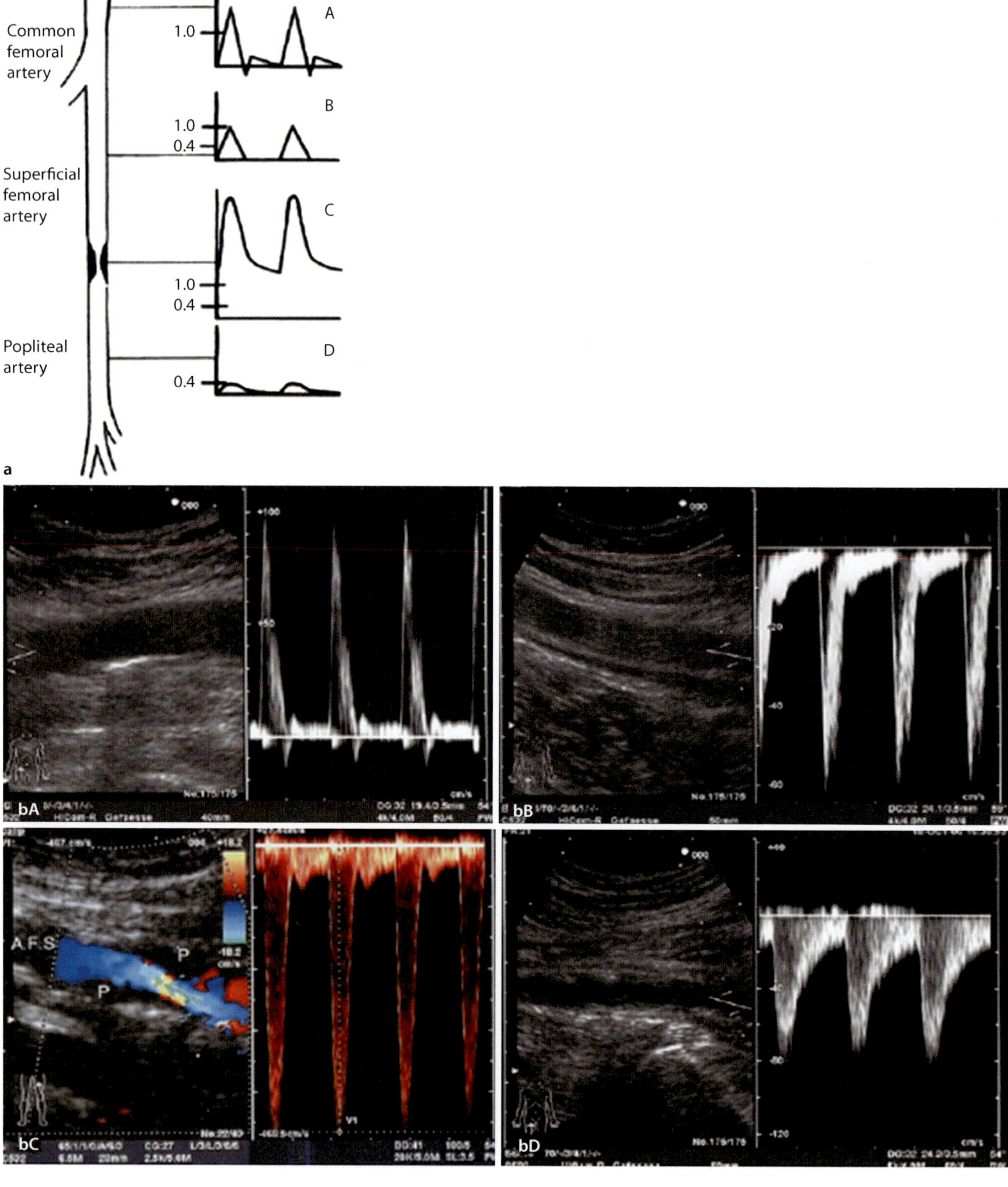

Fig. 2.14 **a** Diagram of Doppler waveform changes induced by superficial femoral artery stenosis at different levels of the lower extremity arterial tree. **bA** Nearly normal triphasic waveform from common femoral artery (far upstream of the stenosis). **bB** Prestenotic waveform from proximal superficial femoral artery with slightly reduced peak systolic velocity (PSV) and reduced or absent early diastolic dip but steep systolic upstroke. **bC** Monophasic flow profile with more than doubling of intrastenotic PSV compared to prestenotic PSV. **bD** Monophasic poststenotic waveform from popliteal artery with delayed systolic upstroke and low PSV (damped waveform)

The changes depicted by (color) duplex ultrasound at the site of stenosis are known as direct stenosis criteria and the poststenotic changes in the flow profile as indirect stenosis criteria. For the leg arteries, the stenosis criteria are as follows:

- Direct stenosis criteria:
  - Absolute intrastenotic PSV > 180 cm/s
  - Focal increase in PSV, expressed as intrastenotic-to-prestenotic PSV ratio
    - PSV ratio > 2 indicates >50% stenosis (diameter reduction)
    - PSV ratio > 4 indicates >75% stenosis (diameter reduction)
  - Perivascular vibration
- Indirect stenosis criteria:
  - Flow profile:
    - Damping (triphasic/monophasic)
    - Delayed systolic rise

Note, though, that the indirect criterion of monophasic flow merely indicates a change from high-resistance to low-resistance flow due to peripheral vasodilation. Several (physiologic and pathologic) factors can alter the normal **triphasic waveform**:

- Physiologic:
  - Muscle activity
- Pathologic:
  - Fever
  - Hypercirculation
  - Downstream infection
  - Vasodilation in response to upstream occlusion

Duplex ultrasound using the direct stenosis criteria has 83–99% accuracy in identifying hemodynamically significant stenosis and occlusion of the aortoiliac and femoropopliteal arteries compared with angiography (◘ Tables 2.7 and 2.20). In a study of 125 patients with stage II-IV peripheral arterial occlusive disease (PAOD) presenting with typical symptoms, conducted by the author's group (1998), (color) duplex ultrasound detected hemodynamically relevant steno-occlusive lesions with 96% sensitivity, 98% specificity, and 97% accuracy compared with angiopgraphy. In this study population, 31 percent of the patients had femoropopliteal steno-occlusive disease, 12% pelvic level involvement, 18% lesions in the arteries below the knee, and 39% had multilevel disease.

In color duplex imaging, the subtle flow acceleration associated with mild to moderate stenosis is displayed in brighter shades of red or blue (primarily within the stenosis jet) or suggested by color aliasing (when a low PRF is used). With increasing stenosis severity, retrograde flow components associated with eddy currents and flow separations are depicted as color changes. High-grade stenosis with turbulent flow is characterized by a mosaic of colors and aliasing. Color duplex imaging performed with adequate settings thus enables rapid localization of a stenosis and semiquantitative estimation of its severity.

Precise stenosis quantification, however, requires spectral Doppler analysis, which is highly sensitive in depicting the hemodynamic changes occurring in the prestenotic, intrastenotic, and poststenotic arterial segments (◘ Table 2.9).

Proximal to a high-grade stenosis, flow may become less pulsatile due to changes in peripheral resistance. In the spectral display, however, the steep systolic rise remains unchanged (in contrast to a postocclusive waveform). The closer the sample volume is placed to a high-grade stenosis or occlusion, the less the prestenotic waveform is affected by collateral flow. When no hemodynamically significant collaterals arise between the sample volume and the flow obstruction, there may be very pronounced pulsatility or even to-and-fro flow (thump pattern; see ◘ Fig. 1.46).

Flow acceleration increases with the degree of stenosis (as predicted by the continuity equation), eventually resulting in loss of the triphasic flow profile. Depending on the degree of stenosis, the poststenotic Doppler waveform will show a decreased PSV, a delayed upstroke, and reduced pulsatility or even monophasic flow (◘ Table 2.9). In addition, flow becomes turbulent. In larger arteries such as the iliac and femoral arteries, high-grade stenosis may also be suggested by the so-called confetti phenomenon outside the blood vessel (due to tissue vibration) or by high-frequency Doppler signals, the so-called seagull's cry.

The loss of pulsatility distal to a high-grade stenosis (◘ Fig. 2.14) or occlusion is due to a decrease in peripheral resistance (widening of collateral vessels, reduced arteriolar tone) and a pressure gradient across the stenosis. The pressure difference between the heart and the periphery is no longer equalized during a single cardiac cycle and there may be flow throughout diastole.

Calcified plaque with acoustic shadowing may preclude direct color duplex evaluation of a stenotic segment. In this situation, the examiner should compare prestenotic and poststenotic Doppler waveforms (◘ Table 2.10). If there is no change in PSV or the character of the waveforms between the prestenotic and poststenotic sampling sites, the plaque does not cause hemodynamically relevant luminal narrowing (see ◘ Fig. 2.64 (Atlas)).

2.1.6.1.5 Stenosis Grading: Ultrasound Versus Angiography

Most studies comparing duplex or color duplex ultrasound and angiography in patients with PAOD show good agreement between the two modalities with sensitivities and specificities of 85% to 99% (◘ Table 2.7). More recent studies report values of over 90%, but earlier studies describe surprisingly good results for conventional duplex ultrasound as well: as early as 1986 Jäger et al. found 96% sensitivity and

Table 2.9 Grading of peripheral artery stenosis (Figs. 1.46, 2.14, 2.20, and 2.21). The degree is defined as the percentage reduction in vascular cross-sectional area. The criteria are not fully applicable in branching vessels. There are no strict boundaries between the different degrees of stenosis as the hemodynamic effects of a stenosis depend on a complex interaction of different factors (modified according to Wolf and Fobbe 1993; Cossman et al. 1989; Polak et al. 1991)

Stenosis degree	(Color) duplex (intrastenotic)	(Color) duplex (just distal to stenosis)	Waveform far distal to stenosis	Waveform proximal to stenosis	PSV ratio[a]
No stenosis	Triphasic waveform (PSV <150 cm/s)	Clear spectral window Markedly pulsatile flow Steep systolic upslope	Unchanged	Unchanged	<1.5
20–50% Low-grade stenosis	Increase in PSV (150–200 cm/s)	Only mild turbulence Moderate spectral broadening may occur	Same as prestenotic	Normal	1.5–2
51–75% Moderate stenosis	Further increase in PSV (200–350 cm/s) Slight reduction in pulsatility	Eddy currents Possibly slight turbulence Partial filling-in of systolic window	Slightly reduced pulsatility	Normal	2–4
76–95% High-grade stenosis	Very pronounced increase in PSV (>350 cm/s) Reduction in pulsatility Monophasic	Considerable turbulence Complete filling-in of systolic window Monophasic flow	Longer systolic acceleration time Reduced pulsatility	Amplitude normal or slightly reduced (compared to other side) Pulsatility may be reduced upstream of collateral origins	>4
>95% Subtotal occlusion	Marked increase in PSV (> 4 m/s) and end-diastolic velocity (depending on collateralization) Monophasic	Pronounced turbulence Completely filled-in systolic window Monophasic	Flattened systolic peak Considerably reduced pulsatility Monophasic	Reduced amplitude Prestenotic pulsatility increased directly before stenosis but reduced upstream of collateral origins	>4
Occlusion	No flow signal detectable	Very reduced flow in distal segment Marked damping of waveform Monophasic	Very flat systolic peak Monophasic	Low amplitude Thump pattern immediately before occlusion: increased pulsatility, small complex with large negative component Decreased pulsatility upstream of collateral origins	

[a]PSV ratio: intrastenotic peak systolic velocity divided by prestenotic peak systolic velocity

Table 2.10 Duplex ultrasound of the peripheral arteries – intrinsic limitations of the method

Technique	Limitations
B-mode	Calcified plaque: posterior acoustic shadowing Edema: scattering
Doppler	Calcified plaque: posterior acoustic shadowing Maximum flow velocity detectable: limited by PRF

81% specificity for the demonstration of abnormal changes in the pelvic and leg arteries by duplex ultrasound compared with angiography. It is noteworthy that the sensitivity is the same and the specificity higher compared with the agreement between two radiologists interpreting the same angiograms (97% sensitivity, 68% specificity).

While many investigators conclude that duplex ultrasound is a valid method for the detection and grading of significant (femoropopliteal) stenosis (>50%), it is noteworthy that they use either absolute peak systolic velocity (PSV) or the PSV ratio (intrastenotic PSV divided by prestenotic PSV)

with different cutoff velocities for defining 50% or 70% stenosis (◘ Fig. 2.21).

An examiner using **absolute PSV rather than the PSV ratio** for grading stenosis must be aware that the intrastenotic PSV reflects not only the degree of stenosis but also the effects of **various other factors**:

- Systolic blood pressure
- Poststenotic PSV (varies with magnitude of collateralization)
- Vessel wall elasticity (medial sclerosis – higher pulsatility)
- Sympathetic tone, outflow restistance, peripheral vasodilatation
- Collateral function:
  - Artery in which PSV is measured functions as a collateral: PSV↑
  - Artery in which PSV is measured is bridged by a collateral: PSV↓

Because the effects of these influencing factors, particularly those of collateralization (◘ Fig. 2.16b), are difficult to estimate, the PSV ratio allows more reliable stenosis grading (see ► Sect. 1.2.3) than absolute intrastenotic PSV (Ranke et al. 1992) (◘ Fig. 2.18). The PSV ratio, in turn, is a measure of the PSV increase at the site of stenosis relative to the normal prestenotic segment and therefore cannot be used at sites of bifurcation, where the hemodynamic situation in the prestenotic segment is different and hemodynamic effects of flow in the other branching vessel are difficult to estimate. A case in point is the femoral artery bifurcation: in a patient with higher-grade stenosis at the origin of the superficial femoral artery, the PSV ratio calculated with use of the PSV in the common femoral artery as the prestenotic value will not yield consistent results. This is because blood flow velocity in the common femoral artery is affected by blood flow in the profunda femoris artery, which in turn increases with the extent to which the latter functions as a collateral to bridge the obstructed superficial femoral artery. Therefore, absolute PVS appears to be a better velocity criterion for grading stenosis at this site.

Most authors investigating absolute velocity parameters for stenosis grading in the femoral bifurcation used **ROC curve analysis to define PSV cutoffs**. For the origin of the profunda femoris artery, for instance, a PSV threshold of 180 cm/s was found to accurately identify hemodynamically relevant stenosis (>50% stenosis) (Strauss et al. 1991). Later investigators applied absolute PSV cutoffs for stenosis grading in the entire femoropopliteal territory. These studies used different cutoffs and reported the following results:

- PSV cutoff of 150 cm/s: 94.5% sensitivity and 99% specificity (Khan et al. 2011)
- PSV cutoff of 180 cm/s: 66% sensitivity and 80% specificity (Ranke et al. 1992)
- PSV cutoff of 200 cm/s: 70% sensitivity and 96% specificity (Leng et al. 1993)

Some authors used surprisingly low cutoff velocities for the detection of therapeutically relevant stenosis (>70%). One study, for instance, found 89% sensitivity and specificity for a PSV cutoff of 200 cm/s (Khan et al. 2011), while another study reported 74% sensitivity and 83% specificity for a cutoff of 250 cm/s (Favaretto et al. 2007) (see, however, ◘ Fig. 2.16b).

For **stenosis grading based on focally increased blood flow velocity**, PSV ratios of 2 and (3-)4 have emerged as cutoffs for 50% and 75% stenosis, respectively (Khan et al. 2011; Ranke et al. 1992). Studies reported in the literature investigated PSV ratios ranging from 1.5 to 2.4 to identify 50% stenosis compared with angiography. For a PSV ratio of 1.5, Khan et al. (2011) reported 90.8% sensitivity and 97% specificity. For a ratio of 2, Polak et al. (1990) found 88% sensitivity and 95% specificity, while Aly et al. (1998) found 92% sensitivity and 99% specificity. For the highest PSV ratio of 2.4, Ranke et al. (1992) reported 87% sensitivity and 94% specificity. Most studies found the best results for identification of >50% stenosis when using a PSV ratio > 2 (Alexander et al. 2002; Flanigan et al. 2008; Kohler et al. 1987; Sensier et al. 1996). For identification of >70(−75)% stenosis, most investigators use velocity ratios of 3.5–4.0 (Alexander et al. 2002; Favaretto et al. 2007; Legemate et al. 1991; Polak et al. 1990; Schlager et al. 2007), while Khan et al. (2011) propose a surprisingly low ratio of 2. One factor accounting for this low ratio appears to be the choice of the prestenotic sampling site (segmental classification).

2.1.6.1.6 Role of Collateralization in Stenosis Grading

Throughout its course, the superficial femoral artery gives off arteries supplying muscles. These arteries can be recruited as collaterals in patients with steno-occlusive disease in this vascular territory, giving rise to intricate hemodynamic patterns and variability in blood flow directions and velocities, which must be taken into account when interpreting Doppler waveforms (◘ Fig. 2.15). Good collateral circulation reduces blood flow in the main artery, resulting in a lower intrastenotic peak systolic velocity (PSV) than in a stenosis of the same degree with poor or absent collateralization (◘ Fig. 2.16b).

The pressure gradient across a higher-grade stenosis leads to pressure reversal in muscle arteries arising distal to the stenotic segment. These arterial branches in turn are supplied by collateral pathways bridging the obstructed main artery, resulting in reversed blood flow into the main artery, where pressure and blood flow are reduced due to the obstruction. Therefore, PSV and pulsatility in the poststenotic segment will be higher distal to the origin of a muscle artery recruited as a collateral than proximal to it.

Collateralization also affects blood flow velocities in the prestenotic segment of the main artery (femoral artery). Good collateralization results in a higher PSV in the main artery upstream of the origin of relevant collaterals than when measured closer to the stenosis and downstream of the collateral origin (see ◘ Figs. 1.46 and 2.16b). This must be taken into account when choosing the prestenotic spectral Doppler sampling site for PSV measurement. Using the higher, more proximal prestenotic PSV to calculate the PSV

2

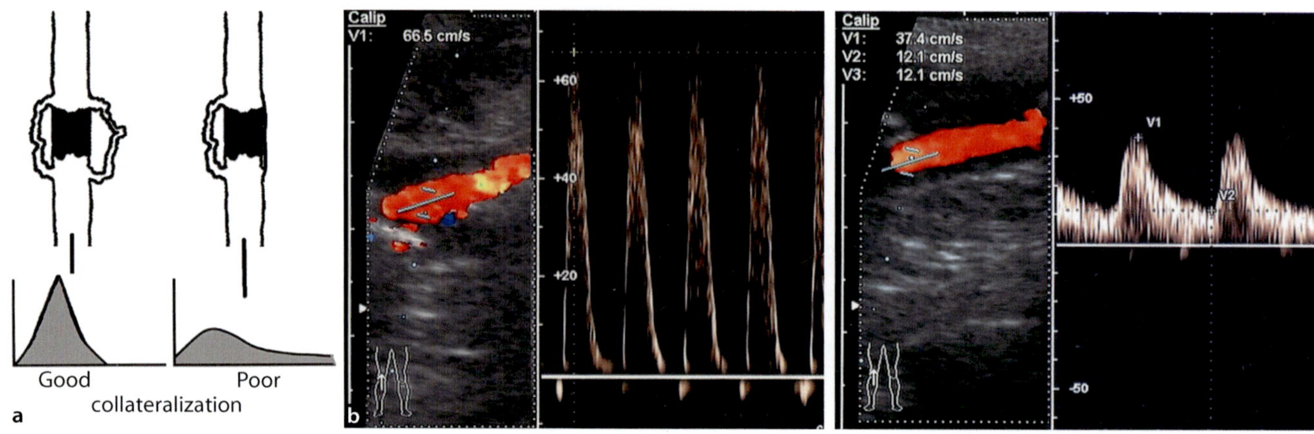

■ **Fig. 2.15** **a** With poor collateralization, the Doppler waveform obtained in the postocclusive segment (right) is damped with a large diastolic component, resulting from distal dilatation in response to chronic peripheral ischemia. With increasing collateralization, blood flow distal to an occluded segment becomes more pulsatile (left), approaching normal flow when there is optimal collateralization and postocclusive pressure approximates preocclusive pressure. **b** The pulsatility of the Doppler spectrum recorded distal to an occlusion is determined by the magnitude of collateral flow. Good collateral pathways can compensate for an occluded main artery and ensure adequate perfusion, at least at rest. For instance, if an isolated occlusion of a pelvic artery or the superficial femoral artery develops slowly over years, one may occasionally obtain a triphasic waveform from the popliteal artery, but with reduced PSV and delayed acceleration. Conversely, the poorer the collateral situation, the more monophasic the waveform and the lower the PSV (relative to end-diastolic flow velocity) become. The first example illustrates the findings in superficial femoral artery occlusion with good collateralization (left): the Doppler waveform from the popliteal artery shows pulsatile flow with short retrograde flow in early diastole and zero diastolic forward flow (ABI of 0.8). The second example (right) shows a monophasic waveform from a patient with poor collateralization of superficial femoral artery occlusion: it is characterized by persistent diastolic flow and a low PSV (ABI of 0.5)

ratio for stenosis grading results in lower PSV ratios and explains why some investigators found lower cutoff ratios for relevant stenosis (e.g., Khan et al. 2011). For consistency of results, it is therefore important to always **measure prestenotic PSV 2–5 cm proximal to the obstructed segment of the main artery** and distal to the origins of relevant collaterals (■ Fig. 2.16b). If this recommendation is followed, the continuity equation applies and an increase by a factor of 4 identifies stenosis with 75% cross-sectional area reduction (which is inversely related to PSV). Note though that this is only an approximation based on the assumptions that hold for the behavior of Newtonian fluids.

Little or no attention has so far been paid to how the site of prestenotic PSV measurement can affect stenosis grading. This is one factor explaining why different PSV ratios have been proposed as cutoffs for stenosis grading in this vascular territory. And what is more, some investigators even deliberatedly aimed at using a prestenotic sampling site farther away from the stenotic segment (Polak et al. 1990; Khan et al. 2011).

A final aspect to be considered is that, because collaterals divert blood away from the obstructed main artery, **absolute intrastenotic PSV may be lower** than expected from the degree of luminal narrowing alone (see study results discussed in the preceding section). Blood flow in the main artery between the origin of a collateral and an obstruction decreases as flow in the collateral increases (Schäberle et al. 2013). Ignoring the effect of good collateralization on intrastenotic PSV in high-grade stenosis (■ Fig. 2.16b) can lead to underestimation of stenosis severity when an absolute PSV cutoff >180 cm/s is used. This pitfall can be avoided by using PSV ratios instead.

2.1.6.1.7 Effects of Collateralization on Pre- and Postocclusive Spectral Doppler Waveforms

In the peripheral arteries, postocclusive perfusion pressure is determined by preocclusive systemic pressure and, above all, by flow resistance in the collateral circulation (■ Fig. 2.16a). Collateral resistance, in turn, depends on the number and size of collateral vessels, the length of the occluded segment to be bridged, and blood viscosity. When collateral resistance is low, the effect on peripheral perfusion is less dramatic, and there is only moderate peripheral vasodilatation. As a result, postobstructive flow remains pulsatile, and a fairly normal triphasic Doppler waveform is obtained. Whether the postocclusive waveform becomes monophasic thus depends on the degree of stenosis or length of occlusion and collateralization. Both the Doppler waveform and the ankle-brachial index (ABI) thus reflect not only the severity of steno-occlusive disease but also the magnitude of collateralization. Better collateralization (e.g., at the pelvic level) results in less abnormal spectral Doppler findings.

This also explains why the postocclusive Doppler waveform correlates well with the ABI and the severity of the patient's clinical condition. A damped but still triphasic postocclusive waveform suggests that, at least at rest, peripheral perfusion is still adequate. These patients also have a longer walking distance. The spectral Doppler findings, along with the ABI, can thus help differentiate pain due to PAOD from other underlying causes.

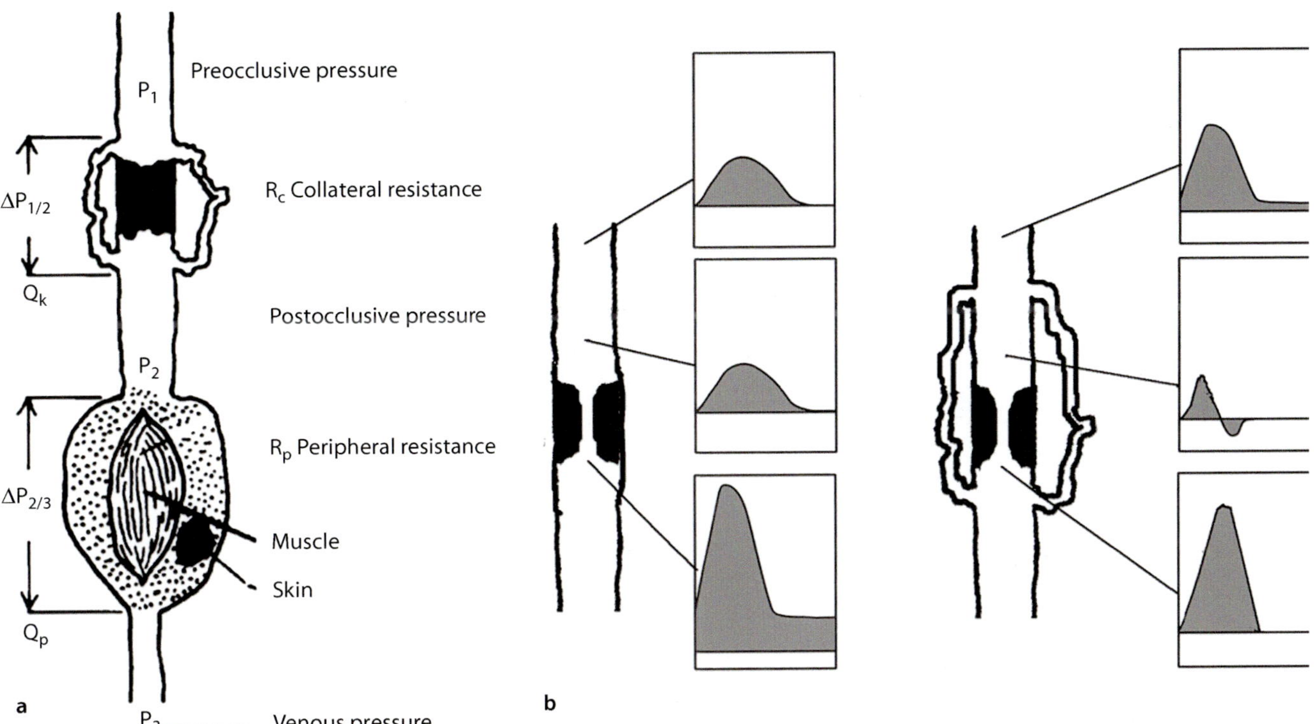

Fig. 2.16 Effects of collateralization on spectral Doppler findings in and around steno-occlusive arterial lesions. **a** Postocclusive arterial pressure depends on the degree of stenosis or length of occlusion as well as on collateral resistance. Collateral resistance is low when there is good collateralization, which in turn results in higher postocclusive pressure in the main artery. With good collateralization, the postocclusive waveform is less abnormal with a higher peak systolic velocity (PSV) and low end-diastolic velocity (EDV). A nearly normal triphasic waveform may be seen in patients with pelvic artery occlusion and good collateralization (from Rieger and Schoop 1998). **b** With little or no collateralization (or in bypass graft stenosis), the prestenotic waveform will show a reduced PSV. In this situation, flow in the prestenotic segment is less affected by compensatory peripheral vasodilation, and a knocking waveform (thump pattern) may be obtained in very high-grade stenosis (left diagram). In case of good collateralization, PSV proximal to the origin of a collateral vessel is relatively normal; however, in patients with reduced peripheral perfusion and compensatory vasodilation, there will be some diastolic flow transmitted through the collateral. Flow is more pulsatile between the origin of a collateral and the stenosis; some to-and-fro flow may be seen immediately proximal to a high-grade stenosis (right diagram). If there are no collaterals, intravascular pressure leads to a higher intrastenotic flow velocity (left). The lower pressure in a collateral vessel diverts blood flow from the stenotic artery. The resultant decrease in pressure in the main artery reduces intrastenotic flow velocity compared with the velocity expected in a stenosis of the same degree without collateral circulation (right). This is why the severity of a stenosis using absolute PSV may be underestimated if the effects of collateralization are ignored. The intrastenotic-to-prestenotic PSV ratio is independent of the magnitude of collateralization (see Fig. 1.46)

Spectral Doppler interrogation provides a wealth of information reflecting the complex hemodynamic situation around a stenotic or occluded arterial segment. With the development of collateral pathways in patients with chronic vascular obstruction, postocclusive flow becomes more pulsatile (Fig. 2.15). Collaterals also affect flow velocity and the flow profile upstream of the stenosis. How collaterals influence the waveform depends on where they arise and enter relative to the site of Doppler sampling. In the prestenotic segment proximal to the origin of collaterals, loss of peripheral resistance results in a monophasic waveform with persistent diastolic flow through the collaterals. However, in contrast to the poststenotic situation, PSV is high and there is a steep systolic upstroke. A prestenotic waveform from the segment between the origin of a collateral and a high-grade stenosis will show more pulsatile flow (Fig. 2.16) because resistance is higher than upstream of the collateral origin (see Fig. 1.46).

2.1.6.1.8 Plaque Configuration and Stenosis Degree

Systematic differences in stenosis grading between angiography and color duplex ultrasound may result from ignoring the effect of plaque configuration (concentric versus eccentric). Stenosis in the common femoral artery is typically due to eccentric plaque. When an eccentric plaque causes 50% diameter reduction, the corresponding cross-sectional area reduction is only 50% (Figs. 2.17 and 5.27) as opposed to 75% when the stenosis is caused by concentric plaque with the same diameter reduction. Hence, a concentric plaque has a greater hemodynamic and clinical effect than an eccentric plaque. This difference in terms of hemodynamic relevance is reflected by the fact that the increase in intrastenotic PSV is twice as high (PSV ratio of 4 versus 2) (Fig. 2.17d). In other words, the increase in PSV within the stenosis reflects the cross-sectional area reduction (Fig. 2.18). The hemodynamic stenosis severity

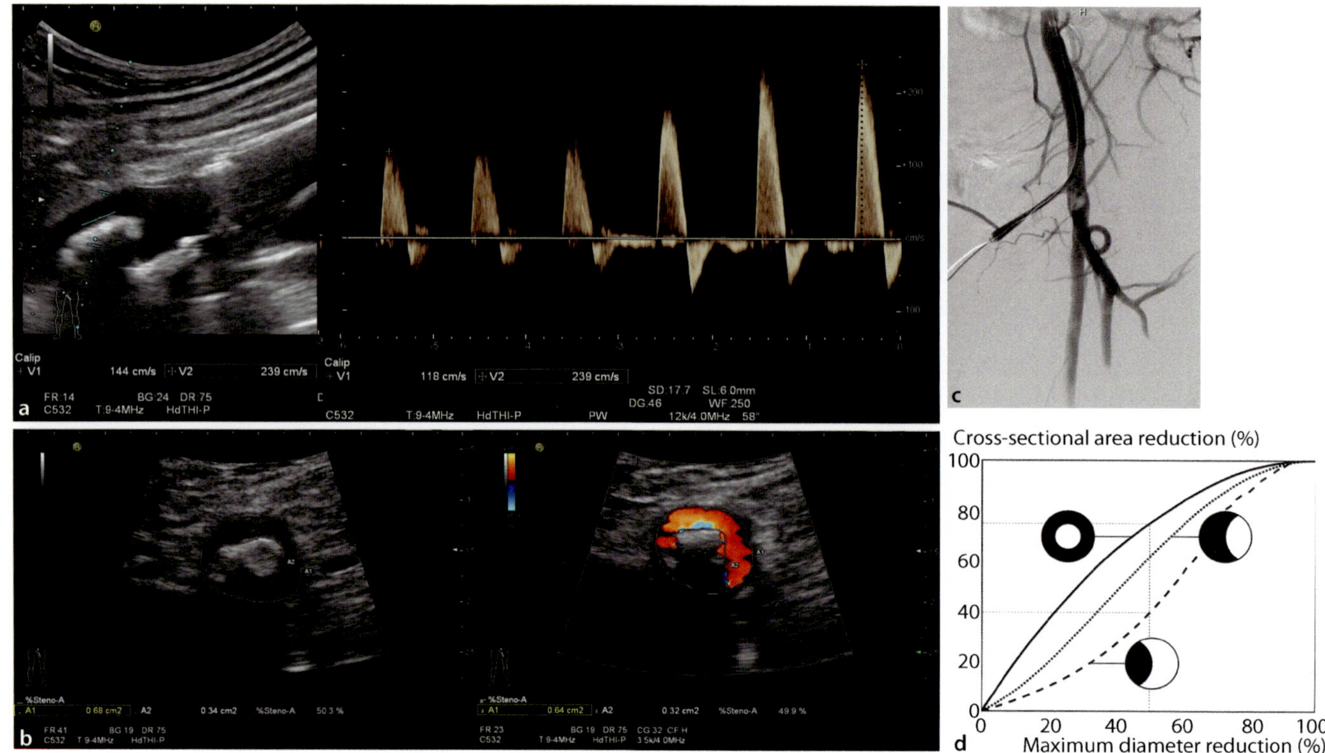

Fig. 2.17a–d Effects of plaque configuration. **a** Common femoral artery stenosis with an intrastenotic peak systolic velocity (PSV) of 220 cm/s. The longitudinal gray-scale image shows luminal narrowing caused by eccentric posterior wall plaque with the appearance suggesting high-grade stenosis, while the PSV is consistent with 50–60% stenosis. A PSV ratio of 2 is calculated from the intrastenotic PSV of 220 cm/s and the prestenotic prestenotic PSV of 110 cm/s, which corresponds to focal doubling of blood flow velocity and indicates 50% stenosis. The waveform was obtained by moving the transducer along the artery and includes the sites of prestenotic and intrastenotic PSV measurement. **b** Gray-scale and color duplex images of the same stenosis as in **c**. The gray-scale image shows eccentric, calcified plaque on the posterior wall. Planimetric measurement of the cross-sectional area reduction yields 50% luminal reduction (measured using the built-in software: 0.68 cm^2 cross-sectional area of the vessel – 0.34 cm^2 cross-sectional area of plaque → 50% area occlusion). While the method yields a correct estimate in this case, it is discouraged, and hemodynamic stenosis grading based on spectral Doppler interrogation should be preferred. Good plaque delineation in the gray-scale image as in this example (left) is rarely accomplished, and activation of the color flow mode does not improve differentiation of plaque from flowing blood. On the contrary, color duplex is prone to color spillover, obscuring plaque and the vessel wall. The perpendicular insonation angle for adequate visualization of the plaque area in the transverse view is a poor Doppler angle (close to 90°). A higher gain setting is not an option either and would even increase color blooming. **c** The anteroposterior angiogram does not allow adequate identification of this stenosis, and the only hint of luminal narrowing caused by the eccentric plaque at this site is some brightening in the otherwise opacified vessel. In a lateral view, this plaque **b** would mimic high-grade stenosis. Technically, only oblique rather than lateral angiographic projections can be obtained in this territory. **d** Diagram illustrating the relationship between cross-sectional area reduction and diameter reduction as a function of plaque configuration (concentric – eccentric). Diameter reduction is the basis for stenosis grading in angiography, while the cross-sectional area reduction, which determines the hemodynamic relevance of a stenosis (see Fig. 5.27), is the basis for sonographic stenosis grading. The drawing illustrates that 50% diameter reduction (in angiography) corresponds to 75% cross-sectional area reduction when caused by a concentric plaque versus 50% reduction when caused by an eccentric plaque. Grading by spectral Doppler measurement would yield a PSV ratio of 4 for the circumferential stenosis, corresponding to a higher-grade stenosis, and a PSV ratio of 2 for the eccentric stenosis, corresponding to a lower-grade stenosis (according to the continuity equation). In both cases, angiography would yield a 50% stenosis in terms of diameter reduction. As the cross-sectional area reduction is what determines the hemodynamic effects of a stenosis and hence the patient's clinical symptoms, the hemodynamic stenosis grade determined by ultrasound is a more adequate measure of the clinical relevance of a stenosis (see ► Sect. 1.2.3)

determined by duplex ultrasound is thus a more adequate measure of the plaque-related blood flow obstruction and also of the patient's clinical situation than angiography, which solely relies on morphologic appearance.

Angiographic stenosis grading is additionally limited by the fact that it often relies on a single (anteroposterior) projection, while exact grading requires two planes, especially when stenosis is caused by eccentric plaque. This limitation is especially relevant in the angiographic evaluation of the common femoral artery, where stenosis is typically caused by posterior wall plaque and even relevant stenosis may be missed when only anteroposterior projections are obtained. Despite these limitations, even scientific studies still use angiography as the gold standard and report poor agreement of duplex ultrasound with anteroposterior angiograms (Schlager et al. 2007). Overall, though, duplex ultrasound is judged to provide adequate accuracy for detecting >50% stenosis in the routine clinical setting.

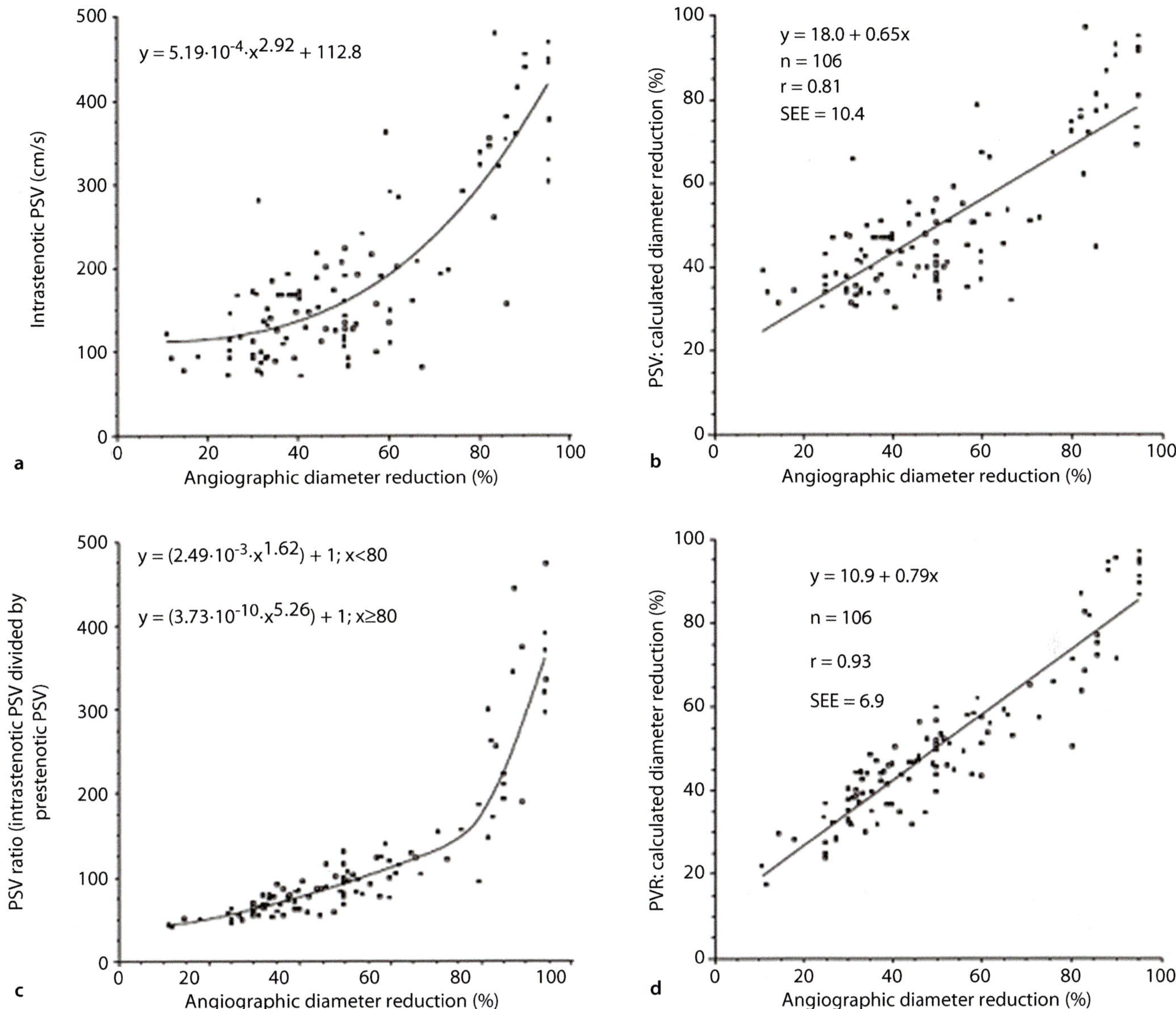

Fig. 2.18a–d Correlation of absolute intrastenotic peak systolic velocity (PSV) (**a, b**) and of the PSV ratio (intrastenotic PSV divided by prestenotic PSV) (**c, d**) with the percentage diameter reduction at angiography (graphs from Ranke et al. 1992). **a** Correlation of intrastenotic PSV and angiographic diameter reduction (%) in 106 femoral artery stenoses using a PSV cutoff of 180 cm/s for >50% stenosis (correlation $r = 0.81$). **b** Linear regression analysis of percentage diameter stenosis calculated from PSV versus angiographic diameter stenosis. **c** The PSV ratio (PVR) correlates better with angiographic diameter reduction ($r = 0.93$) because it is less susceptible to variations in systemic factors (systolic blood pressure) or other effects such as vessel wall elasticity. According to this analysis, the best results were achieved using a PSV ratio cutoff of 2.4, which identified >50% stenosis with 87% sensitivity and 94% specificity. **d** Linear regression analysis of percentage diameter reduction calculated from the PSV ratio (PVR) versus angiographic diameter reduction

It is not surprising that two imaging modalities based on different principles yield discrepant results. Angiography (but also IA DSA and X-ray densitometry) is primarily based on morphologic features, while duplex ultrasound assesses the hemodynamic significance of a stenosis. In addition to the limitations already mentioned, other drawbacks include that angiograms depict only the perfused lumen and not the vessel wall and that the angiogram reduces the three-dimensional lumen to the two dimensions of the film. Specific drawbacks in the iliofemoral territory include limited evaluability of the femoral bifurcation due to superposition and underestimation of stenosis caused by posterior wall plaque, which is common at the pelvic level and in the femoral bifurcation and is difficult to assess on anteroposterior views (see Figs. 5.27, 5.14, and 2.55 (Atlas)). Despite its limitations, however selective angiography continues to be the gold standard against which new methods are evaluated.

2.1.6.1.9 Profunda Femoris Artery

Absolute peak systolic velocity (PSV) thresholds of 180 cm/s or greater have been proposed for stenosis grading in arterial bifurcations (e.g., origin of profunda femoris artery) (Fig. 2.19), where the more reliable PSV ratio with focal doubling of intrastenotic PSV relative to prestenotic PSV does not apply

2

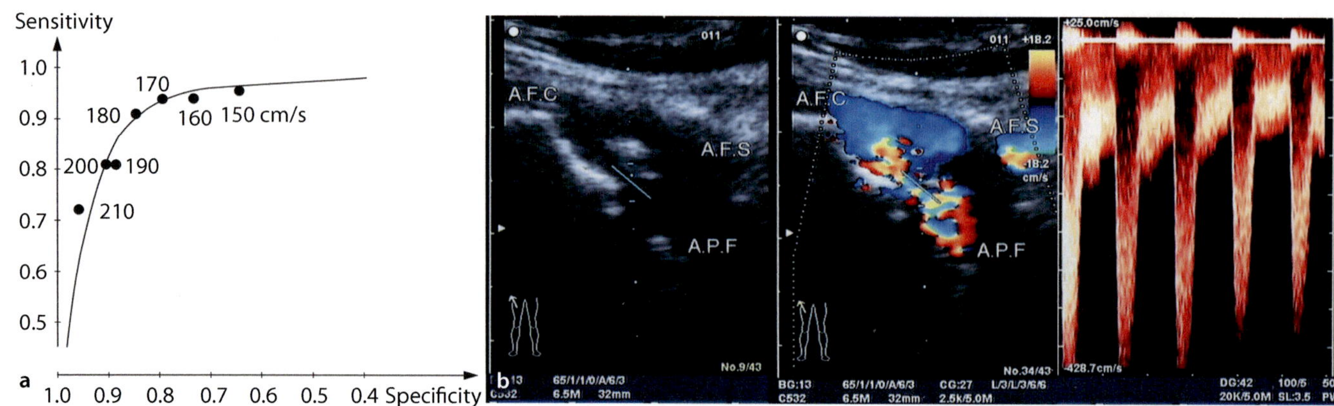

Fig. 2.19 **a** Profunda femoris artery stenosis: ROC curve for determining the sensitivity and specificity of different intrastenotic peak systolic velocity (PSV) cutoffs in the profunda femoris artery measured by duplex ultrasound in comparison with angiography. **b** Stenosis at the profunda femoris origin is suggested by aliasing in the color flow image and confirmed by spectral Doppler interrogation (monophasic flow with a PSV of 403 cm/s). The gray-scale and color flow images show the femoral bifurcation with the common femoral artery (A.F.C), superficial femoral artery (A.F.S), and profunda femoris artery (A.P.F) in one scan plane. While evaluation of the superficial femoral artery is impaired by acoustic shadowing due to plaque, presence of a second stenosis in this artery is suggested by aliasing (blue indicates flow away from the transducer, toward the periphery)

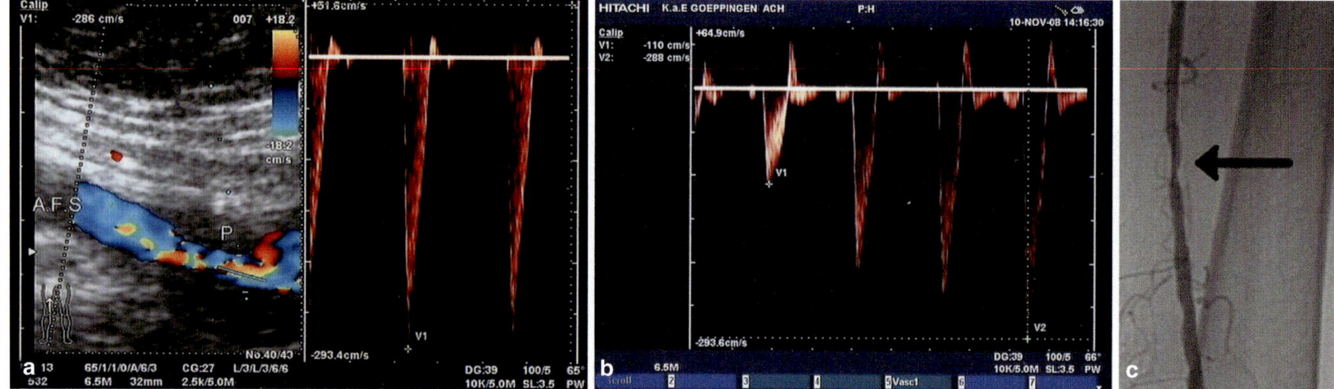

Fig. 2.20a–c Grading of superficial femoral artery stenosis. **a** Hypoechoic plaque (P) causes 50–70% stenosis of the superficial femoral artery. Spectral Doppler measurement yields an intrastenotic peak systolic velocity (PSV) of 290 cm/s (sample volume placed in the stenotic jet identified by aliasing in the color flow image). **b** A continuous Doppler tracing was obtained from the superficial femoral artery (A.F.S.) by moving the tilted transducer (acute Doppler angle) across the skin starting 2 cm proximal to the stenosis. This Doppler tracing yields a PSV of 290 cm/s in the stenotic jet versus 110 cm/s in the prestenotic segment. The PSV ratio calculated from these values (intrastenotic to prestenotic PSV) is greater than 2 but less than 4, indicating 50–70% stenosis. The stenosis is not a high-grade stenosis, which is why the Doppler waveform shows normal triphasic flow (no arteriolar dilatation and hence adequate peripheral perfusion). **c** Angiogram confirms 50–70% stenosis

(▶ Sect. 1.2.3). The indirect signs of hemodynamically relevant stenosis (pre- and poststenotic waveform changes) discussed above (▶ Sect. 2.1.6.1.4) can be used as supplementary criteria.

The **main trunk of the profunda femoris artery** is of particular significance in the diagnostic evaluation of patients with steno-occlusive disease of the superficial femoral artery, for several reasons: it is the most important collateral and concomitant profunda femoris involvement is common. At the same time, blood supply to the calf and foot can be improved by a minor surgical intervention (profunda femoris repair, TEA). Stenotic lesions at the **origin of the profunda femoris artery** are therefore important to identify but may be obscured on angiograms by superimposed vessels. Reliable angiographic assessment is only possible when an additional oblique projection is obtained (◻ Fig. 2.20).

A study conducted by the author's group (Strauss and Schäberle 1988) investiged the hemodynamics at the origin of the profunda femoris with determination of the degree of stenosis from PSV and found a positive predictive value (PPV) and a negative predictive value (NPV) of 86% and 91%, respectively, compared with angiography as the reference method. ROC analysis identified a PSV of 180 cm/s as the optimal cutoff for differentiating normal flow and low-grade stenosis from higher-grade stenoses (>50%) (◻ Figs. 2.20 and 2.21).

As already discussed above, interpretation of flow velocities must take into account **whether the artery being examined acts as a collateral.** As the main collateral in occlusion of the superficial femoral artery, the profunda femoris may show an increase in mean flow velocity of over 100% at its origin without itself being stenosed. Moreover, flow in a

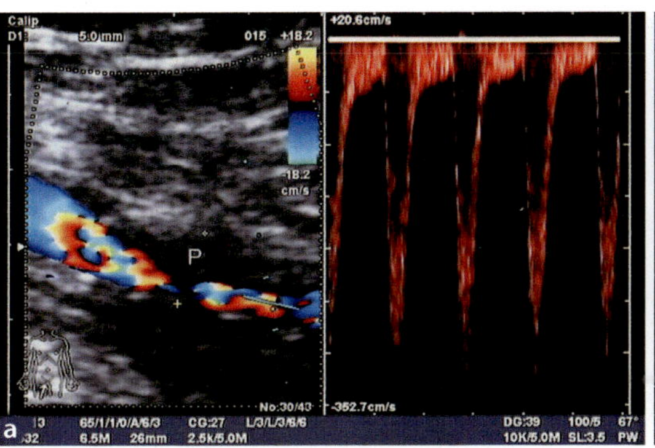

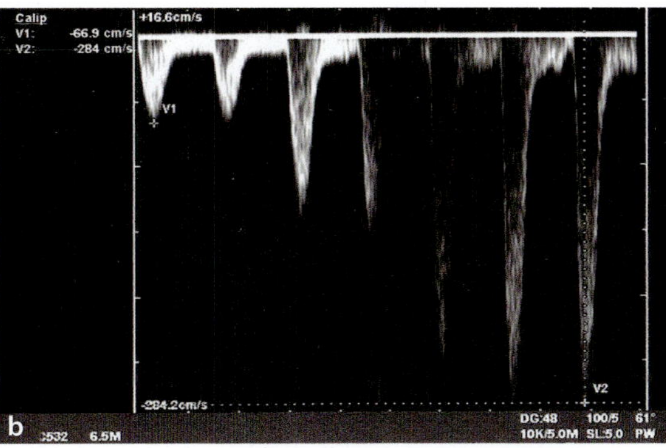

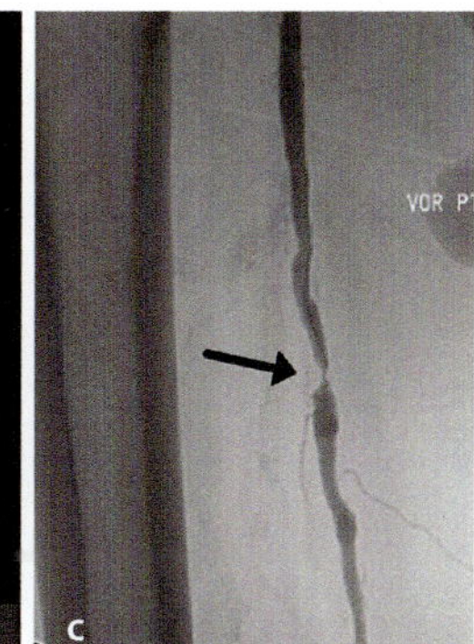

Fig. 2.21a–c Grading of high-grade stenosis. **a** Hypoechoic plaque (P) causes high-grade stenosis with a PSV of almost 4 m/s and monophasic flow. Similar constellation as in Fig. 2.20, except that the stenosis is high-grade. **b** Continuous spectral Doppler imaging as described in Fig. 2.20 reveals an increase in PSV from 60 cm/s to over 3 m/s in the stenosis, corresponding to a PSV ratio > 4, which indicates high-grade stenosis. **c** Angiogram confirms high-grade stenosis of the superficial femoral artery

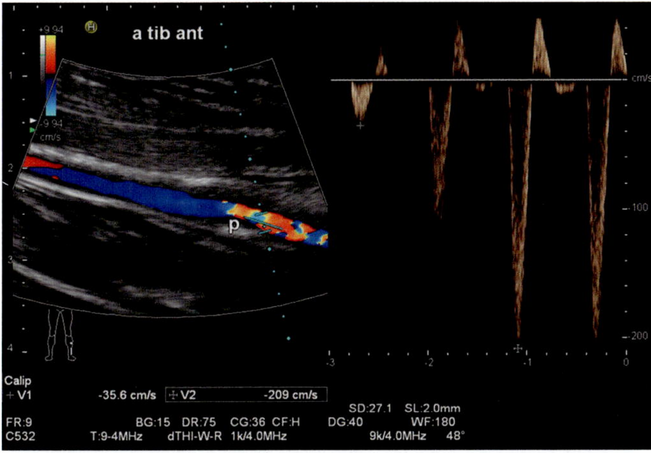

Fig. 2.22 Stenosis of the anterior tibial artery (at mid-calf level) with an intrastenotic PSV of 209 cm/s. Due to wide interindividual variation in blood flow velocities below the knee, absolute PSV is no valid criterion for stenosis grading in this territory. The PSV ratio (calculated from 209 cm/s within the stenosis (right portion of waveform) and 36 cm/s in the prestenotic segment (left portion of waveform)) is >5, corresponding to >80% stenosis

collateral artery bridging an occluded segment is less pulsatile because peripheral resistance is decreased. In this situation, only an increase in absolute PSV above a threshold (defined by comparsion with angiography) and a monophasic flow profile are valid criteria for diagnosing a stenosis.

2.1.6.1.10 Spectral Doppler Imaging below the Knee

Normal peak systolic velocity (PSV) decreases as one progresses down the leg (Table 2.5), and there is wide interindividual variation in PSV in the arteries below the knee. This is why no absolute PSV cutoffs for diagnosing hemodynamically relevant stenosis (>50%) or higher-grade stenosis in this segment have been identified by ROC analysis. Instead, intrastenotic-to-prestenotic PSV ratios should be calculated for stenosis grading below the knee (Fig. 2.22).

The site of occlusion in a below-knee artery can be narrowed down by analyzing and comparing Doppler waveforms from the proximal and distal segments (e.g., tibiofibular trunk or proximal anterior tibial artery and main artery at ankle level; see Figs. 2.68 and 2.69 (both Atlas)). Use of the indirect stenosis criteria discussed above can also facilitate and shorten the sonographic examination of the **calf arteries, which are less amenable to ultrasound evaluation**. The search for steno-occlusive lesions or the evaluation of potential bypass targets below the knee begins with a Doppler interrogation of the dorsalis pedis and posterior tibial arteries. The Doppler waveforms from these sites are compared with a waveform from the popliteal artery. The examiner then proceeds to obtain Doppler waveforms from the proximal calf arteries for comparison with the waveforms from the ankle area to narrow down sites of obstruction. Finally, if relevant for treatment planning, the examiner can try and localize individual lesions (stenosis or occlusion). If the calf arteries are examined to identify the site of distal anastomosis for a crural bypass graft once occlusive disease of the popliteal artery and trifurcation has been confirmed, the examiner first identifies the artery with the highest blood flow in the ankle area. This artery is then continuously scanned from the ankle upward using low-flow settings to detect the slow flow in the calf arteries (similar to venous flow), searching for lesions that might preclude its use as a bypass target and identifying the most suitable site for the distal anastomosis. At the same time, the candidate artery is screened for a greater than 100% increase in PSV, which indicates a hemodynamically relevant stenosis (Fig. 2.24), even in vessel segments distal to an occlusion, possibly rendering it unsuitable for use as a bypass target.

Ultrasound examination of the arteries below the knee is limited in patients with extensive atherosclerotic disease or longstanding diabetes with severe medial sclerosis. In these patients, calcified lesions may produce acoustic shadowing, precluding long segments of the arteries from being evaluated for the presence of stenosis or occlusion. When acoustic shadowing occurs, stenosis grading becomes inaccurate and the length of an occluded segment can be misinterpreted. Acoustic shadowing is a problem that cannot be overcome by the use of ultrasound contrast agents. Good knowledge of the

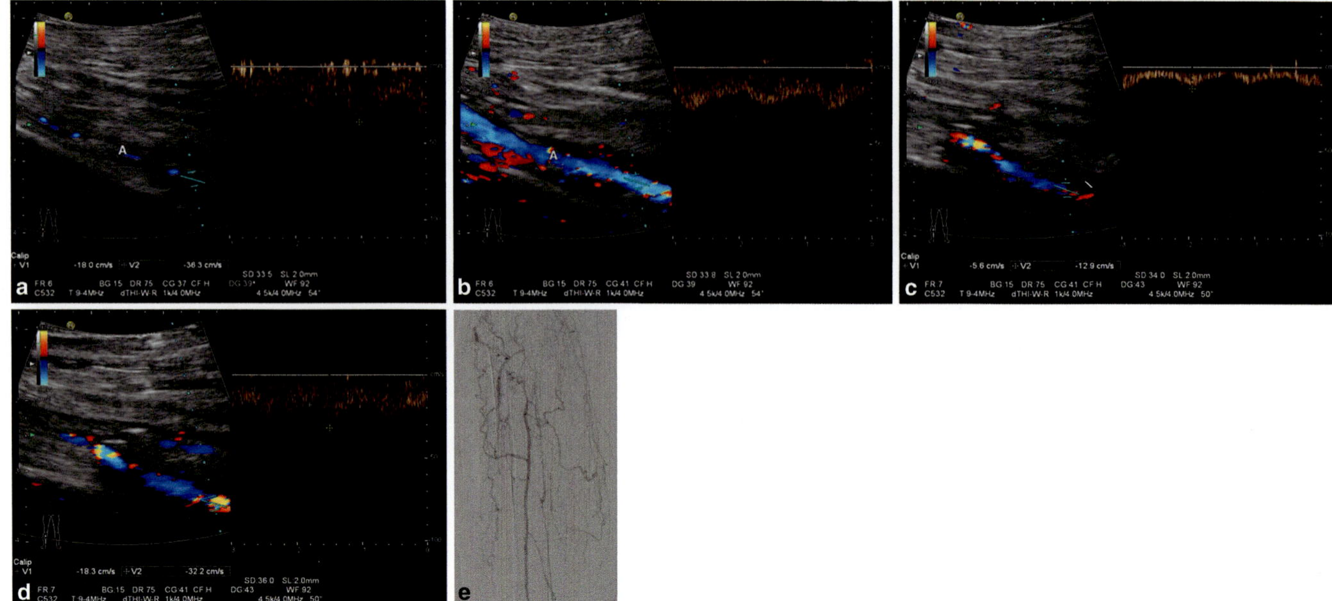

Fig. 2.23 **a** Sonographic examination of the fibular artery in a patient with a long history of diabetes mellitus and popliteal artery occlusion. Hardly any flow signals are apparent in the color flow image (despite adequate PRF and gain settings). In such a situation, it is often possible to demonstrate flow in a spectral tracing recorded with higher gain; in the example the waveform shows postocclusive flow. It is also helpful to overmodulate receive gain (artifacts in waveform). **b** Color flow image (nearly identical view) after echo enhancer administration shows flow almost throughout the artery. Contrast-enhanced ultrasound (CEUS) with a low mechanical index (MI) is not helpful because even simultaneous B-mode imaging often fails to provide adequate resolution for sonoanatomic identification of the arteries below the knee (see Figs. 2.70 (Atlas), 5.19, and 5.59 (Atlas)). Therefore, it is recommended to perform CEUS using the conventional color duplex mode (without lowering transmit gain). Great care is necessary to accurately identify the main arteries sonoanatomically and avoid the pitfall of mistaking a collateral with good color filling for a patent main artery. **c, d, e** The distal fibular artery is patent but multiple focal stenoses (with PSV ratios up to 2, consistent with <50% luminal narrowing) are noted in this segment. For illustration, the examples show an increase in PSV from 12 cm/s (**c**) to 36 cm/s (**d**), corresponding to approx. 60% stenosis. Because the distal fibular artery is imaged approx. 45 s after injection of the echo enhancer (and the microbubbles are rapidly destroyed due to the use of normal transmit gain), the enhancing effect is already fading and there is poorer color filling. Overall, the examination reveals no higher-grade stenosis, suggesting that the fibular artery is a suitable recipient vessel for a bypass graft. A stenosis below the knee identified by CEUS can be graded using the PSV ratio. In the case presented here, the angiogram (**e**) confirms the fibular artery to be the only patent major artery below the knee and to be suitable to receive a bypass graft. Color duplex ultrasound often allows better stenosis grading based on the PSV ratio than survey angiograms based on morphology (which tend to be degraded by poor opacification distal to an occlusion)

sonoanatomy of the calf vessels is important to accurately assess vascular disease in this territory and to minimize the risk of misinterpretation that may result from mistaking a collateral for a main calf artery.

2.1.6.1.11 Role of Contrast-Enhanced Ultrasound

Contrast-enhanced ultrasound (CEUS) of the peripheral arteries may be helpful in patients with poor insonation conditions or for better detection of slow-flow or low-flow states. An example is the evaluation of the arteries below the knee to search for additional steno-occlusive lesions in patients with proximal occlusion, which may be indicated to identify a patent crural or pedal target artery for bypass grafting. A full CEUS evaluation of the arteries below the knee may require repeated injection or continuous infusion of contrast microbubbles to ensure adequate enhancement throughout the examination. This is necessary because the image quality of B-mode imaging with low mechanical index (MI), which is normally used for CEUS to delay destruction of the microbubbles, is too poor for this vascular territory. Performing CEUS with standard power output (▶ Sects. 1.1.5 and 6.1.2.1.2; Fig. 2.70 (Atlas)) requires repeated administration of smaller doses to compensate for rapid microbubble desctruction (Fig. 2.23b, c). Injection of a larger dose or first-pass imaging does not overcome this problem because it is associated with color blooming, which obscures the vessel wall. Shortly after injection, dilution of the microbubbles results in good color filling of the lumen. Conversely, if the dose is too low, there will be poor color filling of the patent lumen.

Few scientific data are available on how contrast agents can improve the sonographic diagnosis. In a small study of 14 patients, Ubbink et al. (2002) found diagnostic confidence to increase from 56% to 91% after contrast administration compared with standard color duplex ultrasound in **postocclusive below-knee arteries** (poor visibility, slow flow, low flow) (Fig. 2.23). In a multicenter study including a total of 82 patients (Sidhu et al. 2006), the percentage of poorly visualized vascular segments was found to decrease from 40.7% to 7.4% when SonoVue was given at a dose of 2.4 mL. A subgroup analysis of agreement with different reference methods (angiography, CT angiography, magnetic resonance imaging) showed that the diagnostic accuracy of color duplex imaging increased from 30.7% to 68.9% after administration of the contrast agent. A limitation of this study is the use of different ultrasound equipment and the diversity of vascular territories investigated (ranging from carotid to peripheral arteries). The subgroups are not well defined in terms of accuracy of the method in different body regions. Most notably, it would have been desirable to have separate results for the calf arteries, as this is the only peripheral vascular territory for which a supplementary CEUS examination appears to have some justification. Using the ultrasound strategy presented above, an ultrasound contrast agent is only necessary in those cases where the standard technique fails to unequivocally identify a suitable target vessel for a planned bypass onto a calf artery. This is typically the case in long-standing diabetes mellitus with medial sclerosis, where acoustic shadowing obscures long vessel segments. However, medial sclerosis impairs CEUS evaluation as well. Overall, therefore, the use of microbubble contrast agents in patients with PAOD has not met initial expectations. In the clinical setting, CEUS is used only in very specific circumstances. The high resolution afforded by state-of-the-art ultrasound equipment allows reliable evaluation of most patients using standard color duplex imaging. And in those instances where evaluation is degraded by artifacts, the problem is rarely overcome even when using CEUS.

2.1.6.1.12 Identification of Pedal Target Artery for Bypass Grafting

Duplex ultrasound is an excellent supplement to angiography in identifying a suitable pedal artery or segment for distal bypass grafting. The arteries below the knee can be examined with a high-frequency transducer (10 MHz), providing excellent spatial resolution and making ultrasound superior to angiography in searching for a patent bypass target in this vascular territory. Poor opacification of calf and pedal arteries often limits angiographic evaluation in patients with proximal occlusion (◘ Fig. 2.71 (Atlas)). A potential bypass target artery is evaluated for plaques in the B-mode, and a spectral Doppler tracing is obtained to establish patency of the pedal arch (Hofmann et al. 2004). Only a few studies have investigated the role of duplex imaging in diabetics with primary peripheral occlusion or diabetic foot syndrome (Boström et al. 2002; Dyet et al. 2000; Schneider and Ogawa 1998). The results are difficult to compare because the patient populations investigated are very heterogeneous in terms of clinical stage and severity of macroangiopathy. What is noteworthy about these studies is that in a large proportion of patients, results for the calf arteries were inconclusive (29%), the calf arteries were not examined systematically (22%), or ultrasound failed to visualize these arteries (13%). The fibular artery, often the only patent calf artery in diabetics, was found to be the most difficult to evaluate by ultrasound.

Detection of an isolated stenosis in the plantar arch remains a problem because continuous evaluation of these arteries is not always possible. This is why duplex imaging alone cannot be used to decide whether the posterior tibial artery or the dorsalis pedis artery is more suitable to receive the bypass graft. The hope of overcoming these limitations by contrast-enhanced ultrasound (CEUS) has not been fulfilled. Ultrasound microbubbles produce excessive enhancement of collaterals (blooming effect), leading to poorer identification of the main calf arteries (Dyet et al. 2000; Ubbink et al. 2002).

2.1.6.1.13 Multilevel Obstruction

The direct stenosis criteria discussed above apply when a single stenosis or occlusion is present but may lead to misinterpretation in patients with multilevel steno-occlusive disease. The hemodynamic situation around a second, more distal stenosis is influenced by the flow effects of the upstream stenosis. The pressure drop across the more proximal stenosis results in a lower peak systolic velocity (PSV) upstream of the second stenosis, and the intrastenotic PSV in the second stenosis is lower than in an isolated stenosis causing the same degree of luminal narrowing (◘ Fig. 2.24c). Hence, the PSV of 180 cm/s proposed as a cutoff for 50% stenosis in case of isolated stenosis will underestimate the distal stenosis in patients with multiple steno-occlusive lesions.

For this reason, the only reliable way to grade the more distal stenosis in these patients is to use the PSV ratio (e.g., doubling of PSV) rather than absolute PSV (◘ Table 2.7). Study results confirm that the lower PSV at the site of more distal stenosis in limbs **with multilevel steno-occlusive disease** markedly reduces the sensitivity of duplex ultrasound using the criterion of absolute PSV (Bergamini et al. 1995), while other studies show the detection and grading accuracy to be the same for sequential and isolated stenoses when the PSV ratio is used (Sensier et al. 1996; Aly et al. 1998).

However, as noted above, stenosis grading based on the PSV ratio becomes rather unreliable for stenoses located at arterial origins, where the prestenotic segment has a different diameter and different hemodynamics.

Finally, the examiner must bear in mind that, in patients with multilevel obstruction, the poststenotic Doppler spectrum is also influenced by distal runoff. For instance, the waveform will be more pulsatile if there is high resistance due to severe obstruction distal to the sampling site (◘ Fig. 2.24a, b).

2.1.6.1.14 Arterial Occlusion

An occlusion is characterized by the absence of flow signals in color flow and spectral Doppler imaging. Note, however, that absence of flow signals may also be due to inadequate instrument settings (gain, PRF) or acoustic shadowing caused by calcified plaque (◘ Table 2.10). The problem of posterior acoustic shadowing due to calcifications in the vessel wall is mainly encountered in diabetic patients with medial sclerosis and can be overcome by comparing spectral Doppler findings upstream and downstream of the calcified segment (monophasic profile downstream of occlusion) and searching for collaterals arising upstream of the obstruction and re-entering the main artery downstream (◘ Fig. 2.25).

Duplex ultrasound allows highly accurate determination of occlusion length (◘ Fig. 2.25e). A study of our group

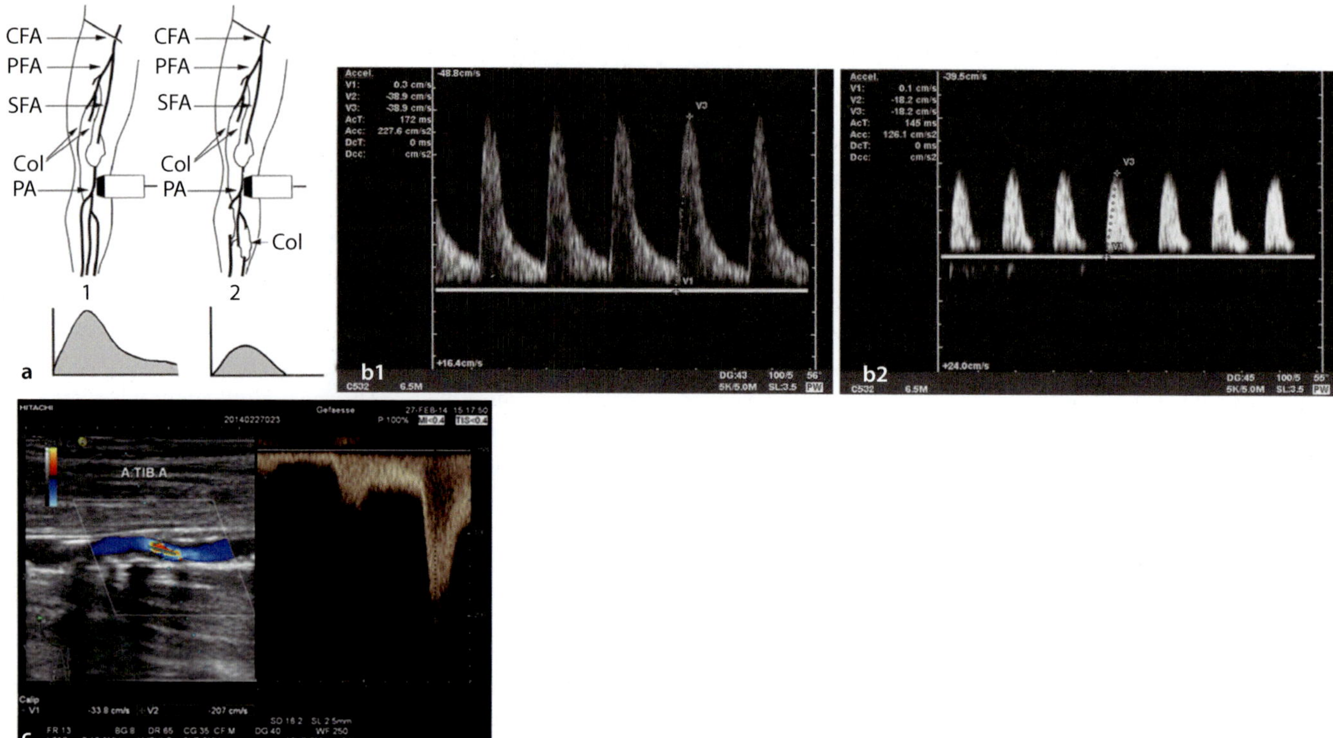

Fig. 2.24 **a** Diagrams illustrating the effects of peripheral outflow on popliteal artery spectral Doppler tracings in superficial femoral artery occlusion bridged by collaterals. When outflow is poor due to occlusion of a calf artery (right), higher outflow resistance leads to a more pulsatile postocclusive waveform; when the calf arteries are patent, peripheral widening leads to a monophasic waveform (left) (CFA, common femoral artery; PFA, profunda femoris artery; SFA, superficial femoral artery; PA, popliteal artery; Col, collaterals). **b** Illustration of the effects of differences in peripheral outflow on spectral Doppler findings in the popliteal artery in two patients with superficial femoral artery occlusion and comparable collateralization. **b1** In the first case, the calf arteries are patent and there is good peripheral outflow. There is an acceleration time of 172 ms, a peak systolic velocity (PSV) of 39 cm/s, and an end-diastolic velocity (EDV) of 8 cm/s (corresponding to left drawing in **a**). **b2** In the second case, all three calf arteries are occluded, and the foot is supplied through collaterals. Here, a knocking waveform (thump pattern) is obtained from the popliteal artery. In this case, acceleration time is 145 ms with a PSV of 18 cm/s. Flow is more pulsatile due to higher outflow resistance (corresponding to right drawing in **a**). **c** Anterior tibial artery stenosis in a patient with superficial femoral artery occlusion. The Doppler waveform (from left to right) shows a typical postocclusive pattern in the prestenotic segment (delayed systolic rise, monophasic flow, PSV of only 34 cm/s); therefore, absolute intrastenic PSV (200 cm/s) is an unreliable criterion for grading the anterior tibial artery stenosis in this patient. The PSV ratio of 8 (intrastenotic PSV of 207 cm/s divided by prestenotic PSV of 34 cm/s) corresponds to >80% stenosis

including 40 legs with femoropopliteal occlusion demonstrated 0.96 correlation between angiography and duplex ultrasound. The length of the occluded segment was less than 5 cm in 21%, 5–10 cm in 54%, and over 10 cm in 25% of cases. Pelvic artery occlusion (n = 30) was correctly identified by duplex ultrasound in all patients; however, due to the poorer insonation conditions at this level, the distal extent of the occluded segment was sometimes overestimated by several centimeters ("dead water zone"). A similar correlation (R = 0.95 in 98 extremities) between sonographic and angiographic measurement of occlusion length was reported by the authors of another study (Karasch et al. 1993).

Slow postocclusive flow may lead to **overestimation of occlusion length**, in particular when collateralization is poor. Further downstream, sonographic evaluation may improve again, as the flow situation in the main artery normalizes through re-supply via collaterals. In vascular regions difficult to evaluate by conventional sonographic methods, intravenous administration of an echo enhancer may improve detection of flowing blood (Langholz et al. 1992). In the routine clinical setting, though, contrast-enhanced ultrasound (CEUS) is rarely used for peripheral artery examinations.

A low PRF and high gain are needed to detect the slow flow downstream of an occlusion and to correctly identify the **distal end of the occluded segment**.

An occlusion, like a high-grade stenosis, influences preocclusive and postocclusive Doppler waveforms. If no color flow option is available, the examiner can approach the occluded zone by sampling spectral Doppler information at both ends. Flow signals from collaterals coursing parallel to the occluded artery may be misinterpreted as patency shortly before the refilled segment of the main artery is actually reached, giving rise to **underestimation of the length of the occluded segment**. Collaterals entering the main artery can be identified by an apparent sudden flow acceleration resulting from the different insonation angle and above all by the change in flow direction indicated by the Doppler signal (Fig. 2.25e). Once a site of origin or re-entry of a collateral has been identified, a

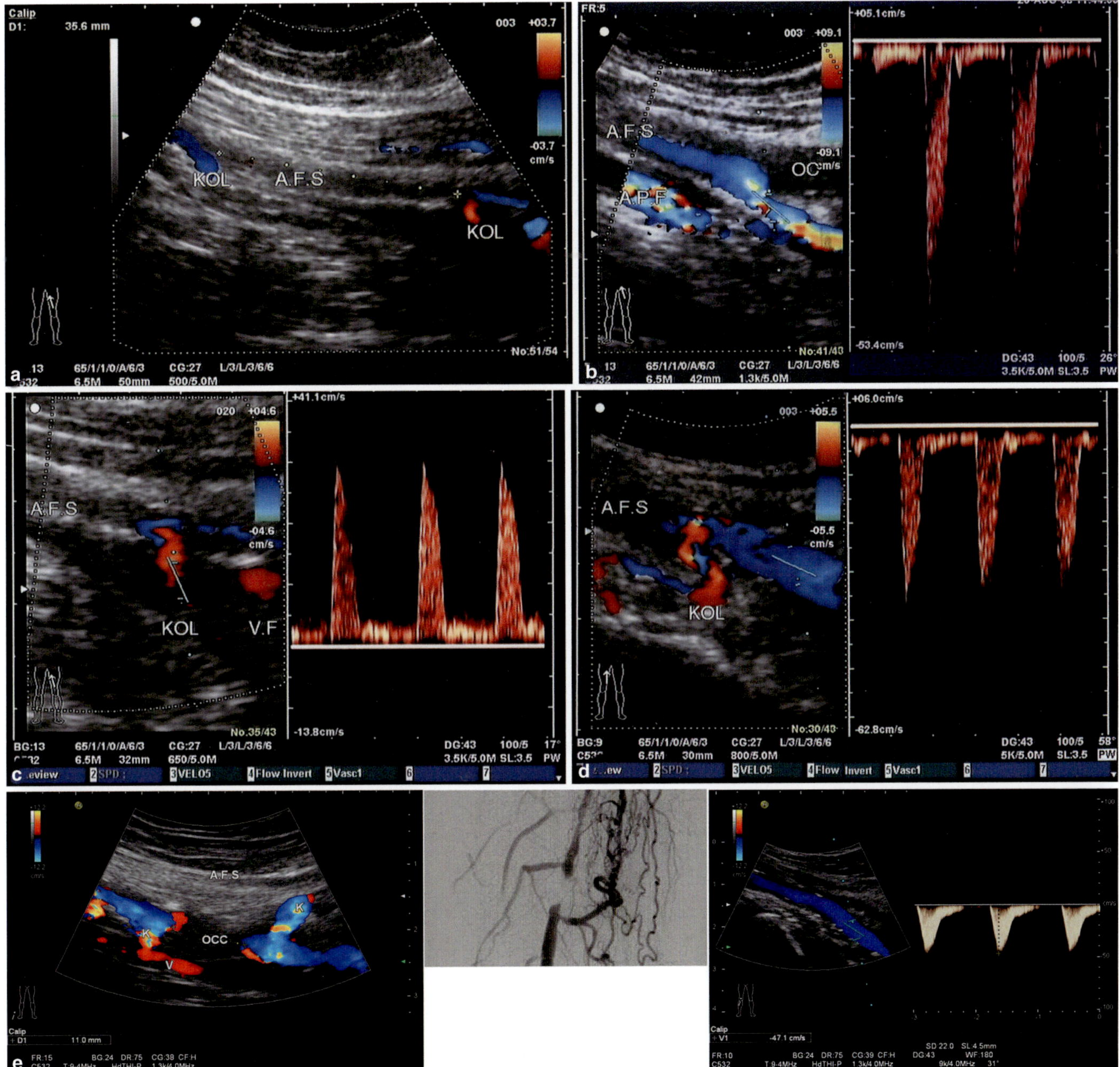

Fig. 2.25a–e Superficial femoral artery occlusion. **a** Exact determination of the length of an occluded segment is important for therapeutic decision making (PTA vs. bypass grafting). First, the length is estimated in the duplex mode using a low PRF to also detect slow flow (3.5 cm in the example shown). Supplementary evaluation for collaterals arising from or entering the main artery is recommended to confirm the measured length, especially when calcified plaques cause acoustic shadowing and impair evaluation of the main artery. The image shows a dilated collateral segment (KOL) proximal to the occlusion (blue, flow away from transducer, left part of image) and another collateral segment refilling the superficial femoral artery (red, flow toward transducer, right part of image). **b** Detailed evaluation of collaterals: the dilated collaterals indicate the beginning and end of the occluded segment (transducer moved to focus on the sites of origins of collaterals). The Doppler waveform from the origin of the collateral shows pulsatile flow with a velocity of 50 cm/s, indicating good inflow into the collateral system (aliasing in the color flow image is due to small Doppler angle and does not indicate stenosis in this case). **c** Detail showing the collateral resupplying the superficial femoral artery 3.5 cm distal to the occluded segment. Flow is toward the transducer (red) with a PSV of 30 cm/s. **d** Doppler waveform from the superficial femoral artery segment (A.F.S.) resupplied by the collateral (KOL) distal to the occluded segment. The postocclusive waveform shows rather high pulsatility with a small diastolic flow component and early diastolic decrease in flow velocity (resulting from the reflected pressure wave), a PSV of almost 40 cm/s, and a rather steep systolic upstroke, consistent with adequate compensatory collateral circulation. The good collateral flow in this case maintains nearly normal pressure in the postocclusive segment, which ensures adequate peripheral perfusion at rest without a need for arteriolar dilatation. The findings (sonographic length of occlusion) would theoretically justify an attempt at PTA (if clinically indicated), but in this case favor a conservative strategy: ultrasound indicates good collateral circulation, while the relationship between the occluded segment and the collateral resupplying the main artery distal to the occlusion suggests that there is a risk that the collateral may become occluded during PTA. **e** Different patient with short occlusion (OCC) of the superficial femoral artery. The length of the occluded segment and the collateral origins (K) exactly match the angiographic findings prior to PTA (V = femoral vein). Retrograde flow in the collateral distal to the occlusion (displayed in blue, away from transducer) refills the superficial femoral artery. The Doppler waveform from the distal popliteal artery (rightmost image) gives an estimate of the adequacy of collateralization (PSV, pulsatility)

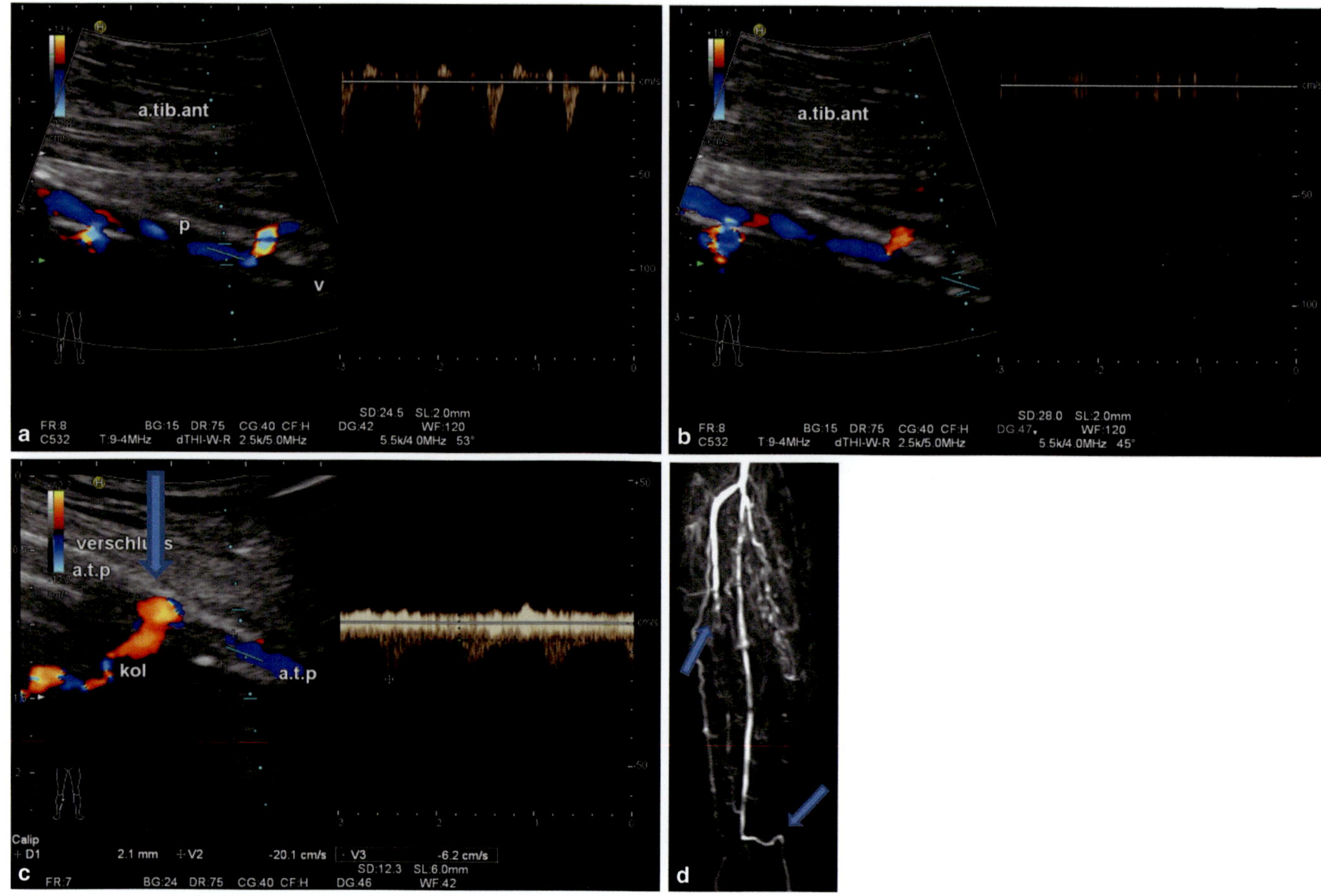

Fig. 2.26 **a, b** Occlusion of the anterior tibial artery (v in **a**) in a patient with a long history of diabetes mellitus. The Doppler waveform obtained directly upstream of the origin of the last strong collateral arising proximal to the occluded segment shows triphasic flow (compare waveform obtained with sample volume placed in the occluded segment (**b**)). **d** The MR angiogram provides an overview of the occlusions below the knee for documentation. The upper arrow indicates the proximal end of the occluded anterior tibial artery segment, the lower arrow indicates refilling of the posterior tibial artery at the ankle level (compare detail resolution of ultrasound with clear visualization of collaterals and of the plaque causing luminal narrowing). The anterior tibial artery is occluded down to the ankle level. **c** Occlusion of the posterior tibial artery (a.t.p) with refilling above the ankle level by a strong collateral (kol) (arrow). The Doppler waveform from this segment shows monophasic flow. This indirect criterion suggests upstream occlusion, which can then be confirmed by direct sonographic evaluation of the proximal segment

Doppler waveform obtained with angle correction will identify stenosis obstructing collateral flow. Spectral Doppler characterization of postocclusive flow is also important for therapeutic decision making (medical treatment or repair).

For correct interpretation and localization of steno-occlusive lesions below the knee (Fig. 2.26), it is crucial to identify the courses of the main arteries by following them downward in their sonoanatomic locations (▶ Sect. 2.1.6.1.4). In addition, the accompanying veins can be used as landmarks. This is important in order not to mistake an enlarged branch that has been recruited as a collateral for the (occluded) main artery. Ultrasound identification of segmental occlusion in this territory may be seriously degraded by medial sclerosis with acoustic shadowing in patients with a long history of diabetes mellitus. In such cases, indirect evidence of occlusion may be obtained by comparing proximal and distal waveforms.

The flow rate downstream of multilevel occlusions with poor collateralization may occasionally drop below the limit of detection of (color) duplex imaging – even when a high-resolution transducer is used and settings are adjusted. In these cases, spectral Doppler interrogation with high gain and a low PRF can often detect any residual flow that may still be present.

2.1.6.2 Arterial Embolism

Arterial embolism with ischemia is typically of cardiac origin (80–90%). The remaining cases are accounted for by arterio-arterial emboli, chiefly arising from a partially thrombosed aneurysm and rarely from an atherosclerotic lesion.

The site and length of occlusion are identified by the absence of flow signals in spectral Doppler or color duplex ultrasound. In the less common case of subtotal embolic occlusion, some residual flow will be detected along the hypoechoic thromboembolus near the wall (see Figs. 2.84 and 2.85 (both Atlas)). An embolic occlusion is suggested by the demonstration of a **hypoechoic and homogeneous mass** in the vessel lumen, **good delineation of the wall** with preservation of its smooth contour, and the absence of plaques.

Embolic occlusions typically occur at bifurcations, where the embolus creates a nidus for the formation of appositional thrombi that may extend proximally to the site of the nearest hemodynamically significant branching. Flow proximal to an occlusion is known as stump flow, which is very pulsatile with a markedly reduced peak systolic velocity (PSV), giving rise to a knocking waveform. Any residual flow along a thrombus is typically also relatively slow. A hemodynamic pattern similar to that caused by stenosis, with high PSV, may be seen when the thrombus is short. The distal end of the occlusion is identified using a low PRF and high gain in order not to miss the slow flow in the postembolic segment (due to poor collateralization). In addition to identifying and characterizing the embolic occlusion, **searching for the source of the embolus** (◘ Fig. 2.27) is an integral part of the examination (echocardiography, duplex ultrasound of the aorta and peripheral arteries). In the peripheral arteries, the search should focus on a possible popliteal artery aneurysm.

2.1.6.3 Aneurysm

2.1.6.3.1 True Aneurysm

An aneurysm is an abnormal, local dilatation of an artery to at least twice its normal diameter. The most commonly affected arteries are the abdominal aorta and the popliteal artery. Popliteal aneurysms account for 85% of all peripheral artery aneurysms and are found in up to 1% of men aged 65 to 80 (Trickett et al. 2002). They are bilateral in 53% of cases, and 14% of patients have a concomitant aortic aneurysm (Diwan et al. 2000). Peripheral aneurysms of the femoral and iliac arteries are predominantly seen in patients with dilated angiopathy (Schuler et al. 1993). An aneurysm is identified **on transverse gray-scale images** as a **saccular or spindle-shaped dilatation** of the vessel lumen. **Mural thrombi** in the aneurysm are often apparent through their slightly higher echogenicity relative to flowing blood and are confirmed by **the absence of color flow**. Thrombotic deposits can cause stenosis, in particular when they occur at the distal end of an aneurysm. Absence of flow signals suggests a completely thrombosed aneurysm. Angiography is not the method of reference for assessing a partially thrombosed aneurysm while computed tomography (CT) depicts the morphology and extent of an aneurysm but provides no hemodynamic information. Patients with an isolated occlusion in the popliteal territory should undergo an ultrasound examination to rule out a thrombosed aneurysm or vascular compression syndrome prior to a radiologic intervention.

Popliteal artery aneurysms can occlude or rupture. A popliteal aneurysm containing thrombotic deposits can cause embolic occlusion of peripheral vessels, which in the worst case may lead to limb amputation.

Surgery is indicated when the diameter of the aneurysm exceeds 2 cm (Robinson and Belkin 2009; Michaels and Galland 1993) and also for smaller ones when they are saccular or contain thrombotic deposits (◘ Fig. 2.27). This is because thrombotic aneurysms in the knee area are exposed to greater shear stress when the knee is bent and therefore have a higher risk of embolism even when they are small. While, in general, popliteal artery aneurysms <2 cm are managed conservatively and monitored, 18–35% become symptomatic and may require surgery even before they reach a size of 2 cm.

Overall, in patients with popliteal artery aneurysm, the risk of rupture is less relevant than the risk of peripheral embolism arising from thrombus, and diameter is not the main criterion in identifying candidates for surgical repair. Detection of **mural thrombus** is thus the primary diagnostic task in these patients. Even a small popliteal artery aneurysm should be operated on if partial mural thrombosis is demonstrated (◘ Fig. 2.27c, d).

Duplex ultrasound is the method of choice, yielding reliable information on the diameter of the aneurysm, its shape, and the presence of thrombosis (see ◘ Figs. 2.87 (Atlas) and 2.27). This information allows identification of surgical candidates and planning the surgical procedure. An aneurysm is superficial and can be examined with a high-resolution transducer. The diameter is measured, and thrombotic material in the lumen is identified (absence of color flow) in transverse orientation, while the shape is assessed in the longitudinal plane.

2.1.6.3.2 Pseudoaneurysm

A pseudoaneurysm (also known as false aneurysm) is an encapsulated extravascular collection of blood that communicates with the feeding artery through a hole in the arterial wall. It is a typical complication of arterial puncture performed for diagnostic angiography or interventional procedures and is observed in up to 6% of individuals undergoing percutaneous transluminal angioplasty (PTA) or cardiac catheterization. The incidence of this complication depends on various factors, including the diameter of the catheter and introducer sheath used, periprocedural anticoagulation, obesity, puncture-related problems, and inadequate compression (Hust and Schuler 1992; Moll et al. 1991; Corriere and Guzman 2005). A suture aneurysm is a pseudoaneurysm developing after vascular surgery, in particular after bypass operations. Other operations near the poplitel artery such as arthroscopic meniscal surgery can also damage the arterial wall and thus give rise to a pseudoaneurysm (Schäberle et al. 1995).

Pseudoaneurysms must be differentiated from perivascular hematoma with transmitted pulsation (see ◘ Fig. 2.79 (Atlas)), but this is difficult on clinical grounds (Thomas et al. 1989). With duplex ultrasound, a pseudoaneurysm can be differentiated from hypoechoic, perivascular structures such as hematoma, seroma, or lymphocele by the demonstration of the characteristic to-and-fro flow pattern (◘ Fig. 2.28a, b). This finding is pathognomonic and requires no angiographic confirmation. To-and-fro flow occurs in the neck of a pseudoaneurysm due to changing pressures: intraluminal pressure is high during systole, and blood flows through the narrow neck into the aneurysm at a rather high velocity. Under the reversed pressure conditions during diastole, the blood flows back into the feeding artery at a slightly lower flow rate. Reflux is typically turbulent.

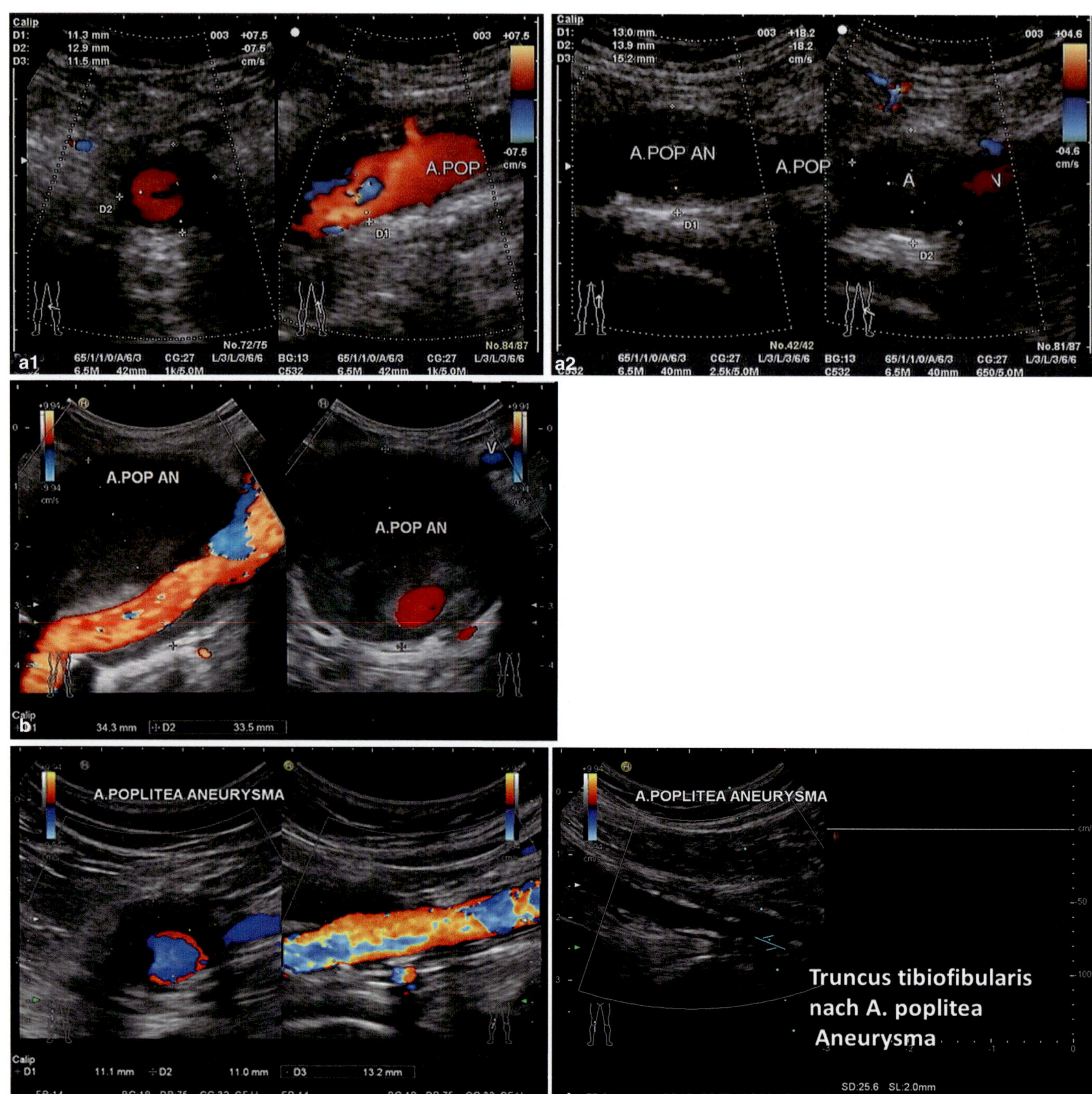

Fig. 2.27 **a** Serial ultrasound of small popliteal artery aneurysm. **a1** Small, partially thrombosed aneurysm of the popliteal artery with a maximum diameter of 13 mm. When thrombus is present, even a small aneurysm like this can cause embolism with occlusion of a lower leg artery (due to shear stress and kinking of the artery when the knee is bent). For this reason, surgical repair is indicated. Color duplex imaging with a low PRF allows good delineation of the patent lumen in transverse and longitudinal planes. Calipers indicate the total luminal diameter. **a2** Same popliteal artery aneurysm 6 months later (patient refused surgery). There is a slight increase in aneurysmal diameter to 15 mm, and complete thrombosis of the aneurysm (A.POP.AN) and trifurcation has occurred. The longitudinal image (left) shows the transition from the normal arterial lumen to the aneurysm. **b** Large popliteal artery aneurysm (diameter of 3.4 cm). The aneurysm is thrombosed except for the width of the normal popliteal artery lumen (A.POP AN). This aneurysm would escape angiographic detection. The aneurysm compresses and displaces the popliteal vein (V). There is a clear indication for surgical repair in this case. **c, d** Small popliteal artery aneurysm (maximum diameter of 13 mm), again with partial thrombosis except for the width of the normal arterial lumen, shown in transverse and longitudinal orientation (**c**). The aneurysm is the cause of embolic occlusion of the tibiofibular trunk in this patient (**d**). More proximally, the origin of the anterior tibial artery is patent (not shown)

Peripheral pseudoaneurysms have traditionally been treated surgically. An alternative treatment is ultrasound-guided compression of the neck to induce clotting of the aneurysm. This alternative option has become possible because ultrasound enables very precise localization of the aneurysm neck relative to the skin surface (Fellmeth et al. 1991; Hust et al. 1993).

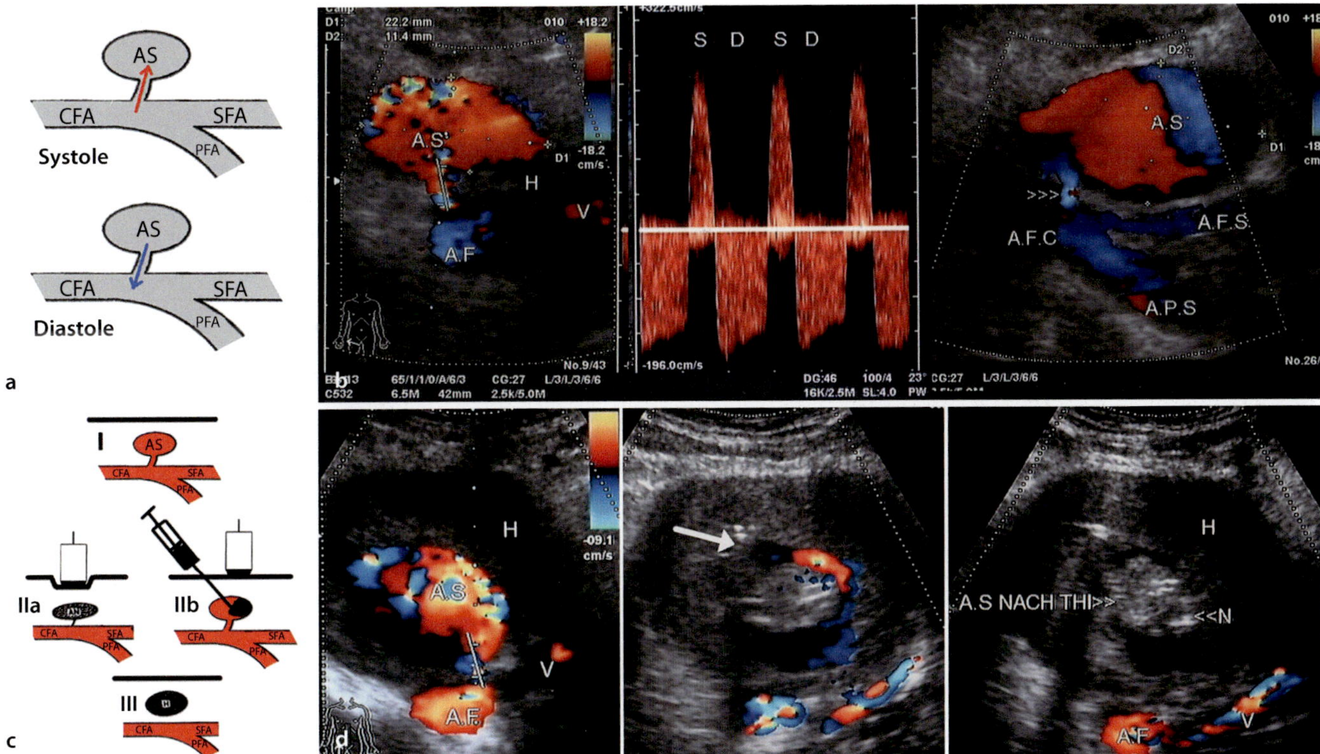

Fig. 2.28a–d Pseudoaneurysm or false aneurysm. **a** Diagrams illustrating blood flow in the neck of a pseudoaneurysm. The alternating flow directions result from blood entering the aneurysm sac (AS) during systole and flowing back into the feeding artery during diastole (CFA, common femoral artery; SFA, superficial femoral artery; PFA, profunda femoris artery). **b** Pseudoaneurysm measuring 22 × 11 mm. The left image shows blood flow during systole (sample volume in the neck). Blood flow is toward the transducer (red). In addition, there is aliasing. The right image (longitudinal view) shows the situation during diastole (aneurysm neck indicated by arrowheads). Flow is away from the transducer (blue). The spectral waveform from the aneurysm neck shows high-frequency inflow of blood during systole (2.5 m/s) and pandiastolic flow (D) from the aneurysm sac (below the baseline, away from transducer). (A.F.C. = common femoral artery; A.F.S. = superficial femoral artery; A.P.F = profunda femoris artery; V = femoral vein; H = hematoma). **c** Illustration of ultrasound-guided compression of the aneurysm neck (IIa) and ultrasound-guided thrombin injection (IIb). These two ultrasound-based techniques have now largely replaced surgical repair, which has become the exception. Pressure is applied with the transducer under real-time monitoring until complete or nearly complete hemostasis has occurred (indicated by absence or near absence of flow signals), which may take 10–45 min. If residual flow persists in the aneurysm, a compression bandage will usually lead to complete thrombosis by the next day. For thrombin injection treatment (IIb), a needle is advanced into the lateral third of the aneurysm for dropwise thrombin injection (5000 IU in 2–5 mL saline solution), both under ultrasound guidance. Fast injection and needle placement near the neck must be avoided to minimize the risk of thrombin spilling into the arterial circulation. **d** Treatment of pseudoaneurysm by thrombin injection. The color duplex image (left) depicts flow in a pseudoaneurysm arising from the femoral artery (A.F.). The aneurysm is surrounded by hematoma (H) (sample volume in aneurysm neck). The next image shows nearly complete thrombosis of the aneurysm after injection of 2000 IU thrombin (in 2 mL saline solution) following ultrasound-guided insertion of the needle (bright echo in the left portion of the aneurysm, indicated by arrow). The final image (right) shows the situation after repositioning of the needle (N) and injection of a second, small amount of thrombin: complete hemostasis of the aneurysm is indicated by the cessation of color flow within the sac. Patent femoral artery (A.F.) and vein (V) posterior to the aneurysm

Thrombosis occurs after 10–30 min of compression with the transducer (see Fig. 2.94 (Atlas)).

Published studies on ultrasound-guided compression treatment of pseudoaneurysm (Krumme et al. 1995; Lange et al. 2001) report success rates of 66–86% after compression for an average of 30–44 min (Coley et al. 1995) and a recurrence rate of 4%. Compression treatment fails in most patients on anticoagulation treatment. In contrast, **ultrasound-guided thrombin injection** for induction of thrombosis has success rates of 93–100% (3% recurrence rate) and is also successful in most patients on anticoagulation treatment (Table 2.11; Vicente and Kazmers 1999;

Table 2.11 Ultrasound-guided diagnostic and therapeutic vascular interventions

Pathology	Interventional treatment/measure
Pseudoaneurysm (typically iatrogenic)	Compression of aneurysm neck Thrombin injection
Postoperative fluid collection around grafts	Ultrasound-guided puncture for diagnosis and possibly treatment: infection, abscess, seroma, lymphocele, graft reaction?

Wixon et al. 2000; Corriere and Guzman 2005). Thrombin treatment of pseudoaneuryms has a complication rate of up to 4%. The most dreaded complication is severe limb ischemia due to distal thrombin migration (up to 2%), which may even result in amputation of the affected limb. Inadvertent occlusion of a distal artery during thrombin treatment requires immediate heparin administration and prompt initiation of intra-arterial thrombolytic treatment. The risk of thrombin migration can be minimized by a meticulous technique with slow instillation of the highly concentrated thrombin solution (e.g., 5000 IU in 5 mL) starting in the periphery of the aneurysm sac.

Sonographically, the neck of a pseudoaneurysm is identified by spectral Doppler interrogation, which will demonstrate forward and reverse flow components as blood enters the aneurysm during systole and exits during diastole. This to-and-fro flow pattern causes a characteristic audible Doppler signal (steam engine sound). Although ultrasound is impaired by hematoma and scattering due to edema, the needle for thrombin instillation can be reliably placed because it is easily recognized by its high echogenicity within the hypoechoic or anechoic pseudoaneurysm. Rapidly moving the needle tip back and forth will help in locating the needle and checking for correct positioning. Injection results in instantaneous thrombosis around the needle tip and, if the solution is injected slowly, will prevent escape of thrombin into the bloodstream. Spilling into distal arteries can occur only if the needle is mistakenly placed in the neck or if thrombin is injected as a bolus. Case reports exist of thromboembolic complications with severe limb ischemia finally resulting in amputation. Some authors therefore recommend starting injection near the wall; however, areas near the neck will thrombose spontaneously once the aneurysmal sac has been obliterated.

Thrombin injection has the advantage of rapidly inducing hemostasis, while compression therapy is less expensive and has the added benefit of reducing the aneurysm volume, leaving a smaller hematoma that produces less swelling and pressure (◘ Fig. 2.28c). In patients on anticoagulation or clopidogrel therapy, hemostasis can be induced by thrombin injection but not by compression treatment. The only pseudoaneurysms difficult to treat by thrombin injection are those with a large defect in the feeding artery and aneurysms with very turbulent, circulatory blood flow in the sac (see ◘ Figs. 2.81 and 2.79 (Atlas)), which washes away the thrombin before a clot begins to form at the needle tip.

2.1.6.4 Rare Stenosing Arterial Diseases of Nonatherosclerotic Origin

The popliteal artery is a common site not only of atherosclerotic stenosis and occlusion or embolism but also of rare vascular disorders, in particular compression syndromes. Nonatherosclerotic vascular conditions include:

- Embolism
- Aneurysm
- Intimal dissection
- Arteritis
- Vessel wall tumor
- Vascular compression syndrome (entrapment syndrome)
- Adventitial cystic disease

◘ Table 2.12 Duplex ultrasound in nonatherosclerotic vascular disease

Ultrasound technique	Structures that can be evaluated/ Findings
B-scan (morphology)	Vessel lumen (thrombotic deposits) Vessel wall (cysts, concentric inflammatory wall thickening; differential diagnosis: plaques) Perivascular structures (external compression)
Doppler (hemodynamics)	Stenosis (hemodynamic significance of narrowing caused by perivascular or mural structures) Functional test (plantar flexion: increase in stenosis severity) Occlusion (collaterals)

Antiography or venography (the traditional gold standards) may be limited in identifying the cause of vascular compression (see ◘ Figs. 2.91, 2.92, 2.93, 2.94, and 2.95 (all Atlas)), especially when occlusion has already occurred.

(Color) duplex imaging provides information on the degree and hemodynamic relevance of luminal narrowing and enables evaluation of the vessel wall and perivascular structures, thus allowing identification of the underlying cause in patients with nonatherosclerotic vascular disease (◘ Table 2.12).

Suspected compression of an artery by muscular structures (entrapment syndrome) can be confirmed by functional tests, and its hemodynamic significance can be determined by spectral Doppler (see ◘ Figs. 2.31, 2.94 (Atlas), and 2.95 (Atlas)). In addition, duplex imaging can identify vascular complications of compression such as development of mural thrombosis or postocclusive aneurysm and occlusion.

Many nonatherosclerotic conditions **predominantly affect the popliteal artery**, owing to its close proximity to the joint and muscles in the popliteal fossa. Duplex ultrasound should be the first-line modality to search for the underlying cause and initiate proper therapeutic management in patients with isolated popliteal artery occlusion (angiography or magnetic resonance angiography). One possible cause is complete thrombosis of an aneurysm. The popliteal artery is the second most common site of aneurysm after the aorta. In a study of 1190 patients with stage II–IV PAOD according to Fontaine, angiography demonstrated isolated popliteal artery occlusion in 51 patients.

The subsequent ultrasound examination of these popliteal occlusions identified atherosclerotic changes with severe plaque as the **cause of occlusion** in 47% of cases. Embolic occlusion was sonographically diagnosed in 21.5% and was characterized by a fairly homogeneous content of the occluded lumen and good delineation of the wall without major plaque. Thrombotic aneurysms accounted for 27.5% of the isolated popliteal artery occlusions and an entrapment syndrome for the remaining 4%.

The differential diagnosis includes advential cystic disease and entrapment syndrome. Advential cystic disease has an incidence of 1 per 1200 to 2000 patients presenting with intermittent claudication (Choschzick et al. 1997) but rarely causes popliteal artery occlusion. A similar incidence is reported for entrapment syndrome.

Our analysis of 12,500 duplex ultrasound examinations of the popliteal fossa (1993–2004) in patients with typical symptoms of PAOD identified the following rare vascular conditions:

- Entrapment syndrome: 12 patients (0.1%), including:
  - Occlusion of the popliteal artery: four patients, among them three with malformation of the medial head of the gastrocnemius muscle or popliteal artery (Insua I) and one with poststenotic aneurysm and additional compression of the popliteal vein due to atypical attachment of the popliteal muscle
  - Compression and stenosis of the popliteal artery during plantar flexion: seven patients (Insua I)
  - Compression of the popliteal artery and vein through hypertrophic heads of the gastrocnemius muscle without malformation: one patient
- Adventitial cystic disease: six patients (0.05%)
- Traumatic intimal dissection: two patients (0.02%)
- Tumor compression: one patient (0.01%)
- AV fistula of the popliteal artery (traumatic, large flow volume): one patient (0.01%)
- Large pseudoaneurysm with compression of artery and vein (iatrogenic after arthroscopic meniscal resection): one patient (0.01%)

2.1.6.4.1 Adventitial Cystic Disease

Adventitial cystic disease is a rare condition in which cystic structures in the outer wall layer of arteries close to joints (Leu et al. 1977) and very rarely of veins cause variable stenosis according to their state of filling. A total of 400 cases of adventitial cystic disease have been reported in the literature. An understanding of the etiology and pathophysiology of this rare condition is necessary to ensure adequate treatment and minimize the risk of recurrence. While various underlying mechanisms have been proposed, there appears to be agreement that adventitial cysts arise from mesenchymal cell formations dispersed to the arterial adventitia near joints during embryonic development. The most likely candidates are ectopic synovial cells, and the popliteal artery is the most commonly affected vessel. Adventitial cysts are filled with a mucinous, viscous fluid and resemble articular ganglions in terms of fluid and wall composition (Flanigan et al. 1979; Vasudevan et al. 2005; Levien and Benn 1998).

Isolated or multiple adventitial cysts can occur and they may be uniloculated or multiloculated. The **clinical manifestation and ischemic symptoms vary widely**, and occasionally there is a rapid succession of asymptomatic intervals and episodes during which the walking distance is reduced to a few meters. This pattern is due to the variable vessel compression resulting from **changes in cystic filling** (■ Fig. 2.29). As a result, there are periods during which the clinical examination is normal, and patients may have a long history before the correct diagnosis is made. An early report postulated a communication with the knee joint to explain the variable filling of adventitial cysts (Flanigan et al. 1979), and some later investigators identified a channel-like communication on imaging studies (Chiche et al. 1994; Ortmann et al. 2009) or during surgery (Tsilimparis et al. 2007; Campbell and Milliar 1985). We may assume, though, that most advential cysts do not communicate with the joint space. Ultrasonography provides direct evidence of the cysts and thus confirms the preliminary diagnosis made on the basis of the clinical presentation and/or angiographic findings. Moreover, ultrasound identifies the cysts and their variable size even during asymptomatic periods, and spectral Doppler interrogation enables precise determination of the degree of stenosis. The ultrasound findings thus provide the basis for therapeutic decision making.

In the **(color) duplex examination**, other hypoechoic lesions in the popliteal fossa **must be differentiated** from adventitial cysts by carefully evaluating their relationship to the vessel wall:

- Aneurysm of the popliteal artery (true/false)
- Hematoma, seroma, abscess
- Hemangioma
- Baker's cyst
- Dissection with thrombosis of false lumen
- Tumor
- Venous aneurysm

The typical hourglass configuration characterizing the angiographic appearance of arterial stenosis caused by an adventitial cyst may be absent or just barely visible as a subtle impression during asymptomatic periods. Therefore, a luminographic technique such as angiography is of limited diagnostic value in patients with suspected adventitial cystic disease, and other modalities including duplex ultrasound, magnetic resonance imaging (MRI), and CT angiography have higher diagnostic accuracy when this condition is suspected. With its high spatial resolution and flexibility, **duplex ultrasound is the method of choice** and is even superior to MRI (Brodmann et al. 2001; Schäberle 1996). In CT, problems may sometimes arise in differentiating adventitial cystic disease from other conditions such as popliteal artery aneurysm (Brodmann et al. 2002), arterial dissection with a thrombosed false lumen, or even atypical Baker's cysts. A very rare differential diagnosis is adventitial cystic disease of the popliteal vein (see ■ Fig. 3.96 (Atlas); Dix et al. 2006).

■ Ultrasound-Guided Treatment

Local surgical enucleation of the cysts from the arterial wall and resection of the affected arterial segment with replacement

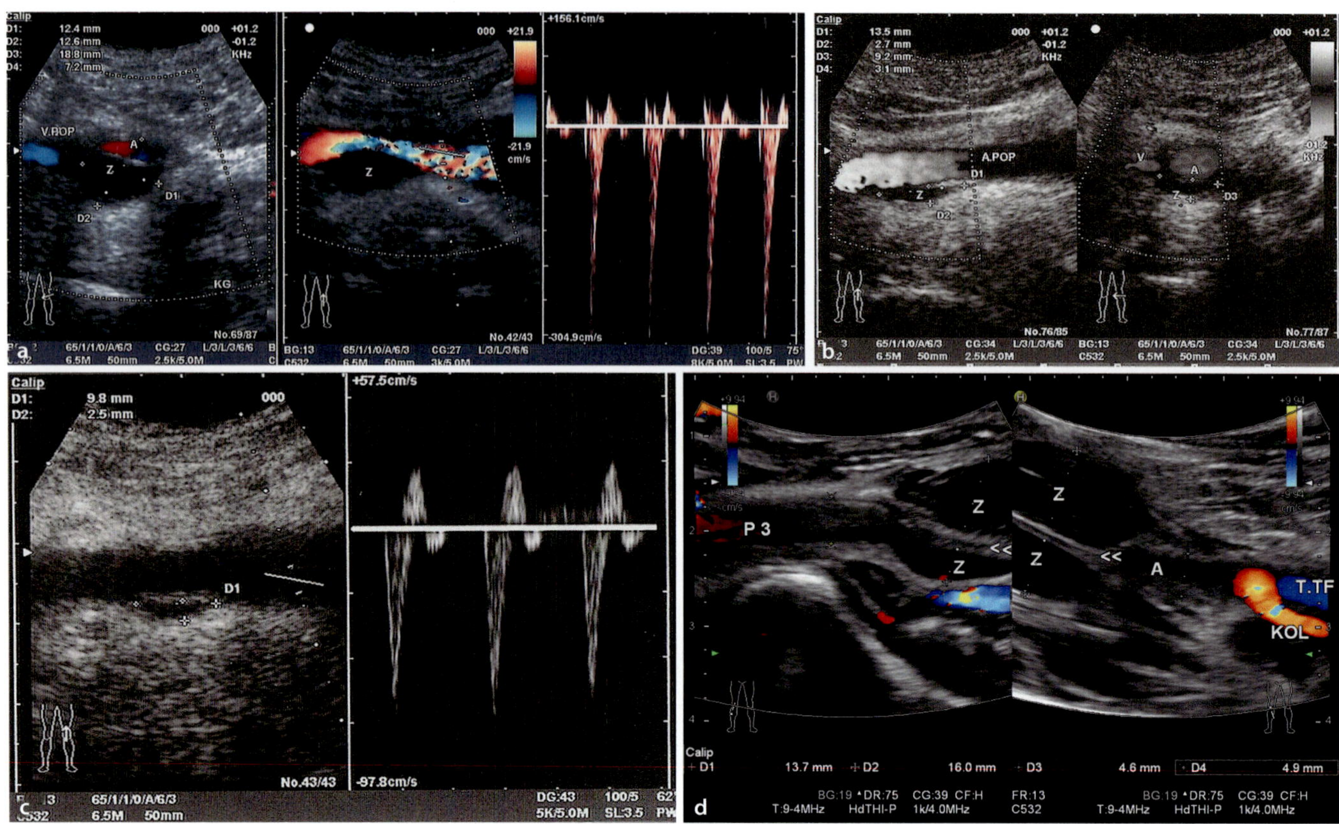

◘ **Fig. 2.29a–d** Adventitial cystic disease. **a–c** Variable cyst size. **a** This patient with intermittent claudication of variable severity due to adventitial cystic disease (Z) shows a highly variable cyst size over a period of 2 weeks. The transverse view (left) demonstrates compression of the popliteal artery with a residual lumen of 20–30%. Aliasing in the longitudinal image and a peak systolic velocity (PSV) of 3 m/s confirm stenosis due to cystic compression. **b, c** The cyst has become so small that it is easily overlooked on routine ultrasound if one is unaware of the earlier findings (**b**, longitudinal view on the left, transverse view on the right). The diameter of the cyst has decreased from 1 cm to 2.7 mm, and the arterial lumen is no longer compromised (not seen angiographically). The Doppler waveform is normal. **d** Patient with multiple adventitial cysts. The composite B-mode image shows compression of the popliteal artery (P3 segment) by multiple cysts anterior and posterior to the affected segment. The cysts cause occlusion of a 3-cm segment of the popliteal artery, indicated by absence of color flow (<<). This sonographic finding is an indication for resection of the compromised arterial segment and insertion of a venous bypass graft. The anterior tibial artery (KOL) is filled by collaterals and in turn provides collateral flow to the tibiofibular trunk (T.TF) through retrograde flow proximally

by a venous bypass graft have the best outcome with the lowest recurrence rates. There is no evidence that one is superior to the other (Tsilimparis et al. 2007; Hong et al. 2007).

Percutaneous **aspiration of the cyst fluid** guided by ultrasound or CT is **controversial**. On the one hand, aspiration is low in complications, and several authors report successful treatment without recurrence (Do et al. 1997; Colombier et al. 1997; Schäberle 1996, Schäberle et al. 2013) for follow-up periods of up to 11 years (Keo et al. 2007). On the other hand, the cyst fluid may be too viscous for aspiration (Wilbur and Spigos 1986; Cassar and Engeset 2005) or the cysts recur after initially successful aspiration (Ortiz et al. 2006; Sys et al. 1997; Holden et al. 2008; Sieunarine et al. 1991). Recurrence is not surprising considering that aspiration alone does not eliminate the postulated communication of adventitial cysts with the knee joint (Cassar and Engeset 2005). Even if the communication is obliterated or does not exist, synovial cells in the cyst wall can secrete fluid that refills the cyst.

Pretherapeutic ultrasound and other imaging modalities can help the physician select the most suitable treatment from the different options available and identify patients in whom ultrasound-guided aspiration may be justified. Enucleation without resection of the affected popliteal segment is promising only when high-frequeny ultrasound demonstrates a single cyst without signs of secondary intimal damage or even small thrombotic deposits. Otherwise, resection of the affected segment with vein graft interposition is preferable. In the author's experience, **ultrasound-guided aspiration** is promising only if the following conditions are met (Schäberle et al. 2013):

- Presence of one or at most two adventitial cysts without secondary intimal damage (thickening) of the affected arterial segment and sonographic exclusion of a communication between the cyst and the knee joint space (using a high-resolution transducer)
- Aspiration with a large needle (14 G) to maximize the chance of completely removing the cyst fluid
- Injection of a small amount of sclerosing agent (e.g., 2–3 mL of 96% ethanol) might be considered to lower the risk of recurrence (after a communication with the knee has been ruled out)

Ultrasound- or CT-guided aspiration aims at relieving compression-related symptoms, leaving the mucin-producing cyst wall and a possible communication with the joint in place. Therefore, the available evidence regarding freedom from recurrence after aspiration treatment must be interpreted with caution. On the other hand, spontaneous resolution confirmed by imaging has been reported (Pursell et al. 2004) and may be attributable to cyst rupture (Lossef et al. 1992). The author also saw a patient with spontaneous resolution of both reactive effusion and advential cyst fluid after arthroscopy with repair of a bucket handle meniscal tear. As a result, the moderate luminal narrowing of the popliteal artery caused by the cyst resolved as well, leaving the patient without symptoms for a follow-up period of 5 years. Two of three patients in whom the author performed initially successful ultrasound-guided aspiration (Schäberle 1996) were asymptomatic for a 5-year follow-up period (see ◘ Fig. 2.92 (Atlas)). The third patient had recurrence with marked refilling of the cysts at 6 months and underwent surgical enucleation.

Cyst aspiration can be performed when desired by the patient or justified on the basis of clinical considerations even if the above conditions are not met. Percutaneous cyst aspiration is uncomplicated and can be performed as an outpatient procedure. Prior aspiration treatment has no effect on the outcome of subsequent surgical resection (Asciutto et al. 2007; Keo et al. 2007). While the exact recurrence rate is unknown due to the rarity of advential cysts, a rough estimate is that recurrence-free cure can be achieved in approx. 60% of cases.

In patients presenting with knee problems (simultaneous Baker's cyst), diagnostic arthroscopy with therapeutic management of other conditions should be performed prior to vascular surgery and may also lead to shrinkage of adventitial cysts. The postulated communication between adventitial cysts and the knee joint space is not compatible with the high intracystic pressure (i.e., higher than systolic blood pressure) that is required to compress the arterial lumen (valve mechanism, inflammatory secretion of the cyst wall?).

2.1.6.4.2 Popliteal Artery Entrapment Syndrome

Entrapment of the popliteal artery was first described in 1879 by a medical student in Edinburgh. Few data are available on the incidence of this syndrome, but it seems to be more common than assumed in the past. A study performed in members of the Greek army reported an incidence of 0.17% (Bouhoutsos and Daskalakis 1981), while an autopsy study found an incidence of 3.5% (Gibson 1977). In the above-quoted analysis of our group (► Sect. 2.1.6.4), the incidence was 0.1% in **symptomatic patients** with clinical stage II or III disease. The lower incidence of popliteal entrapment in symptomatic patients appears to be attributable to the fact that the malformation of the medial head of gastrocnemius, which causes the **entrapment constellation** (see ◘ Fig. 2.96 (Atlas)), may be present without causing symptoms. Close examination of the popliteal fossa occasionally reveals an entrapment constellation as an incidental finding in patients evaluated for other reasons (e.g., suspected thrombosis, preoperative vein mapping prior to varicosis surgery). These individuals are completely asymptomatic, and even extreme plantar flexion does not compress the popliteal artery (no published data on such cases exist). Consequently, there is no risk of arterial wall damage or popliteal artery occlusion, and no treatment is required.

Intermittent claudication, chiefly associated with walking uphill, is the **cardinal clinical symptom**. Paresthesia and rest pain or trophic disorders have been observed but are uncommon. Both our results and published data indicate that thrombosis or segmental arterial occlusion is already present at the time of diagnosis in 50–70% of patients. Bilateral involvement was reported to occur in 30–50% of cases but was seen in only one patient (9%) of our series.

The popliteal artery courses through the center of the intercondylar fossa together with the popliteal vein and the tibial nerve and gives off a variable number of branches along this course (sural arteries). An atypical course of the popliteal artery, and possibly of the popliteal vein as well, or abnormal attachment of the medial head of the gastrocnemius muscle can lead to compression of the vessels during muscle contraction.

Compression of the popliteal artery during plantar flexion temporarily reduces distal blood flow. This in turn can cause intermittent claudication, often becoming apparent only during activities involving extreme plantar flexion, such as walking upstairs. Compression can cause secondary vessel wall damage with intimal and medial proliferation. Intimal damage may give rise to the formation of mural thrombi with subsequent complete occlusion, while compression of the artery may lead to poststenotic dilatation. The mural thrombi developing in the aneurysm may cause arterial embolism with occlusion of peripheral vessels.

Insua et al. (1970) distinguish four types of popliteal artery entrapment syndrome based on the relationship between artery and muscle:

- In **types I and Ia**, the popliteal artery courses on the medial side of the medial head of the gastrocnemius muscle. Type I refers to a malformation of the artery (◘ Fig. 2.30: I), type Ia to the malformation of the medial head of the gastrocnemius (◘ Fig. 2.30: II), which attaches to the femur more laterally and cranially than under normal conditions, thereby displacing the artery from its normal path. Sonographically, these two types are suggested by the demonstration of muscle tissue between the artery and vein, which usually course through the popliteal fossa together (see ◘ Fig. 2.94 (Atlas)).
- In **types II und IIa**, the artery and vein have a normal course but are compressed by structures crossing the popliteal fossa (◘ Fig. 2.30: III and IV) (abnormal attachment of a lateral extension of the medial gastrocnemius head, abnormal course of plantar muscle).

Rarely, a well-developed gastrocnemius can cause intermittent claudication. During contraction, the hypertrophied heads compress the popliteal artery and occasionally the vein as well.

2

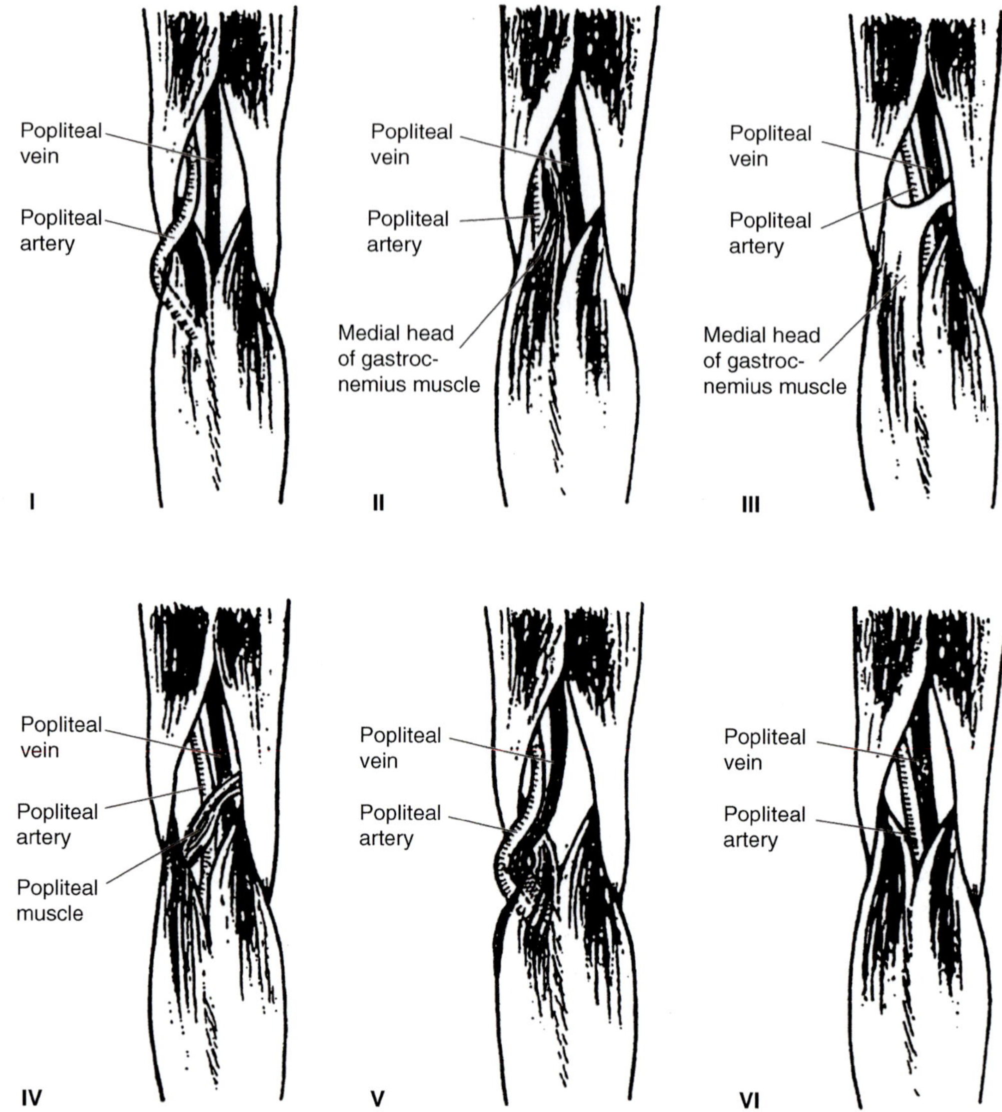

Fig. 2.30 Classification of popliteal artery entrapment syndrome (modified from Insua). **I** The popliteal artery courses medially over the posterior aspect of the normal attachment of the medial head of the gastrocnemius to return to its normal course in front of the muscle (corresponding to Insua type I). **II** The medial head of the gastrocnemius attaches more cranially and laterally, thus forcing the popliteal artery to take an abnormal course around the head (see Figs. 2.31 and 2.94 (Atlas); corresponding to Insua type Ia); the popliteal vein may be compressed as well. **III** The attachment of the medial head of the gastrocnemius has an accessory lateral extension, or the plantar muscle takes an abnormal course. The path of the popliteal artery is normal, but the artery and vein may be compressed to variable degrees, depending on the strength of the muscle fibers (see Figs. 3.98a (Atlas)) coursing to the lateral femoral condyle (corresponding to Insua types II and IIa). **IV** The popliteal artery and vein can be compressed by the popliteal muscle, an abnormal branch of the tibial nerve, or a fibrous ligament (according to Rich). **V** In rare cases, the popliteal vein follows the artery along its abnormal path and is compressed as well. Only one case of an isolated abnormal course of the popliteal vein has been reported so far. **VI** Normal course of the popliteal artery and vein through the popliteal fossa with compression of both vessels by a well-developed gastrocnemius muscle during muscle contraction, giving rise to intermittent claudication or venous congestion (see Figs. 2.95 and 3.98b (both Atlas))

Younger persons presenting with typical claudication should be examined for the presence of popliteal entrapment. This is done sonographically by carefully following the course of the popliteal artery, evaluating its relationship to muscular structures (Fig. 2.30) and performing **the plantar flexion test.** The latter is done using real-time ultrasound to observe the effects of increasing plantar flexion: these may include displacement of the artery from its course in the B-mode and hemodynamic signs of luminal narrowing due to compression of the artery in the spectral Doppler tracing (Table 2.13; Fig. 2.31).

A complete examination always includes the (asymptomatic) contralateral popliteal fossa since the condition is **bilateral** in up to 80% of cases.

Angiography does not yield any relevant additional information that may affect therapeutic management (Table 2.14), especially since ultrasound also demonstrates secondary wall damage and longer-term complications of intermittent vascu-

Table 2.13 Nonatherosclerotic vascular disease: different sites of involvement compared with atherosclerotic disease (intima)

Feature	Site and type of vascular disease
Wall thickening with luminal narrowing (adventitia, media)	Adventitial cystic disease: adventitial cysts in arteries near joints Preferred site: popliteal artery
	Arteritis: wall thickening, media (concentric) Medium-sized and large arteries
Focus of ultrasound examination: morphology (hemodynamics)	
Vessel compression (by perivascular structures)	Popliteal artery entrapment syndrome
	Thoracic outlet syndrome (subclavian artery, axillary artery, axillary vein)
Focus of ultrasound examination: hemodynamics in functional tests (morphology)	

lar compression, which are as follows (Figs. 2.31 and 3.98a (Atlas)):

- Mural thrombus formation secondary to local vessel wall lesions
- Poststenotic aneurysm
- Thrombotic occlusion of the damaged or dilated vessel segment

The diagnosis of popliteal artery entrapment syndrome relies on a high index of suspicion when assessing a young patient with isolated popliteal artery occlusion or dilatation (see Fig. 3.98a (Atlas)). Other findings in patients with arterial stenosis due to vascular compression syndrome or other nonatherosclerotic conditions may include poststenotic aneurysmal dilatation caused by increased wall pressure downstream of the stenosis (see Figs. 2.105 and 2.106 (Atlas)).

Therapeutic management consists in division of the structure compressing the popliteal artery. At a later stage, when occlusion has occurred, surgery includes reconstruction of the damaged artery (Steckmeier et al. 1989). In Insua type I popliteal artery entrapment syndrome, the atypically attaching medial gastrocnemius head is divided.

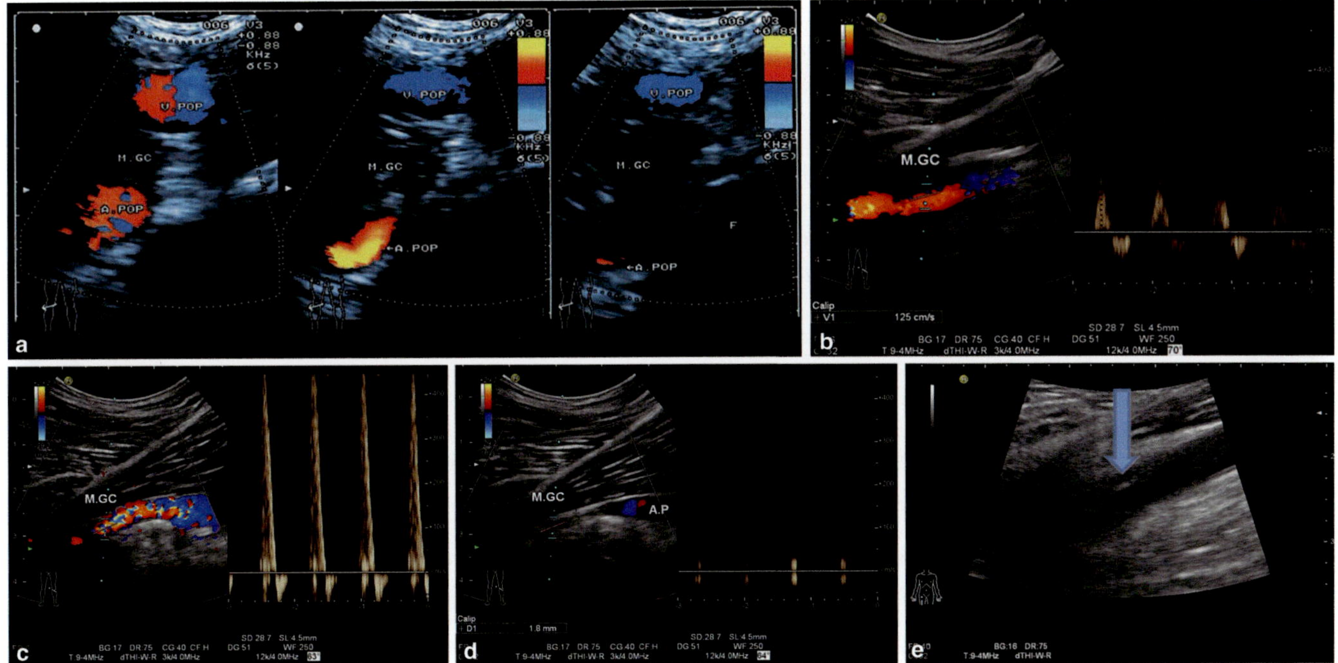

Fig. 2.31 **a** Popliteal artery entrapment syndrome – functional test. 38-year-old athletic man with entrapment syndrome caused by an abnormal gastrocnemius muscle (Insua type I). The transverse images from left to right show progressive compression of the popliteal artery by the gastrocnemius muscle (M.GC) with increasing plantar flexion. The muscle attaches between the popliteal artery and popliteal vein (V.POP) and forces them apart, resulting in subtotal occlusion of the artery (right image). **b–e** Popliteal entrapment syndrome in an 18-year-old male. The examination shows progressive compression of the popliteal artery (A.P) by the medial head of the gastrocnemius muscle (M.GC) with increasing plantar flexion. **b** With the calf muscles relaxed, there is no evidence of popliteal artery stenosis. **c** With the patient beginning to raise the heels off the floor, compression begins to induce stenosis with a PSV of 3 m/s. **d** With the patient standing on tiptoes (full plantar flexion), compression causes occlusion of the popliteal artery. The patient refused surgery. **e** Two years later, the ultrasound examination shows intimal thickening (arrow) of the popliteal artery segment exposed to intermittent compression

Table 2.14 Role of ultrasound in the diagnostic workup of nonatherosclerotic vessel disease prior to surgical repair

Findings/Diagnosis	Diagnostic information provided by ultrasound/supplementary imaging tests
Vascular compression syndrome, adventitial cystic disease	Duplex ultrasound with assessment of morphology and hemodynamics during provocative maneuver: most accurate diagnostic test, method of choice, mandatory in patients with clinical suspicion Optional: angiography – not necessary in: - Adventitial cystic disease without occlusion - Popliteal artery entrapment syndrome without occlusion May be supplemented by MRI, CT angiography
Inflammatory vascular disease	Duplex ultrasound to confirm the diagnosis and prevent unnecessary and contraindicated vessel repair (supplementary CT angiography; sonographic follow-up of immunosuppressive treatment)

2.1.6.4.3 Raynaud's Disease

Raynaud's disease is characterized by intermittent attacks of ischemia of the fingers and toes, typically brought on by cold and enhanced by emotional stress, local compression, and conditions that are associated with an increased sympathetic tone. The vasospasm is relieved by heat or drug treatment. Primary or idiopathic Raynaud's disease (no underlying disease; no occlusion of finger arteries) is distinguished from a secondary form (e.g., in patients with scleroderma or simultaneous finger artery occlusion). Ischemic attacks often occur bilaterally, affecting the second to fifth fingers while in most cases sparing the thumb. The toes are involved in only about 2% of cases. Women are affected two to five times more commonly than men, primarily between the ages of 20 and 50.

The diagnosis of Raynaud's disease chiefly relies on the typical clinical presentation, while further diagnostic tests are only required to identify vasospasm as the underlying cause of the clinical symptoms. Here again, duplex ultrasound has turned out to provide useful information. The examination is performed with exposure to cold to provoke the vasospasm and exposure to heat to relieve the spasm. When exposed to cold, the systolic finger artery pressure in Raynaud's disease drops markedly by 20–50% compared with only up to 10% in healthy persons. Duplex scanning typically demonstrates residual perfusion in the common digital arteries, while there is no or reduced flow in the distal finger arteries during spasm. The vasospasm produces **a markedly pulsatile flow pattern** with a short systolic peak and absence of diastolic flow in the hand arteries and the common digital arteries. Heat exposure induces vasodilatation with hyperemia, which results in pronounced diastolic flow in the proximal finger arteries and distinguishes Raynaud's disease from occlusion of the distal finger arteries. Other helpful diagnostic tests are oscillography and pressure measurement in the finger arteries. Raynaud's disease must be differentiated from vascular disorders of the larger proximal vessels as well as from arterial embolism (popliteal artery aneurysm, aortic aneurysm, thoracic outlet syndrome with poststenotic subclavian aneurysm). This is especially the case if color duplex demonstrates occlusion of interdigital arteries and the clinical picture of trash foot is present.

2.1.6.4.4 Paraneoplastic Disturbance of Acral Perfusion

A tumor can compromise blood flow by the following pathomorphologic and pathophysiologic mechanisms:

- Local displacement and compression (tumors of soft tissue, nerves, vessels, and bones as well as metastases) or tumor infiltration of the vessel wall, which may give rise to arterioarterial embolism
- Paraneoplastic vasculitis
- Paraneoplastic hyperviscosity of the blood and hypercoagulable state

Duplex ultrasound can identify the site of external compression or infiltration of the arterial wall by the tumor and provides information on the hemodynamic significance of the narrowing, which is important for therapeutic decision making. Arteries, with their strong muscle coat and intramural pressure, are much less susceptible to local tumor compression than veins.

2.1.6.4.5 Buerger's Disease

Buerger's disease, or thromboangiitis obliterans, is a chronic nonatherosclerotic endarteritis characterized by inflammation with thrombosis. It has an intermittent course and leads to segmental and multiple occlusions of small and medium-sized arteries of the extremities. As a panangiitis, it can be differentiated from atherosclerosis and other inflammatory vascular diseases. Though the etiology of Buerger's disease is unknown, there is an association between the onset and progression of the disease and cigarette smoking – 93–99% of the patients smoke. Remission is seen in most patients who quit for good. The severity and frequency of disease episodes correlate with the patient's smoking habits.

The clinical symptoms depend on the extent and site of occlusions. Pain at rest and acral necrosis occur at an early stage, while typical intermittent claudication of the calf muscles is less common. The duplex examination can rule out other disorders such as arterial embolism, aneurysms of the aorta and popliteal artery, popliteal artery entrapment syndrome, atherosclerosis, and macroangiopathy. B-mode imaging with a high-resolution transducer will show normal walls of the large arteries without hyperechoic atherosclerotic plaques or thickening. Occlusions primarily involve the arteries below the knee including the pedal arteries, and disseminated occlusion of the interdigital arteries may also be seen. The occluded lumen has low echogenicity. Venous involvement is seen as segmental phlebitis. Demonstration of **corkscrew-like revascularization channels** is diagnostic of thromboangiitis obliterans. The characteristic variation in color is due to tortuosity and merely reflects changing flow direction relative to the transducer rather than true flow reversal (Fig. 2.32). This flow pattern is also

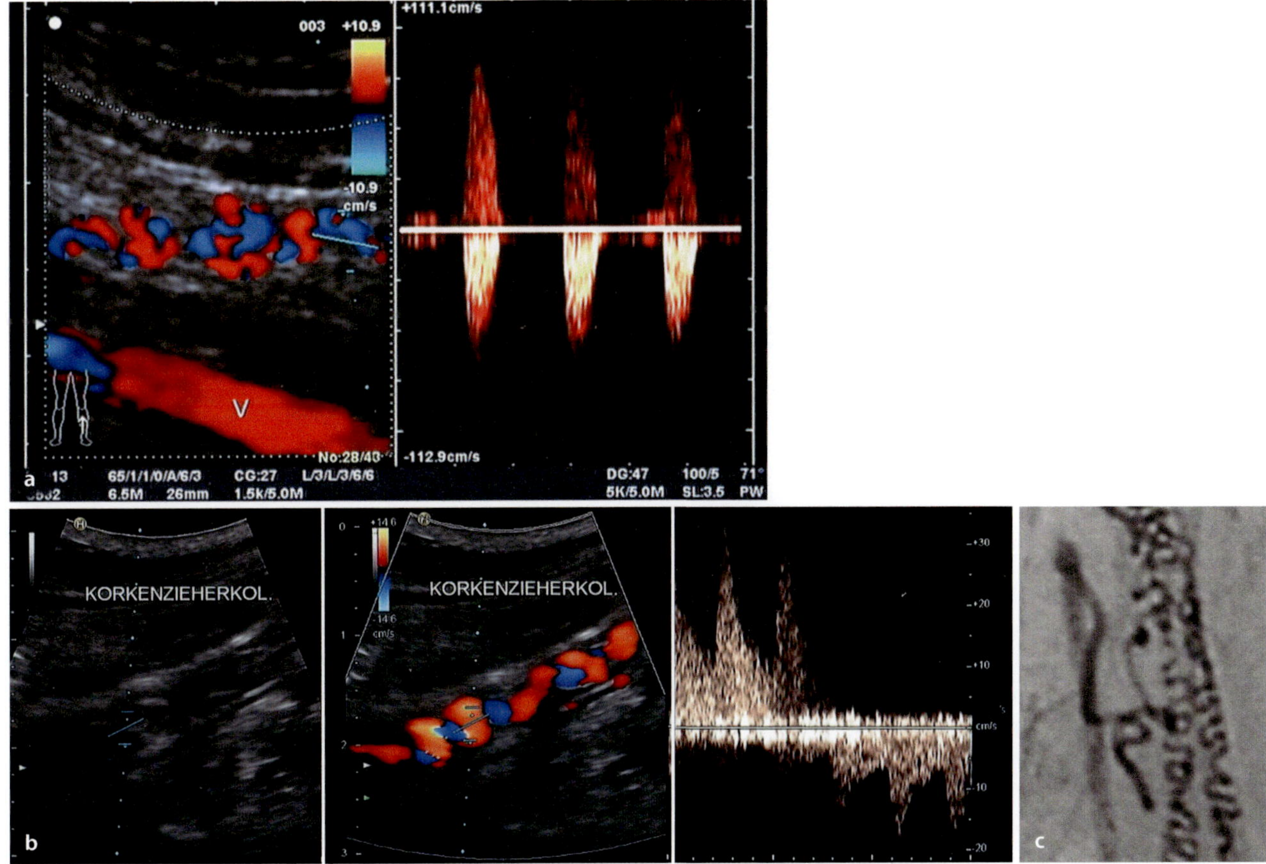

◘ Fig. 2.32 **a** Occlusion of the posterior tibial artery in thromboangiitis obliterans (hypoechoic artery without plaque). The patent vein (V) with flow coded red is seen deep to the occluded artery. A tortuous, recanalized collateral (with sample volume) is depicted close to the transducer with red and blue indicating flow toward and away from the transducer; this is also reflected in the waveform obtained from a short segment of the artery. This flow pattern is typical of a corkscrew collateral and characterizes recanalization in thromboangiitis obliterans. **b** Gray-scale image illustrating poor demarcation of a revascularized artery in thromboangiitis obliterans from surrounding connective tissue and muscle (rather high echogenicity due to septum-like internal structures). Both the color flow image and the spectral Doppler waveform reflect the blood flow pattern in the tortuous transmural revascularization channel. **c** Angiographic appearance of corkscrew collaterals

reflected in the Doppler waveform. Otherwise, there are no specific sonomorphologic findings in Buerger's disease.

2.1.6.4.6 Vascular Inflammatory Disease

Inflammatory vascular disease may be localized or generalized. Primary vasculitis arises in the vessel wall, while **secondary vasculitis** occurs on the background of other systemic diseases (rheumatoid arthritis, collagen disease). The following primary inflammatory vascular diseases are distinguished according to the vessels affected:

- Inflammation of large vessels (giant cell arteritis, Takayasu's arteritis)
- Inflammation of medium-sized vessels (polyarteritis nodosa, Kawasaki's disease)
- Inflammation of small vessels (Wegener's granulomatosis, microscopic polyangiitis, Schoenlein–Henoch purpura, Churg–Strauss syndrome)

The clinical diagnosis is suggested by the symptoms and changes in the organ or body region supplied by the inflamed arteries. These can range from pathognomonic local skin lesions with palpable purpura to organ loss (kidney) or acral ischemia when peripheral arteries are involved. During the active stage of vascular inflammation, most patients have a markedly elevated erythrocyte sedimentation rate (typically above 100 during the first hour) with only a slight increase in C-reactive protein. Additional findings are anemia, mild to moderate leukocytosis, and marked thrombocytosis. Supplementary tests include protein electrophoresis, complement determination, and antibody serology.

Duplex ultrasound allows localization and quantification of vascular constriction, but its foremost role is to noninvasively demonstrate **the typical inflammatory thickening of the vessel wall**. This is done using a high-resolution transducer (7–10 MHz), which will depict the characteristic "**macaroni sign**" (◘ Fig. 2.33) consisting of a higher-level echo from the lumen/intima interface surrounded by a concentric, homogeneous tube-like structure of lower echogenicity (intima-media complex) (see ◘ Fig. 2.100 (Atlas)) (Maeda et al. 1991). If the scanner resolution is not high enough, the macaroni sign may be visualized only in large and medium-sized vessels. With disease progression, wall thickening will lead to the development of concentric and rather long stenoses with subsequent obliteration (◘ Fig. 2.49).

Polyarteritis nodosa is segmental inflammation of medium-sized arteries and is characterized by circumferential

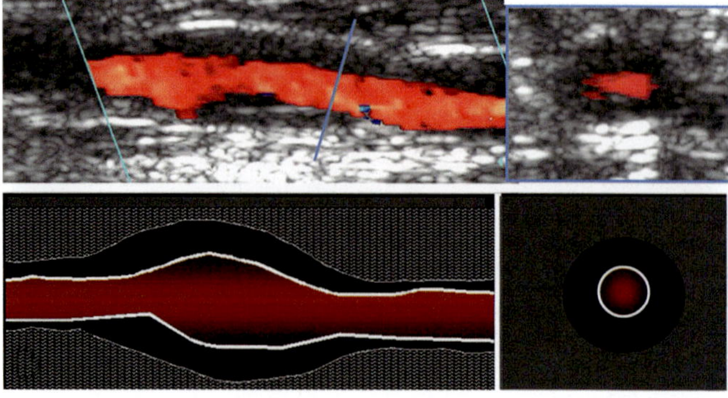

Fig. 2.33 In polyarteritis nodosa, inflammatory thickening of the wall causes circumferential luminal narrowing, which may at times alternate with dilated segments. The diagrams illustrate circumferential arterial wall thickening in longitudinal and transverse orientation (courtesy of K. Amendt)

wall thickening with luminal narrowing or constricted arterial segments alternating with dilated segments (Fig. 2.33).

The sonomorphologic differentiation of intimal thickening and sclerotic changes (calcification) from circumferential thickening of long vessel segments (macaroni sign) in inflammatory disease has important clinical implications. It is highly accurate in superficial vessels (carotid, subclavian, axillary, and femoral arteries), which can be examined with a high-frequency transducer.

Computed tomography (CT) and magnetic resonance imaging (MRI) are the reference methods for the diagnostic evaluation of the vessel wall. Angiographic mapping can identify the segments affected by inflammatory constriction but does not demonstrate wall thickening (see Table 2.14). Duplex ultrasound thus makes an important contribution to the correct diagnosis and treatment of steno-occlusive disease caused by vasculitis, thereby providing a sound basis for initiating proper treatment and sparing patients unnecessary interventions or surgery.

Hypersensitivity vasculitis (antigen-induced immune complex vasculitis) is typically caused by drugs or occurs in association with an infection. It is an arteritis of small arteries and therefore not amenable to sonographic evaluation because medium-sized and large arteries are not involved. In the legs, the clinical manifestations include painful ulcerations, often located on the lateral calf, urticaria, and hemorrhagic necrosis.

2.1.6.4.7 Dissection

Causes of dissection of the peripheral arteries are:

- Spontaneous dissection (very rare)
- Distal extension of an aortic dissection into the pelvic arteries
- Trauma (typically in the popliteal fossa, often involving posterior impact with compression of the artery against bone)
- Iatrogenic injury occurring during catheter-based interventions

Gray-scale ultrasound will demonstrate a thin membrane fluttering in the lumen at different phases of the cardiac cycle. In color flow imaging, dissection may present with different flow directions or different flow velocities in the true and false lumen, indicated by different colors and different levels of brightness, respectively (Fig. 2.34). The diagnosis of dissection is confirmed when different waveforms (with different PSVs) are obtained from the same artery (i.e., the true and false lumen). In addition, waveforms from a dissected artery may reflect superimposed artifacts resulting from oscillation of the dissection membrane. A thrombosed false lumen has low echogenicity and causes eccentric luminal narrowing of a long arterial segment (see Fig. 5.74 (Atlas)). The severity of flow obstruction can be estimated by spectral Doppler interrogation distal to the dissection (Fig. 5.45).

2.1.6.4.8 Arteriovenous Fistulas

An arteriovenous (AV) fistula is a congenital or acquired abnormal direct communication between an artery and a vein. Congenital micro- and macrofistulas occur in association with vascular malformations (hemangiomas). Acquired AV fistulas can develop after penetrating vascular injuries that damage an artery and a vein lying side by side or as iatrogenic complications of interventional procedures or surgery. Spontaneous AV fistulas can develop in the presence of a tumor or aneurysm (large aneurysm penetrating an adjacent vein). These abnormal short circuits between the arterial and venous system are distinguished from AV fistulas created surgically for hemodialysis or other therapeutic purposes (▶ Chap. 4).

Over time, increasing blood flow through an AV fistula can lead to dilatation of the feeding artery and draining vein with arterial complications such as aneurysm formation and venous stasis as late sequelae. Venous stasis leads to edema with tissue damage and crural ulcers. Additionally, large flow volumes across an AV fistula can cause an increased heart rate and cardiac output to maintain arterial pressure, and some patients develop cardiac failure.

Duplex ultrasound identifies an AV fistula by **increased blood flow** in the feeding artery (low-resistance flow) and draining vein. The increase varies with the fistula volume and is most pronounced during diastole. Spectral Doppler imaging will demonstrate arterialized, more pulsatile flow in the draining vein. Ultrasound allows very accurate determination of volume flow through the fistula (calculated from the cross-sectional area of the feeding artery and time-averaged blood flow velocity in comparison to the contralateral artery of the same name). The exact site of an AV fistula can be identified by the presence of perivascular tissue vibration, seen as a mosaic of colors in color duplex imaging, and by the transition from low-resistance to high-resistance flow in the spectral Doppler waveform from the feeding artery (for details see ▶ Sects. 4.1, 4.2, and 4.4 and Figs. 4.7 and 4.8).

2.1.6.4.9 Chronic Recurrent Compartment Syndrome of the Calf

Chronic recurrent compartment syndrome of the calf most commonly involves the anterior compartment. It is an overuse condition causing a rise in intracompartmental pressure

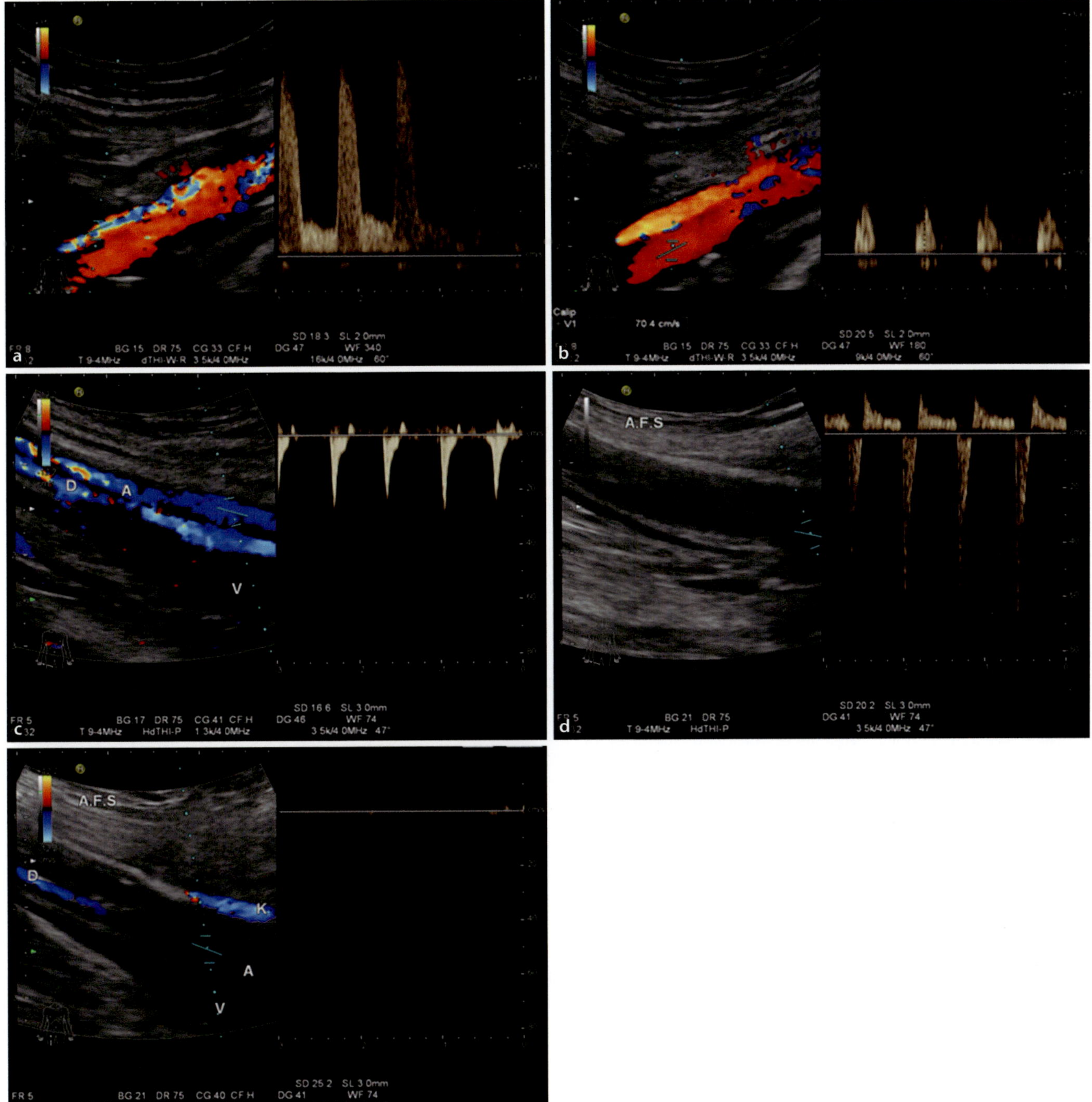

Fig. 2.34 **a, b** Dissection of the external iliac artery after catheter intervention. The lumen of the artery is narrowed by the dissection membrane, and different waveforms are obtained by selectively placing the sample volume in the true and false lumen. **c–e** The dissection flap (D) extends into the proximal superficial femoral artery. Different waveforms are obtained from the false lumen (**c**) and the true lumen (**d**). The artery is occluded distal to the origin of collaterals (K) at the mid-thigh level (**e**)

with subsequent microvascular compromise. Patients present with swelling, tension, and severe pain. Foot pulses are palpable. Muscle damage can lead to an increase in creatine kinase, and intracompartmental pressure, which even during activity is normally below 20 mmHg, can increase two- to fourfold. When duplex imaging is performed after activity to reproduce increased compartmental pressure, the calf veins of patients with chronic compartment syndrome will appear compressed or may be collapsed (at pressures >30 mmHg). At pressures >50 mmHg, arterial flow becomes more pulsatile. With a further increase in pressure, the orthograde diastolic flow component disappears, and finally a line-like artifact will appear in the waveform in late diastole. B-mode imaging will show intrafascial edema in the anterior compartment.

2.1.7 Follow-Up After Surgical and Interventional Treatment

With its proven validity compared with the gold standard and intraoperative findings, duplex ultrasound is an excellent imaging modality for treatment planning in patients with steno-occlusive disease of the pelvic, femoral, and popliteal arteries including the trifurcation and also for surveillance after surgery or endovascular interventions. The duplex ultrasound information on the sites and severity of stenosis or occlusion, in conjunction with the clinical manifestation, helps the physician decide whether conservative management with walking exercises, a radiologic intervention, or surgical repair (TEA or bypass grafting) is the most suitable treatment for the patient.

The surgical procedure and revisions in case of complications can be planned in the infrainguinal arteries with the same accuracy as with angiography (Wain et al. 1999; Ligush et al. 1998). In patients with adequate sonographic visualization, no pretherapeutic angiography is necessary for planning reconstructive procedures in this territory including the P1 segment. Evaluation of the recipient artery is important both in the preoperative workup and in the examination of patients with restenosis or reocclusion after surgery. As this can be done very accurately by duplex ultrasound including evaluation of the trifurcation and segmental evaluation of the arteries below the knee, the indication for a P1 femoral artery bypass can be established without preoperative angiography on condition that an inflow obstruction (at the pelvic level) has been ruled out.

2.1.7.1 Thromboendarterectomy

An important indication for thromboendarterectomy (TEA) is stenosis of the femoral artery bifurcation, which is easily accessible to ultrasound examination. The duplex findings alone can serve to identify candidates for TEA and plan the procedure.

Duplex imaging enables very detailed planning of TEA or profundaplasty for obstructive lesions at the origin of the profunda femoris artery as well as of repeat interventions in patients with complications or recurrent stenosis. Moreover, hemodynamic evaluation by duplex ultrasound provides more valid diagnostic information in this region, where angiography is limited by superimposition of vessels and in the evaluation of stenosis caused by posterior wall plaque.

Ultrasound is also a suitable tool for assessing outcome after surgery, identifying postoperative complications, and detecting recurrent stenosis. For example, in a patient who has undergone surgery for stenosis of the profunda femoris artery to improve its collateral function in superficial femoral artery occlusion, the success of surgery can be confirmed by the sonographic identification of improved flow with higher peak systolic and diastolic velocities in the refilled popliteal artery (◘ Fig. 2.59 (Atlas)). Postoperative complications detectable by high-resolution ultrasound include intimal flaps and constriction at the suture line. Recurrent stenosis after surgical repair can be identified by B-mode imaging and graded by spectral Doppler (◘ Fig. 2.35).

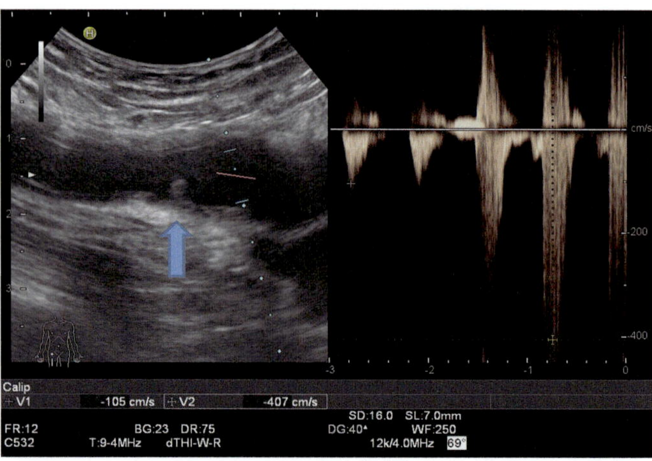

◘ **Fig. 2.35** Restenosis of the common femoral artery after TEA. The gray-scale image demonstrates an intimal flap (arrow) as the underlying cause of stenosis. Spectral Doppler interrogation of this segment with measurement of peak systolic velocity (PSV) gives a PSV ratio of 3.8 (calculated from intrastenotic PSV of 407 cm/s and prestenotic PSV of 105 cm/s), corresponding to 60–70% stenosis

2.1.7.2 Percutaneous Transluminal Angioplasty and Stenting

Percutaneous transluminal angioplasty (PTA) is performed to improve peripheral perfusion by restoring adequate blood flow through a narrowed arterial segment. In patients with occlusion, the therapeutic procedure (PTA or bypass surgery) can be planned beforehand once the length of the occluded segment has been determined. In PTA, atherosclerotic plaques are fragmented and pressed into the arterial wall (◘ Fig. 2.65 (Atlas)), often resulting in intimal or medial tears. The irregular surface is susceptible to the deposition of thrombotic material. A complication of PTA is recurrent stenosis due to fragmented plaques extending into the lumen, dissection, elastic recoil (see ◘ Figs. 5.36 and 5.38), intimal hyperplasia, or progression of atherosclerosis. PTA is also used to dilate residual stenosis persisting after intra-arterial administration of plasmin activators for thrombolytic therapy. Other interventional procedures, apart from standard PTA, include arterectomy, rotational angioplasty, and laser angioplasty.

Duplex scanning is the first-line diagnostic modality to **follow up the outcome of vascular repair** in patients after PTA (with and without stent implantation) or bypass surgery for the early identification of those who require reintervention. A study revealed restenosis in 85% of patients with a postinterventional PSV ratio greater than 2 (Mewissen et al. 1992).

The **role of postinterventional duplex ultrasound** is to detect complications (dissection, aneurysm, perforation) and to identify residual or recurrent stenosis caused by thrombotic deposits or fragmented plaques protruding into the lumen. The morphologic appearance of the wall in the treated segment and hemodynamic information are important for identifying restenosis. Subintimal hemorrhage due to intimal or medial tears may be seen as hypoechoic wall thickening in the treated segment while thrombotic deposits appear as hypoechoic intraluminal areas without color flow.

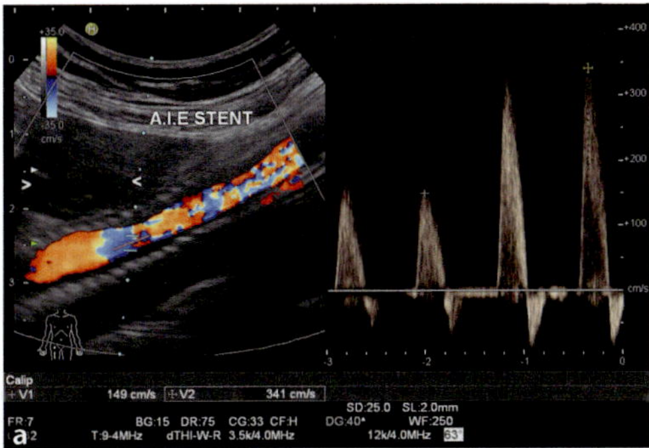

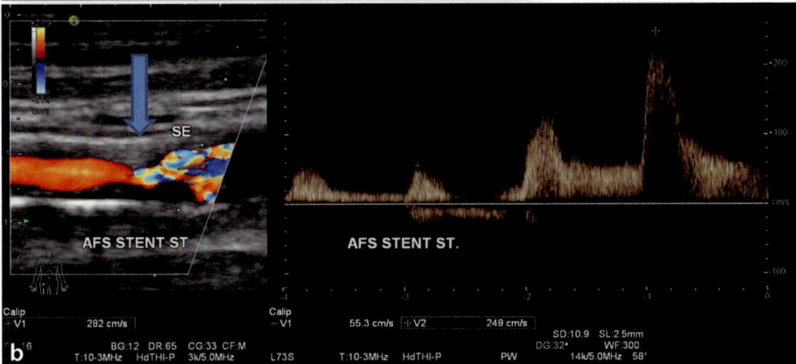

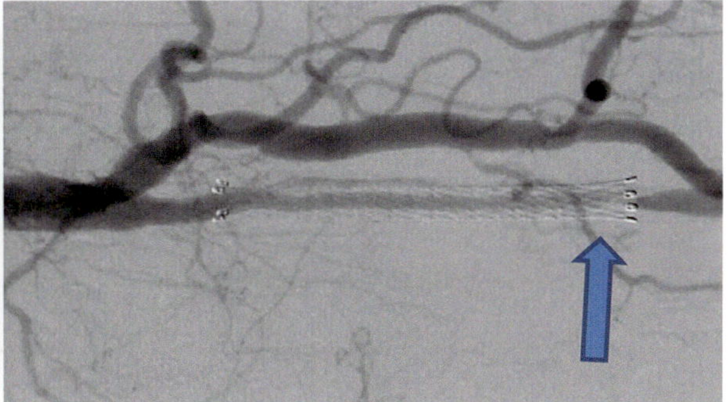

Fig. 2.36 Restenosis after stenting. **a** Patient with in-stent restenosis of the external iliac artery. Hemodynamic grading based on the peak systolic velocity (PSV) ratio indicates 50–60% stenosis (PSV ratio > 2, calculated from intrastenotic PSV of 341 cm/s and prestenotic PSV of 148 cm/s). The waveform was obtained by moving the transducer over the skin, while maintaining a constant Doppler angle, from the prestenotic segment to the site of stenosis (indicated by "> <"). **b** Stent in superficial femoral artery with excessive neointimal proliferation causing circumferential narrowing of a long portion of the stented arterial segment with high-grade stenosis at the distal stent end (arrow; PSV ratio of approx. 5, calculated from intrastenotic PSV of 249 cm/s and prestenotic PSV of 55 cm/s). The angiogram obtained before repeat PTA confirms narrowing of the stent lumen with stenosis at the distal stent end (arrow). The example illustrates the problem of stenosis grading. The intrastenotic PSV of 249 cm/s is low for the degree of stenosis. Good collateralization (flow divider, see angiogram) results in reduced flow and flow velocity in the femoral artery, as reflected by the low prestenotic PSV of 55 cm (see Figs. 2.16b and 1.46b, c and Table 1.10). The PSV ratio of 5, however, is consistent with high-grade stenosis and better reflects the hemodynamic situation here. Conversely, use of absolute intrastenotic PSV alone (cutoffs determined by ROC analysis; see Figs. 2.18 and 2.19) underestimates the severity of stenosis in this case, illustrating the superiority of the PSV ratio over absolute PSV for stenosis grading

A **stent** is identified by its serrated or mesh-like appearance. A focal increase in flow velocity is the most important sign of residual or recurrent stenosis after PTA, stenting (where special attention must be paid to the stent ends), and bypass grafting (primarily at the anastomotic sites) (Fig. 2.36).

In most cases, flow evaluation within a stent requires a higher color gain. Eddy currents and turbulent flow at the proximal and distal ends suggest that the stent does not fit snugly to the wall, which can promote restenosis.

The accurate diagnosis of complications such as arteriovenous (AV) fistula, pseudoaneurysm, and hematoma and the timely identification of residual or recurrent stenosis are crucial for post-PTA patency. A **hemodynamically significant residual or recurrent stenosis** is suggested by focal doubling of the flow velocity within the treated segment. The detection of a hemodynamically significant stenosis by duplex ultrasound is a predictor of patency. The above-quoted study of Mewissen et al. (1992) reported a 1-year patency rate of 83% in the absence of stenosis as opposed to only 15% when a functional stenosis was diagnosed (Mewissen et al. 1992).

Several studies have shown duplex imaging to be more sensitive than angiography in detecting residual stenosis or residual flow disturbance following PTA. In one study, 20% of residual stenoses >50% based on duplex ultrasound were classified as causing <30% diameter reduction at angiography. The sonographic stenosis criteria were PSV >180 cm/s (Fig. 2.37) and an intrastenotic-to-prestenotic PSV ratio > 2.5 (Kinney et al. 1991; Mewissen et al. 1992). The presence of residual stenosis classified as causing >50% diameter reduction by duplex scanning was found to predict late failure (15% success rate) while late patency was observed for <50% diameter reduction (84% success rate). Based on these results, it is recommended to perform a **follow-up duplex scan within 1 month of PTA** to identify patients with residual/recurrent stenosis who should undergo reintervention.

Earlier studies in other vascular territories (carotid artery, renal artery) identified 10–20% higher **PSV cutoffs** (ROC curve analysis) for in-stent restenosis (due to greater wall rigidity and smaller lumen of the stented segment) compared with native arteries. In contrast, more recent studies in stented peripheral arteries suggest that PSV cutoffs should rather be lower than for untreated arteries. These studies report sensitivities and specificities as well as negative predictive values (NPV) and positive predictive values (PPV) on the order of 95% for the following absolute PSV and PSV ratio cutoffs (Baril et al. 2008; Shrikhande et al. 2011):

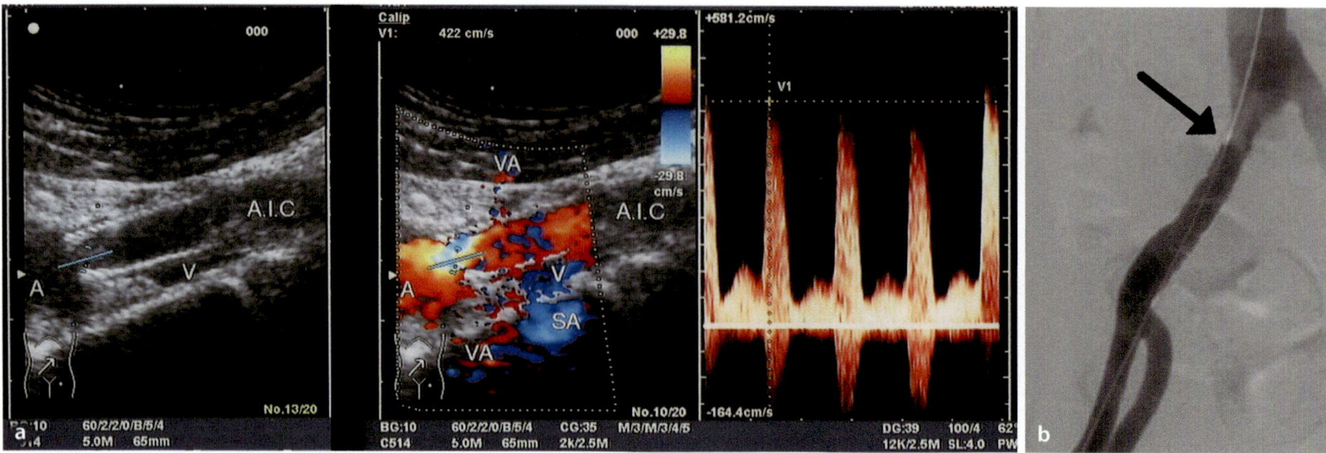

Fig. 2.37 **a** Patient after PTA and stenting of high-grade common iliac artery stenosis. In the gray-scale image (left), the stent is identified by its serrated appearance. The color duplex image shows aliasing at the proximal stent end and backward and forward flow components within the stent (red and blue) (A = aorta, A.I.C = common iliac artery, V = common iliac vein, VA = vibration artifact, SA = mirror artifact). The Doppler waveform from the site of aliasing demonstrates very turbulent flow with a PSV of 422 cm/s, consistent with high-grade stenosis. **b** Angiogram fails to adequately show the stenosis or its cause. The patient underwent repeat PTA on the basis of the duplex ultrasound findings. Following repeat PTA, the patient's clinical symptoms resolved (patient's walking distance before reintervention was limited to 180 m), color duplex confirmed elimination of the stenosis, and the ABI normalized from 0.8 to 1.1

- >50% stenosis: PSV >190 cm/s and PSV ratio > 1.5
- >70% stenosis: PSV >223 cm/s and PSV ratio > 2.5
- >80% stenosis: PSV >275 cm/s and PSV ratio > 3.5

The PSV ratio is a very reliable parameter for identification of in-stent restenosis. However, according to the continuity equation, one would expect the cutoff ratio to be 2 for 50% stenosis and 4 for 75% stenosis. These theoretically predicted PSV ratios are based on the assumption that stenosis is caused by concentric plaque. Hence, the lower actual ratios suggest that in-stent restenosis tends to be caused by eccentric luminal narrowing. Remember that an eccentric stenosis results in a smaller cross-sectional area reduction than a concentric stenosis with the same diameter reduction. Therefore, the hemodynamic effect of an eccentric stenosis is less pronounced and the sonographically measured intrastenotic increase in PSV is smaller (Fig. 2.17d).

2.1.7.3 Bypass Graft Surveillance

The sonographic appearance of a bypass depends on the material used.

The thin wall of **an autologous venous bypass graft** is very difficult to delineate when occlusion has occurred. Such a bypass is easier to identify, in particular in older occlusion, if the examiner has information on its course (anatomic, extra-anatomic). In patients with a venous bypass graft, the entire length must be scanned because the former valves are common sites of stenosis, especially in an in situ bypass with residual valve cusps. An AV fistula developing from a perforating vein that has not been ligated can be identified by the presence of perivascular tissue vibration artifacts in the color duplex mode.

In contrast, the walls of a **synthetic bypass graft** are always clearly seen. A PTFE (polytetrafluoroethylene) prosthesis has a characteristic double-line appearance and a Dacron bypass a sawtooth-like appearance.

In the postoperative evaluation and surveillance of a synthetic graft, special attention must be paid to possible anastomotic stenoses. Narrowing within the bypass is due to neointimal hyperplasia and occurs later. About 20–30% of venous bypass grafts develop strictures on the basis of neointimal hyperplasia within the first year of surgery.

Different factors can cause **occlusion of a bypass** at different times after surgery:

- Immediate postoperative occlusion within the first days after surgery may be due to an inadequate surgical technique, resulting in anastomotic stenosis, or poor distal runoff. Therefore, the examination should include hemodynamic evaluation of the recipient artery.
- Early occlusion, within the first year, chiefly results from neointimal hyperplasia, predominantly causing stenosis at the proximal or distal anastomosis, or from deterioration of the outflow situation due to progression of atherosclerosis distal to the bypass. If the occlusion is due to an impaired inflow secondary to atherosclerotic lesions of the proximal artery with loss of the triphasic waveform, the examiner must carefully evaluate the native artery upstream of the bypass to identify the site of obstruction.
- Late occlusion is predominantly caused by progression of atherosclerosis, especially in the segments close to the bypass ends.

Abnormal fluid around a bypass graft should be punctured under ultrasound guidance for microbiologic testing, in particular in patients with clinical signs of infection. Before puncture, a suture aneurysm should be ruled out by color duplex imaging (see Fig. 2.72 (Atlas)). Hematoma, seroma, and suture aneurysm appear as pulsatile masses at the site of anastomosis, each having a characteristic color duplex appearance, which allows it to be differentiated at a glance.

2.1.7.3.1 Methodological Considerations and Stenosis Criteria

Duplex ultrasound is a valid imaging modality for identifying bypass graft complications (stenosis, occlusion). Published data suggest good agreement with CTA and DSA (Willmann et al. 2004) as well as good interobserver agreement with 85% sensitivity, 93% specificity, and 91% diagnostic accuracy compared with DSA (Ihlberg et al. 1998).

The criteria for grading stenosis severity in a bypass graft are based on those for the native peripheral arteries. However, the hemodynamic changes in a bypass graft may occasionally lead to a monophasic waveform that does not suggest abnormal flow. Eddy currents at the anastomoses cause spectral broadening, which is likewise normal (◘ Figs. 2.41, 2.74 (Atlas), 2.75 (Atlas), and 2.76 (Atlas)).

Normal peak systolic velocity (PSV) is a function of the relative cross sections of the bypass and the proximal and distal native arteries. The complex relationships make it difficult to give a reliable general threshold velocity. Still, one can rule out a hemodynamically significant stenosis with some confidence if PSV at the site of anastomosis is below 2 m/s on condition that there is no size mismatch between the graft and the native artery (◘ Table 2.15).

Flow within a graft is influenced by several factors, which should be borne in mind when interpreting spectral Doppler recordings from within the graft to predict bypass patency. This is especially important in patients with severe atherosclerosis and in assessing bypass grafts onto a calf artery (◘ Fig. 2.43). Pulsatility is physiologically dependent on the demand-oriented widening of the arterioles (monophasic flow). In a bypass, pulsatility is additionally affected by differences in elasticity (depending on the material used for the graft) and an increase in outflow resistance if there is stenosis distal to the bypass (more pulsatile flow). These opposing effects on the flow profile preclude simple monocausal interpretation of the waveform obtained from a bypass graft. Hence, slow flow should prompt an evaluation of both the distal anastomosis and the recipient artery for the presence of stenosis even if the waveform is triphasic (see ◘ Fig. 2.73 (Atlas)).

While a synthetic graft should primarily be searched for stenosis at the proximal and distal ends (the preferred sites of stenosis in this type of graft), the entire length of an autologous venous graft must be examined for stenosis at valve sites (see ◘ Fig. 2.76 (Atlas)). As with native arteries, the examiner can save time by comparing Doppler waveforms from representative sites to narrow down possible sites of stenosis. When scanning an autologous in situ venous bypass immediately after surgery, the examiner must also look for any patent perforating veins, which could give rise to an AV fistula and would thus need to be ligated after having been localized sonographically.

PSV cutoffs ranging from 2 m/s (Passman et al. 1995) to 3 m/s (Westerband et al. 1997) have been proposed to identify stenosis that should prompt graft revision. It should be clear, though, that there is no single PSV cutoff that applies throughout a graft. For example, a PSV of up to 2.5 m/s may be considered normal at the distal anastomosis, especially when there is a transition from a wide bypass lumen to a narrow recipient vessel as is the case with a crural bypass. A PSV of 2.5 m/s is abnormal, however, when it occurs at the proximal anastomosis or within the graft.

Other investigators use the ratio of intrastenotic PSV to PSV in the normal proximal segment to identify hemodynamically relevant bypass graft stenosis. However, the **PSV ratio** (also known as peak velocity ratio/PVR) above which >70% stenosis requiring graft revision is assumed ranges from 3 (Calligaro et al. 1996; Dougherty et al. 1998) to 4 (Idu et al. 1999). Overall, cutoffs proposed for moderate stenosis (50–70%) in a bypass graft range from 2–4 for PSV ratios (Wixon et al. 2000; Mills et al. 2001) and from 2–3.5 m/s for absolute PSV (◘ Table 2.16).

When grading the severity of anastomotic stenoses in synthetic grafts, the PSV ratio must be used with caution due

◘ **Table 2.15** Duplex ultrasound criteria in bypass graft surveillance. Identification of complications: suture aneurysm, abscess, imminent occlusion (failing bypass), stenosis (◘ Figs. 2.38, 2.41, and 2.42)

Method (indirect/direct criteria)	Interpretation of criteria
Single PSV measurement in the bypass graft (indirect sign of flow obstruction/stenosis in the graft)	Reduced PSV in the bypass graft: PSV <45 cm/s suggests failing bypass (exceptions) Distal to stenosis: damped waveform, delayed systolic rise
Analysis of representative spectral waveform (indirect criterion)	Triphasic: good graft function Monophasic: flow obstruction, peripheral vasodilation
Mapping of bypass graft and anastomoses: increased PSV indicates stenosis (direct criterion)	PSV ratio >2: moderate stenosis PSV ratio >4: high-grade stenosis PSV >2–2.5 m/s: moderate stenosis PSV >3–3.5 m/s: high-grade stenosis

◘ **Table 2.16** Stenosis grading in the sonographic surveillance of bypass grafts and therapeutic consequences (Modified from Mills et al. 2001 and Wixon et al. 2000)

Stenosis criteria in bypass graft		Suggested management
Normal	PSV < 200 cm/s PSV ratio < 2	Low risk → follow-up
Moderate stenosis	PSV of 200–300 cm/s PSV ratio of 2–4	Moderate risk → close follow-up, revision in case of progression
High-grade stenosis	PSV > 300 cm/s PSV ratio > 4	High risk (PSV in graft >45 cm/s) → elective intervention Highest risk (PSV in graft <45 cm/s) → urgent intervention

to mismatches in size and elasticity between the bypass graft and the proximal native artery. With these limitations in mind, it may be assumed that a PSV ratio > 2.5 indicates >60% stenosis. Size mismatches between the graft and the recipient artery often result in a flow acceleration downstream of the distal anastomosis, in particular when the anastomosis is located below the knee. Here, an even higher PSV ratio (>3) should be used as a cutoff in order to minimize false-positive results (Polak 1992).

Mapping of an entire bypass graft including the proximal and distal anastomes is very time-consuming. Therefore, protocols have been proposed to make sonographic graft surveillance more efficient. Such protocols rely on the comparison of Doppler waveforms from a few representative sites using the same indirect criteria as in native peripheral arteries (◘ Figs. 2.14, 2.37, 2.38, 2.39, 2.40, 2.41, and 2.43). The flow profile and PSV are evaluated. If there is triphasic flow with a PSV of 55 cm/s or greater in the graft, then higher-grade stenosis within the graft or at the anastomoses is unlikely – especially if the bypass was established for critical ischemia of the leg. In this situation, a stenosis would lead to a monophasic waveform (resulting from reduced peripheral resistance due to demand-adjusted widening of arterioles). If the waveform is not triphasic and flow velocity is slow, the entire bypass must be mapped for the presence of stenosis, with special attention being paid to the anastomoses. However, a monophasic waveform may also be obtained if no stenosis is present in the graft, especially if the bypass was established to improve inflow in patients with multilevel obstruction and there is persistent poor perfusion in the periphery due to additional stenoses more distally. In contrast, an initially triphasic flow profile in a bypass graft that becomes monophasic at later follow-up indicates peripheral vasodilation in response to an **impairment of peripheral perfusion**. This again warrants sonographic evaluation of the entire bypass and the anastomoses. Another possible cause of impaired peripheral perfusion is progressive atherosclerosis with stenotic narrowing of the segments proximal and distal to the bypass graft.

Based on these considerations, a **time-efficient bypass graft surveillance strategy** is proposed (◘ Figs. 2.38, 2.41, and 2.42), which relies on duplex imaging and spectral Doppler interrogation at the following sites (◘ Figs. 2.39 and 2.43):

- Femoral artery bifurcation
- Proximal graft anastomosis with spectral Doppler interrogation
- Distal graft anastomosis with spectral Doppler interrogation including the receiving artery just distal to the anastomosis and the graft just upstream of the anastomosis

Spectral Doppler interrogation of these sites will directly identify most graft complications/stenoses, guiding the examiner to abnormal segments that warrant closer examination (e.g., the feeding artery). Waveforms are obtained by moving the transducer across the proximal and distal anastomoses, and interpretation of the waveforms from these representative sites using the indirect stenosis criteria provides information on inflow and outflow. Comparison of the spectral tracings from the proximal and distal ends of the bypass allows the examiner to suspect or rule out stenosis within the graft (see, however, ◘ Fig. 2.43).

Long-term bypass graft patency depends on the development of stenosis within the graft (predominantly involving the anastomoses) and flow in the recipient artery. Poor runoff affects the blood flow velocity in the graft and, in conjunction with systemic factors such as a hypercoagulable state, can lead to occlusion. Several investigators use PSV as the most important parameter in the surveillance of bypass grafts (Bandyk et al. 1985, 1989; Buth et al. 1991; Calligaro et al. 1996; Grigg et al. 1988; Lundell et al. 1995; Passman et al. 1995). Postoperative mean or median PSVs reported in the literature range from 0.68 to 1.12 m/s (Belkin et al. 1994; Nielsen et al. 1995; Wölfle et al. 1994) and decrease thereafter if the graft remains patent (from 1.125 to 1 m/s after 1 year according to Wölfle et al. and by 30% within the first 6 months according to Nielsen et al. 1993).

A markedly reduced overall PSV in a bypass graft has been proposed as a supplementary indicator of a poor prognosis (Calligaro et al. 1996; Hoballah et al. 1997). Slow flow in a bypass can point to an outflow obstruction caused by stenosis of the distal anastomosis or poor runoff (stenosis of recipient artery, obstructed collateral outflow). Hence, various velocity thresholds have been suggested as predictors of imminent bypass occlusion. Most authors assume that a bypass is likely to fail if blood flow velocity drops below 45 cm/s (Calligaro et al. 1996; Hoballah et al. 1997; Mohan et al. 1995), while others propose thresholds of 40 cm/s (Green et al. 1990) or 55 cm/s (Nielsen et al. 1995). Other data suggest that assuming a single velocity threshold for all types of bypass grafts and recipient vessels is not sensitive and specific enough to identify a failing bypass (Chang et al. 1990; Hoballah et al. 1997; Idu et al. 1999; Mohan et al. 1995; Treiman et al. 1999). Since flow velocity in a bypass is determined by its diameter and by the diameter and outflow of the recipient vessel, crural bypass grafts with far distal anastomoses have slower flow velocities even under normal conditions. Still, slow flow in a bypass is a risk factor for occlusion, especially in patients with other predisposing conditions such as a hypercoagulable state, increased blood viscosity, or low systemic blood pressure. Some authors therefore investigated the predictive power of a prognostic factor combining an increased focal PSV and a low global PSV in the graft (Calligaro et al. 1996). In a study of 85 PTFE grafts, this combined criterion had 81% sensitivity, 93% specificity, a PPV of 63%, and an NPV of 93% (similar results were reported by Green et al. 1990). Other investigators (Hoballah et al. 1997; Mohan et al. 1995) did not confirm these results. In the

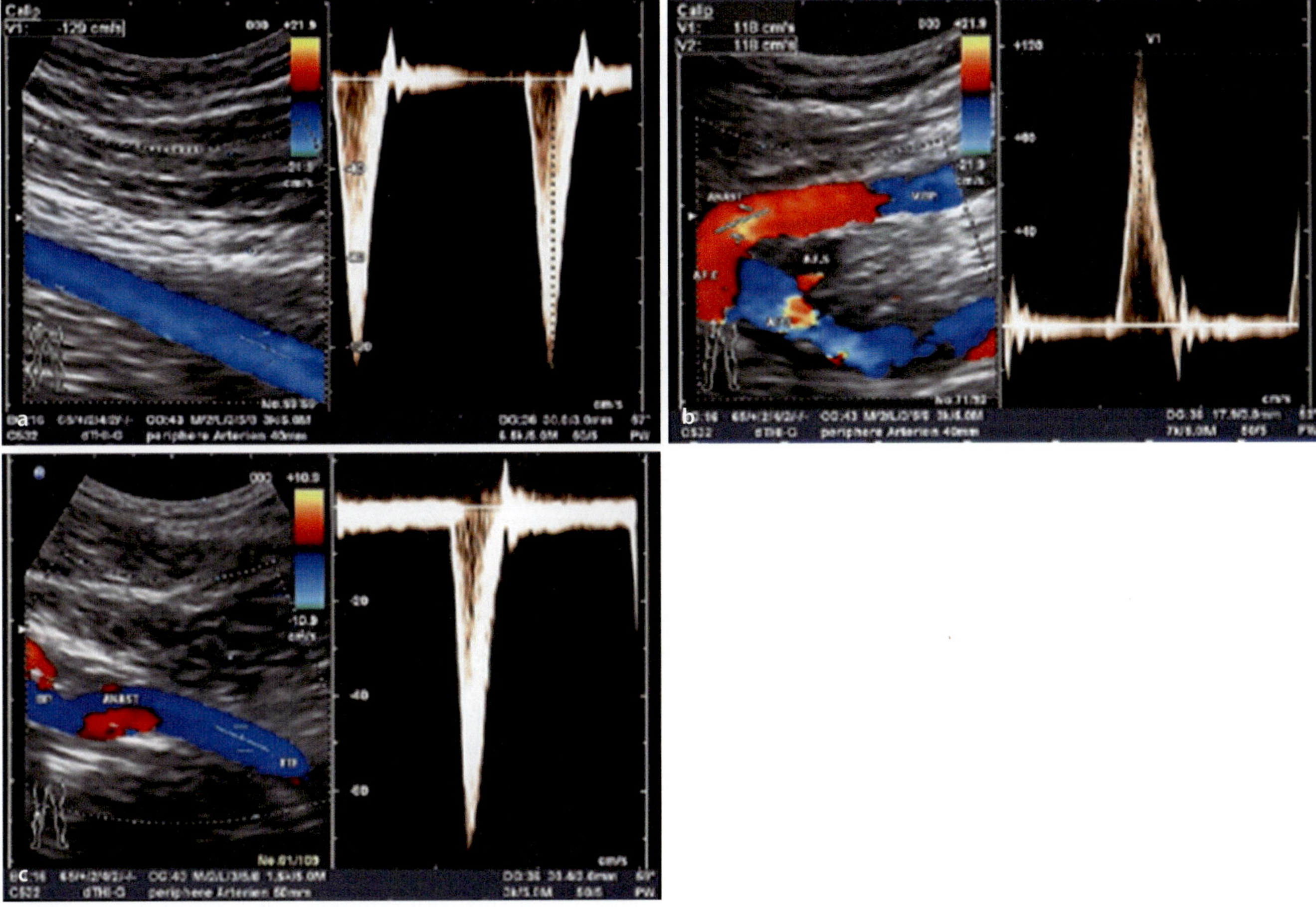

Fig. 2.38a–c Bypass graft surveillance. Duplex examination of a venous femoropopliteal bypass graft (P3 segment). There is no agreement about the need for sonographic venous bypass graft surveillance or the extent of the examination. An efficient procedure is to obtain Doppler waveforms from representative sites to identify those patients who should undergo comprehensive mapping. At a minimum, a Doppler waveform is obtained from an arbitrary site in the main body of the graft (**a**) and interpreted with regard to bypass prognosis and signs of stenosis. A more comprehensive evaluation comprises examination of the proximal and distal anastomoses (where most stenoses occur) and a site within the graft slightly distal to the anastomosis (duplex and spectral Doppler). Signs of abnormal flow should prompt mapping of the entire graft, which may also include evaluation of the inflow artery. **a** The color flow image and waveform from a site within the graft show normal findings. The waveform is triphasic with a PSV of 129 cm/s – there is no sign of bypass graft stenosis and no risk of imminent bypass failure. No further evaluation would be required in this patient. **b** For illustration, the examination proceeds with evaluation of the proximal anastomosis (to rule out anastomotic stenosis or neointimal hyperplasia with relevant luminal narrowing). This is done by placing the sample volume at the origin of the venous bypass graft (V.BP) from the common femoral artery; triphasic Doppler waveform indicates adequate inflow. The profunda femoris artery and superficial femoral artery (A.F.S) arise distally (to the right of the anastomosis). **c** Examination of the distal anastomosis: Doppler waveform from the bypass target artery distal to the anastomosis shows high PSV (70 cm/s), steep systolic upstroke, and pulsatile flow as evidence of good outflow, ruling out relevant proximal stenosis. Overall, there is no evidence of imminent bypass failure in this case

study of Hoballah et al., 24 of 27 patients with bypass occlusion showed no abnormalities in the preceding duplex examination (low flow manifested by PSV < 45 cm/s or threefold focal increase in PSV compared with adjacent segment).

A noteworthy finding is that low-flow bypass grafts identified by duplex ultrasound (drop in blood flow velocity below 45 cm/s) appear to benefit from **maintenance of anticoagulation treatment** (warfarin). While continuation of anticoagulation was found to result in a markedly higher patency rate in low-flow grafts (decrease in occlusion rate from 24% to 4%, $p < 0.0001$), no benefit was observed for high-flow grafts (Brumberg et al. 2008). Surprisingly, graft PSV in this study of 130 bypass grafts was <45 cm/s in 47% of cases.

2.1.7.3.2 Controversy About the Benefit of Duplex Bypass Graft Surveillance Programs

Although studies present conflicting evidence (Wixon et al. 2000; Golledge et al. 1996; Davies et al. 2005), many authors advocate duplex ultrasound surveillance after bypass grafting, at least for vein grafts and during the first postoperative year (Table 2.15) when the risk of occlusion is highest and the prognosis of bypass revision is good (Harris et al. 1988; Passman et al. 1995; Taylor et al. 1990).

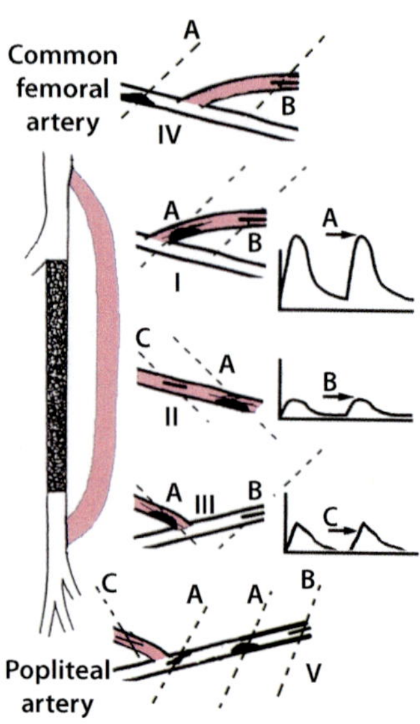

Fig. 2.39 Common sites of bypass graft stenosis and corresponding spectral Doppler changes (A, B) illustrated for femoropopliteal bypass graft bridging occluded superficial femoral artery. **I** Stenosis of proximal bypass anastomosis (A) with poststenotic waveform (B). **II** Stenosis within vein graft (at former valve site) with focal doubling of flow velocity (A) compared with prestenotic waveform (C) and postocclusive flow profile distal to the stenosis (B). **III** Stenosis of distal bypass anastomosis (A) with poststenotic flow profile in the popliteal outflow tract (B). **IV** Stenosis of the native artery proximal to the bypass anastomosis, which is due to progressive atherosclerosis: stenotic waveform (A) in the arterial segment proximal to the stenosis and poststenotic flow profile in the artery distal to the stenosis and in the bypass graft (B). **V** Stenosis of the artery distal to the lower bypass anastomosis: stenotic waveform (A) at the site of stenosis with poststenotic flow profile distally (B) and prestenotic waveform (C) in the proximal arterial segment and in the bypass graft

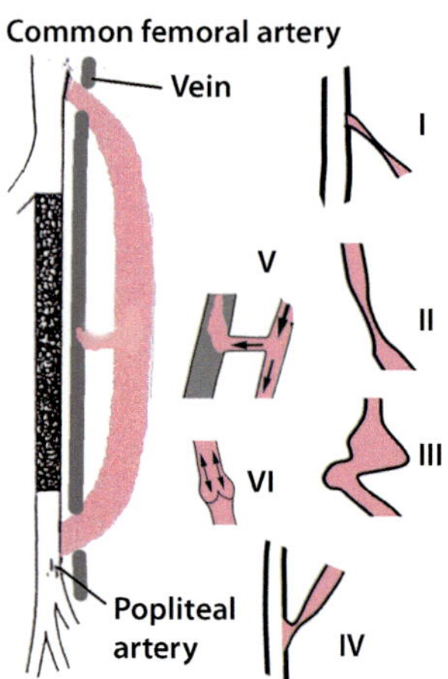

Fig. 2.40 A venous bypass graft is susceptible to a number of specific complications (I–VI), which must be taken into account in bypass surveillance in addition to the preferred sites of stenosis illustrated in Fig. 2.39. **I** A reversed vein graft is prone to stenosis just distal to the proximal stenosis, the narrowest portion of the graft. **II** Scar formation with narrowing at valve sites. **III** Dilatation with elongation and kinking of the graft. **IV** In situ vein graft with a narrow distal end can result in luminal narrowing just proximal to the distal anastomosis. **V** Failure to ligate all perforating veins communicating with an in situ vein can give rise to an AV fistula (between the bypass graft and the venous system). **VI** Residual valve in an in situ vein graft giving rise to graft stenosis or occlusion

Notwithstanding the ongoing controversy, it seems important to document the baseline flow characteristics during the first 3 months after surgery. If there is a decrease in PSV or triphasic flow becomes monophasic over time, this should prompt a search of the graft, the anastomoses, and the inflow and outflow segments for stenosis using the criteria described above.

In a cost-effectiveness analysis, infrainguinal venous bypass graft surveillance with revision for duplex-detected stenoses resulted in a 1-year patency rate of 93% versus 57% for grafts revised after thrombosis (Wixon et al. 2000). The amputation rate was also lower (2% vs. 33%). Especially patients with critical leg ischemia at the time of bypass grafting appear to benefit from sonographic surveillance and graft revision (Visser et al. 2001). In this study, patients in the duplex surveillance group had a major amputation rate of 1.7% compared with 7.7% in patients undergoing surveillance with clinical examination and ABI only. The cost of diagnosis and treatment was only half as high in the duplex group. The subgroup of patients with intermittent claudication at the time of bypass surgery benefited less from sonographic surveillance.

Overall, these findings show a benefit of routine duplex surveillance for patients with autologous vein grafts, while a benefit is less apparent for patients with synthetic grafts. Many studies are limited by the fact that they investigated mixed populations of patients with venous and synthetic bypass grafts. The poorer predictive value of routine surveillance in patients with synthetic grafts seems to be attributable to the complexity of factors that can cause occlusion of these grafts. Often, a stenotic lesion is not detectable and the mechanism of occlusion remains unclear. It is obvious, then, that duplex surveillance can contribute little to the identification of failing synthetic grafts.

A large meta-analysis (Golledge et al. 1996) comparing 2680 duplex surveillance and 3369 nonsurveillance vein grafts showed that routine duplex surveillance improved bypass patency rates but not the (long-term) limb salvage rate.

The Vein Graft Surveillance Randomised Trial (VGST) had great impact regarding the role of routine duplex surveillance in patients with venous grafts (Davies et al. 2005). In this prospective, randomized multicenter trial of 594 patients, no difference was found between clinical and duplex surveillance in terms of primary patency, primary assisted patency, secondary patency, and amputation rates. A limitation of the VGST is that no subgroup analysis was done.

Thus, while there is no added benefit of routine duplex monitoring of leg bypass grafts (as shown by Kaplan–Meier analysis), a duplex ultrasound evaluation is warranted whenever serial clinical examination, pulse status, or the ABI shows deterioration. Moreover, patients with venous bypass grafts who have **a poorer prognosis from the start** also benefit from being enrolled in a **duplex surveillance program**. Several graft-related and patient-related factors contribute to a poorer prognosis (Table 2.17):

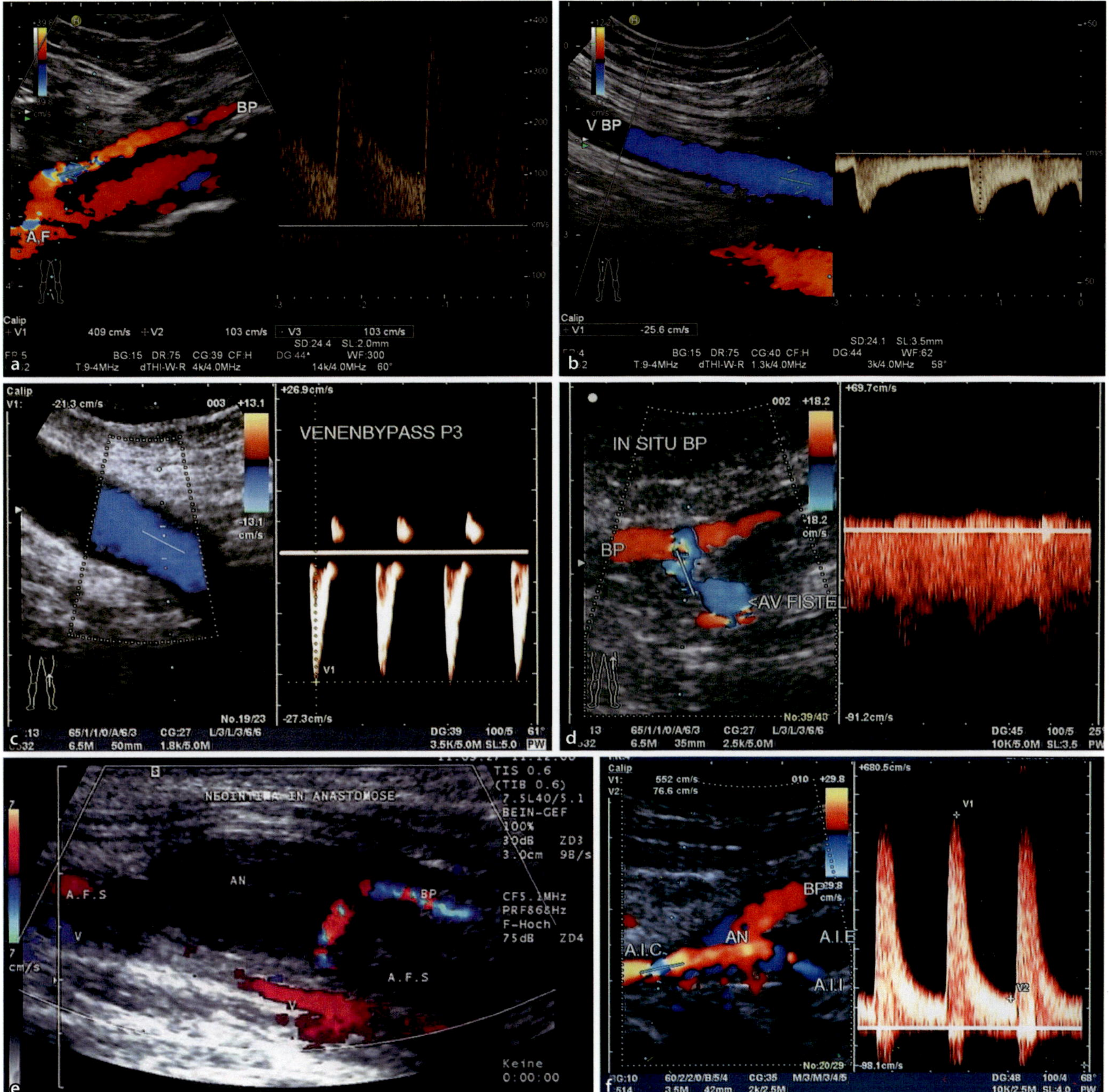

Fig. 2.41 Bypass graft surveillance. **a** Long stenosis in a femorocrural reversed vein bypass graft just distal to the proximal anastomosis (due to use of a small-caliber vein segment for grafting). Spectral Doppler interrogation of the stenotic segment (indicated by aliasing in the color image) demonstrates monophasic flow with a peak systolic velocity (PSV) of 4.1 m/s and an end-diastolic velocity (EDV) of 1 m/s. **b** The Doppler waveform from within the graft downstream of the anastomotic stenosis shows a monophasic, poststenotic pattern with slow flow (PSV of 25 cm/s). **c** If no flow obstruction is present above, within, or below a bypass graft, an altered flow velocity within the graft may be due to a size mismatch between the graft (synthetic or venous) and the recipient artery (e.g., a calf artery). Very slow flow in the absence of upstream or downstream stenosis can occur when a synthetic graft with too large a diameter has been used or a vein graft has become dilated over time (as in the example, where PSV is 21 cm/s). A triphasic waveform obtained in a bypass graft indicates good graft function with adequate peripheral perfusion. In the example, the vein graft anastomosed onto the tibiofibular trunk is dilated to 1.3 cm, and the fibular artery is the only patent calf artery. **d** An in situ vein graft must be scrutinized for the presence of an AV fistula (arising from a nonligated branch or perforating vein), especially if peripheral pulses are poorer than would be expected after a bypass procedure. There is monophasic flow with a large diastolic component in the graft segment proximal to and within the AV fistula due to direct outflow into the venous system (BP = bypass). The site of the AV fistula is marked for ligation. **e** High-grade stenosis at the proximal bypass anastomosis (AN) due to neointimal hyperplasia (hypoechoic). **f** Iliacofemoral bypass graft (BP) with high-grade proximal stenosis in the common iliac artery (A.I.C.) giving rise to a monophasic Doppler waveform with a PSV of 550 m/s. A poststenotic waveform is obtained in the bypass graft (as in **b**). A.I.I. = internal iliac artery; A.I.E. = occluded external iliac artery

2

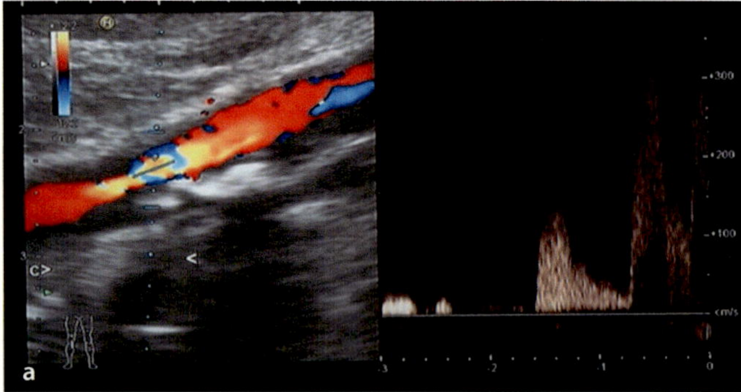

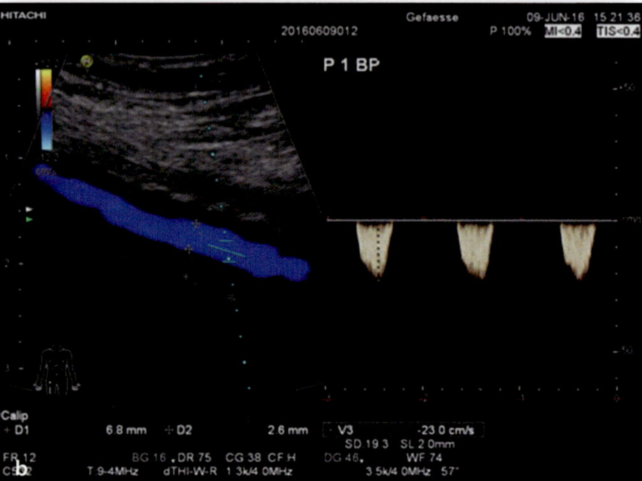

Fig. 2.42 **a** High-grade venous bypass graft stenosis. Stenosis in a vein graft is typically due to scar formatiom at retained valve cusps and is graded most reliably using the peak systolic velocity (PSV) ratio. In the example, the waveform shows the prestenotic situation on the left (PSV < 50 cm/s) and the intrastenotic situation on the right (PSV > 3.5 m/s). **b** Neointima (hypoechoic area around patent lumen) in a synthetic femoropopliteal bypass graft (7 mm in diameter), reducing the patent lumen to 2.6 mm (calipers). Unlike a focal stenosis, a very long segment of luminal narrowing is associated with flow reduction (due to friction) instead of a circumscribed increase in PSV. However, downstream of the narrowed graft, a postenotic flow profile is obtained

- Low-flow bypass and small-caliber vein graft
- Non-great-saphenous vein grafts and composite grafts
- Abnormal intra–/postoperative findings
- Bypass grafting in chronic critical limb ischemia (no alternative options for restoring blood flow)
- Distal-origin bypass in patients with severe inflow atherosclerosis.

Other investigators explored the **benefit of a single duplex follow-up examination** 3–6 months after surgery to estimate bypass prognosis and identify patients requiring revision or continuing duplex surveillance (Mofidi et al. 2007; Tinder et al. 2008). In a study of 365 patients, a single postoperative duplex examination performed 6 months after vein graft bypass surgery to identify grafts at risk (PSV ratio, PSV < 45 cm/s) demonstrated that critical stenosis was associated with much poorer graft patency and that most intermediate lesions identified by early duplex surveillance showed progression (>75%), resulting in graft dysfunction or loss. The 65% of patients without stenosis had a cumulative patency rate of 82% (Mofidi et al. 2009). Tinder et al. (2008) found a similar association between early detection of stenosis and bypass patency in a study of 353 venous bypasses. In this study, patients with normal duplex findings had a cumulative bypass patency rate of 84% at 54 months compared with 62% in patients with stenosis (including mild and moderate stenotic lesions). Investigators reporting angiographic findings for comparison found a surprisingly high percentage of early postoperative stenoses (25–37%) within the first 3 months (neointimal proliferation) despite normal intraoperative completion angiograms. Over time, the rate of de novo stenosis decreased, and patients with early duplex-identified stenosis had a significantly higher occlusion rate (Ihnat et al. 1999; Mercer et al. 1999).

The **decision for bypass revision** is based on the severity of stenosis and poststenotic flow rates; clinical symptoms alone may be misleading as they vary with the patient's disease stage at the time of the bypass procedure (Fig. 2.43). Therefore, demonstration of a higher-grade stenosis by duplex ultrasound should prompt an intervention (typically PTA) to maintain graft patency, even in asymptomatic patients. In estimating the degree of graft stenosis, the proposed threshold velocities must be applied flexibly, taking into account the diameters of the graft and recipient artery. Future studies should establish refined threshold velocities for different types of grafts (autologous vein versus prosthetic grafts, bypass diameter), level of bypass (target vessel above or below the knee), and other factors (status of runoff vessels).

2.1.7.4 Ultrasound Vein Mapping Prior to Peripheral Bypass Surgery

Autologous vein grafts are superior to other materials in peripheral bypass surgery in terms of short-term and long-term patency rates. However, vein preparation may be time-consuming in patients with anatomic variants, such as an aberrant course or duplication, and in obese patients. When the great or small saphenous vein is considered, the superficial course can be identified with a high-resolution transducer (6.5–10 MHz) and marked on the skin before surgery. Moreover, duplicated veins can be localized and the most suitable branch selected for grafting. When an in situ bypass is planned, perforating veins can also be marked for intraoperative ligation to prevent development of an AV fistula. The vein diameter is measured in transverse orientation with the great saphenous vein normally having a diameter of 3–4 mm below the knee; very thin veins (<2 mm) are unsuitable for grafting. If two branches are present, the one with the larger caliber is selected. Finally, preoperative ultrasound avoids unnecessary dissection by identifying unsuitable varicose or postthrombophlebitic veins with thickened walls and sclerosis. Overall, **preoperative sonographic vein mapping for selection of a suitable graft** shortens the length of surgery and can prevent unnecessary incisions and extensive exposure (Figs. 3.81 and 2.67 (Atlas)).

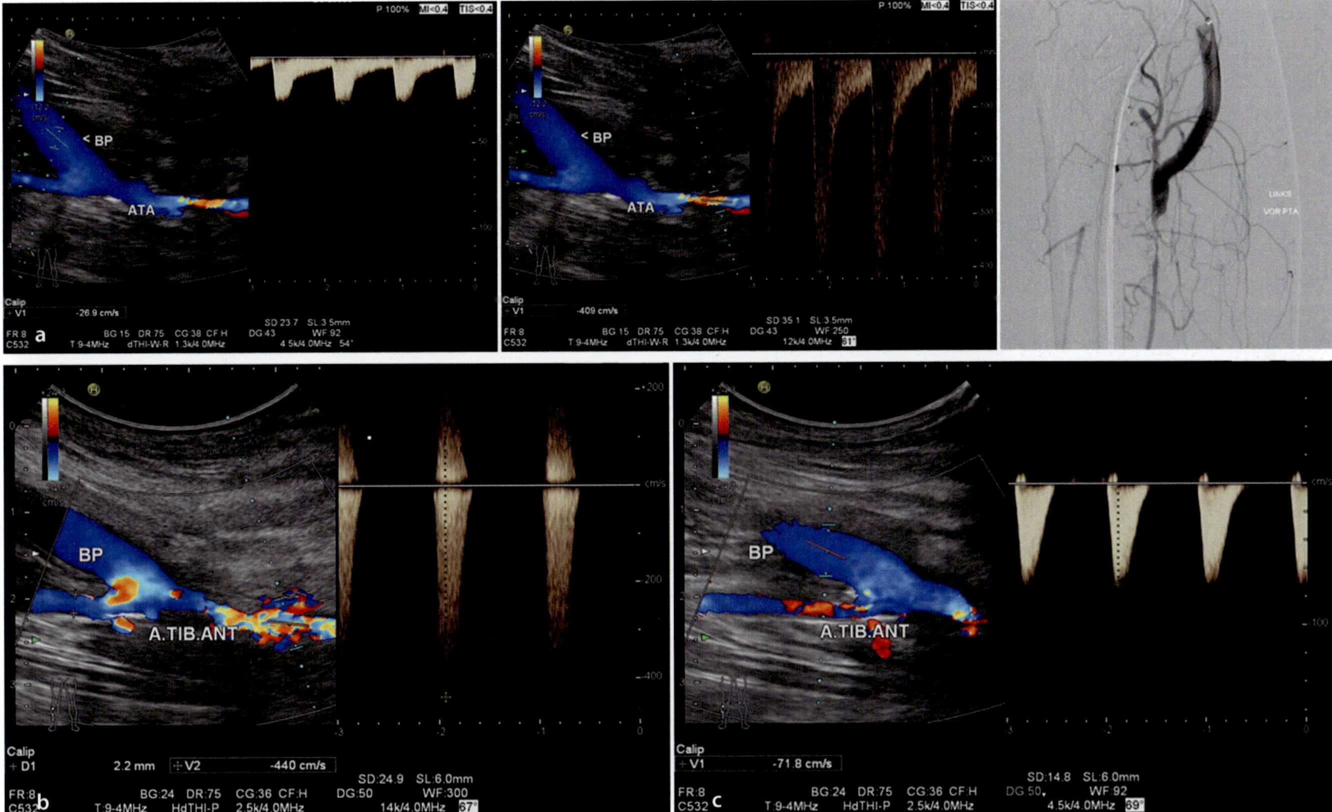

Fig. 2.43 **a** In a crural bypass, a stenosis just below the distal anastomosis has the same significance as an anastomotic stenosis. The color duplex examination reveals high-grade stenosis of the anterior tibial artery (ATA), resulting in slow flow in the bypass (<30 cm/s). These findings suggest a failing bypass and are an indication for graft revision to maintain patency, even in an asymptomatic patient (rightmost image: angiogram obtained during PTA). **b, c** Femorocrural bypass (BP) onto the anterior tibial artery (A.TIB.ANT) with high-grade stenosis (**b**) just distal to the anastomosis (PSV of 440 cm/s). In this case, a single measurement within the graft would have failed as an indirect stenosis criterion because the PSV of 71 cm/s measured in the graft (**c**) in this patient is above the cutoff of 45 cm/s. While the waveform shows adequate, pulsatile flow in the graft and runoff through the proximal anterior tibial artery, this case also underlines that reliance on a single midgraft PSV measurement is an inadequate criterion. PSV in a bypass crucially depends on graft configuration and outflow hemodynamics rather than bypass complications alone

Table 2.17 Differentiated approach to the use of duplex ultrasound in the surveillance of patients with lower extemity bypass grafts. The strategy recommended here has been derived from the conflicting scientific evidence[a] and is based on a single postoperative duplex follow-up examination (after 3–6 months) in all patients, with further ultrasound examinations necessary depending on the type of bypass graft and clinical findings (regular clinical follow-up with ABI at 6-month intervals, duplex ultrasound only in case of bypass deterioration)

Expected benefit of routine duplex surveillance at 6-month intervals	Bypass graft material and perioperative findings
No benefit, except for a single examination 3 – 6 months after surgery	Infrainguinal **synthetic bypass graft** Exception: clinical deterioration (decrease in ABI) → Search for underlying cause using duplex ultrasound
Probably no benefit, except for a single examination 3 – 6 months after surgery	**Venous bypass graft** (in situ, reversed) in patients who meet the following conditions: – Large-caliber bypass graft vein (>5 mm), normal graft vein – **Normal intra-/postoperative completion study** – Bypass grafting performed in patients with stage II PAOD (intermittent claudication) – Good patient compliance
Benefit likely	**Venous bypass graft:** – **Thin bypass vein** – Non-great-saphenous-vein grafts and composite grafts – **Abnormal intra-/postoperative findings** (increased outflow resistance, low flow, poor runoff vessel) – Bypass grafting performed in patients with chronic critical limb ischemia (stage III or IV PAOD) – Poor patient compliance – All distal-origin bypasses with upstream atherosclerosis

[a]Study of Davies et al. (2005) not taken into account because it does not present a subgroup analysis for a differentiated approach

2

2.1.8 Role of (Color) Duplex Ultrasound Compared with Other Modalities: Problems and Pitfalls

In the stepwise diagnostic workup of peripheral arterial occlusive disease (PAOD), the patient's history, clinical examination with evaluation of pulses, and determination of the ankle-brachial index (ABI) should be followed by noninvasive duplex imaging before invasive angiography is contemplated (◘ Fig. 2.7). The clinical stage of PAOD and the sonographic findings are the basis for further patient management, either initiation of treatment or additional diagnostic tests (◘ Tables 2.18 and 2.19).

For example, patients with sonographically diagnosed iliac or femoropopliteal stenosis can undergo diagnostic angiography with PTA standby. In contrast, patients with longer occlusions of the pelvic or thigh arteries and sonographically adequate peripheral runoff with patency of the popliteal artery can be scheduled for bypass surgery without prior angiography if indicated on clinical grounds. Ultrasound alone is also sufficient in patients with a popliteal artery aneurysm.

◘ **Table 2.18** Advantages and disadvantages of duplex imaging

Advantages	Disadvantages
Noninvasiveness Evaluation in different planes Evaluation of – Wall morphology – Surrounding structures – Intraluminal structures – Plaque Stenosis grading based on – Morphology – Hemodynamics Low cost	Documentation of findings Evaluation of collateral pathways Long training period Poor visualization of terminal vascular bed Specific methodological limitations (calcification, air, obesity, edema)

◘ **Table 2.19** Advantages and disadvantages of angiography

Advantages	Disadvantages
Documentation of findings Visualization and evaluation of collateral pathways Adequate evaluation of terminal vascular bed Fairly short training period	Invasiveness and complications (pseudoaneurysm, embolism, bleeding, local thrombosis, AV fistula) Visualization of patent lumen only Projection-related problems: – Stenosis grading – Evaluation of bifurcations Some vascular territories cannot be consistently evaluated in 2 (or 3) planes (iliac artery, femoral bifurcation) No information on hemodynamic relevance of different plaque configurations Nonvisualization: – Vessel wall – Surrounding structures High cost Radiation exposure and contrast medium administration

Patients in whom ultrasound reveals external compression (popliteal entrapment syndrome, adventitial cystic disease) can also be operated on without prior angiography, which provides no additional information and merely serves to document the vascular status. Depicting only the vessel lumen, angiography is inferior to ultrasound in evaluating perivascular structures. A further drawback of angiography is the reduction of the three-dimensional vessel lumen to the two-dimensional plane of the film (see ◘ Fig. 5.27).

With this limitation, the **diameter reduction** randomly depicted in the imaging plane does not necessarily represent the true cross-sectional area reduction, as the wall changes may vary along the length of the stenosis (concentric – eccentric; regular – irregular). Angiographic stenosis severity may thus differ from the degree determined by spectral Doppler, which reflects the hemodynamic effects of the stenosis. Even different ultrasound modes may yield discrepant results regarding the degree of luminal narrowing caused by atherosclerotic plaque because they process different types of information: conventional B-mode imaging relies on the morphologic gray-scale appearance of the arterial lumen in the longitudinal plane, color duplex on the absence of flow signals in the lumen, and spectral Doppler on the hemodynamic effects of the stenotic lesion in terms of flow acceleration. For accurate and reproducible morphologic quantification by both B-mode ultrasound and angiography, it is thus necessary to always evaluate a stenosis in different planes (◘ Table 2.17). This is especially important when assessing the pelvic arteries and femoral trifurcation, where eccentric plaques of the posterior wall are common. The mere morphologic assessment of an eccentric plaque afforded by angiography may overestimate the resulting stenosis compared with its hemodynamic effects, even when evaluated in different planes. Moreover, stenosis caused by eccentric plaque may be overlooked or underestimated if only an anteroposterior angiogram is available.

An aspect that tends to be overlooked in the scientific discussion is that **plaque configuration** (concentric versus eccentric) determines the hemodynamic severity of the resulting stenosis in terms of peripheral perfusion impairment and the patient's clinical symptoms. The hemodynamic severity in turn depends on the cross-sectional area reduction, which is the basis for calculating the sonographic degree of stenosis from intrastenotic flow acceleration (see ◘ Fig. 5.27). Recall that a concentric stenosis that reduces the vessel diameter by 50% reduces the cross-sectional area by 75% as opposed to 50% or less when an eccentric stenosis with the same diameter reduction is present. Sonographically, the former is classified as higher-grade stenosis (PSV ratio of 4 according to the continuity equation) and the latter as 50% stenosis (PSV ratio of 2). Angiographically, the degree of stenosis is 50% in both cases.

At the **origin of the profunda femoris artery**, angiography is additionally limited by the superposition of vessels. Ultrasound is superior in this region when performed with an adequate angle of insonation. In a study of 40 patients who underwent thromboendarterectomy (TEA) for sonographically demonstrated high-grade stenosis of the profunda femoris artery to improve collateralization of superficial femoral occlusion, the high-grade stenosis demonstrated by ultrasound and confirmed intraoperatively was identified definitely by angiography in only 85% of the cases, and there was considerable interobserver variability in stenosis grading.

Catheter-based digital subtraction angiography (DSA) via a transfemoral or transbrachial approach can be regarded as the gold standard on condition that views in two or three planes are obtained and adequate opacification of the distal arteries is ensured. Proper timing taking into account the longer contrast agent transit time to the thigh and foot is important to avoid misinterpretation. **Magnetic resonance angiography (MRA)** using dedicated coils is superior to DSA in evaluating the thigh and foot arteries in patients with reduced contrast agent inflow due to occlusive disease of more proximal arteries (Fellner et al. 1999; Owen et al. 1992; Kreitner et al. 2000). Several investigators demonstrated that MRA allowed good evaluation of distal arteries, including the pedal arch in patients with foot ischemia, and reliable identification of patent runoff vessels in cases where DSA did not allow adequate evaluation for selection of a target artery for pedal bypass grafting (Dorweiler et al. 2002; Kreitner et al. 2000).

For a complete evaluation of the lower extremity arteries, an imaging modality optimized for **visualization of the calf and foot arteries** needs to be supplemented by an additional imaging test for evaluation of the iliofemoral arteries. Noninvasive duplex ultrasound is ideal for the proximal leg arteries and has the added advantage of providing highly valid information on the flow effects of steno-occlusive lesions of the iliac and femoropopliteal arteries. It is therefore conceivable that a noninvasive diagnostic strategy combining (color) duplex ultrasound of the proximal leg arteries with MRA of the calf and pedal arch may in the future replace invasive DSA, which carries a number of risks (related to use of contrast medium, radiation exposure, vascular puncture, and catheterization).

The clinical usefulness of a diagnostic test depends not only on its diagnostic accuracy and the relevance of the results for therapeutic decision making but also on **how efficiently the examination can be performed**. It is theoretically possible to perform a complete duplex scan from the pelvic level down to the pedal arteries including identification of a target artery for bypass grafting (which may require administration of an echo enhancer, especially if a crural bypass is contemplated). Few scientific data are available on the time required for such an examination.

In a study performed by the author, 220 patients with claudication, forefoot lesions, or rest pain were selected for a duplex examination of the leg arteries on the basis of ABI findings. In this preselected population, duplex imaging identified hemodynamically relevant stenosis or occlusion in 93% of cases. Using the above-described protocol (◘ Table 2.1), the examiner first obtained and analyzed Doppler waveforms from the groin at the junction of the external iliac artery and common femoral artery (in comparison with the contralateral leg), followed by evaluation of the profunda femoris origin and superficial femoral artery. Next, spectral Doppler interrogation of the proximal and distal popliteal segments (P1 and P3) of the symptomatic leg was performed. Only if spectral analysis or comparison of the waveforms from the proximal and distal popliteal segments revealed any abnormalities or relevant changes was the proximal arterial segment continuously mapped in the B-mode with continuous spectral Doppler recording (longitudinal plane, sample volume slightly larger than the arterial lumen). Occlusion length was determined taking into account the sites of origin and entry of collaterals. With this protocol, it took on average 5.2 min to establish a diagnosis and to decide on the therapeutic approach (conservative, surgery, PTA) and plan the surgical procedure (TEA or bypass graft including selection of the distal recipient artery). Patients with a long history of diabetes mellitus were not included in this study because severe medial sclerosis with acoustic shadowing makes the sonographic examination more challenging and time-consuming.

This sonographic strategy allows reliable treatment decisions to be made, including selection of a bypass target artery for surgical management of relevant stenosis or **occlusion**, in patients with stage II PAOD and a patent popliteal artery (◘ Table 2.20). In patients with stage III or IV disease and occlusion at the pelvic or thigh level but a patent popliteal segment (from P1 to the tibiofibular trunk), the inflow obstruction above the popliteal artery is eliminated (PTA or bypass), which can be done without examination of the calf arteries. They need to be included in the sonographic evaluation only if the popliteal artery is stenosed or partially occluded and a bypass onto a small artery below the knee is contemplated. Examination of the arteries below the knee by ultrasound is possible but time-consuming, as several authors have demonstrated (Boström et al. 2002; Hofmann et al. 2004). Alternatively, angiography or MRA with dedicated coils can be used. Angiography has several disadvantages including invasiveness, contrast medium administration, and poor visualization of calf arteries in patients with long proximal occlusions. When duplex ultrasound is performed to identify a bypass target below the knee, Doppler waveforms are obtained from the dorsalis pedis and posterior tibial arteries at the ankle level (and possibly also from the distal fibular artery) and are then compared with the waveforms from the P3 popliteal segment or proximal segments of the calf arteries. The artery from which the proximal and distal waveforms are least different is the most suitable target for the planned bypass and should subsequently be mapped to confirm its suitability.

2

Table 2.20 Sensitivities and specificities reported for color duplex ultrasound, contrast-enhanced magnetic resonance angiography (CE-MRA), and computed tomography angiography (CTA) in patients with peripheral arterial occlusive disease (PAOD) using digital subtraction angiography (DSA) as standard of reference

Study/ Meta-analysis	Patient population	Color duplex		CE-MRA		CTA	
		Sensitivity (%)	Specificity (%)	Sensitivity (%)	Specificity (%)	Sensitivity (%)	Specificity (%)
Nelemans et al. (2000)	PAOD, mostly Fontaine stage II	68–82	91–95	78–89	95–98	–	–
Lundin et al. (2000)	PAOD, Fontaine stage II	72	97	81	92	–	–
Koelemay et al. (2001)	PAOD, mostly Fontaine stage II	80–86	97	–	–	–	–
Collins et al. (2007)	PAOD, mostly Fontaine stage II	80–98	89–99	92–99.5	64–99	89–99	83–97

While the studies listed in the table found slightly lower sensitivities for color duplex ultrasound, the method is comparable to DSA in defining the therapeutic strategy in patients with PAOD (Collins et al. 2007; Koelemay et al. 1996)

Sonographic follow-up is useful to monitor the outcome of vascular repair and identify graft stenosis, thus contributing to the timely initiation of therapeutic measures aimed at maintaining graft patency (Table 2.16).

In patients with long-standing stenosis, **extensive collateral pathways** may have developed. The reduced blood flow and altered hemodynamics in the main artery resulting from a division of the blood volume between the collaterals and the obstructed artery can lead to underestimation of stenosis severity when only absolute PSV cutoffs are used for sonographic stenosis grading (see Fig. 2.16a).

Color duplex imaging with a high-resolution transducer enables assessment of collaterals, in particular when the occluded segment is short, and will detect stenosis at the re-entry sites of collateral pathways (see Fig. 2.63 (Atlas)). Nevertheless, angiography is superior to ultrasound in providing a comprehensive overview of collateral circulation around an occlusion. The hemodynamic situation distal to an occluded segment can merely give hints. A relatively high PSV in conjunction with pulsatile flow in the postocclusive segment distal to the re-entry of collaterals suggests good collateralization. PSV alone might lead to misinterpretation and is also increased in diabetics with rigid arterial walls due to medial sclerosis.

When two or more sequential steno-occlusive lesions are present, the more distal ones may be underestimated or difficult to assess, especially in patients with diabetic macroangiopathy. Moreover, the hemodynamic changes associated with diabetic medial sclerosis and peripheral occlusions further impair stenosis grading by duplex ultrasound. Angiographically, such sequential stenoses are identified by their typical goose throat appearance.

When diagnostic ultrasonography and vascular repair are performed by different persons or even by different departments, the lack of continuous documentation of the findings – in particular in patients with complex patterns of vascular lesions – limits the communication of the findings to the surgeon or interventionalist. Therefore, pretherapeutic ultrasound is most valuable when performed by the radiologist or vascular surgeon who also treats the patient and benefits from the additional hemodynamic information. The diagnostic gain also depends on the skills of the examiner, as ultrasound is highly **examiner-dependent**.

2.1.8.1 Comparison of Hemodynamic and Morphologic Imaging Modalities

A systematic review of 48 studies investigating the accuracy of different imaging modalities for detecting significant arterial stenosis (>50%) in patients with symptomatic peripheral arterial occlusive disease (PAOD) was presented by Collins et al. (Collins et al. 2007). Compared with digital subtraction angiography (DSA) as the gold standard, the results were as follws: CT angiography (five studies) had a median sensitivity of 97% (range, 89–100%) and a median specificity of 99.6% (range, 99–100%). Time-of-flight (TOF) magnetic resonance imaging (four studies) had a median sensitivity of 86% (range, 77–100%) and a median specificity of 93.8% (range, 85–98%). MRA using a gadolinium-based contrast agent was found to have a median sensitivity of 94% (range, 85–100%) and a median specificity of 99.2% (range, 97–99.8%). Color duplex ultrasound (7 studies) had a similar diagnostic performance with a median sensitivity of 90% (range, 74–94%) and a median specificity of 99% (range, 89–100%). Duplex imaging and contrast-enhanced MRA were found to have similar sensitivities and specificities of approx. 90% (compared with DSA) in detecting hemodynamically significant stenosis below the knee.

While CT and MRI are also considered noninvasive imaging modalities, color duplex ultrasound is the least invasive method, causing few complications and no patient discomfort (Table 2.21).

Table 2.21 Validity, limitations, and cost of digital subtraction angiography (DSA), color duplex ultrasound, contrast-enhanced magnetic resonance angiography (CE-MRA), and computed tomography angiography (CTA) in patients with peripheral arterial occlusive disease (PAOD). Data are stratified by the segment involved and include diagnostic performance in the identification of wall structures and extramural processes (Modified from Klein-Weigel et al. 2015)

Modality	Aortoiliac PAOD	Femoropopliteal PAOD	Cruropedal PAOD	Plaque morphology and wall structure	Extramural processes
DSA	++ – +++	+++	++ – +++[a]	+	–
Color duplex	++[b]	+++	++[c]	++ – +++	+++
CE-MRA	+++	+++	++[d]	+ – ++[e]	+++
CTA	+++	+++	++ – +	++	+++
Modality	**Degradation by mural calcification or plaque**	**Stent monitoring**	**Examiner dependence**	**Time requirement**	**Cost**
DSA	+ – ++	++ – +++	+	++	+++[g]
Color duplex	++ – +++	+++	++	++[f]	+
CE-MRA	–	+	+	++/+++[g]	++[g]
CTA	+ – ++	++	+	++/+++[g]	++

[a]Diagnostic performance may be reduced in multilevel PAOD, depending on contrast flow selectivity and extent of arterial occlusion
[b]Limited by vascular calcification, bowel gas, and obesity
[c]High for identification of crural/pedal target for distal bypass
[d]Often limited by superposition of veins
[e]Limited by rather poor spatial resolution
[g]Dependent on selectivity, protocol, and postprocessing
[f]Largely dependent on extent of examination, patient-related factors, and technique used

CTA involves high radiation exposure and the use of an iodine-based contrast agent, and stenosis grading may be impaired by calcified plaques or stent-related artifacts. The quality of contrast-enhanced MRA depends on the use of state-of-the-art equipment; general limitations include poor visualization of below-knee arteries unless dedicated coils are used, the susceptibility to artifacts, overestimation of stenosis severity, and venous superimposition, which is most relevant in the periphery. MRI is contraindicated in patients with pacemakers or defibrillators. Gadolinium-based contrast agents should not be used in patients with impaired renal function because they may induce life-threatening nephrogenic systemic fibrosis (Collins et al. 2007).

An experienced examiner is able to assess the arteries below the knee throughout their course using a high-resolution transducer. Extra time is required for the separate evaluation of an occlusion or stenosis. What ultrasound fails to provide is an overview of complex patterns of disturbed perfusion with multiple occlusions of the lower leg arteries that collateralize each other. In this situation, it is often not possible to adequately characterize peripheral outflow.

Acoustic shadowing from calcified plaques may impair the detection and grading of stenosis in small arteries. In such cases, the sonographic search for a patent target artery for a distal bypass is very time-consuming, especially when the indirect stenosis criteria cannot be used due to proximal occlusion or multilevel stenosis. Despite these limitations, some investigators report accuracy rates for the detection of steno-occlusive lesions below the knee that allow surgical planning without prior angiography. According to these studies, preoperative duplex ultrasound alone allows reliable identification of a patent runoff vessel for a planned bypass graft below the femoropopliteal arteries. These patients were found to have the same intraoperative results as well as primary and secondary bypass patency and limb salvage rates as patients undergoing preoperative angiography.

The studies **comparing duplex imaging with DSA** in the assessment of the cruropedal arteries report widely divergent results (Karacagil et al. 1996; Koelemay et al. 1997) with sensitivities and specificities for the detection of occlusion ranging from 50% to 90%. However, the investigators used 5 MHz transducers, which are inadequate for the pedal vessels, and the low resolution may explain the poor results. Other study groups (Boström et al. 2002; Hofmann et al. 2001) describe limitations of nonselective IA DSA in the visualization of the outflow vessels of the foot (see Fig. 2.71 (Atlas)). In a consecutive series of 49 patients reported by Hofmann et al. (2001), the pedal arteries were poorly or not at all visualized by DSA in 32 cases (65.3%). Based on the sonographic evaluation using a high-resolution transducer (13 MHz), all 32 patients underwent pedal bypass grafting with a 2-year patency rate of 69.5%. Boström et al. (2002) compared 157 vascular surgical procedures (32 inguinal TEA, 91 femoropopliteal bypass, 34 femorocrural bypass) performed solely on the basis of the ultrasound findings and 172 procedures (28 inguinal TEA, 144 femoropopliteal and femorocrural bypass) planned on the basis of angiography. The second group included patients with diagnostically inadequate ultrasound examinations (in particular also patients with femorofibular bypass procedures). Cruropedal bypass grafting (ratio of 1:2 [ultrasound versus angiography group]) and femorocrural bypass grafting (ratio of 1:1) were also performed using only the ultrasound findings for planning. The primary patency rate of the bypass grafts was 59% in the ultrasound group versus 64% in the angiography group. In 98% of the patients examined by preoperative ultrasound alone, no intraoperative revision of the planned procedure was necessary (not even on the basis of intraoperative DSA).

In conclusion, there is agreement that duplex ultrasound is a valid method for the localization and grading of steno-occlusive lesions in the iliac, femoral, and popliteal arteries (◘ Table 2.20) and that ultrasound alone provides all the information necessary for selecting the best treatment (medical therapy, PTA, bypass grafting) and for planning bypass procedures including identification of a suitable target vessel in this territory (Boström et al. 2002; Alexander et al. 2002; Ascher et al. 2004; Katsamouris et al. 2001; Lowery et al. 2007). However, there is disagreement regarding its role in **infrainguinal bypass grafting**, with some investigators considering preoperative ultrasound alone to be sufficient (Hofmann et al. 2004; Boström et al. 2002; Mazzariol et al. 2000; Karacagil et al. 1996) and others recommending supplementary IA DSA (Katsamouris et al. 2001). Several studies report comparable infrainguinal bypass patency rates for procedures planned on the basis of preoperative ultrasound versus those planned on the basis of IA DSA (Collins et al. 2007; Koelemay et al. 1996). Some authors conclude that supplementary preoperative IA DSA does not add diagnostic information (Elsman et al. 1995; Aly et al. 1998), not even in patients with complex reconstruction (crural/pedal) (Grassbaugh et al. 2003; Wong et al. 2013). In a large study of 466 patients, Ascher et al. (2002) found preoperative evaluation by color duplex ultrasound to be sufficient for planning the bypass procedure in the majority of cases with only 36 patients requiring a supplementary imaging test (angiography, CTA, MRA). **Contrast-enhanced ultrasound** (CEUS) has not led to the expected improvement in accuracy and stenosis grading. It may be helpful to identify a bypass recipient artery below the knee in an occasional patient with otherwise poor insonation conditions.

Velocity criteria (absolute PSV or PSV ratio) for identification and grading of stenosis need to be refined. The indiscriminate application of a single cutoff, as in some studies, does not take into account, for example, that normal blood flow velocity is lower in the popliteal artery than in the femoral artery or that PSV varies with plaque configuration and the site at which prestenotic PSV for calculation of the PSV ratio is measured.

When all factors affecting the hemodynamic situation evaluated by duplex ultrasound are taken into account, **interventional or surgical revascularization** (PTA, bypass graft) in the iliacofemoropopliteal territory (including the P3 segment) can be performed on the basis of the sonographic findings alone. The sonographic degree of stenosis is a function of its hemodynamic relevance and is a better indicator of the patient's clinical status than estimating stenosis severity on the basis of morphologic appearance alone (plaque). A time-efficient ultrasound protocol based on spectral Doppler interrogation of representative sites and subsequent mapping only of abnormal arterial segments allows sonographic evaluation of each leg including treatment planning in less than 10 min.

When **treatment is planned on the basis of the ultrasound findings**, the examination should ideally be performed by the surgeon or interventionalist treating the patient. This has the added advantage that, during the examination, the physician can ask details about the patient's pain and other symptoms, explain the findings, and discuss the proposed therapy.

2.2 Arm Arteries

2.2.1 Vascular Anatomy

The innominate artery (brachiocephalic trunk) arises from the aortic arch on the right and, behind the sternoclavicular joint, divides into the subclavian and common carotid arteries. On the left, the subclavian artery arises directly from the aortic arch as does the common carotid artery at a more proximal site. Along its course, the subclavian artery first gives off the vertebral artery cranially. Further along the course, the thyrocervical trunk arises, likewise from the posterior aspect, and at once divides into a branch supplying the thyroid and other branches supplying the skin and soft tissue. Together with the brachial plexus, the subclavian artery (◘ Fig. 2.44) passes through the scalene triangle (between the anterior and medial scalene muscles and cranial to the first rib) and arches over the pleural dome, crossing under the clavicle, to continue as the axillary artery. In individuals with a cervical rib, the

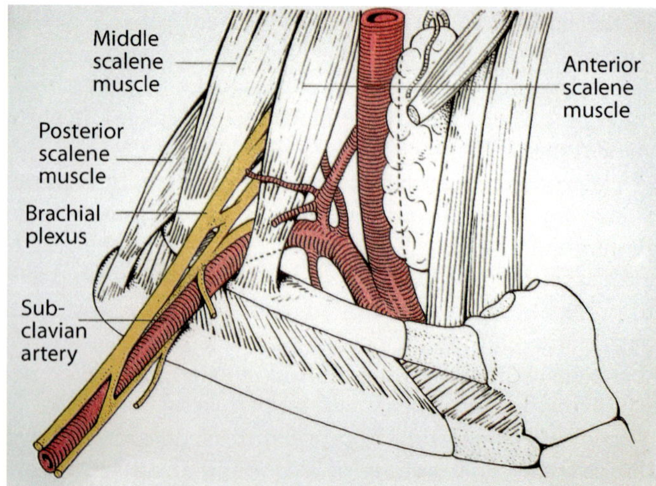

◘ **Fig. 2.44** Course of the subclavian artery through the scalene triangle. The subclavian artery runs between the first rib, medial scalene muscle, and anterior scalene muscle (from Heberer and van Dongen 1993)

subclavian artery is displaced cranially and anteriorly. Distal to the thyrocervical trunk, the internal thoracic (mammary) artery arises and descends behind the anterior chest wall and about one fingerbreadth lateral to the sternum.

The branches of the axillary artery have extensive collateral connections to the branches of the subclavian artery and supply the region of the shoulder girdle. The axillary artery courses along the lower border of the pectoralis muscle through the axilla and continues as the brachial artery. The latter runs through the medial bicipital groove near the humerus to the elbow and divides into the radial and ulnar arteries at the level of the joint space. There are anatomic variants in which the radial artery arises from the brachial artery in the upper arm (approx. 15%) or arises directly from the distal axillary artery (1–3%). In approx. 1% of individuals, the ulnar artery also arises from the axillary artery.

The radial artery continues through the forearm on the ulnar side of the radius to the wrist, where it unites with the deep branch of the ulnar artery to form the deep palmar arch. The radial artery primarily feeds the deep arch and the ulnar artery the superficial arch. The main branches of the superficial arch give off the common palmar digital arteries, which in turn give rise to the proper palmar digital arteries, the main vessels supplying the fingers (Fig. 2.45). A complete connection between the superficial and deep palmar arches is present in only approx. 80–90% of individuals.

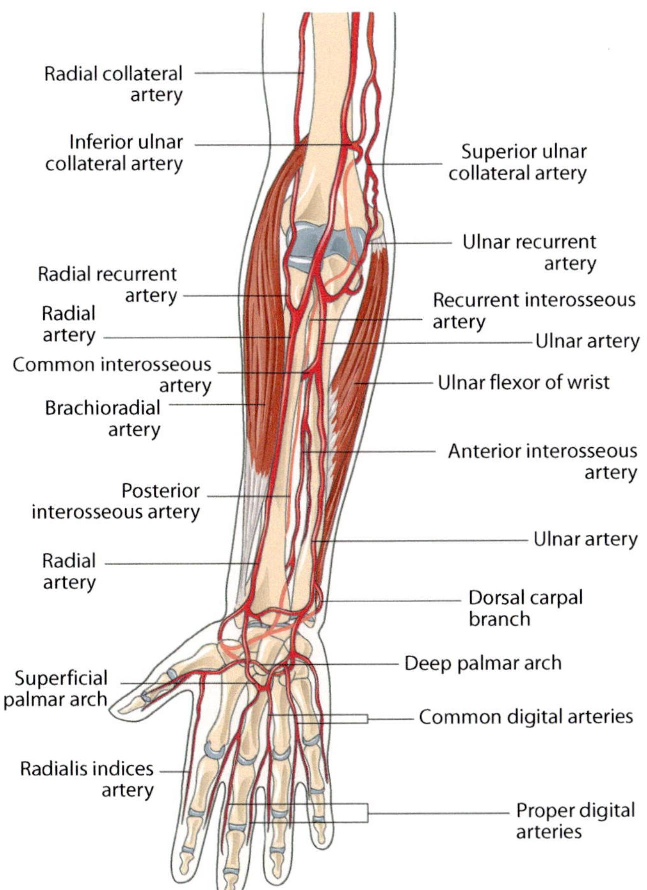

Fig. 2.45 Anatomy of the arm vessels

2.2.2 Examination Protocol and Technique

The subclavian and axillary arteries are scanned at **5–7.5 MHz** while a higher-frequency transducer can be used more distally, where the arteries lie closer to the surface. The finger arteries are examined with a **7.5–10 MHz transducer.** Especially in the supraclavicular fossa, a curved array or sector transducer is better suited than a linear array transducer. The subclavian and axillary arteries are best imaged in the supine position with the examiner behind the patient's head, as for the examination of the carotid arteries. The forearm and finger arteries are examined in the sitting patient with the hand supinated.

The arm arteries are traced along their course from the supraclavicular area to the palmar arch. In the upper arm, the arteries are easily identified by B-mode scanning based on sonoanatomic knowledge. Color duplex can be helpful in identifying the vessels of the palmar arch and fingers. As elsewhere in the body, identification of a vessel is easier with the transducer in transverse orientation. Spectral Doppler imaging is performed in longitudinal orientation using a smaller angle of insonation.

The proximal portion of the subclavian artery is interrogated with the transducer in the supraclavicular position. In evaluating the supra-aortic branches, the examiner should pay special attention to the origin of the vertebral artery, which must be differentiated from the thyrocervical trunk. Rhythmical tapping of the vertebral artery suboccipitally will be transmitted and appear in the Doppler waveform from the proximal segment of the artery.

The axillary artery is identified cranial to the axillary vein with the transducer placed in the infraclavicular fossa and followed along its path to the axilla (Fig. 2.46). The brachial artery is examined in the upper arm from a medial position.

Depending on the clinical question to be answered, special attention must be paid to the presence of aneurysm or stenosis of the subclavian artery. Inconclusive color duplex

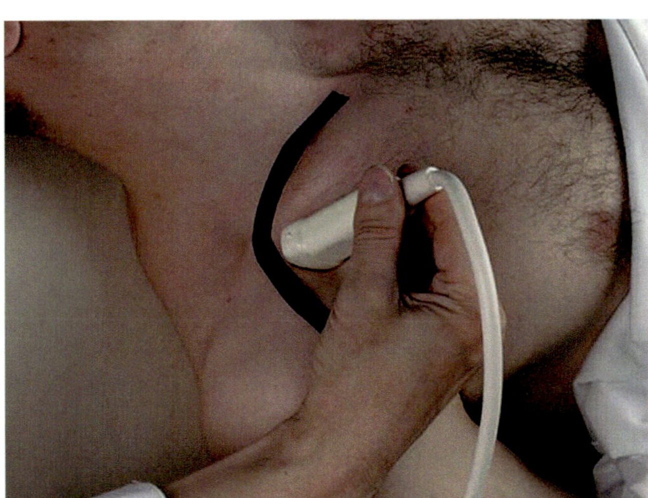

Fig. 2.46 Transducer position for examination of the axillary artery (transducer placed in the infraclavicular fossa) and subclavian artery (course indicated by black line)

findings can be resolved by additional spectral Doppler evaluation. Under normal conditions, the subclavian, axillary, and brachial arteries have a triphasic flow profile (high-resistance flow of arteries supplying soft tissue and skin).

The palmar arch and digital arteries are scanned using a high-resolution probe (>10 MHz), and a complete examination includes color duplex imaging and Doppler interrogation to differentiate thromboembolic disease from vasospastic conditions. A provocative test (heat and cold exposure) may also be helpful for the differential diagnosis.

2.2.3 Clinical Role of Duplex Ultrasound

2.2.3.1 Atherosclerosis

Stenoses of the upper extremity arteries **chiefly affect the proximal subclavian arter**y and are four times more common in the longer left subclavian artery (especially at its origin from the aorta). If a subclavian stenosis or occlusion is suspected, the sonographic evaluation should always include the vertebral artery to identify flow reversal as a sign of the **subclavian steal syndrome**. Prior to coronary bypass surgery, color duplex ultrasound can serve to noninvasively assess the internal thoracic artery as a candidate for grafting. Stenosis of the arm arteries distal to the subclavian artery is rare and typically has no clinical relevance, except in patients with a long history of diabetes mellitus or after creation of a hemodialysis access.

Repetitive trauma to the wrist can damage the distal ulnar artery, which is particularly vulnerable as it passes over the hook of hamate. Damage of the arterial wall can lead to the formation of an aneurysm (◘ Fig. 2.47), which may become partially thrombosed and then embolize to the interdigital arteries.

Besides atherosclerotic conditions and compression of the subclavian arteries, vascular diseases of the upper extremity most commonly involve the finger arteries and palmar arch. The finger arteries can be affected by embolic occlusion, vasculitis, and vasospastic conditions.

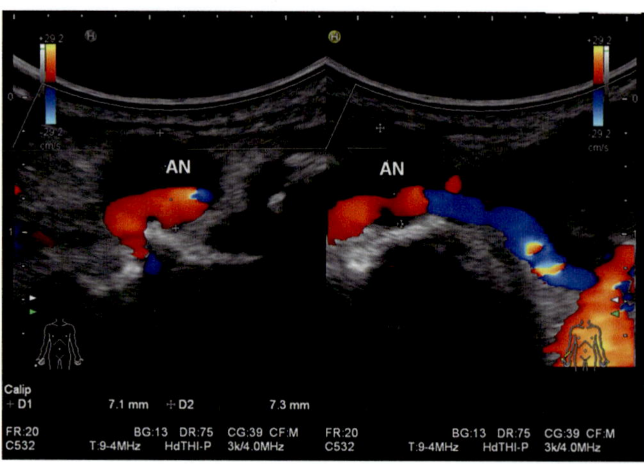

◘ **Fig. 2.47** Partially thrombosed aneurysm (AN) of the distal ulnar artery

2.2.3.2 Vascular Compression Syndromes

Various factors such as abnormal congenital bony and fibromuscular structures and posttraumatic alterations (hyperostosis) are involved in the development of the thoracic outlet syndrome. The nerves and vessels coursing through the narrow space of the upper thoracic aperture may become compressed, injured, or irritated when they have an atypical course or when osseous or fibrous anomalies are present. The clinical manifestation is very heterogeneous and varies with the structure compressed. The vast majority of patients (97%) suffer from neurogenic symptoms due to compression of the brachial plexus.

The most common **vascular symptoms** are insidious episodes of microembolization that may lead to occlusion of the interdigital arteries. Larger emboli, chiefly arising from poststenotic arterial aneurysm (◘ Figs. 2.105 and 2.106 (both Atlas)), may cause occlusion of the major arteries, namely the ulnar, radial, and brachial arteries. The thoracic outlet syndrome predominantly occurs in patients aged 20–50 and affects women at a ratio of 3:2.

Arterial compression syndromes of the thoracic outlet, typically resulting from vascular compromise in certain arm positions, are distinguished from the cervical rib syndrome, which is caused by an accessory rib or a ligamentous or fibrous band arising from the extra rib and ending freely or attaching to the first rib. The prevalence of cervical ribs is reported to be 0.5–1%, but only 5–10% of affected individuals become symptomatic. The diagnosis is primarily radiological. Compression of the subclavian artery mainly occurs at **three sites** where the artery courses through **narrow anatomic spaces**:

- The anterior scalenus muscle gap (scalene triangle)
- The narrow passage between the first rib and clavicle (costoclavicular space)
- The narrow space below the pectoralis minor muscle at its site of attachment to the coracoid process (pectoralis minor space)

As already mentioned, several anatomic variations or pathologic processes can compromise these already narrow spaces, resulting in mechanical irritation or compression of vessels and nerves. Prolonged compression can lead to downstream aneurysm formation with development of mural thrombi and embolism of the arm arteries (see ◘ Figs. 2.105 and 2.106 (both Atlas)).

Compression of neurovascular structures in one of these passageways can cause pain, weakness in the arm and hand, tingling nerve sensations, and other neurosensory disorders or symptoms of vascular compression. Peripheral embolism is the most common vascular complication of thoracic outlet syndrome and is the presenting symptom in 50% of cases (Dunant 1980; Creutzig et al. 1988). Published reports attribute a surprisingly high 70% of all emboli involving the upper extremity to embolic complications of the thoracic outlet syndrome. Most cases of embolism encountered in routine clinical practice are of cardiac origin.

The term **thoracic outlet syndrome** encompasses four neurovascular syndromes distinguished according to the site of vessel or nerve compression:

- **Scalenus anterior or cervical rib syndrome**: In this syndrome, the brachial plexus and the subclavian artery are compressed due to thickening or an abnormal position of the anterior or medial scalenus muscle at its attachment to the first rib, exostosis of the first rib, or a cervical rib. The subclavian vein is not involved as it does not pass through the scalene triangle (◘ Figs. 2.104, 2.105, and 2.106 (all Atlas)).
- **Costoclavicular syndrome**: The narrow passage between the clavicle and first rib is the preferred site of venous compression caused by a sagging shoulder girdle, rib callus, or exostosis. The subclavian artery and the brachial plexus are rarely compressed at this site (◘ Fig. 3.105 (Atlas)).
- **Hyperabduction syndrome**: At the third site, mechanical nerve damage predominates. It is due to compression of the neurovascular bundle by the tendon of the pectoralis minor muscle or the coracoid process when the arms are stretched above the head (◘ Fig. 2.107 (Atlas)).
- **Compression syndrome of the brachial artery***:* The brachial artery passes beneath the bicipital aponeurosis (lacertus fibrosus) in the hollow of the elbow and, in individuals with well-developed biceps and brachial muscles, can become compressed when the elbow is bent.

2.2.4 Documentation

Documentation of the findings is the same as for the leg arteries and comprises longitudinal B-scan views of the subclavian, axillary, and brachial arteries with the corresponding Doppler waveforms obtained with angle correction. An aneurysm is documented in two planes, and its diameter measured in a transverse view. If stenosis is present, the intrastenotic peak systolic velocity (PSV) measured with angle correction is recorded. If no adequate Doppler waveform can be sampled from a central subclavian stenosis, the monophasic waveform distal to the lesion is documented. In patients with a vascular compression syndrome, documentation includes images showing the affected vessel in the compressed state.

2.2.5 Normal Findings

Like the leg arteries, healthy arm arteries show a triphasic flow pattern with rapid forward flow reaching a peak during systole, short reversal of flow during early diastole (due to high peripheral resistance), and slow forward flow during late diastole. Arterial diameters (6–7 mm subclavian artery, 5–6 mm axillary artery) and peak systolic velocities (PSV) decrease toward the periphery (from 80–140 cm/s in the proximal subclavian artery).

2.2.6 Abnormal Findings, Duplex Ultrasound Measurements, and Clinical Role

2.2.6.1 Atherosclerosis

Due to the poor acoustic window in this anatomic region, the diagnosis of a central subclavian stenosis typically relies on indirect criteria with demonstration of monophasic and turbulent flow in the poststenotic segment. In patients with good insonation conditions, the subclavian artery can be followed to its origin from the aorta with a low-frequency transducer, and a stenosis near the origin can be identified directly by spectral Doppler interrogation with angle-corrected PSV measurement.

As in the leg arteries, PSV in the subclavian and axillary arteries shows wide interindividual variation in the normal population. Therefore, focal doubling of PSV is used to identify hemodynamically relevant stenosis. This criterion, however, is not applicable in the proximal subclavian artery and brachiocephalic trunk, the preferred sites of arterial stenosis in the arm. Here, a PSV greater than 2 m/s is assumed to indicate stenosis. The criteria of poststenotic flow in the leg arteries (◘ Table 2.9) can also be used to identify and evaluate steno-occlusive lesions in the arm arteries. However, the waveform obtained downstream of an obstruction does not allow the examiner to differentiate high-grade stenosis from occlusion.

Color duplex ultrasound was reported to have **90% sensitivity** and **99% specificity** for identification of vascular abnormalities in the proximal and middle segments of the arm arteries compared with digital subtraction angiography (Wittenberg et al. 1998). A surprisingly high sensitivity of 91% and specificity of 100% were found for the region near the aortic arch, compared with 93% and 100% in the upper arm and 88% and 98% in the lower arm.

In the **finger arteries**, the examiner must differentiate atherosclerotic and embolic lesions from temporary vasoconstriction in Raynaud's disease (see ◘ Fig. 2.110 (Atlas)). Examination with a high-resolution transducer (8–12 MHz) allows very accurate diagnosis of occlusion and stenosis. Ladleif et al. (1998), for example, reported 86.9% sensitivity and 93.8% specificity with a positive and negative predictive value of 88.4% and 93%, respectively, compared with selective hand angiography. A peripheral blood flow velocity < 15 cm/s suggests upstream stenosis or occlusion. Overall, an ultrasound examination of the finger arteries is very time-consuming. Incidental findings include arteriovenous malformation and hemangioma.

Interdigital artery occlusion is suggested by the clinical presentation and confirmed by duplex ultrasound. It may be caused by cardiac disease or thoracic outlet syndrome. Moreover, such occlusions may be due to the **hypothenar hammer syndrome** if they involve the ulnar artery territory and the patient has a history of chronic repetitive blunt trauma to the hypothenar region with secondary arterial wall damage. When the latter is suspected (occupational history of repetitive hand and wrist trauma and ischemia of the fourth and fifth fingers), the examiner should look for an aneurysmal dilatation of the distal ulnar artery (◘ Fig. 2.47) in the hypothenar area. Ultrasonography depicts corkscrew-like changes already in early disease and demonstrates the intra-aneurysmal thrombi responsible for embolization to the interdigital arteries as well as the patent lumen in the color duplex mode (see ◘ Fig. 2.109 (Atlas)).

2.2.6.2 Vascular Compression Syndromes

The wide variability of clinical presentations and the problem of definitively confirming the thoracic outlet syndrome by means of provocative maneuvers make it difficult to diagnose this condition. A study in a German population revealed that patients consulted an average of 6.5 specialists before the syndrome was finally diagnosed – after a mean of 4.3 years (Gruss et al. 1989; Gruss and Geissler 1997).

As already mentioned above, several neurovascular compression syndromes of the shoulder girdle need to be considered and differentiated in patients presenting with hand ischemia:

- Cervical rib syndrome
- Scalenus anterior syndrome (arterial: Adson test)
- Scalenus minimus syndrome
- Costoclavicular compression syndrome (venous: hyperabduction test)
- Pectoralis minor syndrome
- Compression syndrome of the brachial artery

Diagnostic workup should begin with a **clinical examination** including determination of pulses, auscultation, and bilateral Doppler blood pressure measurement. Unilateral pulse reduction or obliteration with elevation or abduction of the arm is not a very specific symptom and is seen in 30–60% of young adults without symptoms related to thoracic outlet syndrome. This test merely shows intermittent subclavian artery compression, and a positive test is not diagnostic of a clinically relevant vascular compression syndrome. A clinically more relevant test to reproduce the symptoms of thoracic outlet syndrome is the ninety degree abduction in external rotation (90° AER) test: with the arms in this position, the patient is instructed to make a fist every 2–3 s for 3 min. Most patients will experience fatigue, pain, and heaviness before the end of the 3-min test period. Formication suggests compression of the upper plexus. Additional pain and pallor of the fingers indicate arterial compression.

The diagnosis of thoracic outlet syndrome further requires measurement of the **nerve conduction velocity** of the ulnar and median nerves. Diminished nerve conduction velocity suggests brachial plexus compression, but normal nerve conduction velocity does not rule out thoracic outlet syndrome. Nerve conduction velocities above 65 m/s are normal and velocities below 45 m/s indicate brachial plexus compression (Urschel 1976).

When (color) duplex confirms interdigital artery occlusion, the examiner proceeds to identify the source of embolism, primarily a partially thrombosed aneurysm. Such aneurysms typically develop secondary to compression-induced wall damage in thoracic outlet syndrome or as a result of traumatic damage to the distal ulnar artery in hypothenar hammer syndrome (see ◘ Fig. 2.109 (Atlas)). Intermittent compression in thoracic outlet syndrome may also give rise to intraluminal thrombus formation. The specific type of thoracic outlet syndrome (◘ Fig. 2.48) is diagnosed by ultrasonography of the respective sites of compression as suggested by the patient's history and clinical symptoms using the following **provocative tests**:

- **Adson test** to identify arterial compression in the scalene triangle: the hyperextended head is turned toward the affected side (Schoop 1988) with the neck muscles tensed and possibly with additional hyperabduction and rotation of the arm.
- **Costoclavicular or hyperabduction test** to identify venous compression in the costoclavicular space: gliding of the clavicle over the first rib with the arm hyperabducted narrows the passage, thereby inducing venous compression. However, venous compression in this area is more commonly caused by weak shoulder muscles, which are better identified by a downward pull on the posteriorly turned arm (with the shoulder drawn back, inspiration).

The **provocative maneuver is performed with spectral Doppler sampling** at the target site (◘ Fig. 2.48) or, if this region cannot be interrogated, distal to it. The test is positive if there is flow acceleration in the compressed artery or if an altered flow profile is obtained distal to the compressed segment. The examiner can also move the transducer toward the compressed segment from the periphery, intermittently recording spectral Doppler information. Provocative tests are necessary to diagnose the specific type of compression syndrome and initiate proper treatment, as all of them are rare and the clinical symptoms are often nonspecific. (◘ Table 2.22). If there is occlusion of the forearm or finger arteries, it is crucial to identify the source of embolism. The search should focus on the possibility of a partially thrombosed aneurysm of the subclavian artery, which typically develops on the basis of a scalene muscle or cervical rib syndrome. In rare cases, emboli may arise from thrombotic deposits of the damaged wall of the axillary artery in hyperabduction syndrome. These changes are caused by intermittent compression of the axillary artery and will be identified with the transducer placed in the axilla (see ◘ Fig. 2.107 (Atlas)).

Patients with venous compression and clinical symptoms should initially be treated by physical therapy to strengthen the shoulder muscles or by resection if bony abnormalities such as a cervical rib or exostosis are present.

In thoracic outlet syndrome with compression or mechanical irritation of the arteries or brachial plexus, the first rib should be resected before secondary damage to the vessel wall with development of aneurysm occurs. If secondary damage has already occurred, the affected arterial segments must be resected as well.

The management of patients with thoracic outlet syndrome is prevention-oriented, meaning that the goal is to intervene before compression-related complications such as vascular damage, poststenotic aneurysm, or embolism occur. When a combination of the Adson test with hyperabduction of the arm is performed in normal young individuals, 30%

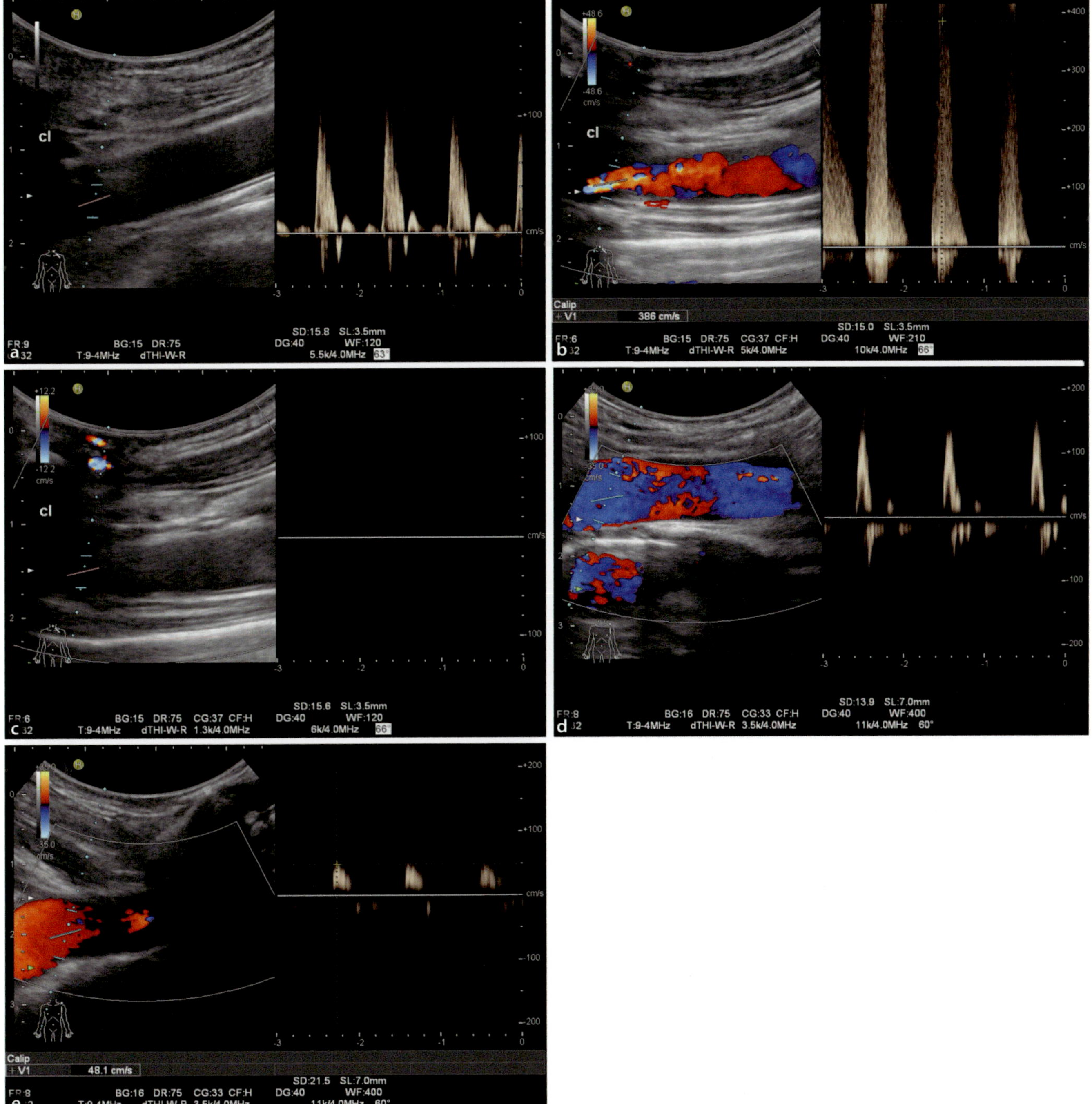

Fig. 2.48a–e Thoracic outlet syndrome caused by exostosis in a patient with a history of clavicular fracture (cl). In the costoclavicular space, compression of the vein is more common than compression of the artery, unless exostosis secondary to fracture is the underlying mechanism. **a** In a relaxed position with the arms at the side, the axillary artery distal to the costoclavicular space shows normal triphasic flow with a peak systolic velocity (PSV) of 100 cm/s (waveform obtained with transducer in infraclavicular fossa). **b** With beginning hyperabduction, flow shows increasing signs of stenosis with aliasing in the color flow image and a PSV of 400 cm/s. **c** With extreme hyperabduction, the clavicular exostosis (cl) completely compresses the axillary artery, seen as absence of flow distally. **d** With the arms at the side (corresponding to **a**), there is normal triphasic flow in the subclavian artery. **e** With hyperabduction, a knocking waveform is obtained from the subclavian artery (prestenotic segment upstream of the exostosis) as a sign of downstream obstruction

will show compression with temporary stenosis of the subclavian artery. Even with these test results, most of them do not develop compression-related complications, and no treatment is warranted. The problem is to identify those individuals in whom the vascular compression that can be reproduced with this provocative maneuver will lead to the rare thoracic outlet syndrome with the above-described vascular complications.

Patients with thoracic outlet syndrome typically do not seek medical attention until vascular complications have developed. In most patients with complications of thoracic

2

Table 2.22 Duplex ultrasound diagnosis of thoracic outlet syndrome in 680 patients presenting with clinical symptoms of arterial/venous compression of the upper extremity (patients seen from 1991 through 2001; diagnosis confirmed by angiography/venography, intraoperative findings)

Type of thoracic outlet syndrome	Number
Cervical rib syndrome (arterial)	3
Scalenus anterior syndrome (arterial) – With poststenotic aneurysm	6 2
Costoclavicular compression syndrome (venous) – With venous thrombosis	8 5
Pectoralis minor syndrome (arterial)	2

outlet syndrome seen by the author, even retrospective analysis of their histories revealed no prior signs or symptoms that might have pointed to the diagnosis.

2.2.6.3 Vascular Inflammatory Disease

Inflammatory disease, such as Takayasu's arteritis (1–3/million/year), is a rare cause of upper extremity ischemia. The arm arteries (subclavian and axillary arteries) are a preferred site of giant cell arteritis, a rare vasulitis primarily affecting the aorta and its primary branches. Rare sites are the pelvic, visceral, coronary, renal, and common carotid arteries. Early differentiation from atherosclerotic steno-occlusive disease is critical for adequate therapeutic management. Timely initiation of cortisone therapy is crucial in autoimmune granulomatous arteritis and is also a prerequisite for successful vascular reconstruction. Without prior or concomitant cortisone treatment, reconstructive measures have a poor outcome, and the risk of early recurrence is high. Most patients responding well to cortisone and showing resolution of inflammatory wall thickening do not require additional vascular repair.

Sonographic demonstration of a thickened vascular wall (>1 mm) with circumferential luminal narrowing of a longer segment than in atherosclerotic stenosis points to an inflammatory process. Wall thickening >1.5 mm is pathognomonic of vasculitis (Schmidt et al. 2008). The thickened wall is of low, homogeneous echogenicity and clearly demarcated from the lumen while an atherosclerotic vessel wall has higher echogenicity and appears inhomogeneous. Duplex ultrasound is the diagnostic modality of choice, allowing identification of the characteristic morphologic changes including assessment of the hemodynamic relevance of luminal narrowing (see ► Sect. 5.8.2) and monitoring of the therapeutic response (Fig. 2.49).

2.2.6.4 Buerger's Disease

Thromboangiitis obliterans (Buerger's disease) of the upper extremity is characterized by multiple segmental occlusions of the palmar and digital arteries. The disease predominantly occurs in men and usually presents before age 40. It is rare in Europe, accounting for 0.5% of all cases of peripheral arterial occlusive disease. In most cases, the occluded arteries show no atherosclerotic lesions. Concomitant thrombophlebitis is common. Ultrasound will typically reveal multiple occlusive lesions characterized by low echogenicity and absence of plaque deposits (skip lesions). The vessel diameter of affected segments may be reduced. Chronic disease is characterized by recanalization and the presence of corkscrew collaterals around occluded segments (see Fig. 2.32). At this stage, affected arterial segments appear inhomogeneous on B-mode images, while color flow images depict thin, tortuous collaterals extending beyond the normal diameter of the artery. Collaterals around occlusions are supplied by intact arterial segments (known as Martorell's sign) or by the vasa vasorum of the occluded segment.

2.2.6.5 Raynaud's Disease

Raynaud's disease manifests as episodes of **vasospasms of the fingers and toes**. A primary or idiopathic form is distinguished from secondary Raynaud's disease, which is often related to connective tissue diseases or other underlying causes.

The episodes are typically triggered by cold or stress and manifest as classic tricolor changes of first white (pallor), then blue (cyanosis), and then red (reperfusion hyperemia). This is known as the tricolor sign and allows the diagnosis of Raynaud's disease to be made on the basis of the patient's clinical presentation. The primary role of duplex ultrasound is to differentiate Raynaud's disease from other vascular conditions (see Fig. 2.110 (Atlas)) based on their specific morphologic and hemodynamic changes. Placing the hand in warm water (37°C) during the examination will relieve the vasospasm, allowing differentiation of Raynaud's phenomenon from fixed vascular occlusion. Supplementary tests to rule out morphologic and structural perfusion disorders of the hands and feet include digital photopletysmography and pulse contour analysis (► Sect. 2.1.6.4.6).

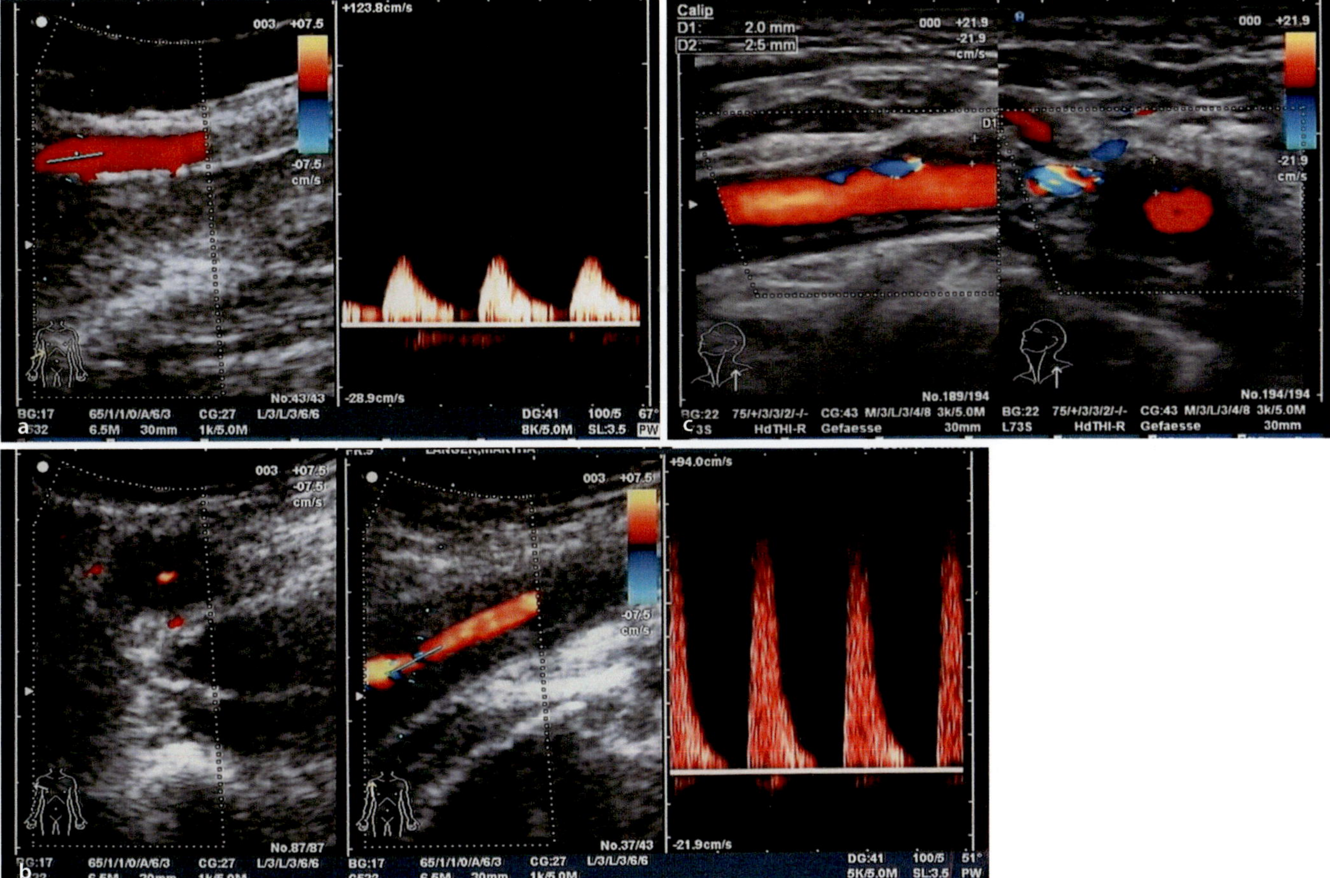

Fig. 2.49 **a** 65-year-old woman presenting with a 5-day history of progressive hand ischemia. The waveform from the brachial artery shows monophasic flow with a reduced peak systolic velocity (PSV) and delayed upstroke, consistent with poststenotic flow. **b** Poststenotic flow in the brachial artery is due to concentric wall thickening of a long segment of the axillary artery (and also of the subclavian artery), causing high-grade stenosis (transverse and longitudinal color flow images). Because of the length of the affected segment, the intrastenotic PSV is only 78 cm/s despite high-grade luminal narrowing. **c** After one month of cortisone treatment, there is only residual circumferential wall thickening without relevant hemodynamic effects

2.3 Atlas: Extremity Arteries

◘ Table 2.23 lists the figures presented in the Atlas. The figures illustrate normal findings, methodology, and vascular diseases of the extremity arteries.

◘ **Table 2.23** Extremity arteries – figures

Table 2.23 (continued)

Entity/Pathology	Figure
Pseudoaneurysm – thrombin injection treatment	Fig. 2.79 (Atlas), page 146
Pseudoaneurysm – challenges for thrombin injection treatment	Fig. 2.79 (Atlas), page 146
Pseudoaneurysm – differentiation from hematoma	Fig. 2.79 (Atlas), page 146
Suture aneurysm	Fig. 2.80 (Atlas), page 146
Pseudoaneurysm – compression therapy/thrombin injection	Fig. 2.81 (Atlas), page 147
Large pseudoaneurysm with multiple perforation – thrombin injection	Fig. 2.81 (Atlas), page 147
Internal iliac artery – pseudoaneurysm, thrombin injection	Fig. 2.82 (Atlas), page 148
Arteriovenous fistula	Fig. 2.83 (Atlas), page 148
Popliteal artery occlusion – atherosclerosis versus embolism	Fig. 2.84 (Atlas), page 149
Embolic occlusion	Fig. 2.85 (Atlas), page 149
Arterial occlusion in deep leg vein thrombosis and patent foramen ovale	Fig. 2.86 (Atlas), page 150
Bilateral popliteal artery aneurysm	Fig. 2.87 (Atlas), page 150
Small popliteal artery aneurysm with arterioarterial embolism	Fig. 2.88 (Atlas), page 151
Pseudoaneurysm following arthroscopy	Fig. 2.89 (Atlas), page 152
Aneurysm of posterior tibial artery	Fig. 2.90 (Atlas), page 152
Adventitial cystic disease	Fig. 2.91 (Atlas), page 153
Adventitial cystic disease – treatment by ultrasound-guided aspiration	Fig. 2.92 (Atlas), page 154
Adventitial cystic disease – differentiation from dissection	Fig. 2.93 (Atlas), page 154
Entrapment syndrome	Fig. 2.94 (Atlas), page 155
Entrapment syndrome	Fig. 2.95 (Atlas), page 156
Entrapment constellation	Fig. 2.96 (Atlas), page 156
Dissection	Fig. 2.97 (Atlas), page 157
Progressive ischemia due to venous outflow obstruction (extensive venous thrombosis)	Fig. 2.98 (Atlas), page 157
Cardiac causes of abnormal spectral Doppler findings	Fig. 2.99 (Atlas), page 158
Vasculitis	Fig. 2.100 (Atlas), page 158
Inflammatory vascular disease	Fig. 2.101 (Atlas), page 159
Subclavian artery stenosis due to atherosclerosis	Fig. 2.102 (Atlas), page 159
Axillary artery stenosis due to atherosclerosis	Fig. 2.103 (Atlas), page 160
Distal axillary artery stenosis in arteritis	Fig. 2.103 (Atlas), page 160
Cervical rib syndrome	Fig. 2.104 (Atlas), page 161
Subclavian artery compression by cervical rib	Fig. 2.104 (Atlas), page 161
Aneurysm of subclavian/axillary artery	Fig. 2.105 (Atlas), page 162
Thoracic outlet syndrome with poststenotic dilatation	Fig. 2.106 (Atlas), page 163
Pectoralis minor syndrome	Fig. 2.107 (Atlas), page 163
Takayasu's arteritis with subclavian artery occlusion	Fig. 2.108 (Atlas), page 164
Aneurysm of the ulnar artery (hypothenar syndrome)	Fig. 2.109 (Atlas), page 164
Interdigital artery occlusion – Raynaud's disease	Fig. 2.110 (Atlas), page 165
Radial artery occlusion with peripheral ischemia	Fig. 2.111 (Atlas), page 165

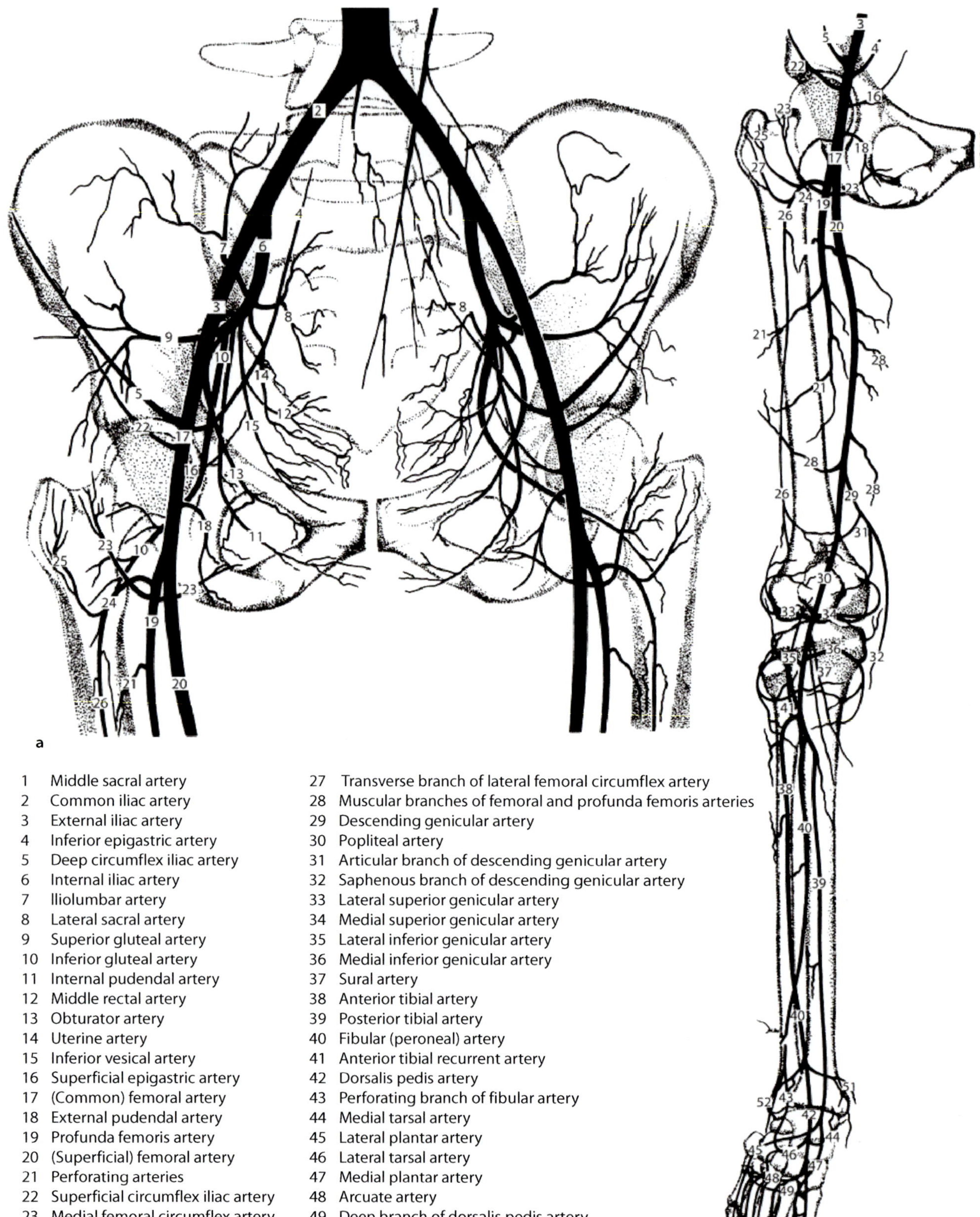

1 Middle sacral artery
2 Common iliac artery
3 External iliac artery
4 Inferior epigastric artery
5 Deep circumflex iliac artery
6 Internal iliac artery
7 Iliolumbar artery
8 Lateral sacral artery
9 Superior gluteal artery
10 Inferior gluteal artery
11 Internal pudendal artery
12 Middle rectal artery
13 Obturator artery
14 Uterine artery
15 Inferior vesical artery
16 Superficial epigastric artery
17 (Common) femoral artery
18 External pudendal artery
19 Profunda femoris artery
20 (Superficial) femoral artery
21 Perforating arteries
22 Superficial circumflex iliac artery
23 Medial femoral circumflex artery
24 Lateral femoral circumflex artery
25 Ascending branch of lateral femoral circumflex artery
26 Descending branch of lateral femoral circumflex artery
27 Transverse branch of lateral femoral circumflex artery
28 Muscular branches of femoral and profunda femoris arteries
29 Descending genicular artery
30 Popliteal artery
31 Articular branch of descending genicular artery
32 Saphenous branch of descending genicular artery
33 Lateral superior genicular artery
34 Medial superior genicular artery
35 Lateral inferior genicular artery
36 Medial inferior genicular artery
37 Sural artery
38 Anterior tibial artery
39 Posterior tibial artery
40 Fibular (peroneal) artery
41 Anterior tibial recurrent artery
42 Dorsalis pedis artery
43 Perforating branch of fibular artery
44 Medial tarsal artery
45 Lateral plantar artery
46 Lateral tarsal artery
47 Medial plantar artery
48 Arcuate artery
49 Deep branch of dorsalis pedis artery
50 Dorsal and plantar metatarsal arteries, dorsal and plantar digital arteries
51 Medial malleolar branch
52 Lateral malleolar branch

Fig. 2.50 (Atlas) Vascular anatomy.
a Pelvic arteries.
b Leg arteries (courtesy of Eastman Kodak Company)

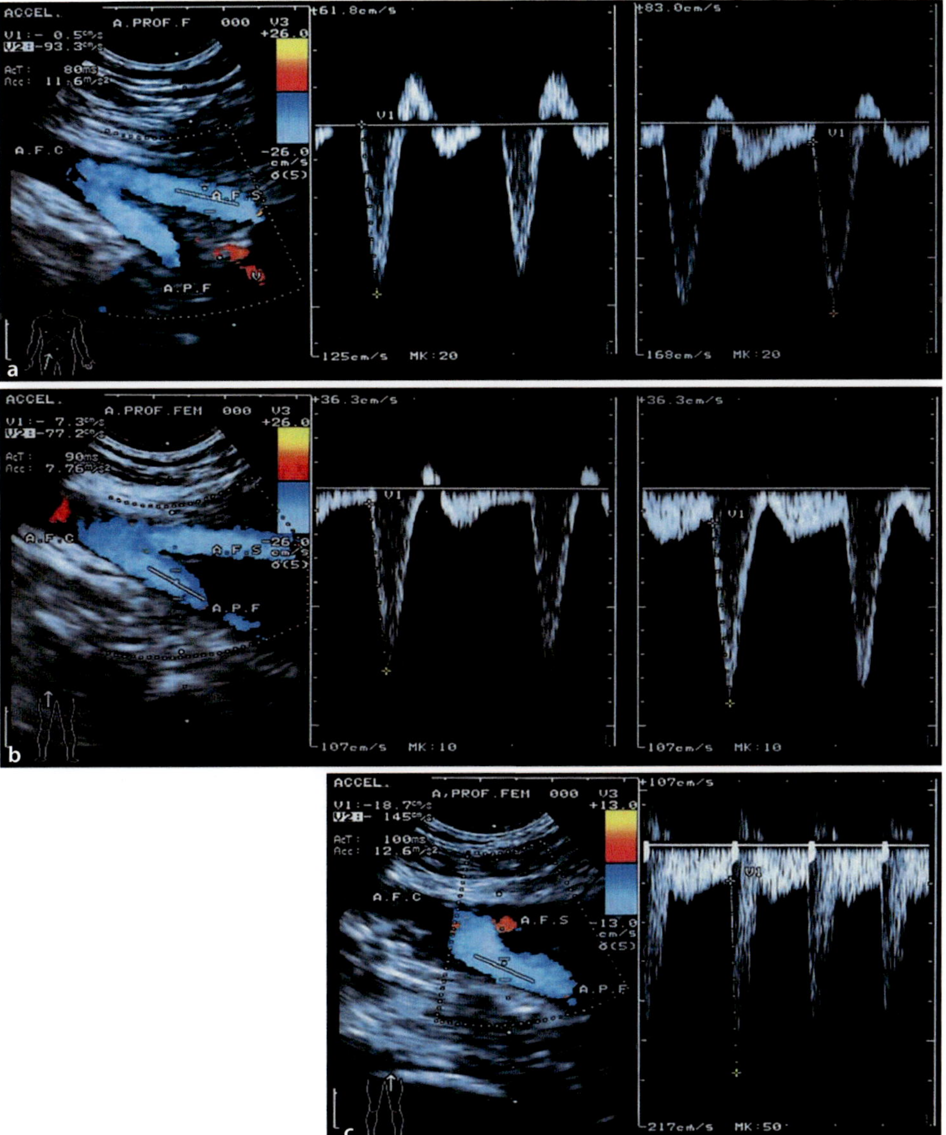

Fig. 2.51 (Atlas) Femoral bifurcation – normal blood flow.

a Gray-scale and color duplex imaging supplement each other: along the course of an artery, some segments may be better appreciated in the B-mode image, others in the color flow mode. In the example, the superficial femoral artery (A.F.S) and profunda femoris artery (A.P.F) are insonated with a smaller angle, improving their visualization in the color mode, whereas wall structures perpendicular to the ultrasound beam (here: common femoral artery, A.F.C, left part of image) are seen more clearly in the B-mode image. Ultrasound pulses striking the vessel wall at a perpendicular angle produce a detailed image of the wall, which is a strong reflector. In contrast, a smaller angle between the direction of flowing blood and the beam is necessary to ensure accurate spectral Doppler measurement and reliable evaluation of blood flow. Although all extremity arteries have a triphasic pulsatile flow profile under normal conditions, resulting from the high peripheral resistance at rest, different spectral waveforms may be obtained, depending on the territory supplied by the artery interrogated. High-resistance flow as in the superficial femoral artery, which mostly supplies skin and subcutaneous tissue and only some muscle tissue, gives rise to a pulsatile, triphasic waveform with zero flow in end diastole. The example shows the femoral bifurcation with the Doppler sample volume placed in the superficial femoral artery (A.F.S). Blue indicates arterial flow away from the transducer, red the flow in the superficial femoral vein toward the transducer. The corresponding Doppler tracings illustrate the hemodynamic situation at rest (left waveform) and after exercise (right waveform). Peak systolic velocity (PSV) increases from 90 cm/s at rest to 141 cm/s after exercise (ten tiptoe movements). The increased muscular blood demand during exercise is met by a decrease in peripheral resistance and is reflected in the Doppler waveform by an increase in end-diastolic velocity (EDV) from 0 (left waveform) to 16 cm/s (right waveform).

b Femoral bifurcation: The profunda femoris (A.P.F) supplying more muscle tissue has a slightly less pulsatile flow but the profile is still triphasic. At rest (left waveform), PSV is 77 cm/s and EDV is 7 cm/s. After exercise (right waveform), PSV increases to 90 cm/s with EDV doubling to 15 cm/s. The color change from red, to black, to blue reflects the change in flow direction relative to the ultrasound beam (toward transducer: red; away from transducer: blue) (A.F.S = superficial femoral artery; A.F.C = common femoral artery).

c In patients with occlusion of the superficial femoral artery (A.F.S), the profunda femoris is the main collateral to bridge the occluded segment and supply the superficial femoral territory. When the profunda femoris artery is recruited as a collateral, the higher flow volume in the profunda femoris circulation may result in a 40–60% increase in blood flow velocity without this indicating stenosis at its origin. In the example shown, a PSV of 145 cm/s and an EDV of 18 cm/s are measured in the profunda femoris artery (A.P.F) bridging the occluded superficial femoral artery. Reversed flow due to eddy currents at the origin of the occluded superficial femoral artery is displayed in red (knocking waveform)

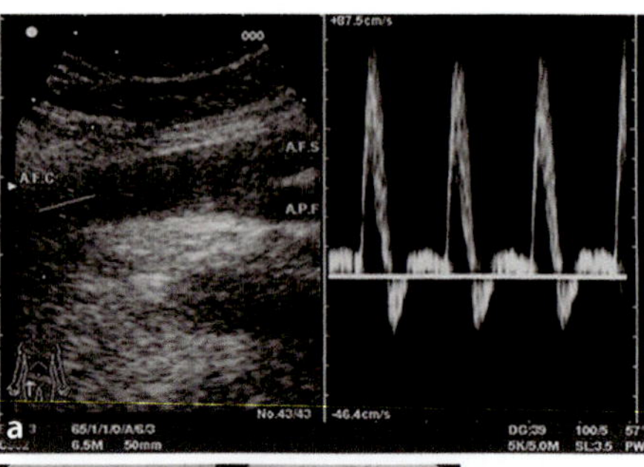

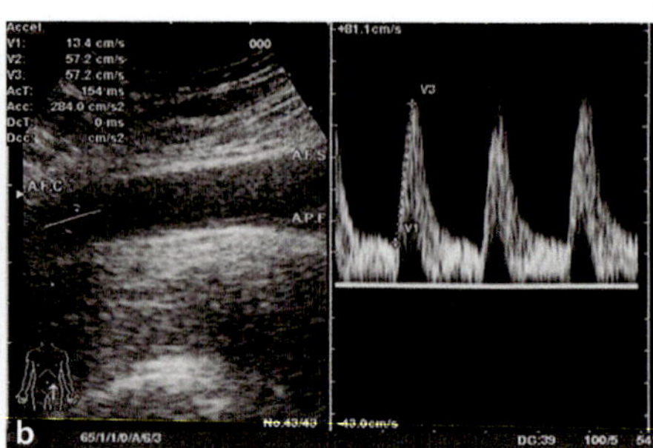

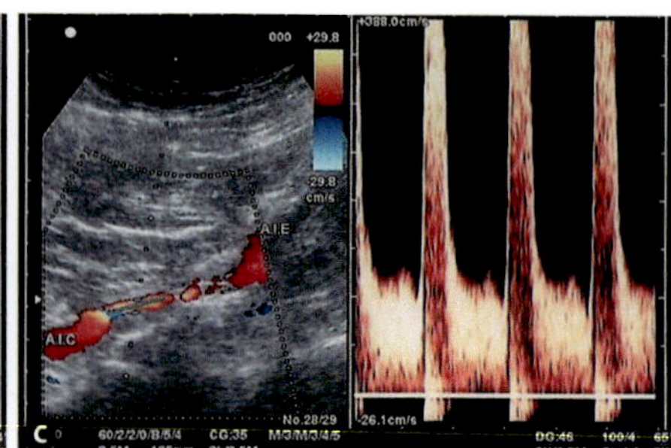

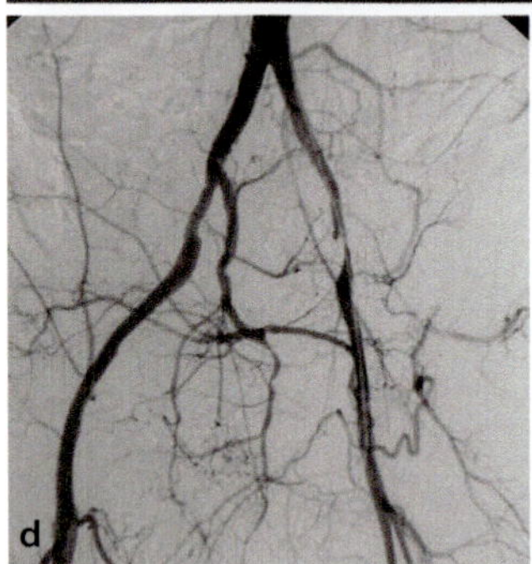

Fig. 2.52a–d (Atlas) Pelvic artery stenosis.
a In evaluating a patient with suspected flow obstruction at the pelvic level, the examiner first obtains Doppler tracings from both common femoral arteries to compare these with regard to triphasic flow, steep systolic upslope, and peak systolic velocity (PSV). Reliable Doppler shift analysis requires an insonation angle below 60°. In this example, the angle is 50° on the right and 54° on the left. The Doppler waveform from the right groin shows triphasic flow with a systolic upslope and a PSV > 80 cm/s.
b The waveform from the left common femoral artery illustrates postocclusive flow with a monophasic profile, reduced PSV (57 cm/s), and delayed systolic rise.
c The monophasic flow profile is due to high-grade stenosis of the common iliac artery (A.I.C) caused by plaque, mainly of the posterior wall. Sonographic signs of stenosis in this case are aliasing in the color duplex image and a Doppler-derived PSV of over 4 m/s. Due to aliasing, the velocity peaks are cut off, and PSV must be interpolated (approx. 4.5 m/s). The simplified Bernoulli equation, P = 4 x (PSV x PSV), yields a maximum pressure gradient of 81 mmHg across the stenosis, resulting in a poststenotic decrease in systolic velocity.
d Angiogram demonstrates the high-grade iliac artery stenosis as a filling defect in the lumen

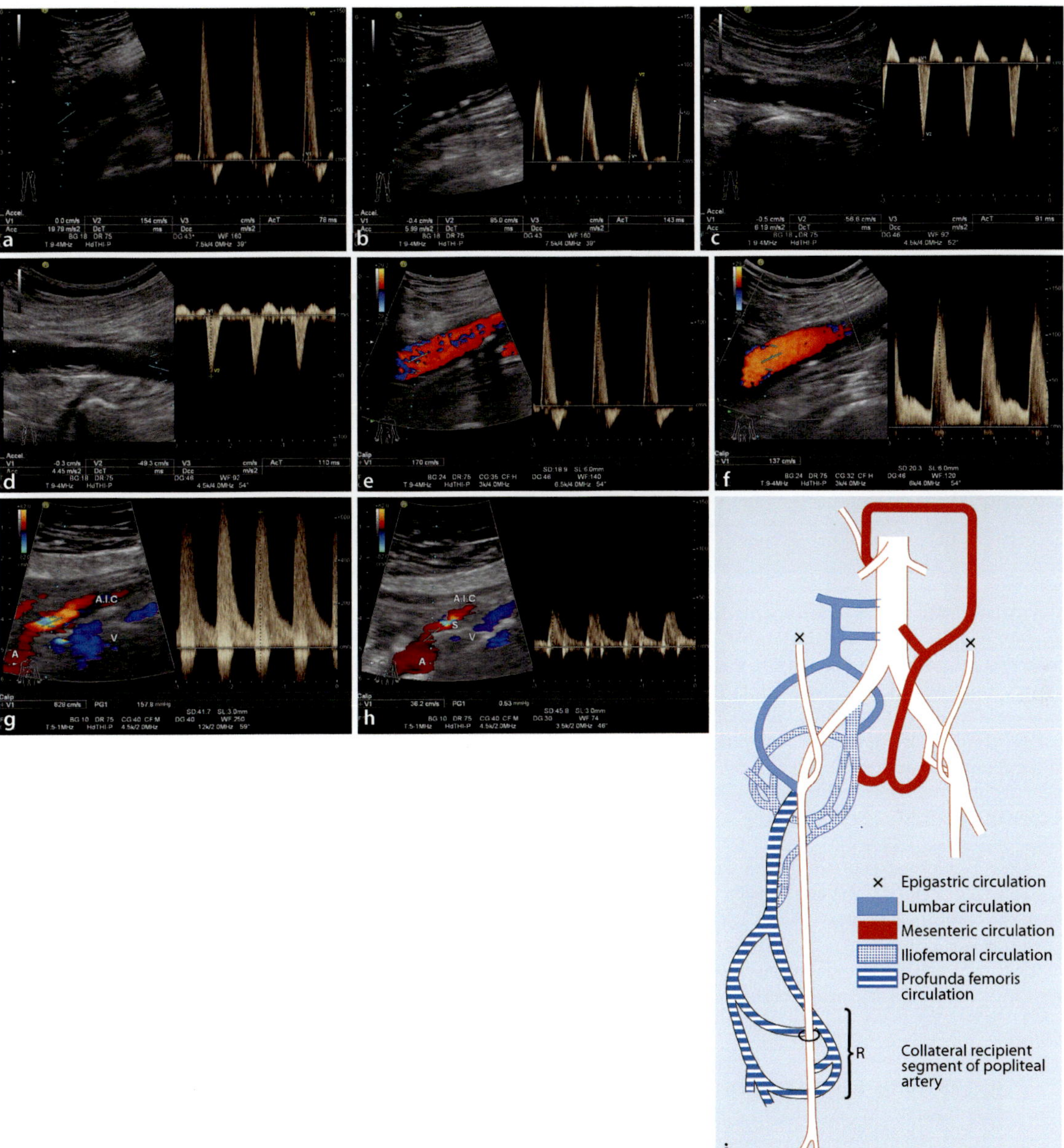

Fig. 2.53a–i (Atlas) Iliac artery stenosis with good collateralization – Doppler waveform analysis.
a–i Ultrasound protocol based on segmental spectral Doppler evaluation illustrated in a 58-year-old patient with stage IIa peripheral arterial occlusive disease (PAOD) and a walking distance of >1 km. The patient has high-grade common iliac artery stenosis with very good collateralization and an ankle-brachial index (ABI) of 0.9 (versus 1.1 on the left).
a The Doppler waveform from the right groin is triphasic. The peak systolic velocity (PSV) is 154 cm/s with an acceleration time of 75 ms.
b A triphasic Doppler waveform is also obtained from the left groin; however, the PSV is 85 cm/s and systolic rise is delayed with a prolonged acceleration time of 143 ms.
c Triphasic Doppler waveform and PSV of 60 cm/s in the right popliteal artery.
d Triphasic Doppler waveform with a lower PSV of 50 cm/s in the left popliteal artery. Overall, the velocity peaks are slightly damped compared with the waveform from the contraleral popliteal artery (**c**). To ensure reliable acoustic and visual spectral analysis as illustrated here, it is important to perform spectral Doppler imaging with small angles of insonation (<50°).
e On the left side, blood flow begins to return to normal 1 min after activity, as shown by the triphasic waveform. Only PSV (170 cm/s) is still slightly higher compared with the situation at rest (compare waveform obtained 5 min after activity in **a**).
f The Doppler waveform obtained from the right proximal common femoral artery 1 min after rapidly walking a distance of 50 m shows monophasic flow and a delayed systolic rise. These findings indicate that flow has not yet returned to normal, and a longer period of rest is necessary before a triphasic waveform is obtained (**b**).
g High-grade common iliac artery stenosis with a PSV of 6 m/s. The pressure gradient across the stenosis, calculated using the simplified Bernoulli equation, is 4 x (PSV x PSV) = 4 x (6 x 6) = 144 mmHg.
h In the common iliac artery just upstream of the stenosis, a PSV of 40 cm/s is measured, corresponding to a 15-fold PSV increase in the stenosis, consistent with subtotal occlusion.
i Diagram of collateral pathways that can be recruited to bridge arterial obstruction at the pelvic and thigh levels. The better the collateral circulation, the less marked the changes in the postocclusive Doppler waveform

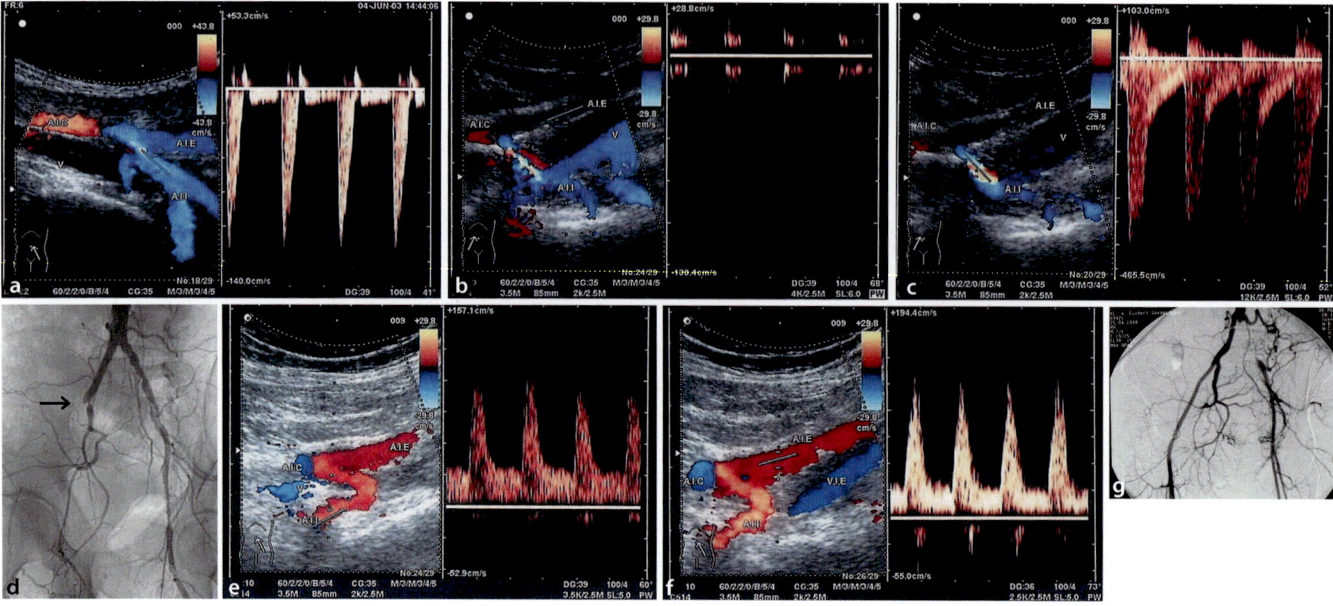

Fig. 2.54a–g (Atlas) Iliac artery – stenosis/occlusion and collateral pathways.
a The iliac bifurcation with the origin of the internal iliac artery (A.I.I) is situated at the deepest point of the true pelvis. The internal iliac artery courses posteriorly (blue, away from transducer, toward periphery). The waveform shows a pulsatile profile but with diastolic flow because the internal iliac artery empties into the pelvic vessels. The color change from red to blue in the bifurcation is due to the changed flow direction relative to the ultrasound beam. With the high PRF selected to depict fast arterial flow, no flow signals are obtained from the iliac vein (V) posterior to the artery (A.I.E = external iliac artery; A.I.C = common iliac artery).
b, c 54-year-old patient with intermittent claudication with a short walking distance and erectile dysfunction (see ► Chap. 7) due to external iliac artery occlusion (Doppler waveform with wall pulsation but no flow signals) and concomitant high-grade internal iliac stenosis (aliasing and peak systolic velocity (PSV) of 4 m/s).
d Oblique angiographic projection showing right-sided external iliac artery occlusion and internal iliac artery stenosis. The internal iliac artery stenosis on the left is obscured by superimposed structures.
e In common iliac artery occlusion, the internal iliac artery supplies the external iliac artery and shows retrograde flow (red, toward transducer). No flow signal in the common iliac artery (A.I.C).
f The refilled external iliac artery (A.I.E) is depicted with normal flow toward the periphery (red). The waveform is monophasic, consistent with postocclusive flow.
g Angiogram showing common iliac artery occlusion

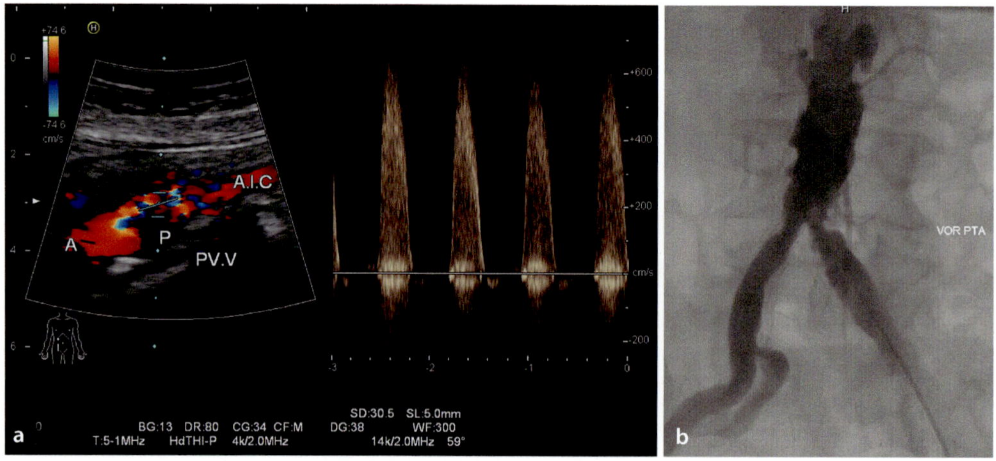

Fig. 2.55a, b (Atlas) Common iliac artery stenosis.
a Stenosis of the iliac and common femoral arteries is typically caused by eccentric plaque on the posterior wall, and angiographic grading is difficult when only an anteroposterior view is obtained. In the example, ultrasound demonstrates high-grade stenosis at the origin of the common iliac artery with aliasing and a Doppler-derived PSV of 6 m/s.
b The angiogram suggests a stenosis with 50–60% diameter reduction at the origin of the common iliac artery. The angiographic underestimation of stenosis in this territory underlines the importance of obtaining different angiographic projections for adequate diagnostic evaluation – even if a segment appears fairly normal or shows only mild to moderate stenosis. This is also important to ensure comparability of angiography and ultrasound

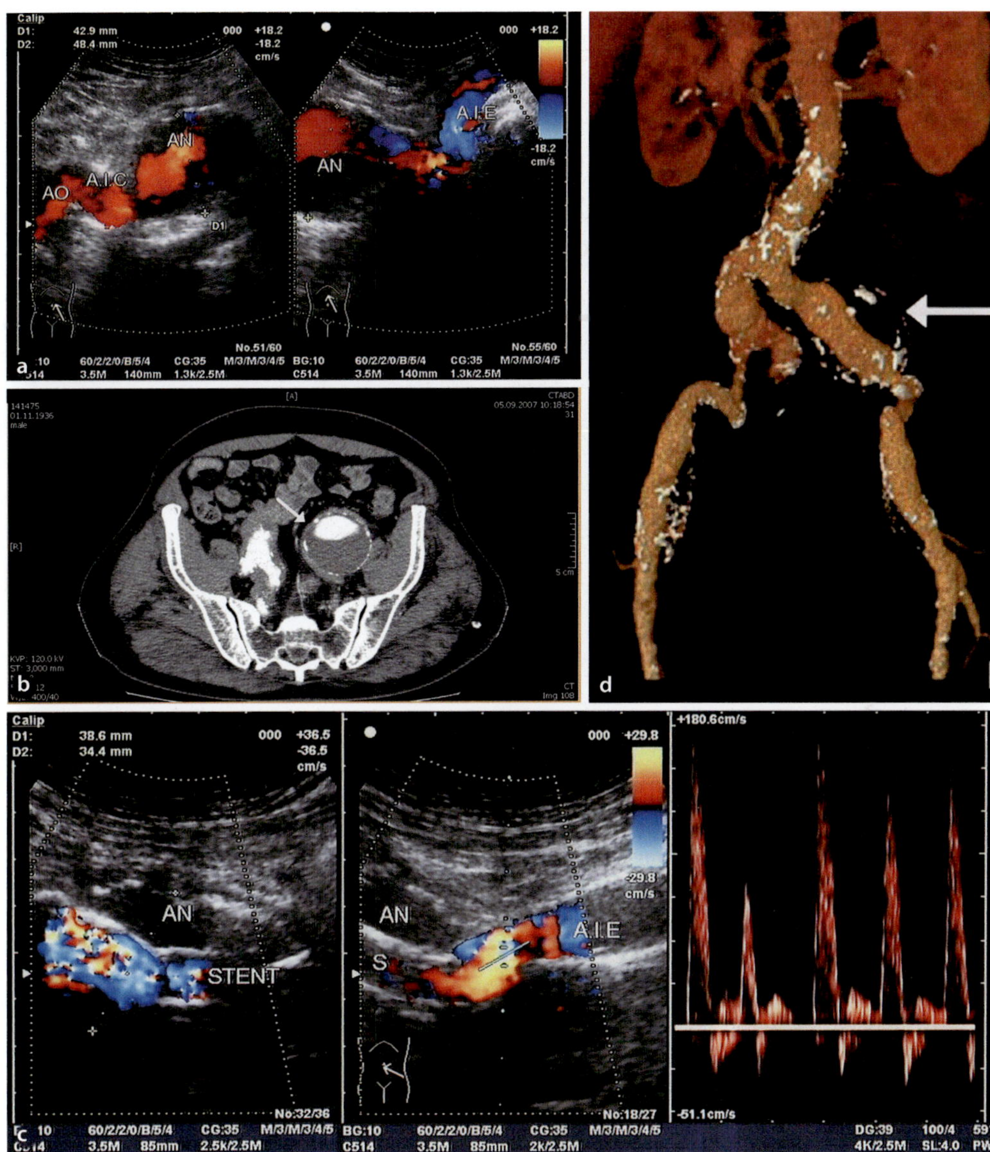

Fig. 2.56a–d (Atlas) Iliac artery aneurysm – stenting.
a Partially thrombosed common iliac artery aneurysm. The left image shows the origin of the common iliac artery from the aorta (AO) and the aneurysm (AN). The right image shows the partially thrombosed aneurysm (AN) and the iliac bifurcation (A.I.E.= external iliac artery).
b CT scan showing the partially thrombosed iliac artery aneurysm.
c Color duplex imaging after endovascular repair with a covered stent demonstrates normal flow in the stent. No signs of endoleak or stenosis. The waveform shown is from the distal stent end.
d CT angiography (3D reconstruction) confirms elimination of the iliac artery aneurysm (arrow) after stent placement

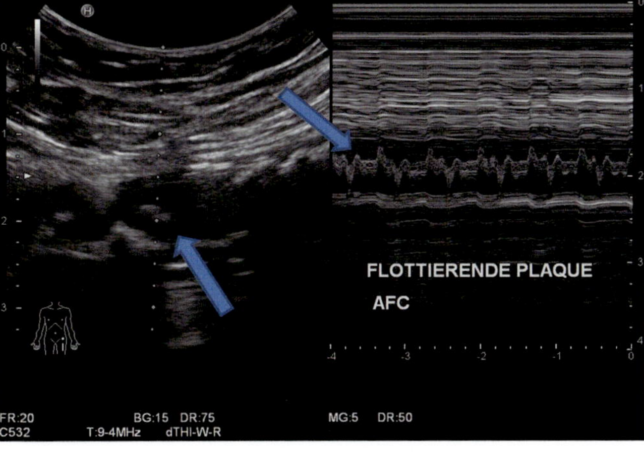

Fig. 2.57 (Atlas) Floating plaque in common femoral artery in a patient with blue toe.
Multiple plaques in the common femoral artery in a 72-year-old patient with blue toe. The peripheral arteries, unlike the carotid arteries, rarely harbor embolizing plaques that give rise to thromboembolic complications. Therefore, the presence of plaque alone does not prove that it is the cause of embolism, and the examiner has to look for other possible sources (cardiac thrombus, partially thrombosed aneurysm). In unclear cases, as in the example shown here, the time-motion mode can demonstrate plaque motion (arrow). Demonstration of plaque floating in the bloodstream is an indication for local TEA even if the stenosis caused by the plaque is of little hemodynamic relevance

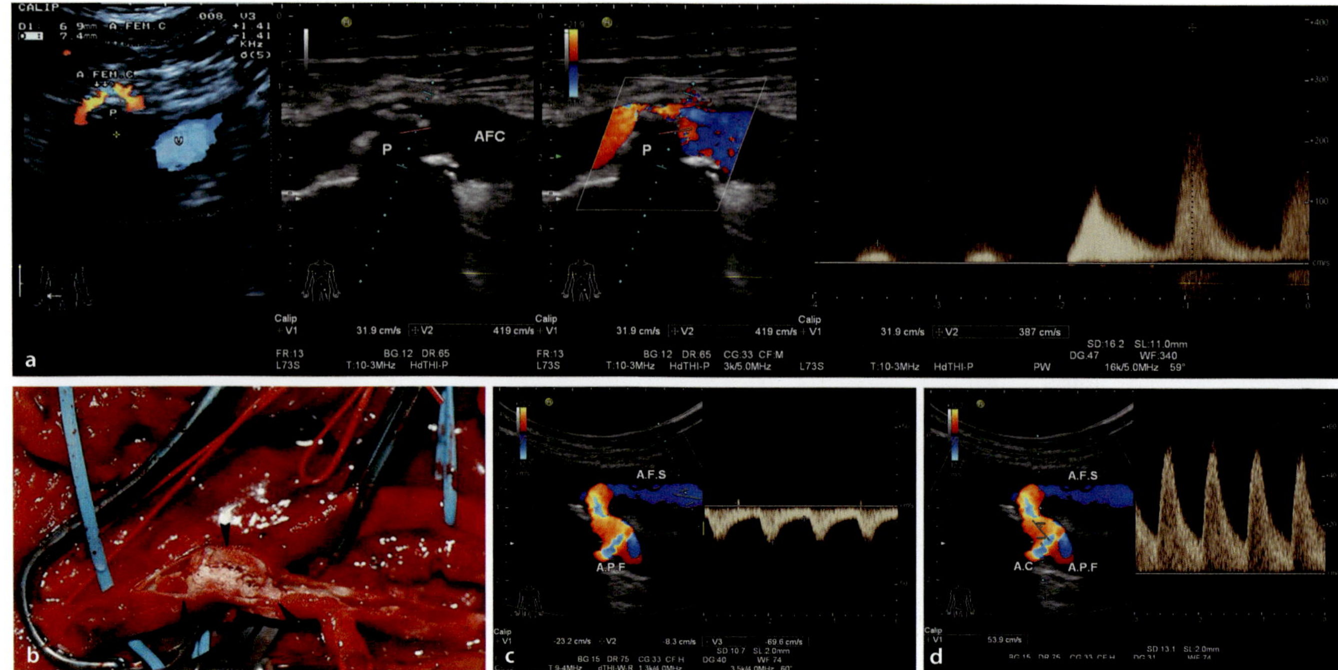

Fig. 2.58 (Atlas) High-grade stenosis/occlusion of common femoral artery.

a High-grade stenosis of the common femoral artery caused by eccentric posterior plaque just upstream of the origin of the profunda femoris artery. The ratio of intrastenotic to prestenotic peak systolic velocity (PSV ratio) is 10.

b Intraoperative site showing the characteristic "cauliflower" appearance of eccentric posterior wall plaque. A segment from the common femoral artery to the profunda femoris artery has been incised longitudinally. The lumen of the superficial femoral artery is also narrowed and the artery is clamped off at its origin. A curved clamp is in place around the proximal end of the common femoral artery. Eccentric posterior wall plaque typically occurs in the common femoral and external iliac arteries and may be difficult to appreciate on anteroposterior angiograms (see Fig. 2.17).

Common femoral artery occlusion – collateralization.

c, d Occlusion (absence of flow signals) of the common femoral artery with refilling of the superficial femoral artery (A.F.S; forward flow coded in blue, away from transducer) via the profunda femoris artery (A.P.F), which shows flow reversal at its origin (red, toward transducer). These findings indicate good collateralization (PSV of 53 cm/s). The profunda femoris artery is supplied by the femoral circumflex artery (A.C). The Doppler waveform shows postocclusive flow (monophasic, delayed systolic rise). In addition, there is plaque with posterior acoustic shadowing in the common femoral artery (see Fig. 2.11)

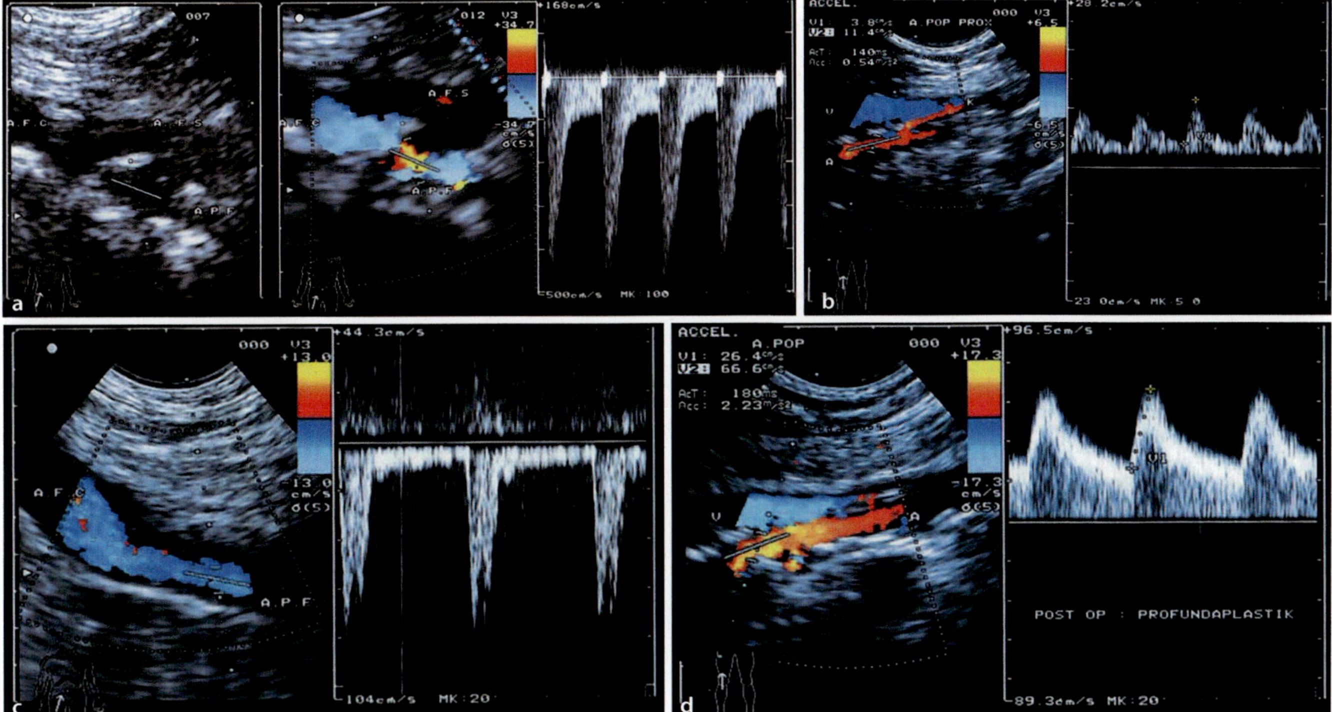

Fig. 2.59a–d (Atlas) Stenosis at origin of profunda femoris artery – TEA.
a High-grade stenosis of the profunda femoris artery (A.P.F) with a monophasic flow profile and a peak systolic velocity (PSV) of 480 cm/s and end-diastolic velocity (EDV) of 90 cm/s. In the color duplex image (middle section), the flow acceleration produces aliasing. The superficial femoral artery (A.F.S) is occluded; only the distal end (about 1 cm) is patent, but the slow flow is not detected with the high PRF used, and only some retrograde flow (red) is recorded. The gray-scale image (left section) depicts plaques of different echogenicity with marked wall irregularities. Some of the plaques produce posterior acoustic shadowing (A.F.C = common femoral artery).
b As a result of the proximal occlusion of the superficial femoral artery and the high-grade stenosis in the main collateral (profunda femoris), the blood volume in the refilled popliteal artery is markedly reduced. This is reflected by the small lumen of the popliteal artery with chronic narrowing and the markedly reduced flow velocity (PSV of 11 and EDV of 3 cm/s). In this image (obtained with the transducer in the popliteal fossa), a collateral arising from the posterior aspect is seen (K). In addition, the popliteal vein (V), which runs posterior to the popliteal artery (A), is depicted closer to the transducer (blue).
c The patient underwent femoral profundaplasty with severing of the ipsilateral superficial femoral artery. Following surgical elimination of the stenosis, the treated segment of the profunda femoris artery (A.P.F) has a PSV of 80 cm/s and EDV of 10 cm/s. The diastolic flow component and the reduced pulsatility are due to collateral flow in the profunda femoris and the altered wall elasticity of the patched segment (A.F.C = common femoral artery).
d Improved perfusion, following profunda femoris repair for superficial femoral occlusion, is reflected in the waveform obtained from the refilled femoral artery at about the same site as the preoperative waveform presented above, now showing a PSV of 66 cm/s and EDV of 26 cm/s. The postocclusive flow character is due to persistent superficial femoral artery occlusion

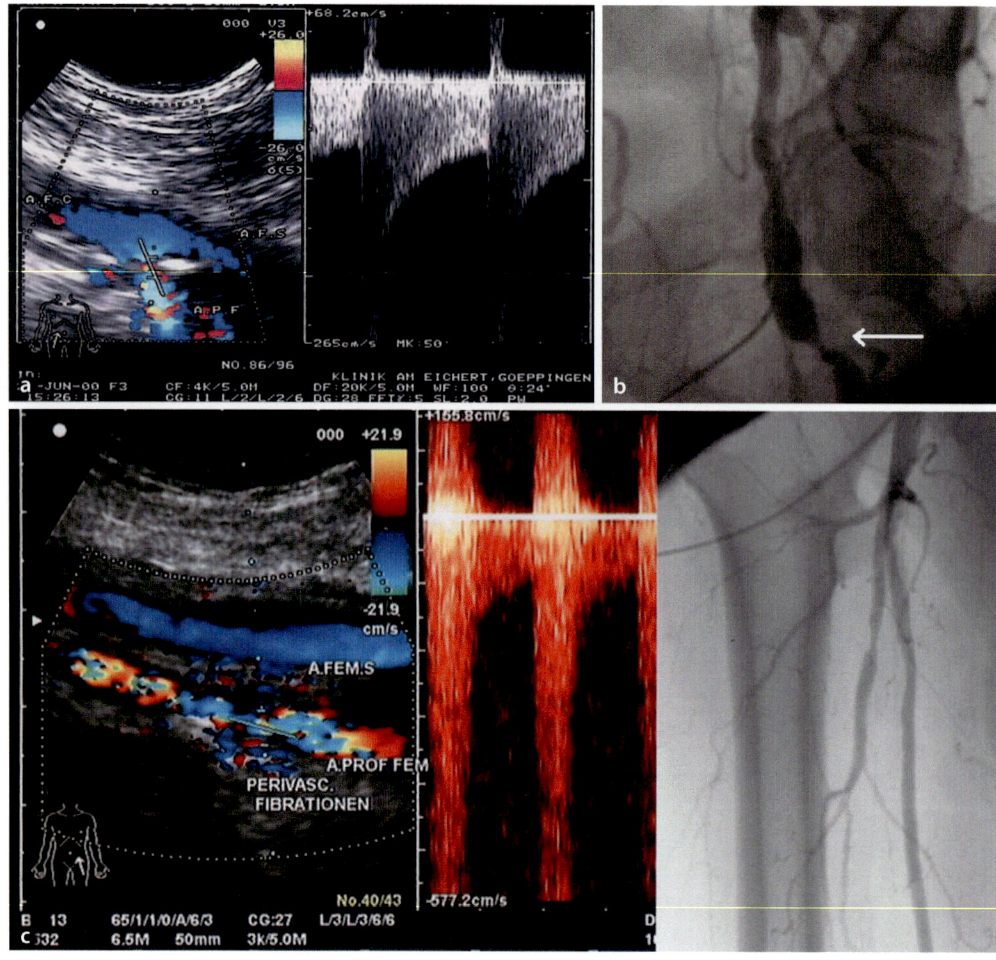

Fig. 2.60a–c (Atlas) Stenosis at origin of profunda femoris artery (recurrence).
a Duplex ultrasound has become the method of choice for diagnosing and grading stenosis of the profunda femoris artery, as anteroposterior angiograms are limited for various reasons: the femoral bifurcation may be obscured by overlying vessels, variants in the course of the artery may not be assessable, and stenosis caused by posterior wall plaque is difficult to grade. In this patient with prior TEA of the common femoral artery, aliasing in the color flow image and a peak systolic velocity (PSV) >3 m/s with a monophasic flow profile indicate recurrent high-grade stenosis.
b The corresponding angiogram depicts the stenosing plaque at the origin of the profunda femoris artery. Recurrent stenosis and wide lumen of the common femoral artery following TEA.
Distal profunda femoris stenosis.
c Distal profunda femoris artery stenosis becomes relevant and requires treatment if it involves the main branch of the artery, which courses parallel to the superficial femoral artery and may thus be recruited as a collateral in superficial femoral artery occlusion. The color flow image (left) shows high-grade stenosis of the profunda femoris artery approximately 4 cm from its origin with a Doppler-derived PSV > 5 m/s. The proximal segment of the superficial femoral artery (A.FEM.S.) is patent. The angiogram confirms the more distal stenosis of the profunda femoris artery and a patent proximal superficial femoral artery with an occlusion in the lower thigh. The angiogram also allows clear differentiation between the main trunk of the profunda femoris, which is relevant as a collateral in superficial femoral artery occlusion, and a second branch arising posteriorly. The latter plays no role as a collateral in superficial femoral artery occlusion; it supplies the upper thigh muscles and receives the circumflex artery (providing arterial flow in case of occlusion of the common femoral or external iliac artery). In a patient with superficial femoral artery occlusion, the sonographic examination cannot be confined to the origin of the profunda femoris but must include a length of 7–8 cm to also identify any relevant stenosis more distally

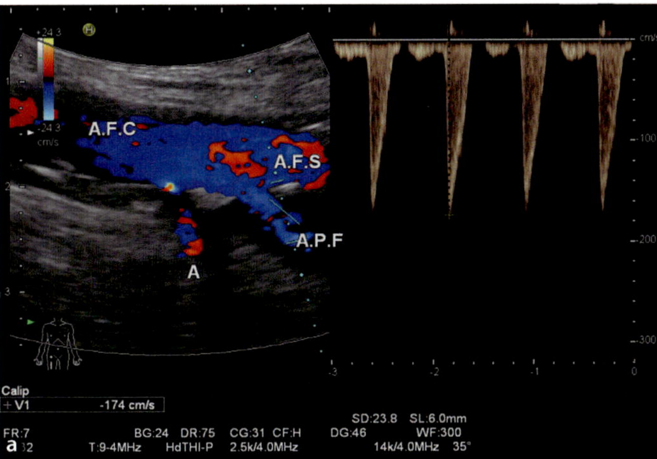

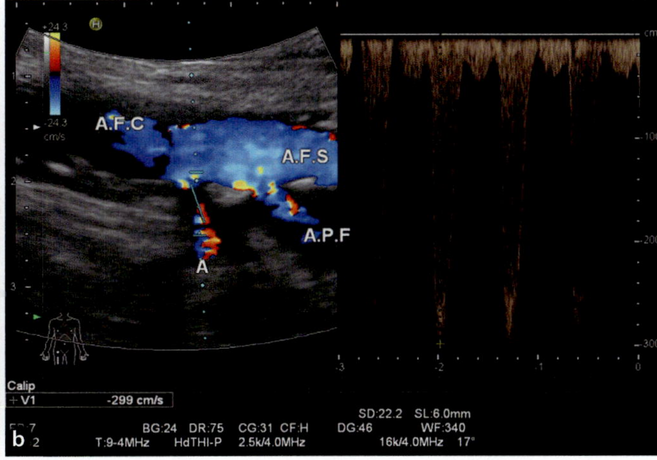

Fig. 2.61a, b (Atlas) Profunda femoris artery – variable origin and branching pattern.
a Two profunda femoris branches arise from the common femoral artery (A.F.C) – a proximal branch (A) supplying the upper thigh and a second branch (A.P.F) supplying the distal thigh muscles. The second branch, with its proximal segment coursing parallel to the superficial femoral artery, can be recruited as a collateral when the superficial femoral artery becomes occluded. Therefore, stenosis of the distal profunda branch (PSV of 170 cm/s) must be ruled out in patients with superficial femoral artery occlusion. If there is stenosis of this branch, TEA is indicated (for further illustration of the situation, see angiogram, Fig. 2.60c (Atlas)). The second or main profunda femoris branch has a variable origin and can arise from the posterior, posterolateral, or lateral aspect of the common femoral artery and rarely from the medial side. Alternatively, a single profunda femoris can arise from the common femoral artery and then divide into two branches.
b Stenosis of the proximal profunda femoris branch (A) (PSV of 3 m/s) has no therapeutic relevance (no collateral function). However, this branch is often easier to identify because it arises from the posterior aspect of the common femoral artery

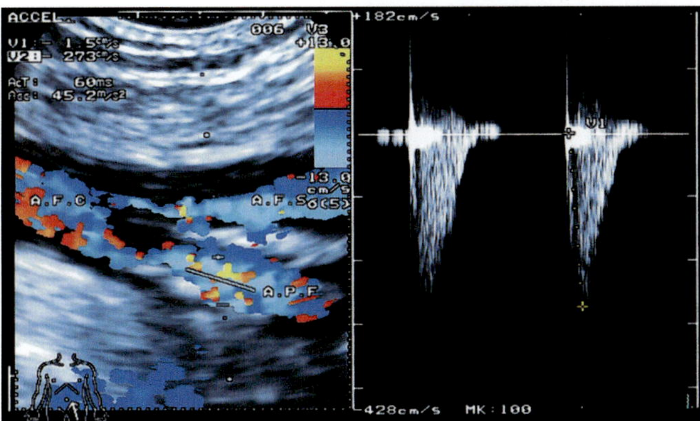

Fig. 2.62 (Atlas) Stenosis at origin of profunda femoris artery in diabetes mellitus.
Plaque with a highly irregular surface causes very turbulent flow, which is reflected both in the color flow image and in the Doppler waveform. Medial sclerosis in diabetes mellitus reduces wall elasticity, resulting in increased pulsatility of blood flow with a higher PSV and smaller diastolic flow components (including the site of stenosis). Therefore, reliance on absolute PSV alone for stenosis grading may result in (slight) overestimation of the severity of stenosis in diabetic patients

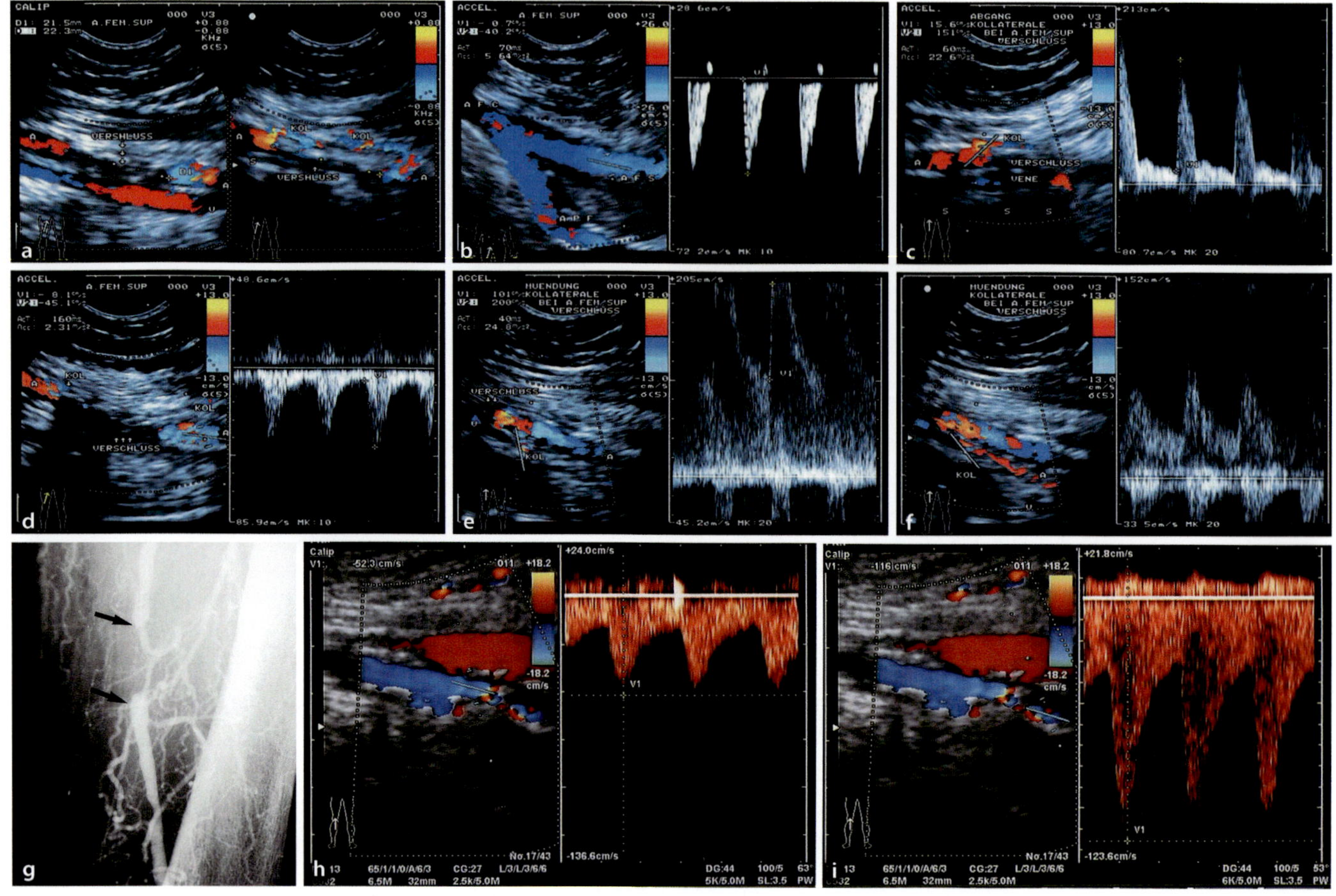

Fig. 2.63a–i (Atlas) Femoral artery occlusion and sequential popliteal artery stenosis.
a Color duplex imaging is superior to conventional duplex in that it enables rapid identification of an occlusion and provides fairly reliable estimates of its length. In the example, there is a 2 cm occlusion of the distal femoral artery just above the adductor canal. The left image shows the proximal and distal ends of the occluded segment with absence of flow signals in between. The absence of flow signals is due to actual absence of flowing blood rather than inadequate instrument setting or calcified plaques, as indicated by the demonstration of flow in the opposite direction in the femoral vein posterior to the artery. Parallel shifting of the transducer leads to the disappearance of the femoral vein from the scanning plane, while the collateral arising from the femoral artery upstream of the occlusion and re-entering downstream comes into view. In the color mode, the collateral (KOL) is depicted closer to the transducer than the occlusion. In this imaging plane, the plaques in the occluded artery cause posterior acoustic shadowing.
b Femoral bifurcation: The Doppler waveform from the proximal superficial femoral artery already suggests a flow obstruction distal to the sample volume. Flow is pulsatile but the early diastolic forward flow component following the dip is absent. In this case, the flow profile cannot be explained by diabetic medial sclerosis. Moreover, peak systolic velocity (PSV) is reduced to 40 cm/s although there is no proximal stenosis. Collateral flow is mainly through the profunda femoris artery (see angiogram).
c Superficial femoral artery occlusion: The Doppler spectrum from the origin of the collateral (KOL) arising from the superficial femoral artery just upstream of the occlusion shows a PSV of 150 cm/s. The higher flow velocity is not due to stenosis at the origin but is attributable to different vessel calibers. The occluded superficial femoral artery is depicted posterior to the collateral and the vein posterior to the artery. Incomplete color coding in the artery and vein is due to plaques (S).
d The postocclusive waveform of the refilled superficial femoral artery shows monophasic flow with a PSV of 45 cm/s.
e, f Just proximal to the refilled segment, two further collaterals (KOL) with flow toward the transducer enter the superficial femoral artery posteriorly. In **f** a long segment of the collateral is depicted in red while the superficial femoral is shown in blue (flow away from transducer). With a PSV of 95 cm/s, this collateral is not stenosed whereas the second collateral (**e**) entering the artery more proximally and medially shows criteria of stenosis at its site of entry on duplex ultrasound and in the Doppler waveform (aliasing, end-diastolic velocity (EDV) of 100 cm/s and PSV >250 cm/s). The occlusion is indicated by arrows in **e**. Retrograde flow components in the superficial femoral artery are displayed in red.
g Angiogram: Confirmation of the 2-cm occlusion of the superficial femoral artery. Also seen are the anterior collateral pathway and the two collaterals entering the posterior aspect of the artery (lower arrow). The latter are supplied by profunda femoris collaterals.
h Serial stenosis in the distal popliteal artery (P3 segment). The Doppler waveform obtained distal to the entry of the collaterals bridging the occlusion shows monophasic postocclusive flow with a delayed systolic upstoke and a PSV of 52 cm/s. The downstream stenosis is indicated by aliasing.
i Direct spectral Doppler interrogation of the suspected stenosis (aliasing) reveals a focal increase in PSV to 116 cm/s. This increase alone does not indicate a relevant stenosis; however, in conjunction with the postocclusive decrease in flow velocity to 50 cm/s between the occluded femoral artery segment and the popliteal stenosis, a 50–60% stenosis is suggested. The PSV ratio is >2

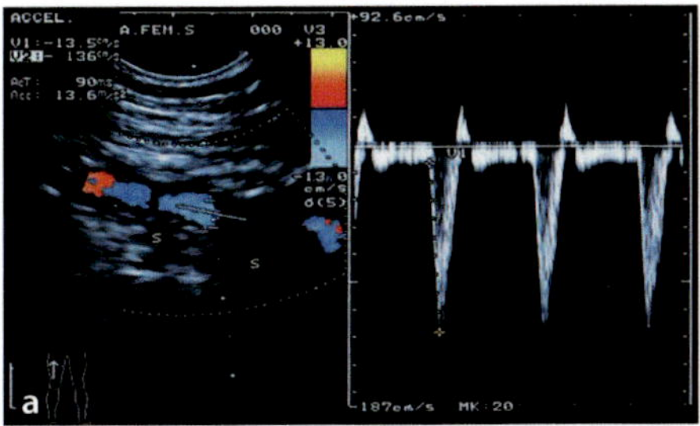

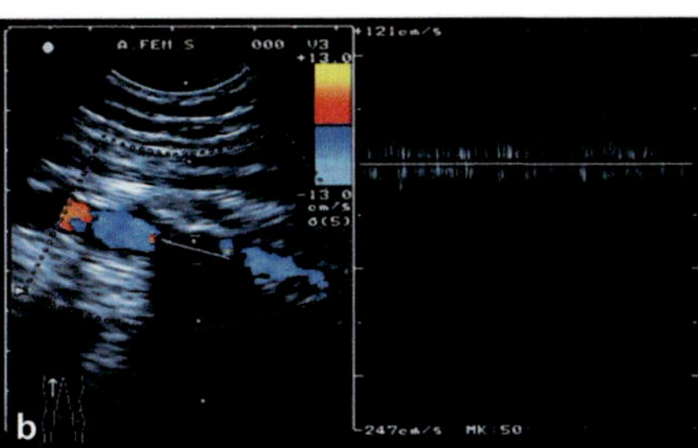

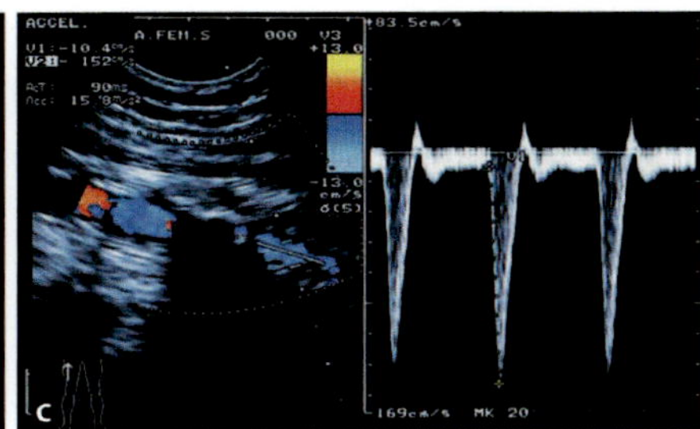

Fig. 2.64a–c (Atlas) Artifact due to acoustic shadowing.
a In contrast to the example presented in Fig. 2.63a–g (Atlas), the absence of flow signals along a 1-cm segment of the superficial femoral artery in this case is not due to occlusion but to acoustic shadowing produced by a calcified plaque. Just proximal to this segment, there is pulsatile, triphasic flow with a PSV of 136 cm/s.
b Neither color duplex nor the Doppler waveform depicts flow in the segment obscured by acoustic shadowing.
c The Doppler waveforms obtained distal and proximal to the obscured segment are identical, excluding a higher-grade stenosis or occlusion of the nonvisualized segment. The slightly higher flow velocity of 152 cm/s may be due to moderate luminal narrowing or a Doppler-angle-related error

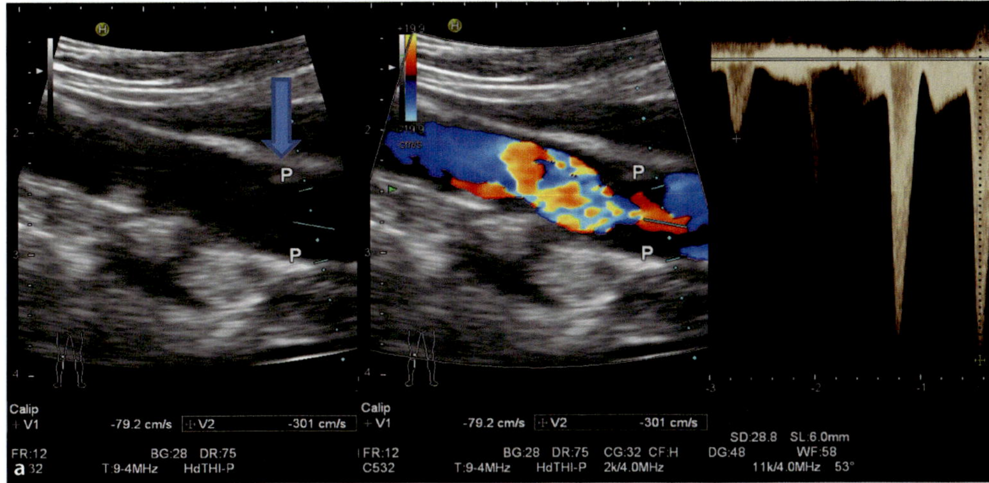

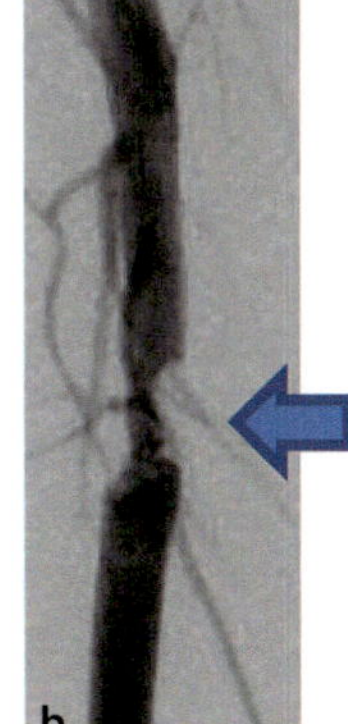

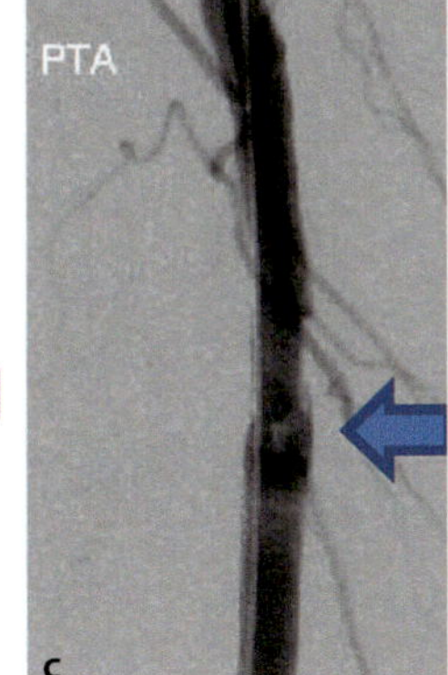

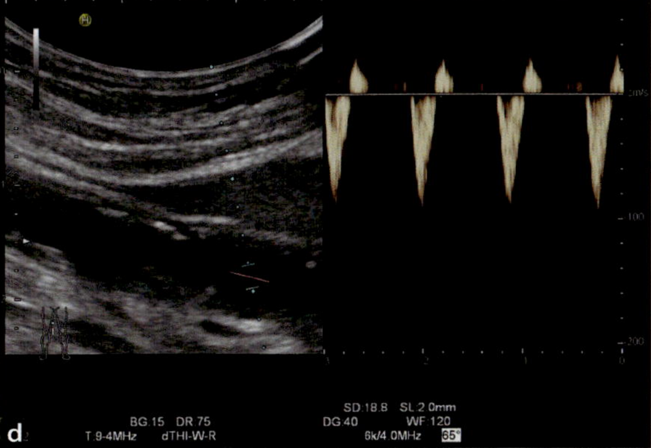

Fig. 2.65a–d (Atlas) Embolizing popliteal artery plaque before and after PTA.
a Very hypoechoic plaque (P), which is indistinct from the lumen in the B-mode image (arrow), in the popliteal artery is the source of embolism in this patient with blue toe. The plaque causes 75% stenosis (calculated according to the continuity equation; intrastenotic PSV of 301 cm/s and prestenotic PSV of 79 cm/s). Aniograms depicting the stenotic segment (arrow) before (**b**) and after (**c**) PTA. Follow-up ultrasound 6 weeks after PTA shows residual plaque pressed into the wall (**d**) without hemodynamically relevant stenosis (PSV of 95 cm/s)

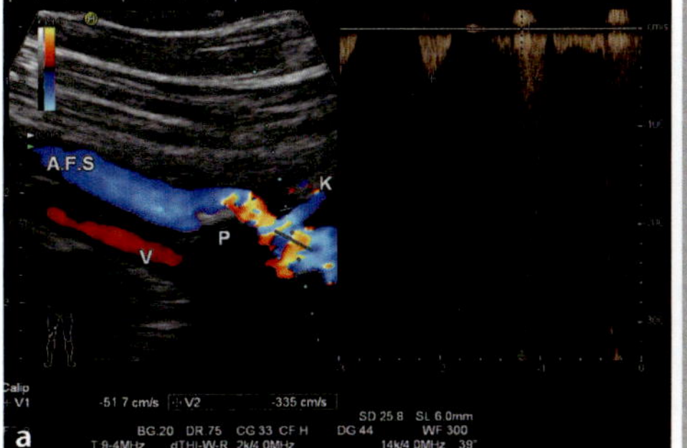

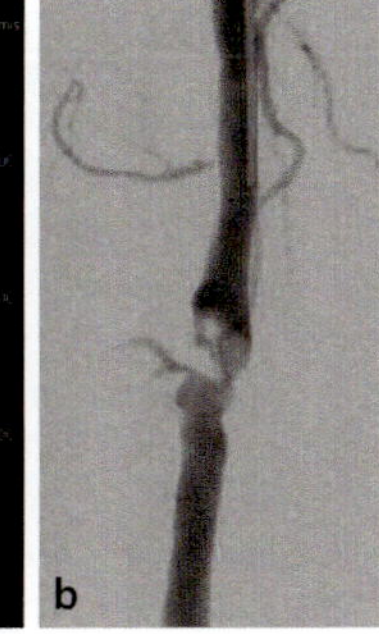

Fig. 2.66a, b (Atlas) Grading of stenosis caused by eccentric plaque.
High-grade stenosis (PSV ratio > 6) of the superficial femoral artery (A.F.S) caused by eccentric plaque (P). Unlike the plaque in Fig. 2.65 (Atlas), the plaque in this example is hyperechoic and calcified. The first collateral (K) re-entering the stenosed artery is seen just distal to the plaque. The ultrasound findings are consistent with the eccentric stenosis seen in the angiogram obtained before PTA (**b**)

2

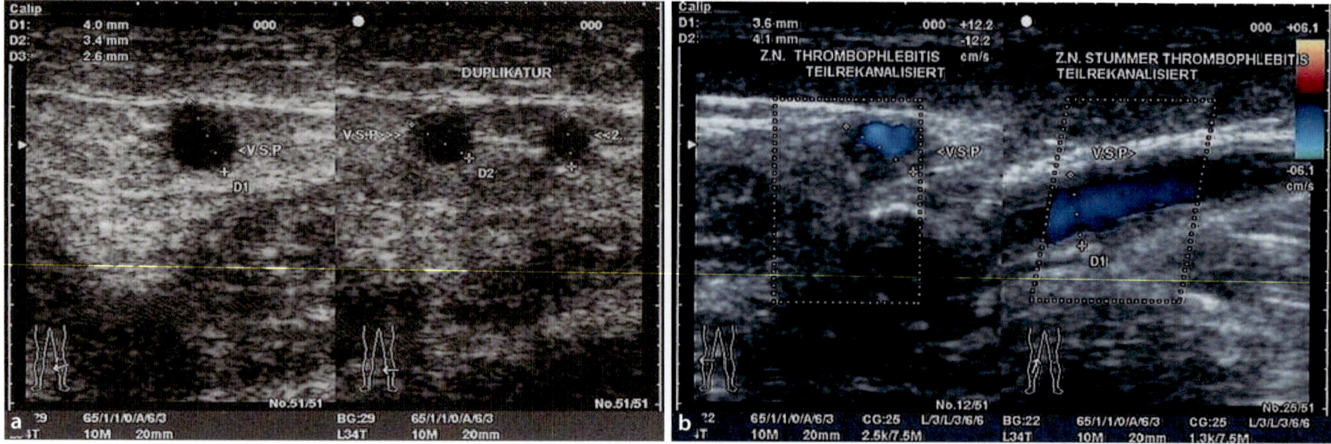

Fig. 2.67a, b (Atlas) **Bypass planning – mapping for suitable vein, target vessel.**
a Ultrasound allows preoperative identification of a suitable vein for bypass grafting. This includes measurement of the diameter, which should be over 2 mm for a crural bypass. Preoperative marking of the course of the selected vein on the skin reduces the length of incision and shortens operation time. In patients with duplication of the candidate vein, the most suitable branch in terms of diameter and course is selected sonographically. The transverse view on the left shows a suitable small saphenous vein with a diameter of 4 mm and the image on the right obtained more distally a duplicated vein with a thicker (3.4 mm) and a thinner branch (2.6 mm).
b Veins with postthrombophlebitic changes are unsuitable for grafting and can be identified by sonography, which will demonstrate a patent lumen with sclerotic wall thickening, as illustrated here for the small saphenous vein. A recanalized thrombophlebitic vein shows the same features as a postthrombotic deep vein: wall sclerosis and thickening, residual thrombi, and valve incompetence. In the example, transverse and longitudinal views (left and right, respectively) depict the thickened hypoechoic wall and flow in the patent lumen of the small saphenous vein (blue)

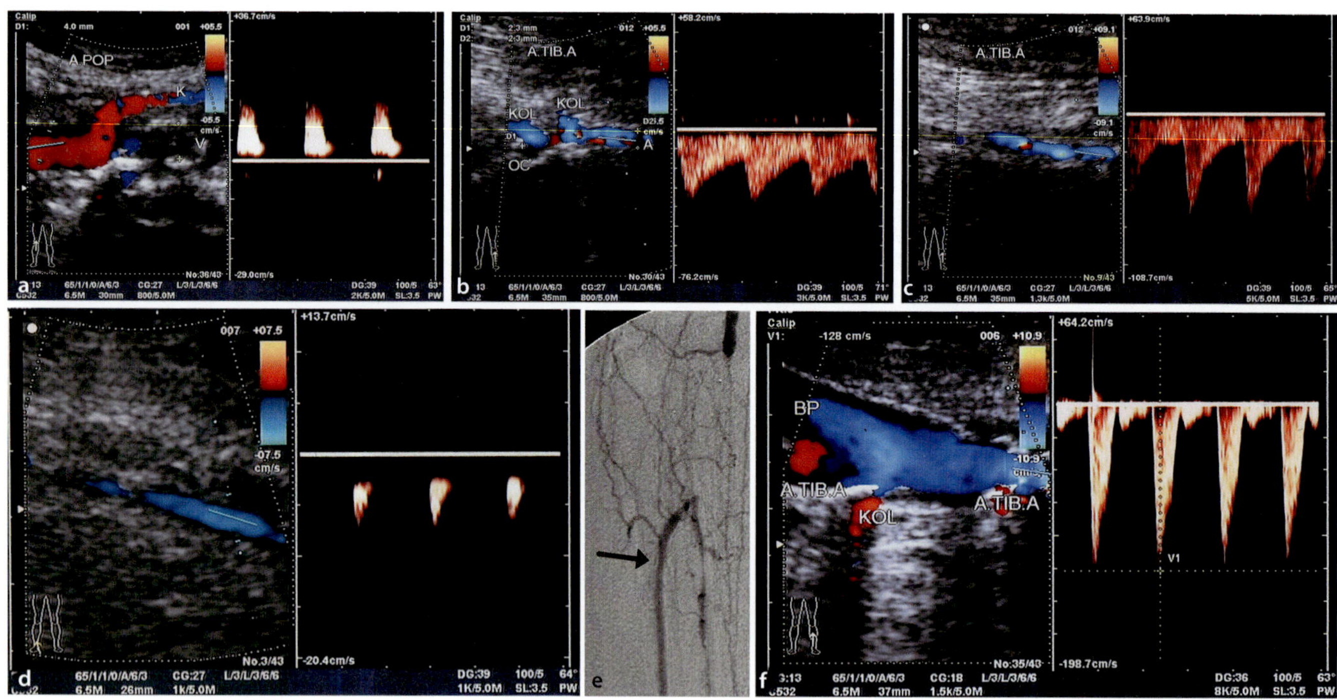

Fig. 2.68a–f (Atlas) **Selection of recipient vessel for distal bypass procedure.**
a Color duplex imaging demonstrates occlusion of the P2 and P3 popliteal segments in a woman with stage IV PAOD. A sural artery provides collateral flow (K). The Doppler waveform shows a preocclusive thump pattern.
b The search for a runoff vessel to position the distal anastomosis of a femorocrural bypass reveals collaterals (KOL) resupplying flow to the proximal tibial artery (A).
c The anterior tibial artery is then followed distally down to the ankle, where a Doppler waveform is obtained. There is no stenosis, and the waveform pattern suggests good peripheral runoff, confirming the anterior tibial artery to be an ideal target vessel for a bypass procedure.
d In contrast, spectral Doppler measurements show the fibular artery and posterior tibial artery (with multiple stenoses and only a short patent segment) to be inadequate target vessels for the planned bypass: high pulsatility and low PSV indicate poor peripheral runoff. In this case, the Doppler findings already show these two arteries to be unsuitable to receive the bypass, and complete mapping is not necessary.
e Angiogram confirms popliteal artery occlusion and suitability of the anterior tibial artery for use in a distal bypass procedure.
f Doppler findings after bypass grafting onto the anterior tibial artery suggest restoration of peripheral perfusion: the anterior tibial artery waveform recorded just distal to the bypass anastomosis shows pulsatile flow and a PSV of 128 cm/s with a short systolic rise time

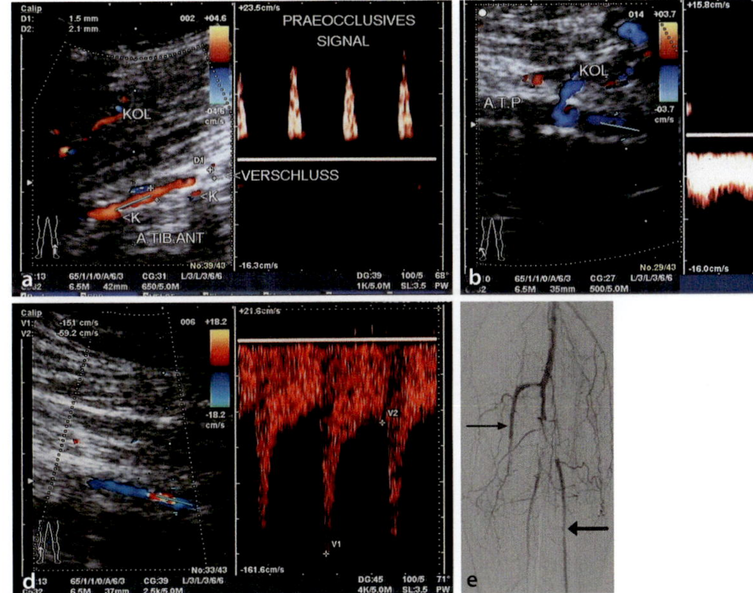

Fig. 2.69a–e (Atlas) Stage IV PAOD with arterial occlusion below the knee.
a Duplex examination before a planned bypass procedure in a woman with stage IV PAOD with occlusion of calf arteries. Color duplex and spectral Doppler reveal only mild to moderate stenoses in the peripheral arteries down to and including the popliteal artery. Below the knee, spectral Doppler analysis demonstrates preocclusive flow (knocking waveform) in the proximal anterior tibial artery between the origin of a collateral (K) and an occlusion demonstrated by color duplex. The diameter (2 mm) of the occluded artery is indicated by calipers. The occlusion extends down to the ankle joint.
b The posterior tibial artery is occluded proximally (3.5 cm in length) with a collateral channel (KOL) providing flow distal to the occlusion. Flow is diminished and very slow with a peak systolic velocity (PSV) of 8 cm/s; the flow pattern resembles that in a vein, but the direction is away from the probe, indicating that an artery is being interrogated. In a situation like this, with occlusion and collateral refilling of the main artery, it is important to continuously image the artery for another 4–5 cm to decide whether distal runoff can be evaluated by spectral Doppler measurement, which will be the case if there is adequate resupply of blood through the collateral pathway.
c More distally, flow is again increased due to inflow from additional collaterals (PSV of 60 cm/s and end-diastolic velocity (EDV) of 25 cm/s; post-occlusive delay in systolic upstroke).
d Two centimeters distal to the waveform presented in **c**, there is aliasing in the posterior tibial artery and Doppler interrogation reveals an increase in PSV of slightly more than 100% (150 cm/s), corresponding to 50–60% stenosis.
e Angiogram confirms occlusions of the anterior tibial artery and proximal posterior tibial artery. The latter is supplied via collaterals distal to the occluded segment. The thick arrow indicates a mildly narrowed segment of the posterior tibial artery (see **d**) and the thin arrow the anterior tibial artery

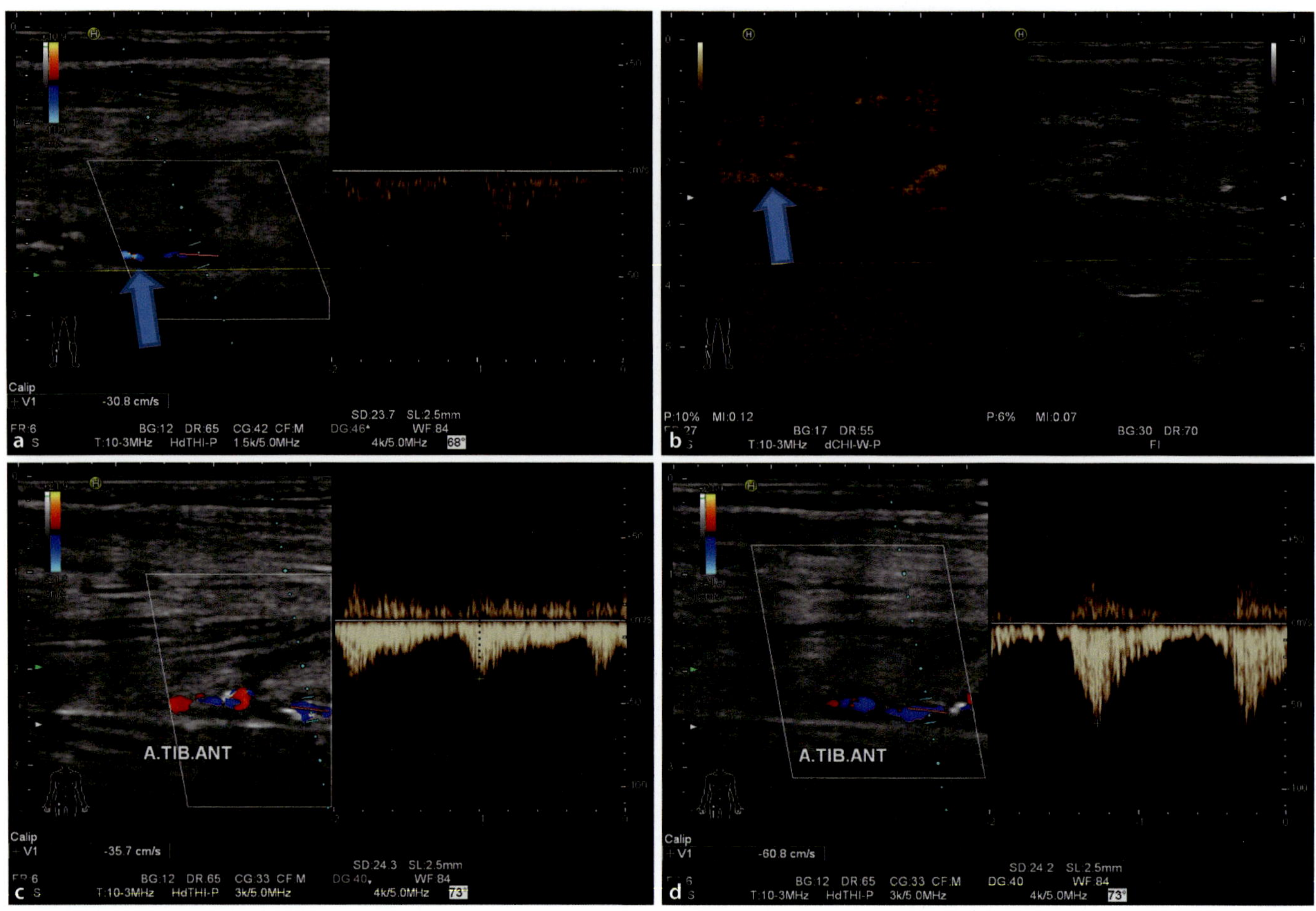

Fig. 2.70a–d (Atlas) Contrast-enhanced ultrasound (CEUS) – bypass recipient vessel in popliteal artery occlusion.
a In this patient with stage IV PAOD, diabetic medial sclerosis, and foot phlegmon, the insonation conditions are very poor as there is scatter due to interstitial fluid accumulation. Even with a low PRF and high gain, only isolated flow signals are obtained from the anterior tibial artery.
b Contrast-enhanced ultrasound (CEUS) performed with low mechanical index (MI; see ▶ Sects. 1.1.5, 2.1.6.1.11, and 6.1.6.1.3) depicts reflections from microbubbles in a long segment of the anterior tibitial artery (arrow). Note, however, that when using CEUS and the artery of interest is difficult to follow in the B-mode image (right), a collateral may be mistaken for the main artery, and it is not possible to detect or rule out stenosis.
c, d Contrast-enhanced color duplex ultrasound performed with normal MI: depiction of the patent anterior tibial artery (**c**) and the abrupt increase in PSV (**d**) allow stenosis detection and grading based on the continuity equation (in the example, there is doubling of PSV, indicating 50% stenosis). However, without use of a low-MI technique, there is rapid destruction of the microbubbles and the diagnostic window is very short (compare intensity of waveforms and color duplex images in **a** versus **c** and **d**)

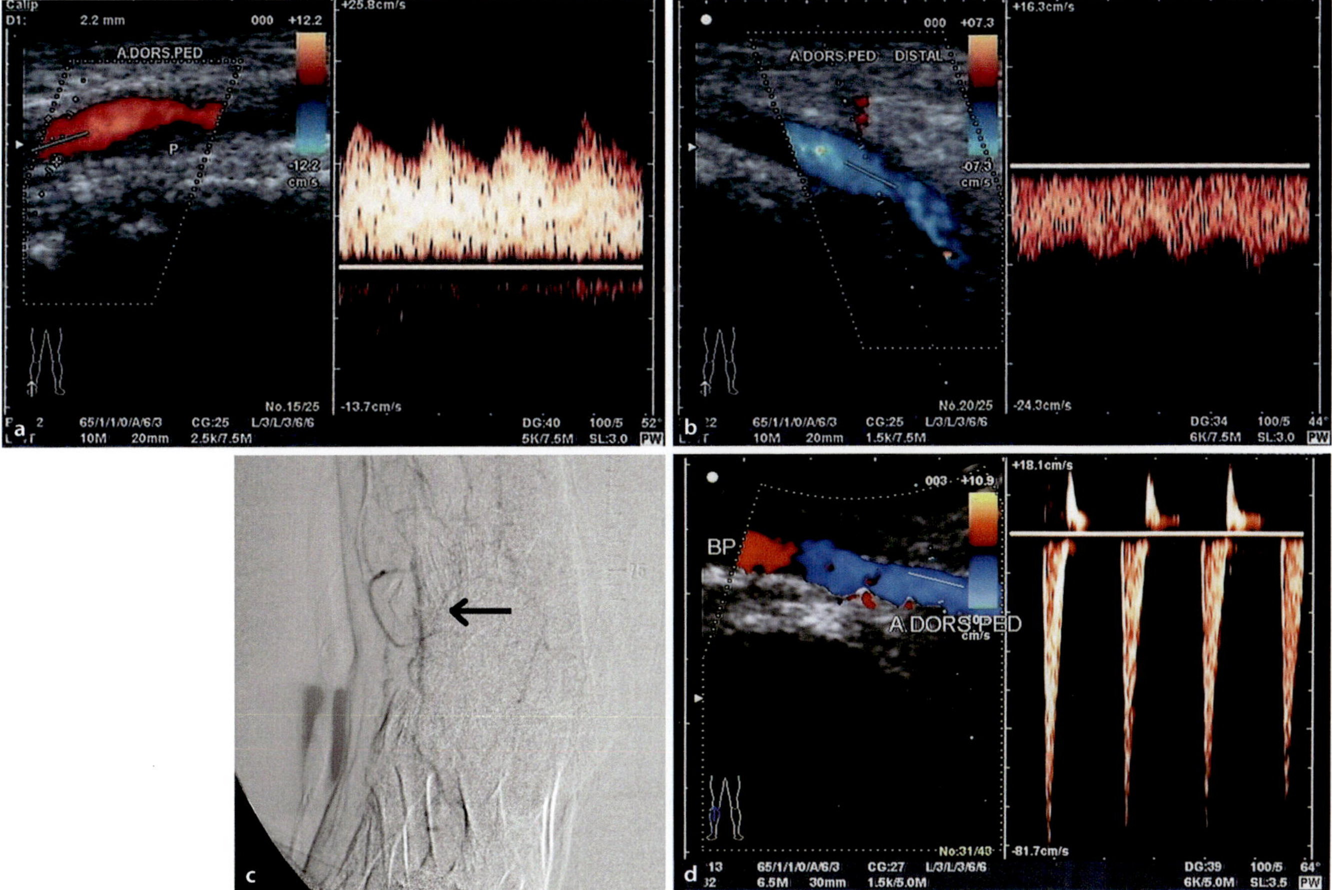

Fig. 2.71a–d (Atlas) Recipient vessel for pedal bypass.
a Slow flow in the superficial pedal arteries is visualized by high-resolution duplex imaging using a high-frequency transducer and a low PRF. Plaques and stenoses are depicted, and a Doppler waveform showing the typical postocclusive monophasic flow, often with an almost venous profile, indicates upstream occlusion. Mean flow velocity or peak systolic velocity (PSV) and the diastolic flow component are other important parameters for determining whether an artery would provide adequate outflow when used as the recipient segment of a planned bypass. This information is important to predict bypass patency prior to surgery. The patient presented has stage IV PAOD with occlusion of all arteries below the knee. The dorsalis pedis artery shows monophasic, postocclusive flow just above the ankle joint. There is some luminal narrowing from a hypoechoic plaque (P).
b Further down, shortly before it enters the arch of foot, the dorsalis pedis artery has an unchanged monophasic flow profile with good perfusion, suggesting that the artery is a suitable candidate for connection of a pedal bypass graft. In this patient, with multiple upstream occlusions, a more pulsatile flow profile would suggest poor outflow.
c Angiogram of the pedal vessels demonstrates patency of the artery though there is poor opacification due to the proximal occlusions. Angiography is inferior to color duplex in predicting whether this artery will ensure adequate runoff for a pedal bypass.
d The venous graft anastomosed onto the dorsalis pedis artery has triphasic flow with a PSV of nearly 80 cm/s, indicating adequate perfusion of the foot without ischemic vasodilatation in the periphery

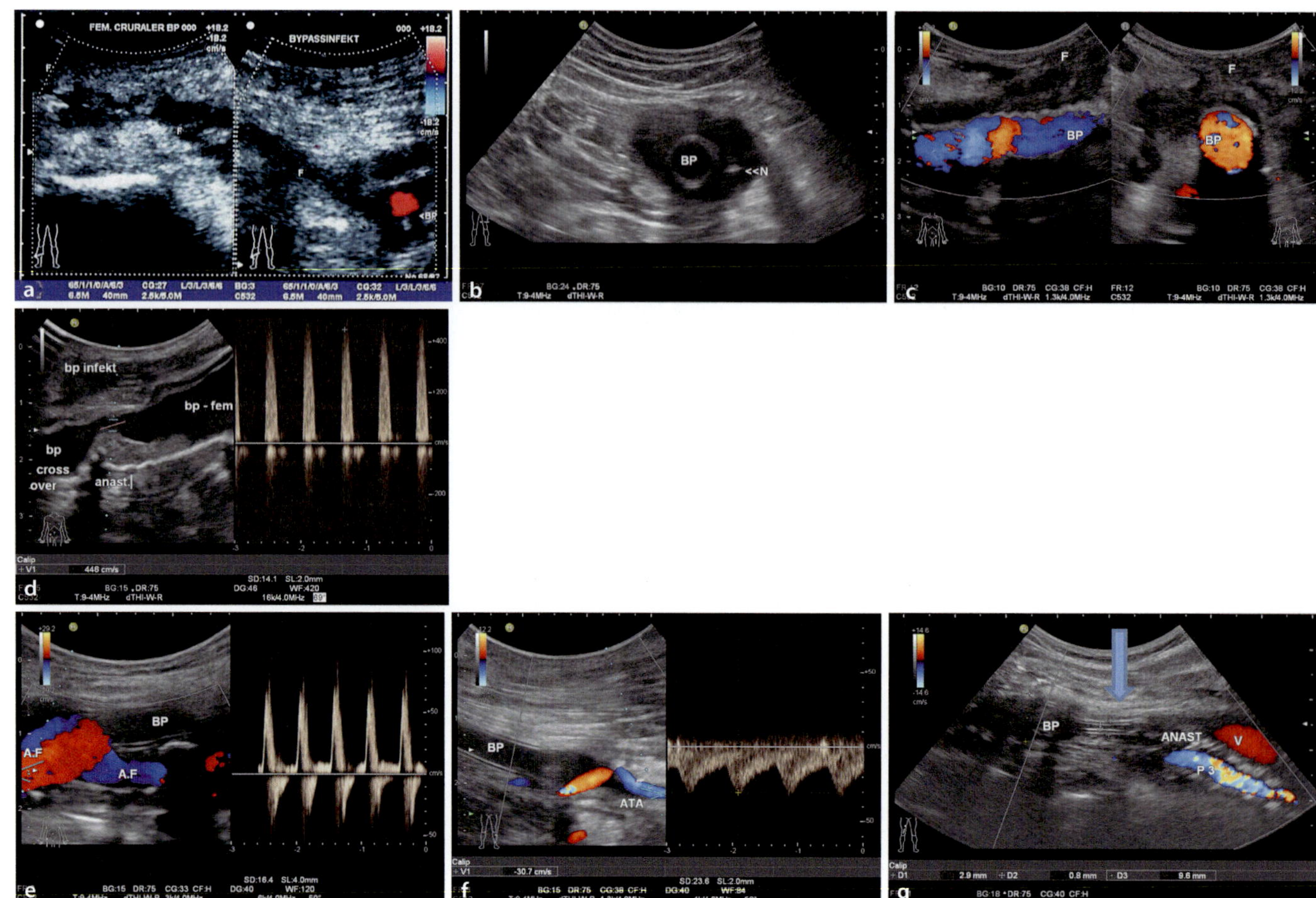

Fig. 2.72a–g (Atlas) Bypass complications: graft infection, graft occlusion.
a A hypoechoic fistula (F) some centimeters in length extends from below the skin to the distal anastomosis of a P2 bypass (composite image), indicating graft infection, although the initial clinical appearance of the wound suggested only a superficial, subcutaneous infection.
b If gray-scale ultrasound depicts elongated hypoechoic to anechoic areas around a bypass graft (BP), an infection of the bypass has to be ruled out, in particular if the respective clinical signs are present. The simplest test is ultrasound-guided aspiration, for which the hyperechoic needle tip (N) is positioned in the hypoechoic zone adjacent to the graft. The needle may have to be moved about a bit under suction to reach a fluid collection.
c Graft infection is often characterized by mixed echogenicity, predominantly low echogenicity, around the graft; if a fistula (F) has formed, a hypoechoic tract extending to the skin level may be identified.
d Infectious thrombosis can cause stenosis or occlusion, especially at the anastomosis (e.g., in a crossover bypass and femoropopliteal graft extension (anast)). In the case presented, there is a peak systolic velocity (PSV) of 450 cm/s (hypoechoic infectious area around the graft). The slightest clinical suspicion of bypass graft infection should prompt a sonographic examination to prevent complications and initiate timely graft revision.
Graft occlusion.
e, f, g When thrombectomy is planned in a patient with a synthetic bypass graft, it is especially important to evaluate inflow and outflow and whether the recipient segment is also occluded and a bypass extension might be necessary. In this patient, the triphasic waveform with an adequate PSV in the inflow tract rules out relevant proximal stenosis (**e**). Outflow can be evaluated by obtaining a waveform from the artery distal to the anastomis. A higher PSV indicates better outflow (**f**); however, PSV also depends on the recipient vessel. In the crural arteries (as in this example of a femoroanterior tibial bypss (ATA)), blood flow is slower than downstream of a popliteal artery bypass. Bypass graft occlusion can be due to external compression as in this case of a bypass graft (BP) onto the P3 segment of the popliteal artery (arrow, see double contour in **g**). External structures compressing a bypass include tendons, scar formation, or excessive longitudinal traction of the graft during implantation. For successful repair in such cases, thrombectomy must include elimination of the external compression

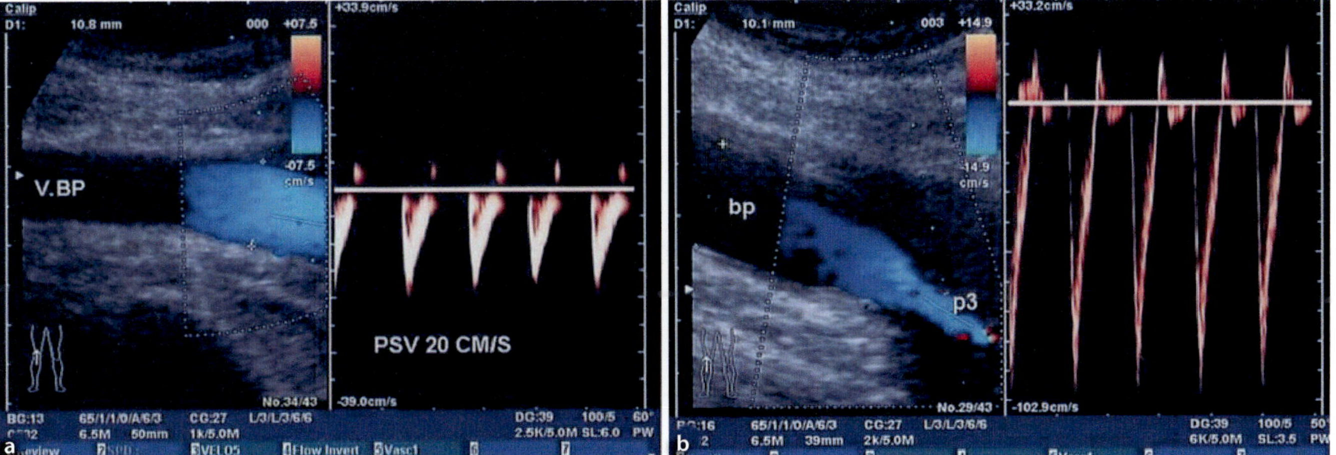

Fig. 2.73a, b (Atlas) Interpretation of Doppler waveforms from within bypass grafts.
a Blood flow velocity within a bypass graft is largely determined by its diameter and that of the distal recipient artery. In the example shown, peak systolic velocity (PSV) in the dilated venous bypass graft (V.BP; diameter of 11 mm) is only 20 cm/s although there is no stenosis proximal to the sampling site. The waveform is pulsatile and exhibits a steep systolic upstroke.
b There is no stenosis at the distal anastomosis with the distal popliteal artery (P3). The focal increase in PSV to 102 cm/s is due to the size mismatch between the dilated graft (bp; see **a**) and the normal-caliber distal popliteal artery. The triphasic and pulsatile waveform recorded in the popliteal artery distal to the anastomosis is that of a normal peripheral artery. In the follow-up of bypass grafts, the examiner should compare the pulsatility and flow velocity with the baseline values determined sonographically within the first 3 months of the bypass procedure

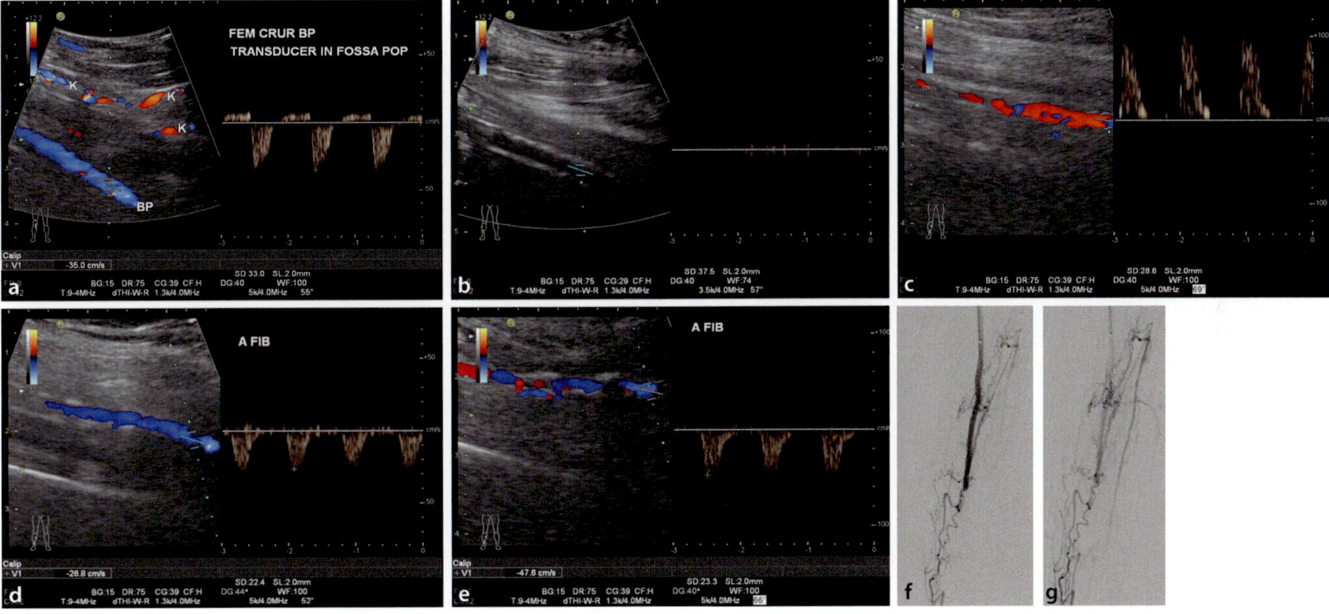

Fig. 2.74a–g (Atlas) Low-flow bypass – failing bypass.
a Patient presenting 2 years after creation of a venous femorocrural bypass onto the posterior tibial artery. A markedly reduced peak systolic velocity (PSV) of 35 cm/s indicates a low-flow bypass at risk for imminent occlusion. In interpreting flow velocities measured in a bypass, however, the examiner must take into account a possible size mismatch between graft and recipient artery. In the case presented here, the pulsatile character of the waveform with to-and-fro flow suggests an increase in peripheral resistance and hence an outflow obstruction.
b In this patient, slow flow and pulsatility in the bypass are due to occlusion of the posterior tibial artery distal to the bypass anastomosis.
c The proximal posterior tibial artery exhibits retrograde flow (red, directed toward the center, PSV of 110 cm/s) and refills the fibular artery via collaterals.
d Blood flow in the fibular artery is orthograde, and the PSV is 26 cm/s.
e More distal spectral Doppler sampling in the fibular artery demonstrates a similar flow character, indicating patency of a long stretch of the artery and absence of high-grade stenosis. These findings suggest that the fibular artery would be a suitable outflow tract for revision of the low-flow bypass. However, because of good collateralization and the patient's multimorbidity including a history of stroke, anticoagulation was initiated instead. The bypass has since been followed up for one year with no evidence of occlusion.
f These sonographic findings (posterior tibial artery patent proximally and occluded downstream of the bypass anastomosis, refilling of fibular artery via collaterals) are confirmed by angiography performed 6 months later for PTA of a new stenosis at the proximal anastomosis (see Fig. 2.75 (Atlas)).
g Later angiogram shows patency of a long stretch of the fibular artery

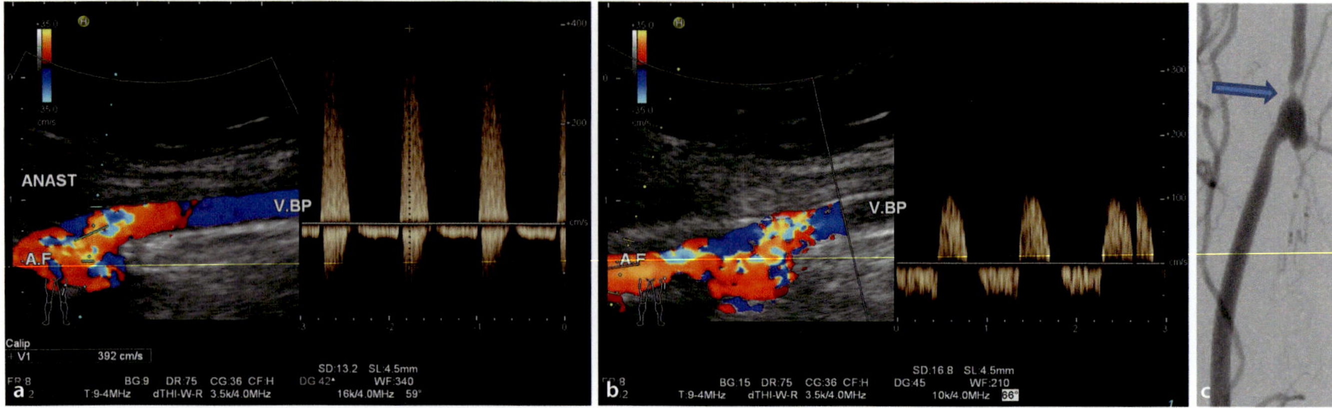

Fig. 2.75a–c (Atlas) Low-flow bypass and new stenosis of proximal anastomosis.
New high-grade stenosis of the proximal anastomosis (**a**) in the patient with low-flow bypass presented in Fig. 2.74 (Atlas)). The PSV ratio is 4 (intrastenotic PSV of 4 m/s and prestenotic PSV of 1 m/s (**b**)). High pulsatility is due to outflow obstruction

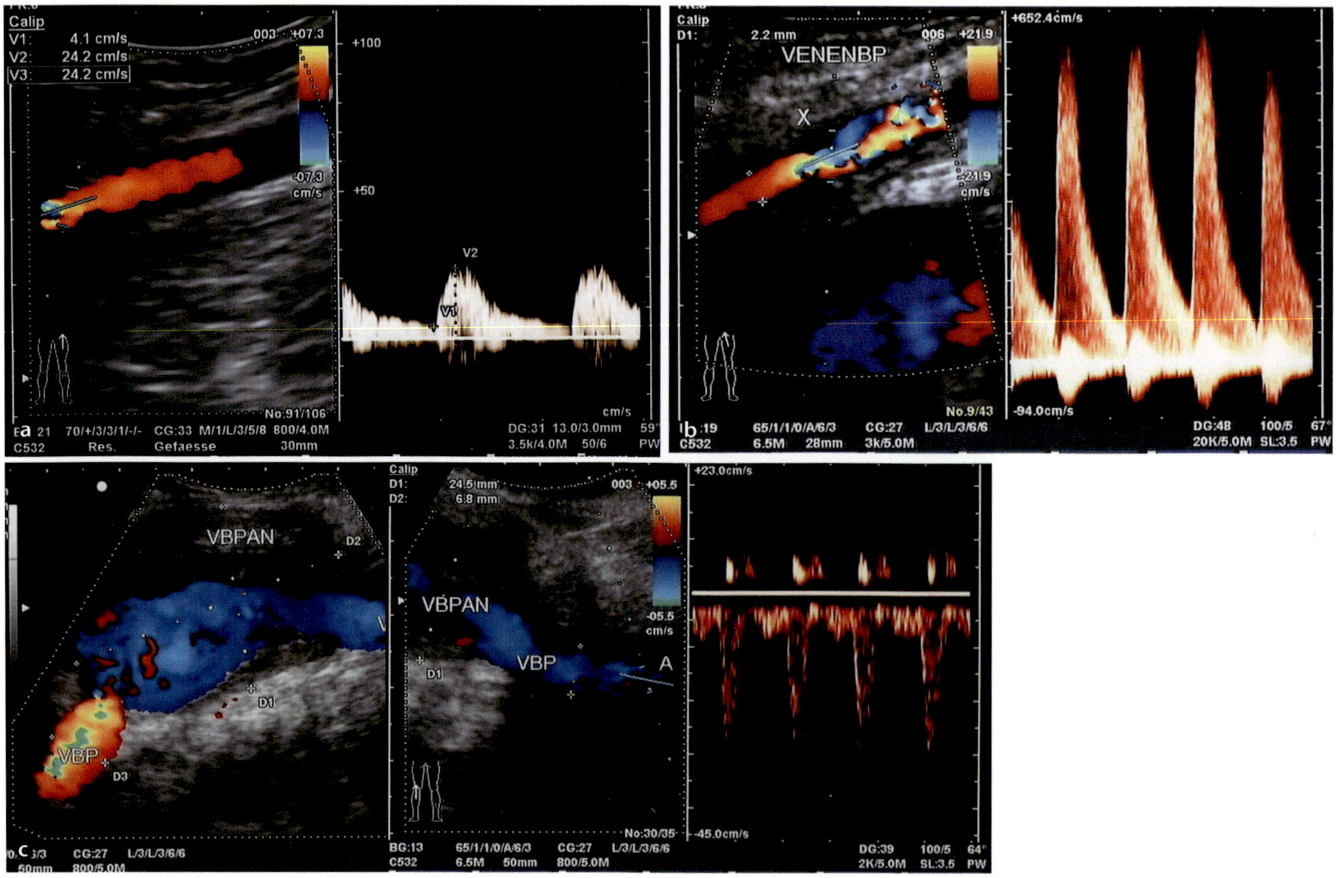

Fig. 2.76a–c (Atlas) Saphenous vein bypass graft – stenosis at valve site.
An autologous bypass graft (great saphenous vein) is more difficult to identify, especially when it is occluded, due to the thin venous wall and the frequent extra-anatomic course. Color duplex helps identify the graft, but spectral Doppler measurement is necessary for quantitative evaluation.
a A postocclusive waveform with a peak systolic velocity (PSV) of 24 cm/s and an end-diastolic velocity (EDV) of 4.1 cm/s obtained in the main body of the graft indicates proximal stenosis.
b While stenosis is rare within a synthetic bypass, the entire length of a venous graft must be carefully scrutinized for the presence of stenosis. In an in situ vein graft, stenosis tends to develop at sites of retained valves. In the example, the color flow image and spectral Doppler measurement reveal a short, high-grade stenosis with a PSV of 6 m/s at the site of a valve leaflet, confirming the stenosis suggested by the postocclusive waveform presented in **a.**
Aneurysmal dilatation of vein graft.
c Aneurysmal dilatation is a late complication of bypass surgery and is often associated with elongation of the graft (VBP). The left color flow image shows a dilated and partially thrombosed venous graft segment (measuring 2.5 × 3.8 cm) 2 cm above the distal anastomosis with the P3 segment of the popliteal artery (VBPAN). The second color flow image shows the site of anastomosis (A), from which the Doppler waveform was obtained

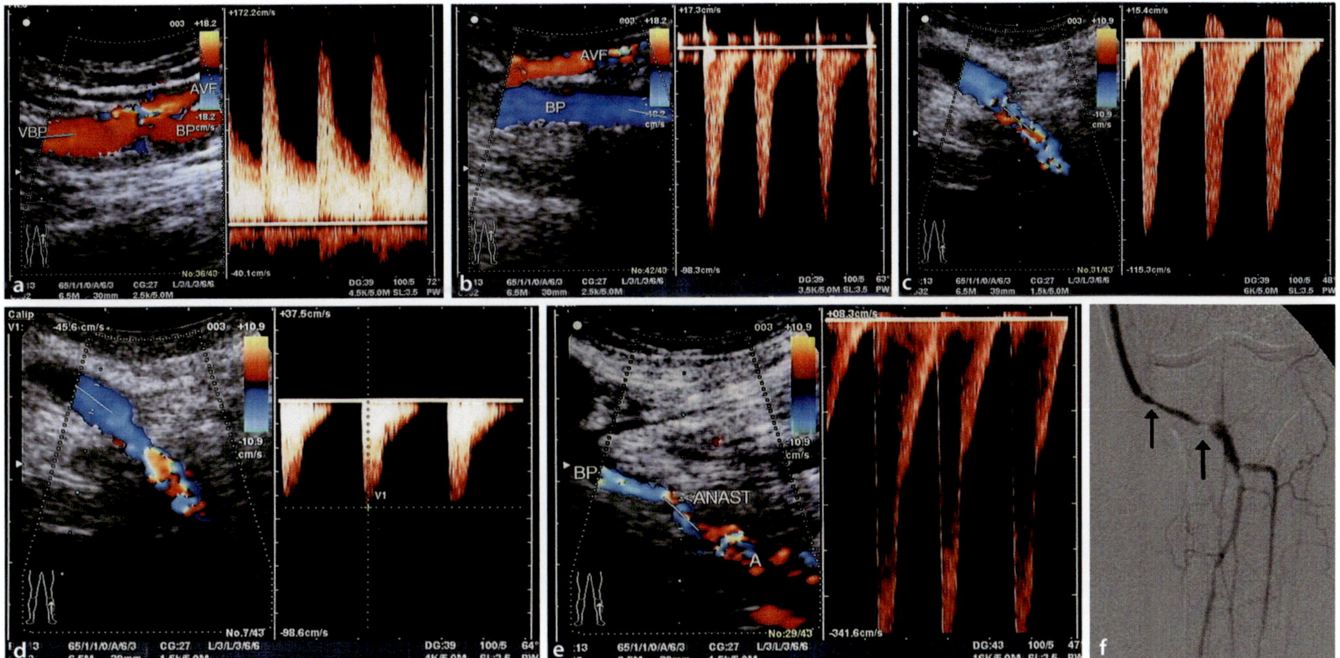

Fig. 2.77a–f (Atlas) In situ vein graft – AV fistula and stenosis.
a Waveform from an in situ vein graft with a steep systolic upstroke but monophasic flow pattern and large diastolic component. The high flow volume in the graft with a peak systolic velocity (PSV) of 150 cm/s and an end-diastolic velocity (EDV) of 50 cm/s is attributable to a distal arteriovenous fistula (AVF).
b Distal to the high-flow fistula (AVF), the flow velocity in the graft (BP) is much lower. Doppler interrogation shows a PSV of 70 cm/s and a monophasic pattern, but with some end-diastolic flow. The waveform is still abnormal, chiefly showing the influence of peripheral vasodilation.
c In addition, there is a stenosis 4 cm proximal to the distal anastomosis at the site of a retained valve leaflet. Stenosis is suggested by a focal increase in PSV to 1 m/s and the monophasic waveform.
d A PSV ratio >2 is calculated (prestenotic PSV of 45 cm/s), corresponding to approximately 50% stenosis. The color duplex image shows aliasing at the site of stenosis. The site of the AV fistula identified by ultrasound was marked on the skin for ligation, while the 50% stenosis was left untreated.
e Over the next 3 months, the patient developed a second, high-grade stenosis at the distal anastomosis (ANAST) with a PSV of >3.5 m/s.
f Angiogram showing the anastomotic stenosis and relative luminal narrowing approx. 3 cm proximal to the anastomosis; the degree of stenosis is difficult to estimate

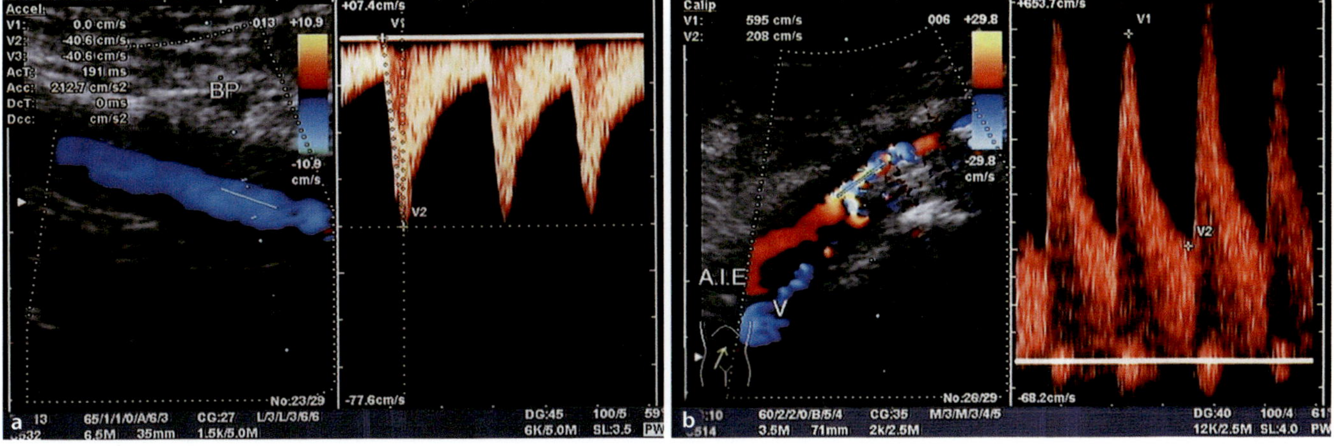

Fig. 2.78a, b (Atlas) Bypass graft – inflow stenosis.
a Inflow stenosis is suggested if, as in this example, spectral Doppler examination of the bypass demonstrates the characteristic features of poststenotic flow including a monophasic waveform with a delayed systolic upstroke, reduced peak systolic velocity (PSV), and persistent diastolic flow. When the waveform from within the graft suggests inflow obstruction, the inflow artery should be followed cranially to identify the site of stenosis.
b High-grade external iliac artery stenosis caused by posterior plaque, suggested by aliasing in the color flow image and confirmed by spectral Doppler interrogation (monophasic flow, PSV of 550 cm/s, end-diastolic velocity of 220 cm/s)

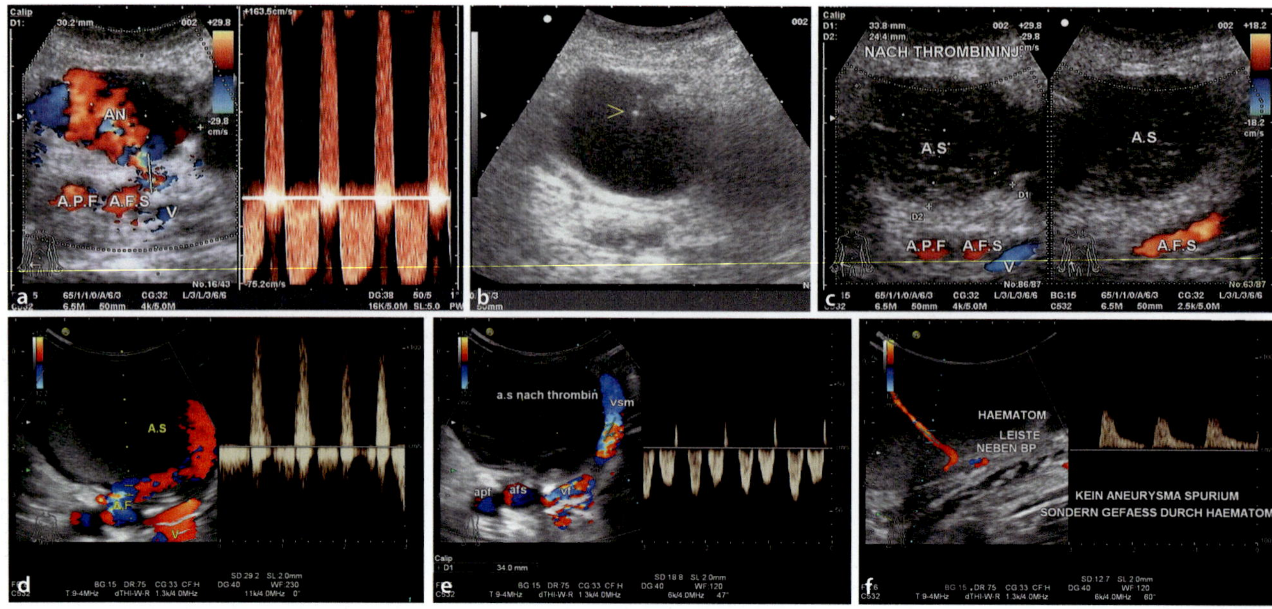

◘ Fig. 2.79a–f (Atlas) Pseudoaneurysm – thrombin injection treatment.
a Transverse view of the thigh reveals a pseudoaneurysm (AN) arising from the superficial femoral artery (A.F.S). With the sample volume placed in the neck, spectral Doppler interrogation reveals the characteristic to-and-fro flow with high-frequency flow into the aneurysm in systole and backward flow into the artery throughout diastole.
b For treatment of the aneurysm by thrombin instillation, a needle is advanced into the aneurysm and the tip positioned between the center of the cavity and the near wall under ultrasound guidance (needle tip identified by bright echo).
c Thrombin is instilled at a dose of 5000 IU dissolved in 2 mL of saline solution. Complete thrombosis of the aneurysm (AN) has occurred after instillation of one to two drops, as demonstrated by cessation of flow within the cavity in the color duplex mode; shown in transverse orientation on the left and in longitudinal orientation on the right (A.F.S = superficial femoral artery; A.P.F = profunda femoris artery; V = femoral vein).
Pseudoaneurysm – challenges for thrombin injection treatment.
d, e Very circulatory and fast flow in a larger aneurysm sac will wash away thrombin from the needle tip and dilute it before a clot can begin to form. Since both spontaneous contrast and color coding show flow directions, the needle can be sonographically guided to a peripheral area with little flow (in the leftmost aspect of the aneurysm in **d**), where a thrombus will begin to form and then enlarge with little risk of thrombin being washed away (**e**). The waveform shows that the color-coded flow adjacent to the thrombosed aneurysm sac is blood flow in the great saphenous vein rather than flow into the aneurysm.
Pseudoaneurysm – differentiation from hematoma.
f Spectral Doppler analysis allows differentiation of a postinterventional hematoma with blood flow in small arteries coursing through it, as in this case, from pseudoaneurysm with to-and-fro flow

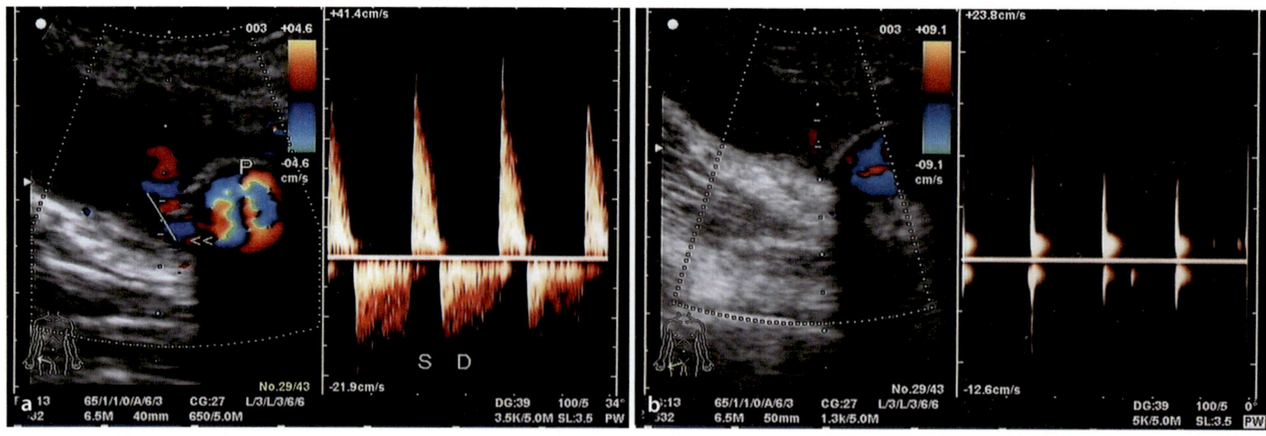

◘ Fig. 2.80a, b (Atlas) Suture aneurysm.
a In patients who have undergone an iliacofemoral bypass procedure, palpation of a mildly pulsatile, protruding mass at one of the anastomoses may suggest a suture aneurysm. In the case presented, the transverse image shows hypoechoic fluid extending laterally from the site of anastomosis. Color duplex imaging demonstrates flow in a portion of the lesion adjacent to the bypass graft. This appearance is also consistent with vibration artifacts. The suspected suture aneurysm is confirmed by spectral Doppler demonstration of to-and-fro flow in the communication between the mass and the anastomosis with a characteristic steam engine sound. This sound is produced by high systolic inflow into an aneurysm and pandiastolic flow reversal.
b Seroma at an aortofemoral bypass anastomosis. The color duplex appearance of a seroma is similar to that of a suture aneurysm (as described in **a**). However, the Doppler waveform recorded at the site of apparent flow (coded red) does not show to-and-fro flow (as in the suture aneurysm) but a signal generated in the seroma by wall motion of the vessel prosthesis. The example nicely illustrates that spectral Doppler analysis can differentiate true flow signals in a pseudoaneurysm from transmitted pulsation (which is also important when examining patients with suspected endoleaks after aortic stenting)

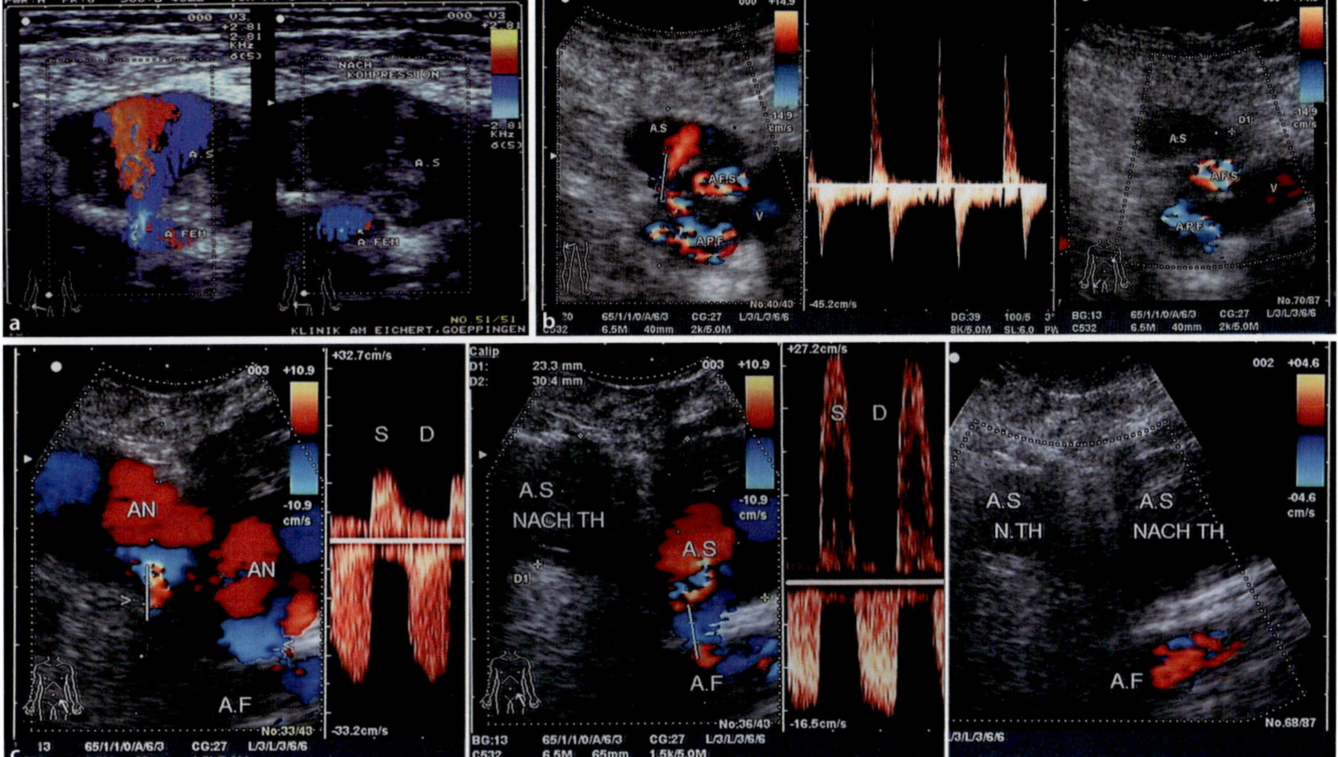

Fig. 2.81a–c (Atlas) Pseudoaneurysm – compression therapy/thrombin injection.
a In the color duplex mode, the examiner identifies the neck connecting the pseudoaneurysm to the femoral artery and then occludes it by exerting pressure with the transducer. During the procedure, which may take up to half an hour, adequate compression is indicated by the absence of flow signals in the neck and cavity. Following the procedure, absence of flow in the cavity demonstrated by color duplex indicates that complete thrombosis has been accomplished. If only partial thrombosis is apparent after the procedure, it is often easier to induce complete thrombosis in a second session on the next day (compression bandage), or complete thrombosis may occur spontaneously. Alternatively, thrombosis of a pseudoaneurysm may be induced by thrombin injection. However, thrombin injection often leaves a larger residual hematoma, which may cause persistent symptoms. Thrombin injection is indicated if the site of the aneurysm precludes compression or in patients with perforated aneurysm or suture aneurysm (which may be infected).
b A small pseudoaneurysm (A.S) measuring only 2 cm but not occluding spontaneously arises somewhat atypically from the profunda femoris artery (A.P.F) approx. 2 cm distal to the femoral bifurcation (left image). With the sample volume placed in the neck, the typical systolic–diastolic to-and-fro flow is recorded. On the medial side of the neck, the superficial femoral artery (A.F.S) and vein (V) are depicted in cross-section. Compression of the neck with the transducer in a more lateral position brings about complete thrombosis of the aneurysm after 15 min (right image).
Large pseudoaneurysm with multiple perforation – thrombin injection.
c A very obese patient developed a large hematoma extending from the left groin to the lower abdomen following angiography with cannulation of the femoral artery (A.F.). Pseudoaneurysm is suggested by the demonstration of flow (AN). The leftmost image shows the sample volume placed in the neck (arrowhead) with the characteristic to-and-fro flow in the corresponding waveform. There is a second aneurysm with a separate communication with the femoral artery (probably due to repeated puncture). The total length of both aneurysms is over 6 cm. The image obtained after thrombin treatment of the upper aneurysm (A.S. NACH TH – middle section) shows the remaining second aneurysm (A.S.) arising from the femoral artery (A.F.). The Doppler waveform from the neck of the second aneurysm also shows the typical to-and-fro flow. Blood flow in the neck is very slow (30 cm/s during systole and 16 cm/s at end diastole), suggesting a large perforation defect. A total dose of 5000 IU thrombin was required to induce closure of both aneurysms, which is very high. Very slow injection was started in the margin to minimize the risk of thrombin escape into the femoral artery. The rightmost image confirms complete thrombosis of both aneurysms and patency of the femoral artery (A.F.) posteriorly. The poor color filling of the femoral artery despite a low PRF is due to scatter by the hematoma. Leg perfusion was normal, and foot pulses were palpable

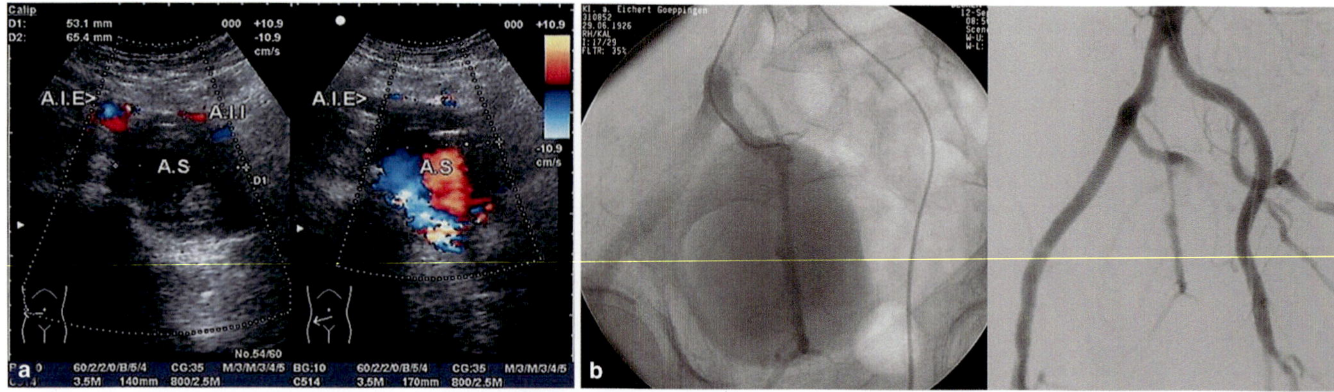

Fig. 2.82a, b (Atlas) Internal iliac artery – pseudoaneurysm, thrombin injection.
a Routine abdominal diagnostic workup prior to gastrectomy for cancer in a 78-year-old patient revealed a large spontaneous pseudoaneurysm (no trauma, no iatrogenic cause) arising from the internal iliac artery and measuring 6 × 6 cm. Under ultrasound guidance, a thin needle is passed somewhat below the iliac bifurcation between the internal and external iliac arteries to puncture the aneurysm for instillation of 5000 IU of thrombin dissolved in 3 mL saline solution. Only marginal thrombosis is achieved (right image). Much of the lumen still shows eddy flow (color coding). Instillation of a second dose of 5000 IU of thrombin into the aneurysm (A.S) results in complete thrombosis (left image). Even at a low PRF, no flow signals are detected in the color duplex mode. There is flow in the external iliac (A.I.E) and internal iliac (A.I.I) arteries. The patient has no clinical symptoms.
b The angiogram obtained prior to thrombin injection (left) shows a large pseudoaneurysm arising from the internal iliac artery (detail with iliac bifurcation in oblique projection). The right angiogram shows the aortic bifurcation and pelvic circulation (both iliac bifurcations) after ultrasound-guided thrombin injection (oblique projection similar to preinterventional angiogram). Absence of contrast medium at the site of the aneurysm confirms that complete thrombosis has occurred

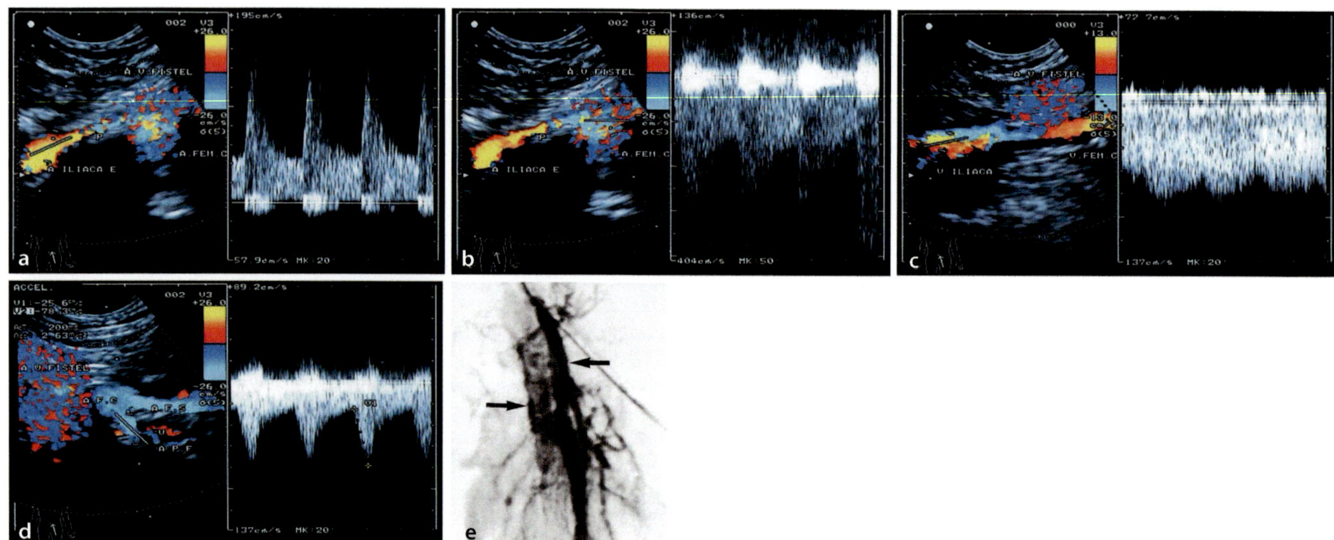

Fig. 2.83a–e (Atlas) Arteriovenous fistula.
a Patient with stage IV PAOD in whom color duplex ultrasound after puncture in the left groin shows a mosaic pattern of colors at the junction of the external iliac and common femoral arteries. The distal external iliac artery shows the high-frequency flow typical of an artery feeding a fistula with a peak systolic velocity (PSV) of 160 cm/s and an end-diastolic flow (EDV) of 50 cm/s (monophasic).
b Just proximal to the mosaic pattern, there is a calcified and stenosing plaque with posterior acoustic shadowing. The high-frequency flow signal from the site of this color pattern (EDV of 80 cm/s and PSV of >400 cm/s) may be related to a stenosis or fistula. The two entities can be differentiated by evaluating venous drainage and the femoral artery distal to this site.
c The iliac vein exhibits the venous flow signal typical of an AV fistula: high-frequency flow (with an angle-corrected velocity of 90 cm/s) with pulsatile variation. Adjustment of the PRF to venous flow leads to aliasing (left side of color flow image).
d The Doppler waveform from the profunda femoris artery distal to the AV fistula has a delayed and flattened systolic upslope and a monophasic profile with a fairly large diastolic flow component. This is a typical poststenotic profile, caused by the puncture-induced AV fistula and the high-grade stenosis resulting from the plaques shown in **a**. For differentiation of the cause of the perivascular vibration artifacts, the downstream circulation must be evaluated (fistula: venous; stenosis: arterial). This case illustrates that vessel manipulation by puncture may not only induce fistula formation but also cause stenosis through detachment of a plaque from the vessel wall.
e Angiogram: Contrast medium outflow in the iliac vein typical of a fistula. Angiography does not allow precise localization of the fistula, nor does it provide definitive evidence for the stenosis in this segment (superimposition). Left arrow indicates the femoral vein, right arrow indicates the femoral artery

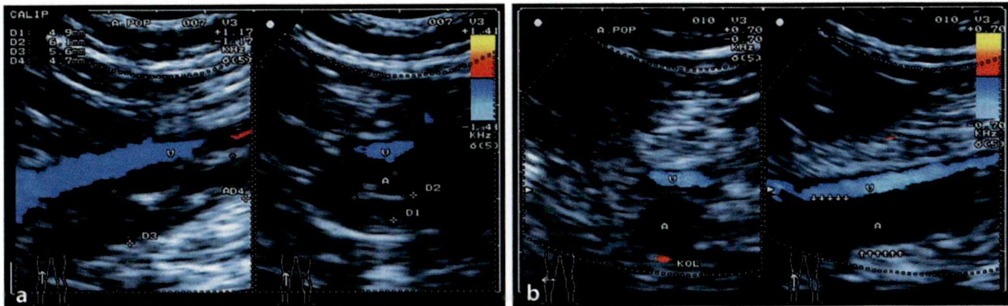

Fig. 2.84a, b (Atlas) Popliteal artery occlusion – atherosclerosis versus embolism.
a Atherosclerotic occlusion of the popliteal artery. The longitudinal view on the left and the transverse view on the right display the popliteal vein (V) in blue close to transducer. Extensive plaque throughout the artery (A) with poor demarcation of the wall contour, in conjunction with the inhomogeneous and partially very hyperechoic vessel lumen, suggests an atherosclerotic process. Based on these ultrasound findings, catheter thrombolysis, possibly with PTA, is not promising. Instead, bypass grafting is indicated, if clinically necessary.
b Embolic occlusion. The lumen of the popliteal artery is filled with a hypoechoic, homogeneous thrombus or embolus. There is good delineation of the vessel wall without signs of plaque. Anterior to the popliteal artery, the popliteal vein is depicted in blue; posterior to it, a red arterial collateral (KOL) is seen

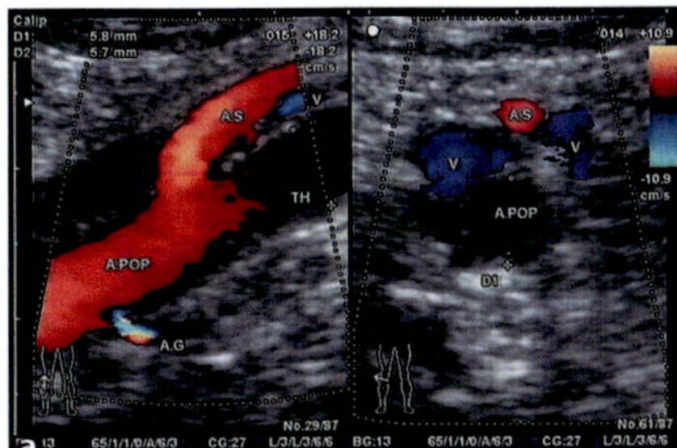

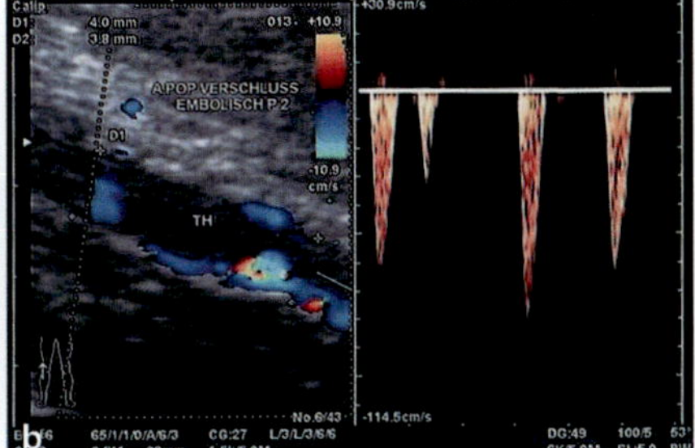

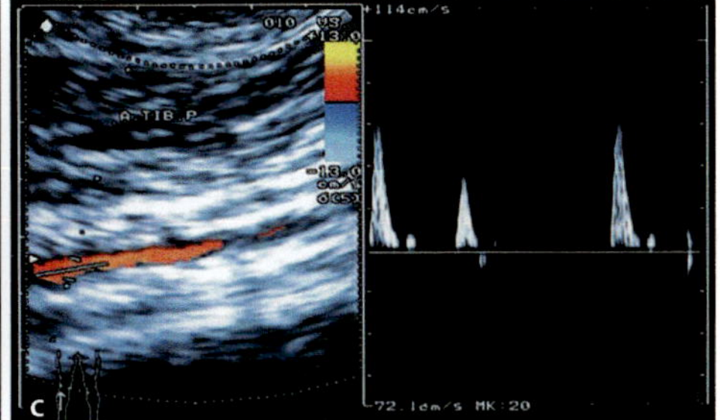

Fig. 2.85a–c (Atlas) Embolic occlusion.
a Emboli grow by thrombotic apposition, extending cranially up to the next branching of a hemodynamically significant collateral, or become lodged in a bifurcation. In the case of embolic popliteal artery occlusion presented here (longitudinal view on the left and transverse view on the right), the artery is patent down to the origin of the sural artery while the distal portion is occluded (TH). The vessel wall is smoothly delineated and shows no atherosclerotic lesions.
b When there is spontaneous partial or complete recanalization of a thromboembolic occlusion, the Doppler waveform at follow-up will show flow signals near the wall. In the example, flow (blue, away from transducer) along the intraluminal thromboembolic material is demonstrated in the distal popliteal artery. The thrombus (TH) is homogeneous and clearly delineated from the wall, which shows no atherosclerotic lesions.
c Although flow is obstructed by the popliteal artery thrombus, the Doppler tracing (arrhythmia) from the patent arteries below the knee shows triphasic flow (as illustrated here for the distal posterior tibial artery). With compensation through collateral perfusion, the flow obstruction in the popliteal artery has only little effect on peripheral perfusion. Complete recanalization of the popliteal artery was observed after another 2 days of heparin therapy

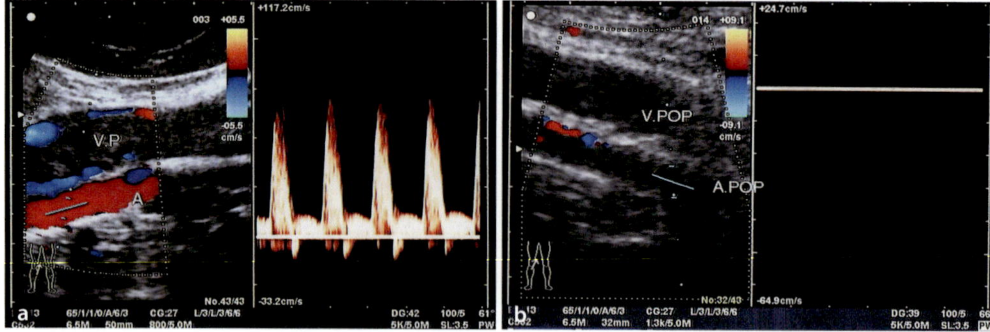

Fig. 2.86a, b (Atlas) Arterial occlusion in deep leg vein thrombosis and patent foramen ovale.
a Deep vein thrombosis of the leg and ipsilateral arterial embolism in a patient with a patent foramen ovale presenting with a 1-week history of calf swelling and acute-onset forefoot ischemia. There is thrombosis of the calf veins and of the popliteal vein with a free-floating thrombus (V.P). The proximal popliteal artery (P1 segment) is patent with high diastolic flow due to low peripheral resistance; regular heartbeat.
b The popliteal artery is occluded distal to the origins of sural branches with residual flow around the thrombus; no plaque is demonstrated. Suspected patent foramen ovale was confirmed by echocardiography

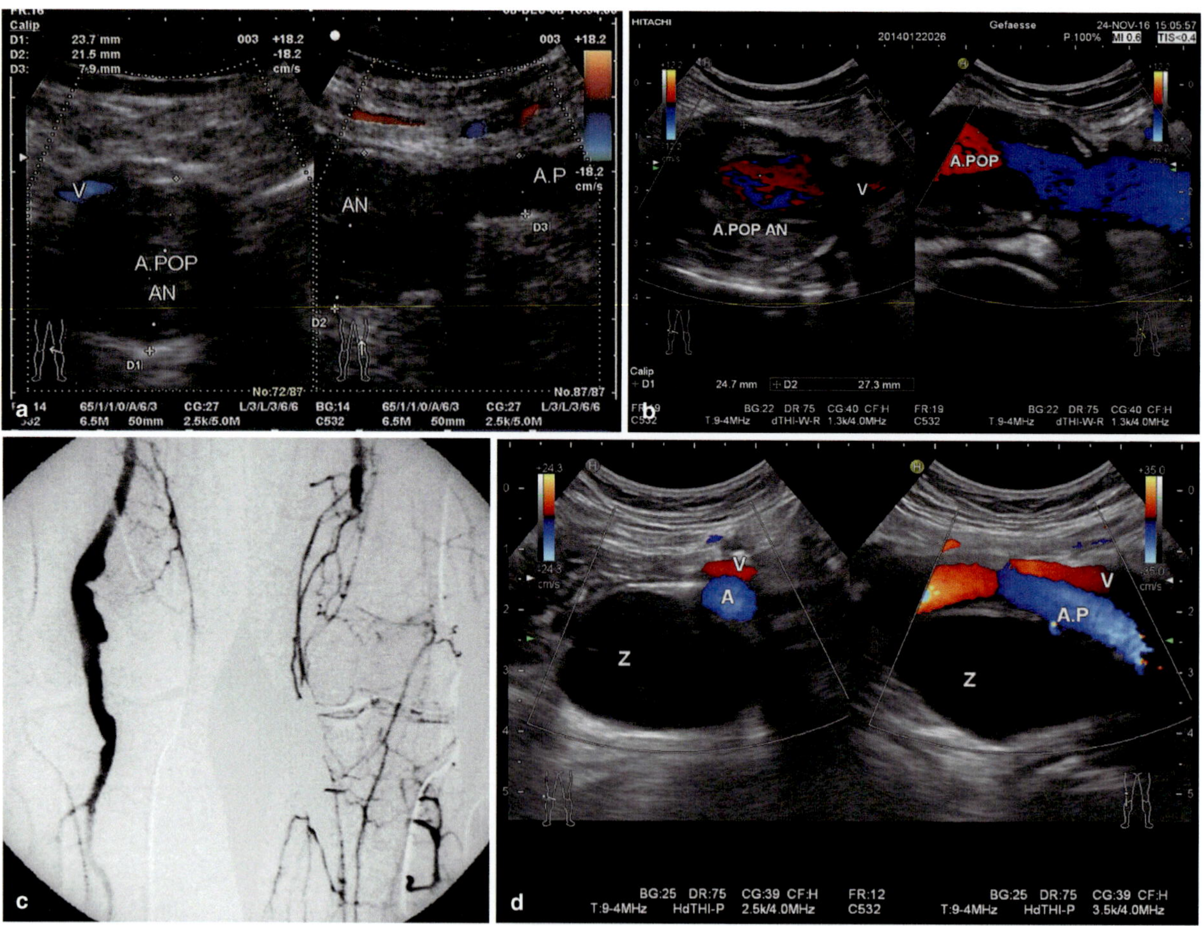

Fig. 2.87a–d (Atlas) Bilateral popliteal artery aneurysm.
a Patient with ischemic rest pain due to occlusion of the left popliteal artery caused by a completely thrombosed aneurysm. Segments of the compressed vein displayed in blue are seen near the transducer. No flow signals are obtained from the lumen of the popliteal aneurysm (transverse view of the aneurysm on the left (A.POP) and longitudinal view on the right).
b The contralateral popliteal artery aneurysm is partially thrombosed leaving a patent lumen (red flow signals) surrounded by hypoechoic mural deposits of the partially thrombosed popliteal artery aneurysm. The diameter of the aneurysm is 2.7 cm (transverse view on the left, longitudinal view on the right).
c Angiogram: Popliteal arteries with occlusion on the left and aneurysmal dilatation on the right. An estimate of the length and diameter of the aneurysms is not possible.
d Medial Baker's cyst (Z) in atypical location must be differentiated from popliteal artery aneurysm and also from adventitial cystic disease

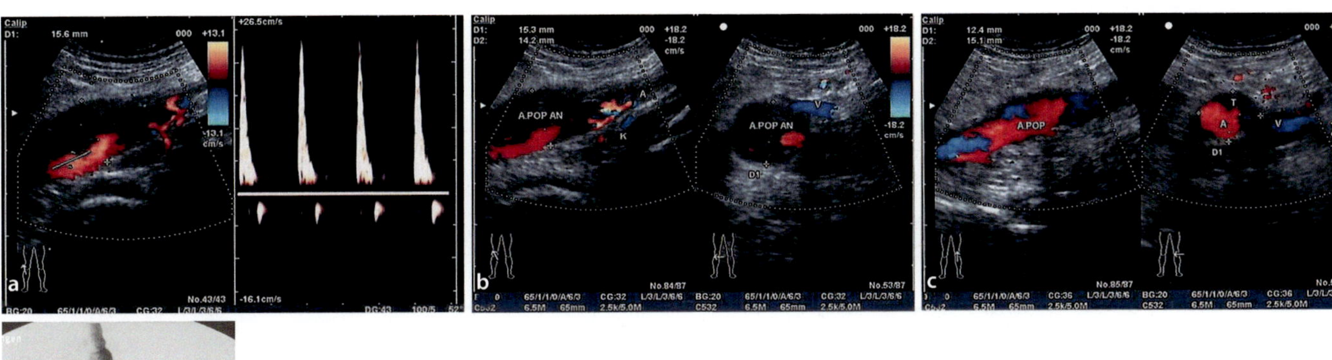

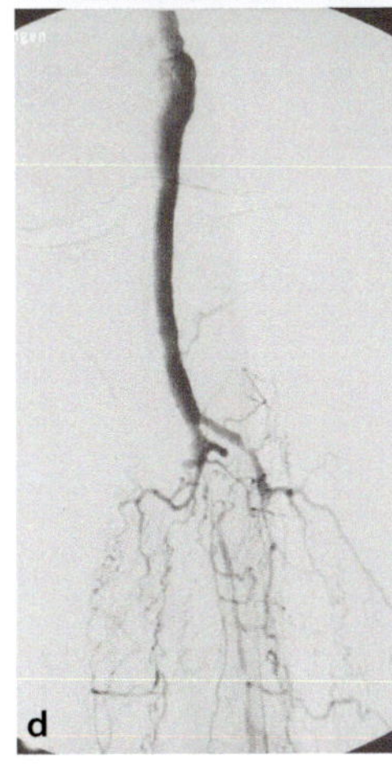

Fig. 2.88a–d (Atlas) Small popliteal artery aneurysm with arterioarterial embolism.
a, b Patient with small popliteal aneurysms on both sides. Ultrasonography demonstrates occlusion of the popliteal artery distal to the aneurysm on the right. The aneurysm is partially thrombosed and has a diameter of 1.5 cm. There is reduced flow through the aneurysm via collaterals (arising from the popliteal artery in the distal aneurysm). The collaterals are patent but outflow is obstructed. This situation is reflected by a thump pattern in the Doppler waveform and a low peak systolic velocity (PSV) of 22 cm/s.
c Images of the left popliteal artery (longitudinal view on the left, transverse view on the right) depict the small aneurysm (diameter of 1.5 cm) with only little thrombosis (clearly seen on the transverse view only) and a patent residual lumen of normal width. The arteries below the knee are still patent. The control examination performed prior to elective aneurysm resection showed an unchanged configuration of the aneurysm, but occlusions of below-knee arteries due to arterioarterial embolism.
d Left-sided angiogram showing below-knee occlusions without significant dilatation of the popliteal artery. Only at the upper margin of the image does the popliteal artery appear somewhat ectatic (corresponding ultrasound images in **c**)

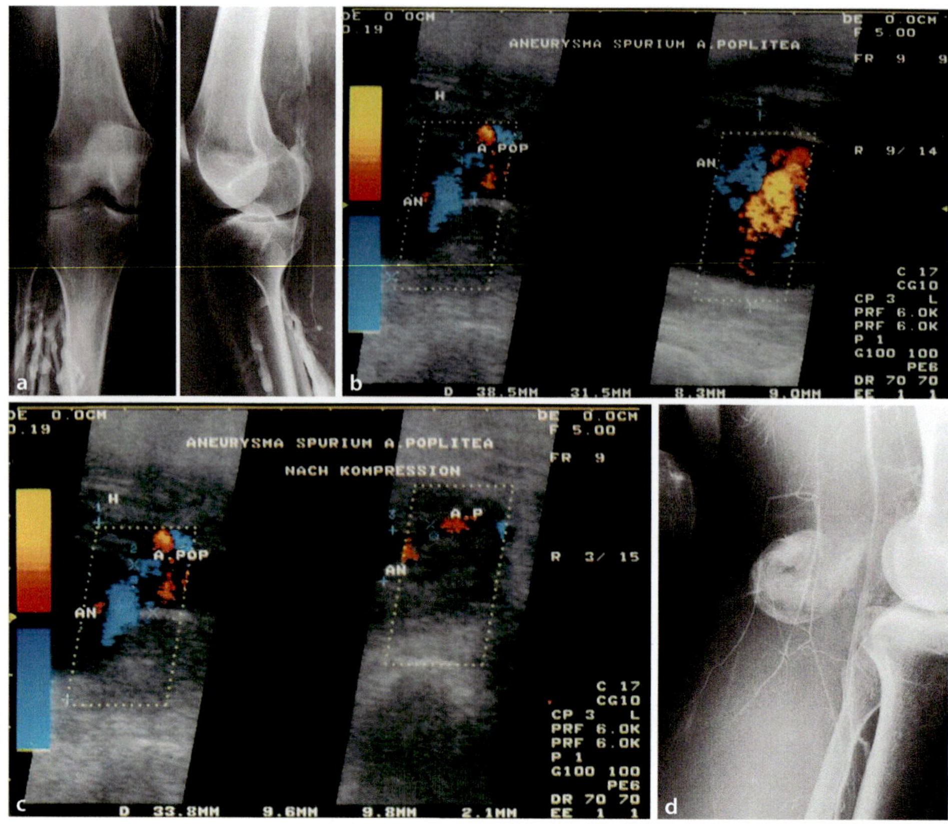

Fig. 2.89a–d (Atlas) Pseudoaneurysm following arthroscopy.
a Iatrogenic damage to the vessels in the popliteal fossa is a rare but serious complication of knee arthroscopy. In the case presented, a large pseudo-aneurysm developed after outpatient arthroscopy with partial resection of the medial meniscus. Venography performed for swelling of the calf showed contrast filling defects in the popliteal vein, which were misdiagnosed as popliteal vein thrombosis.
b Duplex imaging performed after initiation of anticoagulation treatment demonstrates the pseudoaneurysm. In the aneurysm, there is flow toward and away from the transducer (right section). Black areas without flow signals either indicate stasis in the aneurysm or are due to the failure to obtain flow signals at an angle of 90° (cos 90° = 0). The left section depicts the communication between the popliteal artery (A.POP) and the aneurysm (AN) in blue, indicating flow from the artery into the aneurysm. The aneurysm is surrounded by hematoma (H). Ultrasound shows the popliteal vein to be compressed by the aneurysm rather than thrombosed.
c The attempt to induce thrombosis of the aneurysm by compression failed because the neck is too wide and there is no adequate structure against which to compress it. The right section shows persistent flow after attempted compression. Thrombin injection would have been an alternative in this case but experience with this therapy was still limited at the time this patient was treated.
d Angiogram: Pseudoaneurysm of the popliteal artery

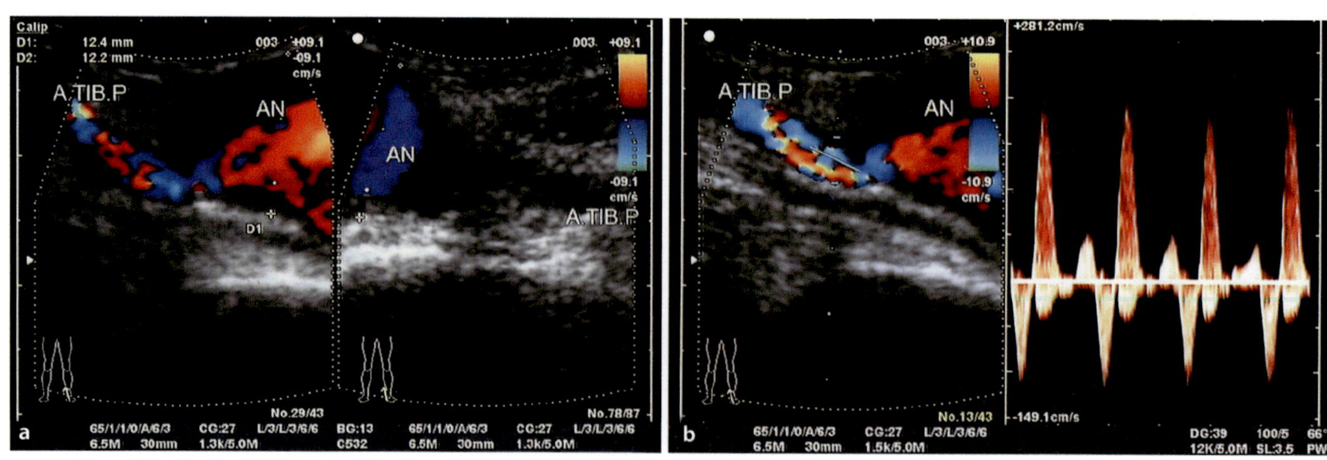

Fig. 2.90a, b (Atlas) Aneurysm of posterior tibial artery.
a Traumatic aneurysm (13 mm in diameter) of the posterior tibial artery just above the ankle joint. There is an abrupt increase in diameter from 2.5 to 13 mm (montage of two adjacent scans showing the aneurysm in the center). The posterior tibial artery is patent proximal to the aneurysm and occluded distal to it (A.TIB.P). A collateral artery arises from the aneurysm.
b The posterior tibial artery has a triphasic flow pattern just proximal to the aneurysm (AN). The distal segment is occluded, and flow is maintained through a collateral arising from the aneurysm. The resulting higher outflow resistance leads to a diastolic to-and-fro flow pattern (normal mid-diastolic flow with reversed early and end-diastolic flow)

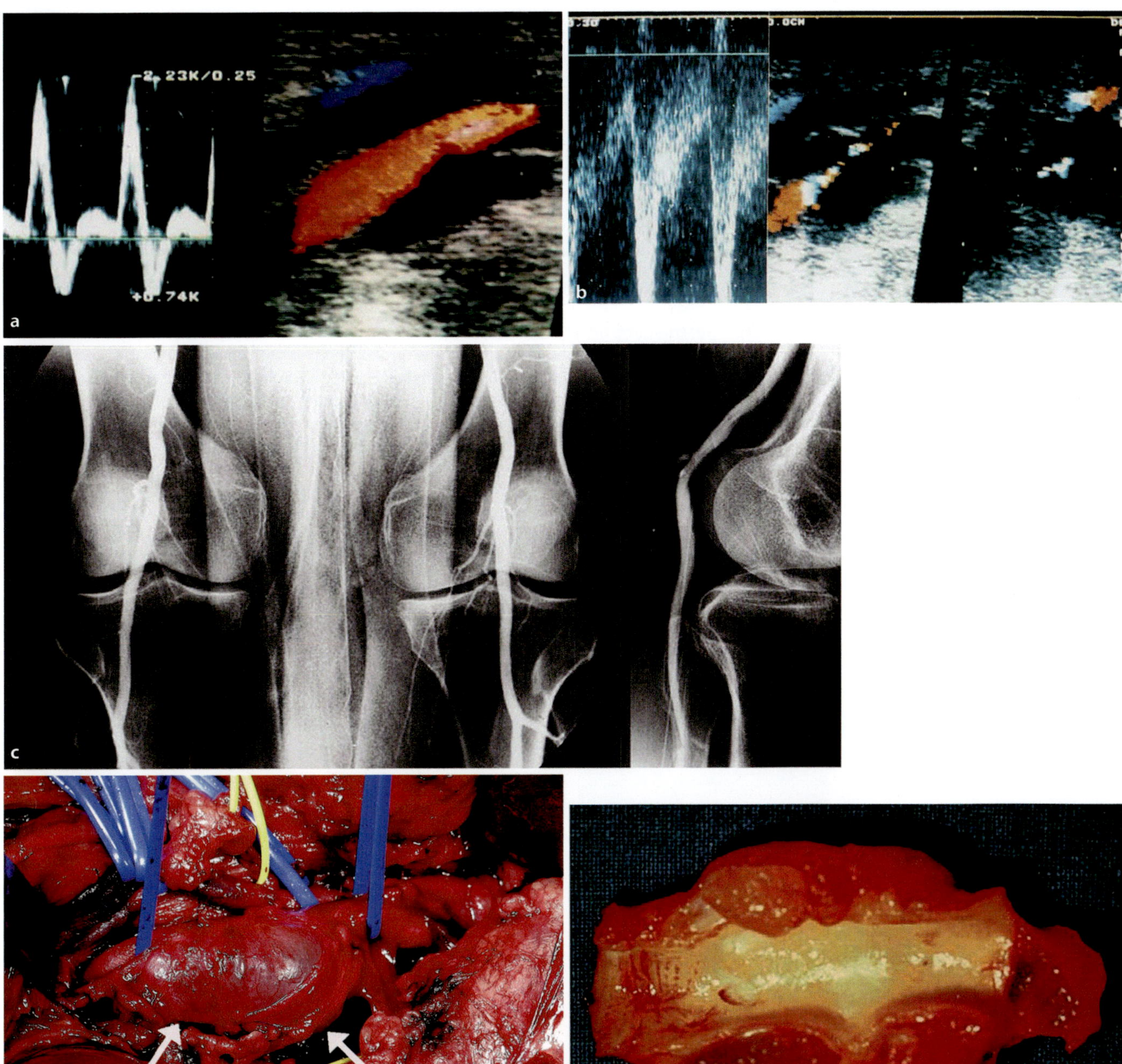

Fig. 2.91a–e (Atlas) Adventitial cystic disease.
a The popliteal artery (red) is surrounded by hypoechoic cystic lesions, which produce slight indentation of the patent lumen but no hemodynamically significant narrowing. The Doppler waveform shows triphasic flow. The patient reports intermittent claudication with a highly variable walking distance.
b Seven days after the first examination, the patient presents with severe claudication and a maximum walking distance of 30 m. Ultrasound shows a markedly increased cyst volume with high-grade stenosis of the popliteal artery (middle section: longitudinal view; right section: transverse view). Color duplex ultrasound depicts a small residual lumen between the cysts with accelerated flow and aliasing. The corresponding Doppler waveform is presented in the inverted mode with arterial flow displayed below the baseline. The waveform indicates stenosis with monophasic flow and a flow velocity of >3 m/s.
c Angiography performed 2 weeks later: Fairly inconspicuous popliteal artery with only slight anterior indentation, identified on a lateral view. The duplex ultrasound examination performed at this time (not shown) demonstrates a markedly increased cyst size without hemodynamically significant stenosis, similar to the situation depicted in **a**.
d Intraoperative view of cystic adventitial degeneration (arrow). Blue slings are placed around the popliteal artery proximal and distal to the diseased arterial segment.
e The therapy of choice is surgical resection of the cyst-bearing arterial segment or enucleation of the cysts if the intima is still intact. In the patient presented here, gross inspection of the surgical specimen shows the adventitial cysts to be filled with gelatinous material

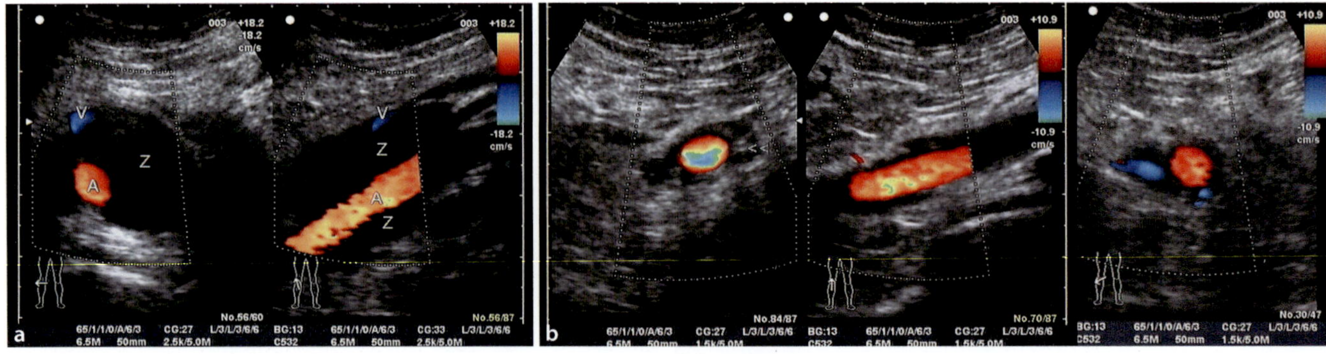

Fig. 2.92a, b (Atlas) Adventitial cystic disease – treatment by ultrasound-guided aspiration.
a 40-year-old patient with intermittent foot pain resembling that of polyneuropathy. Arterial duplex imaging of the popliteal fossa reveals large cysts causing only mild luminal narrowing of the popliteal artery without significant hemodynamic effects. The patient reported no episodes of typical intermittent claudication but variable neurologic signs and symptoms. The neurologic examination revealed slightly reduced peripheral nerve conduction velocity. In patients with adventitial cystic disease, the symptoms vary with the number, size, and location of cysts within the narrow confines of the popliteal fossa. An occasional patient may present with (intermittent) pain due to nerve compression by a large cyst, while the popliteal artery is not compromised. The patient shown has a large cyst (Z), but neither the color duplex images (transverse view on the left, longitudinal view on the right) nor the spectral Doppler interrogation (not shown) suggest significant narrowing of the arterial lumen.
b Because the patient refused an operation, the cyst was drained and sclerosed under ultrasound guidance (transverse and longitudinal views on the left); histologic examination of the gelatinous cyst fluid confirmed adventitial cystic disease. Following ultrasound-guided drainage using a 1.8-mm needle, the cyst was sclerosed with 1 mL of 95% ethyl alcohol to prevent recurrence (needle tip identified by bright echo). The patient's symptoms disappeared after treatment. Right image: Follow-up after 1 month reveals no recurrent or residual cyst; popliteal vein with blue-coded flow lateral to the artery

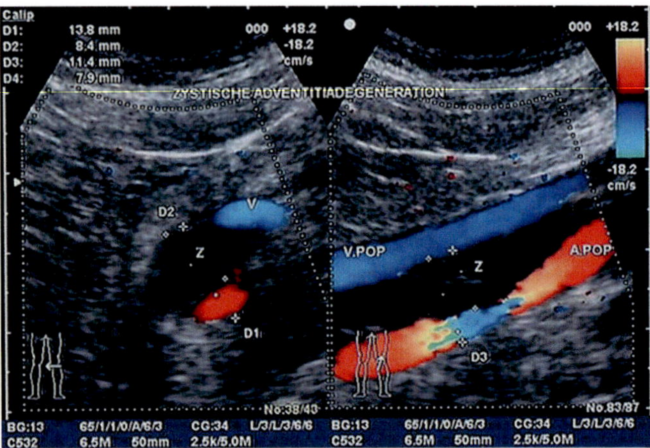

Fig. 2.93 (Atlas) Adventitial cystic disease – differentiation from dissection.
Patients with adventitial cystic disease can have single or multiple cysts with involvement of a long segment of the popliteal artery. When a long segment is involved, as in the case shown here, the condition may be difficult to differentiate from dissection with complete thrombosis of the false lumen (see Figs. 2.97a and 5.74 (both Atlas)). The popliteal artery (A.POP) is shown in transverse orientation on the left and in longitudinal orientation on the right with the cyst (Z) narrowing a long segment of the artery. There is aliasing as a result of cystic luminal narrowing. The popliteal vein (V.POP) is depicted closer to the transducer with flow coded in blue. The diagnosis of adventitial cystic disease was confirmed intraoperatively

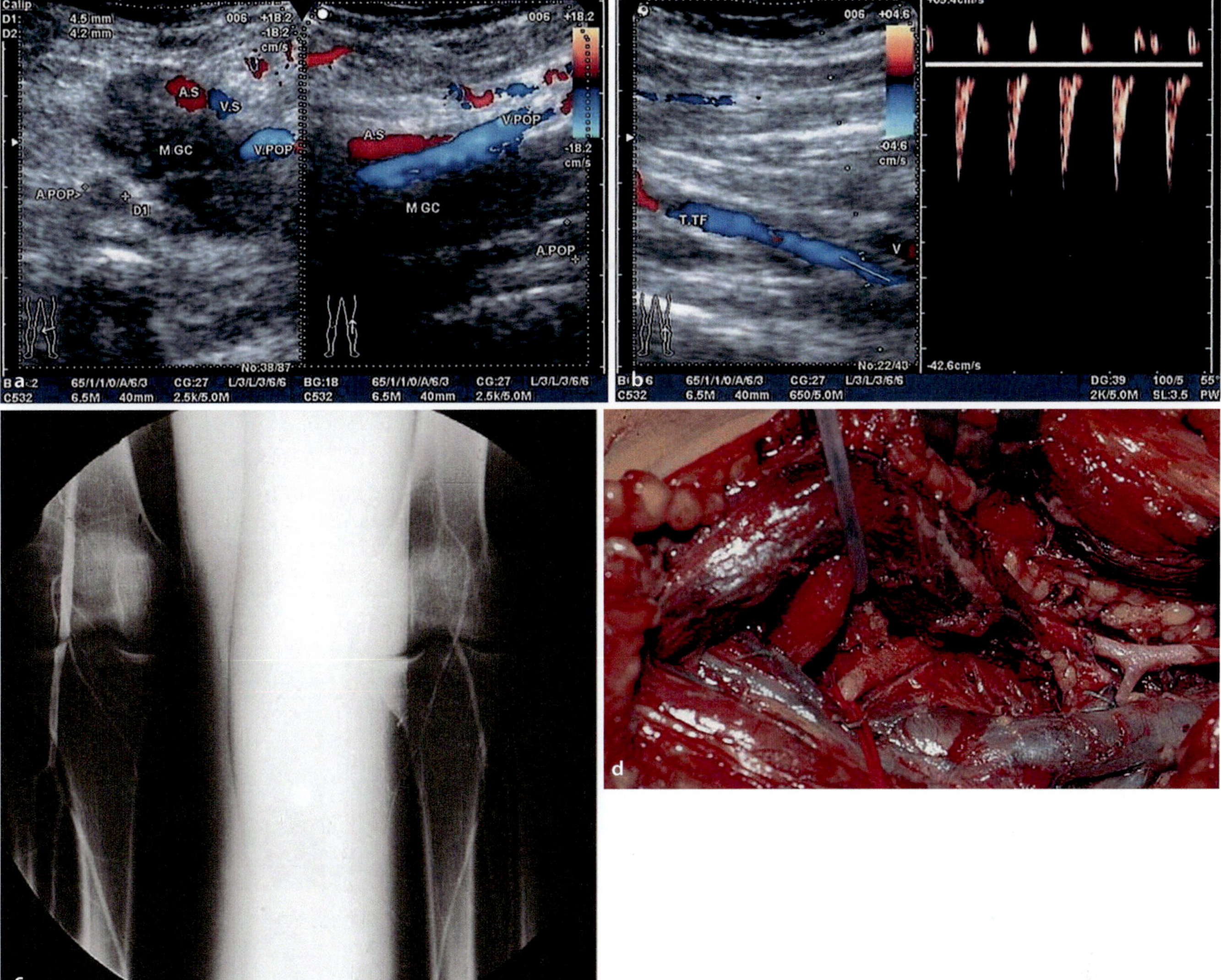

Fig. 2.94a–d (Atlas) Entrapment syndrome.
a Isolated popliteal artery occlusion due to malformation of the medial head of the gastrocnemius muscle forcing the artery to course around the head on the medial side. In this type of malformation, the medial head of the muscle is located between the popliteal artery and vein – which thus do not pass through the popliteal fossa together – and compresses the artery against the femur with each plantar flexion. Intermittent compression damages the vessel wall with deposition of thrombotic material, which may ultimately progress to occlusion. In the case presented, no color duplex signal is obtained from the popliteal artery (A.POP). Posterolateral to the head of the gastrocnemius, the patent popliteal vein (V.POP) is depicted closer to the transducer with a blue flow signal. Posterior to it, the artery (red) supplying the soleus muscle and serving as a collateral and the vein are shown. The arteries recruited as collaterals are markedly dilated due to the chronic occlusion process and may thus be confused with the popliteal artery. The sonoanatomic situation (transverse section on the left and longitudinal section on the right) is as follows: the popliteal artery courses anterior to the popliteal vein and is depicted farther away with the transducer placed posteriorly. The muscle-supplying arteries recruited as collaterals arise from the posterior aspect of the popliteal artery and course posterior to the popliteal vein and are thus closer to the transducer than the vein.
b In this case with good collateralization of a chronic occlusive process, the flow profile in the refilled tibiofibular trunk does not show the typical postocclusive monophasic flow but is triphasic, though damped. Peak systolic velocity (PSV) is just under 20 cm/s. Additional collaterals enter distally. There is no postocclusive peripheral dilatation at rest.
c Angiogram: Short occlusion of the left popliteal artery with refilling at the level of the knee joint cleft (lateral collateral).
d The intraoperative site confirms the ultrasound findings. The popliteal artery and vein do not pass through the popliteal fossa together because the medial gastrocnemius head (transparent sling) attaches between the artery (red sling placed around distal segment) and the vein (at lower margin). The proximal popliteal artery (on the right) gives off the collateral already identified sonographically and coursing parallel to the vein

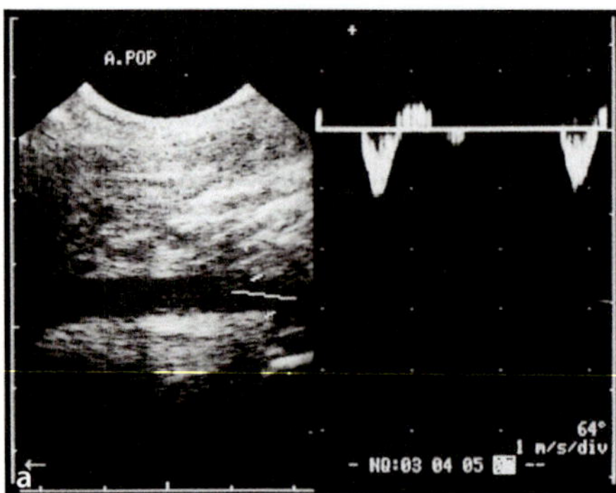

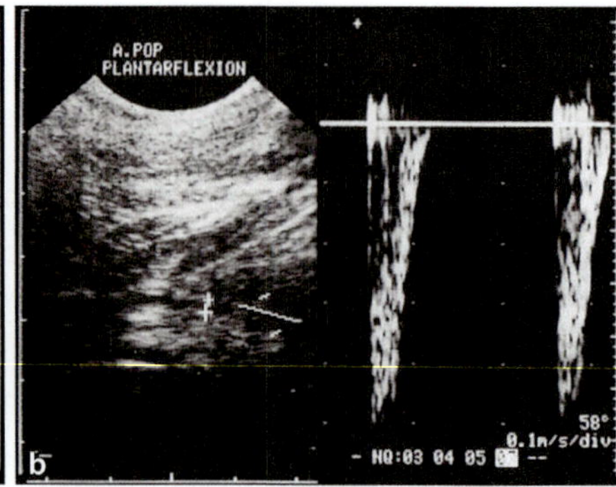

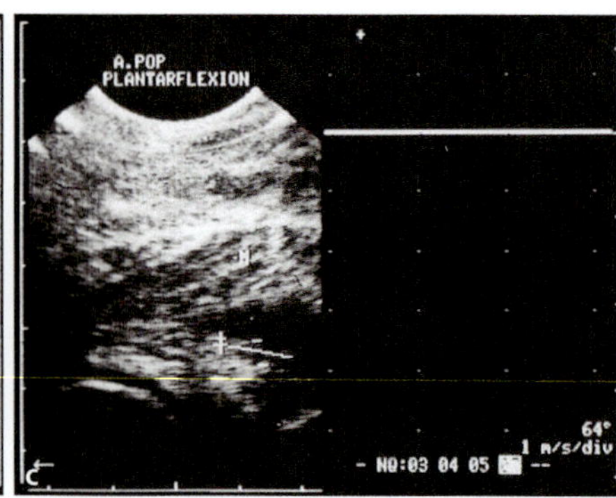

Fig. 2.95a–c (Atlas) Entrapment syndrome.
a Calf swelling with occasional pain in a young patient caused by external compression of the vessels in the popliteal fossa due to a hypertrophied head of the gastrocnemius with normal attachment. The popliteal artery and vein pass through the popliteal fossa together and the vein is already compressed by the relaxed muscle (see Fig. 3.98b, c (Atlas)). The popliteal artery is not stenosed, and a normal, triphasic waveform is obtained.
b Progressive compression of the popliteal artery occurs with increasing plantar flexion, producing a stenosis signal in the Doppler waveform with loss of triphasic flow and a peak systolic velocity (PSV) of 300 cm/s.
c Further plantar flexion leads to complete occlusion of the popliteal artery through muscular compression (see Fig. 3.98 (Atlas) for popliteal entrapment syndrome with arterial and venous compression). This form of entrapment syndrome (type VI; see classification in Fig. 2.30) occurs without malformation and is solely due to a well-developed gastrocnemius muscle (which may result from anabolic intake)

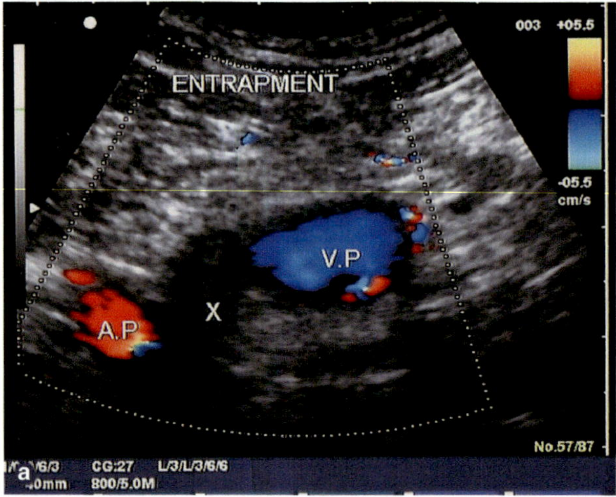

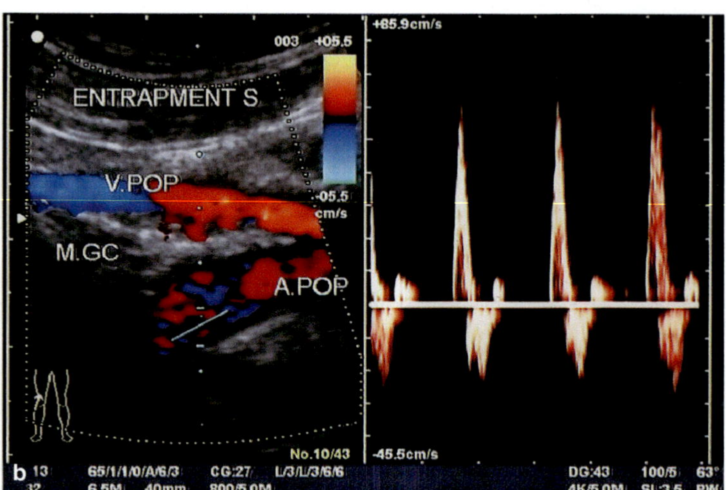

Fig. 2.96a, b (Atlas) Entrapment constellation.
a The image shows the characteristic abnormality of popliteal fossa anatomy predisposing an individual to popliteal entrapment: muscle structures (X) lying between the popliteal artery (A.P) and vein (V.P). This anatomic constellation may be present even if no compression of vascular structures can be elicited by plantar flexion of the ankle. In the literature, only little attention has been paid to this anatomic deviation in asymptomatic individuals, but it explains why popliteal entrapment is much more commonly encountered at autopsy than in the clinical setting. An examiner may see this anatomic constellation during a careful sonographic evaluation of the popliteal fossa in patients examined for other reasons (e.g., suspected venous thrombosis, chronic venous insufficiency). The identification of musculotendinous structures (attachment of medial head of gastrocnemius) between the artery and vein in the popliteal fossa is pathognomonic of this constellation.
b In this case, neither color duplex imaging nor Doppler interrogation shows popliteal artery (A.POP) narrowing during provocative maneuvers (maximum plantar flexion of the ankle). There is normal triphasic flow and peak systolic velocity (PSV) is not increased. The longitudinal view obtained during plantar flexion shows the head of gastrocnemicus (M.GC) between the popliteal artery (A.POP) anteriorly (closer to transducer) and the popliteal vein (V.POP) posteriorly

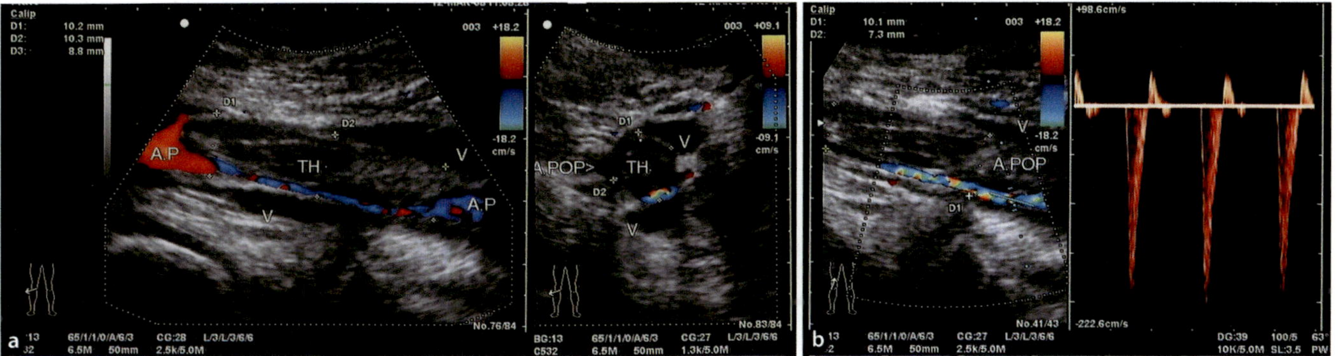

Fig. 2.97a, b (Atlas) Dissection.
a Dissection of the popliteal artery with complete thrombosis of the false lumen (TH) following blunt trauma to the popliteal fossa. Longitudinal view (left) and transverse view (right) show the patent residual lumen of the artery (A.P), which is narrowed by the thrombosed false lumen.
b Peak systolic velocity (PSV) in the compromised popliteal artery segment is increased to 220 cm/s. Calipers indicate the popliteal artery lumen and the thrombosed false lumen in the color flow image. When high-grade luminal narrowing affects a long arterial segment, friction loss is greater and the PSV increase is less marked than in a focal stenosis. The same phenomenon occurs when there is marginal flow in thromboembolic obstruction (see Fig. 2.85 (Atlas))

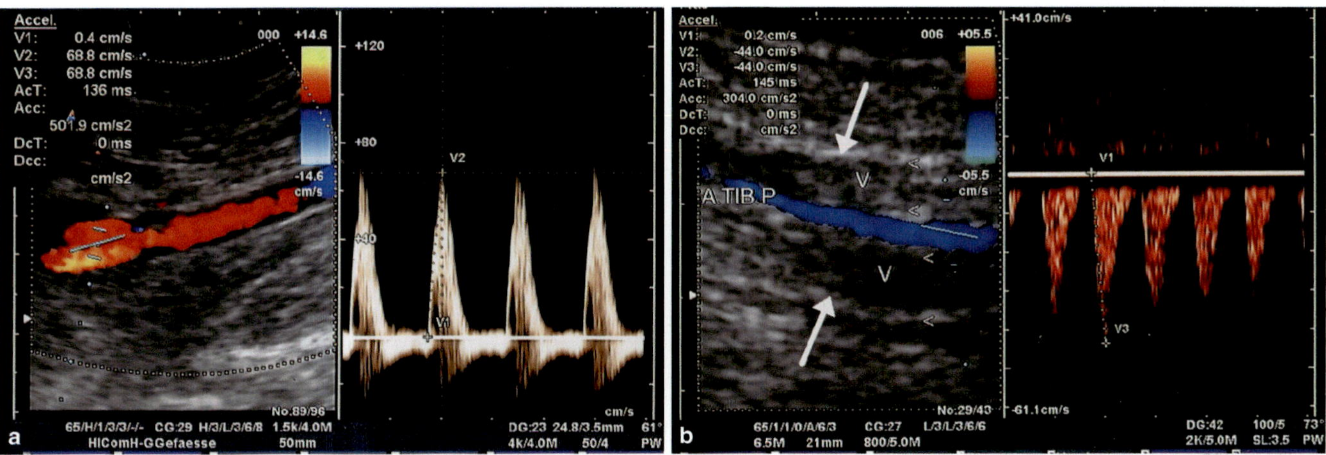

Fig. 2.98a, b (Atlas) Progressive ischemia due to venous outflow obstruction (extensive venous thrombosis).
a 75-year-old woman with a history of PAOD and occlusion of the superficial femoral artery with very good collateral circulation. The Doppler waveform shows triphasic flow with a peak systolic velocity (PSV) of 68 cm/s in the popliteal artery. The most salient feature of postocclusive flow seen in this case is a delayed systolic upstroke with an acceleration time of 136 ms.
b The patient developed secondary peripheral thrombosis ascending to the common femoral vein (level of the inguinal ligament) and presenting with swelling and acute ischemic pain in the forefoot and classic signs of ischemia as well as early ischemic toe necrosis. Duplex imaging reveals no macroangiopathic changes in perfusion compared with her status prior to the onset of thrombosis. Below the knee, the posterior tibial and dorsalis pedis arteries are patent to just below the ankle joint. The Doppler waveform from the posterior tibial artery (same as in the dorsalis pedis artery) is presented, confirming a largely normal PSV (44 cm/s). The longer acceleration time of 145 ms is consistent with postocclusive flow. However, in a patient with foot ischemia, the Doppler waveform should also reflect the flow effects of peripheral dilatation; the pulsatile flow profile seen in this case is due to venous outflow obstruction caused by extensive venous thrombosis. For illustration, the two thrombosed veins (V) are depicted above and below the arteries (venous wall indicated by arrow); also seen is the posterior tibial artery (A.TIB.P). The veins are dilated and no flow signals are obtained despite a low PRF. The dorsalis pedis vein was also thrombosed (not shown).
The ultrasound and Doppler findings show that disease progression with toe necrosis in this patient is attributable to venous obstruction with concomitant extensive thrombosis including the arterioles. This condition cannot be remedied by a femoropopliteal bypass graft. Nevertheless, a bypass procedure was performed in the acute situation, but no improvement ensued. In summary, in this case of stage IIa PAOD, extensive thrombosis led to the clinical and sonographic picture known as phlegmasia coerulea dolens

2

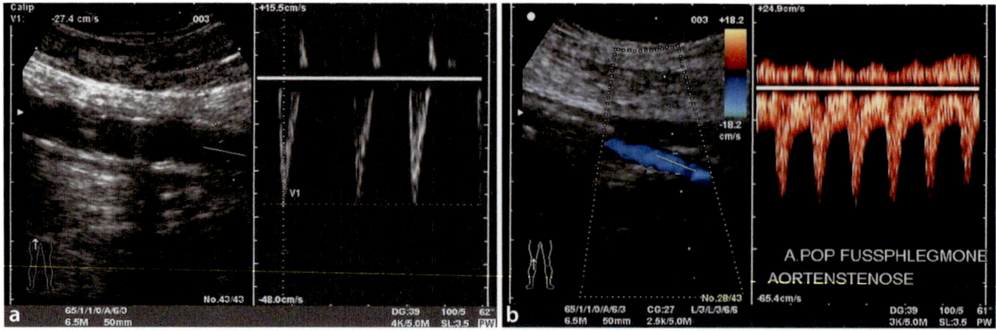

Fig. 2.99a, b (Atlas) Cardiac causes of abnormal spectral Doppler findings.
a Patient with low peak systolic velocities (PSV) at multiple Doppler sampling sites in the leg. As no stenosis is identified, one should consider cardiac insufficiency with reduced cardiac output as a possible underlying cause. If this is the case, PSV will be reduced in all arterial segments. In the example, a PSV of 25 cm/s is measured in the proximal superficial femoral artery and there is plaque, while no stenosis or occlusion is detectable down to the ankle joint.
b In a patient with a higher-grade aortic stenosis, a Doppler tracing from a peripheral artery will show the same poststenotic pattern as distal to a stenosis of a peripheral artery: delayed systolic upstroke, reduced PSV (32 cm/s in the case shown), and monophasic flow. In this case, a foot phlegmon further contributes to the changes in the spectral waveform from the popliteal artery

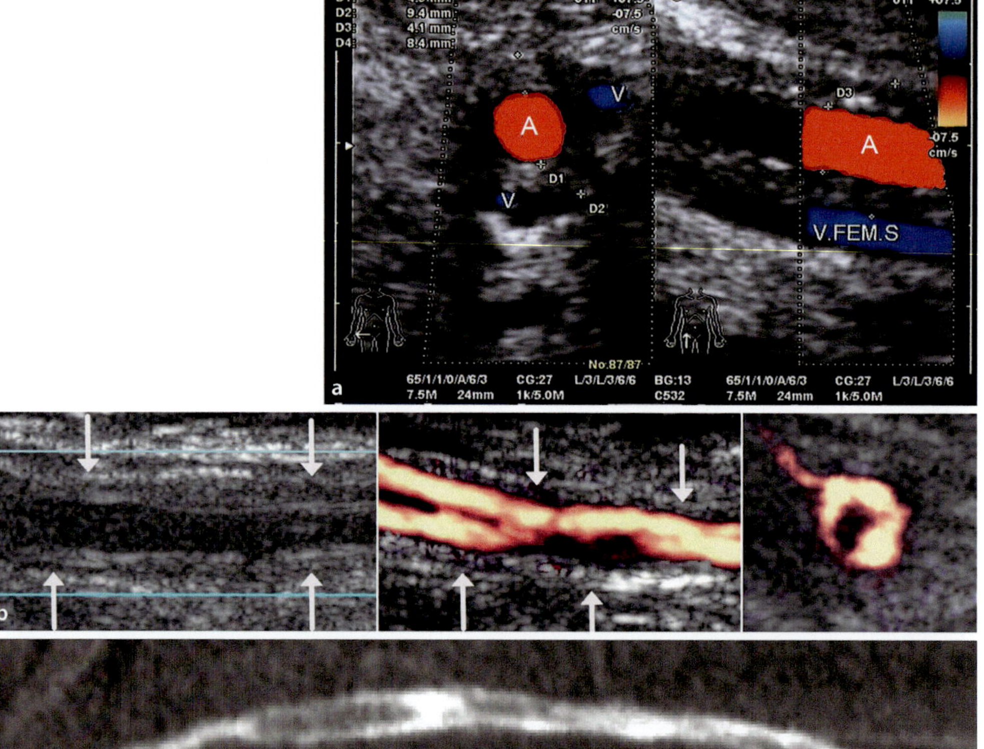

Fig. 2.100a–c (Atlas) Vasculitis.
a Vasculitis of the femoral artery (longitudinal view on the right, transverse view on the left) with concentric hypoechoic inflammatory thickening of the media in a patient with concomitant atherosclerosis. The atherosclerotic plaques on the luminal side are seen as hyperechoic deposits on the thickened wall.
b Calf artery (posterior tibial artery) in polyarteritis nodosa with circumferential wall thickening (conventional longitudinal view and power mode images in longitudinal and transverse orientation).
c Angiogram of the same artery as in **b** (Figs. **b** and **c** courtesy of K. Amendt)

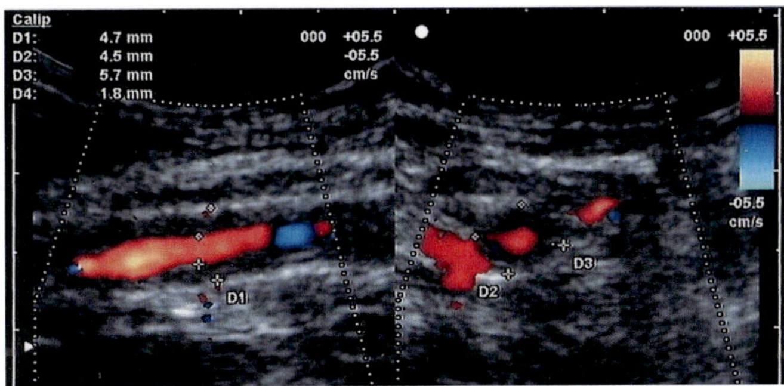

Fig. 2.101 (Atlas) Inflammatory vascular disease.
Vascular inflammation – Takayasu's arteritis of the subclavian and common carotid arteries or polyarteritis nodosa of the extremity arteries – leads to concentric wall thickening with a centrally perfused lumen. It is identified on ultrasound by the macaroni sign. There is a normal echo reflected from the wall interface while the remainder of the arterial wall is depicted as a concentric, hypoechoic structure (wall thickening) over a long segment without signs of atherosclerotic plaques. Progressive inflammatory wall thickening may ultimately lead to occlusion of the affected vessel. Aneurysmal changes may also occur. The longitudinal view on the left and the transverse view on the right show the concentric wall thickening of an artery below the knee in a patient with polyarteritis nodosa. (Due to reflux caused by postthrombotic venous changes, the veins depicted to the left and right of the artery are likewise displayed in red)

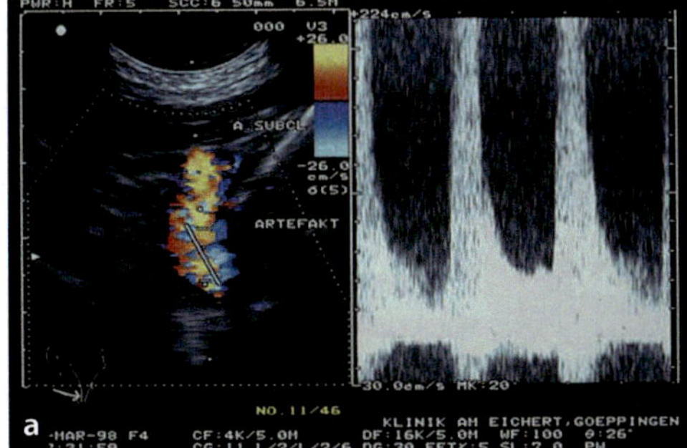

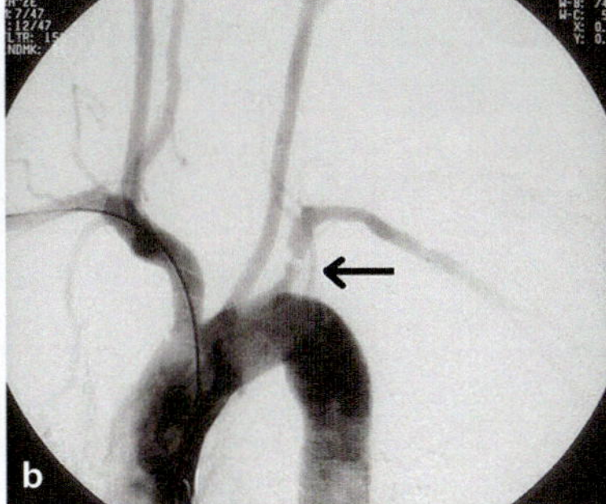

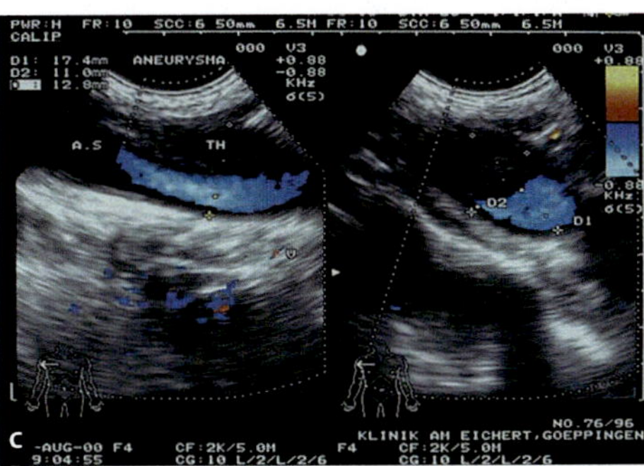

Fig. 2.102a–c (Atlas) Subclavian artery stenosis due to atherosclerosis.
a Scanning of the left subclavian artery from the supraclavicular position demonstrates direct signs of stenosis: increased peak systolic velocity (PSV), aliasing, and perivascular vibration artifacts. Atherosclerotic stenosis of the arm arteries typically occurs at the origin of the subclavian artery and cannot always be identified directly. Instead, the diagnosis has to rely on indirect criteria such as monophasic postocclusive flow.
b Angiogram showing stenosis of the left subclavian artery.
c The additional aneurysm (AN) of the right subclavian artery (longitudinal view on the left, transverse view on the right) is not depicted angiographically (see **b**) due to thrombosis

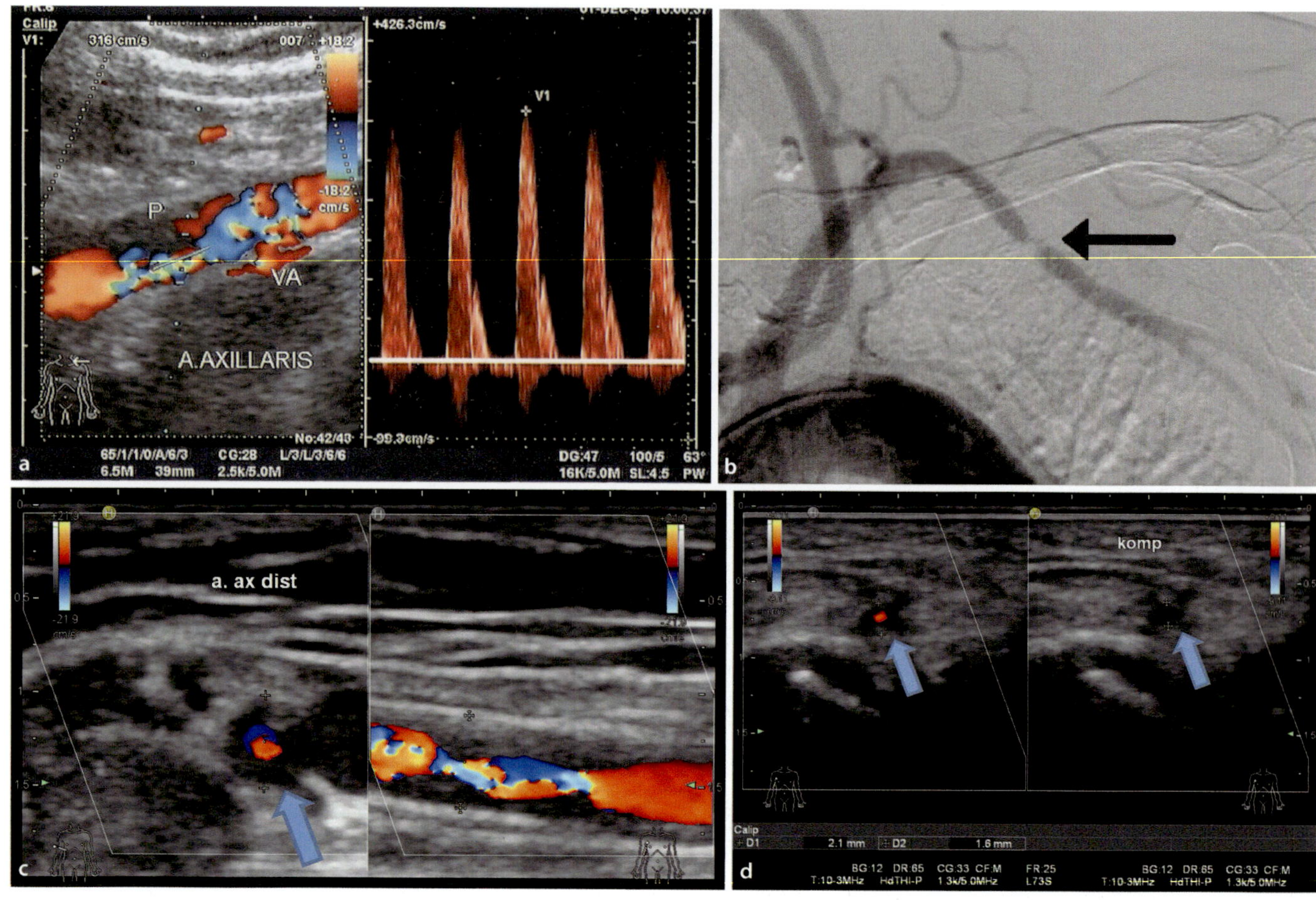

Fig. 2.103a, b (Atlas) Axillary artery stenosis due to atherosclerosis.
a High-grade axillary artery stenosis due to a hypoechoic plaque, revealed by ultrasound with the transducer placed in the infraclavicular fossa. This is a rare case of atherosclerotic plaque distal to the subclavian artery causing peripheral embolism with occlusion of interdigital arteries (ischemia of the 4th and 5th fingers).
b Angiogram showing axillary artery stenosis before PTA.
Distal axillary artery stenosis in arteritis.
c A 69-year-old patient with an 11-year history of immunosuppressive treatment for histologically proven Horton's arteritis developed ischemic symptoms of the hand during long-term cortisone treatment at a dose of 10 mg. Color duplex ultrasound shows only mild concentric wall thickening of the proximal axillary artery but a fairly localized high-grade stenosis with a PSV of 4 m/s (not typical of an acute episode of vasculitis).
d Examination of a temporal artery branch (prior temporal artery biopsy on the same side 10 years earlier) shows concentric wall thickening characteristic of vasculitis. Application of pressure with the transducer (right image) reveals incomplete compressibility of the thickened wall (1.6 mm) and is highly diagnostic of vasculitis

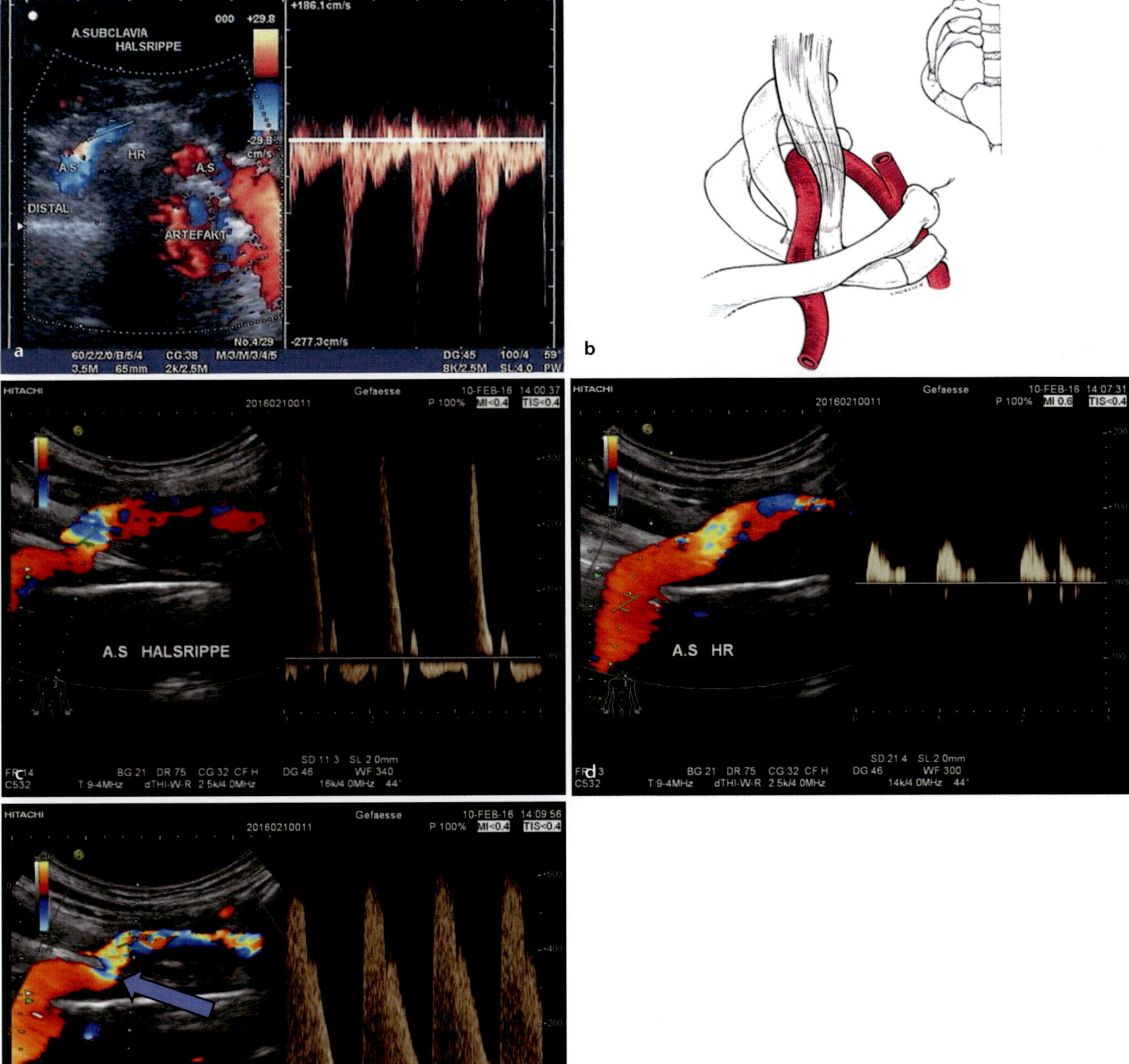

Fig. 2.104a–e (Atlas) Cervical rib syndrome.
a A cervical rib (HR) forces the subclavian artery (supraclavicular transducer position) to take an abnormal, arched course ("the artery is riding the rib"). The patient presented here has moderate stenosis with a peak systolic velocity (PSV) of 2.5 m/s. Due to its abnormal course, the artery is not depicted completely in a single scan plane. Mirror artifacts (with superimposed vibration artifacts) are seen posterior to the proximal subclavian artery.
b Diagram of the mechanism causing the cervical rib syndrome: Displacement and compression of the subclavian artery by the cervical rib (from Heberer and van Dongen 1993).
c–e Subclavian artery compression by cervical rib.
c Strand-like extensions from a cervical rib compress the subclavian artery, resulting in stenosis with a PSV of >3 m/s (sample volume in the compressed arterial segment).
d Flow velocity is reduced in the subclavian artery upstream of the compressed segment.
e Hyperabduction results in more severe compression of the subclavian artery (arrow) by the strand-like extension of the cervical rib with a PSV of >6 m/s indicating subtotal occlusion

2

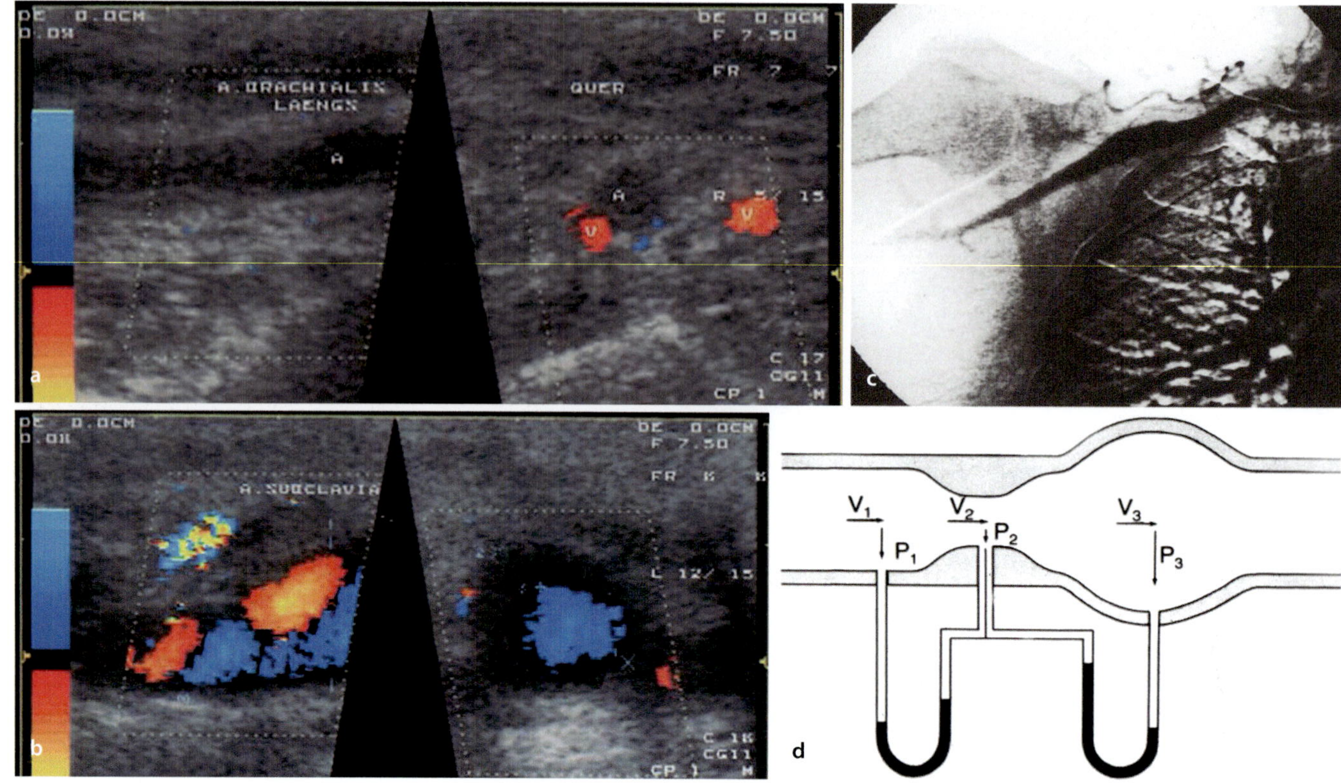

Fig. 2.105a–d (Atlas) Aneurysm of subclavian/axillary artery.
a 62-year-old patient presenting with acute onset of a sensation of cold and pallor of the right hand and increasing pain unrelated to exercise. The radial and ulnar arteries are not palpable. Duplex imaging identifies an occluded brachial artery (A) as the cause of the patient's complaints with the absence of plaques and the hypoechoic homogeneous lumen suggesting an embolic mechanism. The veins (V) are coded red.
b The brachial occlusion in this case is caused by emboli from a 14-mm aneurysm of the subclavian artery at the junction with the axillary artery. Due to mural thrombosis, the patent lumen is only slightly dilatated compared to the proximal, normal vessel segment (hypoechoic rim around the blue, patent lumen of the artery on the transverse scan, right section). The longitudinal view on the left shows the proximal end of the aneurysm with retrograde flow components (eddy currents).
c Angiogram: Due to mural thrombosis, only mild dilatation of the subclavian artery at the junction with the axillary artery is seen angiographically. The aneurysm in this patient is caused by mechanical irritation due to an exostosis of an old clavicular fracture.
d Intravascular pressure on the arterial wall increases downstream of a stenosis. In an artery without pre-existing atherosclerotic damage (e.g., patients with vascular compression syndrome), this increase in pressure can lead to dilatation of the poststenotic segment (see Fig. 2.106 (Atlas))

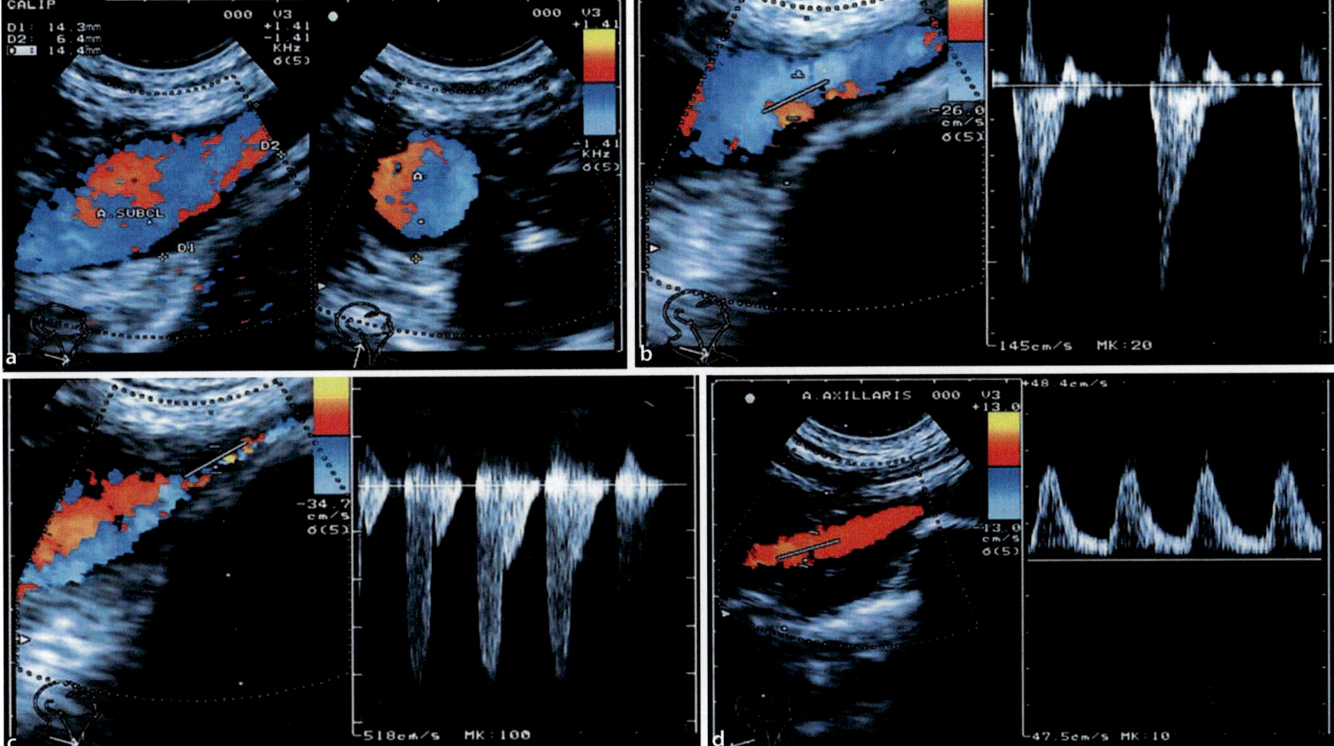

Fig. 2.106a–d (Atlas) Thoracic outlet syndrome with poststenotic dilatation.
a 45-year-old patient with recurrent pain of the right hand during work (painter). With the transducer in the supraclavicular position, the transverse image (right) and the longitudinal image (left) show aneurysmal dilatation of the subclavian artery. No mural thrombi are depicted. The aneurysm has a maximum diameter of 14 mm; eddy currents in the aneurysm give rise to blue and red flow signals.
b The Doppler waveform recorded with the patient lying in a relaxed position (without provocative maneuver) shows disturbed flow but a triphasic profile without signs of hemodynamically significant stenosis.
c Examination during Adson's test reveals compression of the subclavian artery with color aliasing and a peak systolic velocity (PSV) > 400 cm/s in the Doppler waveform (consistent with stenosis). The test is positive for a compression syndrome with poststenotic dilatation.
d Specific anatomic conditions (obesity and short neck) may prohibit proper placement of the transducer during Adson's test. In these patients, compression during provocation can be demonstrated by the presence of the typical poststenotic changes in the Doppler waveform sampled in the axillary artery with the transducer placed in the infraclavicular fossa

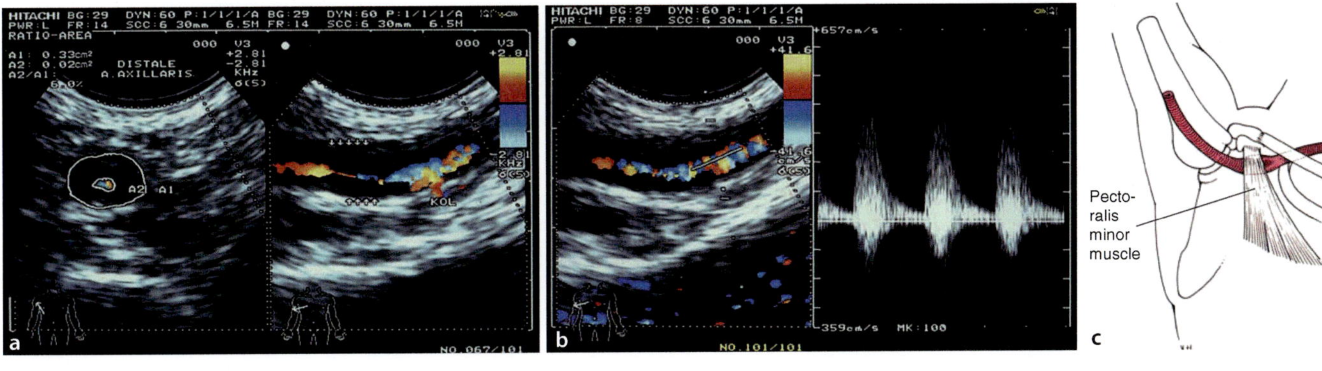

Fig. 2.107a–c (Atlas) Pectoralis minor syndrome.
a Ultrasound imaging of the axillary artery during hyperabduction with the transducer in the armpit reveals compression-induced stenosis as well as complications of long-standing compression syndrome: extensive, though circumscribed, wall damage with thickening and local thrombus formation. Aliasing in the color duplex mode enables differentiation of the perfused lumen from mural thrombus. The outer white line in the transverse view (left) indicates the normal vessel diameter. A low echogenicity and concentric wall thickening as in this case may also occur in vasculitis (which must be considered in the differential diagnosis when patients present with elevated inflammatory markers).
b Doppler waveform showing high-grade stenosis with a flow velocity of over 3 m/s, monophasic flow, and turbulence.
c Diagram of compression of the axillary artery between the pectoralis minor muscle and the coracoid process during hyperabduction (from Heberer and van Dongen 1993)

2

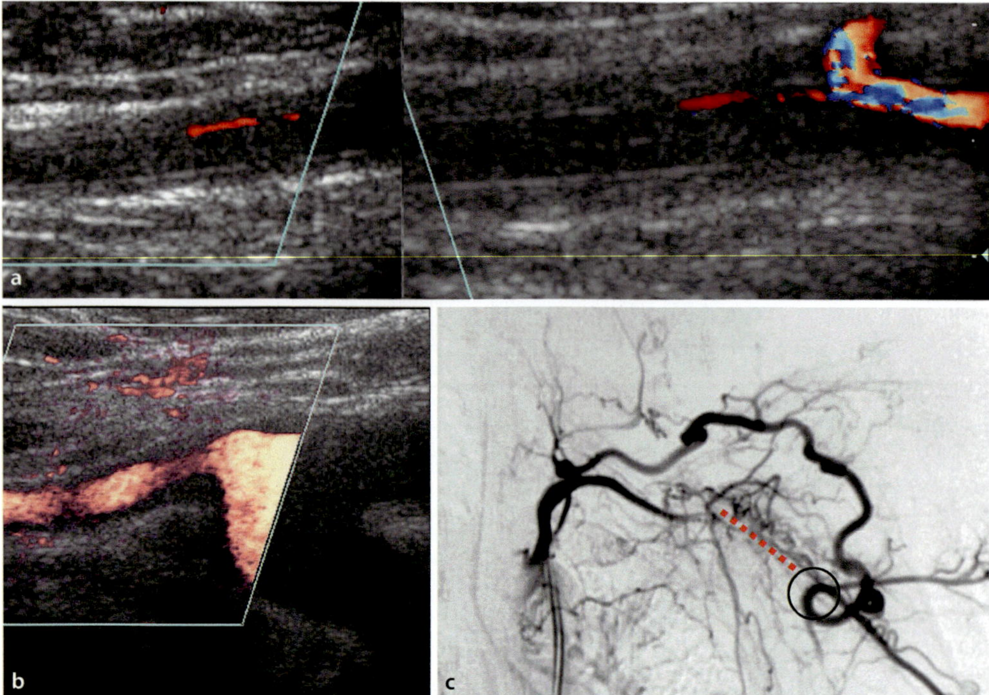

Fig. 2.108a–c (Atlas) Takayasu's arteritis with subclavian artery occlusion.
a Long occlusion of the axillary artery and distal subclavian artery. There is conspicuous circumferential wall thickening of low echogenicity.
b Resupply of the axillary artery through dilated collaterals (right) and inflammatory wall thickening of the axillary artery (left).
c Angiogram showing occlusion of the subclavian and axillary arteries with good collateralization (indicating a chronic process). The circle indicates the site of entry of the collateral into the artery and corresponds to the detail shown in **b**. The dotted red line corresponds to the occluded arterial segment visualized in **a** (courtesy of K. Amendt)

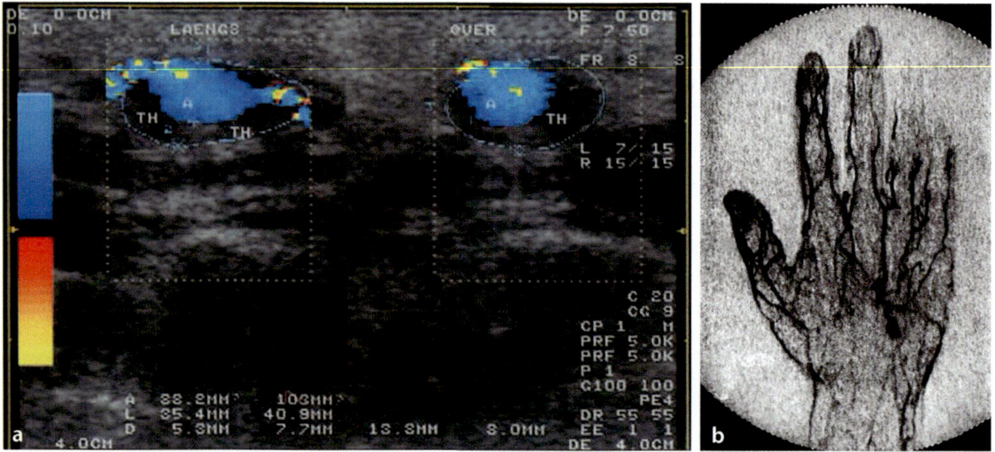

Fig. 2.109a, b (Atlas) Aneurysm of the ulnar artery (hypothenar syndrome).
a Patient with ischemia of the pads of fingers 4 and 5 due to arterial emboli from an aneurysm of the distal ulnar artery proximal to the palmar arch. The extent of the aneurysm is outlined in the color duplex images (longitudinal on the left, transverse on the right) to illustrate the relationship between the overall size of the partially thrombosed aneurysm (20 × 18 mm) and the patent lumen.
b Angiogram: Aneurysmal dilatation with a rather small caliber of the distal ulnar artery at the junction with the palmar arch and peripheral occlusions of the digital arteries of fingers 4 and 5. The largely thrombosed aneurysm of the ulnar artery was confirmed intraoperatively

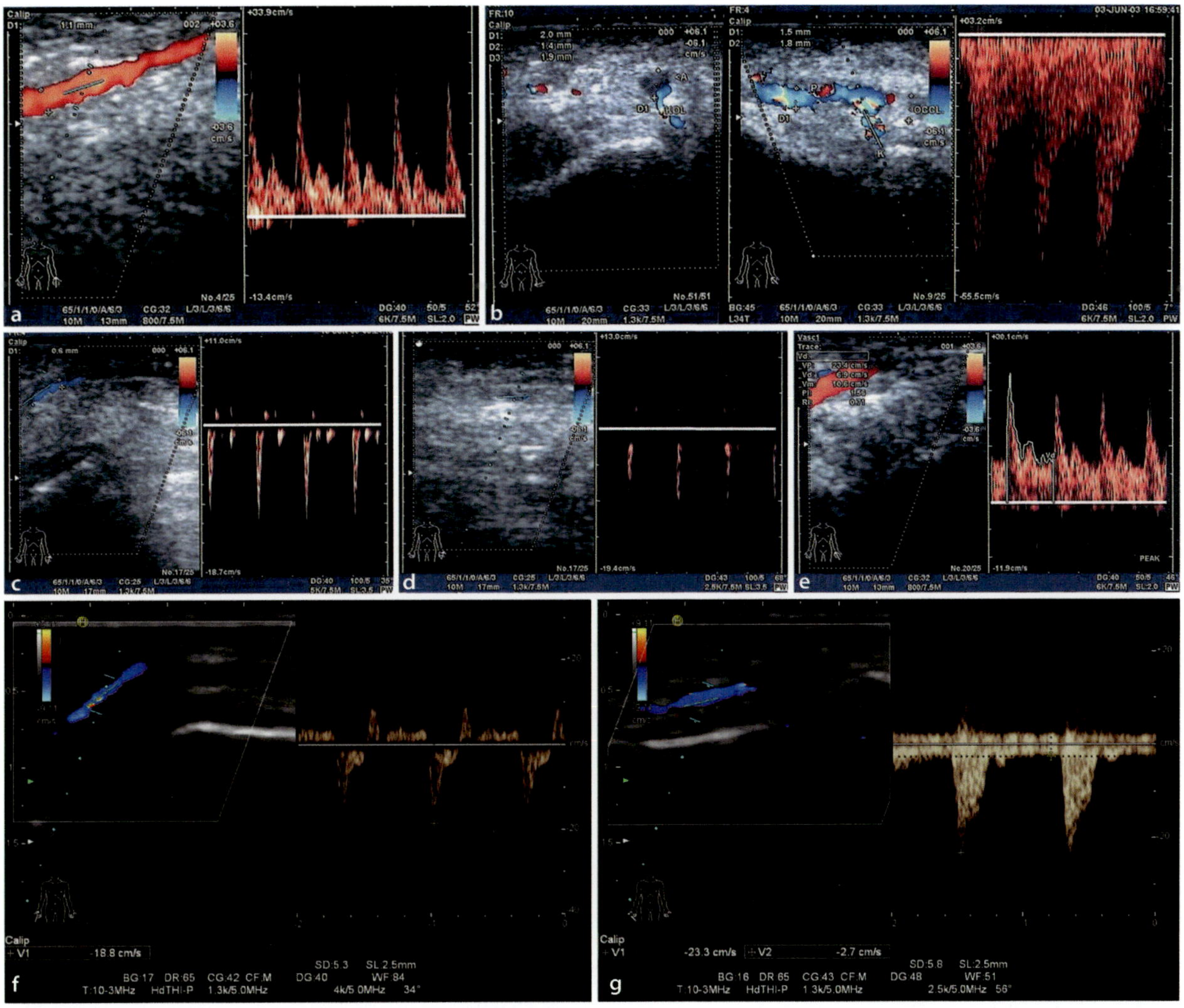

Fig. 2.110a–e (Atlas) Interdigital artery occlusion – Raynaud's disease.
a Interdigital arteries to the right and left of the metacarpal bones scanned from the palm show pulsatile flow (pulsatility varies with sympathetic tone).
b In interdigital artery occlusion, the small collateral vessels show monophasic flow due to peripheral dilatation. The occluded interdigital artery with the origin of a collateral is depicted in transverse orientation in the left section and in a longitudinal plane in the middle section. It has a diameter of 2 mm and a plaque (P) is depicted.
c Color duplex and spectral Doppler show a common digital artery in Raynaud's disease with a diameter of 0.6 mm and very pulsatile flow due to vasospasm (atypically displayed in blue because the transducer had to be rotated to visualize the artery).
d A "knocking" waveform is recorded from the affected distal interdigital artery due to peripheral spasms associated with Raynaud's disease.
e Arterial dilatation induced by bathing of the hand in warm water leads to less pulsatile flow with a large diastolic component.
f, g In patients with vasospasm (**f**), the effect of thermal vasodilation (**g**) can vary considerably (compare **e**)

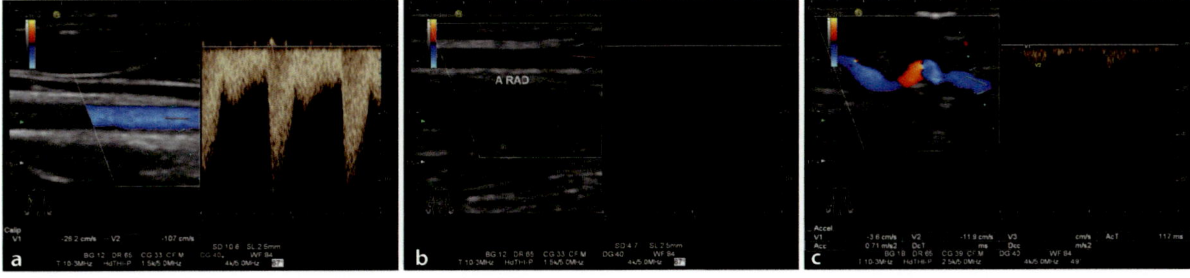

Fig. 2.111a–c (Atlas) Radial artery occlusion with peripheral ischemia.
a Patient presenting with index finger pain after cardiac catheter examination via the radial artery. There is a conspicuously large diastolic component in the brachial artery but with a steep systolic rise (PSV of 107 cm/s, EDV of 27 cm/s: peripheral widening).
b Long radial artery occlusion.
c Poststenotic Doppler waveform from the digital artery of the index finger; despite a patent ulnar artery, collateralization via the palmar arch is inadequate (PSV of 12 cm/s, EDV of 4 cm/s)

Extremity Veins

W. Schäberle, *Ultrasonography in Vascular Diagnosis*, https://doi.org/10.1007/978-3-319-64997-9_3

3.1 Pelvic and Leg Veins

3.1.1 Vascular Anatomy

Three groups of leg veins that are affected by different clinical conditions can be distinguished:

- Epifascial (superficial) veins
- Subfascial (deep) veins
- Transfascial (perforating) veins

The epifascial veins belong to the superficial venous system of the leg and the subfascial veins to the deep venous system with the transfascial or perforating veins establishing connections between these two venous systems. The deep veins accompany the arteries of the same name (◘ Figs. 3.1 and 3.2).

The **iliac vein** runs through the true pelvis posterior to the iliac artery, pierces the inguinal ligament, and then immediately passes to the medial side of the artery, where it continues as the common femoral vein. Just below the inguinal ligament, the great saphenous vein enters the common femoral vein on its anteromedial aspect. The common femoral vein receives the deep femoral vein just after the division of the common femoral artery into the deep and superficial branches. The deep femoral vein runs between the arterial branches of the femoral bifurcation. Distally, the superficial femoral vein courses along the posterior aspect of the artery of the same name. In most individuals, a second, large branch of the deep femoral vein opens into the superficial femoral vein. Different variants exist as to where, how, and how many deep femoral vein branches enter the superficial femoral vein.

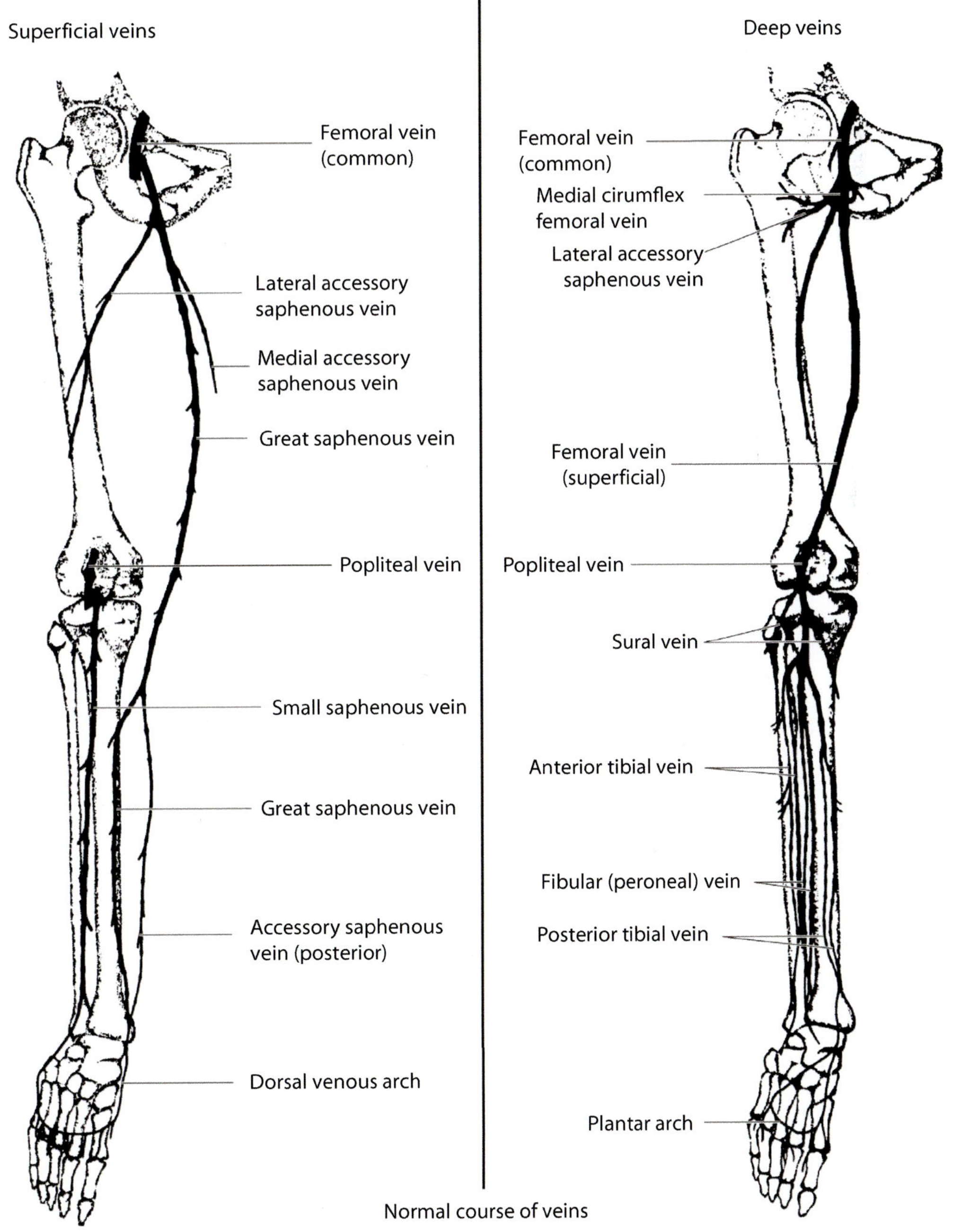

◘ **Fig. 3.1** Radiographic anatomy of the large veins of the leg (Courtesy of Eastman Kodak Company)

3

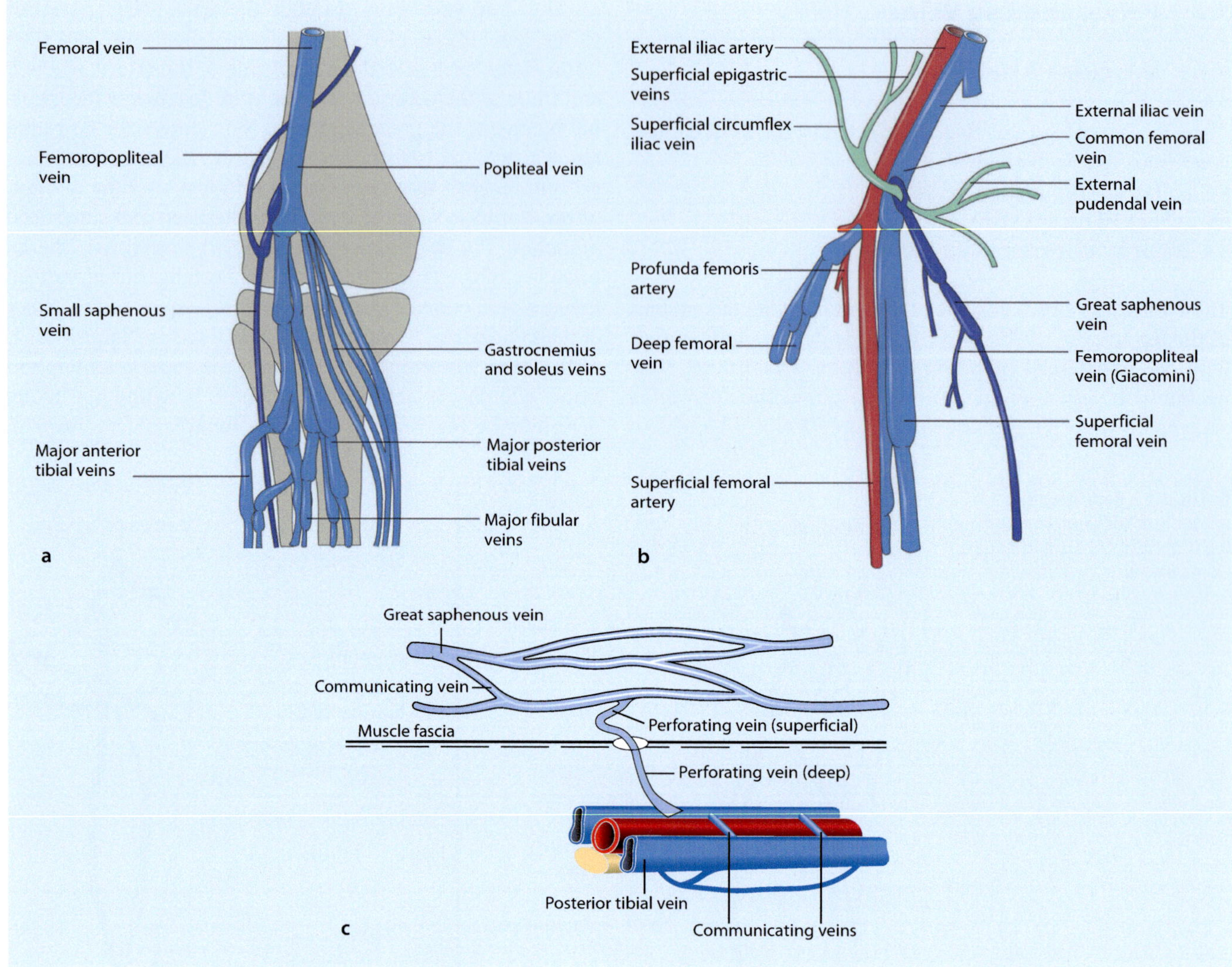

Fig. 3.2 **a** Anatomic relationship between the small saphenous vein and the gastrocnemius veins entering the popliteal vein in the popliteal fossa. The major calf veins converge distally. **b** Diagram of the vessels in the groin. Just below the saphenofemoral junction, the great saphenous vein receives the lateral accessory pudendal vein and the superficial epigastric veins. Farther down, the deep femoral vein joins the femoral vein. The arteries of the same name (red) lie anterolateral to the veins. **c** Perforating veins traverse the muscle fascia to drain blood from the superficial to the deep venous system. Communicating veins connect veins within the same venous compartment

A single **superficial femoral vein** is present in 62% of individuals only, 21% have a duplicated vein, and in another 14%, even three or more branches are present. If there is more than one vein, these may vary in caliber and course lateral or anterior to the artery rather than posterior to it. While the iliac vein has no valves, the superficial femoral vein has four or five valves (Weber and May 1990). After its passage through the adductor canal, the superficial femoral vein becomes the popliteal vein, which runs posteriorly along the artery of the same name (closer to the transducer when scanning from the popliteal fossa). The small saphenous vein joins the proximal popliteal vein (Fig. 3.1) on its posterior aspect at a highly variable level. Just below the saphenopopliteal junction, the small saphenous vein perforates the deep fascia and descends along the back of the calf. The distal popliteal vein receives the calf muscle veins (soleus and gastrocnemius veins) at various levels around the cleft of the knee joint. Just before flowing into the popliteal vein, the proximal small saphenous vein gives off a connecting branch to the deep muscle veins of the thigh, the femoropopliteal vein (Fig. 3.2a).

The **popliteal vein** may be present as a single or duplicated vessel and arises from the union of the posterior tibial and the fibular veins. It receives the anterior tibial vein as the first lower leg vein at a variable level. The main lower leg veins typically follow the arteries of the same name. The anterior tibial veins penetrate the interosseous membrane and course along its anterior aspect. The fibular veins run close to the fibula in the deep crural fascia between the superficial and deep flexors, as do the tibial veins, but on the posteromedial aspect of the tibia.

The **superficial** (**epifascial**) **venous drainage system** consists of two subsystems, that of the **great saphenous vein** and that of the **small saphenous vein**, which receive the larger arch veins and side branches. The great saphenous vein extends from the back of the foot to the medial malleolus and takes a medial course through the lower and upper leg to about 2–3 cm below the inguinal ligament, where it joins the popliteal vein. There is variation in the tributaries to the great saphenous vein below the knee, but these are mainly the following:

- the posterior arch vein, which is connected to the major deep veins, in particular the posterior tibial vein, through the perforating veins (Cockett I, II, and III)
- the great saphenous branch from the back of the foot
- the anterior tributary vein.

In the thigh, connections to the deep venous system are established by Dodd's perforators. Just before its junction with the common femoral vein, the great saphenous vein receives tributary veins from the thigh and lateral branches (lateral and medial accessory great saphenous vein), which then establish connections to the abdominal (epigastric) veins and become important as collaterals in pelvic vein thrombosis (▪ Fig. 3.2b).

The **small saphenous vein** drains the lower leg and arises at the lateral dorsum of the foot, coursing behind the lateral malleolus to the posterior side of the lower leg, where it ascends between the heads of the gastrocnemius and pierces the fascia to join the popliteal vein above the knee joint cleft. The gastrocnemius veins enter the small saphenous vein just before its termination or enter the popliteal vein directly.

In over 90% of individuals, there is a connection between the small saphenous vein (just before its junction with the popliteal vein) and the superficial thigh veins via the subcutaneous posterior femoral vein. This vein may also run as a proximal continuation of the small saphenous vein in those rare cases where the latter does not enter the popliteal vein. The posterior femoral vein may run in the deep or superficial compartment. In the deep compartment, it communicates with the deep femoral veins via muscle veins of the thigh. In many persons, a side branch of the posterior femoral vein courses craniomedially. This branch is also known as the femoropopliteal vein or Giacomini anastomosis. When these veins run in the superficial compartment, they terminate in the great saphenous vein via interconnecting veins; in the deep compartment, they drain into the superficial femoral vein.

Both the great and small saphenous veins have valves. Compared with the deep veins, the superficial veins have thicker walls with a thin muscle layer. The lumen varies with the intravenous pressure and can be compressed by external structures. There is wide variation in the course of individual veins and the connections they form.

The **perforating veins** are transfascial veins that drain blood from the superficial venous system into the major deep veins. About 150 such short veins exist between the superficial and deep venous systems, among which the Cockett groups I–III, the Sherman vein, and the Boyd vein are of clinical importance in the lower leg, the Dodd group in the upper leg, and the May perforator between the small saphenous vein and deep lower leg veins. The clinically most relevant perforators are the veins connecting the posterior arch vein of the great saphenous vein and the posterior tibial veins (Cockett's group and 24-cm perforator). Direct perforating veins connect the great saphenous vein territory with the major deep veins (posterior tibial vein). Indirect perforators connect these territories via the soleus and gastrocnemius muscle veins. Boyd's perforator courses between the great saphenous vein and the posterior tibial vein at the level of the tibial plateau, and a further, more cranial perforator runs into the popliteal vein. Dodd's perforators are the connecting veins at the level of the adductor canal (usually two perforators between the great saphenous vein and the superficial femoral vein). Under normal conditions, valves ensure blood flow from the superficial to the deep venous system, while the blood is propelled toward the heart by muscular contraction with compression of the deep veins. This mechanism prevents backward flow into the superficial veins.

3.1.2 Examination Protocol

3.1.2.1 Thrombosis

3.1.2.1.1 Equipment

The ultrasound examination of the peripheral veins depends on the clinical question to be answered. If the clinical symptoms suggest thrombosis, compression ultrasound of the upper and lower leg veins of the affected side is indicated. In patients with suspected chronic venous insufficiency, the ultrasound examination includes assessment of valve competence by spectral Doppler interrogation during compression and release to elicit reflux. The deep leg veins are scanned using a transducer operating at 5–7.5 MHz, while the pelvic veins and the vena cava are examined at 3.5–5 MHz (depending on the depth of the target vein). The superficial veins and particularly the perforating veins should be imaged at 7.5–10 MHz.

A linear or curved array transducer can be used. To achieve full compression of muscle veins and major lower leg veins in transverse orientation, however, the footprint for compression ultrasound should not be too small. To depict the slow venous flow, scanning is performed with a low wall filter and a low pulse repetition frequency (PRF). Most manufacturers provide a slow flow preset package optimized for imaging the veins.

3.1.2.1.2 Patient Positioning

The inferior vena cava and iliac vein are examined with the patient in the supine position. If there is overlying air, improvement may be achieved by repositioning the patient on the right or left side; bowel gas can be pushed aside by applying pressure with the transducer. The femoral vein is scanned in the supine patient with the knee slightly bent and a slight outward rotation of the leg. An experienced examiner can scan the popliteal vein and lower leg veins with the patient in the supine or semilateral position and the knee slightly bent. Alternatively, the popliteal vein can be examined with the patient in the prone position. However, to avoid collapse of the veins due to hyperextension of the knee, the

3

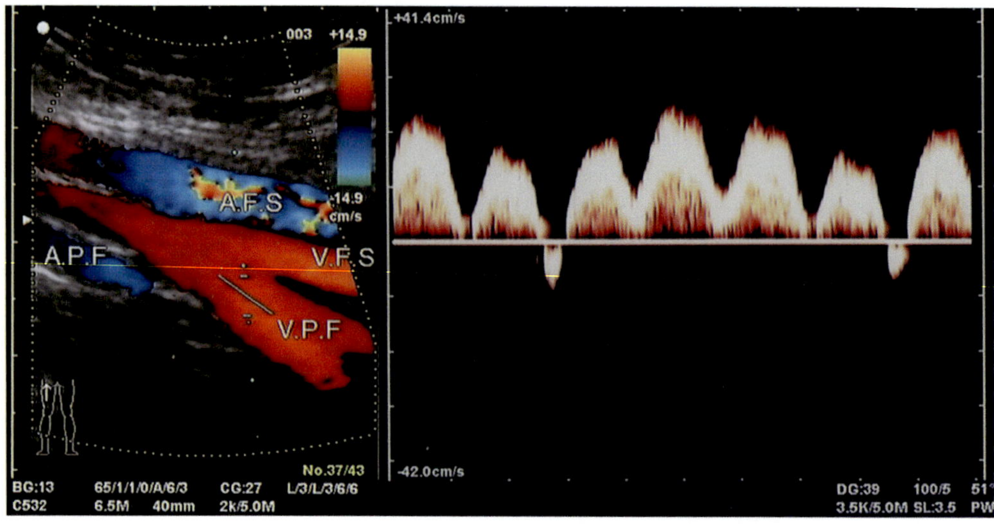

Fig. 3.3 Sonographic anatomy of the junction of the superficial (V.F.S) and deep (V.P.F) femoral veins. There are usually two main branches of deep thigh veins that join with the superficial femoral vein to form the common femoral vein. One passes under the superficial femoral artery just below the femoral bifurcation, and the second (the one seen in the image) enters the femoral vein slightly more distally. Thrombosis of this vein is rare and nearly always involves this more distal branch. The Doppler waveform from the deep femoral vein shows respiratory phasicity and sometimes also cardiac pulsatility (as seen here)

ankle should be slightly elevated by placing a cushion underneath. When the patient is sitting or standing, venous flow is increased and the veins below the knee are easier to identify. However, muscle tone is also increased, making it more difficult to assess vein compressibility. Valve competence in the popliteal vein, the superficial lower leg veins (varicosis), and the perforating veins is best evaluated in the sitting patient. The proximal great saphenous vein and the femoral vein are examined with the patient supine and performing the Valsalva maneuver (like the femoral artery; Figs. 3.3 and 3.69 (Atlas)).

3.1.2.1.3 Examination Technique

In the diagnostic evaluation of thrombosis, the deep veins are continuously scanned from the groin to the ankle and checked for the presence of intraluminal thrombi by intermittent compression (Figs. 3.4 and 3.17). First, the common femoral vein is identified on the medial side of the common femoral artery below the inguinal ligament and followed in transverse orientation down to its junction with the superficial femoral vein. Along the course of the common femoral vein, the terminations of the great saphenous vein and of the deep femoral veins from the upper leg muscles are tested for compressibility as well (Table 3.1 and Fig. 3.2).

At the pelvic level, compression ultrasound does not yield valid results because a continuous structure against which to compress the veins is not available, and the abdominal organs and fatty tissue preclude reliable compression, in particular in obese patients. Nevertheless, compression ultrasound can be performed, especially in slender patients. The arched iliac veins in the true pelvis are tested with the transducer in transverse orientation with additional longitudinal scanning as required. If adequate evaluation of compressibility is not possible in this way, patency must be evaluated by color duplex imaging.

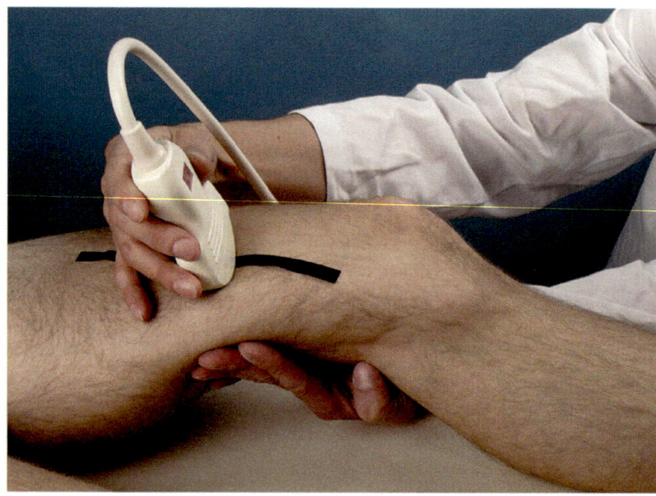

Fig. 3.4 Compression ultrasound applying pressure with the transducer alone is inadequate at the level of the adductor canal. Instead, the examiner must additionally push the vein against the transducer from below with the flat hand

If the scanning conditions are poor, occlusive thrombosis of a **pelvic vein** can be ruled out by spectral Doppler imaging of the junction of the common femoral and external iliac veins, where the insonation window is good. When an obstruction is present, respiratory phasicity of flow is eliminated or reduced compared to the unaffected side. Doppler measurement is performed in the external iliac vein (posterior to the artery) somewhat above the inguinal ligament in the longitudinal plane and with a low PRF. With the patient stretched in the supine position, the common femoral vein segment passing under the inguinal ligament may be compressed, especially in slender patients. In such cases, visualization can be improved by slight outward rotation of the hip joint.

Table 3.1 Ultrasound examination of the leg veins

Ultrasound mode	Parameter	Scan orientation and diagnostic information obtained and documented
B-mode	Scan orientation	Transverse (except for external and internal iliac veins)
	Criteria	Compressibility
		Lumen width
		Wall morphology
		Internal structures
	Note	Reversed compression maneuver in adductor canal
	Documentation	Split image: without/with compression
		Normal findings as outlined in the text, abnormal findings according to the situation
(Color) duplex	Scan orientation	Longitudinal plane, overview in transverse plane
	Criteria	Spontaneous flow, augmented flow (Valsalva, compression-and-release maneuver)
		Color filling of lumen (gaps?)
		Wall contour abnormalities, perivascular structures
	Note	Spectral Doppler always in longitudinal orientation
	Documentation	B-mode image with corresponding waveform, color flow image as needed

Next, with the patient in the supine position, the **superficial femoral vein** is followed down the leg in transverse orientation and is intermittently compressed (every 1–2 cm). The termination of the deep femoral vein is examined by color duplex ultrasound in the longitudinal plane (Fig. 3.3). In the distal segment of the superficial vein, at the level of the adductor canal, compression is difficult due to the absence of a bony structure and the interfering connective tissue. Instead, the examiner must press the muscle and vessels against the transducer from below with his or her other hand to achieve adequate compression (Fig. 3.4).

Below the adductor canal, the **popliteal vein** is scanned from a posterior approach. This part of the examination is performed with the patient supine and the knee slightly bent or in the prone position with a support under the ankles. The bent knee ensures better filling and hence improved visualization. With the knee stretched or even overstretched in the flat position, the popliteal vein is often collapsed or compressed by the surrounding connective tissue structures, pushing the vein against the artery and bony structures.

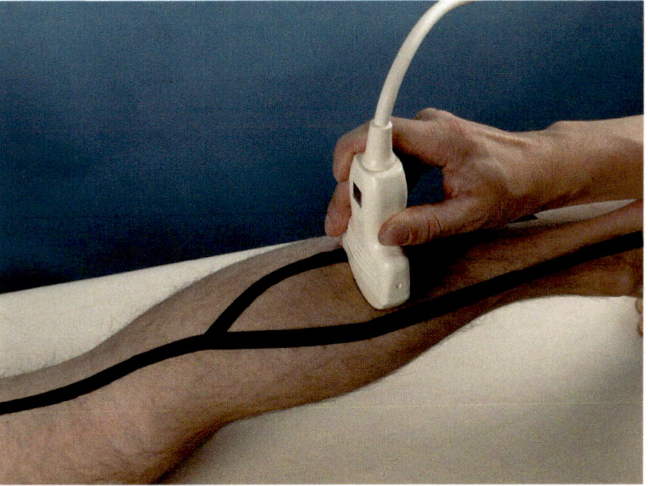

Fig. 3.5 Compression ultrasound of the lower leg veins (course marked). The transducer is positioned on the calf such that the ultrasound beam is perpendicular to the interosseous membrane between the tibia and fibula

Following evaluation of the popliteal vein for compressibility in transverse orientation, it is followed downward to the confluence of the fibular and posterior tibial veins. The anterior tibial vein entering at a higher level is often identified at its point of entry by means of color duplex only. The anterior tibial artery can serve as a landmark for identification of the accompanying anterior tibial veins. Compressibility is then evaluated intermittently while following their course to the ankle from an anterior approach.

For scanning of the **posterior tibial vein**, the transducer is placed on the extensors and then moved so as to achieve a beam direction roughly perpendicular to the interosseous membrane between the tibia and fibula. The procedure for evaluation of the fibular and posterior tibial veins including intermittent testing for compressibility is the same as for the anterior tibial vein, except that the transducer is in a posterior position on the gastrocnemius muscle (Fig. 3.5).

While the popliteal and femoral veins are reliably identified by B-mode ultrasound, the veins below the knee may have to be localized using the arteries of the same name as landmarks, which are visualized by color duplex. The hyperechoic interosseous membrane is an anatomic landmark for identifying the anterior tibial artery and vein coursing in it, whereas the deep crural fascia between the deep flexors and the soleus and gastrocnemius muscles is not always depicted well enough to serve as a landmark for identifying the posterior tibial and fibular veins coursing in it (Fig. 3.6). The fibular vein is easier to identify from the posterior approach, as it courses close to the fibula (and the proximal anterior tibial vein from the anterior approach). Sonographic evaluation for thrombosis can be performed with the patient in the supine or prone position, but better filling facilitates visualization of the veins in the sitting patient.

In addition to the major veins of the calf, evaluation of patients with suspected thrombosis also includes testing the compressibility of the muscle veins (the gastrocnemius veins joining the popliteal vein) and of the soleus veins joining the

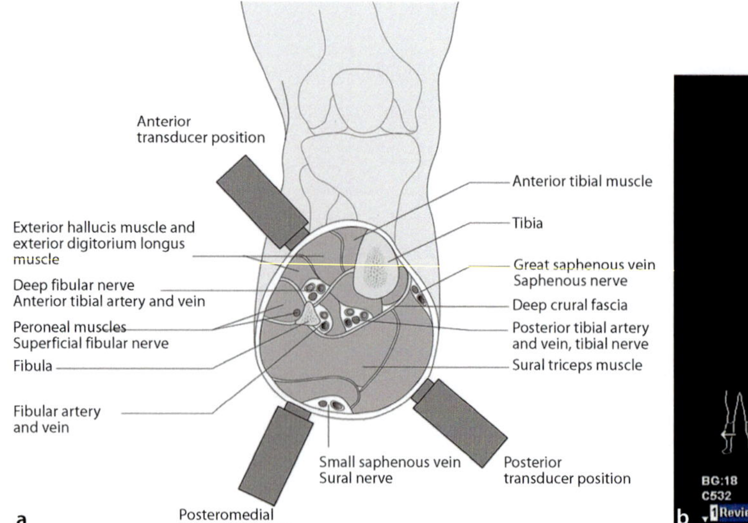

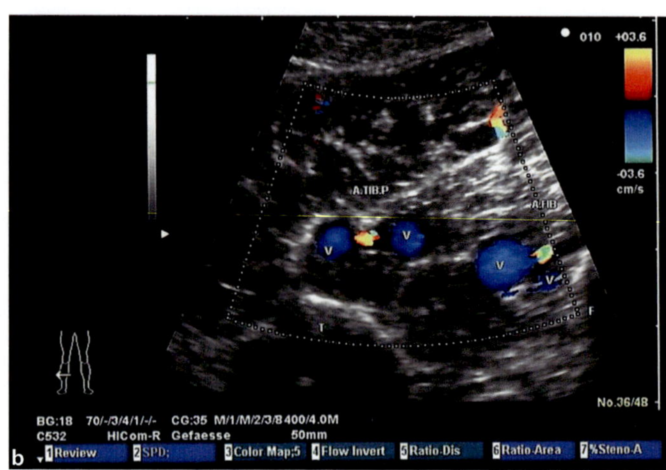

■ **Fig. 3.6** **a** Cross-sectional anatomy of the lower leg and transducer positions. **b** Sonoanatomy of the calf veins with the transducer in the posteromedial position. The transverse view shows the posterior tibial artery and vein (left part of image) somewhat posterior to the tibia (T) and the fibular artery and vein posteromedial to the fibula (F). Blue indicates flow in the veins, red flow in the artery (with some aliasing resulting from the low PRF selected to improve sensitivity to slow venous flow). The artery lies within the slightly hypoechoic deep crural fascia and is accompanied by two veins on the left and right

major calf veins to rule out muscle vein thrombosis (the same applies to the deep femoral vein in the thigh). The muscle veins can be traced in a distal direction from their sites of entry into the main vein, especially when there is adequate venous filling with the patient sitting.

The **ultrasound examination in thrombophlebitis** serves to determine the extent, in particular the cranial extent, and involvement of the deep venous system (inflow into deep venous system). This is done by performing compression ultrasound of the great or small saphenous vein in transverse orientation after identification of the clinically inflamed segment and using the same criteria as in the diagnostic assessment of thrombosis.

In thrombophlebitis, special attention must be paid to the sites of entry of the small and great saphenous veins into the popliteal and common femoral vein, respectively, which are checked for compressibility in the transverse plane.

In patients examined for thrombosis, compression ultrasound is always performed in transverse orientation, for two reasons: it makes it easier to identify the vein and follow its course down the leg and prevents false-negative results during compression. Longitudinally, when pressure is applied, a noncompressible vein may be displaced and disappear from the scanning plane, thereby mimicking compressibility.

3.1.2.2 Chronic Venous Insufficiency and Varicosis

In patients with chronic venous insufficiency of the deep veins or varicosis of the superficial veins, the affected venous segments are evaluated for reflux using provocative maneuvers while recording spectral Doppler information in longitudinal orientation. For identification of valve incompetence of the deep veins, evaluation is performed at representative sites in the common femoral, superficial femoral, and popliteal veins.

Function of the proximal valves is evaluated by spectral Doppler recording in the common and superficial femoral veins in the recumbent patient during increased abdominal pressure (Valsalva's maneuver). Valve incompetence is demonstrated by persistent backward flow to the periphery, indicated by a corresponding color change in the color flow image. If this test is positive for proximal valve incompetence, it is progressively extended to the popliteal vein and below-knee veins to identify the distal end of the incompetent segment.

In patients with competent proximal valves (common femoral and proximal superficial femoral veins), distal insufficiency is identified by the demonstration of persistent flow reversal (over 1 s) in the popliteal vein using spectral Doppler (■ Fig. 3.7) or color flow imaging (in longitudinal orientation) during **compression and release** with the patient sitting or standing. The best results are achieved with maximum relaxation of the calf muscles (■ Fig. 3.7).

Incompetence of the terminal valve of the great saphenous vein is assessed longitudinally during **Valsalva's maneuver** (■ Fig. 3.8). When truncal varicosis is suggested, the great saphenous vein is followed distally to identify the lowest point of incompetence through intermittent Valsalva maneuvers (grading according to Hach). In case of sufficiency of the proximal segment, the extent of distal varicosis of the great saphenous vein is determined by intermittent testing along the vein in the cranial direction (■ Fig. 3.8b: compression of the vein with the thumb distal to the transducer) to identify the proximal and distal points of insufficiency (transition from persistent reflux to absent reflux upon compression with subsequent release) in the sitting or standing patient. This valve function test is also used to diagnose reflux in the small saphenous vein (■ Fig. 3.9).

To assess valve competence of the perforating veins, these are first identified in their typical locations (e.g.,

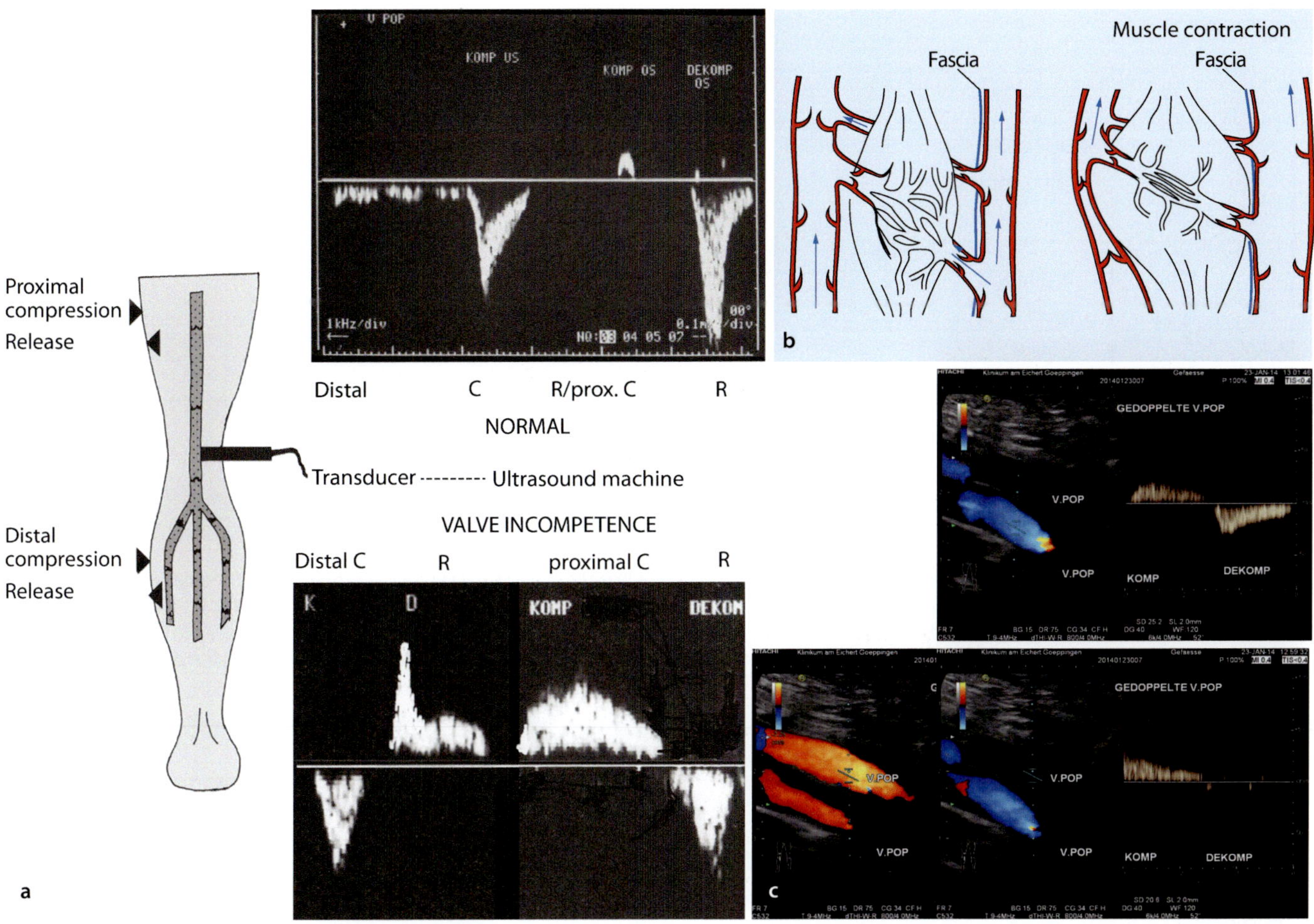

Fig. 3.7 **a** Illustration of the proximal and distal valve function test (alternating compression and release) with spectral Doppler measurement in the popliteal vein. The upper waveform represents the normal findings obtained when there is proper valve closure (distal compression and release on the left; proximal compression and release on the right); the lower waveform shows reflux due to valve incompetence (C = compression; R = release of compression). In individuals with a competent valve, venous flow with normal respiratory phasicity is followed by augmented flow toward the heart upon compression of the vein in the calf distal to the sampling site ("KOMP US" in the upper waveform). No flow signal is recorded upon release of compression (R), consistent with adequate valve closure and absence of reflux. Following compression of the muscle and vein in the thigh, i.e., proximal to the sampling site ("COMP OS" in the upper waveform), there is short reversed flow toward the periphery until the valve closes. Valve incompetence would be associated with persistent reflux. Release of compression in the thigh ("DECOMP OS" in the upper waveform) results in augmented flow toward the heart. When there is unobstructed venous drainage, the waveform shows a steep upstroke. The elicited flow increase is less pronounced when a flow obstruction is present between the sampling site and the site of compression (see Figs. 3.24 and 3.95 (Atlas)). **b** Venous drainage of the legs. The right drawing shows blood flow and valve function during muscle contraction. The contracting muscle squeezes the surrounding veins, propelling the blood in the draining veins toward the center. Competent valves prevent reflux toward the periphery. The valve function test (compression and release) simulates the role of muscle contraction in venous drainage (muscle pump). **c** Color flow images and spectral Doppler waveforms obtained in a patient with a duplicated popliteal vein (one competent/one incompetent branch) nicely illustrate the effect of alternating compression (KOMP) and release of compression (DEKOMP) for identification of valve incompetence. The popliteal vein closer to the transducer has adequate valve function, seen as absence of reflux upon release of compression ("DEKOMP" in the waveform accompanying the two color flow images shown at the bottom). The corresponding color flow image shows no flow in this popliteal vein, consistent with absence of reflux (bottom panel, second color flow image). In the second popliteal vein, there is incompetent postthrombotic valve closure, seen in the waveform (top panel) and the corresponding color flow image with blue-coded flow toward the periphery in the popliteal vein farther away from the transducer upon release of compression ("DEKOMP" in the waveform). During compression of the veins in the calf ("KOMP" in the waveforms), both popliteal veins show flow toward the center (red in the first color flow image in the bottom panel)

Cockett's group in the distal medial lower leg, Boyd's group in the proximal lower leg, or Dodd's group in the upper leg) (Fig. 3.10).

On B-mode images, the perforating veins are identified as hypoechoic, tubular structures passing through the deep fascia from the superficial to the deep veins. Once identified, the valve function test is performed as described in Fig. 3.11.

If there is incompetence, (color) duplex with the sample volume placed in the perforating vein identified by B-mode imaging will demonstrate reflux (retrograde flow from the deep into the superficial system) during compression of the calf just proximal to the sample volume. When the valves function properly, there is no backward flow from the deep to the superficial veins. Compression of the calf will cause

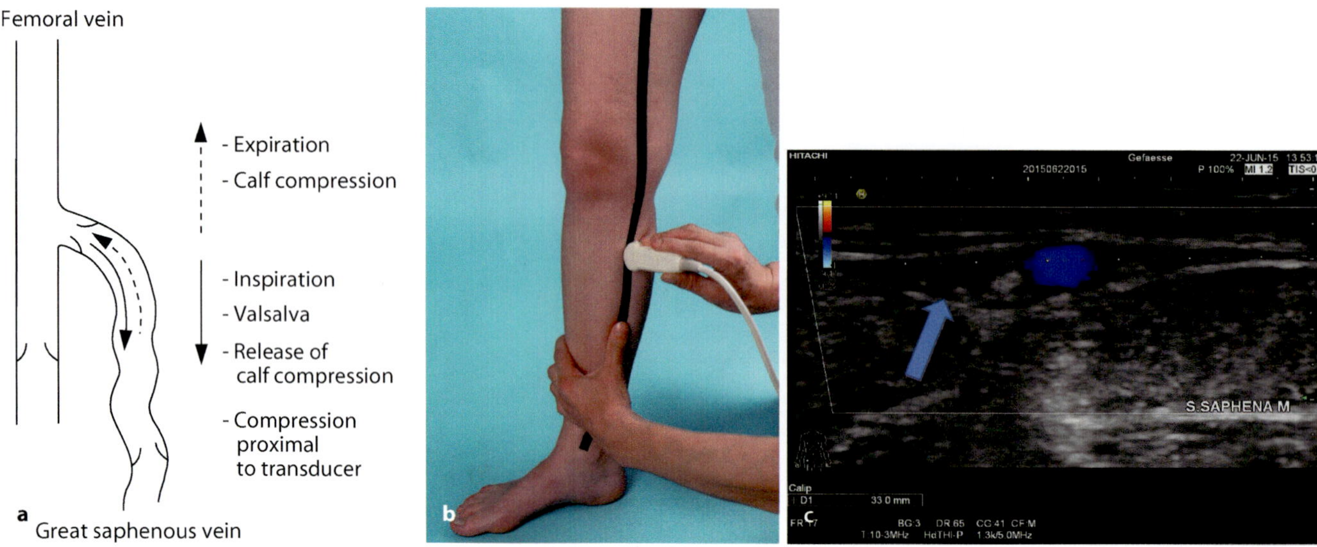

Fig. 3.8 **a** Valve function test in the great saphenous vein. **b** Transducer position for evaluating valve competence of the distal great saphenous vein. Alternating distal compression of the vein and release during recording of the Doppler spectrum is performed with the left thumb. **c** Transverse image of the sonoanatomy of the great saphenous vein (arrow) in the saphenous compartment enclosed by the bright saphenous fascia anteriorly and the muscle fascia posteriorly. This appearance has been referred to as Cleopatra's eye and can help the examiner distinguish the great saphenous vein from branch varices coursing outside this compartment. The great saphenous vein enters the common femoral vein from anteromedially

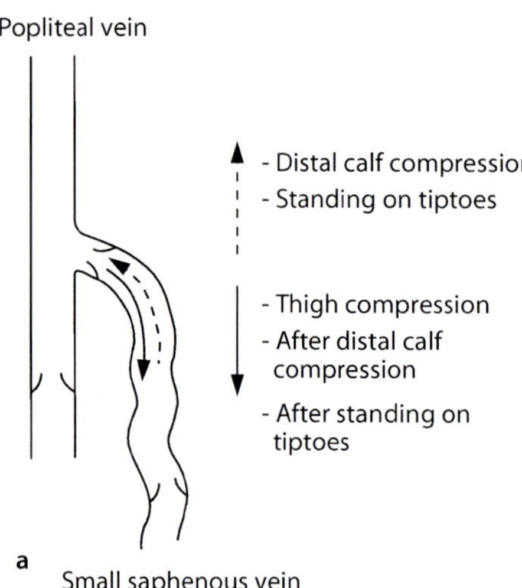

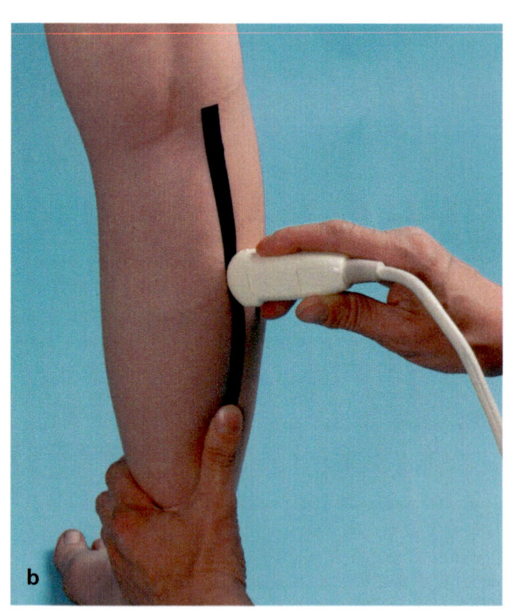

Fig. 3.9 **a** Valve function test in the small saphenous vein. **b** Transducer position for evaluating valve competence of the small saphenous vein (see legend to Fig. 3.8b)

stoppage of flow but no reversal. Application of a tourniquet proximal to the site of evaluation can prevent interference from flow in insufficient superficial veins.

3.1.3 Normal Findings

The leg veins, with their delicate walls and low intraluminal pressure, are fully compressible when pressure is exerted with the transducer. When compressed, normal veins become nearly invisible on ultrasound, or only a hyperechoic reflection indicating the wall but no lumen is seen. The breathing-related intra-abdominal pressure changes lead to **respiratory modulation of venous return** with faster flow during expiration due to lower intra-abdominal pressure (upward movement of diaphragm) and slower flow during inspiration due to higher intra-abdominal pressure (downward movement of diaphragm). This pressure-dependent flow pattern is transmitted through the upper leg veins into the major deep veins in the distal lower leg and into the major superficial veins (great and small saphenous veins) in the recumbent patient. Respiratory phasicity of venous flow may be overridden by cardiac pulsatility (changes in atrial pressure) in the iliac and proximal femoral veins, especially in young patients.

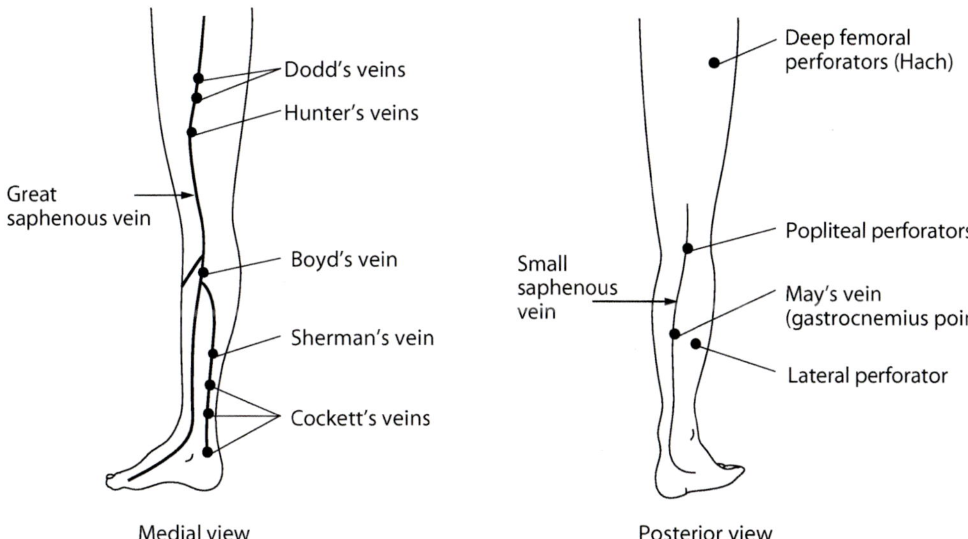

Fig. 3.10 Typical locations of clinically relevant perforating veins

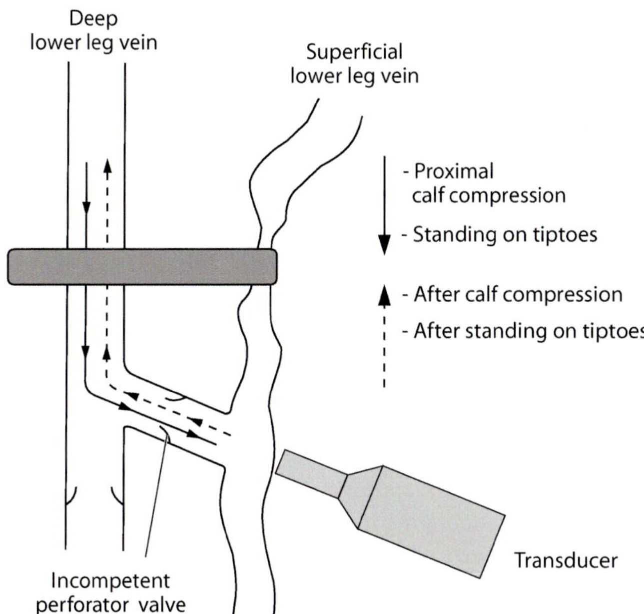

Fig. 3.11 Valve function test in the perforating veins

In summary, the following factors determine venous blood flow:

- Vis-a-tergo
- Variation in intra-abdominal and intrathoracic pressure (suction pump)
- Cardiac suction pump (systole, early diastole)
- Musculovenous pump (requires competent valves): competent perforating veins prevent blood flow into superficial veins; competent valves distal to the contracting muscle prevent backward flow (Fig. 3.7b)

The pocket-like valves ensure undisturbed flow from the periphery to the center. Physiologic backward flow induced by pressure reversal ceases upon closure of the valves (after a short reflux of 0.3 s on average). Valve function tests with manual compression and release simulate the interplay of the muscle pump and venous valves in transporting blood back to the heart.

Therefore, under normal conditions, there should only be a short reflux during Valsalva's maneuver before valve closure. When the compression-and-release test is performed to evaluate peripheral valve competence with spectral Doppler measurement in the popliteal vein, manual compression at the calf level will result in a rapid increase in blood flow velocity (unless there is obstruction of venous flow). Like Valsalva's maneuver, release of compression should lead to short reversed flow until the valve closes. The test will allow more confident assessment and differentiation of normal and abnormal function when performed with the patient sitting and legs dangling (Fig. 3.7).

3.1.4 Documentation

As with the examination protocol, the documentation of findings is dictated by the clinical question to be answered.

3.1.4.1 Deep Vein Thrombosis of the Leg

The findings of sonographic valve function tests performed in patients with deep vein thrombosis (DVT) should be documented without and with compression (ideally split images showing venous flow without and with compression side by side). The sites for which these findings are documented include the common femoral vein at about the level of the termination of the great saphenous vein, the superficial femoral vein somewhat distal to the site of entry of the deep femoral vein, the popliteal vein, and the major veins below the knee from a posterior approach. The findings at these representive sites should be supplemented by images documenting abnormal findings and a Doppler waveform from the junction of the common femoral vein and external iliac vein to document unobstructed venous return at the pelvic level.

When the documentation of findings in patients with suspected DVT relies on duplex ultrasound, it is generally recommended that this should comprise longitudinal images with the corresponding waveforms confirming preserved respiratory phasicity of venous return in the common femoral, superficial femoral, and deep femoral veins near their terminations and in the popliteal vein.

In addition, if DVT is diagnosed, the abnormal findings should be documented (incompressible venous segments) in transverse images obtained with and without compression or waveforms obtained in longitudinal orientation and showing absence of flow or an abnormal flow profile. If color duplex images are stored to document absence of flow, the images must contain information to the effect that adequate instrument settings including a low PRF and adequate gain were used.

3.1.4.2 Chronic Venous Insufficiency and Varicosis

When ultrasound is performed for varicosis or postthrombotic syndrome, documentation should include longitudinal B-mode images (optionally supplemented by color duplex images) with corresponding waveforms from the common, superficial and deep femoral veins and the popliteal vein.

For the common and superficial femoral veins and for the great saphenous vein (near its termination), longitudinal scans with the corresponding Doppler spectra during normal breathing and Valsalva's maneuver are required. Terminal valve function of the popliteal vein and the small saphenous vein is documented on longitudinal scans with the corresponding Doppler spectra obtained during compression and release. Color duplex scans alone are inadequate for documenting reflux because the duration must be quantified to differentiate abnormal reflux from the short backward flow that is normal before valve closure.

3.1.5 Clinical Role of Duplex Ultrasound

3.1.5.1 Thrombosis and Postthrombotic Syndrome

3.1.5.1.1 Leg Vein Thrombosis

The incidence of deep vein thrombosis (DVT) of the legs is 1–2‰ per year and increases with age. Various noninvasive diagnostic tests were developed for the diagnosis of this common condition, which often takes an asymptomatic or unspecific clinical course but has serious early (pulmonary embolism) and late complications (chronic venous insufficiency in about 50% of cases). The tests include plethysmography, thermography, iodine fibrin test, and Doppler ultrasonography (Bollinger and Franzeck 1982; Hull et al. 1984; Kakkar 1972; Lepore et al. 1978; Neuerburg-Heusler and Hennerici 1995; Sandler et al. 1984; Strandness 1977).

The methods are either very time consuming or yield reliable results only in certain venous segments. Continuous wave (CW) Doppler ultrasound used to be the noninvasive modality of first choice in the diagnostic assessment of valvular incompetence of the superficial and deep veins and, as a functional modality, showed good results at the pelvic and thigh levels including popliteal artery thrombosis with reported accuracies of up to 90%. However, isolated venous thrombosis below the knee and central thrombi surrounded by flowing blood are difficult to detect with CW Doppler. A review of 2060 patients who underwent additional venography yielded a sensitivity of 84% and a specificity of 88% for CW Doppler ultrasound in demonstrating venous thrombosis (Wheeler 1985).

Combining morphologic information (B-scan) and functional information (spectral Doppler), duplex ultrasound has gained a central role as a noninvasive modality for venous diagnosis.

Stasis is an important risk factor for the development of DVT in addition to a hypercoagulable state and a damaged vessel wall. Thus, immobilization plays a crucial role in the pathogenesis of thrombosis of the deep veins, which primarily arises in the muscle veins in bedridden patients or patients with cast immobilization of the leg. The risk of thrombosis without heparin prophylaxis is 10–30% in general surgery and as high as 54% in hip surgery (Lippert and Pabst 1985). Venous thrombi are ascending in over 90% of cases and have an annual incidence of 160/100,000 inhabitants in Germany with pulmonary embolism occurring in 60/100,000 inhabitants per year. Thrombosis of the deep pelvic and leg veins is the source of pulmonary embolism in over 90% of cases. The importance of isolated venous thrombosis below the knee should not be underestimated as it may extend cranially and cause pulmonary embolism, though often asymptomatic, in 15–26% of cases (Kroegel 2003). In contrast, iliofemoral thrombosis has a 56–85% incidence of pulmonary embolism. The mortality of pulmonary embolism ranges from 0.1% to 5%, depending on the risk group (Polak 1992).

Data on the incidence of **paraneoplastic thrombosis** vary with the study population investigated. For thrombosis without apparent cause such as immobilization, incidences of 10–34% have been reported in the literature (Silverstein et al. 1998; Goldberg et al. 1987; Aderka et al. 1986; Monreal et al. 1989). Recurrent thrombosis without an apparent cause or thrombophlebitis without varicosis should prompt a search for an underlying malignancy (Prandoni et al. 1992). Pareneoplastic venous thrombi tend to be larger at the time of diagnosis, grow more aggressively, and cause more severe symptoms (Schulman et al. 2000).

Known **risk factors** include immobilization, trauma, pregnancy, intake of oral contraceptives, protein-C and protein-S deficiencies, factor V clotting disorder, hyperhomocysteinuria, and lupus anticoagulant. In addition, an association with atherosclerosis has been proposed (Prandoni et al. 2003) since inflammatory processes play a role in both conditions.

Results on the **distribution of venous thrombosis in the leg** are not very consistent. In a study of 1084 lower extremities with acute venous thrombosis, the thrombosis was localized above the knee in 51%, below the knee in 32%, and in a superficial vein in 17% (Kerr et al. 1990). A venographic study (Schmitt et al. 1977) of DVT showed concomitant involvement of the common iliac vein in 16%, external iliac vein in 33%, common femoral vein in 46%, deep femoral vein in 45%, superficial femoral vein in 65%, popliteal vein in 66%, anterior tibial vein in 73%, posterior tibial vein in 82%, and fibular vein in 77%.

A study investigating 189 venograms in the early 1990s (Cogo et al. 1993) identified isolated calf vein thrombosis in 18% of cases. The vast majority of the 82% of patients with proximal vein thrombosis had popliteal vein involvement, while only 8% were found to have isolated pelvic vein thrombosis. No case of isolated thrombosis of the superficial femoral vein was reported in this study.

The generous use of diagnostic ultrasound in patients with clinically suspected DVT can help reduce the incidence of thrombosis of the pelvic and femoral veins.

The results of a retrospective analysis of **DVT distribution** performed by the author in a patient population with 18% thrombosis prevalence in 2008 confirm that, with generous use of ultrasound, most patients are identified when thrombosis is still confined to the veins below the knee (indication for sonography: swelling of the leg or calf pain for which no other cause was apparent). The analysis included a total of 280 cases of DVT of the legs. Isolated DVT below the knee was present in 63% of cases (including 8% isolated calf muscle vein thrombosis), 23% had extension to the popliteal vein and 11% involvement of the femoral and popliteal vein, while only 3% of patients had isolated or concomitant pelvic vein thrombosis. With one exception, isolated pelvic vein thrombosis extended down to the level of the saphenofemoral junction. There was one case of isolated superficial femoral vein thrombosis, which was seen in a patient with duplication of this vein. In 1.5% of patients, a muscle vein (soleus or gastrocnemius) was the site of origin of popliteal vein thrombosis, as thrombosis was absent in the other major calf veins. Thrombosis of the deep femoral vein with thrombus extension into the common femoral vein accounted for 0.7% of cases.

The high proportion of isolated calf vein thrombosis in this population may be attributable to the fact that symptoms indicative of thrombosis following trauma or surgery of the leg prompted a sonographic examination in all cases, frequently revealing calf vein thrombosis (in particular of the fibular vein or muscle veins).

Also contributing to this distribution is the policy of early diagnosis and treatment of DVT of the legs pursued by the ultrasound laboratory at the author's institution. This helps reduce the number of cases with thrombosis of the popliteal and distal superficial femoral veins, which always arise from ascending calf thrombosis. Our observations therefore underscore the need for always including the calf veins when examining patients for vein thrombosis.

Most thrombi arise in the venous sinusoids of the lower leg muscles or in regions of relatively stagnant blood flow behind the pocket-like valves of the popliteal and femoral veins (◘ Figs. 3.12a and 3.60 (Atlas)). In the majority of patients, DVT of the legs develops in the valves of the calf muscle veins (soleus or gastrocnemius veins) (>50%) or in the valves of the fibular vein. Recirculation in the cusps induces platelet activation and the release of procoagulant substances, which may lead to the formation of a red thrombus. It is estimated that 20–30% of such thrombi undergo spontaneous thrombolysis through the simultaneous activation of the fibrinolytic system and that approx. 50% of the thrombi become organized and thus remain clinically asymptomatic. Approx. 20–30%, however, exhibit appositional growth with extension into the deep venous system, and from there may continue to grow cranially. With further growth in the major deep veins, a thrombus may become free-floating and lead to pulmonary embolism without causing any severe local clinical symptoms such as swelling or pain. Local clinical symptoms leading to the initiation of diagnostic measures may thus not occur – unless a thrombus occludes a main vein or interferes with blood flow by protruding from a muscle or superficial vein into a major deep vein (see ◘ Figs. 3.61, 3.62, and 3.63 (all Atlas)).

Depending on flow in the partially thrombosed tributary vein and the flow obstruction caused by the growing thrombus in the main vein, **further growth is ascending or descending** (◘ Fig. 3.12b). Descending venous thrombosis

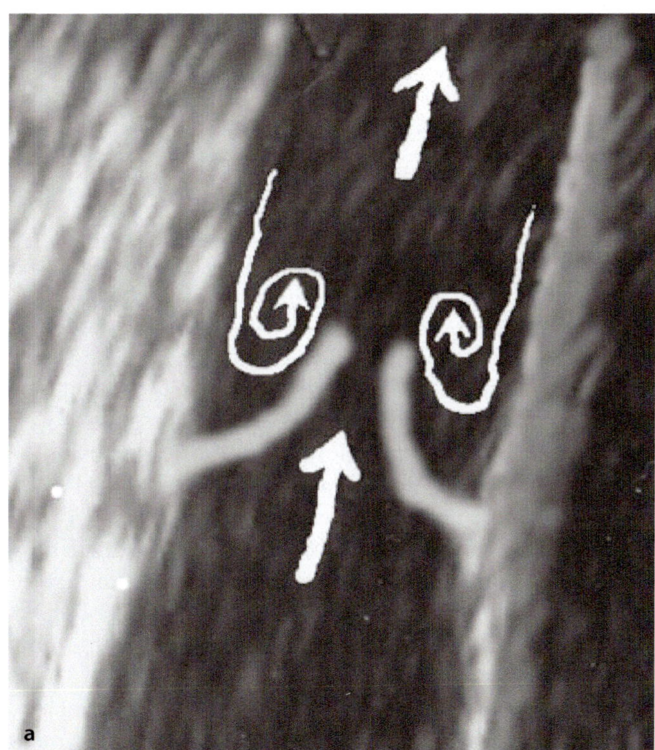

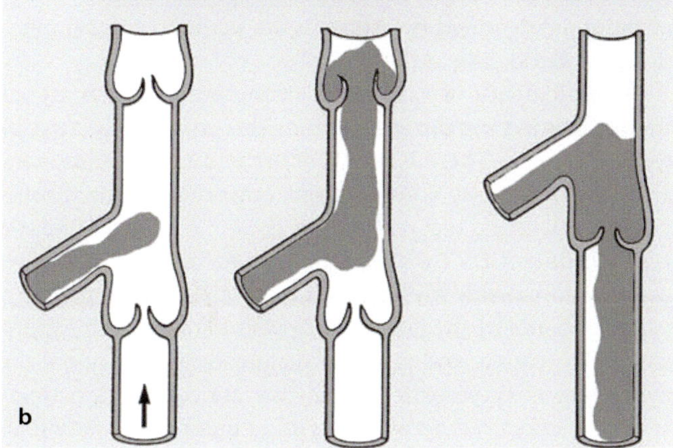

◘ **Fig. 3.12** a Turbulent flow and eddy currents in the pocket-like valves can lead to local stasis with release of procoagulant substances. b Diagram of a thrombus (left) extending from a tributary (e.g., calf muscle vein) into the main vein, where it can ascend (center) or descend (right)

3

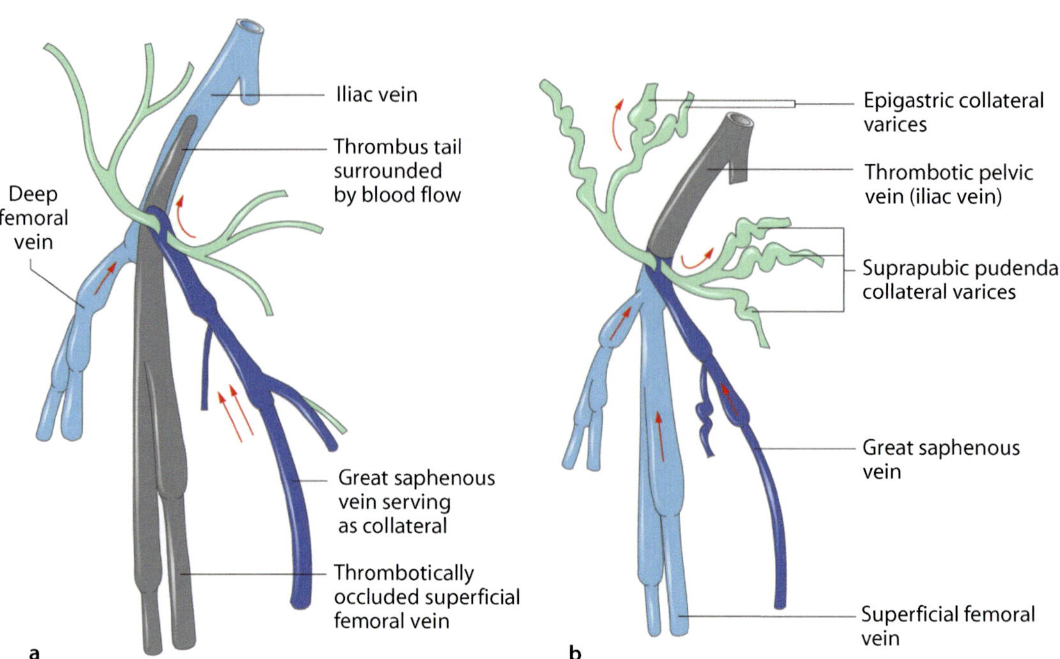

Fig. 3.13 **a** Venous blood flow in thrombotic femoral vein occlusion with venous return from the periphery occurring primarily through the great saphenous vein (indicated by arrows). **b** Collateral pathways in descending (isolated) pelvic vein thrombosis: suprapubic pudendal and epigastric collaterals (see Figs. 3.48 and 3.61 (both Atlas))

is less common, and in primary pelvic vein thrombosis, it is twice as common on the left side. This is attributed to a pelvic vein spur, a connective tissue structure producing chronic wall trauma with luminal narrowing, as the vein is compressed against the spur by the pulsation of the common iliac artery. The spur is difficult to detect on imaging.

In patients with **complete thrombotic occlusion of the deep leg veins**, blood drains through superficial veins, chiefly the great saphenous vein. The increased blood flow from the great saphenous vein stops the growth of most ascending thrombi at the saphenofemoral junction. In the superficial femoral vein, blood from the deep femoral vein stops ascending thrombus growth or surrounds a thrombus extending more proximally (Fig. 3.13a).

In isolated descending pelvic vein thrombosis, the blood is drained through epigastric collaterals or suprapubic pudendal veins (Fig. 3.13b). Sonographically, this collateralization is identified by reflux in the saphenofemoral junction (see Fig. 3.45 (Atlas)).

The incidence of early DVT of the legs is much higher than suspected on clinical grounds due to its fairly asymptomatic course. There is a risk of serious early (pulmonary embolism) and late complications (chronic venous insufficiency with crural ulceration). For these reasons, **diagnostic tests to detect DVT of the legs should be used liberally**, even when patients present with unspecific symptoms. This is underscored by the fact that ultrasound offers an inexpensive, noninvasive, and accurate diagnostic modality for the evaluation of these patients and that anticoagulation treatment can effectively reduce the risk of pulmonary embolism and prevent further thrombus growth.

With most venous thromboses starting to develop below the knee, assessment of the major calf veins and of the muscle veins in this territory is an integral part of diagnostic sonography in these patients.

Ultrasound has the advantage of "illuminating the blind spots" of venography. In the elderly, stasis due to degenerative ectasia of gastrocnemius and soleus veins is a common source of ascending thrombosis. For technical reasons (valve function), this form of calf muscle vein thrombosis and the less common deep femoral vein thrombosis cannot be identified by venography; these veins are not opacified or take up the contrast medium only through retrograde flow. Sonographic data suggest that ascending thrombophlebitis with thrombus extension from muscle or perforating veins into the deep venous system is a much more common cause of DVT than assumed in the past.

The **fibular vein** is a typical source of error in venography, as nonvisualization of this vein may indicate the presence of thrombus, or it may simply be due to limitations of the method. At the same time, the fibular vein is the most common site of isolated venous thrombosis of the calf with ascending thrombus growth. In an analysis of 105 cases of isolated venous thrombosis of the lower leg (without popliteal vein involvement) by our group, the fibular vein alone was affected in 48 instances, the posterior tibial vein in 36, and both veins in 21. Only one case of anterior tibial vein thrombosis, attributable to a large traumatic hematoma of the anterior compartment, was seen. Spontaneous thrombosis of the anterior tibial vein is always caused by descending thrombus growth from the popliteal vein.

Soft tissue lesions such as abscess, hematoma, or perforated Baker's cyst cause similar clinical symptoms but usually have distinct sonographic features allowing them to be differentiated from deep vein thrombosis or to be confirmed by ultrasound-guided biopsy.

Thrombus Organization and Recanalization

Thrombus organization begins on day 3 or 4 with attachment to the venous wall, and ingrowth of capillaries occurs after

8–12 days (Leu 1973). At the end of the first week, lipoblasts and fibrocytes start to induce the formation of collagen fibrils that fill the hollow and intercapillary spaces left after liquefaction and absorption (Rotter 1981). As cellular infiltration is an ongoing process, a thrombus is composed of layers reflecting the different stages of development. Further organization is associated with shrinkage of the vein, which can be seen with ultrasound. Hemolysis with partial degradation of fibrin occurs after days to weeks.

The duration of thrombus organization depends on the vessel diameter and intraluminal pressure and may additionally be affected by external factors such as application of compression bandages. Attachment of the thrombus to the wall by collagen fibers will invariably have occurred by day 8–10. Thrombolytic therapy (e.g., streptokinase) performed at this time or later will recanalize the vessel but cannot prevent venous valve destruction in most cases. When surgical thrombectomy is performed at this stage, only central thrombus portions can be removed, while mural residues remain and may give rise to the postoperative development of recurrent thrombi through appositional growth. Residual thrombotic material near valves induces valve incompetence. Late sequelae are calcifications of the venous wall.

Complete thrombus organization can transform superficial and small veins into strands of fibrous scar tissue. In most cases, however, there will be recanalization of the lumen through the ingrowth of capillaries. The latter dilate and become merged, thereby re-establishing patency over a course of several months. However, recanalization is associated with shrinkage and destruction of the valves as well as fibrosis and thickening of the wall. The main mechanism involved in the recanalization of a thrombosed vein is the high fibrinolytic potential of the venous wall.

Collateralization and recanalization following acute DVT lead to the more or less complete reconstitution of venous drainage. Long segments of an occluded vein are recanalized in most cases (endogenous thrombolysis). Recanalization is a highly variable process: it may begin after 3–4 weeks in small vessels and may take 3–9 months in large veins such as the popliteal and femoral veins. The patency of a deep vein is re-established 3 months after the onset of thrombosis in about half of all cases (Killewich et al. 1989).

Venographic studies show that, within 1 year, complete recanalization occurs in up to 35% of all venous thromboses and partial recanalization in another 55%, with only 10% of patients showing persistent occlusion. The clinical severity of the postthrombotic syndrome mainly depends on the degree of valve incompetence, in particular of the popliteal vein, while a persisting lumen reduction after thrombosis has only a minor effect. Insufficient venous return is further compromised by secondary damage (widening with subsequent valve incompetence) to superficial and perforating veins resulting from the higher pressure and volume overload due to collateral flow (secondary varicosis).

Anticoagulation and compression therapy are major components in the management of thrombosis. The latter serves to limit the extent of progressive dilatation of the collateral veins induced by the increased outflow resistance, in particular during the first 3 months.

3.1.5.1.2 Chronic Venous Insufficiency/Postthrombotic Syndrome

Chronic venous insufficiency (disturbed venous return from peripheral veins) can have the following causes:

- Obstruction of deep veins
- Valve incompetence of deep veins
- Valve incompetence of superficial veins
- Valve incompetence of perforating veins
- Calf muscle pump dysfunction (Fig. 3.14)

The superficial system (varicosis) and deep system (chronic venous incompetence) may develop secondary changes in

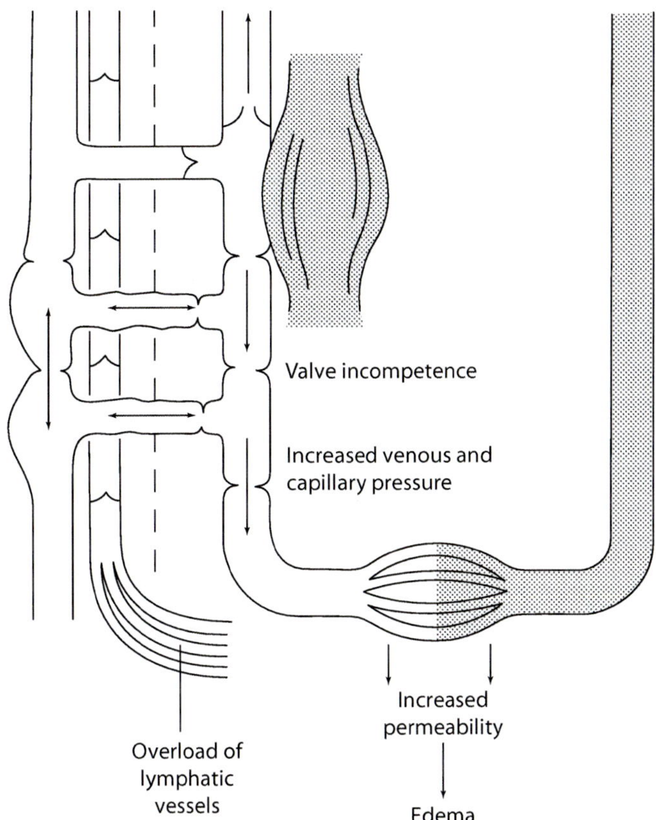

Fig. 3.14 Diagram of the pathophysiological changes occurring in chronic venous incompetence. The drawing represents the superficial venous system on the left and the deep system on the right. When there is valve dysfunction in a major deep vein, the calf muscle pump (compression of the veins) fails to propel the blood toward the center (centripetal), resulting in at least partial reversal of flow toward the periphery (centrifugal). The ensuing recirculation via incompetent perforators and dilated varicose superficial veins further contributes to inefficient drainage. The increase in venous and capillary pressure results in a higher fluid infiltration and permeability of the damaged capillary wall. Interstitial edema in turn can lead to an overload of the lymphatic system, causing lymphatic microangiopathy in severe cases. Extensive and partially indurated edema in severe chronic venous insufficiency is not due to insufficient venous drainage alone but mainly to secondary lymphatic drainage insufficiency (According to Rieger and Schoop 1998)

response to disease of the respective other system. These secondary changes result from the compensatory increase in pressure and volume and may worsen the state of the already compromised venous return.

The morphologic features associated with the postthrombotic syndrome can be demonstrated in part by B-mode ultrasound but above all by venography. The functional parameters reflecting the severity of reflux are reliably determined by duplex ultrasound and play a crucial role in planning treatment (type, extent, and duration of compression therapy).

Ultrasound also has an important role in documenting the status of the venous system after completion of anticoagulant treatment to serve as a baseline in case a patient later develops symptoms suggesting **recurrent thrombosis**. Recent data suggest that patients have an up to 8% risk of recurrence during the first months after the end of anticoagulant treatment and a cumulative 5-year risk of 30%.

Other causes of calf swelling besides acute thrombosis and chronic venous insufficiency include edema of different etiology (cardiac, lymphedema, lipedema). After exclusion of thrombosis and incompetent valves by duplex imaging, sonography can also provide important clues for differentiating lymphedema and lipedema. Lymphedema is characterized by the presence of primarily longitudinal, anechoic clefts (due to fluid collections) in the thickened subcutaneous tissue, while in lipedema such clefts are absent, and the subcutaneous layer appears rather uniform.

3.1.5.2 Varicosis

Varicosis of the great or small saphenous vein is caused by valve incompetence. In the primary form this is due to constitutional or external factors. In secondary varicosis, on the other hand, the valves of the superficial system fail due to pressure and volume overload resulting from disease (e.g., thrombosis) of the deep venous system. Causes of valve incompetence are:

- Destruction (postthrombotic)
- Dilatation with incomplete coaptation
  - Weakness of the venous wall (acquired, congenital)
  - Pressure overload
  - Volume overload (secondary, varicosis)
- Anomalies

Four grades of varicosis of the great saphenous vein are distinguished according to Hach, depending on the length of involvement from its termination to its origin (◘ Fig. 3.15). Grade I is varicosis of the terminal valve, grade II extension to the distal thigh, grade III to the proximal calf, and grade IV complete incompetence of the vein down to the ankle.

Primary superficial varicosis can in turn lead to pressure and volume overload of the deep venous system with **secondary damage** resulting from the formation of pathways of venous reflux. In this situation, the blood draining through the deep veins reaches a proximal point of insufficiency in the superficial system (typically the terminal valve of the

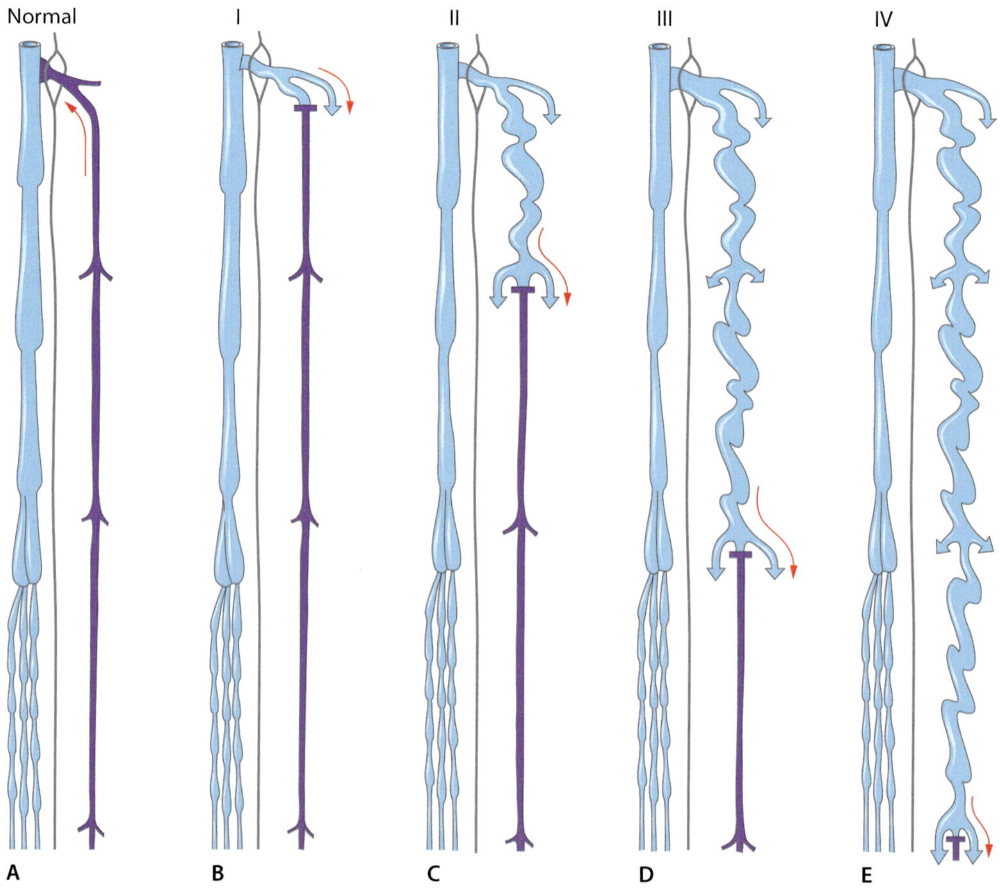

◘ **Fig. 3.15** Grades of truncal varicosis of the great saphenous vein according to Hach: **A** Normal blood flow toward the heart in the great saphenous vein. **B** Grade I: incompetent terminal valve of great saphenous vein, possibly with concomitant lateral branch varicosis of accessory veins. **C** Grade II: varicosis of great saphenous vein in upper leg, possibly with concomitant lateral branch varicosis. **D** Grade III: varicosis of great saphenous vein extending to proximal lower leg, possibly with concomitant varicosis of anterior or posterior tributary vein of lower leg. **E** Grade IV: varicosis of great saphenous vein extending down to ankle region with more or less severe lateral branch varicosis

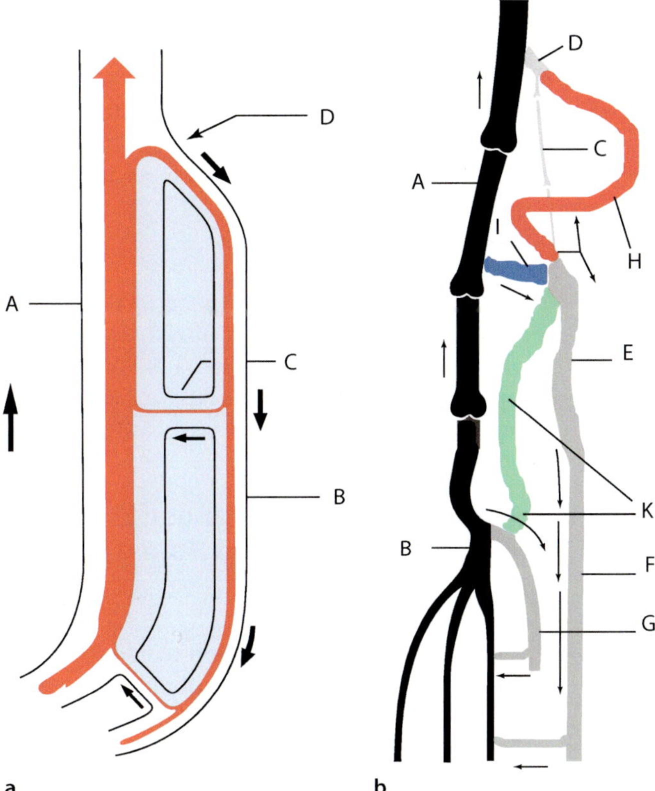

■ **Fig. 3.16** **a** Diagram of the recirculation pathway in superficial venous insufficiency. Part of the blood draining toward the heart in the deep venous system (**A**) flows back to the periphery through an incompetent terminal valve (**D**) or through incompetent superficial veins (great or small saphenous vein; **B**). The blood is then recirculated from the superficial to the deep venous system via perforating veins (**C**), resulting in volume overload of the deep (**A**) leg veins (according to Rieger and Schoop 1998). **b** Diagram of the different forms of incomplete varicosis of the great saphenous vein (red: lateral branch type, anterior variant; blue: perforator type; green: lateral branch type, posterior variant). **A** femoral vein; **B** popliteal vein; **C** competent (intact) proximal portion of the great saphenous vein; **D** terminal valve of great saphenous vein; **E, F** varicose segments of the great saphenous vein in the distal thigh and lower leg; **G** small saphenous vein; **H** lateral accessory saphenous vein; **I** Dodd perforator (incompetent); **K** medial accessory saphenous vein and Giacomini anastomosis (reflux through an incompetent connection between the small saphenous vein, femoropopliteal vein, medial accessory saphenous vein, and great saphenous vein). The proximal point of insufficiency is the transition from the competent to the incompetent great saphenous vein segment (arrows) (see ■ Figs. 3.77 and 3.80 (both Atlas))

great saphenous vein) and then flows back down to the distal point of insufficiency (defined as the highest competent valve or the deepest incompetent valve). At this point, the blood flows back into the deep system and toward the heart (■ Fig. 3.16a). The resulting overload of the perforating and deep veins induces secondary valve incompetence in these veins. When the deep vein valves are competent, this condition is referred to as compensated recirculation and when they become incompetent as decompensated recirculation.

Complete truncal varicosis of the great saphenous vein is characterized by reflux in the saphenofemoral junction (i.e., the terminal valve of the great saphenous vein is incompetent). The ensuing pressure buildup causes secondary failure of distal valves (peripheral varicosis, grading according to Hach, ■ Fig. 3.15).

In **incomplete varicosis** of the great saphenous vein, the proximal valves initially tend to be competent, while the first dysfunctional valve (i.e., the **proximal point of insufficiency**) is more distal. Below this point, the valves of the great saphenous vein are incompetent. In incomplete varicosis, the insufficient junction between the superficial and the deep venous system may involve the perforating veins, a branch of the great saphenous vein, or both. Incompetence of one or more perforating veins is the most common form. In this case, some of the blood entering the superficial system through the incompetent perforator flows into the distal portion of the great saphenous vein below this junction to then re-enter the deep system through a distal perforator.

In the second type, a varicose branch is responsible for reflux between the deep venous system and the proximal point of incompetence of the great saphenous vein (■ Fig. 3.16b). In most cases (55%), the incompetent branch is the lateral accessory saphenous vein (anterior variant); less commonly it is the medial accessory saphenous vein. In the posterior variant, the medial accessory saphenous vein establishes an incompetent venous communication with the proximal small saphenous vein via the femoropopliteal vein (Giacomini anastomosis). In this form of incomplete distal great saphenous vein varicosis, the incompetent Giacomini anastomosis connects the great and small saphenous veins.

Careful sonographic evaluation of the extent of varicosis with identification of the upper and lower points of insufficiency, secondary involvement of the deep venous system, and the presence of recirculation pathways is crucial for selecting the most suitable treatment (obliteration, surgery, compression) (see summary of the components of a comprehensive sonographic evaluation at the end of this section and ■ Table 3.6). **Surgery is performed to remove** the insufficient portion of the affected deep vein between the upper and lower insufficiency points, sparing uninvolved venous segments for later arterial reconstruction. Incompetent superficial segments and perforating veins will invariably lead to recurrent varicosis if they are not removed. This is why precise determination of the distal point of insufficiency and the identification of insufficient perforating veins is crucial for successful surgical management. Duplex ultrasound is the method of choice and gold standard for this indication.

Thrombophlebitis is a typical complication of varicosis and is diagnosed by B-mode sonography using the same criteria as in the assessment of DVT. Since thrombophlebitis often extends beyond its clinically apparent boundaries, identification of the proximal thrombus end by imaging is clinically relevant to rule out involvement of the deep system.

Moreover, further progression of thrombophlebitis into the deep system must be prevented by high ligation of the saphenofemoral junction in cases where the disease process already extends close to the deep veins. Alternatively, transient anticoagulation in combination with local symptomatic measures can be performed to prevent further progression.

B-mode ultrasonography is the most suitable imaging modality both to identify the upper end of the thrombus for the initiation of adequate therapeutic management and to follow up therapy.

A retrospective analysis of the ultrasound findings in 363 patients with thrombophlebitis demonstrated growth of the thrombus into the deep venous system over an observation period of 10 days in 11% of the cases. Seventy percent of these cases were accounted for by great saphenous vein thrombophlebitis with thrombus growth into the common femoral vein (Foley et al. 1989).

Other ultrasound studies of thrombophlebitis show thrombotic involvement of the deep venous system in 11–44% of patients, which is a much higher rate than suspected on the basis of the clinical appearance (Blättler 1993; Blättler et al. 1996; Gaitini 1990; Gaitini et al. 1988; Lutter et al. 1991; Jorgensen et al. 1993; Ascer et al. 1995). Since therapeutic management must encompass the deep veins in these patients, the indication for ultrasonography of the deep leg veins should be established generously.

In patients presenting with chronic venous insufficiency, the question to be answered is whether the condition is due to great or small saphenous vein varicosis or whether it exists in the context of the postthrombotic syndrome. As the therapeutic consequences are different, adequate diagnostic workup always includes evaluation of the morphologic and functional status of the major deep veins. Primary valve incompetence of the superficial veins (varicosis) without involvement of the deep veins is treated by surgical removal of the affected superficial vein segments to prevent dermatologic damage as well as secondary involvement of the deep leg veins due to pressure and volume overload (so-called Trendelenburg private circulation; Hach and Hach-Wunderle 1994). In secondary valve incompetence of the superficial veins with simultaneous deep vein involvement (postthrombotic), on the other hand, excision of the varices will not provide much improvement with regard to venous return. With few exceptions, surgery is not indicated in this situation. Instead, patients, including those operated on, are treated by a rigorous compression regimen (which must also be continued after surgery).

Incomplete recanalization or **nearly complete postthrombotic occlusion** of deep veins is a contraindication to the surgical removal of incompetent superficial vein segments. Tailoring therapeutic procedures to the individual patient relies on precise information regarding the localization and extent of morphologic and hemodynamic abnormalities. Duplex ultrasound is superior to all other imaging modalities in providing this information. To obtain all relevant diagnostic information in patients with varicosis, the ultrasound examination should include the following components:

- Evaluation of major superficial veins (great and small saphenous veins), terminations, recirculation pathways (truncal insufficiency)
- In patients with incomplete truncal varicosis:
  - Determination of the upper point of insufficiency
  - Determination of the lower point of insufficiency
- Identification of incompetent perforating veins
- Demonstration of secondary major vein insufficiency/valve incompetence of major deep veins
- Identification of variant terminations of superficial veins. Morphologic variants
- Detection of (residual) thrombus in the superficial and deep venous systems
- Quantification of poor venous return

If sclerotherapy is planned for the treatment of varicosis of a side branch or mild truncal varicosis, ultrasound can also serve to guide insertion of the thin cannula for injection of the sclerosing agent, particularly in obese patients, and to assess outcome.

3.1.6 Duplex Ultrasound: Diagnostic Criteria, Indications, and Role

3.1.6.1 Thrombosis

The most important sonographic criterion of acute deep or superficial vein thrombosis is incompressibility of the vein when applying pressure with the transducer in transverse orientation (Figs. 3.17, 3.18, 3.19, and 3.21).

Additional sonographic findings supporting the diagnosis of acute deep vein thrombosis (DVT) are:

- Widening of the lumen (other than breathing-related diameter variation)
- Abnormal intraluminal structure of low echogenicity (but more echogenic than flowing blood), may appear inhomogeneous
- Absence of extravascular causes (perivascular structures) of disturbed venous drainage

A fully compressed vein is no longer visible. Only a high-resolution transducer will depict the thin venous wall as an echogenic line within the muscle tissue. Incomplete compressibility indicates a thrombus surrounded by flowing blood (adherent to wall, floating) or partial recanalization after thrombosis with residual thrombus or severe wall sclerosis preventing full compression (Figs. 3.18 and 3.19).

The **examination** is usually performed with the patient lying on the examination table. Having the patient sit or stand may augment blood flow and improve evaluation of the calf veins. In the calf, the presence of a fresh thrombus improves visualization because the hypoechoic dilated vein is more conspicuous than a collapsed vein or a small, thin-walled vein with normal blood flow. A positive compression ultrasound result is nearly 100% specific for DVT of the leg. A negative result can rule out thrombosis in the thigh and in the popliteal fossa with acceptable accuracy. Some uncertainty remains in below-knee thrombosis, even with additional use of color Doppler imaging. If the findings are equivocal and the clinical presentation is highly indicative of thrombosis (high pretest likelihood), additional diagnostic tests should be performed including venography, a D-dimer test or repeat ultrasound after 5 days.

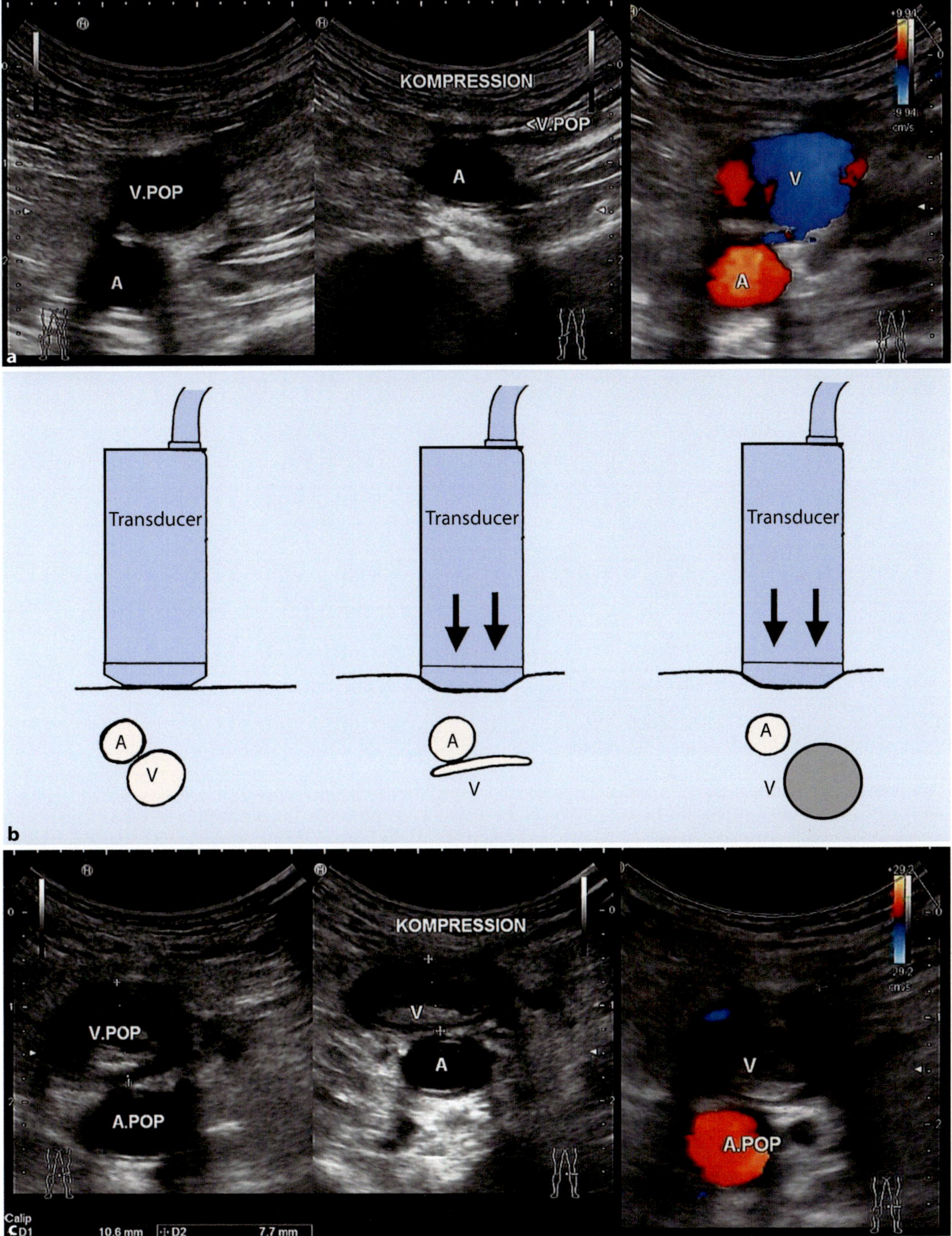

Fig. 3.17 **a** Normal compression ultrasound of the popliteal vein (transducer in popliteal fossa): the vein and artery have similar diameters, and the walls are clearly delineated from surrounding fatty connective tissue (left gray-scale image). Applying pressure with the transducer (right gray-scale image) results in complete compression of the popliteal vein (<V.POP) – the lumen is no longer visible and the delicate walls are just barely distinct from the surrounding tissue. In the color flow image (right), flow in the popliteal artery is encoded in red (A). In the popliteal vein, the main flow direction is encoded in blue (V). There is also some flow in the opposite direction (coded in red) from venous branches joining the popliteal vein at these sites. **b** Diagram of compression ultrasound. A patent vein is completely compressible and virtually disappears when pressure is exerted with the transducer (second drawing). A thrombosed vein retains its shape upon compression (right drawing), while a partially thrombosed or partially recanalized vein can be compressed to some degree. A very fresh thrombus in a large vein may also be compressible to some extent, while the vein itself often has a wider lumen than the unaffected vein or the accompanying artery. A more or less hyperechoic intraluminal structure may be visualized (see Fig. 3.25). **c** Acute thrombosis of the popliteal vein. The fresh thrombus markedly dilates the lumen of the vein (V.POP) (up to twice the size of the adjacent artery). The predominantly low echogenicity of the lumen clearly differentiates the vein from surrounding fatty connective tissue. Application of pressure with the transducer (right gray-scale image) results in flattening of the thrombus, while the vein itself retains its shape. The color flow image (right; low PRF to detect slow flow) shows no flow in the popliteal vein (V) except for some residual marginal flow (blue). This finding corresponds to the rubber phenomenon in venography (Modified from Schäberle 2014)

3

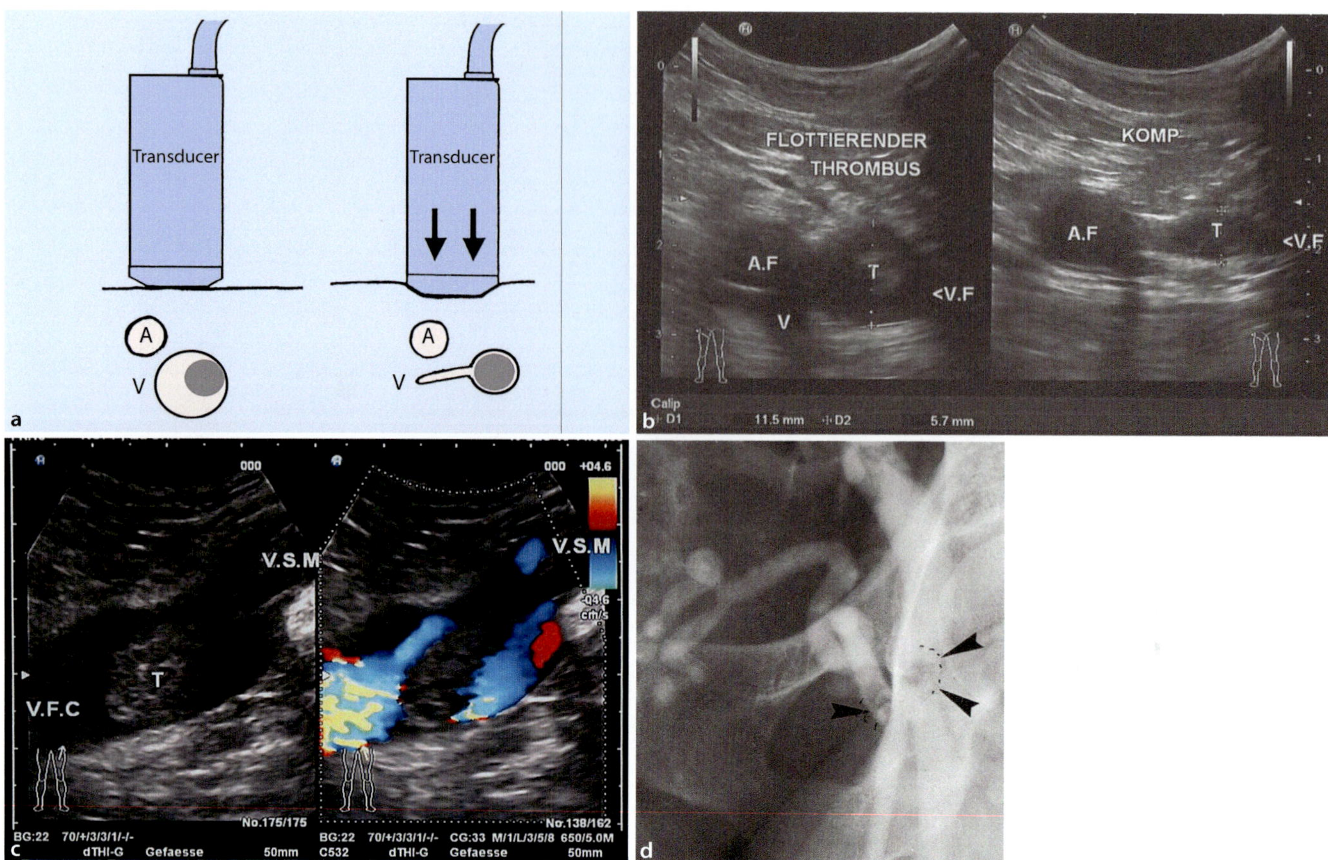

Fig. 3.18 **a** Compression ultrasound findings in partially thrombosed veins. When pressure is applied to a vein containing a mural thrombus surrounded by flowing blood (right drawing), only the patent portion of the lumen is compressible. The delineation of the thrombus within the lumen depends on its echogenicity, which in turn is determined by its composition. **b** B-mode imaging of the femoral vein without compression (left) and with compression (right). Incomplete compressibility of the vein (V.F.) is due to thrombus (T) in the center of the lumen. The thrombus is identified by its higher echogenicity compared with flowing blood. **c** Gray-scale and color flow images showing floating thrombus (T) extending from the great saphenous vein (V.S.M) into the femoral vein (V.F.C). This thrombus prevents full compression of the vein. **d** Venogram confirming the thrombus

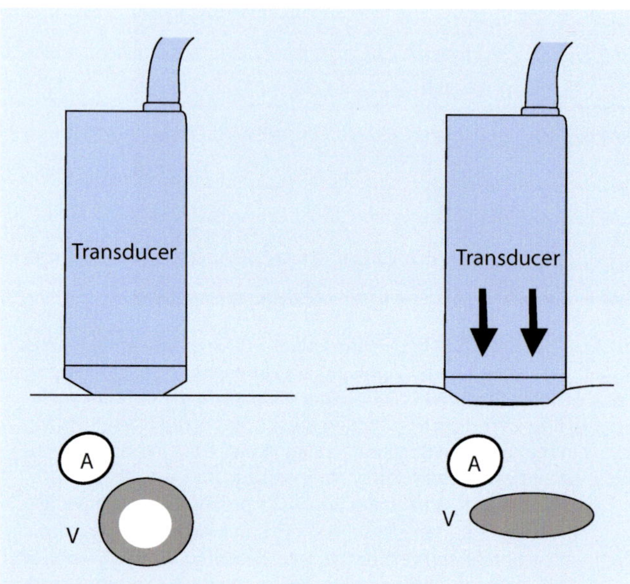

Fig. 3.19 Compression ultrasound of a partially recanalized vein. The extent to which the vein can be compressed depends on the degree of recanalization. Residual mural thrombi prevent full compression (Fig. 3.23)

Incompressibility is a necessary and sufficient criterion for the diagnosis of DVT of the leg. Study results indicate that color duplex imaging does not improve diagnostic accuracy in DVT and tends to be less specific when used alone (i.e., without compression) because slow venous flow or poor imaging conditions below the knee may give rise to false positive findings. Color duplex is required only to diagnose isolated pelvic thrombosis, which is rare. Evaluation of flow in the color duplex mode improves the diagnostic evaluation at the pelvic level, especially in obese patients, in whom compression maneuvers are difficult to perform. Moreover, color duplex imaging enables identification of residual blood flow around a thrombus or floating thrombus and also of recanalized veins, which often have a small lumen (see Fig. 3.23).

Isolated pelvic vein thrombosis is thus the only case in which compression ultrasound alone tends to be unreliable due to the lack of an adequate structure against which to compress the vein and interfering overlying structures. Instead, the diagnosis is based on absent or abnormal flow (compared to the unaffected side) in the Doppler waveform or a gap in color filling in the color duplex mode.

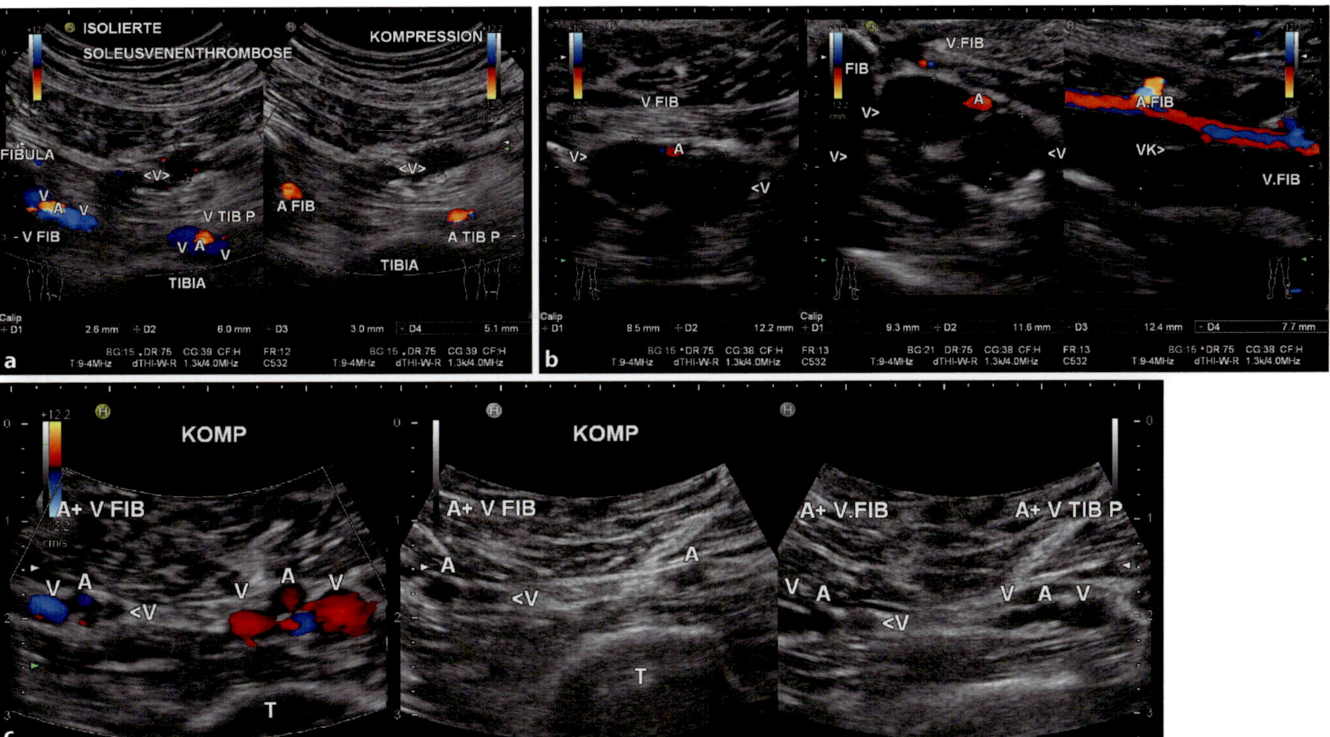

Fig. 3.20 Compression ultrasound findings in different calf veins. **a** Isolated soleus vein thrombosis (<V>) with widening of the affected segment. The lumen is hypoechoic and incompressible (right image). The posterior tibial vein (V TIB P) and fibular vein (V FIB) are patent (left image) and compressible (right image). Color duplex imaging can help the examiner in identifying the main calf veins by first looking for the corresponding arteries, and the evaluation of flow can corroborate the diagnosis made by compression ultrasound. (The images shown are not magnified to illustrate what the examiner will see in the routine clinical situation.) **b** In this example, both branches of the paired fibular vein (V) coursing to the left and right of the artery of the same name, are widely dilated and cannot be compressed (middle image, obtained while applying pressure with the transducer). The diameter is more than twice that of the artery (A), consistent with fresh thrombosis. The intraluminal thrombotic material has low echogenicity and appears homogeneous. The longitudinal color flow image (right) shows no flow in the vein (see Fig. 3.56 (Atlas)), and there is thrombosis at the site of a valve cusp (VK>). **c** Isolated thrombosis of one branch of the paired fibular vein. The thrombosed branch does not collapse (V FIB) when pressure is exerted with the transducer (KOMP, center image), and there is no spontaneous flow in this branch in the color duplex image (left). The shrunken lumen and poor demarcation from surrounding muscle tissue (right image) are signs of older thrombosis. The posterior tibial vein (KOMP, middle image) is compressible, and there is good color filling upon slight manual compression of the calf distal to the transducer (right part of leftmost image) (see Fig. 3.51 (Atlas))

Careful scrutiny of the pelvic axis is indicated if an **abnormal Doppler waveform** with reduced respiratory phasicity and slower flow compared to the contralateral side is obtained **in the distal external iliac vein**. The patient must lie supine with the thigh slightly abducted and externally rotated to ensure undisturbed venous outflow under the inguinal ligament. Flat positioning with the thigh stretched will compress the vein as it courses under the inguinal ligament, reducing or even eliminating respiratory phasicity in the Doppler waveform obtained from this site. However, since even isolated pelvic vein thrombosis typically involves the entire external iliac vein (including drainage through veins of the saphenofemoral junction and abdominal wall), the thrombosis can be demonstrated by B-mode and compression ultrasound above the inguinal ligament. This method of indirect hemodynamic flow analysis in the groin will only miss non-flow-obstructing thrombus (i.e., thrombus extending from the external iliac into the common iliac vein or thrombosis caused by mural thrombi in a partially patent pelvic vein).

The small-caliber vessels below the knee are less well demarcated from the inhomogeneous echotexture of surrounding muscle tissue. Still, the criteria for **isolated vein thrombosis** in this territory are the same as in the thigh.

Better filling of the veins is achieved if the examination is performed in the sitting or standing patient. Since a tubular structure distended by acute thrombosis can be identified more easily than a normal vein, nonvisualization can be interpreted to indicate absence of acute thrombosis. Note, however, that this only holds true for acute venous thrombosis, whereas older thrombi shrink and often become more hyperechoic and inhomogeneous with the venous lumen returning to its normal diameter. Hence, the vein is again more difficult to differentiate from surrounding muscle tissue (Figs. 3.20, 3.50 (Atlas), 3.51 (Atlas), and 3.52 (Atlas)), rendering the method less accurate in identifying older thrombosis below the knee.

Many studies with different study designs conducted in the 1980s and 1990s yielded sensitivities of 88–100% and specificities of >95% for compression ultrasound compared with the then gold standard, venography (Table 3.2). A meta-analysis (with subgroup analysis by site of thrombosis) found >95% sensitivity for the femoropopliteal segment

3

Table 3.2 Studies investigating the diagnostic performance of compression ultrasound, duplex ultrasound, and color duplex ultrasound in larger patient populations with suspected deep vein thrombosis (DVT) of the leg (with venography as the gold standard)

Author/Year	Patients [n]	Thrombosis [n]	Sensitivity [%]	Specificity [%]
Compression ultrasound				
Appelman et al. (1987)	112	52	96	97
Dauzat et al. (1986)[a]	145	100	94	100
Elias et al. (1987)[a]	430	303	98	95
Habscheid et al. (1990)[b]	238	153	96	99
Hobson (1990)	209	–	99	100
Krings et al. (1990)	182	–	95	97
Lensing et al. (1989)[b]	220	66	99	100
Pederson (1991)	215	113	89	97
Herzog et al. (1991)[b]	113	57	88	98
Langholz (1991)	64	25	76	88
Compression ultrasound: analysis of below-knee veins only (thrombosis)[b]				
Habscheid (1990)	37	–	89	99
Elias et al. (1987)	92	–	91	96
Duplex ultrasound				
De Valois et al. (1990)	180	61	92	90
Comerota et al. (1990)	103	44	96	93
Killewich et al. (1989)[b]	47	38	92	92
Van Ramshorst et al. (1991)	117	64	91	95
Schäberle (1991)[b,c]	125	56	97	98
Betzl (1990)	66	–	97	72
Color duplex ultrasound				
Schindler et al. (1990)	97	54	98	100
Grosser et al. (1990)[b]	180	154	94	99
Van Ramshorst et al. (1991)	117	64	91	95
Schönhofer (1992)	100	63	97	98
Miller et al. (1996)	216	98	99	100
Fürst et al. (1990)	102	39	95	99
Persson et al. (1989)[b]	264	16	100	100
Rose et al. (1990)[b]	69	32	79	88
Van Gemmeren et al. (1991)	114	74	96	97
Langholz (1991)	116	65	100	94
Fobbe et al. (1989)	103	58	96	97
Lensing et al. (1989)	220	–	91	99
Krings et al. (1990)	235	–	93	96
Schweizer et al. (1993) (with ultrasound contrast agent)	78	70	96	100

Note that below-knee veins were not included in the examination in all cases
[a]Compression ultrasound, in part, supplemented by CW Doppler
[b]Below-knee veins included in examination and analysis
[c]Compression ultrasound as first-line diagnostic test with optional supplementary duplex ultrasound (primarily to assess pelvic veins and resolve inconclusive findings below the knee)

and 85–90% sensitivity for veins below the knee (Elias et al. 1987; Lensing et al. 1989; Krings et al. 1990; Atri et al. 1996; Habscheid 1990 and 1998; Schäberle 2010). Of note are the studies of Habscheid and Elias et al. because they determined sensitivity and specificity separately for veins below and above the knee. Habscheid (1990) found 88% sensitivity below the knee versus 96% above the knee with 99% specificity for both territories. Elias et al. (1987) found 91% versus 98% sensitivity. These studies have also revealed that venography is a poor gold standard, especially below the knee, where nonvisualization of a vein such as the fibular vein is inconclusive, suggesting either thrombosis or a technical limitation of the method (nonopacification) (◘ Figs. 3.55 and 3.56 (both Atlas)).

In addition to the major veins below the knee (which can be identified using the arteries of the same name as landmarks), the **muscle veins of the gastrocnemius and soleus groups** deserve special attention. They are a common source of DVT, especially in immobilized patients. Stasis of blood flow is common when the muscle veins become ectatic with age. The diagnostic criteria are the same as for thrombosis of the main veins (dilated, incompressible vein, identified as a tubular structure in its typical location in the muscle). Thrombosis of muscle veins below the knee and of the deep femoral vein is rarely detected by venography.

The diagnostic limitations of venography (see ► Sect. 3.1.9) in the evaluation not only of below-knee veins, such as the fibular vein and muscle veins, but also of superficial leg veins led some investigators to abandon venography as the gold standard. Instead, they determined the occurrence of thromboembolic complications in untreated patients (typically at 3-month follow-up) as a measure of the **diagnostic performance of ultrasound**. In other words, they assessed ultrasound in terms of missed thrombosis rather than in comparison to venographic findings. A meta-analysis of 7 studies found a pooled venous thromboembolism event rate of 0.57% (0.25–0.89%) in a total of 4731 patients who did not receive anticoagulation after negative whole-leg compression ultrasound (Johnson et al. 2010). These studies also revealed a difference between outpatients and inpatients (higher prevalence).

In most patients, femoropopliteal thrombosis is due to ascending thrombosis arising in a main vein below the knee or a muscle vein. Surprisingly, a review of therapeutic studies including a total of more than 3500 patients with suspected thrombosis in whom only the territory from the distal external iliac vein (inguinal ligament) to the distal popliteal vein was continuously evaluated using compression ultrasound identified a 3-month thromboembolism rate of only 0.4–2.6% in untreated patients. While this protocol will miss instances of isolated below-knee thrombosis, this has no diagnostic or therapeutic relevance because the clinical course tends to be uncomplicated as long as there is no ascending growth. Nevertheless, various diagnostic algorithms (◘ Fig. 3.21) were proposed to minimize the risk of thromboembolic complications from ascending growth of missed below-knee thrombosis (Bernardi et al. 1998; Cogo et al. 1998; Perrier et al. 1999; Wells et al. 1997) (◘ Table 3.3). Specifically, investigators used the following measures **to supplement diagnostic workup in patients with negative ultrasound findings but clinically suspected thrombosis**:

- Repeat compression ultrasound after 1 week (Cogo et al. 1998)
- D-dimer test for risk stratification before repeat ultrasound (Bernardi et al. 1998)
- Supplementary venography in patients with a relevant risk but negative compression ultrasound (Perrier et al. 1999)
- Repeat compression ultrasound in patients with initially negative compression ultrasound; venography only in patients with a high likelihood of thrombosis based on a set of clinical criteria (Wells et al. 1997).

All of these algorithms were proposed to remedy the diagnostic uncertainty of compression ultrasound in the calf (85–90% sensitivity) by supplementary measures. The most common strategies include the highly sensitive but rather unspecific D-dimer test, repeat ultrasound after 1 week, and venography in high-risk patients (◘ Table 3.3). Based on empirical and clinical experience, patients with suspected venous thrombosis can be assigned to a high-probability or a low-probability group on the basis of their risk factors, the severity of clinical signs, and the likelihood of alternative conditions that may explain their symptoms. This risk stratification guides further diagnostic management if the ultrasound findings are inconclusive. For instance, high-risk patients will undergo supplementary venography or a D-dimer test, while no further diagnostic measures will be taken in patients with a low risk (◘ Fig. 3.21).

Some of the **diagnostic algorithms** proposed in the literature are rather complex. In the hands of an experienced examiner, compression ultrasound yields clinically acceptable results despite its limitations below the knee. In a study of 1265 patients in whom treatment decisions were made on the basis of a complete compression ultrasound examination of the leg veins, 0.3% of patients with negative findings experienced a thromboembolic event during 3-month follow-up (Schellong et al. 2003). This low risk of DVT in patients with negative ultrasound examinations including the calf veins was confirmed in another study, which reported thromboembolic complications in 0.5% of cases (Elias et al. 2003) (see ► Sect. 3.1.9.1 and ◘ Fig. 3.38).

The **diagnostic accuracy of ultrasound including the veins below the knee** is also confirmed by large cohort studies conducted more recently (Stevens et al. 2004; Subramaniam et al. 2005; Sevestre et al. 2009; Stevens et al. 2013). The residual failure rate is less than 1%, which is at the upper limit of the 95% confidence interval. Note, however, that cohort studies often include many patients with a low pretest likelihood of disease. The only study that selectively investigated patients with a high pretest probability (n = 167) (Stevens et al. 2013) found a low thromboembolism rate of 0.6% at 3 months in patients with prior negative ultrasound above and below the knee (see ► Sect. 3.1.9.1).

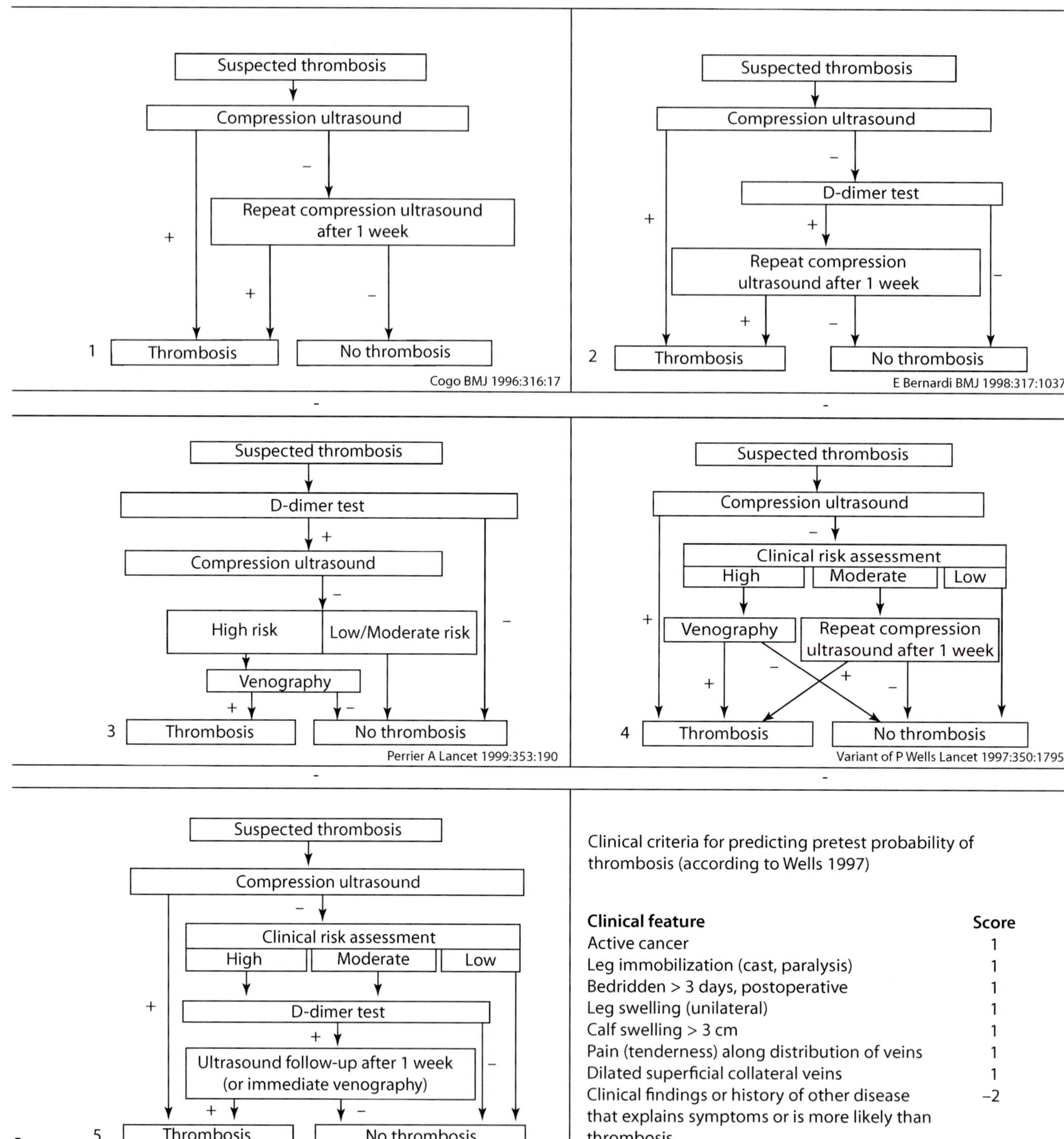

Clinical criteria for predicting pretest probability of thrombosis (according to Wells 1997)

Clinical feature	**Score**
Active cancer	1
Leg immobilization (cast, paralysis)	1
Bedridden > 3 days, postoperative	1
Leg swelling (unilateral)	1
Calf swelling > 3 cm	1
Pain (tenderness) along distribution of veins	1
Dilated superficial collateral veins	1
Clinical findings or history of other disease that explains symptoms or is more likely than thrombosis	–2

Fig. 3.21 **a** Algorithms for the diagnostic management of deep vein thrombosis (DVT) of the legs. The clinical risk of DVT is assessed by means of a scale with a score greater than 2 indicating a high risk of thrombosis and a score of 1 or 2 a moderate risk. Charts 1–4: Algorithms used in prospective studies with compression ultrasound restricted to veins above the knee including the popliteal vein. Chart 5: Diagnostic algorithm with compression ultrasound of the veins above and below the knee and procedure in patients with inconclusive findings below the knee (according to W. Habscheid). No further diagnostic tests are required in patients with a moderate risk and negative ultrasonography of the calf performed by an experienced examiner (see Fig. 3.38). **b** Algorithm for the diagnostic management of DVT using whole-leg compression ultrasound as the only diagnostic test; 3-month thrombosis rate of 0.3% in the group with negative ultrasound findings (Schellong et al. 2003)

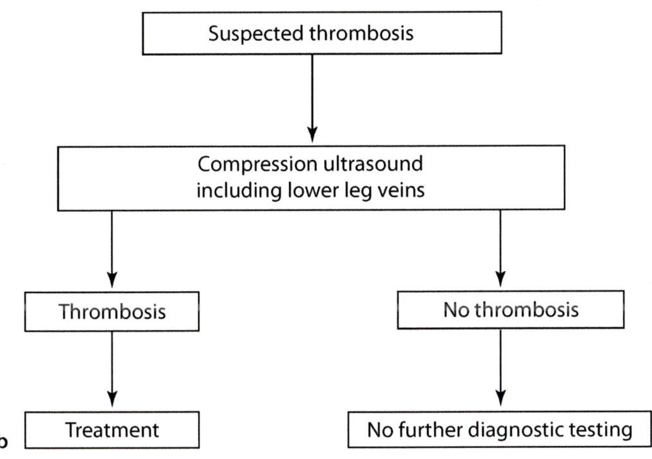

Fig. 3.21 (continued)

The largest database was analyzed in the above-quoted study of Johnson et al. (2010). This meta-analysis of the diagnostic accuracy of a single compression ultrasound examination for ruling out DVT included 7 studies totaling 4731 patients with negative whole-leg compression ultrasound who did not receive anticoagulation. The rate of clinically apparent venous thromboembolism in this population was only 0.57% during 3-month follow-up.

Data on the **outcome of thrombosis** indicate that patients with completely recanalized veins have a lower risk of recurrence than patients whose veins recanalize only incompletely (1.3% versus 23.3%). In a group of 180 patients with residual thrombosis after 3 months of anticoagulation (69% of the total study population), recurrent thrombosis occurred in 19.3% of patients who continued anticoagulation treatment and in 27.2% of patients who discontinued treatment (Siragusa et al. 2008). In the group of 78 patients (31%) without sonographic evidence of relevant postthrombotic residues (complete recanalization), there was only one case of recurrent thrombosis. These results indicate that follow-up ultrasound findings at 3 and 6 months are helpful in identifying patients who might benefit from prolonged anticoagulant treatment.

Another study using serial ultrasound follow-up found a cumulative incidence of postthrombotic states without major postthrombotic residues in 38.8% of cases at 6 months, 58.1% of cases at 12 months, 69.3% at 24 months, and 73.8% at 36 months (Prandoni et al. 2002 and 2009). In this population of initially 313 patients, 41 of the 58 patients with recurrent thrombosis had major postthrombotic residues (hazard ratio of 2.4, 95% confidence interval: 1.3–4.4; $p = 0.004$; patients with residual thrombosis versus patients with early recanalization).

These findings suggest that, in patients with sonographic evidence of **major residual thrombosis**, the risk of recurrent thrombosis can be reduced by prolonging anticoagulation treatment.

Recanalization after an episode of DVT is subject to individual variation, which is why a postthrombotic vein may no longer be compressible and compression ultrasound is less

Table 3.3 Prospective therapeutic studies of patients with clinically suspected deep vein thrombosis (DVT) of the legs and diagnostic workup based on compression ultrasound of the proximal leg veins including the popliteal vein using the algorithms presented in Fig. 3.21a (According to Bounameaux 2002)

Study	Cogo 1998	Bernardi 1998	Wells 1997	Perrier 1999
Diagnostic tests	rCUS	rCUS + DD	rCUS + PP	CUS + DD + PP
Diagnostic algorithm (see Fig. 3.21a)	1	2	4	3
Number of patients	1702	946	593	474
Prevalence of thrombosis	24%	28%	16%	24%
PP	–	–	Score	Empirical
DD	–	Yes	–	Yes
CUS	100%	100%	100%	73%
rCUS	76%	9%	28%	0%
Abnormal rCUS	0.9%	5.7%	1.8%	–
Venography	0%	0%	6%	0.4%
3-month risk of thromboembolism in untreated group	0.7%	0.4%	0.6%	2.6%

CUS compression ultrasound, *rCUS* repeat compression ultrasound, *DD* D-dimer test, *PP* estimation of pretest probability

specific in diagnosing **recurrent thrombosis** (false positive results). There are several sonographic findings that suggest recurrent thrombosis. One is the presence of a markedly dilated, incompressible vein segment (◘ Fig. 3.26c) proximal to a partially recanalized venous segment (with demonstration of flow by color duplex). Another sonographic criterion indicating recurrence is a central flow void that represents a thrombus surrounded by flowing blood (comparable to the rubber phenomenon in venography). In contrast, restored flow in a formerly thrombosed segment tends to occur centrally and take a meandering course (◘ Fig. 3.23). Incompressibility of a previously normal vein segment is nearly 100% diagnostic of recurrent thrombosis but requires meticulous documentation of serial ultrasound findings for comparison (Prandoni et al. 1993). It is therefore recommended to perform a comprehensive color duplex ultrasound evaluation at the end of anticoagulation treatment (usually 6 months after the onset of thrombosis) to establish a new baseline for future examinations, typically when recurrence is suspected on clinical grounds.

Patients with complete recanalization following an episode of acute vein thrombosis and at least partially competent valves (based on duplex testing of reflux) can be allowed to discontinue elastic compression stocking therapy (Ten Cate-Hoek et al. 2010).

3.1.6.1.1 Controversy About the Ultrasound Strategy in Suspected Deep Vein Thrombosis

Abbreviated examination protocols not including the veins below the knee in the diagnostic evaluation of patients with clinically suspected lower extremity deep vein thrombosis (DVT) are mainly used in North America. The rationale for only examining the venous territory from the inguinal ligament to the tibiofibular junction is that the risk of pulmonary embolism from thrombosed veins below this level is very low (<3%) and that postthrombotic changes in the calf veins have little clinical relevance. If the calf veins are not included, then one can just as well restrict compression ultrasound evaluation to two representative sites (**two-point strategy**) without a relevant loss of information. The two sites are:

- the femoral bifurcation (i.e., the segment from the inguinal ligament to the confluence of the superficial and deep femoral veins) and
- the popliteal vein (i.e., from the adductor canal to the tibiofibular junction) (◘ Fig. 3.22).

The justification for the two-point strategy is that isolated femoral vein thrombosis is extremely rare (Frederick et al. 1996; Pezzullo et al. 1996). The junction of the external iliac and common femoral vein is virtually always involved in descending thrombosis, while the popliteal vein is involved in ascending thrombosis arising in a calf vein. Isolated superficial femoral vein thrombosis is virtually confined to individuals with duplication of this vein (see ◘ Fig. 3.58 (Atlas)). In duplication, one branch may be thrombosed and the other patent (Cogo et al. 1998). The other exception is thrombophlebitis with thrombus growth into the femoral vein through a Dodd perforator.

Proponents claim that not including the superficial femoral vein in the sonographic workup of suspected lower extremity thrombosis reduces the examination time by 30–50%. Two large prospective randomized studies (each including approx. 1000 patients) confirm that the rate of thromboembolism is not much higher in patients examined using the **two-point strategy** (◘ Fig. 3.22) plus D-dimer test compared to patients undergoing whole-leg ultrasound (Bernardi et al. 2008; Gibson et al. 2009). In the study of Bernardi et al., the thrombotic complication rate was 1.2% in the whole-leg ultrasound group versus 0.9% in the two-point ultrasound group. In the latter group, ultrasound was repeated after 1 week if the initial examination was negative but the D-dimer test was positive.

In the prospective management study of Gibson et al. (2009), 1002 consecutive patients with suspected DVT underwent clinical probability assessment and a D-dimer test. In this way, 481 (48%) of patients with low clinical probability and normal D-dimer findings were excluded (0.4% thromboembolic complication rate), and the remaining patients were randomized to a complete compression ultrasound examination or a rapid protocol, which examines the veins in the groin and the knee. DVT was confirmed in 23% of the 257 patients who underwent two-point ultrasound and in 38% of the 264 patients who underwent a complete examination. The incidence of venous thromboembolism during follow-up was 2% in the former and 1.2% in the latter.

While detection of isolated calf vein thrombosis remains a problem for the two-point protocol, the risk of thromboembolic complications arising from missed calf vein thrombosis appears to be much lower than expected. In the above-quoted study of Gibson et al. (2009), the rate of missed thromboses was 65%; however, only a small number of additional thromboembolic complications were observed (4 versus 2 patients or 2% versus 1.2%) compared with patients examined by whole-leg compression ultrasound including the calf veins. A higher rate of venous thromboembolism in patients with untreated isolated calf thrombosis was found in the CALTHRO study (Palareti et al. 2010). In this study, ultrasound was positive in 15.3% of 431 patients examined for isolated calf vein thrombosis. While untreated calf vein thrombosis progressed to the proximal main vein (popliteal vein) in only 3.1% of cases, the 3-month thromboembolic complication rate was significantly higher in the group with calf vein thrombosis than in the group without calf vein thrombosis (7.8% versus 0.8%, $p = 0.003$). However, not counting two patients in whom repeat ultrasound after 1 week detected ascending thrombus growth, the difference became barely significant (4.7% versus 0.8%, $p = 0.049$).

The authors of a meta-analysis (Righini et al. 2005) found good safety profiles for complete proximal and distal ultrasound examinations versus examinations limited to the proximal veins with similar pooled estimates of the 3-month thromboembolic rate (0.6% versus 0.4%). However, they also found that calf vein thrombosis accounted for 50%

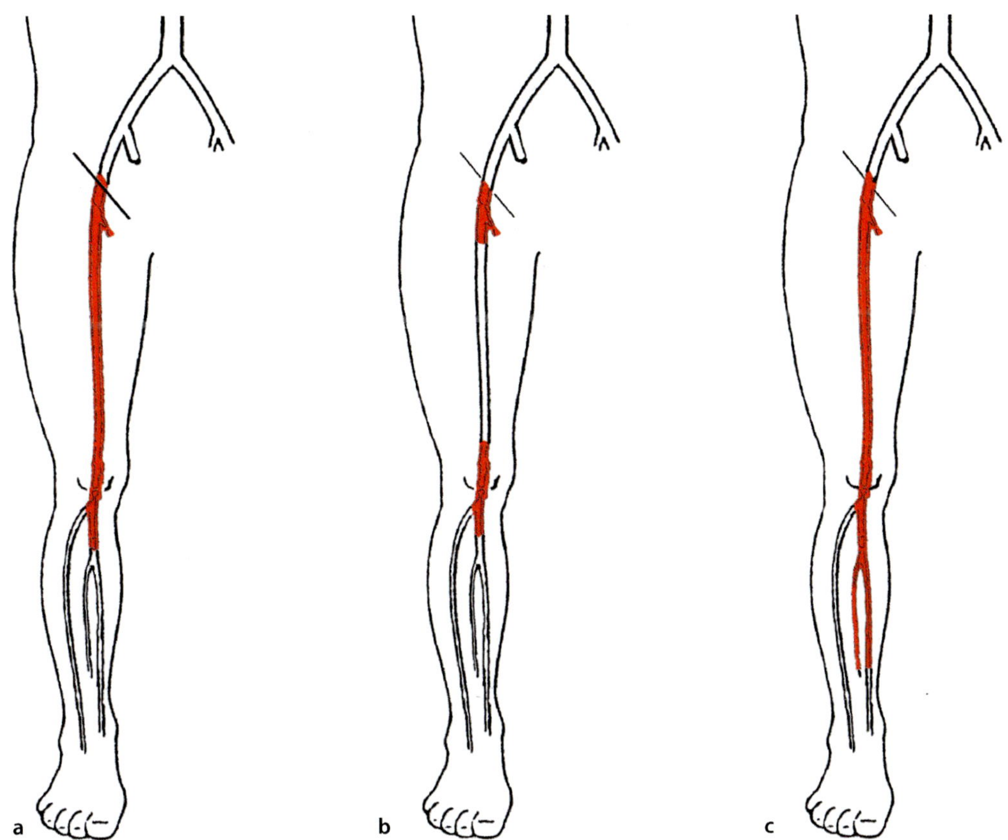

Fig. 3.22a–c Diagnostic evaluation of patients with suspected deep vein thrombosis (DVT) of the legs using compression ultrasound. There is no agreement about the venous segments that should be included in the examination. **a** Compression ultrasound from the inguinal ligament to the distal popliteal vein using a standardized algorithm (see Fig. 3.21); this approach is based on the assumption that calf vein thrombosis rarely causes thromboembolic complications. **b** Reduced examination of the femoral vein (from the inguinal ligament to just below the site of entry of the deep femoral vein) and of the popliteal vein (two-point strategy). This approach assumes that isolated thrombosis of the superficial femoral vein is rare, which is why this vein is not included in the examination. **c** Compression ultrasound from the inguinal ligament to the distal portion of the calf veins (whole-leg strategy). The anterior tibial vein need not be included in the basic examination (except in patients with trauma of the anterior compartment) as no cases of isolated anterior tibial thrombosis have yet been reported

of patients with positive findings in the series undergoing whole-leg ultrasound, concluding that searching for distal deep vein thrombosis potentially doubles the number of patients given anticoagulant therapy and may result in overtreatment.

The controversy about the **clinical and therapeutic relevance of isolated calf vein thrombosis** and its diagnosis is not over. The risk of thromboembolic complications and late valve failure is considered to be low (Moser and LeMoine 1981). Moreover, experience also suggests that many patients with calf vein thrombosis will never develop symptoms. There is only one study showing a significantly increased rate of thromboembolic complications in patients not treated by long-term anticoagulation for calf vein thrombosis (Lagerstedt et al. 1985), and this was in a rather small patient population. Other authors have shown that isolated calf thrombosis will progress proximally into the popliteal vein and farther in about 20% of untreated patients (Kakkar et al. 1969; Langerstedt 1985; Cornus et al. 1999; Gottlieb et al. 2003).

Even less scientific evidence is available on the **significance of muscle vein thrombosis**. In the clinical setting, though, we keep encountering patients with popliteal vein thrombosis that has arisen from isolated soleus vein thrombosis. This is especially common in the elderly, in whom these veins are dilated. The soleus veins drain into the posterior tibial and fibular veins, and thrombus growth into the major deep veins of the calf was observed in 16% of cases. Gastrocnemius veins drain into the popliteal vein, and here, growth into the popliteal vein was observed in only 3% of cases over a period of 2 weeks. This can be interpreted to justify short anticoagulation treatment. Because dilated thrombosed veins are tender, the patient can direct the examiner to the disease focus during the compression ultrasound examination. Dilated calf veins are more conspicuous sonographically, making them easier to identify than normal or collapsed veins (Figs. 3.17 and 3.19).

In conclusion, although **isolated calf vein thrombosis as such rarely causes thromboembolic complication, timely anticoagulation treatment is indicated to prevent proximal progression**. In the German-speaking countries, the general strategy is to include the calf veins in the compression ultrasound examination of patients with suspected

DVT. Evaluation of the calf veins requires little extra time and is also advocated here although the sonographic examination is less reliable below the knee. Negative ultrasound findings in this territory despite a high pretest likelihood of disease may be attributable to poor insonation conditions. In such cases, the risk of thromboembolic complications from proximal propagation of undetected calf vein thrombosis can be minimized by proceeding according to one of the above-discussed algorithms (▣ Fig. 3.21), treating inconclusive findings as if no prior examination of the calf veins took place. The most practical procedure then is to perform a D-dimer test or repeat the ultrasound examination after 1 week.

Another advantage of including the calf veins in the examination is that ultrasound additionally allows evaluation of soft tissue and identification of a ruptured Baker's cyst (▣ Fig. 3.90 (Atlas)), which has a clinical presentation that is surprisingly similar to that of DVT. Other conditions that can be identified by ultrasound include hematoma, fluid collections in muscle compartments after trauma, and abscess.

3.1.6.1.2 Additional Examination of the Asymptomatic Leg

There is also disagreement about the need to examine the asymptomatic leg when deep vein thrombosis (DVT) has been diagnosed in the other. In the past, when the diagnosis of thrombosis mainly relied on venography, the invasiveness of the procedure with radiation exposure and contrast medium administration precluded the additional examination of the asymptomatic leg. This policy was continued even after venography had been replaced by compression ultrasound. The debate about whether or not to examine the contralateral leg as well was stoked by conflicting evidence regarding the incidence of thrombosis in the asymptomatic leg (Scheiman et al. 1995; Strotham et al. 1995). Published incidences range from less than 1% (Cronan 1996, 1997; Naidich et al. 1996; Sheiman et al. 1995) to more than 20%; however, such high rates are mostly found in patients with neoplastic thrombus or in fully immobilized patients. Most cases of contralateral disease involve the calf veins and have a low risk of thromboembolism. Since systemic anticoagulation is initiated for thrombosis of the symptomatic leg anyway, any thrombosis present in the contralateral leg will be simultaneously treated as well. If ultrasound rules out suspected thrombosis in the symptomatic leg, the likelihood of finding a thrombus in the other leg is less than 0.5%. These patients should then undergo venography because the high diagnostic accuracy of compression ultrasound in detecting calf vein thrombosis is limited to symptomatic disease, and when no symptoms are present, the sensitivity drops to less than 60%.

In summary, while the low incidence of thrombus in the asymptomatic leg does not seem to justify its routine examination, the asymptomatic side should be examined in patients with neoplastic thrombosis and in patients who are completely immobilized for an extended period of time.

In patients with **clinically suspected bilateral DVT**, careful evaluation of the clinical symptoms is essential to rule out other more common causes of bilateral disease (lymphogenic or cardiac). In patients with risk factors for DVT (paraneoplasia, immobilization, clotting disorder), the indication for bilateral examination should be established generously.

3.1.6.1.3 Pulmonary Embolism

Pulmonary embolism is sometimes incidentally detected by computed tomography (especially in immobilized ICU patients), or it may present with severe or very sudden symptoms without any prior signs of DVT. Historically, patients with pulmonary embolism were examined by bilateral venography to identify the underlying cause; results of studies from that time indicate that even bilateral venography failed to detect thrombosis in one third of these patients (Cronan 1993; Smith et al. 1994; Stein et al. 1993). As suspected leg thrombosis is asymptomatic in these patients, it is unclear whether compression ultrasound would be helpful in this setting – given its poor sensitivity in the absence of clinical symptoms (<60–70%). Anticoagulation treatment of pulmonary embolism will also have a therapeutic effect on pelvic vein thrombosis, if present. While a large number of sonographic examinations need to be performed to detect pelvic or leg thrombosis in a patient population with pulmonary embolism (although it is the most likely cause of embolism), the author nevertheless recommends bilateral compression ultrasound to identify the site of thrombosis in these patients. Depending on the findings, additional compression treatment may have to be instituted, one reason being to prevent the development of postthrombotic syndrome. The detection of a free-floating thrombus by color duplex imaging can affect the therapeutic regimen despite the controversy about immobilization in this situation.

The poor performance in detecting DVT after clinically suspected pulmonary embolism also shows that ultrasound or venography of the legs cannot replace **CT** for the **exclusion of pulmonary embolism** in this setting (Killewich et al. 1993; Sheiman et al. 1999). Contrast-enhanced spiral CT is the method of choice for ruling out pulmonary embolism. It is an open question, however, whether a CT scan is also necessary for confirmation and assessment in patients who have clinical signs and symptoms of pulmonary embolism and DVT of the leg and in whom thrombosis has been confirmed by compression ultrasound and anticoagulation treatment has been initiated. The necessity depends on the clinical severity of pulmonary embolism (Rosen et al. 1996; Goodman and Lipchick 1996).

The risk of inadvertently **inducing pulmonary embolism when performing compression ultrasound** in patients with DVT must be taken seriously and implies that compression must be performed gently at the proximal end of a thrombus, especially when dealing with a free-floating thrombus. Many examiners with a long experience in evaluating venous thrombosis (Perlin 1992; Schroeder and Bealer 1992) have probably witnessed the (luckily very rare) occurrence of pulmonary embolism while performing a compression ultrasound examination. There are even some anecdotal case reports of examinations in which the migration of thrombotic material from the proximal thrombus end was actually documented (◘ Fig. 3.80 (Atlas)). In all published reports, the pulmonary embolism induced by compression ultrasound was asymptomatic. The true prevalence of (small) pulmonary embolisms following compression ultrasound is difficult to estimate, even more so as thrombi extending above the knee are associated with spontaneous, clinically irrelevant, and asymptomatic pulmonary embolism in >50% of cases (Cronan 1993).

Chest ultrasound has over 90% accuracy in diagnosing pulmonary embolism, including small peripheral defects (Mathis et al. 2005). The detection of peripheral embolism by the sonographic identification of defects near the pleura has no prognostic implications for recurrent embolism or death in clinically asymptomatic patients with deep vein thrombosis; this is why routine chest ultrasound (Egbring and Görg 2007) or other tests for diagnosing pulmonary embolism are not necessary in this setting.

3.1.6.1.4 Diagnostic Tests Supplementing Compression Ultrasound

In patients with inconclusive sonographic findings, the D-dimer test is of limited value. The test has very low specificity (approx. 50%), and D-dimer levels are also elevated in patients with other conditions in which coagulation is activated such as surgery, bleeding, sepsis, trauma, pregnancy, and inflammation. The sensitivity of the D-dimer test is very high (about 95%) in extensive thrombosis, but may be as low as 65% in isolated calf vein thrombosis (depending on the assay used), which is also more difficult to detect by ultrasound (Jennersjo et al. 2005).

Venography is still used as the gold standard but also has poorer performance in the calf, for several reasons: nonopacification of the fibular veins may be due to thrombus or technical limitations, and adequate opacification of all vein segments of interest fails in about 10–20% of cases. Evaluation for muscle vein thrombosis is time-consuming or impossible.

For these reasons, patients in whom the venogram does not allow adequate evaluation of all relevant vein segments in the calf should undergo a supplementary ultrasound examination (see ◘ Figs. 3.55 and 3.56 (both Atlas)). A thrombus in a duplicated vein may also escape detection by venography (◘ Figs. 3.57 and 3.58 (both Atlas)).

While studies have demonstrated no advantage of **color duplex ultrasound** over compression ultrasound in diagnosing acute DVT of the legs, it is helpful in evaluating recanalization and in identifying thrombus surrounded by flowing blood (◘ Fig. 3.23) or free-floating thrombus. If a fresh thrombus is partially surrounded by flowing blood, color duplex imaging will detect flow signals along the vein wall (between the thrombus and the wall). This is distinct from early recanalization, which is characterized by flow confined to the center of the vein or a meandering flow pattern (◘ Fig. 3.23).

The supplementary diagnostic information provided by color duplex ultrasound in acute DVT of the leg can be summarized as follows:

- Detection of residual flow near the wall
- Identification of collaterals
- Evaluation of veins at the pelvic level
- Demonstration of recanalization
- Direct visualization of patent calf veins

At the pelvic level, where it is not always possible to reliably test compressibility of veins (no abutment, obesity), color duplex ultrasound can be used instead to evaluate flow: the absence of flow signals (color flow imaging and spectral Doppler analysis) indicates pelvic vein thrombosis; conversely, color duplex demonstration of blood flow with normal respiratory phasicity in the Doppler waveform indicates patency despite incompressibility.

If the main calf veins are difficult to delineate from surrounding muscle tissue by color duplex imaging, the examiner can try and detect spontaneous or augmented venous flow along the accompanying arteries. Venous flow is augmented by compressing the leg below the point of examination. Collateral circulation will be detectable in patients with longer-standing thrombosis (dilated veins with spontaneous flow signals in the deep and superficial compartments). The presence of collateral pathways is an additional criterion for differentiating older and more recent thrombosis and recurrence (see ◘ Figs. 3.51 and 3.53 (both Atlas)).

Documentation of the patency of all relevant veins by duplex ultrasound is time-consuming and would prohibit the liberal use of ultrasound advocated by the author. Therefore, all ultrasound laboratories should implement a standardized and efficient algorithm for the diagnostic management of patients with suspected acute DVT. This can be done using compression ultrasound, which enables examination of both legs in approx. 10–15 min.

In conclusion, the indications for compression ultrasound and (supplementary) color duplex ultrasound in the diagnostic workup of patients with suspected DVT of the leg may be summarized as follows:

- Indications for gray-scale ultrasound/compression ultrasound:
  - Evaluation of thrombosis (exclusion, confirmation, extent, age) with localization and differentiation (main veins, muscle veins)
  - Thrombophlebitis (extent, thrombus protrusion into major deep vein)
  - Follow-up (spontaneous resolution, thrombolysis, thrombectomy)
  - Differential diagnosis: identification of perivascular structures compressing the vein (Baker's cyst, soft tissue tumor, hematoma, abscess, wall tumor)
- Indications for color duplex ultrasound:
  - Follow-up after thrombosis (spontaneous or thrombolysis-induced recanalization)
  - Pelvic vein thrombosis
  - Floating thrombus
  - Chronic venous insufficiency/postthrombotic syndrome (valve incompetence of deep leg veins: severity of reflux, extent, degree of recanalization)

3

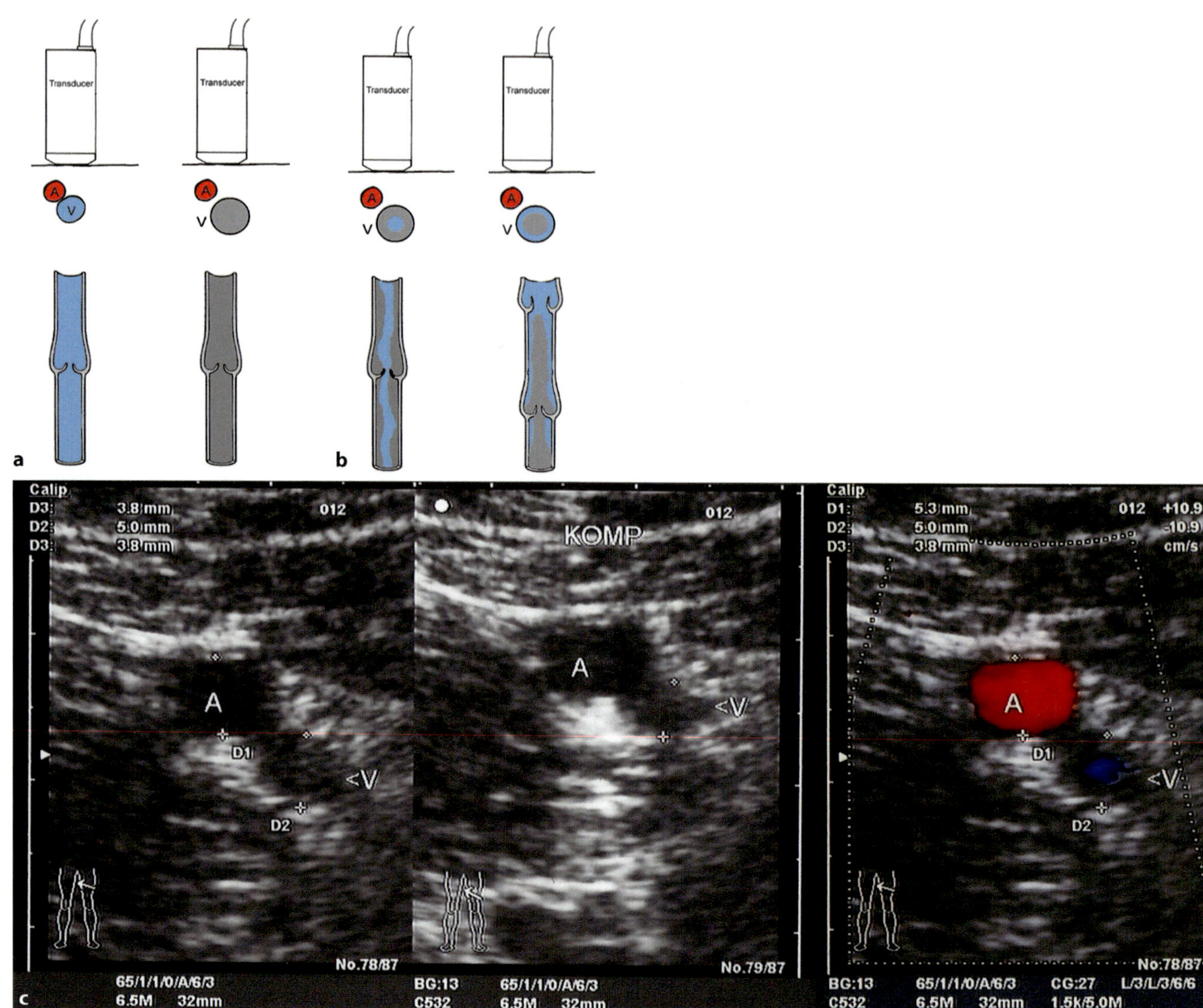

Fig. 3.23a–e Diagnostic role of color duplex imaging in deep vein thrombosis (DVT). **a** Color duplex imaging does not significantly improve diagnostic accuracy compared with compression ultrasound, providing no additional information for ruling out thrombosis (left drawing) or detecting occlusive thrombosis (right drawing) (see Fig. 3.17). **b** Color duplex offers advantages in detecting recanalization and estimating its degree (left drawing) because it depicts spontaneous or augmented flow (e.g., Valsalva maneuver); it also offers advantages in identifying nonocclusive mural thrombus or free-floating thrombus (right drawing) by detecting flow signals around the thrombus (again, this may require a provocative maneuver). Settings must be adjusted to depict slow flow (low PRF). **c** Ultrasound examination performed 6 months after an episode of acute DVT of the leg: in the left image (without compression), the shrunken lumen of the femoral vein (<V) is less clearly delineated from surrounding muscle and connective tissue compared with the lumen of the artery (A). The second image, obtained while applying pressure with the transducer, shows incomplete compressibility of the vein (see Fig. 3.19) with a diameter reduction from 5 to 3.8 mm (calipers). The color duplex image (right) reveals the cause of poor compressibility (see **b**) in this patient: there is only a small recanalized channel with flow coded in blue in the center of the superficial femoral vein (V). The thin recanalization channel indicates a high residual thrombus burden, which can be calculated from vein diameters measured with and without compression as follows: residual vein thrombosis (RVT) = 3.8 mm × 100/5 mm = 76% (for more details see Fig. 3.24b). **d** Longitudinal view (left) and transverse view (right) of thrombus in the popliteal vein (V.POP) partially surrounded by flowing blood. All features of acute thrombosis are present: hypoechoic, markedly dilated vein, good demarcation from perivascular connective tissue, and marginal flow. These features differentiate this case from older thrombosis with partial recanalization (corresponding to the rubber phenomenon in venography). **e** Transverse view (left) and longitudinal view (right) of popliteal vein thrombosis with beginning recanalization (6 weeks after onset): there are flow signals in the center of the lumen (meandering flow and multiple recanalized channels are also present). The Doppler waveform from this segment reflects the flow obstruction due to extensive residual thrombosis: flow is slow and respiratory phasicity is lost

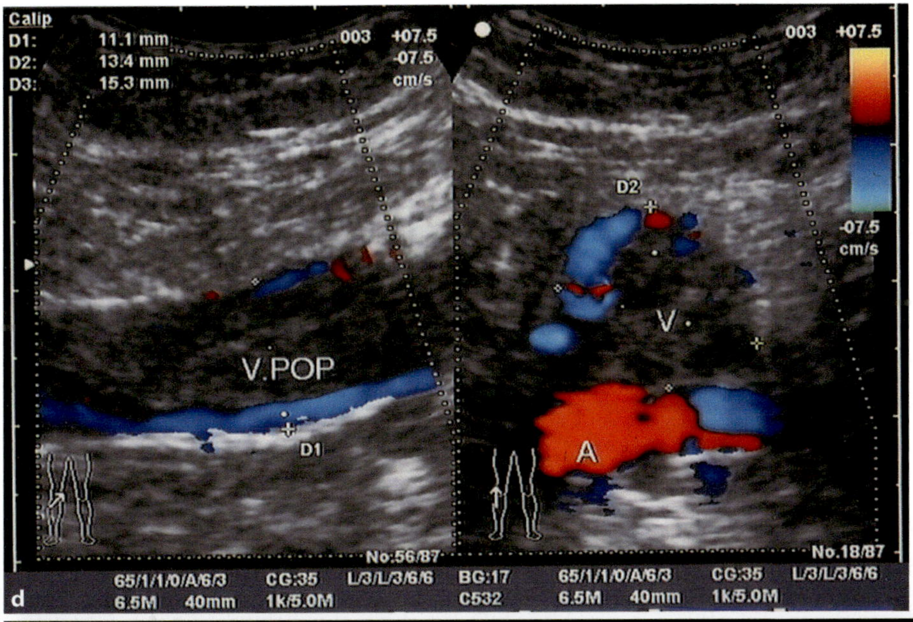

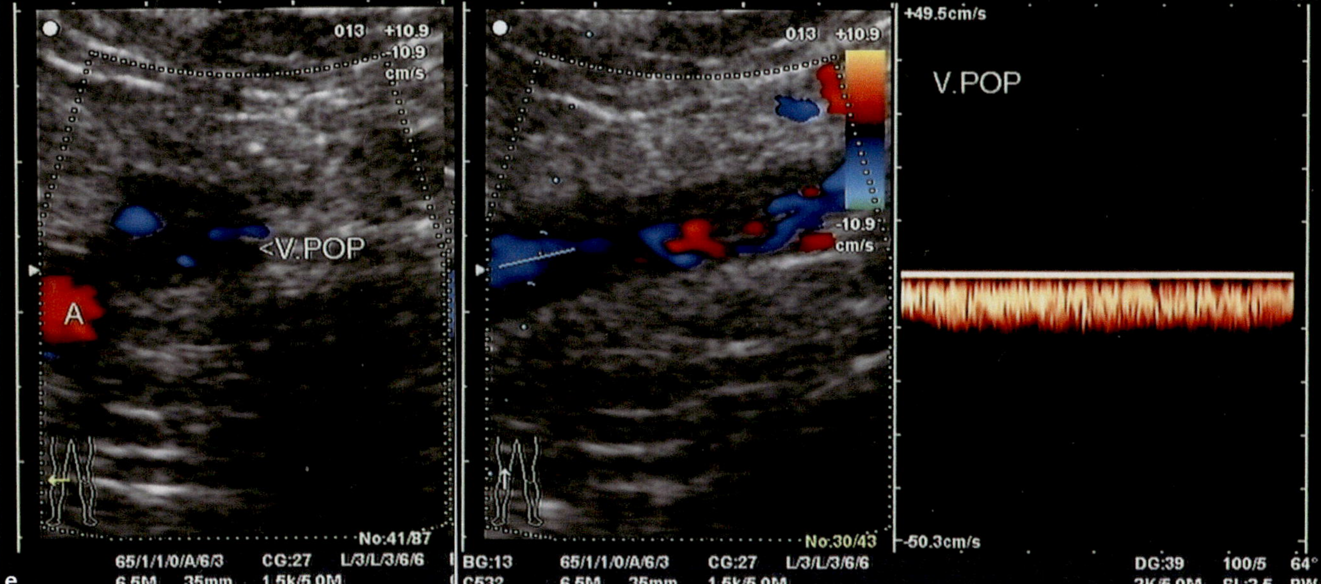

Fig. 3.23 (continued)

- Varicosis (extent, severity of reflux, secondary incompetence of main veins; preoperative evaluation: determination of upper and lower points of insufficiency, identification of incompetent perforating veins)
- Vein mapping prior to bypass surgery (suitability of saphenous vein for venous bypass grafting)
- Venous aneurysm (size; configuration: spindle-shaped, saccular, intraluminal thrombosis)

Spectral Waveform Criteria

Obstruction of venous return (thrombosis, external compression) leads to increased intravascular pressure distal to the obstruction, demonstrated by duplex ultrasound as slower flow (see Fig. 3.24a).

The increased venous flow resistance associated with occlusion, compression, or persisting postthrombotic obstruction eliminates the respiratory phasicity of venous drainage (resulting from changes in intra-abdominal pressure). This loss is reflected in the Doppler waveform as a constant flow velocity in the vein distal to the obstructed segment and as a reduced flow velocity, which is best appreciated by comparison with the other leg (Fig. 3.24a). The following criteria, known from CW Doppler ultrasound, indicate **venous obstruction** (Figs. 3.24a, 3.44 (Atlas), 3.46 (Atlas), and 3.49 (Atlas)):

- Zero flow in the thrombotically occluded vein
- Decreased flow velocity with reduction or elimination of respiratory phasicity due to proximal thrombus or compression of the vein by surrounding structures

- Flow signal not modulated by respiration, possibly of high frequency, in partially thrombosed or compressed vessel segments or along thrombus surrounded by flowing blood (differential diagnosis: flow signal from collateral vein not subject to respiratory phasicity)
- Augmented flow (compression and release) abnormally reduced when thrombosis or flow obstruction is present distal or proximal to the sampling site

3

3.1.6.1.5 Thrombus Age

Initial hopes of determining thrombus age by means of sonomorphologic criteria and using this information for making better treatment decisions (surgery, thrombolysis, anticoagulation) have been disappointed. What is possible though is to differentiate very recent thrombi from much older ones (◘ Fig. 3.25 and ◘ Table 3.4) and differentiate them based on increasing inhomogeneity and echogenicity of the thrombus and shrinkage of the vein diameter (◘ Figs. 3.26 and 3.50 (Atlas)). In general, however, there is wide interindividual variation in thrombus development, and the criteria are not reliable enough for therapeutic decision-making. This holds true especially for the clinically relevant identification of thrombi that are still amenable to recanalization measures, i.e., thrombi not older than 1 week. Nevertheless, the sonomorphologic criteria can contribute to the therapeutic decision in individual cases. For instance, a homogeneous thrombus of lower echogenicity in a markedly dilated vein with good demarcation of the wall and thrombus portions surrounded by flowing blood is more likely to respond to thrombolytic therapy and will undergo rapid recanalization.

Older thrombosis is characterized by progressive narrowing of the venous lumen and a loss of wall conspicuity (◘ Fig. 3.26a and ◘ Table 3.4). The poorer delineation from surrounding muscle tissue and increasing echogenicity of the thrombus contribute to a lower accuracy of ultrasound in diagnosing older thrombosis, especially in the calf. Following the acute stage, early recanalization can also be demonstrated by color flow imaging. When the recanalized lumen is still small, sparse and slow venous flow may be depicted after augmentation (calf compression, Valsalva's maneuver) even if spontaneous flow is not detectable with the transducer set to detect slow flow. Both gray-scale ultrasound and color duplex imaging (with assessment of reflux severity) allow evaluation of venous drainage, which may be compromised by poor recanalization or postthrombotic changes. The findings may range from complete recanalization with a normal sonographic appearance of the venous wall to persistent thrombotic occlusion with luminal narrowing, residual thrombi of various size, wall sclerosis, and synechia.

If the sonographic examination shows not only postthrombotic changes but also newly obstructed venous segments (hypoechoic thrombus and dilatation of the vein compared with the accompanying artery), this is a sign of recurrent thrombosis (◘ Fig. 3.26c) – especially if the proximal thrombus end is surrounded by flow. In contrast, flow signals in the center of a thrombosed vein depicted by color duplex indicate older thrombosis with beginning recanalization. Impaired venous drainage due to thrombus surrounded by flow or residual thrombus in a recanalized vein with a narrow lumen is identified by the absence of respiratory phasicity in the Doppler waveform (◘ Figs. 3.23 and 3.28).

3.1.6.1.6 Recurrent Thrombosis

Following completion of treatment after a first episode of deep vein thrombosis (DVT) in an unselected patient population, the risk of recurrence was found to be 13% after 1 year, 23% after 5 years, and 30% after 10 years (White 2012). In another study, 50% of patients had residual thrombosis after 1 year (Piovella et al. 2002).

Although postthrombotic veins have several characteristic features including persistent occlusion with shrinkage of affected veins, partial recanalization with irregular and meandering flow, or residual thrombus with poor differentiation from perivascular tissue, they cannot always be differentiated from acute recurrent DVT with confidence. To improve differentiation, it is helpful to obtain a detailed

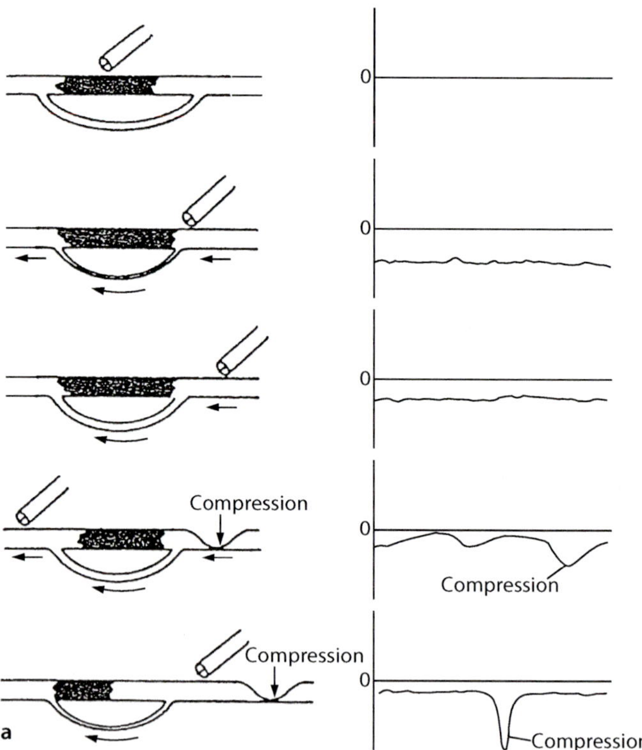

◘ **Fig. 3.24** **a** Diagrams of Doppler waveforms obtained at different sampling sites relative to flow-obstructing venous thrombosis without and with flow augmentation (manual compression) (see ◘ Fig. 3.44 (Atlas)). **b, c** Quantification of residual thrombus burden after deep vein thrombosis (DVT). **b** Calculation of percentage residual vein thrombosis (RVT) (Siragusa et al. 2011). The left drawing illustrates the situation for a large residual thrombus burden (vein diameter with compression ≥40%; see ◘ Fig. 3.23c) and the right drawing the situation for a small residual thrombus burden (vein diameter with compression <40%). **c** Calculation of residual thrombus thickness from the anteroposterior diameter measured without and with application of pressure with the transducer (Prandoni et al. 2002 and 2004). Recurrent DVT is defined as a diameter increase of ≥4 mm

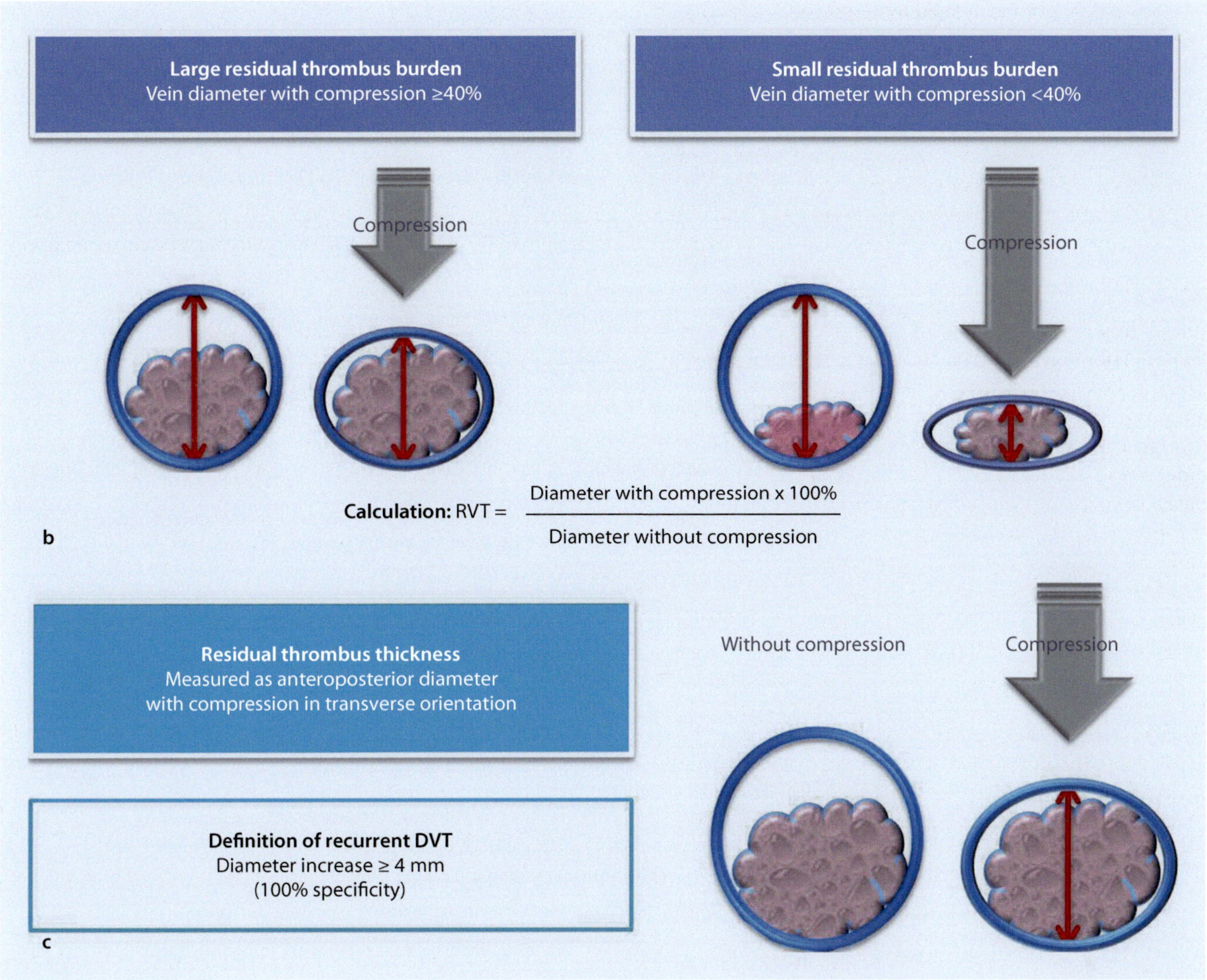

Large residual thrombus burden
Vein diameter with compression ≥40%

Compression

Small residual thrombus burden
Vein diameter with compression <40%

Compression

Calculation: RVT = $\frac{\text{Diameter with compression x 100\%}}{\text{Diameter without compression}}$

b

Residual thrombus thickness
Measured as anteroposterior diameter
with compression in transverse orientation

Definition of recurrent DVT
Diameter increase ≥ 4 mm
(100% specificity)

Without compression

Compression

c

Fig. 3.24 (continued)

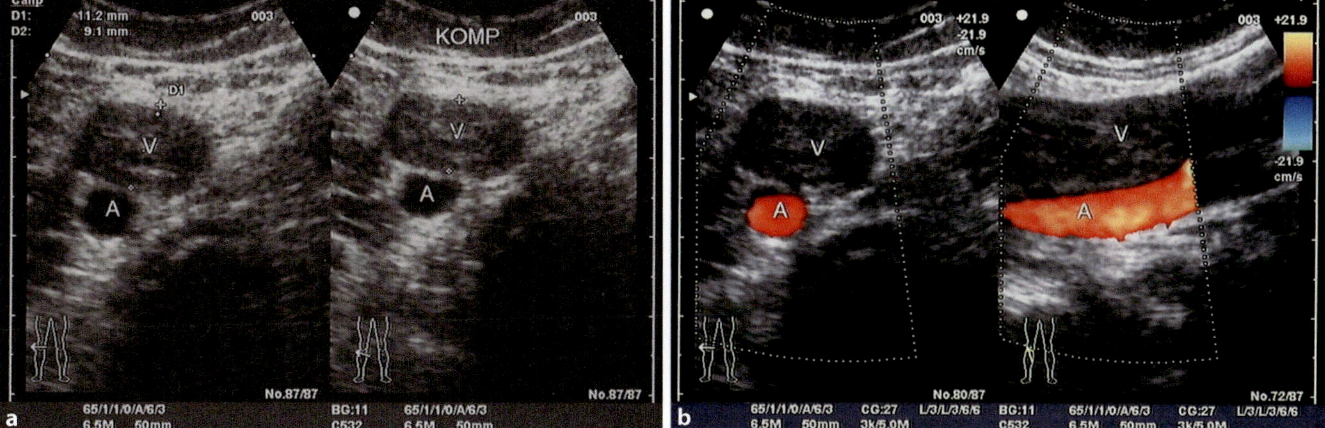

Fig. 3.25 **a** Acute thrombosis of the popliteal vein (V), which is dilated by the thrombus (compare diameter of the accompanying artery (A)). The wall of the thrombosed vein is sharply demarcated from the surrounding tissue. The thrombus is identified in the gray-scale image as intraluminal hypoechoic, homogeneous material. The right image obtained during compression with the transducer shows that the soft clot is still somewhat compressible (with a diameter reduction from 11 to 9 mm). **b** Color duplex imaging (transverse view on the left, longitudinal view on the right) shows no spontaneous or augmented venous blood flow, indicating occlusive thrombosis

3

Table 3.4 Sonographic findings in the diagnostic evaluation of deep vein thrombosis (DVT) and estimation of thrombus age

Presence of thrombus/thrombus age	Ultrasound findings
Normal vein (no thrombosis)	Complete compressibility of vein Thin wall Breathing, Valsalva's maneuver, and distal compression elicit identical changes in flow on both sides No elicitation of retrograde flow in valve function test (indicating adequate valve closure)
Acute thrombus (<8 days)	Incompressibility of vein Vein diameter at least twice that of accompanying artery Flow signals near the wall if thrombus is still surrounded by blood or if a free-floating thrombus is present Thrombus tending to be homogeneous and hypoechoic Good delineation of vessel wall, in part with hypoechoic halo No collaterals detectable by color duplex imaging
Older thrombus (>2–3 weeks)	Total occlusion: – Incompressibility of vein – Diameter less than twice that of accompanying artery – No flow signals, thrombus tends to become more hyperechoic and inhomogeneous – Poor delineation of vessel wall, hyperechoic halo may still be present Partial occlusion: – Partial compressibility of vein – Diameter comparable to that of accompanying artery – Signs of marginal and central recanalization – Collaterals begin to form
Postthrombotic lesions	Persistent occlusion: – Reduced venous lumen (same as or smaller than the diameter of accompanying artery) – Vessel wall poorly demarcated from surrounding soft tissue – Fully developed collateral vessels Partial recanalization: – Meandering flow pattern in center of vein – Little or no respiratory phasicity of blood flow – Short residual occlusions – Sclerotic thickening and rigidity of vessel wall; incomplete compressibility Recanalization: – Flow signal throughout lumen – Sclerotically altered wall segments alternating with sonographically normal segments – Identification of incompetent valves using Valsalva's maneuver or valve function test (compression and release) – Variable lumen with widened and narrowed segments

status of residual thrombosis, ideally after the completion of anticoagulation treatment, to serve as a new baseline in case of future recurrence. Criteria of recurrence on compression ultrasound include incompressibility of a previously normal segment and a marked increase in the thrombus burden (Piovella et al. 2002; Prandoni et al. 2002; Siragusa et al. 2011). Prandoni et al. (2002) reported 99% sensitivity for the diagnosis of recurrent thrombosis in the proximal deep veins.

Still, compression ultrasound may not allow confident diagnosis of recurrent DVT in 30% of cases (Tan et al. 2010), and the residual thrombus burden after a thrombotic event is at times difficult to define and to quantify. Moreover, investigators differ in how they define recurrent DVT or measure residual thrombus. While some investigators report residual thrombus thickness as the anteroposterior vein diameter in mm (Prandoni et al. 2002), others calculate a percentage thrombus burden from vein diameters measured with and without compression (Siragusa et al. 2011) (see Figs. 3.23c and 3.24b). If the sonographic findings are inconclusive, the same strategy as in the diagnosis of primary DVT may be used – either a supplementary D-dimer test and clinical risk assessment according to Wells (see Fig. 3.21) or a repeat ultrasound examination in conjunction with a repeat D-dimer test.

Another option to differentiate older residual DVT from acute recurrence is magnetic resonance direct thrombus imaging (MRDTI) (Westerbeek et al. 2008).

3.1.6.2 Chronic Venous Insufficiency

While thrombosis can be evaluated by B-mode imaging alone, Doppler ultrasound is necessary for the hemodynamic assessment of the severity of poor venous drainage in patients

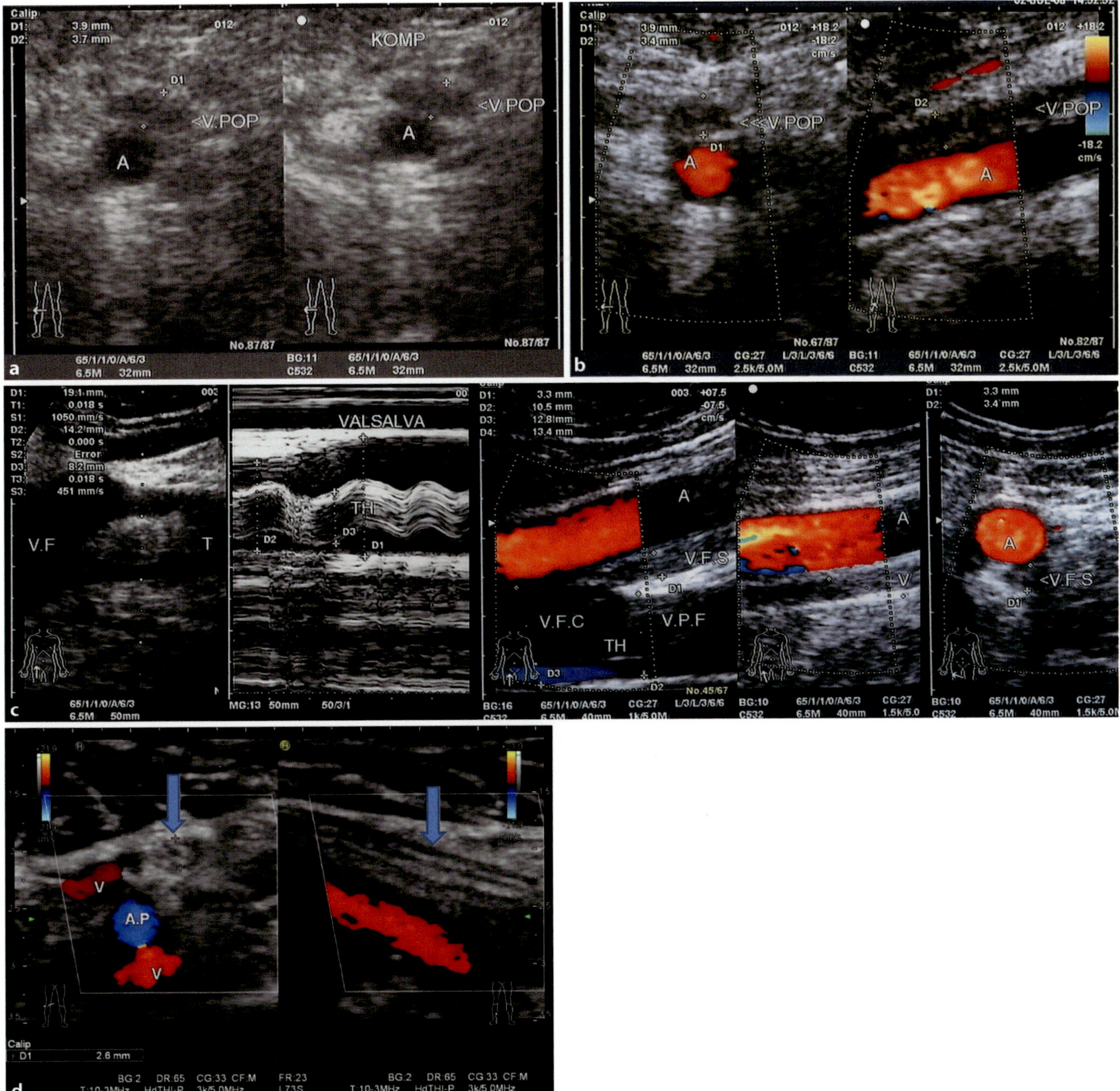

Fig. 3.26 **a** Older thrombosis (>3 months) of the popliteal vein. Transverse views of the vein obtained without compression (left) and with compression (right). The wall of the thrombosed popliteal vein (V.POP) is blurred and difficult to delineate from surrounding tissue. The vein has decreased in diameter (and is smaller than the accompanying artery). At this stage (after fibroblast invasion), the thrombus cannot be compressed with the transducer (lumen diameter of 3.9 and 3.7 mm without and with compression, respectively). **b** Transverse (left) and longitudinal (right) color duplex images fail to depict flow in the popliteal vein (V.POP), confirming occlusive thrombosis. The blurred wall and poor delineation from surrounding tissue are most obvious in the longitudinal image. Red-coded flow indicates the accompanying popliteal artery (A). **c** Patient with recurrent mild swelling of the leg 1 year after an episode of deep vein thrombosis (DVT). The color flow images show persistent complete occlusion of the superficial femoral vein (thin vein with poorly differentiated wall and higher echogenicity in the color flow images (V.F.S, V)). The first color flow image additionally shows a fresh appositional thrombus (TH) extending from the old thrombosis into the common femoral vein (V.F.C) and deep femoral vein (V.P.F). The appositional portion has low echogenicity and is attached to the wall anteriorly with flow posteriorly (blue). It is well delineated from the wall and causes marked dilatation of the vein. The grays-scale image (leftmost scan) shows a free-floating component (3 cm in length), and the time-motion scan next to it shows the floating thrombus to be highly mobile within the dilated vein (during Valsalva's maneuver). There is a risk of pulmonary embolism, and anticoagulation treatment should be resumed promptly. **d** Older thrombosed veins must be differentiated from nerve strands running parallel to vessels, such as the tibial nerve coursing along the popliteal vein (V). A longitudinal image obtained with a high-resolution probe typically allows identification of the cordlike bundles of nerve fibers (arrow), thus distinguishing a nerve from an old thrombosed vein

3

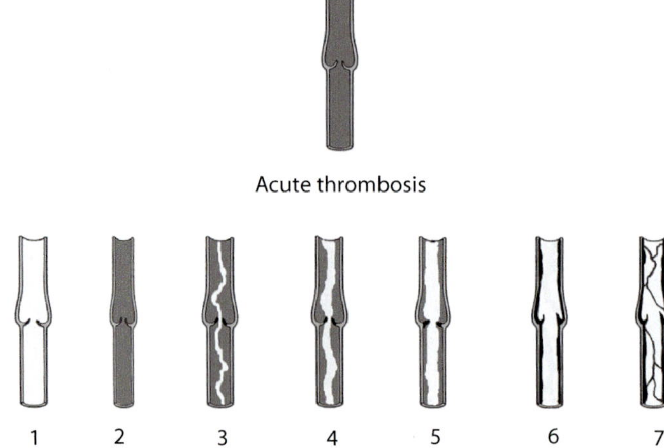

◘ **Fig. 3.27** Persistent venous changes following deep vein thrombosis (DVT). **1** Complete recanalization, only valve damage. Normal gray-scale and compression ultrasound findings of the vein. **2** Persistent occlusive thrombosis. Sonographically, the vein typically has a reduced lumen (diameter no larger than that of the accompanying artery), contains material of higher echogenicity, and cannot be compressed. **3** Narrow recanalized lumen. The recanalized vein is often missed by B-mode or compression ultrasound; color duplex imaging is usually required to demonstrate flow in the vein (and Valsalva's maneuver or compression may be necessary to augment flow). **4** Recanalization with residual mural thrombus. Visualization of the recanalized vein may be poor on gray-scale images, and the vein is not fully compressible. **5** Recanalization with persistent wall thickening. In most cases, the patent lumen is sonographically delineated from the thickened wall, and the vein can be compressed, but full compression is prevented by the thickened wall. **6** Recanalization with wall sclerosis. Hyperechoic wall, possibly with focal posterior acoustic shadowing, on B-mode imaging and incomplete compressibility due to thickened, sclerotic wall. **7** Intraluminal synechia and membranes, which are hyperechoic and slightly mobile when the vein is compressed. The membranes, typically with concomitant wall sclerosis, preclude complete compression of the vein

with chronic venous incompetence. A high-resolution transducer depicts venous wall sclerosis by an increase in echogenicity and thickening of the wall in the presence of a patent lumen and also identifies valves damaged and immobilized by the sclerotic process. Nevertheless, B-mode imaging alone is insufficient in evaluating the postthrombotic patient because a recanalized vein will have a normal sonomorphologic appearance in about 30% of cases (◘ Fig. 3.27). The other 70% show wall irregularities and thickening, a strand-like vein with a smaller lumen, or a vein that has become dilated after recanalization due to the pressure and volume overload resulting from incompetent valves (see ◘ Figs. 3.69, 3.73, and 3.74 (all Atlas)). If recanalization is delayed, serial ultrasound will show residual mural thrombi or a thickened wall, from which residual thrombus cannot be differentiated. The affected vein cannot be fully compressed, and color flow images will depict a narrow lumen with flow signals surrounded by an inhomogeneous area of mixed low and high echogenicity extending to the perivascular connective tissue (◘ Fig. 3.28).

Compressibility of the postthrombotic vein increases with the degree of recanalization, while residual intraluminal structures (◘ Fig. 3.29a), which are inhomogeneous and mostly hypoechoic relative to the surrounding connective tissue, prevent full compression. Especially the postthrombotic femoral vein may be difficult to identify since all that may remain is a cord-like structure visible on B-scan ultrasound. For this reason, it is helpful to use the accompanying artery as a landmark. A recanalized femoral vein with incompetent valves will dilate during Valsalva's maneuver (◘ Table 3.5 and ◘ Fig. 3.73 (Atlas)).

Hence, B-mode ultrasound alone does not allow reliable evaluation of the recanalization process as it does not depict flow in sclerotic segments, and wall sclerosis may preclude compression of the vein (◘ Table 3.5 and ◘ Fig. 3.73 (Atlas)).

The clinical severity of the postthrombotic syndrome is chiefly influenced by the degree to which venous return is compromised, which in turn varies with the degree of thrombosis and recanalization as well as with the presence of collateral pathways. Valve incompetence in the main veins determines the extent of reflux, which correlates well with the extent of the initial thrombosis. Duplex ultrasound studies demonstrate abnormal reflux after recanalization of thrombotic deep vein segments in approx. 45–70% of cases after 1–3 years, while normal findings with complete recanalization and preserved valve function are seen in 12–30% patients (Johnson et al. 1995; Markel et al. 1992), and 10–20% of vessel segments remain completely obstructed (Johnson et al. 1995).

Venous reflux is measured with a Valsalva maneuver to evaluate proximal valve function and the compression test to evaluate distal insufficiency. The increase in intra-abdominal pressure induced by the Valsalva maneuver produces a short, physiologic backward flow with a mean duration of 0.3 s (◘ Fig. 3.29b–e). Reflux persisting for over 1 s is abnormal. Studies in patients with stage II or III chronic venous insufficiency found sensitivities of 77–91% and specificities of 85–100% for reflux assessment by duplex ultrasound (Araki et al. 1993; Neglen and Raju 1992). Moreover, the duplex findings correlated better with the clinical stage than did ascending venography.

Ultrasound with a Valsalva maneuver can be performed in the recumbent patient, while the **compression-release test** has 10% higher diagnostic accuracy when performed with the patient sitting or standing. The vein is compressed manually distal to the ultrasound probe or in a standardized manner using a cuff for compression. Standardized spectral Doppler recordings for evaluation of reflux in the popliteal vein are obtained upon sudden deflation of a blood pressure cuff placed around the calf and inflated to 100 mmHg. Sonographic evaluation with use of standardized provocative maneuvers ensures interindividual comparability in the setting of scientific studies. The compression-release test reproduces the flow variations resulting from contraction-induced compression of muscle veins (muscle pump).

Because the main veins are also embedded in the muscle, contraction not only propels blood toward the heart but also induces flow toward the periphery, which is prevented by competent valves. In patients with incompetent perforators,

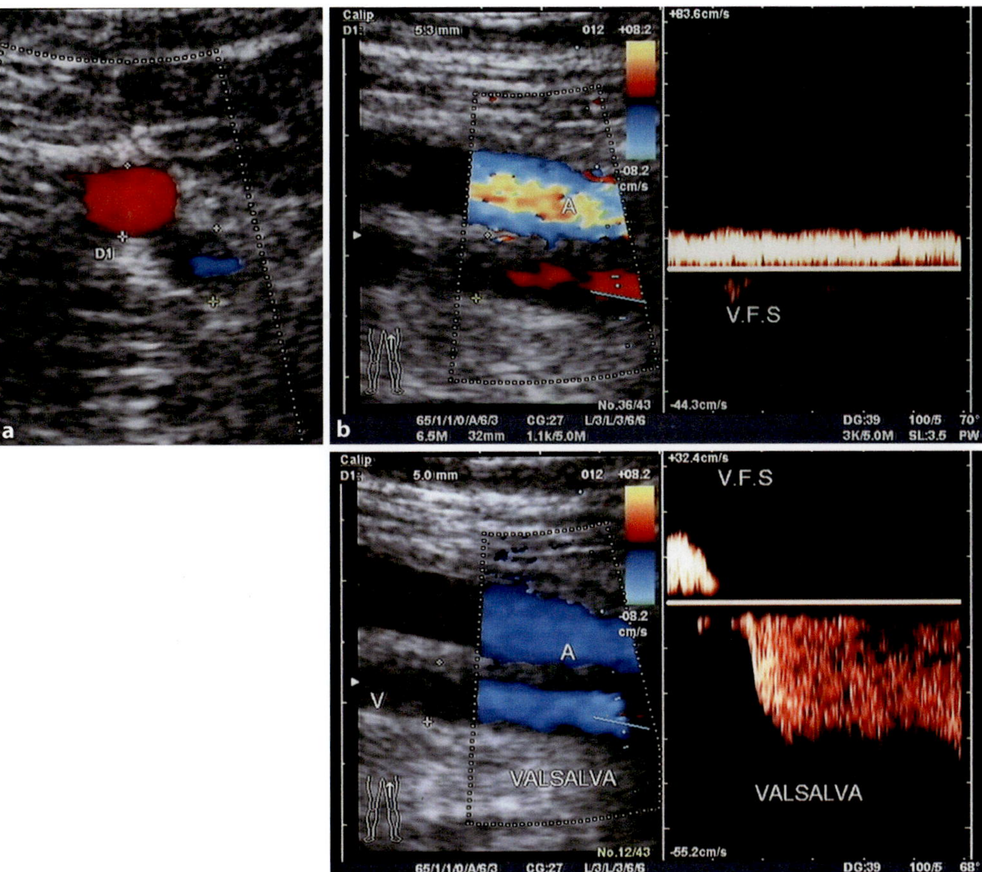

Fig. 3.28 **a** Transverse image shows the artery with red-coded flow and the femoral vein posterolaterally (indicated by calipers). The center of the vein is recanalized (blue-coded flow) and surrounded by an inhomogeneous, thickened wall with areas of high and low echogenicity. Residual mural thrombus cannot be differentiated from the wall, and the wall is poorly delineated from surrounding connective tissue. **b** The longitudinal color flow image shows flow in the center of the recanalized venous lumen (red, toward transducer) and extensive residual mural thrombosis. The low PRF chosen to depict slow venous flow causes aliasing in the accompanying popliteal artery (blue, flow away from transducer). **c** Flow reversal in the vein elicited by Valsalva's maneuver (blue, away from transducer) indicates incompetent valves. In the corresponding waveform (right), the flow reversal is seen as persistent flow below the baseline (away from transducer)

the muscle pump is also responsible for abnormal reflux from the deep into the superficial veins (Figs. 3.7b and 3.14). Therefore, incompetent valves reduce the efficiency of the muscle pump because venous pressure, which normally decreases with muscle activity, remains unchanged or drops only a little. These complex interactions must be taken into account when selecting a site for placing the Doppler sample volume and also in interpreting the flow data obtained.

In **severe valve incompetence**, as in the postthrombotic syndrome, reflux can be induced not only by Valsalva's maneuver but also by normal inspiration or deep inspiration in the horizontal position (Fig. 3.75 (Atlas)). Under normal conditions, the craniocaudal pressure gradient ensures rapid valve closure during inspiration and thus prevents reflux. In patients with incompetent valves, the pressure gradient results in reflux persisting until the patient begins to expirate (reversal of pressure).

Pressure and volume overload occurring **distal to postthrombotic veins** can lead to secondary damage through hyperextension of valvular rings in formerly unaffected vessel segments (Killewich et al. 1989). The same pathomechanism leads to secondary, nonpostthrombotic valve incompetence of the deep veins in patients with a long history of truncal varicosity (Trendelenburg private circulation; Fig. 3.30). In this secondary form, as in primary chronic venous insufficiency of the deep leg veins, B-mode images show dilatation of the affected vein but no wall thickening or inhomogeneous structures within the lumen. Moreover, the vein can be completely compressed. Under good insonation conditions, mobility of the valve can be demonstrated, distinguishing this condition from the postthrombotic syndrome with valve immobility due to fibrotic thickening (Figs. 3.29 and 3.43 (Atlas)).

Different **patterns of reflux** can be observed, depending on the underlying mechanism of valve incompetence (Evers and Wuppermann 1995, 1997). Reflux in postthrombotic valve incompetence sets in immediately with the provocative maneuver (without signs of valve movement), increases rapidly, peaks during the first seconds, and then decreases (type B). Reflux will be less severe than expected when overall flow is reduced due to incomplete recanalization and flow obstruction caused by residual thrombosis (Fig. 3.31). In primary chronic venous insufficiency and primary varicosis, abnormal reflux is slightly delayed compared with physiologic reflux, continuous (see Fig. 3.74 (Atlas)), and slower (type A).

In patients with complete valve failure due to severe venous dilatation, however, even primary chronic venous insufficiency of the superficial or deep venous system results in immediate high-frequency reflux.

Reflux velocity can be used as a semiquantitative measure of postthrombotic valve damage. It increases during the first year and then reaches a plateau. In addition, the velocity and duration of reflux are influenced by secondary postthrombotic changes caused by pressure and volume overload.

3

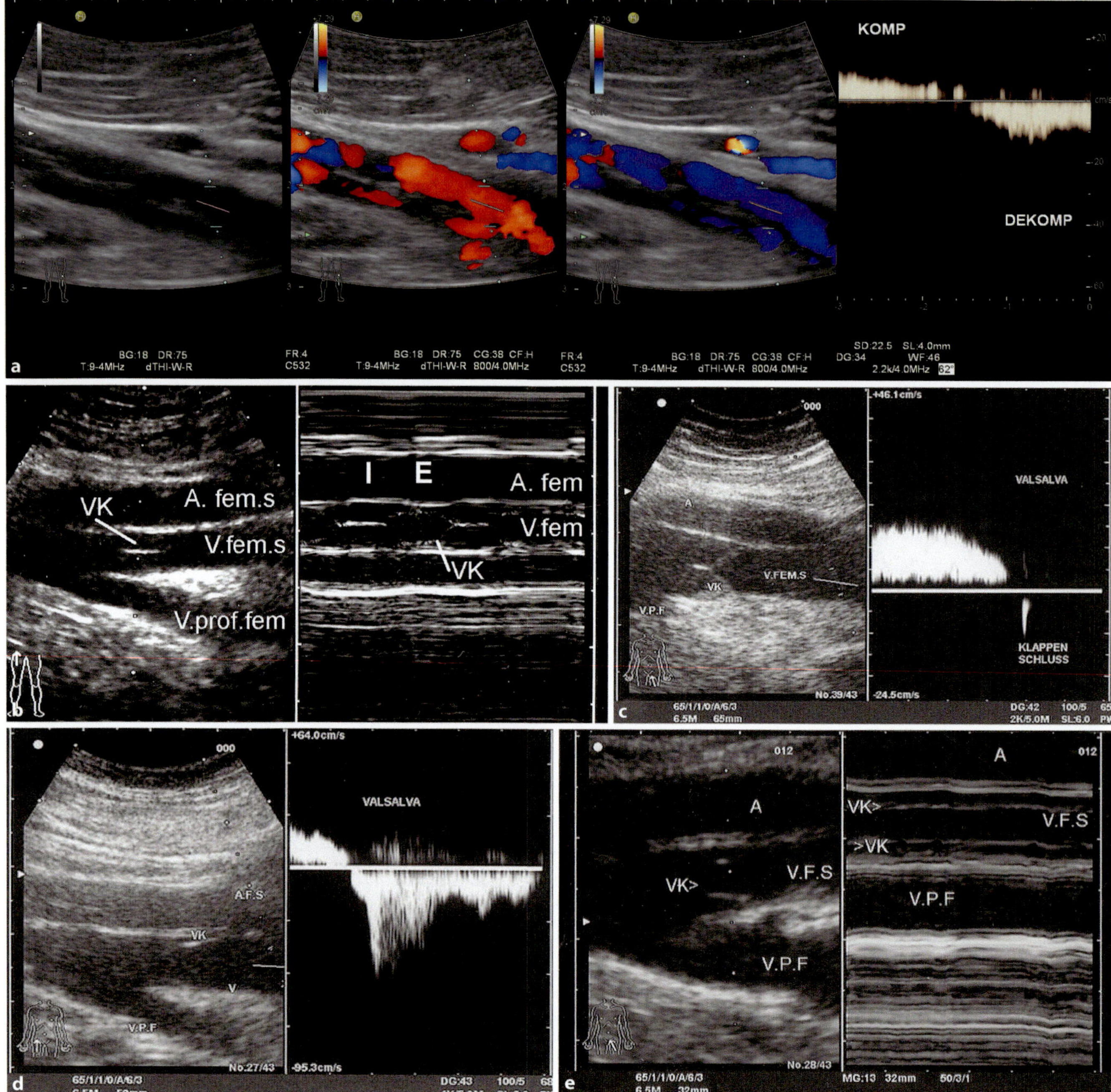

◘ Fig. 3.29 **a** Intraluminal synechia (◘ Fig. 3.73 (Atlas)) seen as hyperechoic reflections from the lumen. Such strands obstruct flow and can cause severe valve incompetence by adhering to valve cusps. **b** A time-motion scan obtained with the ultrasound beam through the valve leaflets allows good evaluation of valve motion: the leaflets (VK) are open and close to the wall during expiration (E), and they are closed during inspiration (I) as a result of the increased intra-abdominal pressure, preventing reflux of the venous blood (closed leaflets seen in the center of the lumen). **c** Imaging during Valsalva's maneuver demonstrates adequate valve closure (VK) in the superficial femoral vein (V.FEM.S), indicated by a short flow reversal (flow toward the periphery) just before valve closure and by cessation of reversed flow upon complete closure. **d** Postthrombotic damage, with sclerotic fixation of the valve leaflets to the wall, results in failure of the valve (VK) to close and is indicated by persistent reflux (flow away from transducer, toward the periphery) during Valsalva's maneuver. **e** In this patient, the corresponding time-motion scan shows failure of the damaged valve (VK) to close because of postthrombotic adhesion to the wall and sclerotic rigidity (compare normal valve closure in **b**)

3.1.6.3 Varicosis

The variability of venous reflux patterns makes it necessary to establish the following data to identify candidates for varicose surgery and to select the most suitable approach and extent of the operation (see ► Sect. 3.1.5.2):

- Terminal competence/incompetence of the great and small saphenous veins
- Proximal and distal points of insufficiency in patients with major vein insufficiency (to spare adequate vein segments for future bypass procedures)

Table 3.5 Ultrasound findings in patients with the postthrombotic syndrome (see Figs. 3.23 and 3.27)

Ultrasound technique	Sonographic criteria and findings
B-mode imaging (normal in 30–40% of patients)	Narrowing of vessel lumen
	Blurred wall structure
	Thickened wall
	Wall sclerosis, intramural calcifications
	Intraluminal connective tissue strands, synechia
	Echogenic vessel lumen
	Not fully compressible
Color duplex imaging	Degree of recanalization
	Incompetence of major veins
	Better visualization of wall sclerosis and of postthrombotic wall lesions
	Identification of collaterals
	Incompetence of superficial veins (secondary)
	Perforator incompetence

- Identification of incompetent perforators (to minimize risk of recurrence) and status of the deep venous system (Wong et al. 2003)
- Exclusion of secondary, postthrombotic varicosis (presence of residual thrombi obstructing flow?)
- Exclusion of arterial obstruction (risk of disturbed postoperative wound healing)

Valve function of superficial veins is evaluated in the same way as in the deep venous system, namely by spectal Doppler imaging during provocative maneuvers. While flow reversal is also seen in color flow images, only spectral Doppler permits accurate measurement of reflux duration. Clinically, it is important to identify the proximal extent of venous insufficiency (Fig. 3.16a). In complete varicosis of the great saphenous vein, the proximal point is identified by repeated Doppler sampling during Valsalva's maneuver beginning at the saphenofemoral junction. The vein is then followed down the leg, repeating this test until the distal point of insufficiency is identified (transition from reflux to normal flow). This point determines the **grade of great saphenous vein varicosis** according to Hach (Figs. 3.15, 3.16, and 3.32). In Hach grades I to III, varicose side branches often enter the vein at the level of the distal point of insufficiency.

A short reflux (<0.3 s) before valve closure is normal in the main veins, while reflux with backward flow persisting for >0.5 s is abnormal according to the criteria of the Union Internationale de Phlébologie (UIP). Investigators meanwhile may advocate different cutoff values for different vein segments, with some regarding reflux durations of up to 1 s as normal (Coleridge-Smith et al. 2006).

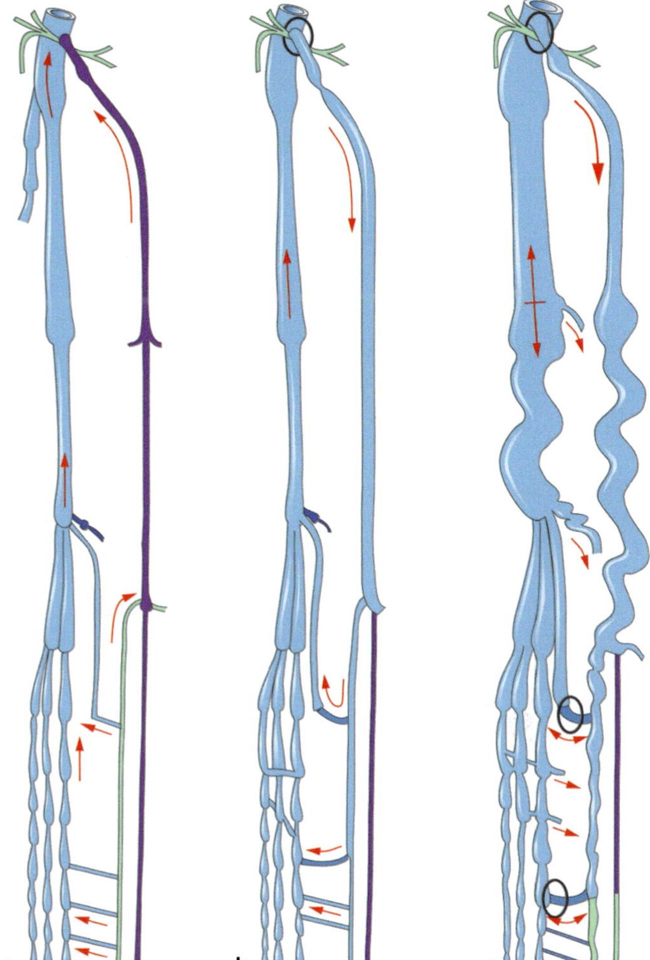

Fig. 3.30a–c Development of chronic venous insufficiency with valvular incompetence of the deep veins secondary to truncal varicosity of the great saphenous vein. **a** Physiologic blood flow direction in deep and superficial veins (red arrows). Perforating veins drain the blood from the superficial to the deep venous system. **b** Truncal varicosis of the great saphenous vein is associated with retrograde flow through perforators back into the superficial venous system. This hypercirculation (Trendelenburg private circulation) is compensated as long as the valves of the deep veins remain competent, but it leads to dilatation of superficial side branches and perforators as well as volume overload of the deep veins. **c** Hypercirculation eventually becomes decompensated as a result of volume overload, leading to dilatation and subsequent valve failure of the deep veins. This valve failure in turn leads to pressure-induced dilatation and secondary valve incompetence of further perforating veins (Cockett's, Boyd's, and Dodd's perforating veins). Finally, the muscle pump becomes ineffective, resulting in full-blown drainage insufficiency

Clinically apparent varicose changes of the great saphenous vein are often restricted to the lower leg. Nevertheless, duplex imaging frequently also reveals incompetence above the knee, where dilatation of the great saphenous vein is less pronounced due to the lower intravascular pressure. A study by our group including 103 patients with great saphenous vein varicosis demonstrated involvement of the saphenofemoral junction in 66% of the patients with clinically normal findings of the

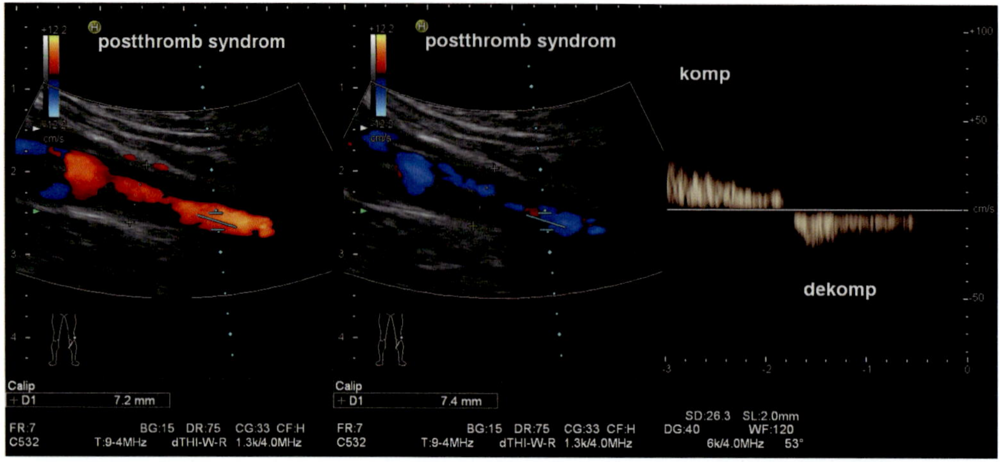

Fig. 3.31 Patient with postthrombotic syndrome and extensive residual thrombus following an episode of acute three-level thrombosis. The residual thrombus leaves only a narrow patent channel, resulting in flow obstruction with slower flow in the popliteal vein. In the valve function test with manual compression and release of the calf, this is reflected in a reduced blood flow velocity during compression (left color flow image with red-coded flow) and less marked reflux (in terms of duration and magnitude) upon release of compression (blue-coded flow in right image) than expected in severe valve incompetence

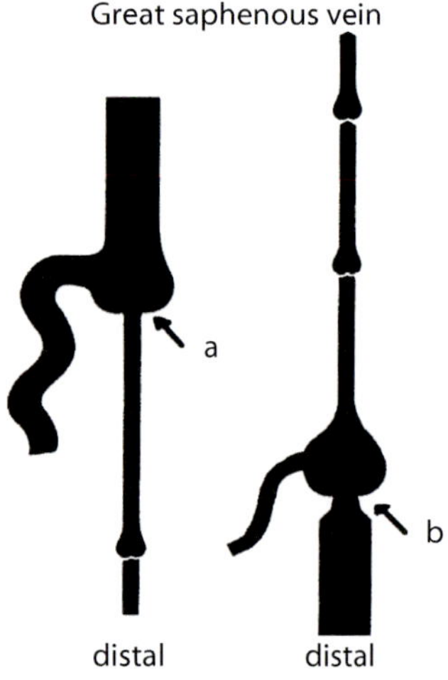

Fig. 3.32 Valve incompetence of major superficial veins. Left drawing: distal point of insufficiency (a) with pressure-induced dilatation of a side branch or perforating vein (varicose degeneration) joining the main vein at this level. Normal vein segment with functioning valves distal to this point. Right drawing: proximal point of insufficiency (b). Normal vein with competent valves proximal to the point of insufficiency and valve incompetence distal to it

thigh. Therefore, evaluation of the junction is mandatory even if clinical signs of varicosis are only apparent below the knee.

In patients who have undergone stripping of the great saphenous vein, a remaining stump can be identified with Valsalva's maneuver, but several years after surgery, it cannot always be reliably differentiated from neoreflux or neovascularization (Turton et al. 1999).

In **incomplete great saphenous vein varicosis**, only the distal valves are incompetent while the terminal and preterminal valves are intact. It is important, especially in incomplete great saphenous vein varicosis, to identify the upper and lower points of insufficiency so that competent vein segments can be spared in case they are required for future bypass graft procedures.

Four main types of incomplete truncal varicosis are distinguished:

- In incomplete varicosis of the **perforator type** with an intact saphenofemoral junction, distal incompetence of the great saphenous vein originates from an insufficient perforating vein, e.g., a Dodd vein in the upper leg (see Fig. 3.80 (Atlas)).
- In incomplete varicosis of the **lateral branch type** with proximal competence, the distal great saphenous vein varicosis is maintained by varicosis in a side branch, e.g., an insufficient lateral accessory vein in the thigh (see Fig. 3.77 (Atlas)).
- In the **posterior type**, venous incompetence involves the small saphenous vein and femoropopliteal vein, from where it extends to the great saphenous vein via an accessory branch of the latter (Giacomini anastomosis) (see Figs. 3.16b and 3.65 (Atlas)).
- **Distal varicose lateral branches** such as veins communicating between the great and small saphenous veins can maintain secondary varicose changes of the distal saphenous vein.

Preoperative identification of the upper point of insufficiency in distal varicosis by **duplex imaging** is important to ensure complete surgical removal of the incompetent vein segments, thereby preventing recurrence and sparing competent venous segments for possible later bypass procedures. The dilated varicose segments are identified in the standing patient, followed to the point of insufficiency, and marked on the skin. Surgeons will benefit most from real-time sonographic evaluation of venous morphology and function if they perform the examination themselves.

In incomplete distal great saphenous insufficiency, the Valsalva test yields no valid results because the proximal valves still function properly. Instead, the compression-and-release test is performed with the patient standing. The incompetent great saphenous vein depicted by B-mode ultrasound is followed upward to identify the proximal point of insufficiency for tailoring the surgical procedure. Divisions into arch veins can thus be identified by duplex imaging as well and evaluated for incompetent valves. The ultrasound examination thus enables accurate identification of all incompetent venous segments prior to surgery.

The examination should include the perforating veins, which can be identified in their typical locations (Cockett's, Boyd's, and Dodd's perforators). Perforator competence is evaluated by duplex ultrasound using the compression-and-release test in the standing patient. Evaluation may be easier when a tourniquet is applied to stop blood flow in the superficial veins. Identification of incompetent perforators is important in order to eliminate them as potential sources of recurrent varicosis (◘ Figs. 3.10 and 3.33).

Perforator incompetence is suggested by reflux from the deep into the superficial veins in the compression-and-release test (◘ Fig. 3.11). Incompetent perforating veins arising from the great saphenous vein below the knee are identified by B-mode imaging as slightly tortuous, tubular structures coursing to the posterior tibial vein territory in the transfascial compartment (see ◘ Fig. 3.79 (Atlas)). Competent perforating veins are usually so small that they will not be detected unless a thorough search is done with a high-resolution transducer and the patient in the standing position.

In a comparative study, 95.5% of a total of 252 incompetent perforating veins diagnosed by color duplex ultrasound were confirmed intraoperatively. In comparison, venography identified only 65% of these incompetent perforating veins (Stiegler et al. 1994). The accuracy of palpation alone is 49% and that of CW Doppler 75%.

The ultrasound examination for **incompetence of the small saphenous vein** is also performed with the patient standing. If the deep veins are still competent, however, insufficiency can only be evaluated by using the compression-and-release test and not the Valsalva maneuver, unless there is simultaneous valve incompetence of the femoral and popliteal veins (◘ Fig. 3.33). After identification of the highly variable saphenopopliteal junction, spectral Doppler is obtained while performing the compression test using the other hand or a cuff to compress the vein distal to the transducer. The course of the small saphenous vein is then traced downward with repeated compression to identify the distal point of insufficiency. Valve incompetence is suggested by dilatation – primarily in the popliteal fossa – and a tortuous course resulting from elongation of the vein.

It is very important to include the deep venous system in the preoperative workup to rule out secondary postthrombotic major vein insufficiency. The latter is a contraindication to surgery because interruption of collateral pathways (involving the great saphenous vein) would result in further deterioration in patients with existing postthrombotic flow obstruction due to occlusive residual thrombi.

3.1.6.3.1 Treatment Options

During **endovenous interventions**, such as radiofrequency ablation or intravascular laser therapy, ultrasound is used to monitor correct positioning of intraluminal probes. In foam sclerotherapy, ultrasound allows real-time monitoring of the spread of the sclerosant, and foam migration into the deep venous system can be prevented by compressing the terminal portion of the vein being treated.

In endovenous radiofrequency ablation, the introducer sheath is advanced from a distal access using ultrasound guidance and placed in the great saphenous vein just below the site of entry of the superficial epigastric vein (see ◘ Fig. 3.82 (Atlas)) to prevent occlusion of this vein during treatment. Ultrasound enables good visualization of the superficial epigastric vein in this area as it extends cranially from the saphenofemoral junction. The saphenous side branches arising more distally, in particular the lateral and medial accessory veins, will be obliterated by the thermal energy applied during radiofrequency ablation. The intervention is performed under tumescent anesthesia, which is applied under sonographic guidance and serves to compress the target vein, thereby ensuring a good energy transfer to the vein wall, and also to protect the surrounding structures from heat damage.

Tumescent anesthesia is performed by injecting tumescent fluid (modified Klein's solution) around the vein once the catheter is in place. This is done under ultrasound guidance and serves to create a circumferential fluid layer of 4–5 mm around the vein and compress it (target diameter for the great saphenous vein: 4–6 mm) (see ◘ Fig. 3.82 (Atlas)). These conditions have been shown to ensure nearly pain-free endovascular laser treatment. Although the tumescent solution spreads within the saphenous compartment, it is necessary to inject the fluid along the course of the vein every few centimeters, starting proximally and using ultrasound for guidance.

Duplex ultrasound has an important role in identifying **contraindications to endovenous ablation treatment (laser or radiofrequency) or conditions requiring a modified approach**:

- Chronic or acute phlebitis, which may hinder advancement of the ablation probe (see ◘ Figs. 3.65 and 3.80 (both Atlas))
- Anatomic variants that preclude passage of the ablation probe. The catheter used in the Venefit procedure (formerly known as VNUS ClosureFast) has a lumen allowing ultrasound-guided insertion of a guidewire via a distal introducer sheath for advancement of the radiofrequency probe to the saphenofemoral junction.
- Identification of varicose veins that are too close to the skin surface (to prevent skin burns, the distance should be at least 1 cm following injection of Klein's solution)
- Aneurysmal dilatation of the great saphenous vein (>2.5 cm).

Sonographic evaluation after endovenous laser or radiofrequency ablation of the saphenous vein aims at ruling out thermal damage and thrombosis of the common femoral

3

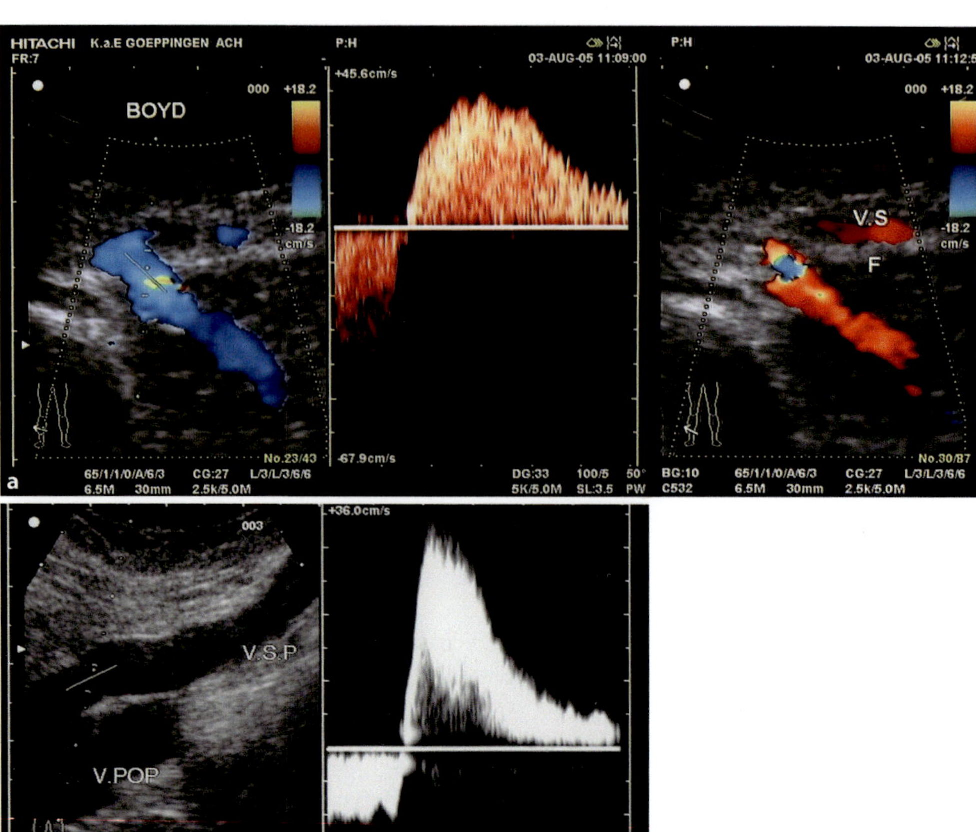

Fig. 3.33 **a** Valve incompetence of a Boyd perforator in the calf. The valve function test reveals normal flow from the superficial to the deep venous system (leftmost image, blue-coded flow) and flow reversal upon release of compression (rightmost image, red-coded flow) (F = fascia, V.S = great saphenous vein). The Doppler waveform shows persistent reflux from the deep into the superficial system (flow above the baseline, toward the transducer). **b** The Doppler waveform from the saphenopopliteal junction (sample volume as indicated in the longitudinal view obtained with the transducer in the popliteal fossa). There is flow toward the heart during manual compression of the calf (away from transducer, below the baseline) and persistent retrograde flow upon release (above the baseline), indicating severe valve incompetence

vein or popliteal vein. Successful closure of the varicose vein is seen as thickening and thrombosis without flow (see Fig. 3.83 (Atlas)).

Approx. 3 days after treatment, all patients should undergo a duplex ultrasound evaluation for thrombosis and thermal damage and signs of thrombus growth in the common femoral vein and popliteal vein (Lawrence et al. 2010).

The so-called **CHIVA technique** is an alternative strategy that aims at hemodynamic correction by interruption of recirculation pressure loops, while sparing the saphenous veins for venous drainage. Sites of recirculation from the deep system into the superficial veins are identified by duplex imaging and marked for open surgical ligation. Outcome is evaluated by duplex ultrasound to ensure that all recirculation routes have been eliminated and that flow in all patent veins is from the superficial into the deep system.

Recurrent varicosis is the occurrence of varicosis at a new site or in a varicose vein segment previously treated by sclerotherapy or endovenous ablation. Recurrent varicosis in the strict sense cannot occur after varicose vein resection or crossectomy with great saphenous vein stripping. In this situation, varicosis can recur if the residual saphenous stump is too long and veins terminating proximally connect to this stump or to a saphenous branch. Thus, when a patient presents with suspected recurrence, the first diagnostic step is to evaluate the saphenofemoral junction using duplex imaging. Valsalva's maneuver is performed to identify any incompetent lateral branches entering the residual great saphenous vein and connecting to a more distal superficial vein and to determine whether a persisting lateral or medial accessory branch is present that has undergone varicose degeneration (Table 3.6).

A limitation of duplex ultrasound is that it does not always allow reliable differentiation of a residual saphenous vein trunk from neoreflux or neovascularization (see Fig. 3.84 (Atlas)).

3.1.6.4 Varicophlebitis

Varicophlebitis is defined as **thrombotic inflammation of a varicose superficial vein** and is a typical complication of varicosis. Thrombophlebitis is an inflammation of a previously healthy vein and typically occurs as a paraneoplastic complication. The clinical relevance of varicophlebitis has long been underestimated. Its most serious complication **is thrombus extension into the deep venous system**, typically through the junction of the great saphenous vein (Fig. 3.34) or small saphenous vein and less commonly through perforators.

The risk of progression of superficial thrombophlebitis into the deep venous system is 16% with 70% of cases accounted for by thrombus extension via the saphenofemoral junction and 20% by progression through perforators (Chengelis et al. 1996).

The possible complications of deep vein thrombosis and a relatively high risk of pulmonary embolism (caused by free-floating components; Bergquist 1986) have led to adoption of

Table 3.6 Pretherapeutic ultrasound examination in varicosis: relevant diagnostic information to be obtained for adequately planning the therapeutic strategy

Duplex ultrasound findings	Therapeutic relevance
Incompetent great saphenous vein/saphenofemoral junction vs. peripheral/lateral branch varicosis	Stripping/ligation/endovenous intervention
Secondary varicosis with (postthrombotic) incompetence of the deep leg veins	Compression treatment, surgery in exceptional cases only; ulcer: perforator dissection, division of fascia
Upper and lower points of incompetence in incomplete saphenous vein varicosis	Sparing of relevant competent vein segments for possible later bypass graft operations
Incompetent perforating veins	Ligation of incompetent perforators identified by ultrasound for prevention of recurrent varicosis
Postthrombotic syndrome with partial or complete occlusion by residual old thrombus	Contraindication to varicose surgery (impaired venous drainage would deteriorate further)
Exclusion of PAOD/arterial occlusion (using time-efficient protocol)	Prevention of disturbed postoperative wound healing

Table 3.7 Classification of varicophlebitis and recommended treatment based on extent defined by compression ultrasound

Extent of phlebitis	Recommended treatment
Varicophlebitis of a lateral branch or of the great saphenous vein below the knee	Local anti-inflammatory treatment, anti-inflammatory medication, possibly short-term anticoagulation
Varicophlebitis of the great saphenous vein in the thigh but far below the saphenofemoral junction or ascending small saphenous vein thrombosis with extension above the level of the May perforator	2–4 weeks of anticoagulation with low-dose heparin
Thrombophlebitis ascending to the junction or close to the junction (proximal 5–10 cm) of the great or small saphenous vein	Crossectomy, severing of the great saphenous vein or small saphenous vein; anticoagulation treatment alone in exceptional cases only
Thrombus extends beyond the saphenofemoral or saphenopopliteal junction with DVT of variable severity	Anticoagulation with low-molecular-weight heparin and overlapping change to phenprocoumon (6 months)
Varicophlebitis with secondary DVT resulting from thrombus extension through an incompetent perforator ("collar stud thrombosis")	Anticoagulation with low-molecular-weight heparin and overlapping change to phenprocoumon (6 months)

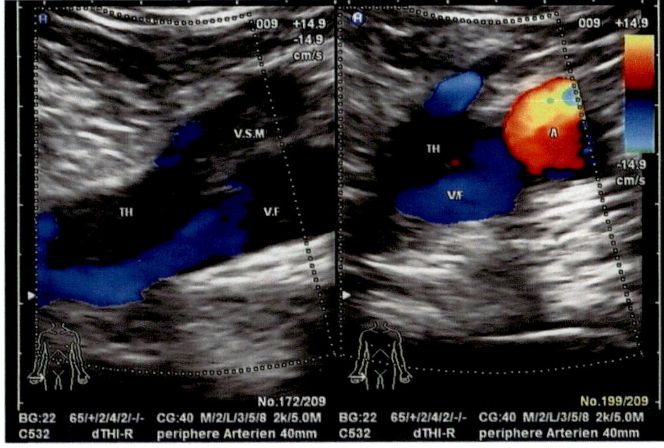

Fig. 3.34 Longitudinal and transverse images of thrombophlebitis of the great saphenous vein (V.S.M) with thrombus (TH) adhering to the wall and extending 1.5 cm into the common femoral vein (V.F)

a more aggressive therapeutic strategy in patients with superficial varicophlebitis extending close to the saphenous junction. The foremost aim in the management of varicophlebitis is to prevent deep vein thrombosis (DVT) and the attendant risk of embolic complications, which is why a therapy-oriented classification system appears reasonable (Table 3.7).

The need to perform ultrasound in all patients with clinically manifest disease arises from the fact that patients with clinical signs of calf varicophlebitis (classic signs of inflammation such as redness or pain, tumor) often have disease extending above the knee even when the thigh appears normal. Ultrasound is performed to define the proximal extent of thrombophlebitis as a basis for planning treatment. A study reports propagation into the deep venous system in 10–25% of cases (Uthoff et al. 2010), causing symptomatic and asymptomatic pulmonary embolism in 4% and 33% of cases, respectively.

In the Prospective Observational Superficial Thrombophlebitis (POST) study (Quéré et al. 2012), a complete sonographic exploration of the deep venous system in more than 800 patients with proven thrombophlebitis revealed DVT in nearly a quarter of the study population. In this subset, DVT was contiguous with superficial vein thrombosis in 42% of patients and noncontiguous in another 42%. Five patients had isolated contralateral DVT.

Therefore, the workup of these patients should always include **compression ultrasound evaluation of the deep venous system** with special attention to possible extension of thrombosis through incompetent perforators. Concomitant DVT of the calf is seen in up to 20% of patients and is especially common in patients with paraneoplastic thrombophlebitis.

3

3.1.7 Rare Venous Disorders

3.1.7.1 Venous Aneurysm

For a long time, the term aneurysm was only used to refer to local widening of arteries, while the venous counterpart was described as ectasia or aneurysmal dilatation. Venous aneurysm is now commonly used to designate a marked, localized sacculated or spindle-shaped dilatation of a venous segment (at least 2.5–3 times the normal luminal diameter). Data on the incidence of venous aneurysms are scarce, and most case reports do not mention a size threshold.

Histologically, a venous aneurysm is a **true aneurysm** with a wall consisting of all venous layers but with thinning of the muscle layer. Medial sclerosis may occasionally be present. The etiology is unknown, but various mechanisms have been proposed including embryonal defects, excessive local pressure in narrow anatomic spaces, and trauma (Fischer et al. 1996; Smets et al. 1997; Aldridge and Comerota 1993). Venous aneurysms are very rare (120 case reports or case series in the literature) and mainly occur in the legs, in particular the **popliteal vein**. Aneurysms of leg veins account for approx. 65% of all venous aneurysms, 17% occur in neck veins, and 14% in the arms (overview in Ritter 1993). Leg aneurysms mainly affect the major deep veins but may also occur in the superficial compartment, where they have to be differentiated from varicosis and regional or diffuse phlebectasia, which, when occurring in the calf veins, may take the form of long tubular ectasias (see ◻ Fig. 3.89 (Atlas)).

Most venous aneurysms remain undetected unless there is thrombus formation or pulmonary embolism secondary to local thrombosis and patients undergo workup to identify the underlying cause of embolism. Other complications are due to compression of surrounding structures, typically manifesting as abnormal sensations, and very rarely rupture and hemorrhage. The popliteal vein is the most common site of venous aneurysm in the leg, and mechanical factors are considered major contributing factors to aneurysm formation at this site.

Some venous aneurysms present with calf swelling or are detected incidentally in patients scheduled for treatment of varicosities.

As with arterial aneurysms, **fusiform** or **spindle-shaped** (◻ Fig. 3.35) and **saccular aneurysms** are distinguished. Sonographically, an isolated venous aneurysm must be differentiated from ectatic dilatation, which involves longer segments. While some investigators define venous aneurysm as a permanent and irreversible localized dilation of a deep vein to two times (McDevitt et al. 1993) or three times its normal diameter (Maleti et al. 1997), many case reports give no size definition. When the superficial venous system is affected, an isolated aneurysm must be distinguished from varicose lesions and thromboembolic complications from thrombophlebitis. Only two cases of thromboembolism of superficial venous aneurysm have been reported in the literature (Gillespie et al. 1997; Siani et al. 2010).

There is agreement in the literature that a saccular venous aneurysm should be resected when thromboembolic complications have occurred, while no consistent strategy has emerged for the management of incidental venous aneurysms, especially when they are fusiform. Deep vein aneurysms have been discovered incidentally by ultrasound in nearly all body regions, including the neck veins (see ◻ Fig. 3.100 (Atlas)), the arm veins, and the splenoportal system, but rarely cause thromboembolic complications. Thromboembolism is most common in aneurysm of the popliteal vein, the most commonly affected leg vein. Both the popliteal artery and vein are subject to shear and mechanical stress during knee movement, which promotes the detachment of thrombotic material from popliteal aneurysms. Experimental investigations in models have shown that quasilaminar flow is predominant in fusiform aneurysms while turbulent flow with flow separations occurs in saccular aneurysms (Brunner et al. 1997; Haaverstad et al. 1995). Stasis in dead water zones in an aneurysm can give rise to thrombus formation (see ◻ Figs. 3.35 and 3.85a (Atlas)). Only anecdotal cases of pulmonary embolism caused by venous aneurysms have been reported (Biesseaux et al. 1994; Seino et al. 1994).

3.1.7.1.1 Sonographic Workup

Duplex ultrasound is the method of first choice for the diagnostic workup of thromboembolism. Allowing assessment of overall aneurysm size including thrombosed portions, duplex ultrasound, and in particular color duplex, is superior to venography, which is limited because it is an indirect, luminographic technique. The flexibility of ultrasound permits evaluation of aneurysm shape in different planes and differentiation of spindle-shaped from saccular venous aneurysms (see ◻ Figs. 3.85, 3.86, 3.87, and 3.88 (all Atlas)). True aneurysms of the popliteal vein and other veins must be distinguished from terminally dilated small veins at their sites of entry into larger veins. Here again, ultrasound is superior to all other imaging modalities. However, very careful evaluation in different planes is necessary, particularly of the terminal small saphenous vein and terminations of muscle veins. Distal vein compression to augment flow may be necessary for adequate evaluation. The incidence of spindle-shaped venous aneurysms depends on the size threshold used. When defined as a persistent focal dilatation of at least twice the normal vein diameter, venous aneurysm is not an uncommon incidental finding but is relevant only when its diameter is 2.5 to 3 times that of the normal vein. Many large venous aneurysms (>3 times the normal diameter) appear saccular.

Two factors – aneurysm shape and intra-aneurysmal thrombosis – are crucial for **therapeutic management**. In the superficial popliteal vein, both can be accurately characterized by color flow imaging and compression ultrasound. Blood flow in a nonthrombosed aneurysm can be assessed by gray-scale or color duplex ultrasound in transverse orientation but preferably in longuditinal orientation. At times, spontaneous contrast (known as the cigarette smoke sign) may be present, indicating very slow flow (◻ Fig. 3.35a). Consistent with the above-mentioned experimental model

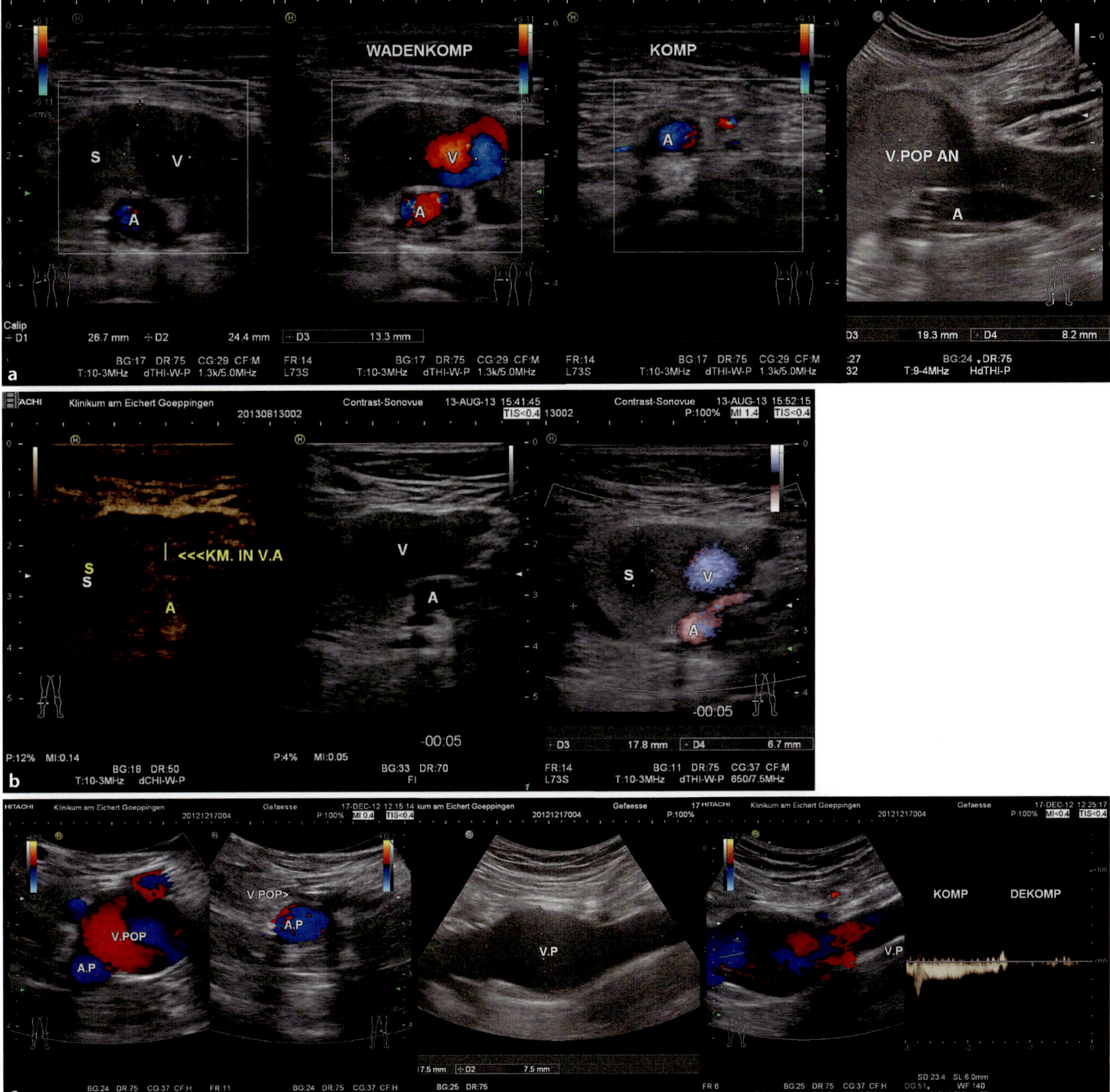

Fig. 3.35 **a** Large saccular aneurysm (26 mm) of the popliteal vein in transverse and longitudinal orientation (leftmost and rightmost images). The appearance in transverse orientation suggests a thrombosed aneurysm cavity (no flow signals due to stasis). The second image (obtained with calf compression (WADENKOMP) to augment flow) still shows no flow in the area of stasis (S). While the absence of flow, even with augmentation, is consistent with partial thrombosis, thrombus is ruled out by complete compressibility of this segment when pressure is applied with the transducer (KOMP, third image). **b** Contrast-enhanced ultrasound (CEUS) provides no additional diagnostic information in this situation. The contrast-enhanced color duplex image (right) suggests absence of flow (even with gentle calf compression) in the area of stagnant blood (S) within the saccular popliteal vein aneurysm (V) already identified by conventional ultrasound. In the CEUS image (left) and the corresponding B-mode image (center section) obtained with a reduced mechanical index (MI), microbubbles are absent from the area of stagnant blood (S) and only distribute in areas of flowing blood (indicated by "KM. in V.A") above the popliteal artery (A). While the CEUS findings are also consistent with a partially thrombosed aneurysm, this is ruled out by complete compressibility (see **a**). However, severe stasis of blood as in this aneurysm is associated with a high risk of thrombus formation. **c** Spindle-shaped aneurysm of the popliteal vein (transverse views on the left and longitudinal views on the right) with an abrupt increase in diameter from 7 mm to 20 mm (in transverse view) just below the saphenopopliteal junction. Complete compressibility reliably rules out thrombus in the aneurysmally dilated segment of the popliteal vein (second transverse view, V.POP>). The Doppler waveform shows no reflux in the compression-and-release test (KOMP/DEKOMP), consistent with competent valves proximal and distal to the aneurysm

studies (Brunner and Hauser 1997), ultrasound can show that quasilaminar flow is predominant in spindle-shaped venous aneurysms, while saccular aneurysms are characterized by turbulent flow and flow separations. Intra-aneurysmal deadwater zones promote **thrombus formation**. Color duplex ultrasound does not allow reliable differentiation of stagnant blood in deadwater zones from areas of thrombosis. Compression ultrasound is required to reliably differentiate stagnant blood from thrombosis in a venous aneurysm.

Stagnant blood in a venous aneurysm also needs to be differentiated from slow flow. This is most reliably done during compression and release applying gentle pressure at the calf level to augment flow. A supplementary option to differentiate stagnant blood and slow flow is **contrast-enhanced ultrasound** (CEUS) (Schäberle 2014). During the venous phase of microbubble inflow, CEUS can impressively reveal areas of turbulent flow and stagnant blood (absence of flow signals) in a saccular venous aneurysm (◘ Fig. 3.35).

3.1.7.1.2 Prevalence of Venous Aneurysms in Ultrasound Studies

The frequency of venous aneurysms in unselected populations is not known, and there are no data on the proportion of symptomatic to asymptomatic venous aneurysms. Two large ultrasound studies of patients presenting with different venous symptoms (mostly workup of varicosis) found a prevalence of asymptomatic aneurysms of the deep leg veins of 0.1% in 3500 patients (Franco et al. 1997) and 0.2% in 3880 patients (Labropoulos et al. 1996). One study reports a surprisingly high prevalence of 1.5% (all body regions) with two thirds accounted for by aneurysms of the deep leg veins (Gillespie et al. 1997). An analysis conducted by our group identified four saccular and four spindle-shaped aneurysms of the popliteal vein (focal diameter increase to at least 2.5 times the normal vein diameter) in 11,500 ultrasound examinations of the deep leg veins performed for suspected thrombosis and varicose workup, corresponding to a prevalence of 0.07% (Schäberle and Eisele 2001). Two of the saccular aneurysms were partially thrombosed and were diagnosed in patients with pulmonary embolism. The other two saccular aneurysms were incidental findings, one of them in a patient with concomitant DVT of the calf. Thus, the prevalence of saccular venous aneurysms requiring treatment was 0.035% in this population (half of them with thrombus and thromboembolic complications). The higher prevalence in patients undergoing ultrasound workup prior to varicose surgery suggests an association of venous aneurysms with degeneration of the superficial venous system. This in turn points to wall degeneration as a possible underlying mechanism, which is confirmed by histologic studies (Sigg et al. 2003; Lev et al. 1952; Friedmann et al. 1990).

3.1.7.1.3 Therapeutic Relevance of Sonographically Detected Venous Aneurysms

Resection is indicated for sonographically detected **saccular aneurysm** regardless of thrombosis or thromboembolic complications. The preferred technique is tangential resection with lateral plication of the venous wall or resection of the aneurysmal wall segment with vein graft interposition or closure by direct suture. However, the question when to treat needs to be reconsidered in view of the fact that more venous aneurysms, often spindle-shaped and typically involving the popliteal vein, are detected incidentally through the wider use of ultrasound in patients with suspected thrombosis. Since local aneurysmal dilatation of a single vein segment does not cause calf swelling (and duplex ultrasound allows adequate evaluation of valve function proximally and distally), the only **justification for surgical elimination is the risk of thromboembolic complications**. To prevent surgical overtreatment in this preventive situation, a risk stratification strategy based on ultrasound findings is warranted. Contrast-enhanced ultrasound (CEUS) is useful in identifying areas of prethrombotic stasis of blood (◘ Fig. 3.35).

In a follow-up study of the analysis already discussed above (Schäberle 2001, 2014), the author's group found no thrombotic components in any of the 13 spindle-shaped aneurysms (>2.5-fold normal vein diameter), and no patient had clinical signs of prior episodes of pulmonary embolism. Assessment of blood flow in these aneurysms by color duplex ultrasound or CEUS revealed mostly laminar flow and no regional stasis of blood. These patients were managed by surveillance (the former policy of anticoagulation treatment was abandoned at the author's institution), and no thromboembolic complications were observed. The eight sonographically detected saccular aneurysms of the popliteal vein included one aneurysm in a patient with complete thrombosis of the popliteal vein and major calf veins. Two of the patients had partially thrombosed aneurysms and pulmonary embolism. Five of the aneurysms were detected incidentally (in patients with swelling). All saccular aneurysms in this series were resected because flow analysis revealed vortexing with areas of stagnant blood or thrombus.

While investigators agree that saccular venous aneurysms should be resected (Gabrielli et al. 2010, 2011; Sessa et al. 2000; Coffman et al. 2000; Uematsu et al. 1999; Gosselin et al. 1997; Labropoulos et al. 1996), there is disagreement regarding the management of spindle-shaped venous aneurysms. Most investigators advocate a conservative strategy along the lines outlined above (Labropoulos et al. 1996; Rubin et al. 1995; Gobin et al. 1997; Sessa et al. 2000). Others recommend surgical resection also for spindle-shaped aneurysms (Tumko et al. 2013; Gabrielli et al. 2012). Anticoagulation treatment is another controversial issue in the management of venous aneurysms.

One case of paradoxical embolism has been described (Manthey et al. 1994). Most venous aneurysms are incidentally detected in patients undergoing ultrasound to rule out DVT of the leg. The patients typically report pain and swelling.

In venography, flow phenomena caused by contrast medium in muscle veins entering the popliteal vein in the popliteal fossa and in the small saphenous vein may mimic thrombus, impairing the identification of thrombus and evaluation of its extent in popliteal vein aneurysm.

Ultrasound findings, on the other hand, provide the basis for a differentiated approach to the treatment of the rare popliteal vein aneurysms (incidence of 0.07% of all patients examined for suspected DVT of the leg in our study).

Intraoperative findings and follow-up results confirm the validity of duplex ultrasound, which is the method of first choice in venous aneurysm.

In summary, a conservative strategy is justified if **ultrasound demonstrates a saccular aneurysm** no larger than 2 to 3 times the diameter of the vein proximal and distal to it. For larger spindle-shaped aneurysms, surgical resection may be contemplated, especially if CEUS or color duplex ultrasound with flow augmentation demonstrates stagnant blood within the aneurysm. Conversely, a **saccular aneurysm** should be resected when its size exceeds twice the normal vein diameter (Gabrielli et al. 2012). The need for surgical repair of these aneurysms is also underscored by reported embolic complication rates of 24–32% for (saccular) venous aneurysms (Sessa et al. 2000).

3.1.7.2 Tumors of the Vein Wall

Unilateral venous stasis or disturbed drainage with leg edema of unclear origin can point to a benign or malignant tumor of the vein wall. Such tumors can give rise to appositional thrombus growth as wall compression or infiltration progresses. Ultrasound (possibly supplemented by MRI or CT) allows direct demonstration of the tumor as a circumscribed wall thickening, differentiating it from venous thrombosis and thus providing the basis for establishing the indication for surgical resection. Benign tumors of the vein wall include papillary endothelial hyperplasia, hemangioma, leiomyoma, and fibroma. Malignant tumors are angiosarcoma, leiomyosarcoma, and malignant hemangioendothelioma (◘ Fig. 3.36 and ◘ Fig. 3.97 (Atlas)).

Benign wall tumors are more clearly demarcated sonographically compared with malignant tumors, which tend to infiltrate perivascular connective tissue (Reix et al. 1998; Kutzner and Schneider-Stock 2010). Malignant tumors arising from vein walls in the lower extremity are rare and can be difficult to differentiate from thrombus with both gray-scale and compression ultrasound as well as with other imaging modalities. Misdiagnosis is a common problem, especially in patients with secondary, tumor-induced thrombosis of the peripheral veins, and can lead to initiation of antithrombotic treatment. In a small series of 7 malignant venous tumors, the mean duration from initial symptoms to diagnosis was 7 months (up to 2 years) (Reix et al. 1998).

Histologically, **malignant tumors arising from the vein walls** are divided into two groups: malignant leiomyosarcomas and the less common hemangioendotheliomas. The latter usually have a better prognosis after complete surgical resection as they have a lower tendency to metastasize (Enzinger and Weiss 1993; Sebenik et al. 2005). More commonly than other tumors, leiomyosarcomas arise from larger veins (van Gulik et al. 1991; Gonzales et al. 1965; Dzsinich et al. 1993; Kutzner and Schneider-Stock 2010). A review of a soft tissue tumor registry identified 90 epithelioid hemangioendotheliomas of the venous system (Enzinger and Weiss 1995; Sebenik 2005) but only a few case reports of epithelioid hemangioendotheliomas in larger veins exist (Reix et al. 1998; Weiss and Enzinger 1982; Harris et al. 1989; Schröder et al. 2001; Charette et al. 2001). They typically develop in the smaller veins of soft tissues (Fischer et al. 1982; Kutzner and Schneider-Stock 2010) or parenchymal organs such as the liver, less commonly in major veins (Ferretti et al. 1998; Lau et al. 1998; Delin et al. 1990; Schröder et al. 2001).

Epithelioid hemangioendothelioma can show circumscribed or invasive growth and usually arises from a small vein, rarely from an artery (Traverse et al. 1999) or a thick-walled vein (Charette et al. 2001; Enzinger and Weiss 1995; Kutzner and Schneider-Stock 2010). The tumor tends to grow transmurally without destroying the vessel wall (Kutzner and Schneider-Stock 2010), causing dilatation and obliteration.

Although these tumors are rare, they may be encountered in vascular ultrasound examinations of patients with suspected thrombosis of the legs (see differential diagnostic features in the legend of ◘ Fig. 3.36). With its high resolution, ultrasound is superior to other imaging modalities, and venography may even lead to the misdiagnosis of thrombus because it merely shows a defect in opacification without providing clues to the underlying cause (Schröder et al. 2001; Reix et al. 1998).

Vessel wall tumors must be differentiated from paravascular tumors such as neurogenic tumors, which tend to be spindle-shaped and grow along vessels (◘ Fig. 3.37a).

3.1.7.3 Venous Compression

The venous wall has only a thin muscle layer and is therefore easily compressed by lymphoma (predominantly in the true pelvis and groin), perivascular tumors, hematoma, abscess, and arterial aneurysm (primarily affecting the popliteal artery), causing flow obstruction and clinical signs of thrombosis (◘ Fig. 3.37b). With its ability to visualize both the vein itself and the surrounding structures (see ◘ Figs. 2.87, 2.92, 3.49, and 3.93 (Atlas)), ultrasound will either demonstrate the cause of disturbed drainage directly or provide clues guiding further, more specific diagnostic procedures such as ultrasound-guided aspiration or biopsy.

In rare cases, **popliteal entrapment syndrome** involves both the artery and the vein, for instance in individuals with an ectopic popliteal muscle or pronounced hypertrophy of the heads of the gastrocnemius muscle. In such cases, outflow obstruction can be elicited by active plantar flexion (see ◘ Fig. 3.98 (Atlas) and 2.31).

Only augmented flow elicited by distal compression may be detectable when a vein is compressed by an external structure. Normal respiratory phasicity is lost distal to the flow obstruction. When there is flow in a small residual lumen, spectral Doppler depicts a high-frequency flow signal resembling a stenosis signal (see ◘ Fig. 3.95 (Atlas)).

3.1.7.4 Venous Adventitial Cystic Disease

Venous adventitial cystic disease is very rare, occurring 80–50 times less commonly than its arterial counterpart. As in the arteries, the lesions are histologically true ganglia (in terms of cyst contents and wall composition) in the adventitial layer of the diseased vein. The cysts have been attributed to ectopic synovial cells and compromise the venous lumen (Paty 1992; Schraverus 1997; Chakfe 1997; Hach-Wunderle 2003).

3

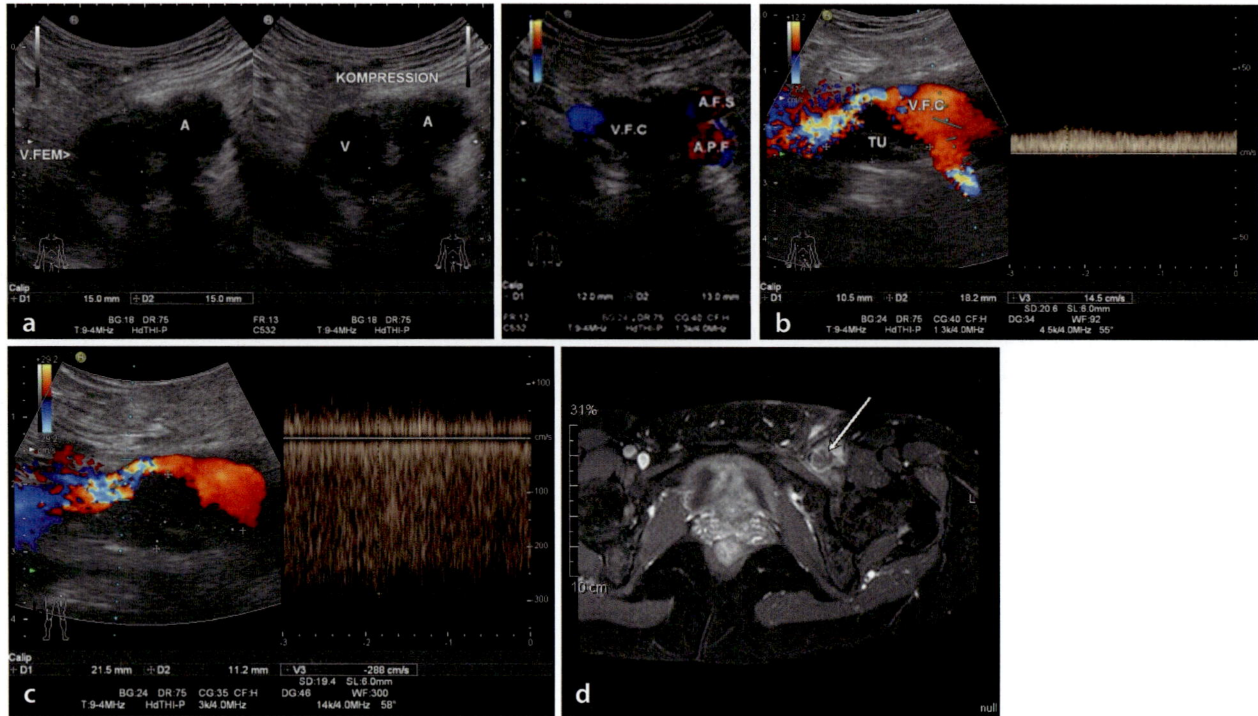

Fig. 3.36 Tumor of the vein wall. **a** Dilated common femoral vein (V.FEM>, indicated by calipers) shown in transverse orientation without and with compression (leftmost and center, respectively). The vein is incompressible but the wall is poorly demarcated from surrounding tissue, which distinguishes tumor from thrombus. The color duplex image (rightmost) shows residual flow along the anteromedial vessel wall, similar in appearance to marginal flow in the presence of a floating thrombus. **b** The longitudinal color flow image shows a short hypoechoic femoral vein segment without flow (1.8 cm in length, calipers) and patency of the vein distally. The Doppler waveform from the patent distal vein segment shows a markedly reduced flow signal with loss of respiratory phasicity, consistent with obstructed venous drainage. The patent lumen is markedly narrowed by the wall tumor. Clinically, the tumor causes only disturbed venous drainage and slight calf swelling. The slow increase in luminal narrowing due to the tumor allowed formation of a collateral pathway via the great saphenous vein with retrograde flow through the deep femoral vein toward the pelvis. **c** Marginal flow along the tumor is consistent with stenosis. However, the flow velocity of 2 m/s is too high for thrombotic stenosis and is only observed when a wall tumor is present or the vein is compressed by an external structure (see Fig. 3.49 (Atlas)). Workup for treatment planning included ultrasound-guided biopsy of a lymph node seen medial to the wall tumor (histology: epithelioid hemangioendothelioma). Overall, the sonographic findings including B-mode appearance, spatial relationships, and hemodynamic information allowed the diagnosis of vein wall tumor to be made before lymph node biopsy was performed. **d** Magnetic resonance imaging of the chest, abdomen, and pelvis performed for tumor staging shows the vein wall tumor (arrow) in the groin

As with arterial adventitial degeneration, compression of the underlying vein and the associated clinical symptoms vary with the filling of the cysts, and the lesions always develop close to a joint. Occasionally, the surgeon will encounter a communication between an adventitial cyst and the joint capsule. Venous adventitial cystic degeneration **most commonly affects the common femoral and popliteal veins.** Depending on the degree of luminal compression, there may be swelling of the leg with a sensation of congestion distal to the lesion, which intensifies during physical activity. Edema usually recedes over night. As with the arterial counterpart, there will be cystic lesions in the venous wall (which may be multiple), seen as luminal narrowing on B-mode ultrasound. The degree of luminal narrowing and the hemodynamic relevance of venous obstruction can be evaluated using color duplex imaging. Venous obstruction is seen as loss of respiratory phasicity and reduced flow velocity in the Doppler waveform obtained distal to the degenerative lesion.

Luminal narrowing varies with cyst size (Fig. 3.96 (Atlas)) and is reflected by a variable increase in flow velocity (Doppler waveform) in the diseased vein segment as well as by a flow signal similar to that seen with a stenosis.

Inconclusive findings should be resolved by computed tomography or magnetic resonance imaging; ascending venography will only show external compression.

3.1.7.5 Differential Diagnosis: Lymphedema, Lipedema

Once duplex imaging has ruled out chronic venous insufficiency as the underlying cause of edema, edema of cardiac origin must be differentiated from lymphedema and lipedema.

Lymphedema has rather characteristic sonomorphologic features including increased echogenicity of the thickened subcutaneous layer and sound scattering with demonstration of anechoic clefts. These clefts tend to be longitudinal in orientation, distinguishing them from clefts in cardiac edema. They represent subcutaneous fluid collections and correlate with the extent of edema. In severe edema, lymphatic fluid can be aspirated from these clefts using ultrasound-guided

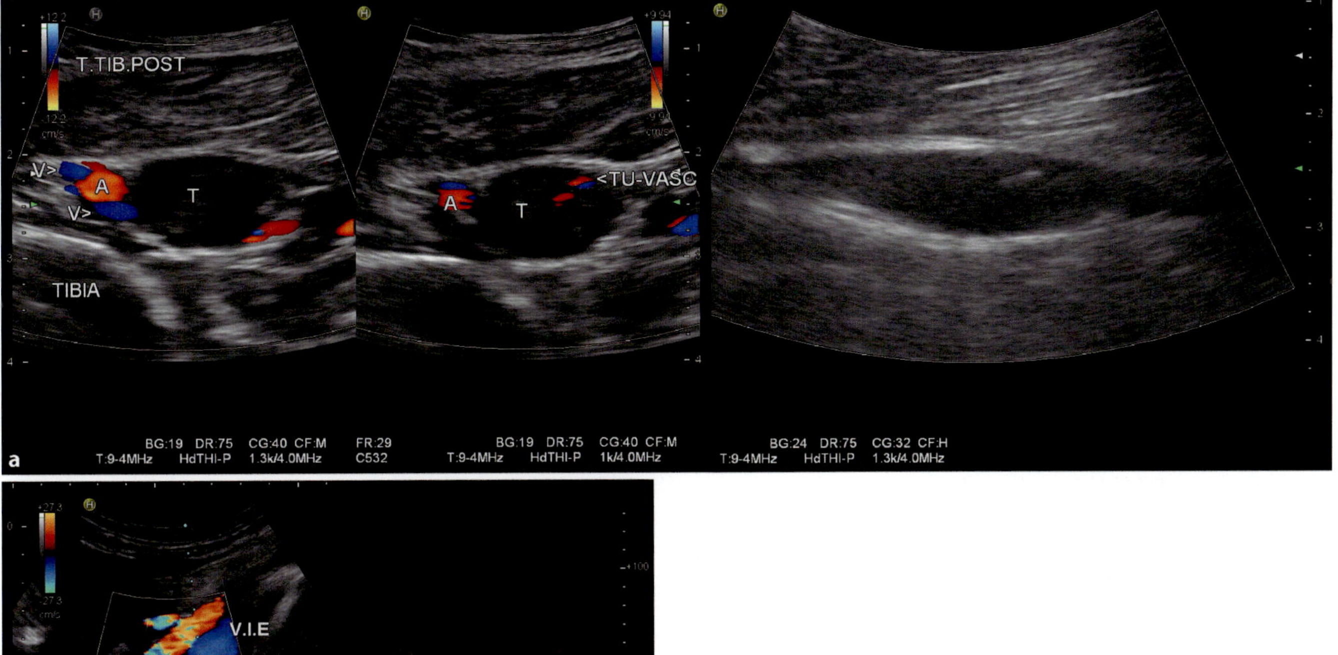

Fig. 3.37 **a** Transverse color flow images without and with compression (left section and center section) and longitudinal image (right section) of a paravascular spinalioma (along posterior tibial artery and vein). **b** Typical waveform showing loss of respiratory phasicity of the external iliac vein (V.I.E) consistent with central outflow obstruction. In this patient obstruction is due to late pregnancy

fine needle aspiration. In patients with chronic proximal lymphatic outflow obstruction, ultrasound may show 2–3 mm wide channels with a hyperechoic margin arranged parallel to the skin surface (Fig. 3.94 (Atlas)). Confusion with blood vessels can be ruled out by color duplex imaging. The channels are most likely dilated, sclerotic lymphatics, which would be consistent with the histologic demonstration of sclerotic transformation of lymphatic vessels (Altdorfer 1976) and with the lymphographic identification of dilated lymphatics (2–3 mm) in lymphangiosclerosis. These channels are distinct from the anechoic or hypoechoic clefts seen more distally in patients with peripheral lymphatic obstruction. The latter are more irregularly arranged and appear more blurred. They contain free lymphatic fluid, or are prelymphatic clefts in lymphedema. The sonographic findings in peripheral lymphedema are less specific, and subcutaneous fluid collections may also be present in other types of edema. Cardiac edema is therefore more difficult to diagnose. While lymphedema is characterized by longitudinal clefts, meshlike patterns may be seen in cardiac edema.

The excess fat in **lipedema** (Fig. 3.94e (Atlas)) is sonomorphologically seen as thickening of the subcutaneous layer with a relatively uniform appearance and partially increased echogenicity ("flurry"). There may be conspicuous, hyperechoic subcutaneous septa but no fluid-containing clefts.

Ultrasound with a high-resolution transducer (between 7.5 and 13 MHz) allows differentiation of phlebedema (no specific sonomorphologic findings in the subcutaneous layer but identification of incompetent venous valves) from edemas of other etiology (with characteristic subcutaneous findings) and also allows inexpensive follow-up of these conditions (Marshall 2008).

3.1.8 Vein Mapping

Autologous saphenous vein grafts have the best patency rate of all materials used in peripheral bypass surgery. However, the vein may be unsuitable for bypass grafting for several reasons (see Fig. 2.67 (Atlas)):

- Small lumen
- Postthrombophlebitic lesions
- Ectatic, varicose degeneration

These criteria can be assessed in the preoperative ultrasound examination by measurement of lumen width, evaluation of valve competence, and visualization of postthrombophlebitic wall lesions (see Fig. 3.81 (Atlas)). The ultrasound examination will thus shorten the length of surgery and prevent unnecessary vein exposure. Moreover, preoperative marking of the course of the vein on the skin helps prevent large incisions and is especially helpful in obese patients. Duplex imaging is highly reliable in identifying suitable vein segments for grafting as demonstrated by intraoperative confirmation of the findings in 98% of cases (Krishnabhakdi et al. 2001).

3.1.9 Diagnostic Role of Ultrasound

3.1.9.1 Deep Vein Thrombosis

The role of a diagnostic method also depends on the availability and diagnostic performance of other tests. Apart from venography, the traditional standard, other modalities used in the diagnostic assessment of patients with suspected deep vein thrombosis (DVT) included thermography, scintigraphy, plethysmography, and CW Doppler. All of these modalities rely on the demonstration of indirect criteria and have low specificity. Moreover, each of them is restricted to a specific vascular territory and none of them enables evaluation of the entire venous system. Scintigraphy is highly sensitive in diagnosing thrombosis of the calf, whereas CW Doppler ultrasound is reliable only in identifying DVT above the knee.

The German guideline on DVT (Hach-Wunderle et al. 2010) derived on the basis of the algorithms presented in ► Sect. 3.1.6.1 (Fig. 3.21) advises a stepwise evaluation of patients with suspected DVT (Fig. 3.38), which is rather cumbersome for routine clinical practice. The generous use of compression ultrasound as first-line test in patients with even a slight clinical suspicion of DVT allows a much more time-efficient examination (<5 min per leg) with less logistic effort than prior stratification and identification of the subset of patients who should have a compression ultrasound examination based on a D-dimer test and pretest likelihood of disease (assessed using the Wells score). At the same time,

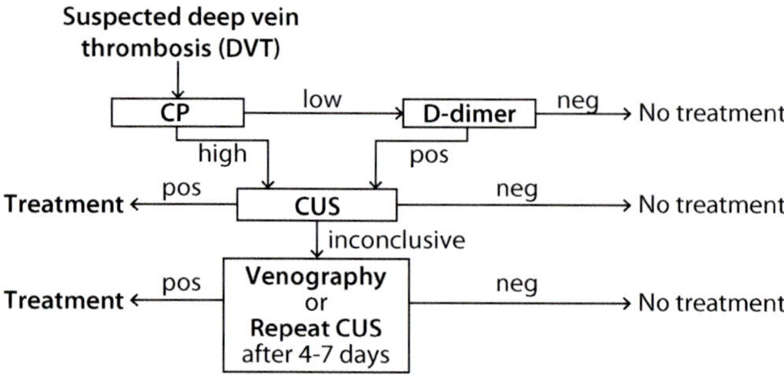

Fig. 3.38 Guideline-based diagnostic algorithm in patients with suspected deep vein thrombosis (DVT) (Hach-Wunderle et al. 2010)

the sonographic B-mode evaluation can identify other causes that might explain the patient's clinical symptoms.

Similar conclusions in terms of practical implementation of the guideline were reached by the authors of a survey of 326 German centers examining a total of 4976 consecutive patients with suspected DVT over a 3-month period (TULIPA registry (Thrombosis and pulmonary embolism in out-patients); Gerlach et al. 2009). A total of 1388 patients were diagnosed with DVT using imaging without a prior D-dimer test or clinical probability assessment (95.9% ultrasound and 5.8% venography; however, the latter was used as first-line imaging test in only 1.6% of cases). In a representative subset of patients who were initially negative for DVT, follow-up revealed DVT in 0.4% of cases. These excellent results were achieved although most centers followed their routine procedure, which included imaging as the first-line diagnostic test, rather than adhering to the recommended diagnostic algorithm.

Therefore, **compression ultrasound** should be the first-line imaging modality in patients with **clinically suspected DVT of the leg.** It has several advantages but also some disadvantages.

- Advantages:
  - Highly valid method above and below the knee
  - Direct evaluation of the extent of DVT
  - Direct thrombus visualization (muscle vein thrombosis, thrombophlebitis)
  - No special equipment needed (5-MHz transducer)
  - Concomitant evaluation of soft tissues
  - Easy and fast to perform
- Disadvantages:
  - Examiner dependence
  - Poor documentation
  - Poor visualization and compressibility of proximal pelvic vein segments

The high diagnostic accuracy of compression ultrasound with nearly 100% sensitivity and specificity in assessing the veins above the knee, the popliteal vein, and the proximal segments of the calf veins ensures a confident diagnosis, provided the scanning conditions are adequate. For calf vein thrombosis, studies report a lower sensitivity of 85–90%. Here, additional venography should be performed if the sonographic findings are inconclusive and the patient has a high risk of thrombosis or if ultrasound visualization is inadequate. Alternatively, the D-dimer test can be used, which is highly sensitive but not very specific. Due to the low specificity, a positive D-dimer test is of little use, especially in postoperative patients with suspected thrombosis. In conjunction with compression ultrasound, however, a negative test result rules out DVT.

Venography is not necessary in patients with patent femoral and popliteal veins on compression ultrasound. Instead, these patients can undergo **close serial sonographic surveillance** for early detection of popliteal extension of calf thrombosis missed due to poor scanning conditions in the initial examination. The high specificity of compression ultrasound results in a high positive predictive value, i.e., an abnormal finding (noncompressibility of the vein) is diagnostic of DVT of the leg.

While being highly accurate in symptomatic patients with suspected DVT, duplex imaging has a **lower accuracy** in detecting **suspected symptomatic recurrent thrombosis** and in screening asymptomatic high-risk patients for thrombosis (patients who have undergone orthopedic, urologic, or general surgery).

Such screening examinations in high-risk patients are nevertheless justified clinically as 17–20% of patients develop DVT of the leg after hip or knee replacement despite antithrombotic prophylaxis (Hamulyak et al. 1995). A review of 11 studies performed in asymptomatic patients after hip and knee surgery found a sensitivity of only 62% for compression ultrasound but a specificity of 97% for identifying femoropopliteal venous thrombosis (Wells et al. 1995). An even lower accuracy was found for the diagnosis of DVT below the knee (Lensing et al. 1997).

In neurosurgical patients, ultrasound was found to have a sensitivity of only 56% in asymptomatic proximal thrombosis and only 50% in distal thrombosis compared with venography (Jongbloets et al. 1994; Lausen et al. 1995).

Most venous thrombi in asymptomatic patients cause no or only very short occlusion and, in the presence of postoperative edema, are easily overlooked. Venography is superior, especially in depicting minute clots in the pocket-like valves of the femoral and popliteal veins. The poor results in asymptomatic high-risk patients are also due to a lack of compliance and a less thorough examination in this patient population. The results may be improved by exploiting the flexibility of ultrasound and testing the compressibility of poorly visualized vessel segments with different transducer orientations.

Mural thrombi in a partially compressible vein can be identified if the vein is insonated through the artery, which can thus serve as an acoustic window, provided that it is free of atherosclerosis. The clinical relevance of such thrombi is controversial but they may be the source of further thrombus growth. Therefore, despite the limitations just outlined, postoperative patients should be assessed by compression ultrasound of the deep leg veins prior to mobilization.

The term "**free-floating thrombus**" is based on the venographic appearance of a thrombus component surrounded by flowing blood: the convoluted tail suggests a swimming motion, but this is due to thrombus growth in the blood stream and merely gives the thrombus the appearance of floating. Floating thrombi were considered to carry a high risk of embolism and therefore used to be operated on much more frequently in the past. Ultrasound and CT studies suggest that actual movement of floating thrombi is overestimated due to their morphologic structure. A truly floating thrombus can be identified by real-time ultrasound and documented in the time-motion mode. Floating thrombi are diagnosed three times more often by venography than by ultrasound and even less frequently by CT (Gartenschlager et al. 1996). This overestimation of floating thrombi is also confirmed by the author's experience. For these reasons, a floating thrombus should only be diagnosed if an unattached thrombus segment is seen on gray-scale ultrasound, color duplex scanning demonstrates a thrombus tail several centimeters in length, or the thrombus is surrounded by flowing blood on all sides (without wall adherence) and appears to float in the center of the vessel with respiration or during a gently performed Valsalva maneuver (◘ Figs. 3.26c, 3.59 (Atlas), and 3.61 (Atlas)).

The high diagnostic accuracy of compression ultrasound that can be achieved with state-of-the-art equipment is both a blessing and a curse: while early anticoagulation treatment prevents ascending progression of calf vein thrombosis, it means overtreatment and exposure to unnecessary risks for patients whose calf vein thrombosis would never ascend further even without treatment and thus would not cause thromboembolic complications or other late sequelae.

The simultaneous visualization of perivascular structures by ultrasound enables the **differentiation of abnormal soft tissue changes** that may cause thrombosis-like clinical symptoms. A hematoma occurring after trauma or in association with a coagulation disorder is seen as a hypoechoic area more or less clearly delineated from the surrounding muscle. If the findings are inconclusive or abscess is suspected, the diagnosis can be confirmed by ultrasound-guided puncture.

Baker's cysts are caused by the escape of synovial fluid. They are located in the popliteal fossa and typically arise from the medial knee joint space. Depending on their size, they cause swelling and tension. Cyst rupture is associated with acute pain of the calf and is demonstrated on ultrasound as an anechoic, leaking fluid collection under the fascia. Ultrasound-guided aspiration confirms the diagnosis and also leads to rapid improvement or complete elimination of the complaints.

In patients diagnosed with a soft tissue tumor, ultrasound additionally provides direct information on vein compression by the tumor and allows hemodynamic assessment of the outflow obstruction. The sonographic examination thus enables precise preoperative determination of the **extent and localization of disturbed drainage** and identification of possible vascular infiltration, which is important for surgical tumor removal. The sonographic workup of thrombosis includes the search for a tumor to exclude a paraneoplastic origin, especially in older patients. The site of compression of a vein by a lymphoma can be identified, and the severity of the outflow obstruction estimated from spectral Doppler interrogation (spontaneous and augmented flow) distal to the compressed vein.

Venous compression syndromes of the upper and lower extremities can be diagnosed sonographically by assessing flow patterns elicited by provocative tests.

3.1.9.1.1 Ultrasound Versus Venography

Before they became widely accepted, both compression ultrasound and duplex ultrasound had to prove their diagnostic performance in relation to venography, the traditional gold standard, which in turn was never validated in comparison with another modality. While opacification of the veins by the contrast medium enables direct assessment of the lumen, venography provides no information on perivascular abnormalities. Moreover, filling defects may give rise to misinterpretation because they may be due to occlusion

3

or methodological limitations, especially below the knee (see ◘ Figs 3.55, 3.56, and 3.57 (all Atlas)). The veins below the knee are depicted incompletely in 15% of cases and inadequately in 4% (Schmitt 1974, 1977). Angiographic assessability of the leg veins depends on the venous segment, and ranges from 61–96%. Repeat venography in patients with clinical signs of venous thrombosis of the leg performed due to progression of symptoms within 5 days of a negative initial venography enabled definitive diagnosis of thrombosis in 1.3% of cases (Hull et al. 1981).

These results call into question the suitability of venography as the gold standard in the diagnosis of thrombosis. In a study performed by our group in 159 patients with clinically suspected deep vein thrombosis (DVT) who were independently examined by duplex scanning and venography (Schäberle and Eisele 1991), venography yielded inconclusive or false results or, due to methodological limitations, failed to identify the cause of leg swelling in a total of 21 cases. In these cases, duplex scanning demonstrated an AV fistula, thrombophlebitis, muscle vein thrombosis, and venous compression by pelvic tumors, Baker's cysts, or arterial aneurysms. In five instances, venography yielded false-negative results compared to ultrasound (deep femoral vein thrombosis; complete thrombosis of one branch of a duplicated superficial femoral vein; below-knee venous thrombosis, predominantly in patients with thrombosis of one branch of paired major veins; mural thrombosis of venous aneurysm). False-positive venograms were seen in three cases (compression of the popliteal vein and proximal veins below the knee by a ruptured Baker's cyst and a large false aneurysm; misinterpretation of filling defect). The ultrasound findings were confirmed intraoperatively or through additional examinations. In this study, venography had an accuracy of 95% compared to duplex ultrasound (and the results of further diagnostic tests).

In a large study of 430 consecutively examined patients, the 5% discrepancy between venography and ultrasound (including the veins below the knee) is attributed to false-negative venograms, which are represented in the study as false-positive ultrasound findings (Elias et al. 1987). Some of the false-negative venograms were retrospectively accounted for by sonographically identified venous thrombi below the knee and misinterpretation of filling defects.

Complete evaluation of all deep veins below the knee is often not possible by venography because thrombi producing complete occlusion of small veins are missed as they are not apparent as filling defects. Ultrasound can supplement venography and provide useful additional information:

- Evaluation of the deep femoral vein
- Identification of muscle vein thrombosis
- Thrombosis of veins entering the saphenofemoral junction
- Demonstration of thrombus in an unopacified calf vein
- Visualization of the thrombus end (in segments with reduced contrast medium flow/long thrombotic segments)
- Evaluation of surrounding soft tissues

The limitations of venography have led some investigators to abandon venography as the gold standard for assessing the diagnostic performance of ultrasound. Instead they measure performance as the incidence of new thromboembolic complications after an initial negative ultrasound examination.

Earlier studies still using venography as the gold standard found sensitivities and specificities of compression ultrasound ranging from 87% to 100% (◘ Table 3.2). In one of these studies, performed by our group and including 131 legs with clinically suspected DVT (confirmed by venography in 73 legs) in 125 patients (72 women, 53 men; mean age 55 ± 18.5 years), ultrasound had a sensitivity of 97% and a specificity of 98% (Schäberle and Eisele 1991). Discrepancies between ultrasound and venography mainly concerned the venous territory below the knee.

3.1.9.1.2 Ultrasound for Follow-Up and Therapeutic Decision Making

The **high risk of appositional thrombus growth** with propagation into a major deep vein secondary to superficial thrombophlebitis was first truly recognized and documented by ultrasonography. High ligation of the saphenofemoral junction aimed at preventing further appositional growth and pulmonary embolism is indicated if thrombosis extends to the terminal portion of the saphenous vein or if a thrombus protrudes from a superficial vein into a major deep vein. Patients with thrombosis confined to more peripheral segments are treated by short-term anticoagulation. Unlike venography, ultrasound enables very reliable evaluation of the extent of phlebitis (Barrelier 1993; Schuler et al. 1995; Schönhofer et al. 1992). Since thrombophlebitis occasionally correlates with occult deep vein thrombosis (DVT) below the knee, especially in paraneoplastic disease, this should be confirmed or ruled out by ultrasound (Jorgensen et al. 1993).

Precise determination of **thrombus age** is crucial for selecting the most promising treatment (thrombolysis, surgery, or conservative management). Thrombus age is often underestimated if based on the clinical findings and history alone. Venography chiefly relies on indirect criteria (collateralization) to estimate thrombus age, while the morphologic appearance is of limited value in venographic age determination. The ultrasonographic evaluation of thrombus morphology provides the most reliable data for estimating thrombus age despite the variations that exist in echotexture and extent of venous dilatation in relation to thrombus genesis and localization (Fobbe et al. 1991).

Early recanalization (occurring spontaneously or induced by thrombolytic treatment) is suggested by the presence of spontaneous or augmented flow in the venous lumen. Incompetent valves in recanalized thrombotic veins are identified by functional tests (Valsalva's maneuver, compression-and-release test). Wall irregularities and hyperechoic deposits as well as a rigid vessel wall in the compression test already suggest the postthrombotic syndrome in the gray-scale scan. Noninvasive color duplex imaging can be repeated any time and is thus an excellent modality for **monitoring the response to thrombolysis and deciding when treatment can be discontinued**. Moreover, color duplex can be used to evaluate the outcome of thrombectomy and to quantitatively estimate the flow volume after the creation of a bucket handle shunt, which is done by determining blood flow in the common femoral artery proximal to the shunt and comparing it with the contralateral side.

Close sonographic follow-up of the natural history (or of patients undergoing heparinization with subsequent phenprocoumon versus patients treated by thrombolysis or thrombectomy) provides data for a critical appraisal of these therapies and may lead to changes in established therapeutic strategies. The fact that patients undergoing thrombolytic therapy for more than 5 days develop valve incompetence casts doubt on this approach, although it leads to recanalization (but fairly late). Moreover, one must take into account the increasing bleeding risk associated with longer thrombolytic therapy. Valve damage occurs with increasing thrombus organization; the valves immobilized by residual thrombotic material can be depicted in the recanalized veins if the scanning conditions are good. Comparative studies of the late outcome of thrombolytic therapy in subgroups stratified by thrombus age, treatment duration, and thrombus localization in comparison with the natural history would be desirable but would require a complex study design.

The sonographic examination yields very detailed information on the **extent and localization of thrombosis**. It provides direct evidence as to whether a thrombus is localized in a calf muscle vein or a main vein or if a thrombus protruding into the femoral vein originates from the great saphenous vein or from the deep femoral vein. Pulmonary emboli may arise from the proximal deep femoral vein, especially if an appositional thrombus protruding into the common femoral vein is dislodged. Venographically, the deep femoral vein is often not depicted or only after retrograde contrast filling, which does not occur in most patients with competent valves. In contrast, ultrasound enables good visualization of the proximal deep femoral vein (4 cm) and its termination.

Another, though rare, source of embolism is thrombus in the terminal segment of the internal iliac vein. This site should be assessed by color duplex imaging for the presence of a floating thrombus, particularly in patients with pulmonary embolism and no evidence of thrombosis elsewhere. However, sonographic assessment of this venous segment is limited in obese patients or when there is scattering and acoustic shadowing due to overlying bowel gas. If visualization of the pelvic veins is limited, occlusive pelvic vein thrombosis can be ruled out indirectly by Doppler interrogation of the common femoral vein and comparison with the contralateral waveform.

Patients with descending pelvic vein thrombosis, but without extension into the femoral vein (either naturally or because descent has been stopped by heparin and compression treatment), are not expected to develop postthrombotic syndrome following recanalization because the iliac veins have no valves.

The initial expectation that sonographic evaluation of thrombus morphology might allow identification of patients likely to benefit from short immobilization for prevention of pulmonary embolism has not been fulfilled. It has emerged, though, that preventive immobilization is not necessary when nonimmobilized patients develop thrombosis, even if a free-floating thrombus is present or thrombosis extends to the pelvic level (formerly classified as high-risk thrombosis). In contrast, immobilized patients (e.g., ICU) developing acute thrombosis have a high risk of pulmonary embolism when they are mobilized.

Ultrasound, not involving radiation exposure and not requiring contrast medium administration, is the **method of choice in pregnant women, children and adolescents, and in patients allergic to contrast medium**. Another advantage of this noninvasive modality is the short examination time of <5 min per leg in the diagnostic workup of suspected DVT. Some extra time is required for assessing valve function in patients with the postthrombotic syndrome and varicosis.

While the detection and evaluation of thrombosis by ultrasound is highly examiner-dependent, the **learning curve is steep**, and performance improves rapidly. In a study of 99 patients using venography as reference standard, the initial sensitivity of duplex ultrasound was 67% in the thigh and 57% in the calf, increasing to 100% and 79%, respectively, after the first 50 examinations. Specificity was already over 95% when the study began, indicating that the pathognomonic criteria for thrombosis are highly accurate (Leutz et al. 1994).

As with arterial aneurysms, the extent, localization, and presence of mural thrombosis of **venous aneurysms** can be assessed more reliably using ultrasound compared with radiographic techniques that rely on the opacification of the patent lumen (angiography, venography). The decision for conservative management or surgical resection is mainly based on the presence of partial thrombosis, the shape of the aneurysm, and its extent.

3.1.9.2 Chronic Venous Insufficiency

In patients with the postthrombotic syndrome, duplex ultrasound is a highly valid modality both for depicting morphologic changes of the venous wall (B-scan) and for identifying insufficiency of the main vein (Doppler). Recanalization is visualized with a high degree of accuracy and drainage insufficiency is evaluated semiquantitatively by measuring flow velocity and the duration and magnitude of reflux. Differentiation of reflux from persisting occlusion has important prognostic implications. Careful documentation of the findings is crucial for comparison and diagnosis of recurrent thrombosis at follow-up. In the occasional patient, venography is required to confirm morphologic wall changes and recurrent thrombosis. Venography is also required for documentation when providing expert opinion.

Noninvasive duplex imaging would also be a suitable modality for determining functional parameters in monitoring the response to pharmacologic treatment. To establish a basis of comparison for the definition of abnormal functional parameters, **various duplex parameters** were determined in 30 subjects **with normal vessels** (18 men, 12 women; mean age 34.7 ± 7.3 years). Mean values were calculated for each leg from five individual measurements. The measurements were performed with the subjects in the flat supine position and the feet lowered 10° after a 15-min period of rest. The following values were measured in the common femoral vein just above the saphenofemoral junction (n = 60 legs):

- Diameter: 11.7 ± 2.1 mm during expiration,
  12.4 ± 2.2 mm during inspiration

- Planimetrically determined cross-sectional area: 1.07 ± 0.28 cm^2 during expiration, 1.16 ± 0.31 cm^2 during inspiration
- Peak flow velocity: 23.5 ± 8.3 cm/s during expiration; mean flow velocity averaged over 3 respiratory cycles with normal inspiration depth and abdominal breathing: 7.7 ± 1.9 cm/s.

During Valsalva's maneuver the femoral vein cross-sectional area increased to 1.82 ± 0.6 cm^2. The mean intraindividual diurnal variation in the cross-sectional area from morning to evening was 19.2% in expiration and 17.7% in inspiration. Peak expiratory flow velocity varied by 18.9% and mean flow velocity by 17.3%. Measurements performed on different days demonstrated a variation in the cross-sectional area of 24.6% during expiration and of 27.8% during inspiration while peak expiratory flow velocity varied by 24.7% and mean flow velocity by 21.4%. Other diameters determined in the 30 subjects were 8.9 ± 1.8 mm in the superficial femoral vein just after the origin of the deep femoral vein and 8.7 ± 1.6 mm in the popliteal vein at about the level of the knee joint cleft. The mean diameter of the great saphenous vein measured just below its termination in standing subjects was 5.6 ± 1.9 mm.

The parameters show **wide intra- and interindividual variation** in repeat measurements performed on the same day or from day to day. Blood flow velocity as well as the diameter and cross-sectional area of large veins vary with breathing. Our results are confirmed by Marshall (1990), Hirschl and Bernt (1990), and Ludwig (1991), who report similar variations in diameter and cross-sectional area. Even with incorporation of respiratory variations in venous cross-sectional area (mean cross-sectional area = 1/3 × (2 × area in expiration + area in inspiration)) into the equation, the **mean flow rate determined for the common femoral vein** just above the saphenofemoral junction (calculated as mean cross-sectional area multiplied by mean flow velocity, V_{mean}) was found to be rather high at 503 ± 137 mL/min.

Measurement of venous blood flow is **very inaccurate** compared with measurement of arterial blood flow (see ► Sects. 1.1.2.4 and 6.1.3.2) because venous diameter measurement is subject to errors that are difficult to control. The diameters of large veins vary with breathing and the proximal iliac vein even shows pulsatile diameter variation. These variations are difficult to quantify and respiratory maneuvers do not easily lend themselves to standardization. The large veins are typically not circular but elliptical.

Another source of error is the use of high-pass filters that eliminate slow venous flow components from the Doppler spectrum, resulting in overestimation of mean blood flow velocity. In the above-described measurement series in 30 subjects with normal vessels, comparison of flow in the common femoral artery and in the common femoral vein just proximal to the saphenofemoral junction surprisingly showed mean venous flow to be 21% faster than arterial flow. In a series reported by Ludwig (1991), blood flow in the common femoral vein was approx. 32% higher than in the artery.

The potential errors, along with the wide physiologic variation in vein diameters and cross-sectional areas, appear to preclude the use of these parameters for monitoring the response to pharmacologic treatment. Other studies, however, suggest that such parameters (Jäger et al. 1986; Eichlisberger and Jäger 1989), when measured serially, can indeed be used to identify physiologic variations or to objectively monitor the effectiveness of pharmacologic therapies aimed at altering venous tone.

The **severity of drainage insufficiency** in chronic venous incompetence can be evaluated more reliably on the basis of morphologic criteria depicted by venography compared to the wall changes seen on gray-scale ultrasound. Although dilatation in primary chronic venous incompetence or shrinkage of the vessel lumen in the postthrombotic syndrome with wall thickening, sclerosis, residual thrombi, or persistent occlusion are important descriptive criteria, the severity of drainage insufficiency can be evaluated more reliably using hemodynamic parameters such as magnitude, type, and duration of reflux. Moreover, postthrombotic gray-scale sonography shows normal vein morphology in 20–30% of cases.

Since there will be no persisting incompetence of the major veins after DVT in approx. 20–30% of cases (probably because some valves retain their function), the evaluation of reflux by duplex imaging identifies those cases with persistent insufficiency that require treatment with compression stockings. Wearing of compression stockings reduces postthrombotic trophic skin damage but does not affect the rate of recurrent thrombosis.

Disadvantages of ultrasound are the lack of full documentation of the findings and the greater examiner dependence. It is limited in the presence of large edemas or vessel and soft tissue calcifications and if the scanning window is small or inadequate due to surgical wounds, skin defects, or overlying bowel gas. A patient's inability to cooperate and thoracic breathing can lead to misinterpretation of Doppler waveforms; no cooperation is required in compression ultrasound.

The wall changes associated with recanalization after thrombosis make the vessel more resistant to compression, and they may mimic acute thrombus if too little pressure is applied. The question as to whether there is recurrent thrombosis or appositional growth on the basis of earlier thrombosis with or without partial recanalization may be difficult to answer using venographic and sonographic criteria. **Fresh**, nonoccluding **thrombotic deposits are differentiated from older, mural residues of thrombotic material** by searching for other residual changes in the form of wall thickening or incompetent proximal valves, which can be identified during Valsalva's maneuver. The demonstration of flow signals near the wall suggests a fresh thrombus surrounded by flowing blood while meandering flow in the center of the vessel is a sign of early recanalization (◘ Figs. 3.23 and 3.28).

CT and MRI allow assessment of the veins in the arms and legs, but they are mainly used to evaluate the venous system in the pelvis. Although ultrasonography is a highly accurate method providing extensive information on venous abnormalities, the examiner must always retain a critical stance and be aware of its limitations, which may make it necessary to order supplementary diagnostic tests in individual cases.

3.1.9.3 Varicosis

Color duplex ultrasound is a valid diagnostic tool for determining the extent of venous varicosis (upper and lower points of insufficiency) and identifying **incompetent perforators** prior to surgery. Duplex ultrasound was found to have significantly higher sensitivity than venography in identifying incompetent perforators (96% vs 65%; Stiegler et al. 1994) although only venograms with good image quality were included in the analysis. Venograms of poor quality depicted only 16% of the insufficient perforators identified sonographically.

The sonographic examination enables differentiation of primary from secondary, postthrombotic varicosis. Duplex ultrasound is thus superior to all other imaging modalities in establishing the indication for surgery and planning its extent. Apart from cosmetic reasons, treatment of varicosis primarily aims at preventing secondary incompetence of major veins. **Duplex ultrasound** is the most reliable imaging modality for determining the proximal and distal points of insufficiency and for identifying incompetent perforating veins, which must be eliminated to interrupt extrafascial recirculation pathways. In addition, precise determination of the disease extent allows sparing nonvaricose vein segments, which are thus available for possible later **arterial reconstruction**. The exact disease extent determined by duplex ultrasound, in particular involvement of the saphenous vein, is important for choosing between sclerotherapy and surgical stripping, and duplex ultrasound is the only modality that allows adequate identification of candidates for endovascular interventions. At the same time, ultrasound is a useful tool for guiding such interventions.

In patients with varicosis complicated by **thrombophlebitis**, duplex ultrasound is the preferred method for identifying the proximal end of the thrombus, which determines whether anticoagulant therapy or high ligation of the saphenofemoral junction is indicated. Moreover, it serves to exclude concomitant involvement of the deep venous system. By demonstrating varicose as well as postthrombophlebitic changes in **vein mapping** prior to bypass procedures, ultrasonography can help to identify suitable segments for grafting, and these can be marked on the skin prior to surgery.

3.2 Arm Veins and Jugular Vein

3.2.1 Vascular Anatomy

As in the leg, superficial and deep veins can be distinguished in the arm. The most important superficial vein is the cephalic vein, which has a crucial role in establishing a hemodialysis access. It courses from the wrist to the bend of the elbow on the radial side of the arm and continues on this side to the shoulder, from where it passes anteriorly to the infraclavicular fossa. The deep veins accompany the arteries of the same name and have multiple connections with the superficial veins. The deep veins of the lower arm join at the bend of the elbow to continue as the brachial vein. The latter often has multiple branches and courses along the medial aspect of the humerus to the axilla. The axillary vein begins at the lower border of the teres major muscle as the continuation of the basilic vein, from where it passes to the clavicle. It receives the cephalic vein at the level of the infraclavicular fossa. Proximal to the clavicle, the axillary vein continues to the superior vena cava as the subclavian vein. Along its course, the subclavian vein relates anteriorly with the clavicle and subclavius muscle and above with the subclavian artery. Inferiorly, the vein rests on the first rib. The subclavian vein passes in front of the scalene triangle (in front of the scalenus anterior) and unites with the internal jugular vein to form the brachiocephalic vein (◘ Fig. 3.39).

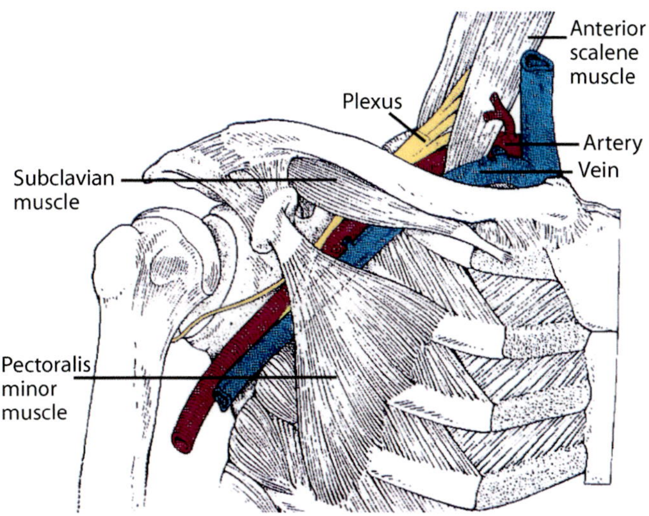

◘ **Fig. 3.39** Anatomy of the subclavian and axillary veins (From Heberer and van Dongen 1993)

3.2.2 Examination Protocol and Technique

The subclavian, axillary, and brachial veins are examined with a 7.5 MHz transducer. These veins are scanned with the examiner positioned at the patient's head. Morphologic assessment and the compression test are performed as with the deep leg veins. Note, however, that the compression test is reliable only for the axillary and brachial veins but not for the subclavian vein when interrogated from the supraclavicular approach. First, the axillary vein coursing below the artery is tested for compressibility in transverse orientation with the transducer in the infraclavicular fossa. Next, a Doppler waveform is obtained in the longitudinal plane to rule out central outflow obstruction due to thrombosis or compression. The further course of the vein is traced, and compressibility of the brachial vein is tested in the upper arm from medially pressing the vein against the humerus.

The subclavian vein is scanned longitudinally from the supraclavicular position with recording of a Doppler waveform and evaluation of the termination of the jugular vein. The internal jugular vein can be followed in transverse orientation as it courses parallel to the carotid artery. Intermittent compression is performed to rule out thrombosis. The color duplex mode in longitudinal orientation enables assessment of recanalization, identification of central thrombi surrounded by flowing blood, and detection of partial thrombosis after implantation of a portal catheter, central venous catheter, or pacemaker probe.

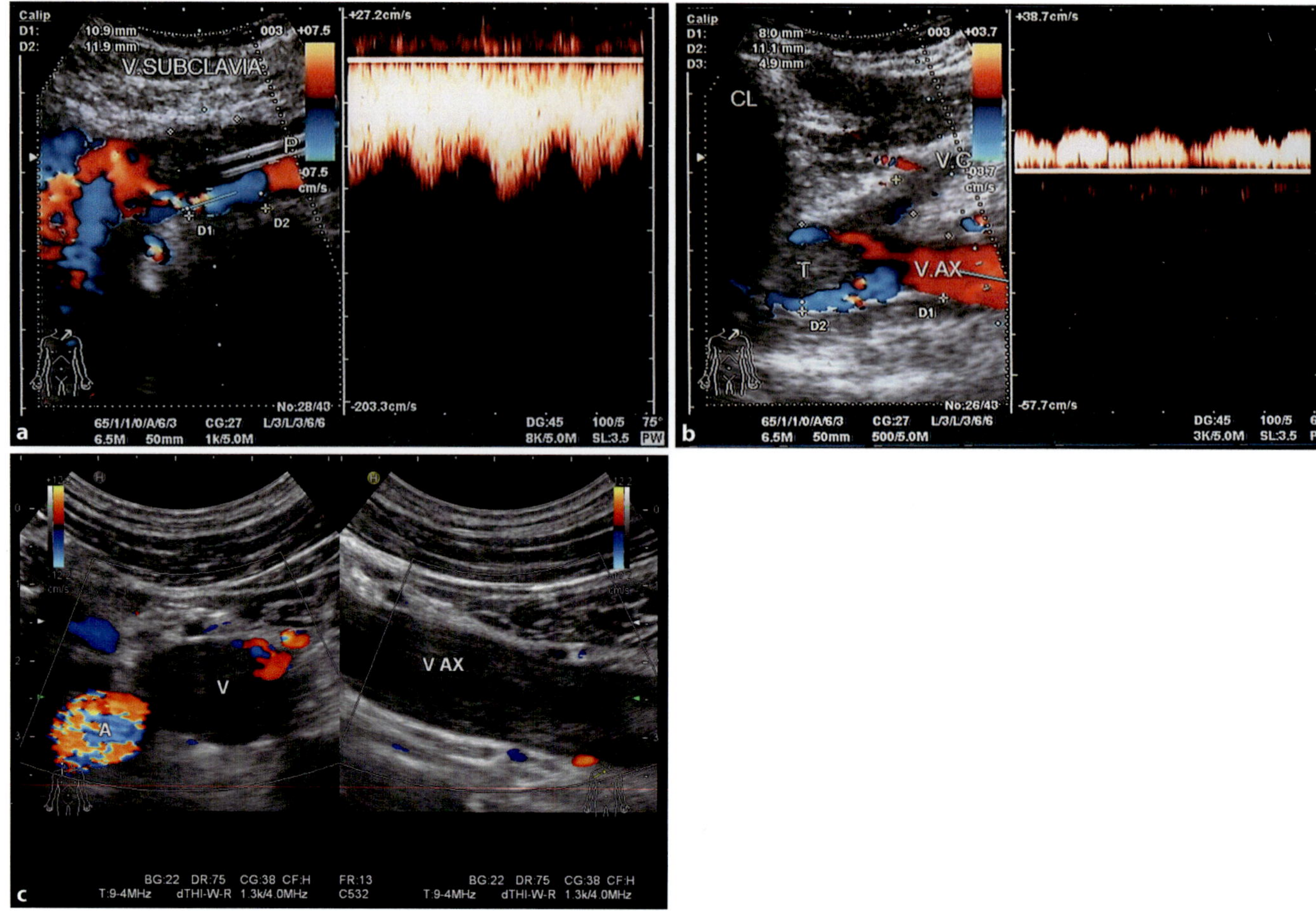

Fig. 3.40 **a** Thrombus (T) surrounded by flowing blood in the subclavian vein; the thrombus in this patient is due to the thrombogenic effect of an implanted venous access port (P). **b** The port tube inserted through the cephalic vein (V.C., occluded by suture) extends to the site of the thrombus, which is surrounded by flowing blood and extends into the axillary vein (V.AX.). The blood flow direction distal to the thrombus is normal (red, toward transducer), but flow is markedly disturbed by the thrombus: flow velocity is reduced to 10 cm/s, and both cardiac pulsatility and respiratory phasicity are lost. The cephalic and axillary veins are indicated by calipers; CL = clavicle. **c** Color duplex ultrasound shows paraneoplastic thrombosis of the axillary vein (transverse view on the left, longitudinal view on the right). In this territory, compression ultrasound would have been possible as well to confirm thrombosis (compression of vein against the ribs). The axillary vein courses inferior to the artery

3.2.3 Normal Findings

As with the pelvic and leg veins, undisturbed flow in the arm veins shows respiratory phasicity. In addition, flow in the subclavian and axillary veins varies during the cardiac cycle (W-shaped profile with two peaks, one during systole and a second upon opening of the atrioventricular valves; markedly reduced flow during atrial contraction with short transient reflux). The typically elliptical lumina of the subclavian and axillary veins show respiratory diameter variations on longitudinal and transverse views (see Fig. 3.99 (Atlas)).

3.2.4 Documentation

The findings in the subclavian, axillary, and brachial veins are documented by storing longitudinal images and the corresponding angle-corrected waveforms. If venous thrombosis has been demonstrated, additional transverse views of the diseased vessel segment without and with compression are documented.

3.2.5 Clinical Role

Thrombosis of the arm veins is rare compared with venous thrombosis of the legs and is most commonly caused by

- Paraneoplasia (Fig. 3.40c)
- Obstructed drainage in the narrow costoclavicular space (see Fig. 3.105 (Atlas))
- Tumor compression in the thoracic outlet
- Thrombogenic effects of portal catheters, central venous catheters, or pacemaker probes in the axillary and subclavian veins (Fig. 3.40a,b)
- Thrombosis of deep major veins secondary to phlebitis (iatrogenic) (rare).

The **narrow costoclavicular space** through which the vein must pass is formed by the first rib, the clavicle, and the subclavian muscle. Venous drainage may be obstructed when the already narrow passage is constricted further by weak shoulder muscles, rib callus, or exostosis. Obstruction can be reproduced during the examination by hyperabduction of the arm. If the hyperabduction test demonstrates an outflow obstruction in the costoclavicular space following recanalization after thrombolytic therapy, resection of the first rib may be contemplated.

Ultrasound can be used to evaluate **patency** prior to insertion of a **pacemaker probe** or **central venous catheter**, especially in patients with clinical signs or a history of previous venous thrombosis of the upper extremity. Prior to placement of a central venous catheter in the jugular vein, ultrasound can additionally serve to identify the correct vessel in order to preclude misplacement or complications in patients with an abnormal course of the vein.

The risk of pulmonary embolism in venous thrombosis of the arm is very low. Clinically relevant postthrombotic damage is unlikely because there is good collateralization. Nevertheless, early examination by noninvasive duplex ultrasound is indicated in patients with clinical signs of thrombosis to initiate full-dose heparin treatment and thus stop further progression. Thrombophlebitis is typically caused iatrogenically and is rarely associated with thrombus extension into major deep veins.

3.2.6 Duplex Ultrasound Findings and Their Diagnostic Significance

The ultrasound criteria of thrombosis are the same as in deep vein thrombosis (DVT) of the legs: the vein appears markedly dilated and contains homogeneous or inhomogeneous structures, it cannot be compressed, and (color) duplex imaging depicts either no flow signals or, if a central thrombus is present, only flow near the wall. Any intraluminal or external obstruction of venous drainage **eliminates cardiac pulsatility and eliminates or reduces respiratory phasicity** of blood flow in the vein. Therefore, in cases where methodological limitations prohibit adequate evaluation of the subclavian vein from the supraclavicular position, a Doppler waveform from the axillary vein (from the infraclavicular fossa) can rule out significant flow obstruction.

Apart from the subclavian vein, the easily accessible axillary vein may be affected by thrombosis because blood from the arms is emptied into this vein through thoracic wall collaterals. Compression ultrasound is used to exclude thrombosis of the axillary vein (with the transducer in the infraclavicular fossa) and of the peripheral veins. As already mentioned, the compression test is unreliable in the subclavian vein, and blood flow has to be demonstrated directly by obtaining a Doppler waveform. Sonographically, thrombophlebitis can be distinguished from deep thrombosis on the basis of the course of the vessel affected and its relationship to anatomic landmarks (accompanying artery of the same name).

In an earlier series of 610 patients with arm swelling analyzed by the author (1994 to 1998), the duplex ultrasound examination revealed arm vein thrombosis in 96 cases. In 61 of the patients, thrombosis was attributable to paraneoplasia, a central venous catheter, or a pacemaker probe. Nine of the remaining 35 patients, in particular younger ones, underwent thrombolytic therapy, which led to recanalization in seven cases. Subsequently, flow obstruction was demonstrated in the **costoclavicular space** by duplex imaging with **provocative maneuvers** in five of the seven patients (◘ Figs. 3.105 and 3.106 (Atlas)).

In the **hyperabduction test**, the arm on the affected side is raised above the head while the Doppler spectrum is recorded in the axillary vein with the transducer in the infraclavicular fossa. Note, however, that there may be some physiologic flow obstruction during extreme hyperabduction, especially in slender patients. A more reliable way of demonstrating clinically significant narrowing of the passage between the clavicle and the first rib is to use a modified "apron grip" test, which involves spectral Doppler measurement in the axillary vein while pulling down the arm while it is turned backward and rotated to the side. Flow reduction with elimination of cardiac and respiratory fluctuation is abnormal (see ◘ Figs. 3.105 and 3.106 (both Atlas)).

The **underlying mechanism** is complex. Typically, however, the **clinical symptoms** are caused by weakness of the shoulder muscles. Normal muscle tone elevates the clavicle above the neurovascular bundle. If the muscles are too weak, however, the bundle is compressed by the movement of the clavicle over the first rib during abduction with rotation.

Obstruction in the costoclavicular space primarily affects the vein while the scalenus and cervical rib syndromes do not affect venous drainage as the subclavian vein passes in front of the scalenus anterior muscle. The **costoclavicular compression syndrome is primarily treated by physical therapy** aimed at strengthening the muscles of the shoulder girdle. The outcome can be followed up by duplex imaging. If the symptoms persist after physical therapy, or after recanalization following thrombolytic therapy of compression-induced thrombosis, resection of the first rib may be contemplated.

Color duplex imaging allows reliable evaluation of both spontaneous and thrombolytic **recanalization after arm vein thrombosis** and identification of abnormalities persisting after thrombosis such as luminal variations, residual mural thrombi, or wall sclerosis (see ◘ Fig. 3.107 (Atlas)).

3.2.7 Diagnostic Role of Duplex Ultrasound Compared with Other Modalities

Duplex ultrasound is comparable to the traditional gold standard, venography, in evaluating the arm veins for thrombosis, as their superficial course provides good insonation conditions. It is superior to venography in evaluating the wall of the axillary vein for postthrombotic lesions persisting after recanalized thrombosis. Moreover, spectral Doppler interrogation yields highly accurate information on the hemodynamic effects of vein compression by tumor or in the costoclavicular compression syndrome, especially when assessing flow in the vein distal to the outflow obstruction during provocative maneuvers (respiratory phasicity, cardiac pulsatility). Since sonographic evaluation of the thoracic outlet is limited, CT is superior in assessing tumor-related inflow obstruction. As in the legs, venography is superior in evaluating the extent of collateralization. In controlled studies using venography as the reference modality, duplex ultrasound was found to have 94% sensitivity and 96% specificity in detecting arm vein thrombosis (Koksoy et al. 1995; Haire et al. 1991).

3

3.3 Atlas: Extremity Veins

▪ Table 3.8 lists the figures presented in the Atlas. The figures illustrate normal findings, methodology, and vascular diseases of the extremity veins.

▪ **Table 3.8** Extremity veins – figures

Table 3.8 (continued)

Entity/pathology	Figure
Postthrombotic syndrome – residual lesions/synechia	Fig. 3.73 (Atlas), page 243
Postthrombotic residues – wall sclerosis	Fig. 3.73 (Atlas), page 243
Degrees of valve incompetence	Fig. 3.74 (Atlas), page 244
Respiratory phasicity and cardiac pulsatility of reflux in severe valve incompetence	Fig. 3.75 (Atlas), page 245
Truncal varicosis of great saphenous vein (distal extent)	Fig. 3.76 (Atlas), page 245
Incomplete truncal varicosis of great saphenous vein	Fig. 3.77 (Atlas), page 246
Truncal varicosis of small saphenous vein	Fig. 3.78 (Atlas), page 246
Valve incompetence of perforating vein	Fig. 3.79 (Atlas), page 247
Thromboembolism from great saphenous vein and Dodd perforator incompetence	Fig. 3.80 (Atlas), page 247
Recanalized great saphenous vein after thrombophlebitis	Fig. 3.81 (Atlas), page 248
VNUS closure of great saphenous vein	Fig. 3.82 (Atlas), page 248
Follow-up of VNUS closure	Fig. 3.83 (Atlas), page 248
Follow-up after endovenous varicose treatment	Fig. 3.83 (Atlas), page 248
Recurrent varicosis	Fig. 3.84 (Atlas), page 249
Venous aneurysm	Fig. 3.85 (Atlas), page 249
Venous aneurysm with thrombus	Fig. 3.86 (Atlas), page 250
Venous aneurysm and deep vein thrombosis of leg	Fig. 3.87 (Atlas), page 250
Saccular popliteal vein aneurysm	Fig. 3.88 (Atlas), page 251
Venous ectasia of the calf	Fig. 3.89 (Atlas), page 251
Differential diagnosis of venous thrombosis – Baker's cyst	Fig. 3.90 (Atlas), page 252
Differential diagnosis of calf vein thrombosis – hematoma	Fig. 3.91 (Atlas), page 252
Calf swelling due to torn muscle	Fig. 3.91 (Atlas), page 252
Calf swelling due to popliteal fossa tumor	Fig. 3.92 (Atlas), page 253
Calf swelling due to subfascial abscess	Fig. 3.93 (Atlas), page 253
Edema of various etiologies, lymphoma, lymphedema, lipedema	Fig. 3.94 (Atlas), page 254
Calf swelling caused by edema	Fig. 3.94 (Atlas), page 254
Vein compression by Baker's cyst	Fig. 3.95 (Atlas), page 255
Adventitial cystic disease of the popliteal vein	Fig. 3.96 (Atlas), page 255
Venous wall tumor	Fig. 3.97 (Atlas), page 256
Entrapment syndrome	Fig. 3.98 (Atlas), page 256
Axillary vein – normal findings	Fig. 3.99 (Atlas), page 257
Thoracic outlet obstruction	Fig. 3.100 (Atlas), page 257
Jugular vein aneurysm	Fig. 3.101 (Atlas), page 257
Jugular vein thrombosis – central venous catheter	Fig. 3.102 (Atlas), page 258
Axillary vein thrombosis – thrombolytic therapy	Fig. 3.103 (Atlas), page 259
Recanalization	Fig. 3.104 (Atlas), page 259
Costoclavicular compression syndrome with thrombosis	Fig. 3.105 (Atlas), page 260
Costoclavicular compression syndrome	Fig. 3.106 (Atlas), page 261
Follow-up of subclavian vein thrombosis after pacemaker implantation	Fig. 3.107 (Atlas), page 262
Thrombophlebitis of arm veins	Fig. 3.108 (Atlas), page 262

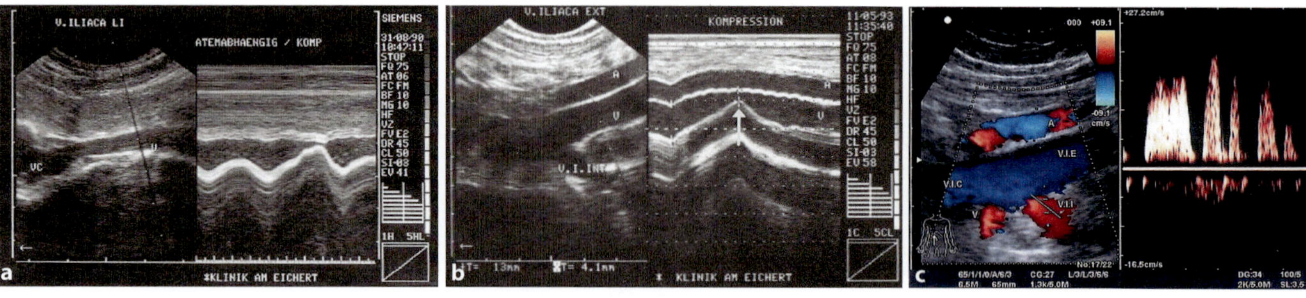

Fig. 3.41a–c (Atlas) Pelvic veins – normal ultrasound findings (see Fig. 2.2).

a Like in the vena cava (VC), blood flow in the iliac veins is subject to respiratory phasicity. The resulting variation in diameter is apparent in the time-motion mode (right part of **a**). In slender individuals, the iliac vein is also compressible (KOMP).

b Compression ultrasound of pelvic veins is reliable only in slender patients. Therefore, incompressibility is not a reliable indicator of thrombosis in this territory, while compressibility rules out thrombosis. The example illustrates compressibility in the time-motion mode (arrow).

c The pelvic veins (common iliac vein/V.I.C and external iliac vein/V.I.E) take an arched course through the true pelvis posterior to the arteries of the same name (A). The internal iliac vein (V.I.I) enters the common iliac vein on its posterior aspect at its lowest point (flow toward transducer, coded in red). There is respiratory phasicity of venous flow, and younger individuals (as in this case) sometimes also show cardiac pulsatility. In addition, a second pelvic vein (red) enters the common iliac vein (blue) slightly above the internal iliac vein

Fig. 3.42 (Atlas) Venous Doppler waveform.
Just below the inguinal ligament, the common femoral vein (V.F.C) divides into the deep femoral vein (V.P.F) and the superficial femoral vein (V.F.S). Flow in the veins is characterized by respiratory fluctuation when no proximal obstruction (thrombus, compression) is present. The Doppler waveform illustrates the respiratory variation in flow velocity in the deep femoral vein. Venous flow velocity decreases with increasing intra-abdominal pressure during inspiration. In this young woman, there is additional cardiac modulation of venous flow, which even perists during expiration. With the PRF adjusted to venous flow, the femoral artery close to the transducer shows aliasing (A) and reversed flow in diastole (arrows)

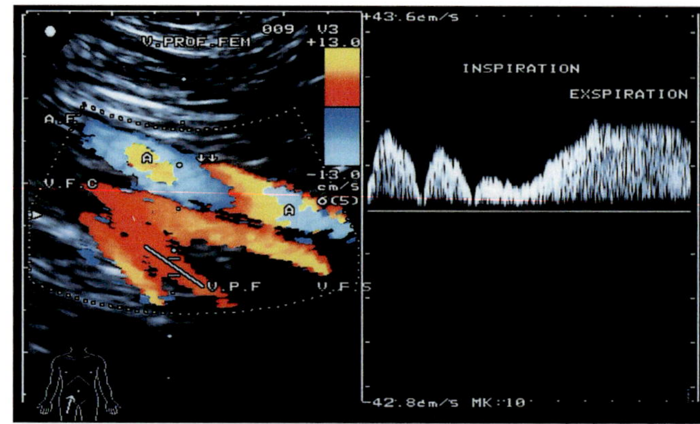

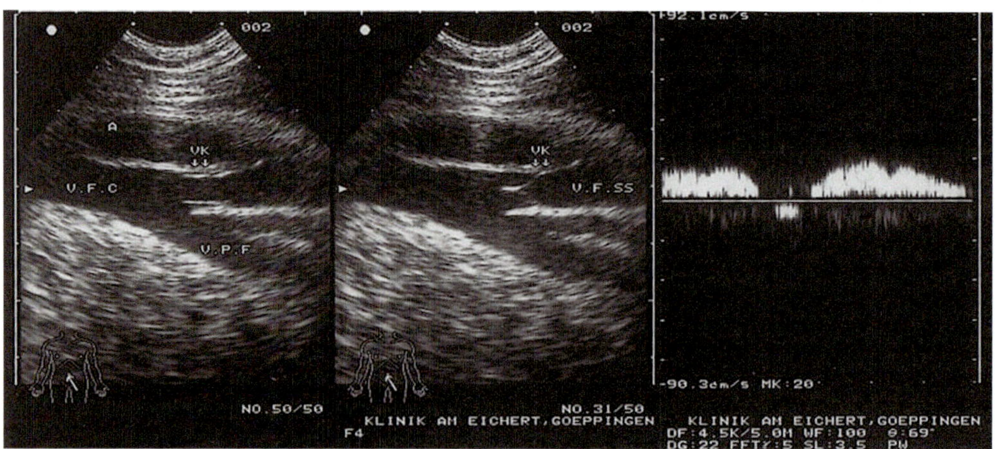

Fig. 3.43 (Atlas) Normal valve function – gray-scale imaging.

a Under good insonation conditions, normal valve function is apparent on gray-scale imaging. The valve (VK) depicted in the superficial femoral vein (V.F.S) just before it receives the deep femoral vein (V.P.F) is shown during expiration (valve open) in the left gray-scale image and during inspiration (valve closed) in the right image. The cusps prevent backward flow toward the periphery during the inspiration-induced increase in intra-abdominal pressure. The respiratory variation in blood flow is documented in the Doppler waveform. Flow toward the transducer is increased in expiration and decreased in inspiration. Flow may even drop to zero, and the short transient reflux until valve closure may be absent if the sample volume is placed near a valve

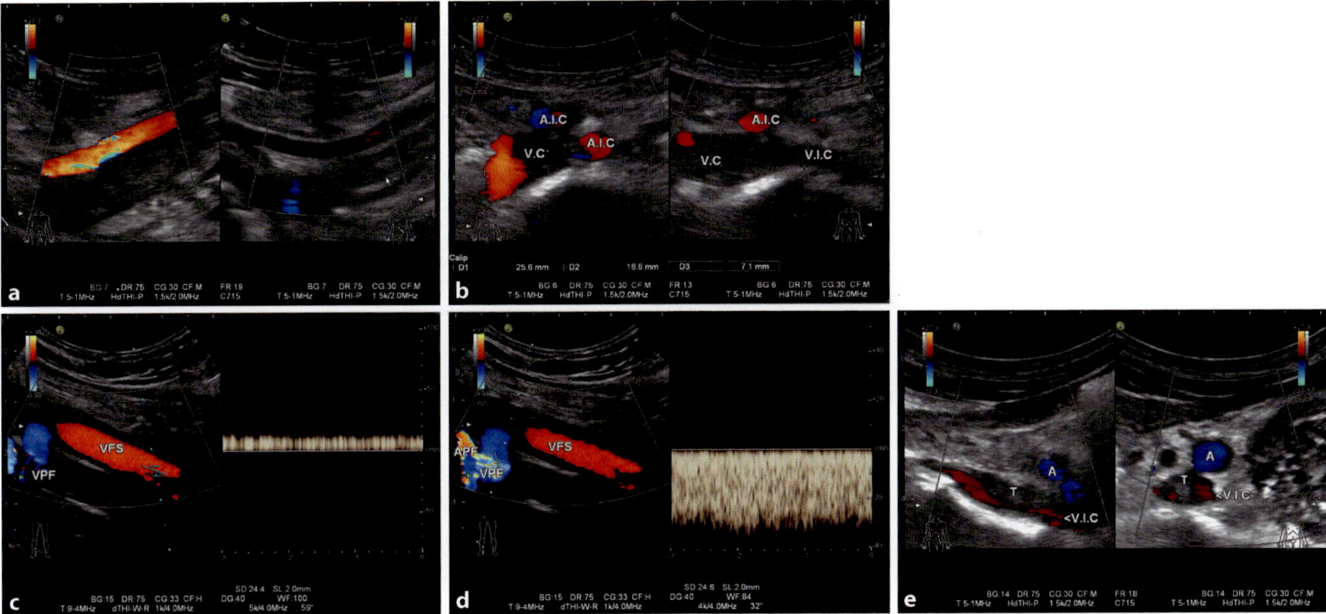

Fig. 3.44a–e (Atlas) Pelvic vein thrombosis.
a The left iliac vein coursing posterior to the iliac artery (red) has low echogenicity and is markedly dilated. These findings, along with the absence of flow signals, indicate acute thrombosis.
b The thrombus protrudes into the vena cava (V.C), and there is marginal blood flow along the thrombus entering from the right iliac vein (A.I.C = common iliac artery).
c Proximal venous stenosis leads to reduced flow and loss of respiratory phasicity in the left superficial femoral vein (VFS) (Fig. 3.24).
d With thrombosis extending into the common femoral vein, collateral flow occurs through the deep femoral vein (VPF), where flow is retrograde (blue, away from transducer), and through pelvic collaterals.
e Beginning recanalization with blood flow toward the heart (red) along the thrombus (T) in the common iliac vein (V.I.C)

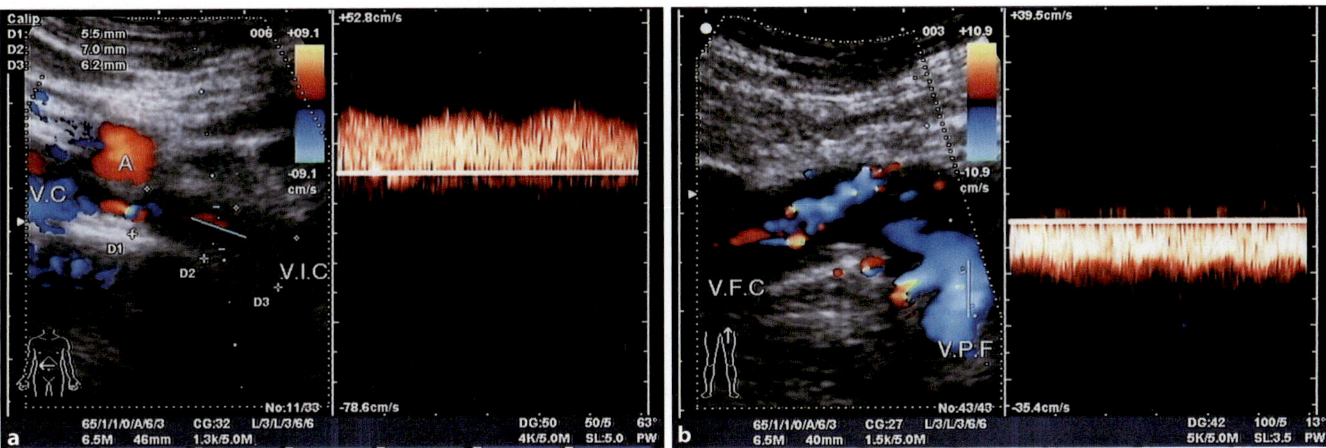

Fig. 3.45a, b (Atlas) Pelvic vein thrombosis – beginning recanalization.
a Follow-up ultrasound after acute thrombosis shows a shrunken lumen of the common iliac vein as well as flow signals, indicating beginning recanalization (smaller diameter compared with recent thrombosis). Flow in the vena cava (V.C) is displayed in blue (due to transducer position) (A = aorta).
b Retrograde flow in the deep femoral vein (V.P.F; blue, away from transducer; below the baseline in the Doppler waveform) indicates inadequate or absent drainage at the pelvic level, which is due to descending pelvic thrombosis in the case presented here

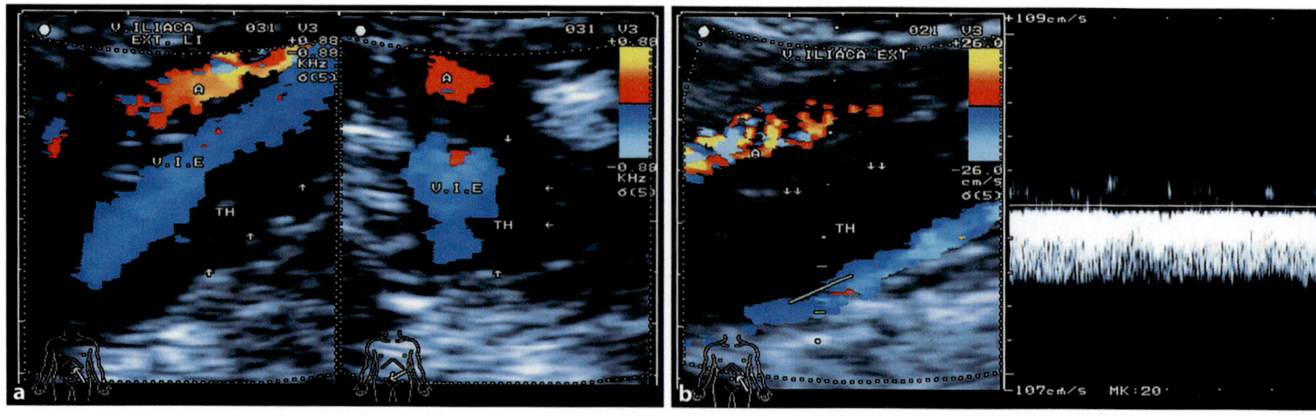

Fig. 3.46a, b (Atlas) Pelvic vein thrombus surrounded by flowing blood.
a In this young woman with scintigraphically proven pulmonary embolism, ultrasound showed patent deep leg veins, while there were thrombi in the iliac vein. Unlike recanalization with central flow signals (as shown in Fig. 3.45 (Atlas)), the fresh thrombus (TH) in the external iliac vein (V.I.E) is attached to the wall and surrounded by flowing blood.
b More proximally, close to the junction with the internal iliac vein, the thrombus is surrounded by flowing blood posteriorly. The flow obstruction produces a high-frequency, continuous signal (with loss of respiratory phasicity) typical of venous stenosis. The peak flow velocity is 50 cm/s. With the PRF adjusted to venous flow, there is aliasing in the artery anterior to the vein. The thrombus is indicated by arrows. The Doppler waveform from the uninvolved common femoral vein distal to the thrombus is not shown. The patent lumen of the common femoral vein is relatively wide, and respiratory phasicity is only slightly reduced. A thrombus in an otherwise patent lumen as in this case may be overlooked if only the waveform from the common femoral vein is analyzed, even if it is compared with the contralateral waveform and valve function is evaluated. Routine venography may likewise fail to identify such mural thrombi in an otherwise patent iliac vein or to differentiate them from flow phenomena

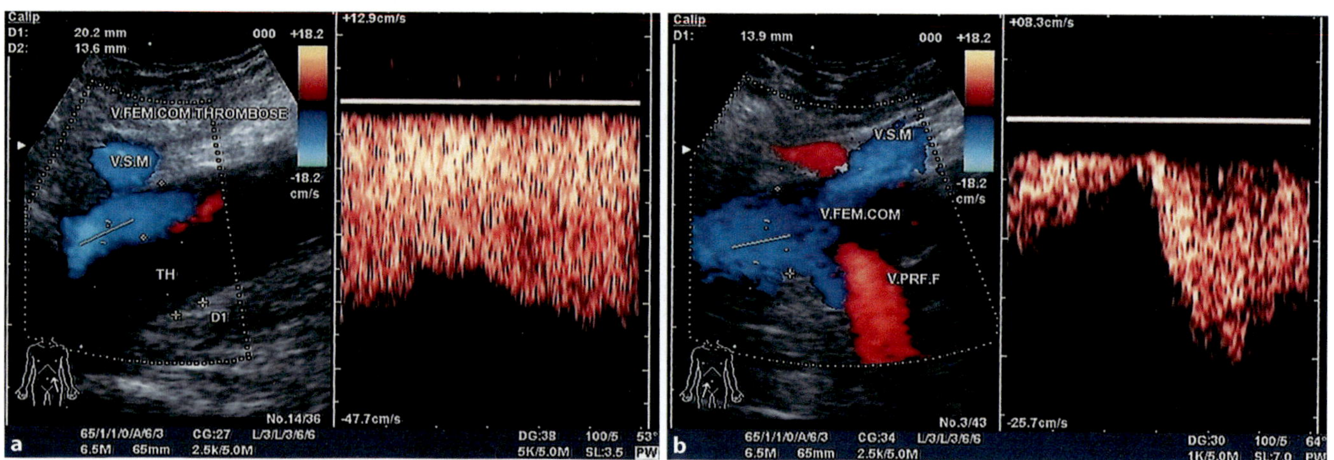

Fig. 3.47 (Atlas) Loss of respiratory phasicity due to obstructed venous drainage.
a Flow obstruction in a partially thrombosed vein eliminates or reduces respiratory phasicity and results in a higher-frequency flow signal in the Doppler waveform, unless the blood is drained through collaterals (similar to the situation in arterial stenosis).
b Since some residual respiratory variation may still be present, the waveform should be compared with the other side. In the example, respiratory phasicity is markedly reduced on the affected side compared with the contralateral side. The common femoral vein (V.FEM.COM, blue) receives the great saphenous vein (V.S.M, blue) and a deep femoral vein (V.PRF.F) displayed in red (flow toward transducer)

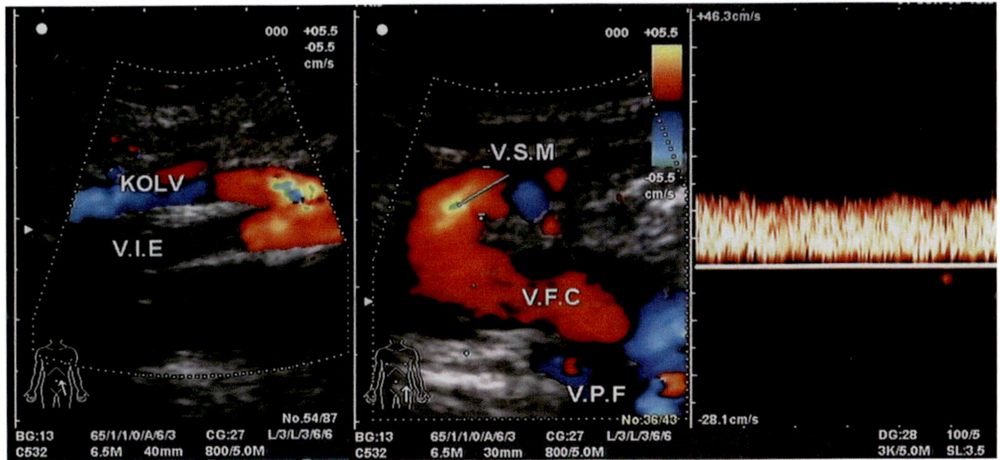

Fig. 3.48 (Atlas) Collateral circulation in pelvic vein thrombosis (see Fig. 3.49 (Atlas)).
The degree of recanalization is not always easy to estimate in older thrombosis of the external iliac vein. The shrunken vein is more difficult to evaluate along its course into the true pelvis and must be differentiated from collaterals such as the epigastric veins, which arise at the level of the inguinal ligament and, when dilated, may be of similar size as the shrunken external iliac vein (left color flow image). Retrograde flow in the saphenofemoral junction (right image, V.S.M) indicates outflow obstruction of the pelvic veins; the course of the abdominal wall collaterals can be followed using color duplex ultrasound. The Doppler waveform (right) also shows retrograde flow toward the transducer in the great saphenous vein

Fig. 3.49 (Atlas) External pelvic vein compression by lymphoma.
Leg swelling and widening of major veins secondary to obstructed venous drainage at the pelvic level due to external compression of the external iliac vein (V.I.E) by lymphoma (L). (V.I.I = internal iliac vein). The Doppler waveform shows high flow velocity of 170 cm/s in the external iliac vein and loss of respiratory phasicity

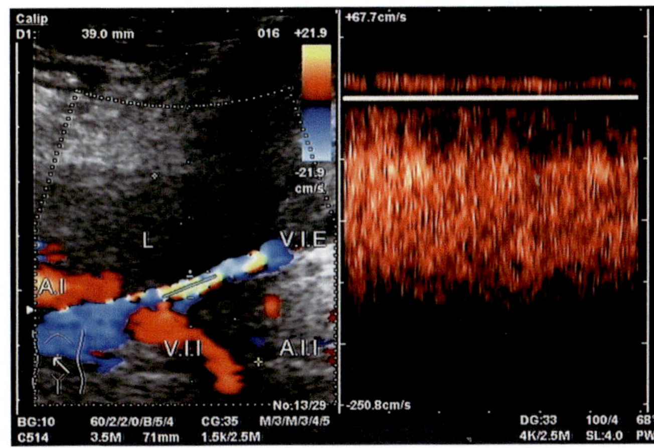

Fig. 3.50 (Atlas) Criteria for estimating thrombus age.
The major signs of acute deep vein thrombosis (DVT) of the legs are marked dilatation of the vein and good delineation of the homogeneous, often hypoechoic, thrombosed venous lumen from perivascular connective tissue. The two images obtained in the same patient show acute DVT with the venous lumen dilated to well over twice that of the accompanying artery in the right leg (right image) and an old thrombosis of the common femoral vein already partially recanalized in the area of the femoral bifurcation at the same level on the left (V.F.C, flow displayed in blue). (A.F.C = common femoral artery; A.P.F = deep femoral artery; A.F.S = superficial femoral artery)

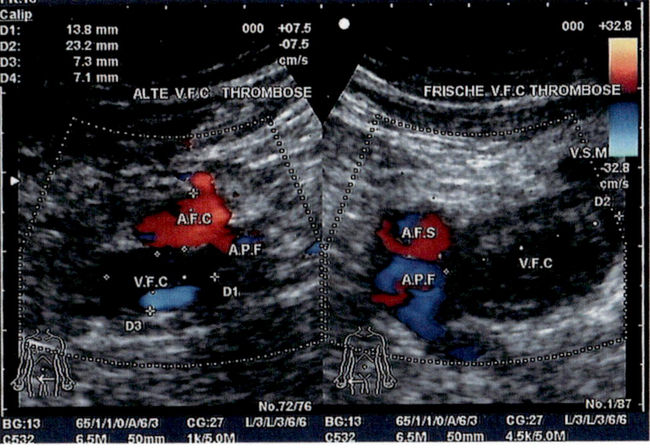

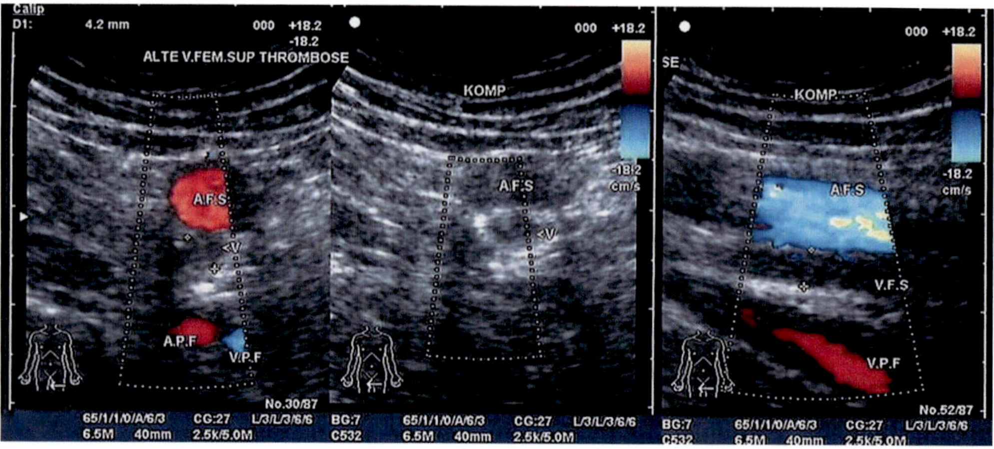

Fig. 3.51 (Atlas) Older femoral vein thrombosis.
Older thrombosis is associated with shrinkage of the lumen (relative to the corresponding artery). The image on the left shows the thrombotically occluded superficial femoral vein (V) posterior to the superficial femoral artery (A.F.S, red). Demarcation is much poorer than in acute thrombosis. The image obtained with application of pressure (middle section) shows incompressibility of the vein depicted posterior to the artery. The longitudinal image (right section) of the occluded superficial femoral vein (V.F.S) shows absence of flow in the vein posterior to the artery shortly before receiving the deep femoral vein (V.P.F). The deep femoral vein is recanalized with flow toward the transducer coded in red. However, marginal hypoechoic thrombosis still persists along the patent venous lumen

Fig. 3.52 (Atlas) Calf vein thrombosis.
With a satisfactory acoustic window, fresh venous thrombosis below the knee is easily identified as a hypoechoic tubular structure within the soft tissue in the typical anatomic location of the vein. The lumen is wider than that of the corresponding artery. The fibular artery and vein course along the medial aspect of the fibula. Compression ultrasound and color duplex imaging are highly accurate in differentiating between patent and thrombotic segments. The image on the right shows one patent vein and one thrombosed vein, and the left image shows thrombosis of both fibular veins, while both adjacent posterior tibial veins are patent (blue-coded flow)

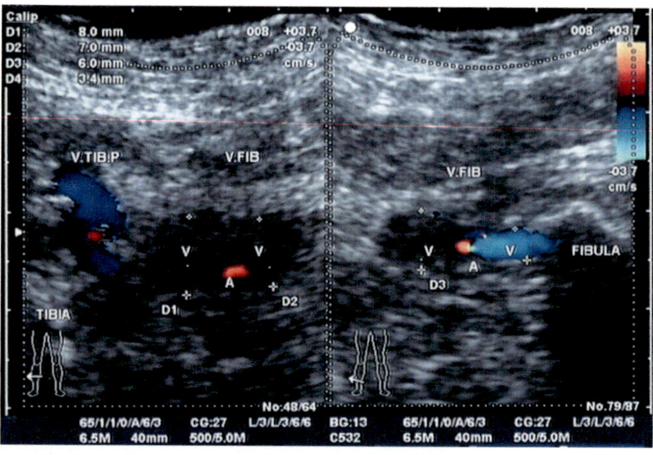

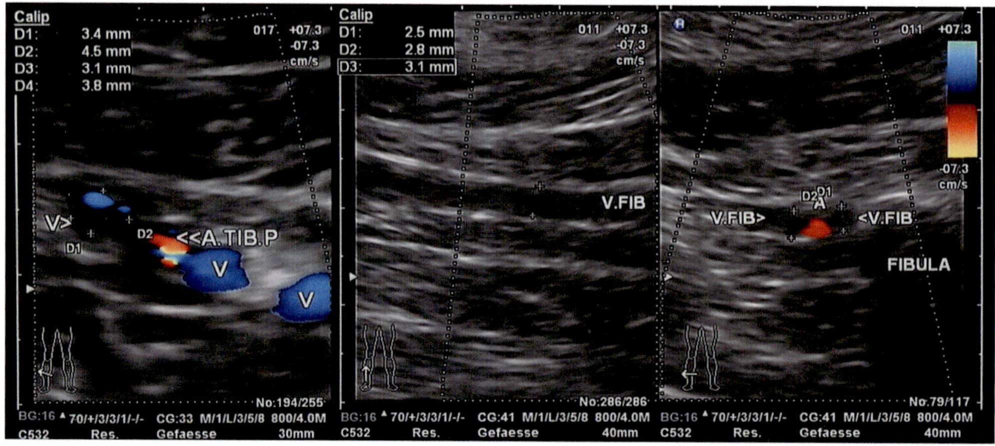

Fig. 3.53 (Atlas) Older calf vein thrombosis.
Following acute thrombosis, recanalization may set in early as indicated in the example by partial recanalization (blue) of the left posterior tibial vein (left section; diameter of the vein indicated by calipers). On the other hand, recanalization may occur late or not at all, which is indicated by a shrunken lumen without flow signals, shown here for the fibular vein (V.FIB) on longitudinal and transverse views (middle and right sections). Older thrombosis is characterized by more echogenic thrombus and shrinkage of the venous lumen, which is more difficult to distinguish from surrounding muscle and fatty connective tissue. The examples illustrate the difficulties encountered in diagnosing older thrombosis both in partial recanalization and in completely occluded postthrombotic veins with shrunken lumina

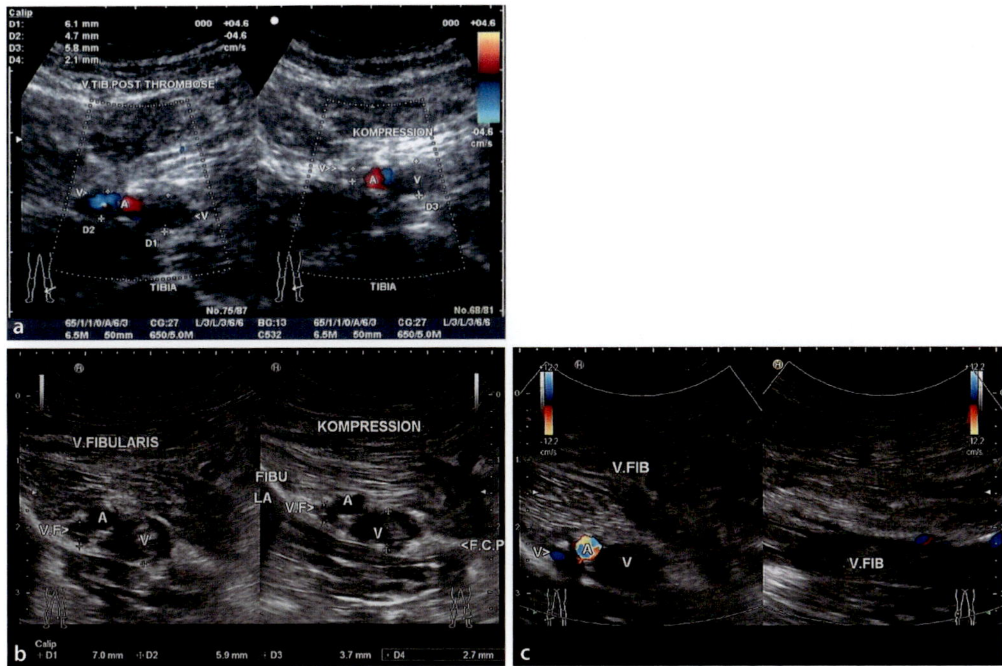

■ **Fig. 3.54a–c (Atlas) Recurrent thrombosis after recanalization.**
a The posterior tibial vein to the right of the artery (A, red) is markedly dilated (6.1 mm) and shows no flow, suggesting acute thrombosis. The vein to the left exhibits flow coded in blue with a surrounding hypoechoic margin corresponding to wall thickening as a sign of recanalized thrombosis. Compression ultrasound (right) shows only little compressibility of the thrombosed vein. No venous flow signals are depicted to the left of the artery during compression. However, the vein is not fully compressed. There is a hypoechoic area in the connective tissue corresponding to the postthrombotically thickened walls. The vein is surrounded by hyperechoic connective tissue of the deep crural fascia, and the tibia is depicted farther away from the transducer.
b,c Recurrent calf vein thrombosis after partial recanalization.
b Partial recanalization and recurrent thrombosis in the paired veins coursing to the right and left of the artery of the same name (A). Ultrasound images obtained without compression (left) and with compression (right) show residual thrombosis with partial recanalization in the fibular vein (indicated by "V.F>") to the left of the artery, close to the fibula, while there is acute recurrent thrombosis of the fibular vein (V) to the right of the artery. Residual thrombosis results in poor demarcation of the lumen from the wall and incomplete compressibility (with reduction of the lumen from 3.7 to 2.7 mm in the compression image (calipers). The fibular vein with acute thrombosis (V) shows some deformability although it is occluded and the lumen is widened by the thrombus (F.C.P = deep crural fascia).
c Color duplex imaging shows blood flow (blue) filling approx. half the lumen of the older, partially recanalized fibular vein ("V>"), while there is no flow in the other, markedly dilated and acutely thrombosed fibular vein (indicated by "V" in the transverse image (left) and "V.FIV" in the longitudinal image (right). Aliasing in the artery is due to the low PRF chosen to depict slow venous flow (■ Fig. 3.54b, c adapted from Schäberle 2014)

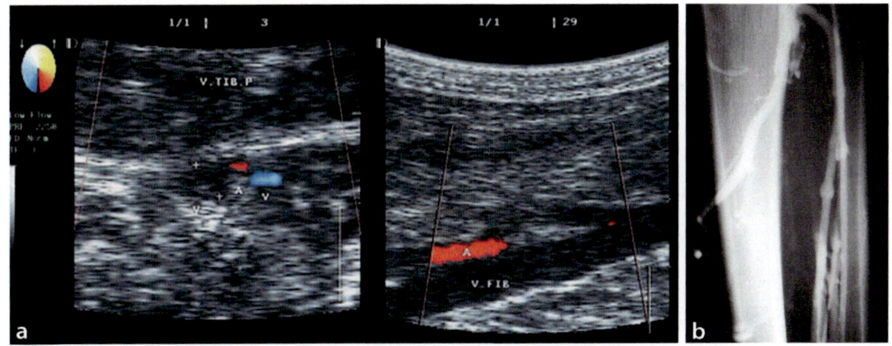

■ **Fig. 3.55a, b (Atlas) Diagnosis of calf vein thrombosis – ultrasound versus venography.**
a Isolated calf vein thrombosis of a single vein group may be overlooked or misinterpreted on venography. Moreover, small filling defects may be difficult to assign to a muscle vein or a major vein. B-mode ultrasound identifies acute thrombosis of a calf vein as a hypoechoic tubular structure along the artery of the same name, which can serve as a landmark. Color duplex imaging corroborates the diagnosis by the failure to demonstrate flow when performed with a low PRF. When only little residual flow is present, augmentation by manual compression distal to the transducer may be necessary to obtain a flow signal. The left image shows a patent posterior tibial vein (V) with blue-coded flow to the right of the red artery (A), while the second vein (V) to the left of the artery is thrombosed. The marked dilatation of the vein (to more than twice the width of the arterial lumen) and the low-level echo of the thrombus suggest acute thrombosis. The longitudinal image (right) shows the fibular vein to be thrombosed as well. The lumen is much wider than that of the corresponding artery (A) with flow depicted in red. The thrombosed vein is hypoechoic and homogeneous, clearly demarcating it from the surrounding soft tissue.
b Venogram: Filling defect in the posterior tibial vein. The fibular vein is not depicted

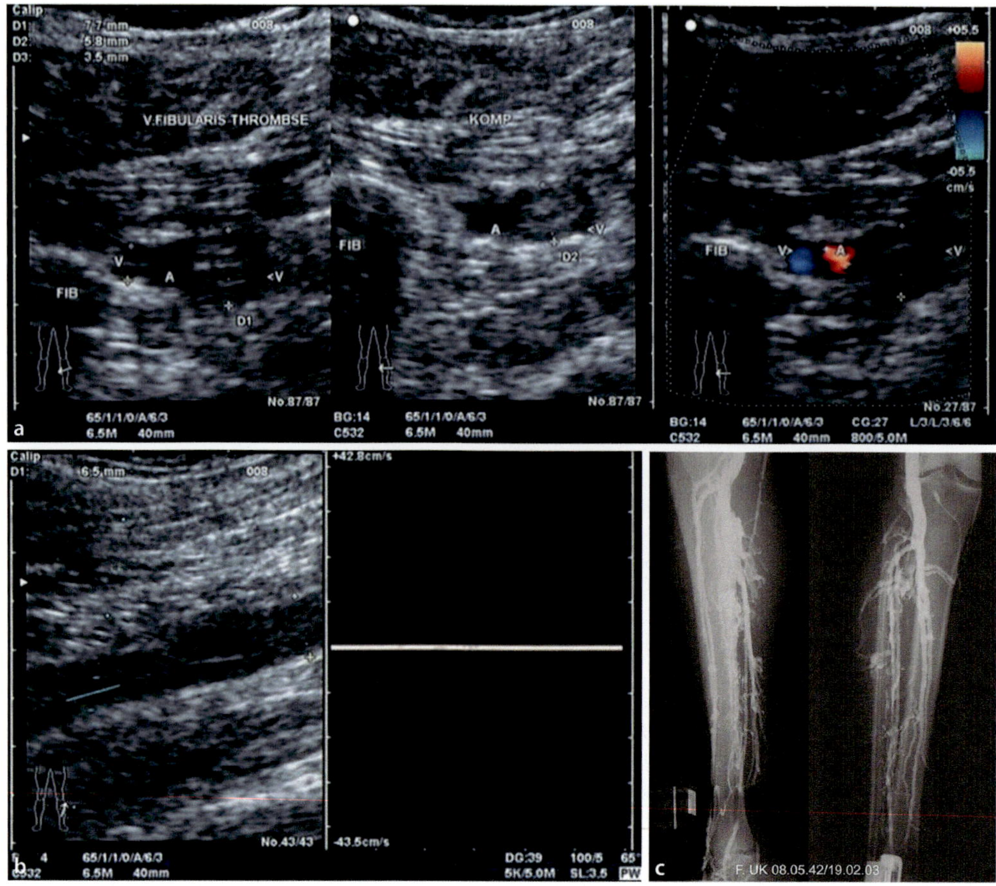

Fig. 3.56a–c (Atlas) Isolated fibular vein thrombosis – venography.
Venography is limited in the evaluation of the fibular veins. A filling defect in this vein may be due to a technical limitation or thrombosis.
a Sonographic examination identifies one thrombosed and one patent fibular vein. The transverse view (left section) depicts round, tubular structures to the left and right of the artery and the fibula (FIB) to the left. The veins are indicated by calipers: the thrombosed vein (right) is markedly dilated compared with the patent fibular vein (7.7 mm versus 3.5 mm). The image obtained while compression is being applied (middle section) no longer shows the fibular vein to the left of the artery (A), indicating complete compressibility. The vein to the right shows only little compressibility (diameter reduced from 7.7 to 5.8 mm), consistent with acute thrombus. The color duplex image (right section) depicts the patent vein in blue to the left of the artery (red), the thrombosed vein (V) to the right (marked with calipers). The thrombosed vein is hypoechoic, markedly dilated, and shows no flow.
b Longitudinal duplex image of the markedly dilated vein with the Doppler waveform confirming absence of blood flow. The clot immobilizes a valve in the center of the image.
c The venogram fails to depict the fibular veins. Based on the duplex sonographic demonstration of one patent and one thrombosed fibular branch, this example nicely illustrates that absence of contrast filling may be due to thrombosis or technical limitations of the method

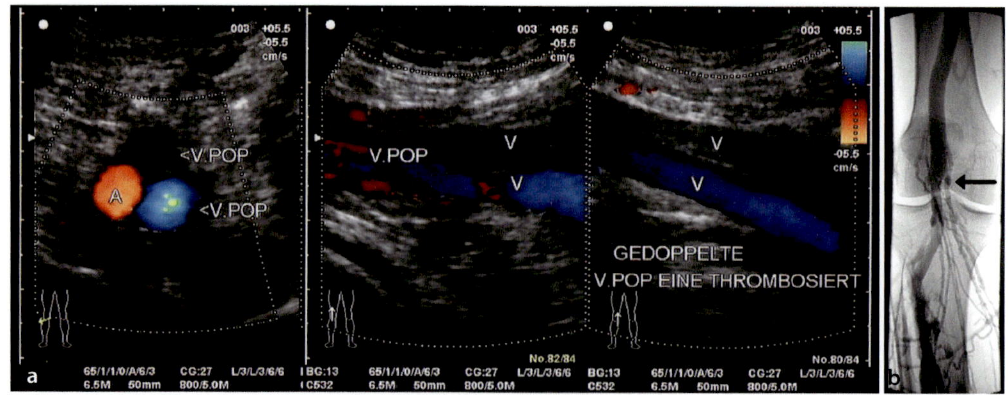

Fig. 3.57a, b (Atlas) Diagnosis of thrombosis – ultrasound versus venography.
a Transverse image (left) and longitudinal images (middle and right) of a duplicated popliteal vein with one patent and one thrombosed branch. Flow in the patent branch is coded blue. The first of the two longitudinal views shows the junction where the two branches (V) unite to form a single vein (V.POP).
b Venogram showing normal appearance of the common popliteal vein segment and the patent branch of the paired segment. As there is a smooth transition from the doubled popliteal segment to the single branch, there is no chance of identifying the thrombosed, second popliteal vein by venography

Fig. 3.58 (Atlas) Duplicated femoral vein.
A duplicated femoral vein with one patent branch and one completely occluded branch is a pitfall in venography. Color duplex imaging shows a perfused vein (V) to the left of the artery (A) and a markedly dilated vein (V) without flow to the right. The image obtained with compression (right) demonstrates complete compressibility of the vein to the left of the artery with only little compression of the vein to the right, which is still apparent as a hypoechoic tubular structure

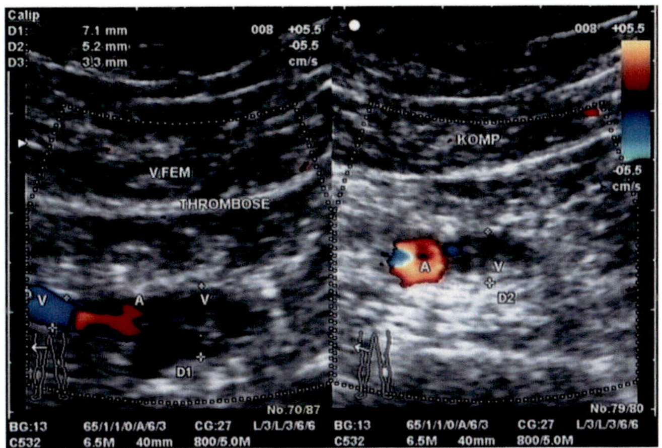

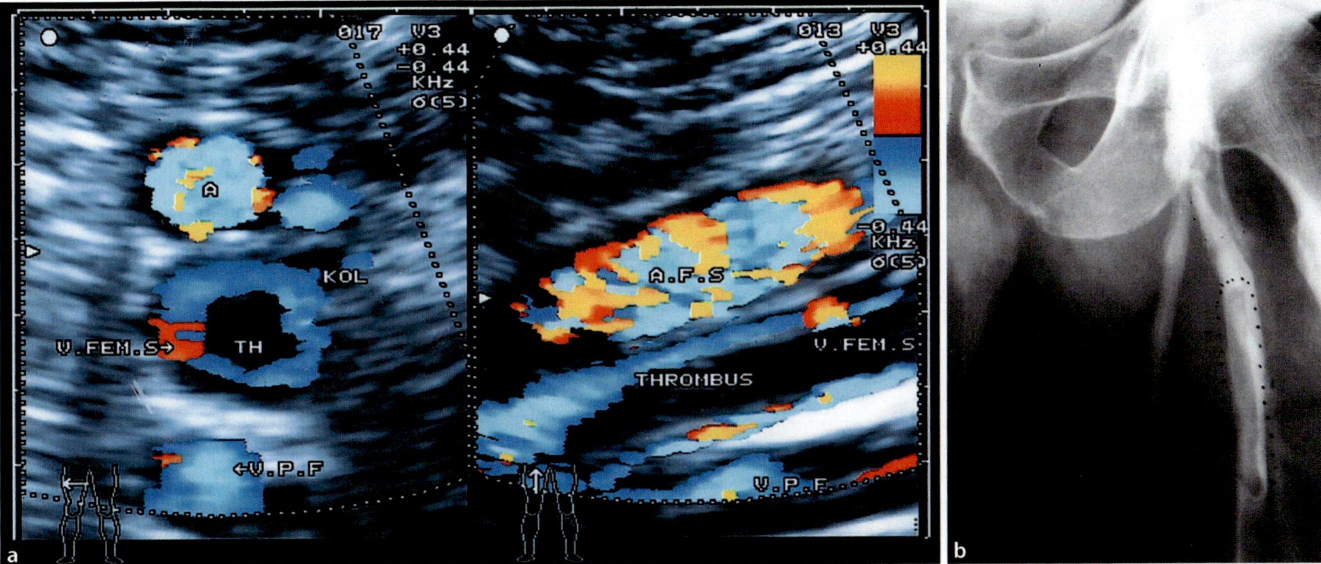

Fig. 3.59a, b (Atlas) Free-floating thrombus of femoral vein.
a Free-floating thrombus in the superficial femoral vein (V.FEM.S); transverse view on the left and longitudinal view on the right. A circular flow signal around a thrombus in a color flow image is diagnostic of free-floating thrombus (TH) and enables determination of the extent of the floating component. The slow flow around the floating tail proximal to the occlusion may be difficult to depict despite adequate instrument settings (high gain, low PRF). The problem may be overcome by having the patient perform a Valsalva maneuver to augment flow. Instrument adjustment to slow venous flow leads to aliasing in the superficial femoral artery (A, anterior to the vein). Collaterals with flow in blue (KOL) are depicted anterolaterally and the deep femoral vein (V.P.F) posteriorly.
b Venogram: The femoral vein is thrombosed; a second plane is necessary to estimate the length of the floating tail

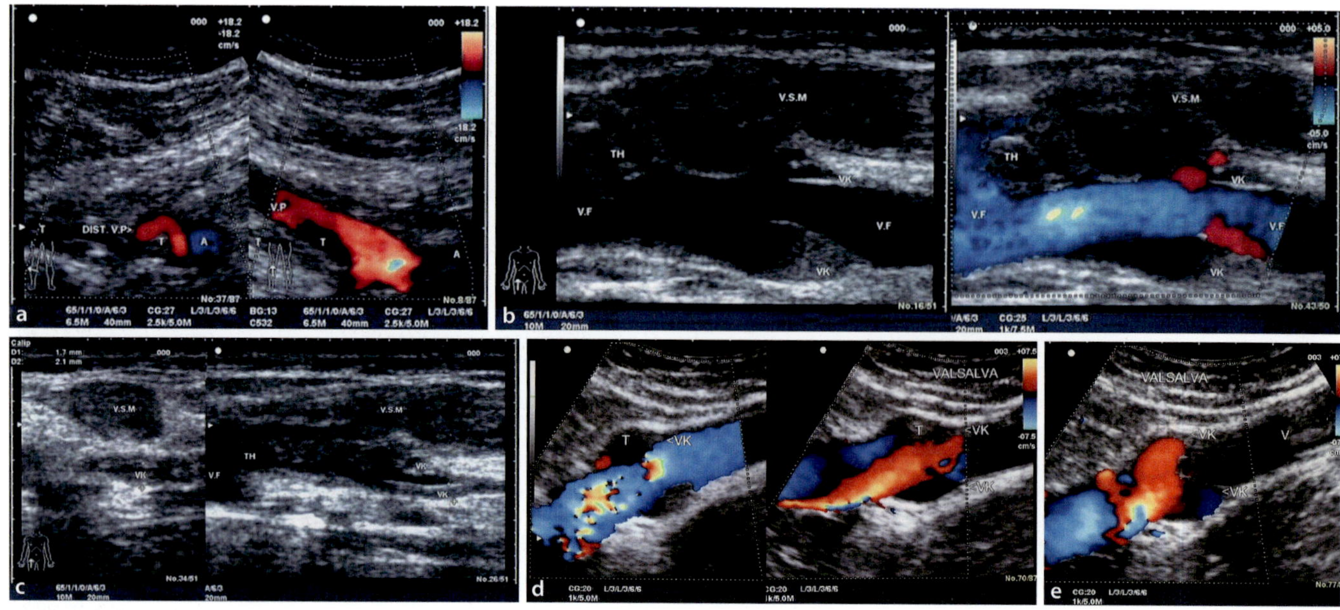

Fig. 3.60a–e (Atlas) Asymptomatic venous thrombosis developing in valve pockets.
a Ultrasound has much lower sensitivity in asymptomatic thrombosis than in symptomatic thrombosis. This is due to the fact that thrombus surrounded by flowing blood may be overlooked in calf vein segments notoriously difficult to scan, especially if there is only little dilatation and partial compressibility, or if clot is confined to valve pockets. The transverse (left) and longitudinal views (right) depict the distal popliteal vein with a patent lumen (red, flow toward transducer) but with absent color coding at the valve. Color duplex scanning facilitates the identification of such subtle abnormalities in problematic areas. However, to rule out flow phenomena as a possible cause of the filling defect, the thrombus must be confirmed by compression ultrasound of this vein segment.
b Duplex scanning performed in a clinically asymptomatic patient prior to stripping of varicose veins demonstrates thrombophlebitis of the great saphenous vein (V.S.M) with thrombus (TH) protruding into the common femoral vein (V.F). The gray-scale image (left) shows a hyperechoic structure in a valve (VK) somewhat distal to the saphenofemoral junction. In the color flow image (right), absence of color coding indicates the thrombus (TH) including its valvular component, which prevents proper opening of the valve (despite flow augmentation by manual thigh compression). Red color in the valve area indicates eddy flow (Fig. 3.12a), particularly in the pocket of the valve (VK) depicted closer to the transducer. To rule out a flow-related cause of this subtle change in the color coding, the thrombus must be confirmed by compression ultrasound.
c The images obtained with compression (transverse view on the left and longitudinal view on the right) show incompressibility of the great saphenous vein (V.S.M) and incomplete compression of the femoral vein at the level of the thrombotic valve (residual incompressible diameter of 2 mm, see markings). The example illustrates two major sources of thrombosis of the principal deep veins: thrombus development in a valve pocket (for its pathogenesis see Fig. 3.12a) and extension of thrombi from superficial or muscle veins.
d Thrombus in a venous valve pocket (illustrated for the great saphenous vein in the thigh) can lead to stasis of blood flow and thus become a nidus for venous thrombosis or thrombophlebitis. Absence of flow signals due to stasis can be differentiated from true thrombus using compression ultrasound or using color duplex imaging with a very low PRF (aliasing in the vein in left section) during Valsalva's maneuver or distal compression. In case of thrombosis, the valve leaflets (VK) will not move and Valsalva's maneuver will not elicit flow between the venous wall and the leaflet of the incompetent valve (right section).
e Adequate valve closure. The example shows an incompetent saphenofemoral junction with an incompetent arch vein, while the great saphenous vein valves above the knee are competent. The proximal valves are incompetent, and the image depicts the first competent valve, indicated by adequate closure with Valsalva's maneuver. Retrograde flow causes flow signals extending into the valve pockets during closure (distal point of insufficiency). There is no flow distally, except for a minimal, thin stream coded in red and indicating minimal leakage of the valve; this is no evidence of relevant valve incompetence (VK = valve leaflet)

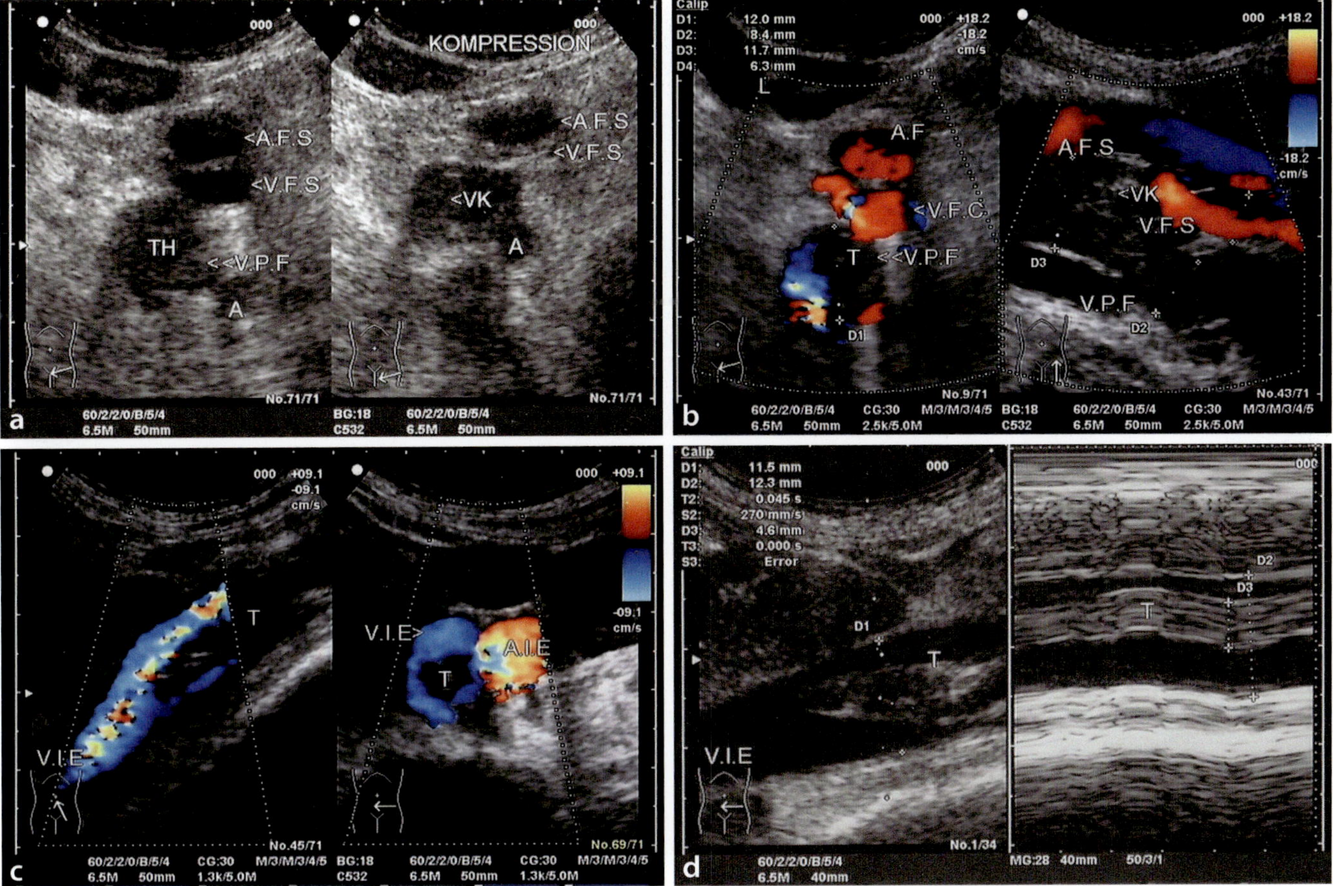

■ **Fig. 3.61a–d (Atlas) Pelvic vein thrombosis secondary to ascending deep femoral vein thrombosis.**
a Compression ultrasound (transverse image on the right) reveals compressibility of the superficial femoral vein (V.F.S), while the deep femoral vein is not compressible (TH in V.P.F).
b Color flow images (transverse section on the left and longitudinal section on the right) show flow in the superficial femoral vein (red) and no thrombosis; the deep femoral vein (V.P.F) joins the superficial vein posteriorly. Also depicted are the superficial femoral artery (A.F.S) anterior to the vein and the profunda femoris artery posteriorly.
c The thrombus (T) extends into the external iliac vein (V.I.E) and is surrounded by flowing blood.
d The time-motion display documents floating of a long thrombus tail (T) in the external iliac vein (■ Fig. 3.13)

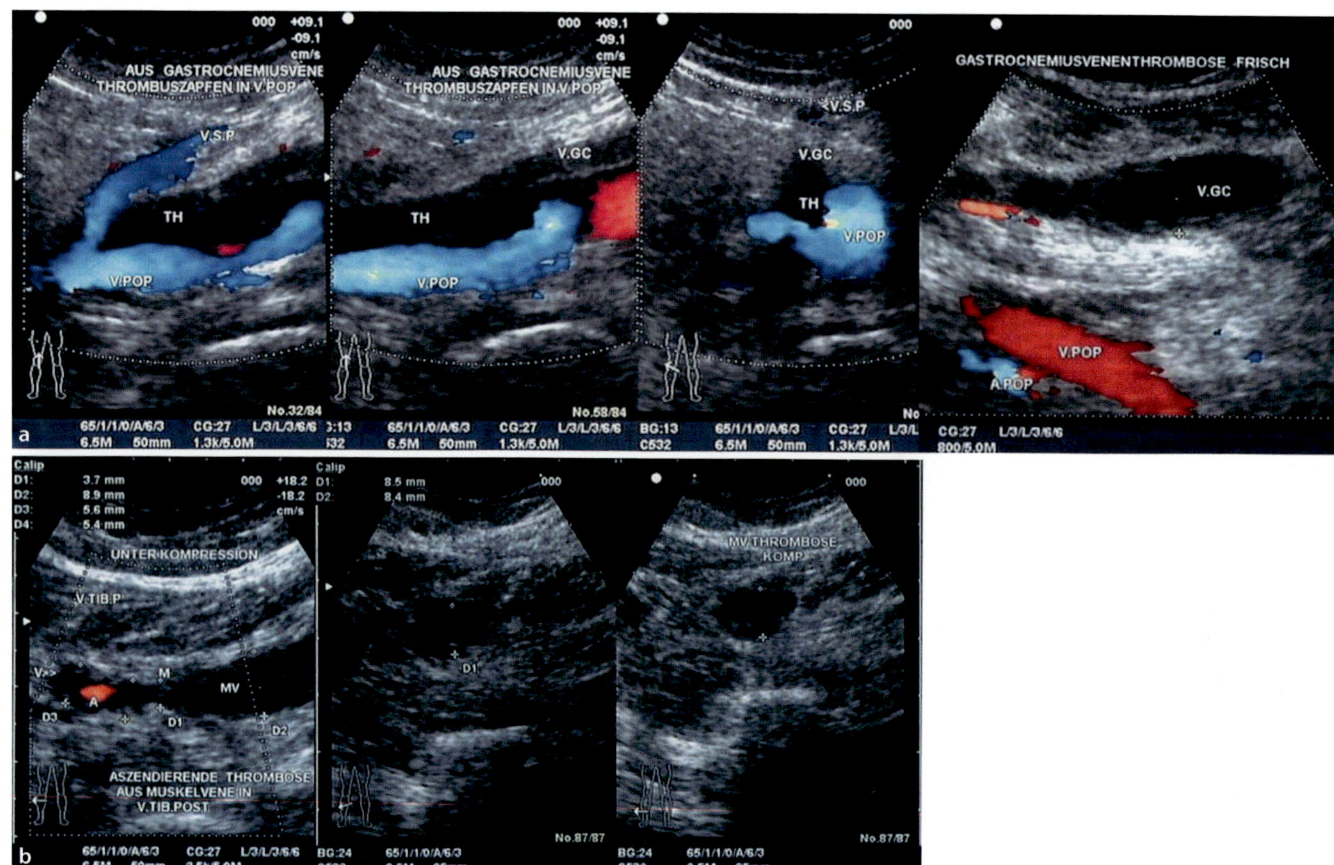

Fig. 3.62a, b (Atlas) Calf muscle vein thrombosis with thrombus extension into popliteal vein.
a The two longitudinal views (leftmost and left center) and the transverse view (right center) show a gap (TH) in the color-coded flow in the popliteal vein (V.POP). An ascending thrombus (TH) protrudes into the popliteal vein from a thrombosed gastrocnemius vein (V.GC). More cranially, the small saphenous vein (V.S.P) is depicted with blood flow in blue. The mural thrombosis ascending from the gastrocnemius vein into the popliteal vein ends at the saphenofemoral junction (leftmost and left center). The gastrocnemius vein thrombosis cannot be traced further distally (rightmost section).
b Muscle vein thrombosis below the knee is suggested by the depiction in the soleus or gastrocnemius muscle of hypoechoic tubular structures that cannot be compressed. The veins are markedly dilated, making them more conspicuous than normal muscle veins. The distinction between muscle vein thrombosis and thrombosis of a major calf vein is made sonoanatomically. The major veins run parallel to the lower leg arteries of the same name. The transverse image (middle section) depicts a hypoechoic structure in the soleus muscle. Noncompressibility of the vein confirms muscle vein thrombosis (right section). The oblique color duplex image on the left depicts the thrombosed soleus vein (MV, labeled as D2) on its course from the mid-calf to the knee, where it enters (labeled as D1) the posterior tibial vein. There is appositional thrombus growth into the posterior tibial vein, which is thrombosed up to the tibiofibular junction, while it is compressible somewhat distal to the entry site of the muscle vein. The image on the left was obtained during compression and depicts the hypoechoic, noncompressible posterior tibial veins (labeled as D3 and D4) to the left and right of the posterior tibial artery (red)

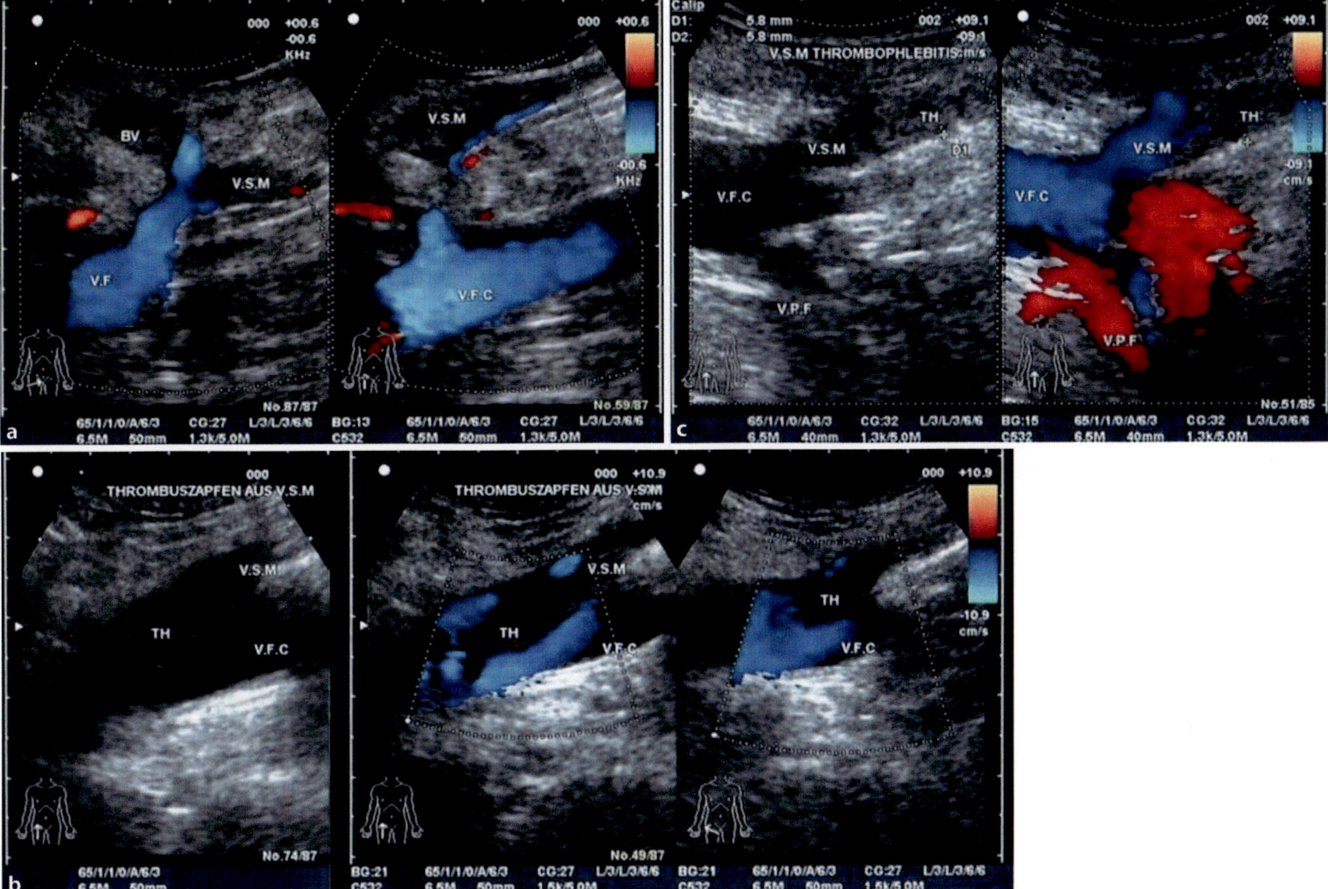

Fig. 3.63a–c (Atlas) Thrombophlebitis of great saphenous vein with thrombus extension into femoral vein (natural history).
a The proximal extent of thrombophlebitis may be greater than suggested by the clinical findings. The patient shown presented with reddening along the course of the great saphenous vein up to the mid-thigh, while color duplex imaging (transverse view on the left and longitudinal view on the right) demonstrates gaps in the color coding extending up to 1.5 cm below the saphenofemoral junction. The longitudinal view depicts flow in blue along the thrombus. Ultrasound also demonstrates thrombophlebitic involvement of the clinically normal anterior tributary vein (BV). In this situation, surgical ligation is indicated to prevent further thrombus growth into deep veins.
b Ascending thrombophlebitis can extend into a deep vein in the form of a cone-shaped thrombus. The gray-scale image (left section) already depicts a slightly more hyperechoic thrombus (TH) protruding into the anechoic lumen of the common femoral vein (V.F.C) from the great saphenous vein (V.S.M). In the color flow image (right), the thrombus (TH) protruding into the common femoral vein is identified by the absence of color in the blue-coded lumen.
c Based on the duplex findings, high ligation of the great saphenous vein was indicated but was refused by the patient. In this case, the course of endogenous thrombolysis under heparin therapy can thus be followed. After 3 weeks, the thrombus in the great saphenous vein has receded to 1 cm below the junction. The image on the left demonstrates the thrombus (TH) in the lumen of the great saphenous vein (V.S.M). The color flow image on the right depicts flow in the great saphenous vein in blue (away from transducer, toward center) and a branch of the deep femoral vein (V.P.F) coming from posteriorly with flow toward the transducer coded in red

3

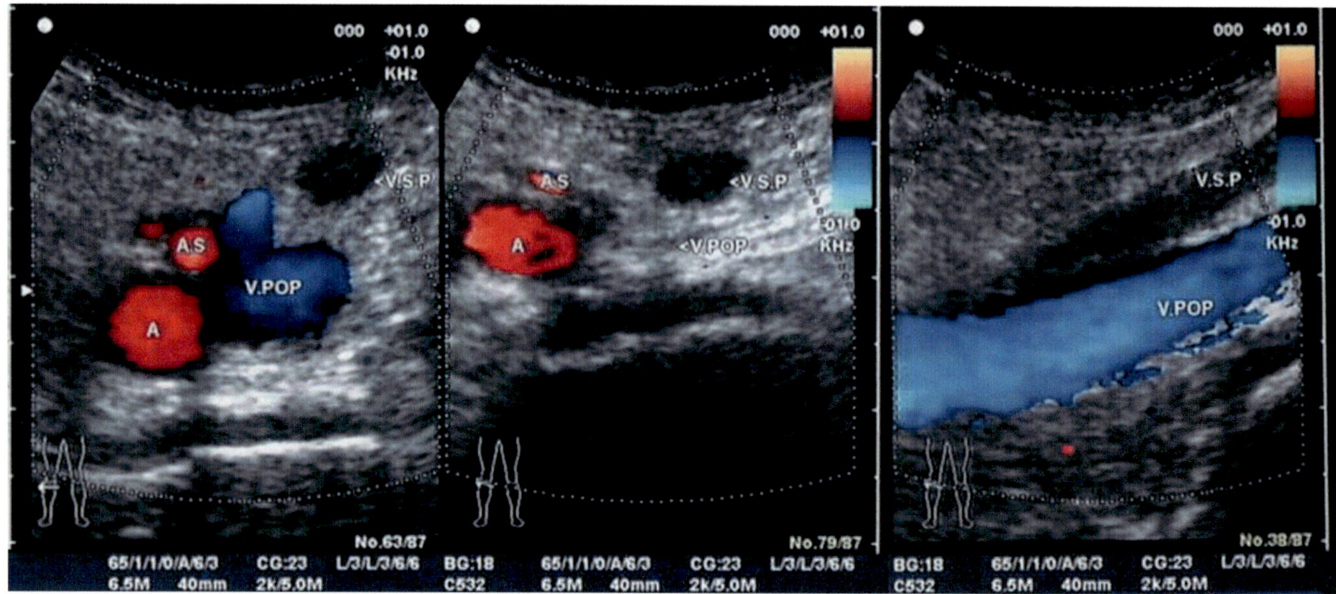

Fig. 3.64 (Atlas) Thrombophlebitis of small saphenous vein.
Patients with thrombophlebitis of the small saphenous vein often present with unspecific clinical symptoms that may mimic deep vein thrombosis (DVT). For this reason, diagnostic evaluation of patients for exclusion of DVT must also include the small saphenous vein. The transverse view on the left depicts the small saphenous vein (V.S.P) as a nonperfused hypoechoic tubular structure posterior to the popliteal vein (V.POP). The image obtained with compression (middle section) shows incompressibility of the vein. The longitudinal image (right section) depicts the small saphenous vein (V.S.P) without flow to the level of the saphenopopliteal junction. There is no thrombus extension into the popliteal vein (V.POP), seen as complete blue color filling of the popliteal vein

Fig. 3.65 (Atlas) Femoropopliteal vein.
The femoropopliteal vein (V.FP) passes posteriorly from the small saphenous vein (V.S.P, dilated by fresh thrombus) just below the saphenopopliteal junction. Despite thrombophlebitis of the small saphenous vein distal to the site of entry of the femoropopliteal vein, proximal compression and release elicits reflux at the saphenopopliteal junction due to femoropopliteal valve incompetence (orthograde venous drainage through the femoropopliteal vein)

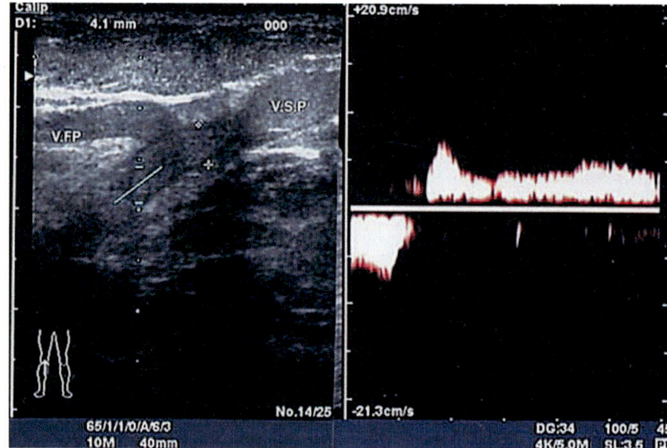

Fig. 3.66 (Atlas) Thrombosis arising from thrombophlebitis extending through perforator.
Extension of thrombophlebitis into the deep venous system can also occur through a perforating vein. In the case presented, extensive thrombophlebitis of the great saphenous vein (V.S.M) gives rise to a thrombus extending through a perforating vein (PV) into the posterior tibial vein (V.TIB.P), where it causes a circumscribed thrombosis 3 cm in length. Next to the vein, the artery is depicted with flow in red. The great saphenous, perforating, and posterior tibial veins are markedly dilated by the thrombus and not compressible (right image). The hyperechoic reflection indicates the site at which the vein pierces the fascia (F)

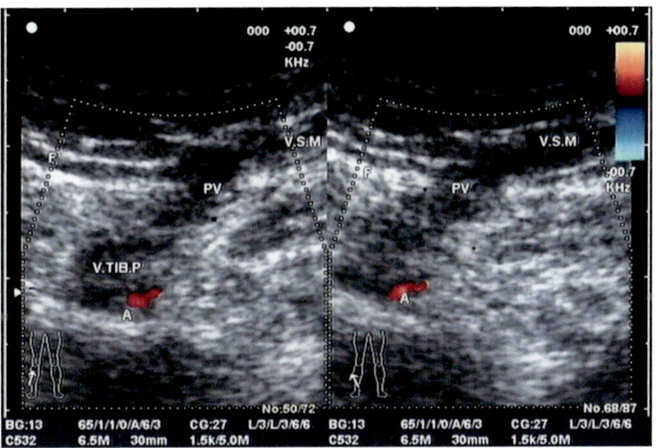

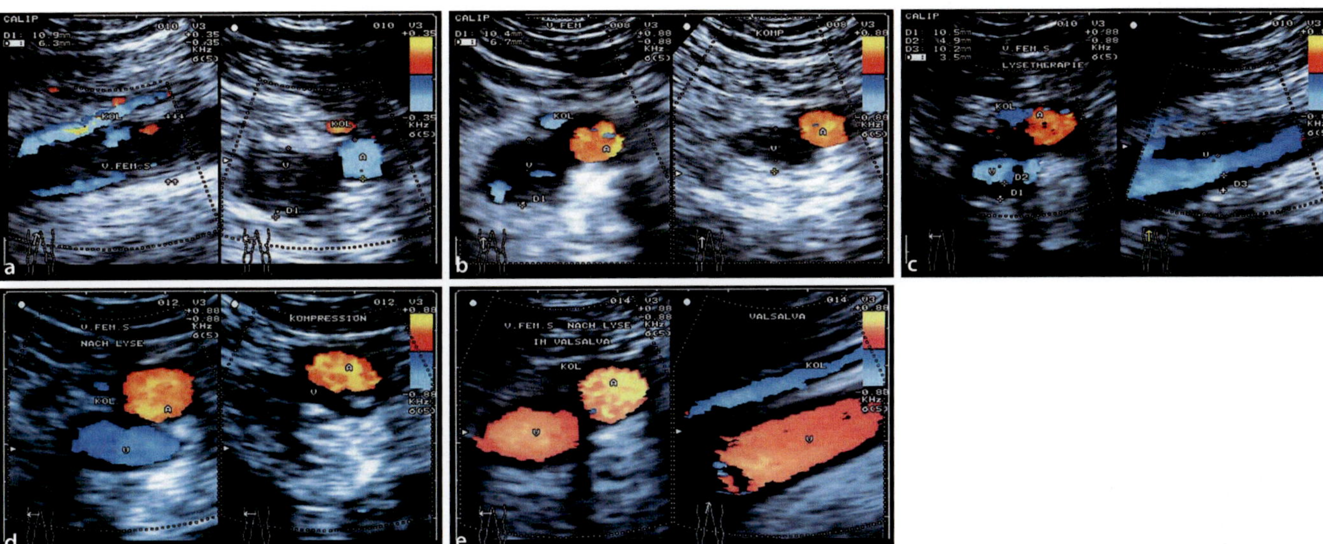

Fig. 3.67a–e (Atlas) Monitoring of thrombolytic therapy.
a Marked dilatation of the superficial femoral vein (compared with the accompanying artery) and the hypoechoic, homogeneous thrombus with a just barely visible hypoechoic halo suggest acute thrombosis. The transverse view depicts a collateral (KOL) with flow in red anterior to the superficial femoral artery (A). The longitudinal view on the left shows a more proximal segment of the superficial femoral vein (V). Proximal to the site of entry of a collateral vein, the thrombus in the superficial femoral vein is surrounded by residual flow near the walls (blue).
b After three cycles of thrombolytic therapy with streptokinase, there is flow in the center and periphery of the lumen of the superficial femoral vein (V), indicating beginning recanalization. The image was obtained in the same plane as the transverse image in (**a**) but with the transducer angled superiorly. The image on the right shows that flow signals disappear from the collateral vein and the partially recanalized femoral vein upon compression. The patent lumen collapses and only the thrombosed portion is still visible.
c Complete recanalization of the vein after another three cycles of thrombolytic therapy. The transverse view (left) and the longitudinal view (right) depict only some residual mural thrombus of low echogenicity around the patent lumen. The collateral (KOL, blue) anterior to the superficial femoral vein (V, blue) is also still present.
d After another cycle of thrombolysis, the residual mural thrombi have almost completely dissolved. Upon compression (right section) of the vein (V), only a thin, hypoechoic band is depicted posterior to the artery, indicating reactive inflammatory wall thickening and intimal edema.
e Despite complete recanalization following streptokinase therapy, Valsalva's maneuver elicits persistent reflux. Valve damage in this patient is due to the delay of more than 10 days between the onset of thrombosis and complete recanalization. The image on the left demonstrates blood flow in the same direction (coded red) in the vein (V) and the corresponding artery (A). The image on the right shows flow toward the heart (blue) in the competent collateral vein (KOL) during Valsalva's maneuver. This forward flow in the competent collateral is induced by the calf muscle pump because some patients inadvertently also contract their muscles during Valsalva's maneuver

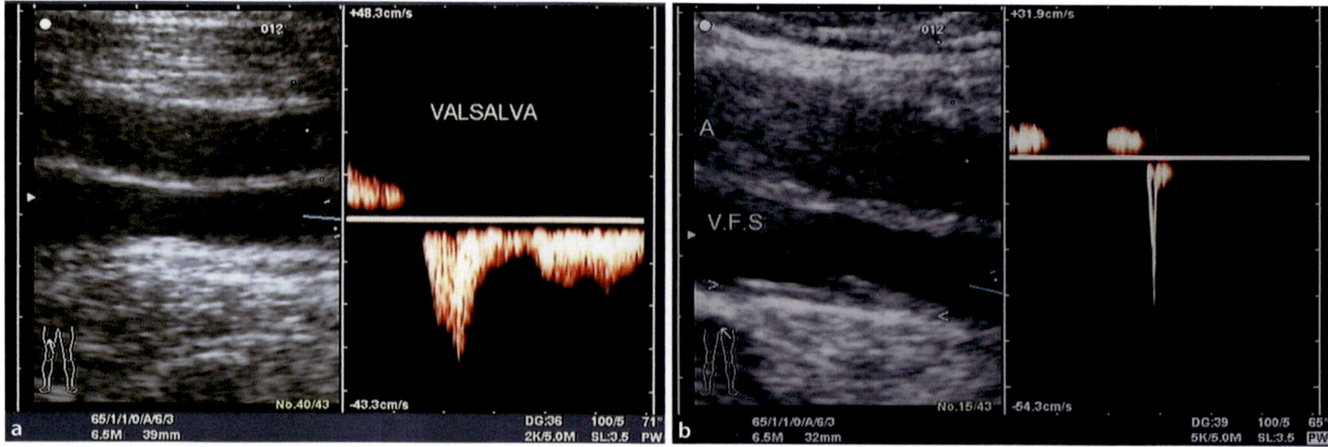

Fig. 3.68a, b (Atlas) Postthrombotic syndrome – valve function.
a The severity of insufficient venous drainage depends on the degree of recanalization and the development of postthrombotic valve incompetence of major veins. If there is complete recanalization, the veins may appear perfectly normal on B-mode ultrasound with valve dysfunction being the only postthrombotic sequela.
b Conversely, there may be normal function of individual venous segments, which will prevent reflux, even if B-mode images show vascular wall changes (sclerosis, thickening). In the example, Valsalva's maneuver elicits only a short reflux before valve closure (Doppler waveform) although B-mode imaging demonstrates postthrombotic wall thickening

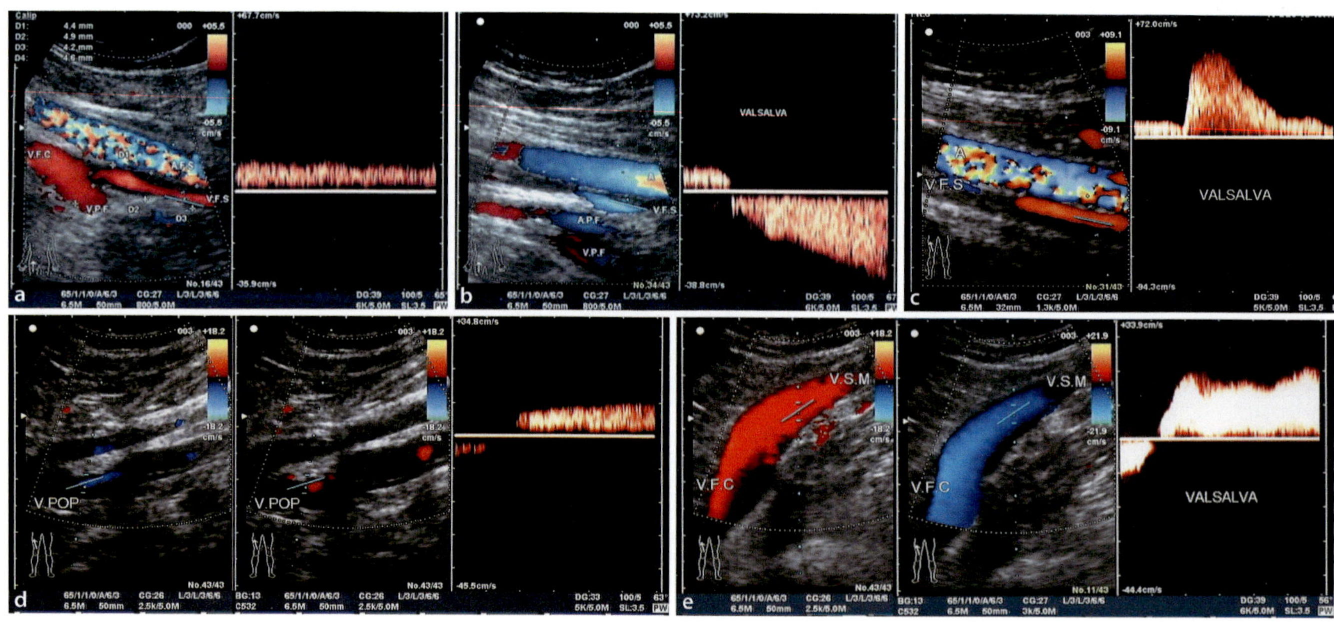

Fig. 3.69a–e (Atlas) Postthrombotic syndrome – recanalized lumen.
a In about 10% of cases, thrombosis leads to permanent damage of the vein (see Fig. 3.51 (Atlas)), depicted sonographically as a hypoechoic, tubular strand with a thin caliber adjacent to the artery. In most cases, however, there is postthrombotic recanalization but often with a smaller lumen. In the example shown, the superficial femoral vein is patent 4 months after thrombosis, but only trickling flow is present. Hypoechoic thrombotic wall deposits and sclerotic wall lesions persist. Aliasing in the superficial femoral artery closer to the transducer confirms the PRF to be adequate for the detection of slow venous flow. There is continuous venous flow due to loss of respiratory phasicity, indicating persistent flow obstruction in the recanalized vein.
b Flow in the superficial femoral vein (V.F.S) during Valsalva's maneuver is coded in blue (away from transducer), and the Doppler waveform shows reversed flow.
c–e Postthrombotic syndrome – paradoxical flow during Valsalva's maneuver.
c When Valsalva' maneuver elicits increased flow rather than flow reversal in a recanalized vein (here the superficial femoral vein), this indicates flow through dilated collaterals. In the example, Valsalva's maneuver induces blood flow from the incompetent great saphenous vein into the femoral vein via incompetent perforating veins. The resulting flow increase in the superficial femoral vein (Doppler waveform) indicates poor recanalization of the femoral vein and above all of the popliteal vein (see **d**) and persistent severe obstruction of peripheral venous drainage. While the paradoxical flow pattern indicates pathology in the case presented here, the examiner must be aware that such a pattern may also occur because some patients inadvertently also contract their leg and in particular their calf muscles when performing Valsalva's maneuver.
d In more distal, partially recanalized vein segments such as the popliteal vein (distal to the Dodd perforators, through which the blood enters the deep system), Valsalva's maneuver induces typical to-and-fro flow with flow reversal (spontaneous flow in the left image, augmented flow in the right image).
e Valsalva's maneuver reveals severe terminal valve incompetence of the great saphenous vein (reflux in the Doppler waveform)

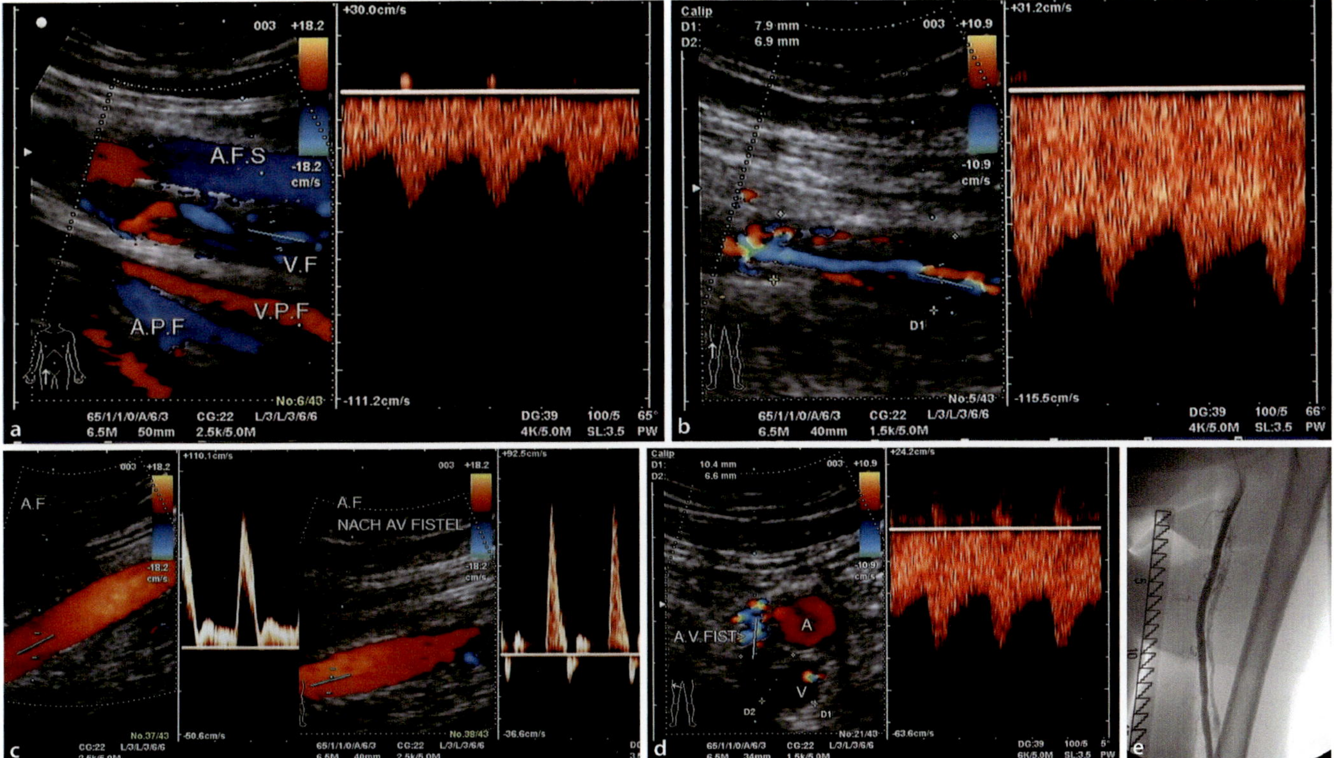

Fig. 3.70a–e (Atlas) Postthrombotic recanalization with arteriovenous fistula.
a Patient with venous thrombosis of the thigh showing the typical signs of early recanalization (color duplex) after 4 months: meandering flow and flow signals mostly confined to the center of the vein. The Doppler waveform obtained from the partially recanalized vein shows retrograde pulsatile flow. A possible cause is an arteriovenous (AV) fistula; in this patient, retrograde flow is due to occlusive thrombosis proximally.
b In the distal femoral vein, color duplex ultrasound also shows signs of recanalization with residual mural thrombus, with the Doppler waveform demonstrating high-frequency flow toward the periphery.
c To search for the AV fistula, the length of the femoral artery is scanned from proximal to distal with continuous Doppler recording. A sudden change to more pulsatile flow indicates the site where to look for the AV fistula. The Doppler waveform on the left was obtained in the femoral artery, upstream of the AV fistula, and the one on the right downstream of the fistula.
d Transverse image of the AV fistula between the superficial femoral artery (A) and the femoral vein (V). The sample volume is placed in the fistula, and the Doppler waveform shows the typical pulsatile flow pattern of a fistula; however, the frequency is lower than expected. The femoral vein is still largely thrombosed, but some flow is present, suggesting recanalization (next to the "V"). The communication between the AV fistula and the recanalized venous lumen is not visualized because it does not lie in the scan plane.
e Angiogram simultaneously depicts the artery and a thin stream in the vein with flow directed toward the periphery. The preceding color duplex examination provides the explanation for this phenomenon

3

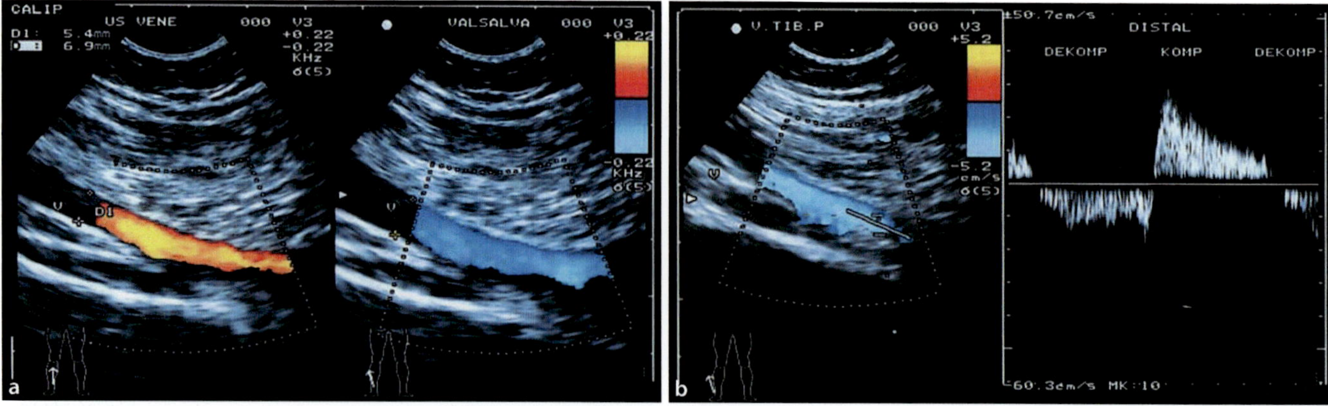

Fig. 3.71a, b (Atlas) Chronic venous insufficiency.
a Primary chronic venous insufficiency of the deep leg veins differs from the postthrombotic syndrome in that valve failure is due to venous dilatation. The delicate venous walls are free of deposits and therefore easy to compress. In the example shown, valve incompetence of the proximal posterior tibial vein is associated with persistent reflux during Valsalva's maneuver, indicated by the color change from red to blue. In patients with severe dysfunction of all venous valves proximal to the transducer, even deep abdominal inspiration can induce reversed flow, and normal rhythmical inspiration and expiration may induce to-and-fro flow.
Valve incompetence of calf veins.
b Determination of the duration of reflux from the Doppler waveform enables differentiation of short physiologic reflux prior to valve closure from persistent reflux due to incompetent valves. Blue indicates reflux in the posterior tibial vein away from the transducer. Repeated and somewhat longer manual compression and release of the distal calf lead to alternating flow toward the transducer during compression (KOMP) and away during release (DEKOMP)

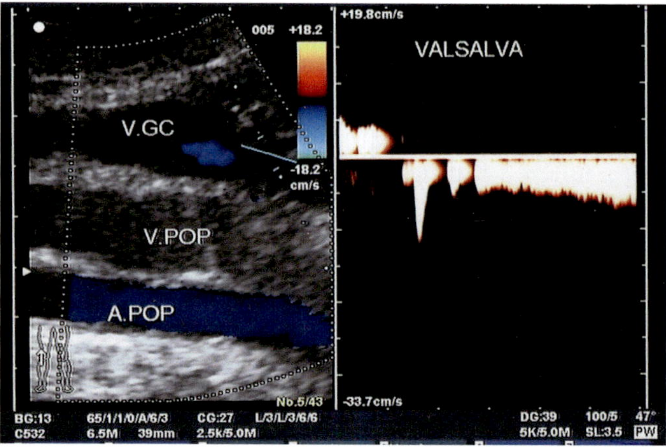

Fig. 3.72 (Atlas) Dilated muscle veins.
Patient with crural ulcer but without signs of insufficiency of the great saphenous vein in the thigh. There is valve incompetence of the superficial femoral vein and the proximal popliteal vein with good valve closure in the major veins distally. Valsalva's maneuver reveals valve incompetence with persistent reflux (Doppler waveform) in a dilated gastrocnemius vein (V.GC). The color duplex image (left) shows no flow in the popliteal vein (V.POP) with Valsalva's maneuver, indicating competent valves. The crural ulcer in this patient was caused by incompetent indirect perforating veins (not shown) and healed after elimination of the incompetent perforators identified by ultrasound (several weeks of prior compression therapy had no effect). Such dilated gastrocnemius and soleus veins can cause stasis of blood flow, giving rise to calf thrombosis with extension into the popliteal vein

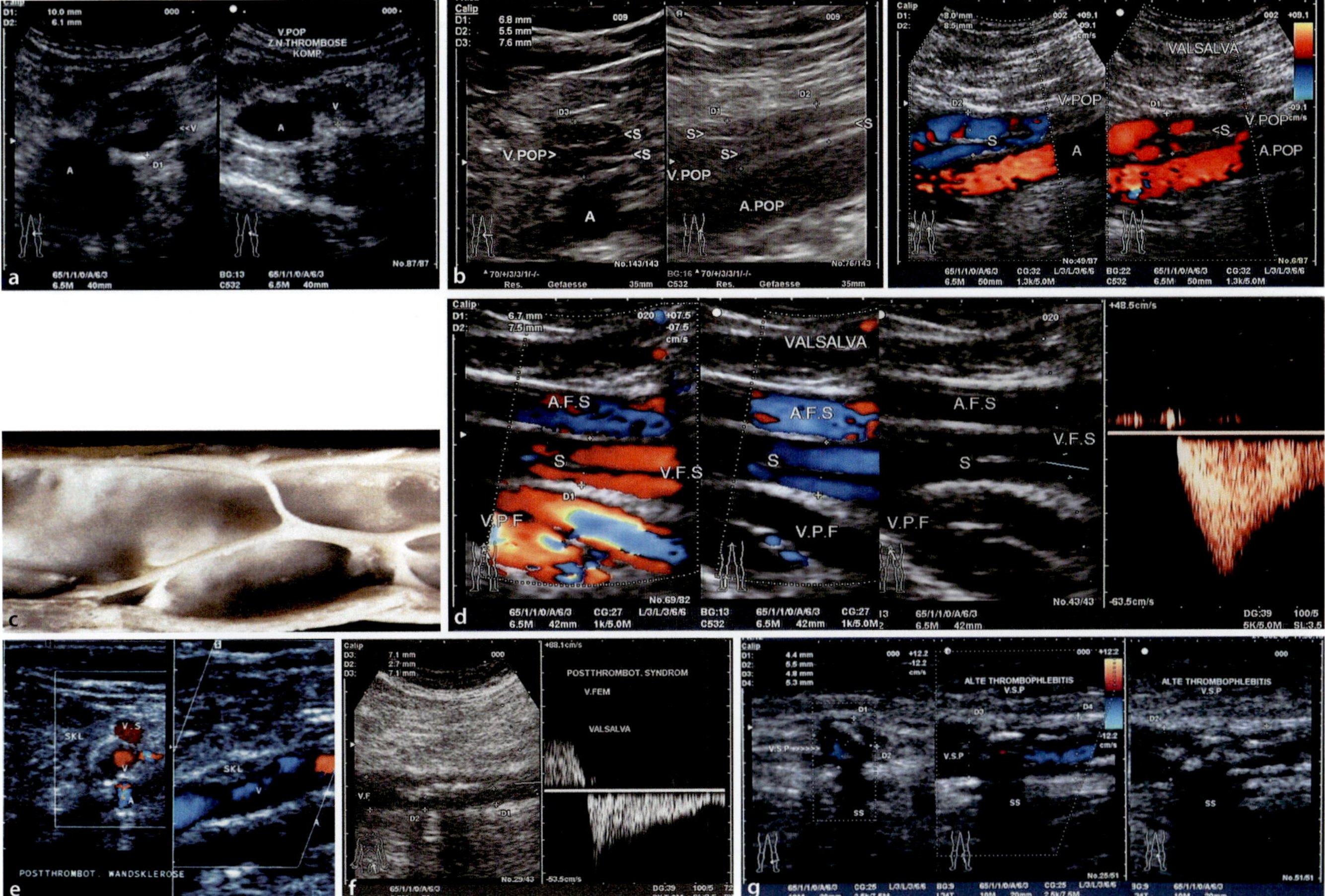

Fig. 3.73a–g (Atlas) Postthrombotic syndrome – residual lesions/synechia.
a Patient with severe postthrombotic syndrome. Incomplete compressibility (right image) of postthrombotic veins may be due to residual thrombus or synechia. The image obtained without compression (left) depicts hyperechoic thread-like structures in the partially recanalized (more hypoechoic) lumen. These structures, which may occasionally have a honeycomb appearance, are sclerotic strands persisting after thrombosis. The image on the right shows these structures in longitudinal orientation.
b The transverse and longitudinal gray-scale images (left) show the recanalized popliteal vein (V.POP) with postthrombotic wall sclerosis and synechia (S). The longitudinal color flow images (right) reveal postthrombotic reflux in the recanalized popliteal vein (V.POP). The first color flow image (without Valsalva's maneuver) shows the blood in the popliteal vein (blue) draining between the strands (S). They appear as membraneous structures within the lumen and are identified by the absence of color-coded flow. During Valsalva's maneuver (second color flow image), the flow direction in the vein is the same as in the adjacent popliteal artery (from the center toward the periphery, displayed in red).
c Recanalized postthrombotic vein with severe wall sclerosis and postthrombotic strands.
d Intraluminal synechia (S) extend to the proximal superficial femoral vein (V.FS). The left color flow image shows the recanalized superficial femoral vein with blood flow toward the heart (red). The right color flow image shows reversed flow (blue) along the strands (S) toward the periphery with Valsalva's maneuver. There is normal valve closure in the deep femoral veins (V.PF) without reflux (A.FS = superficial femoral artery). The gray-scale image depicts synechia in the recanalized lumen, and the Doppler waveform shows slow flow due to obstruction by the strands and marked reflux elicited by Valsalva's maneuver (flow away from transducer, toward the periphery).
e–g Postthrombotic residues – wall sclerosis.
e The popliteal vein is completely patent, but there is postthrombotic wall sclerosis depicted as hyperechoic thickening of the wall (SKL, longitudinal view on the right). The transverse image on the left also depicts more hypoechoic areas in the lumen, corresponding to residual thrombotic deposits on the wall or wall thickening. These abnormalities appear to the left of the recanalized patent lumen (with flowing blood displayed in red) and farther away from the transducer. The more superficial small saphenous vein appears normal shortly before it joins the popliteal vein.
f Postthrombotic wall lesions can lead to wall sclerosis and calcifications with acoustic shadowing on ultrasound. The Doppler waveform shows reflux due to incompetent valves.
g Vasosclerotic changes with wall thickening and calcification may also occur after thrombophlebitis. In the example, the longitudinal view on the right shows the hyperechoic sclerotic wall lesions with intraluminal deposits in the small saphenous vein. There is posterior acoustic shadowing (SS) due to partial calcification. The longitudinal image in the middle and the transverse image on the left depict flow (blue) in the thin recanalized lumen of the postthrombophlebitic small saphenous vein

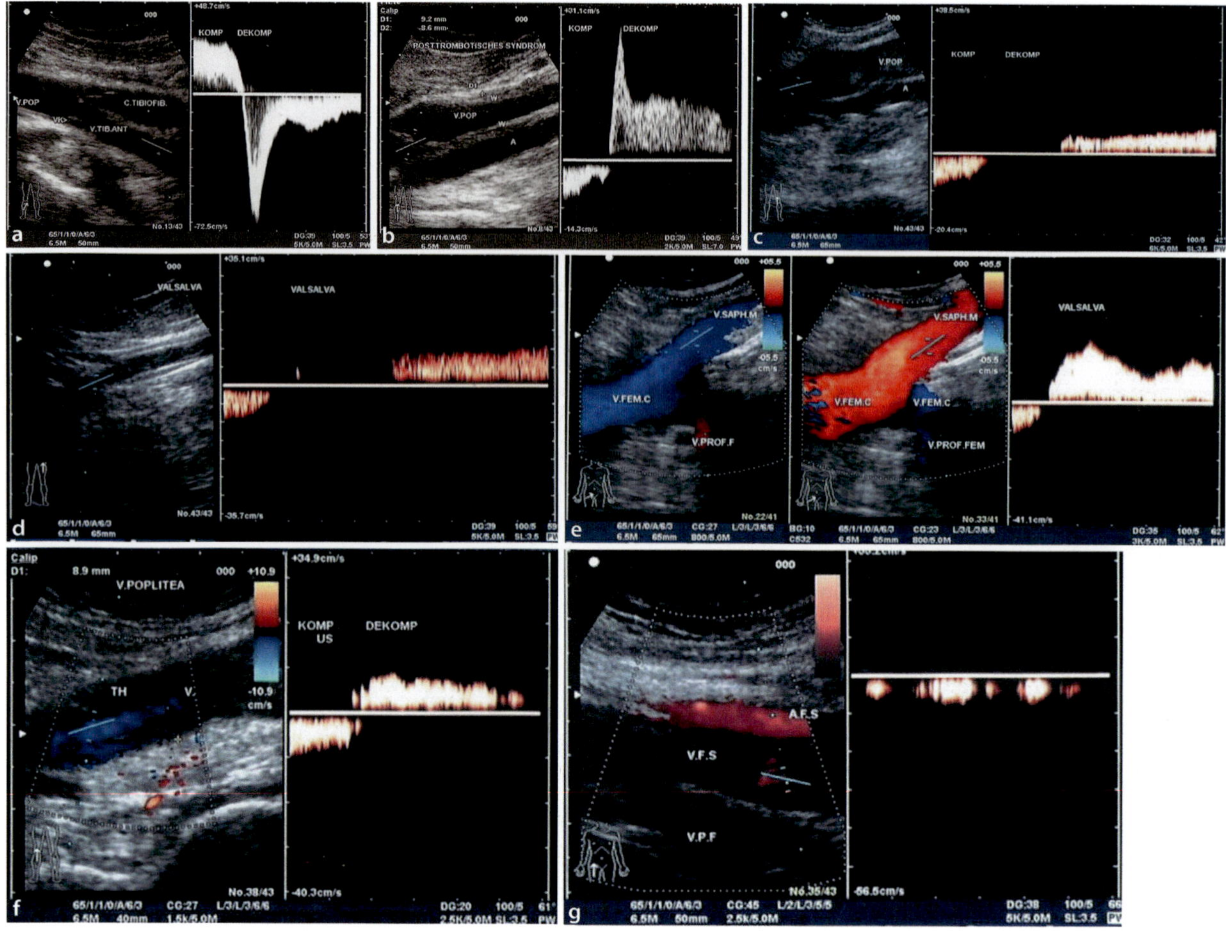

Fig. 3.74a–g (Atlas) Degrees of valve incompetence.
a Postthrombotic thickening of a venous valve (VK) with adhesion to the wall prevents closure, which is indicated by reflux during Valsalva's maneuver or the valve function test (compression and release). Postthrombotic sclerosis and valve incompetence of the popliteal and calf veins cause immediate backward flow upon compression of the calf (KOMP) with subsequent release (DEKOMP) as a sign of complete valve failure. Once the blood column expulsed from the calf has flowed back, a decrease in the reflux signal induced by release of compression is noted. The example illustrates valve incompetence of the anterior tibial vein (V.TIB.ANT) before it enters the popliteal vein (V.POP).
b The popliteal vein also shows postthrombotic valve adhesion and wall sclerosis (W), reflected sonographically as hyperechoic wall thickening (wall near transducer). The Doppler waveform from the popliteal vein (V.POP) depicts the prompt and pronounced reflux (toward transducer) upon release of compression (DEKOMP) as a sign of complete valve failure.
c Primary chronic venous insufficiency with preservation of some residual valve function due to dilatation is indicated by delayed reflux upon Valsalva's maneuver or release of compression. This is illustrated in the example by delayed reflux (toward transducer) with a lower but constant flow in the popliteal vein.
d A similar pattern of backward flow is seen in this case of varicosis of the great saphenous vein with early, mild valvular incompetence. There is delayed but constant reflux through the leaking valve after Valsalva's maneuver.
e Marked varicose dilatation produces severe valve incompetence without residual function, as in the postthrombotic syndrome, resulting in immediate and pronounced reflux with high-velocity flow toward the periphery during Valsalva's maneuver.
f The reflux resulting from postthrombotic valve incompetence is additionally influenced by flow obstruction due to residual thrombus. In the example, the popliteal vein is still partially thrombosed (TH) with only slow spontaneous flow. Compression (KOMP) of the calf induces constant flow from the periphery to the heart, while the backward flow occurring upon release of compression (DEKOMP) is less pronounced and less persistent than would be expected in extensive, recanalized thrombosis. The reduced backward flow is due to flow obstruction by residual thrombus.
g When the ultrasound examination is performed with a high-resolution transducer and low PRF or in the power mode (for detection of slow flow), even slight reflux through a small leak in a valve leaflet during prolonged Valsalva's maneuver can be detected. The power mode image on the left shows only little flow (red) directly behind the leaking valve leaflet in the proximal superficial femoral vein. In such situations, the sample volume must be placed close to the valve to depict the slight reflux during Valsalva's maneuver (flow toward periphery, away from transducer). As only little blood leaks back into the vein, no flow signals are detectable elsewhere in the vein. Such slight leakage as in this case should not be overinterpreted as valve incompetence but merely illustrates the high sensitivity of high-resolution ultrasound to low flow. However, repeat Doppler sampling along the course of the vein with provocative maneuvers is necessary to definitely rule out clinically relevant reflux. Anterior to the vein, the superficial femoral artery (A.F.S, red) is depicted; and posterior to it, the deep femoral vein (V.P.F, without flow signals during Valsalva's maneuver)

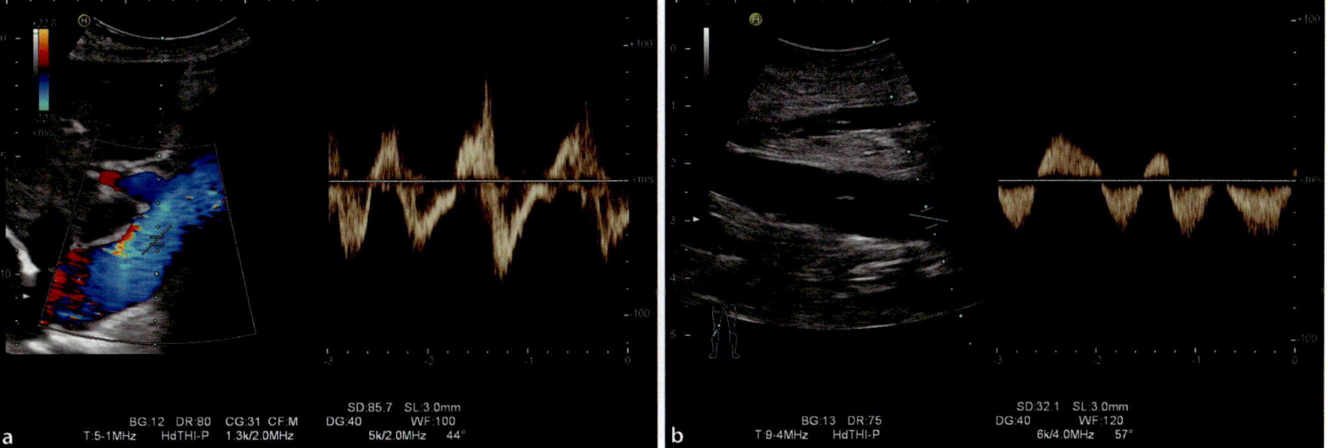

Fig. 3.75a, b (Atlas) Respiratory phasicity and cardiac pulsatility of reflux in severe valve incompetence.
a Severe obstruction of venous drainage in the vena cava with to-and-fro flow modulated by cardiac pulsatility.
b Doppler waveform obtained in a postthrombotic popliteal vein (synechia) with severe valve incompetence of the entire deep vein system of the leg in a patient with concomitant cardiac inflow obstruction and tricuspid insufficiency. In this situation, there is two-and-fro flow with reflux (absolute arrhythmia) and both respiratory phasicity and cardiac pulsatility

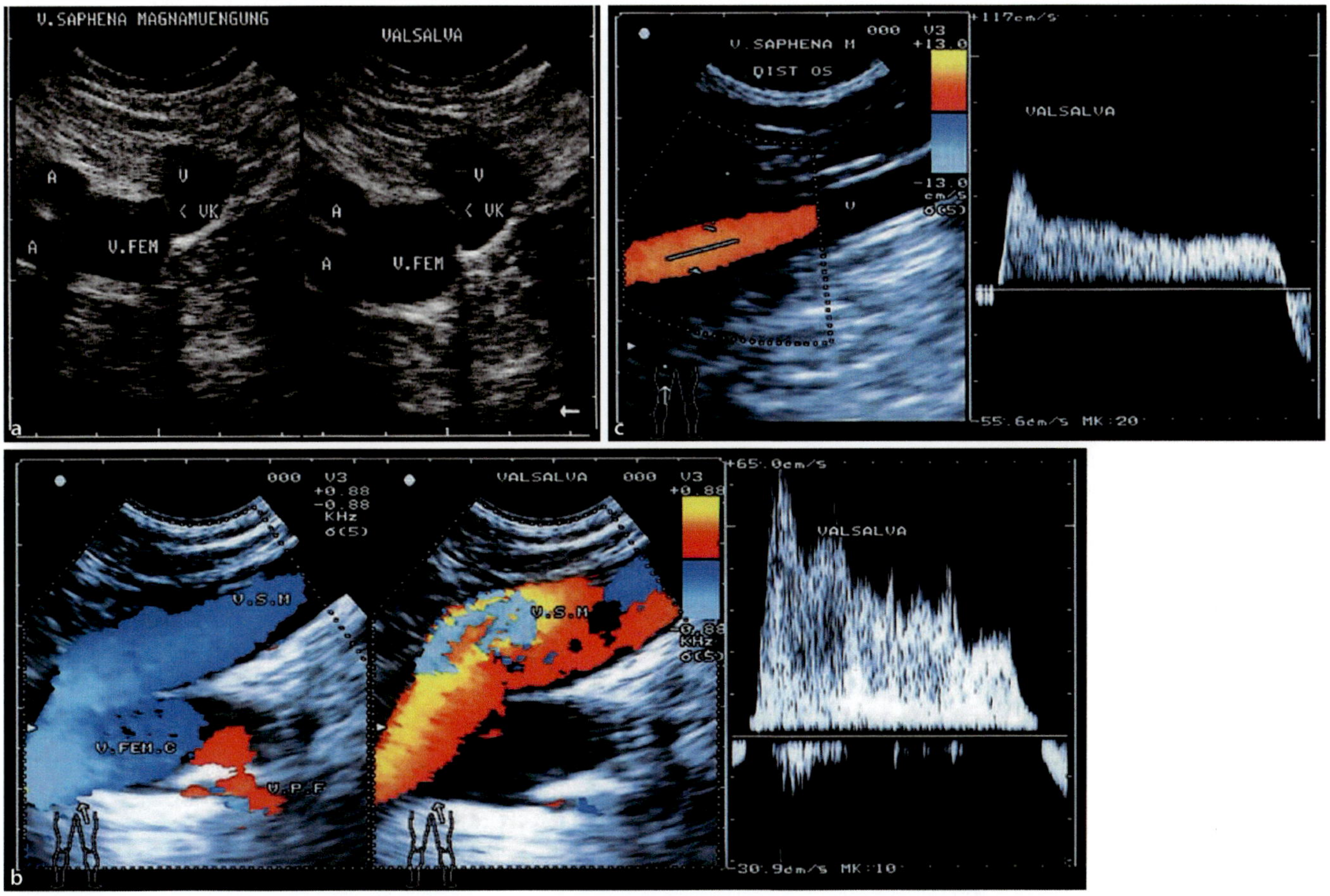

Fig. 3.76a–c (Atlas) Truncal varicosis of great saphenous vein (distal extent).
a The transverse B-mode images show dilatation of the proximal great saphenous vein during Valsalva's maneuver with the incompetent valve leaflet turning distally and thus becoming visible (VK).
b Incompetent terminal valve of the great saphenous vein. The image on the left shows blood flow toward the heart (blue). The great saphenous vein (V.S.M) courses close to the transducer, and a deep femoral vein (V.P.F) with flow displayed in red is seen entering the common femoral vein (V.FEM.C) posteriorly. Valsalva's maneuver (second color flow image) induces reflux (red) with aliasing due to the low PRF adjusted to slow venous flow. Proper valve closure in the common femoral vein prevents reflux into the deep venous system. The Doppler waveform recorded in the saphenofemoral junction during Valsalva's maneuver shows flow to the periphery (toward transducer).
c The distal point of insufficiency of the great saphenous vein for grading according to Hach is identified by determining reflux during Valsalva's maneuver (toward transducer) in the color duplex mode or in the Doppler tracing obtained along the course of the vein from the thigh (V) to the calf

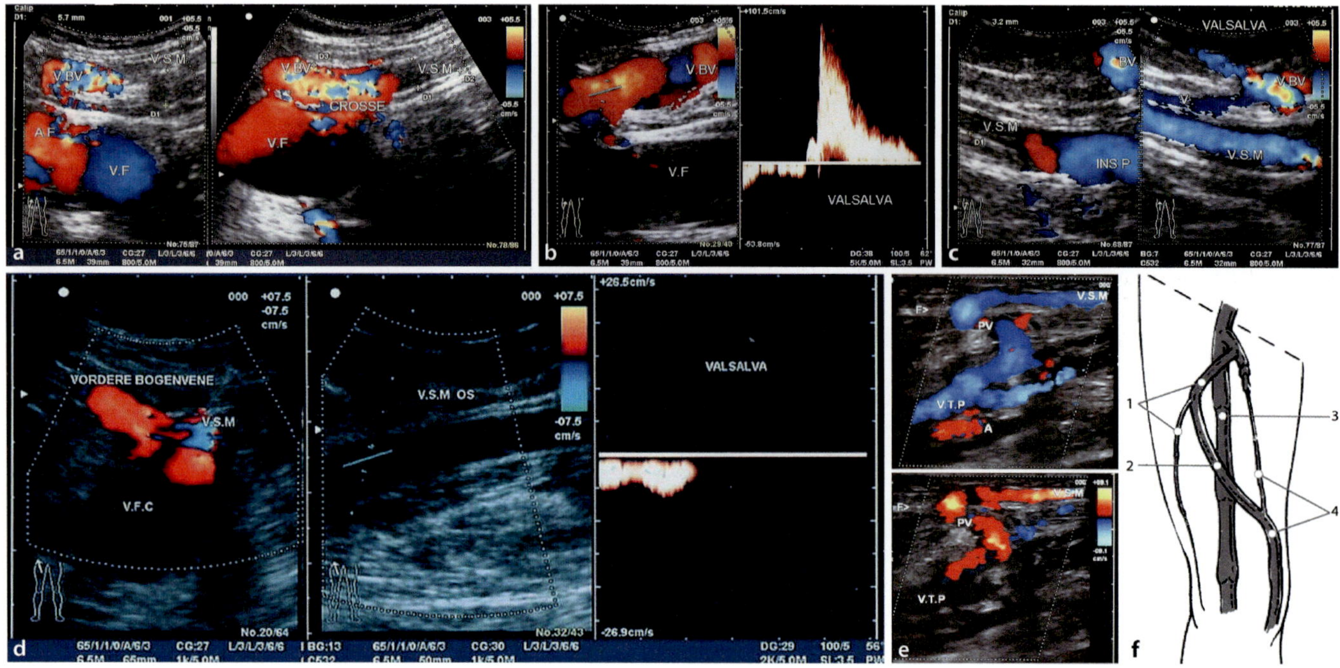

◘ Fig. 3.77a–f (Atlas) Incomplete truncal varicosis of great saphenous vein.
a Transverse view on the left and longitudinal view on the right (or rather oblique view) show reflux in the lateral accessory saphenous vein (V.BV = arch vein) in the right groin, induced by Valsalva's maneuver. Absence of flow in the proximal great saphenous vein (V.S.M, marked by calipers) during Valsalva's maneuver indicates competent valves in this segment. The incompetent accessory saphenous vein joins the competent great saphenous vein just below the saphenofemoral junction and the incompetent terminal valve (V.F = femoral vein).
b Flow into the periphery (toward the transducer) induced by Valsalva's maneuver is seen in the lateral accessory saphenous vein (arch vein) in the color flow image (red) and in the Doppler waveform (see ◘ Fig. 3.16).
c Longitudinal image depicting the accessory saphenous vein (V.BV = arch vein) and great saphenous vein (V.S.M) including the vein connecting the two (V = bucket handle anastomosis) in one plane. The right image shows reflux in this venous system upon Valsalva's maneuver: flow toward the periphery coded in blue (away from transducer) in the arch vein, the connecting vein, and the great saphenous vein. The valves of the great saphenous vein are incompetent up to this level (proximal point of insufficiency). The left image (composite image of proximal segment) again shows the upper point of insufficiency of the great saphenous vein (V.S.M, marked by calipers); there is no flow in the competent proximal segment of the great saphenous vein. At the proximal point of insufficiency (INS P), the bucket handle anastomosis (V) enters laterally.
d Neither color duplex nor the Doppler waveform shows flow reversal just below the saphenofemoral junction with Valsalva's maneuver, confirming competence of the proximal great saphenous vein.
e Insufficient Cockett I perforators in the calf. The perforating vein establishes a transfascial connection (F) between the great saphenous vein (V.S.M) and the posterior tibial vein (V.T.P). When the calf is compressed (left image), there is flow toward the center (blue) in the great saphenous vein, posterior tibial vein, and perforating vein (from the superficial into the deep venous system). The right image shows reversed flow (from deep into superficial system, encoded in red) upon release of compression, indicating incompetence of the perforating vein. The great saphenous vein is also incompetent distal to the incompetent perforator (reflux, red), while the posterior tibial vein is competent, as indicated by the absence of flow reversal upon release of compression.
f Diagram of incomplete truncal varicosis of the great saphenous vein of the lateral branch type: 1 = lateral accessory saphenous vein; 2 = bucket handle anastomosis; 3 = superficial femoral vein; 4 = great saphenous vein. The great saphenous vein is competent proximally (above the site of entry of the bucket handle anastomosis) and insufficient distally

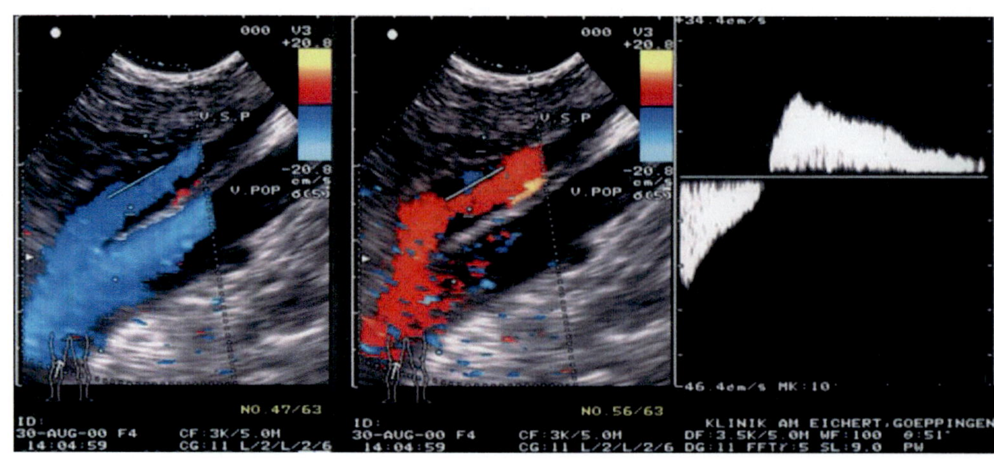

◘ Fig. 3.78 (Atlas) Truncal varicosis of small saphenous vein. The Doppler waveform from the saphenopopliteal junction (V.S.P = small saphenous vein, V.POP = popliteal vein) shows normal flow toward the heart during calf compression and high-velocity reversed flow upon release of compression. In the color flow images, flow reversal in the small saphenous vein is indicated by red color coding (flow toward the periphery, right image), while the absence of flow in the popliteal vein suggests competent valves here

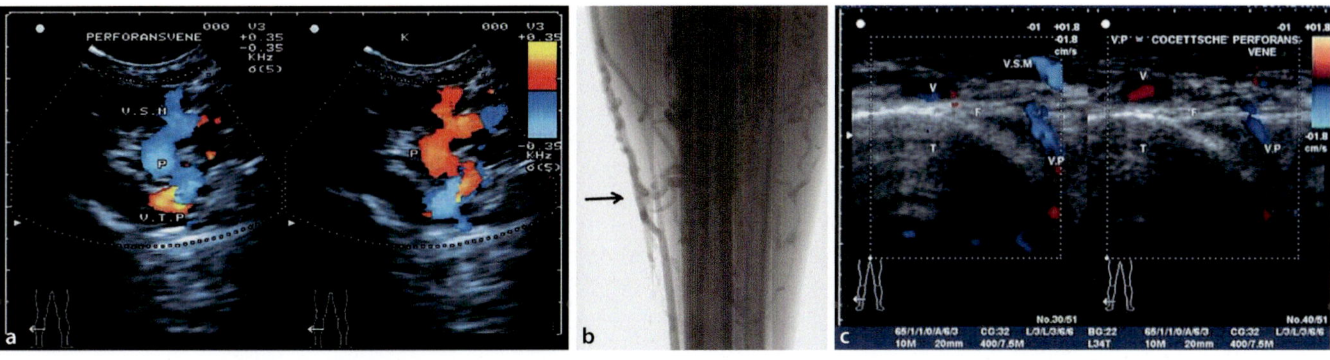

Fig. 3.79a–c (Atlas) Valve incompetence of perforating vein.
a Incompetent perforating veins are identified by looking for transfascial tubular structures originating from branches of the great or small saphenous vein in transverse orientation using a high-frequency transducer. In the example, compression of the calf proximal to the transducer with application of a tourniquet to stop blood flow in the superficial veins induces retrograde flow (displayed in red) from the posterior tibial vein (V.T.P) into the great saphenous vein (V.S.M) with a return to forward flow (blue, away from transducer) upon release of compression. Reflux from the deep venous system into the superficial system in this test confirms perforator incompetence (see Fig. 3.77e (Atlas)).
b Venogram showing incompetent perforator between the great saphenous vein and the posterior tibial vein.
c Valve incompetence leads to widening of the vein, making it much easier to identify an abnormal perforating vein than a normal one. A very thin perforating vein (V.P) in the calf is depicted crossing the fascia (F). During compression, there is flow in the perforating vein (V.P), coded in blue, from the superficial into the deep system and no reflux upon release of compression. The image on the left depicts a perforator, the image on the right an additional Cockett perforator slightly more distally. Between the fascia (F) and the skin, the great saphenous vein and lateral branch veins (V) are depicted

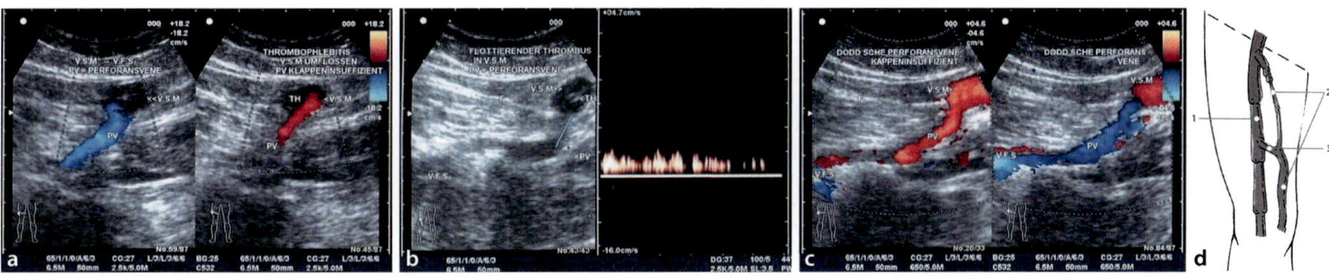

Fig. 3.80a–d (Atlas) Thromboembolism from great saphenous vein and Dodd perforator incompetence.
a Patient with thrombophlebitis clinically extending to the knee and sonographic demonstration of a thrombus in the great saphenous vein with proximal extension to the level of the mid-thigh. The proximal end (3 cm) is surrounded by flowing blood. At this level, the transverse view depicts a Dodd perforator (PV) with normal flow into the deep venous system and an increase in flow velocity upon compression of the great saphenous vein just above the thrombophlebitic segment. Release induces reflux into the superficial system (displayed in red, right image), indicating valve incompetence of the perforating vein. Absence of color indicates the thrombus in the great saphenous vein (TH).
b B-mode image depicting the thrombus (TH) in the great saphenous vein (V.S.M). The Doppler waveform from the perforating vein demonstrates reflux from the superficial femoral vein (V.F.S) upon release of compression.
c Valsalva's maneuver inadvertently dislodged the thrombus in the great saphenous vein, inducing asymptomatic pulmonary embolism. Scintigraphy showed a small perfusion defect in the right lower lobe. Following this incident, the great saphenous vein was patent in the area of the Dodd perforator with antegrade flow from the great saphenous vein (V.S.M) into the superficial femoral vein (V.F.S) and persisting reflux after a provocative maneuver as definitive evidence of perforator incompetence (PV, coded red, toward transducer).
d Diagram of incomplete truncal varicosis of the great saphenous vein of the perforator type: 1 = superficial femoral vein; 2 = great saphenous vein (competent above the perforator, incompetent below); 3 = Dodd's perforating vein

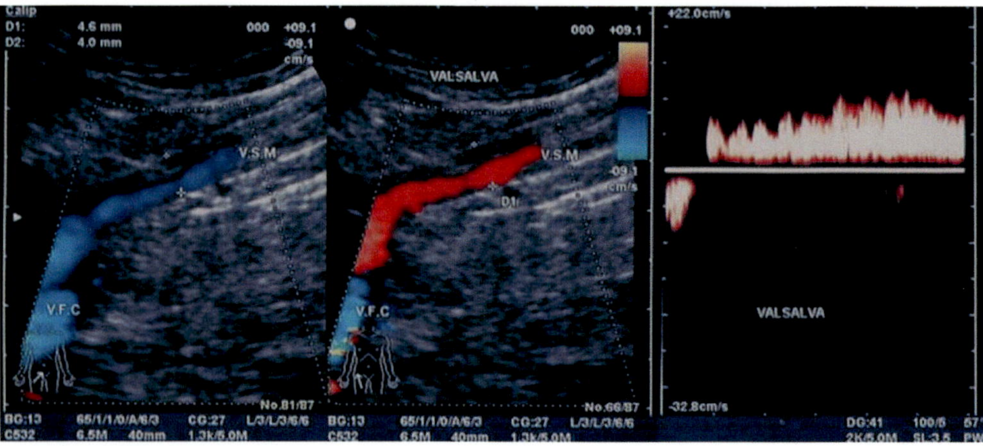

Fig. 3.81 (Atlas) Recanalized great saphenous vein after thrombophlebitis.
Only about half of the lumen of the great saphenous vein (V.S.M) is patent just below the junction with the common femoral vein (V.F.C) and shows normal flow displayed in blue (lumen indicated by calipers). There is reflux in the great saphenous vein during Valsalva's maneuver (red). In addition, hypoechoic areas are depicted along the patent lumen. The Doppler waveform demonstrates reflux during Valsalva's maneuver. Identification of venous segments with postthrombophlebitic changes is important in preoperative vein mapping because they cannot be used for bypass grafting

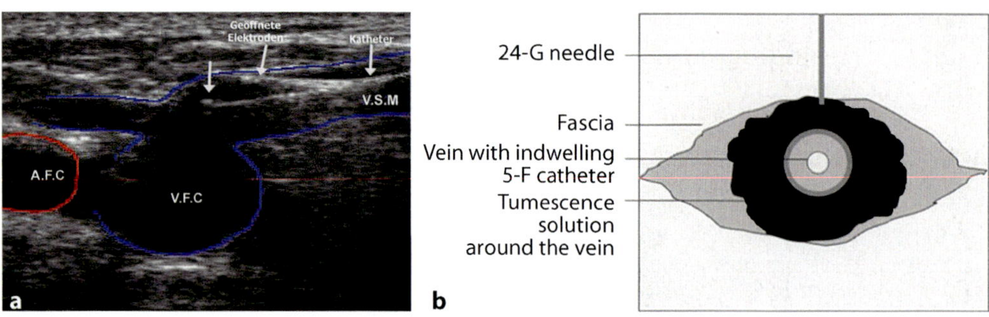

Fig. 3.82a, b (Atlas) VNUS closure of great saphenous vein.
a Endovascular obliteration of the great saphenous vein by laser or radiofrequency ablation involves insertion of a catheter with an electrode into a peripheral vein. Under ultrasound guidance, the catheter is advanced to the saphenofemoral junction, placing the tip just below the site of entry of the epigastric vein. The femoral vein, great saphenous vein, and epigastric vein are encircled by a blue line; the catheter and open electrode are indicated by arrows as they are advanced to the target site in the great saphenous vein (*V.S.M*) (Image courtesy of D. Tsantilas).
b Following intravascular insertion of the probe for laser treatment, a 24-G needle is placed adjacent to the great saphenous vein for tumescent anesthesia. The amount of tumescent solution injected with ultrasound guidance aims at compressing the vein to a final diameter of 4–5 mm and creating a circumferential fluid layer of at least 5 mm to prevent thermal damage of the tissue around the vein

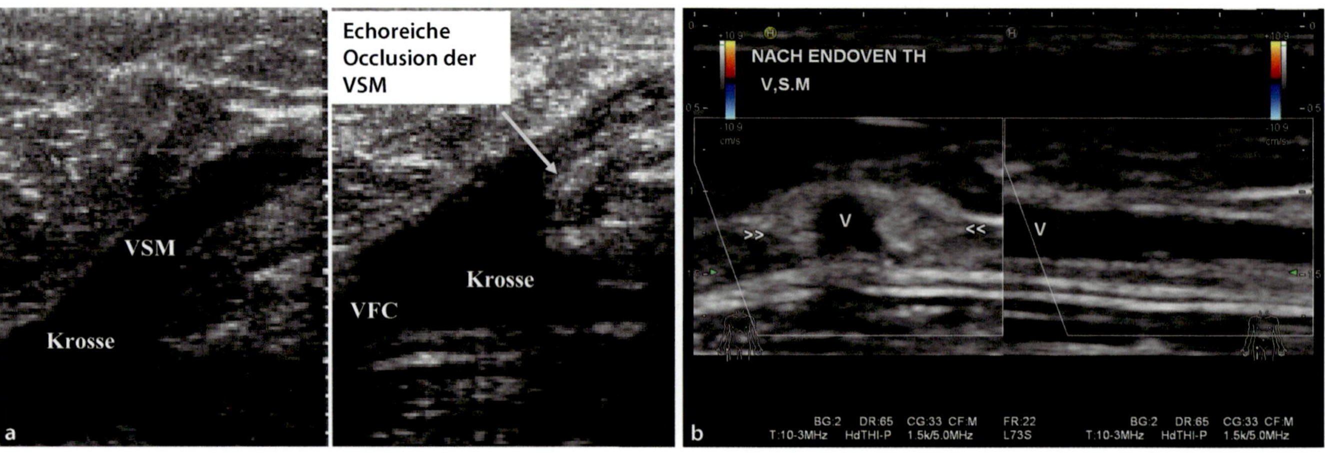

Fig. 3.83a, b (Atlas) Follow-up of VNUS closure.
a The left image shows the patent lumen of the great saphenous vein (VSM) at the level of the saphenofemoral junction (Krosse) before obliteration; the right image shows the shrunken and hyperechoic lumen (arrow) of the great saphenous vein below the junction, confirming successful occlusion in conjunction with noncompressibility (image courtesy of D. Tsantilas).
Follow-up after endovenous varicose treatment.
b In a patient presenting with disturbed sensation along the course of the distal saphenous nerve, the ultrasound examination reveals hyperechoic connective tissue around the occluded great saphenous vein due to heat exposure during endovascular radiofrequency treatment for varicosis 8 days earlier. The vein appears to have shrunken (distinguishing the effect of treatment from thrombophlebitis), and the wall is blurred

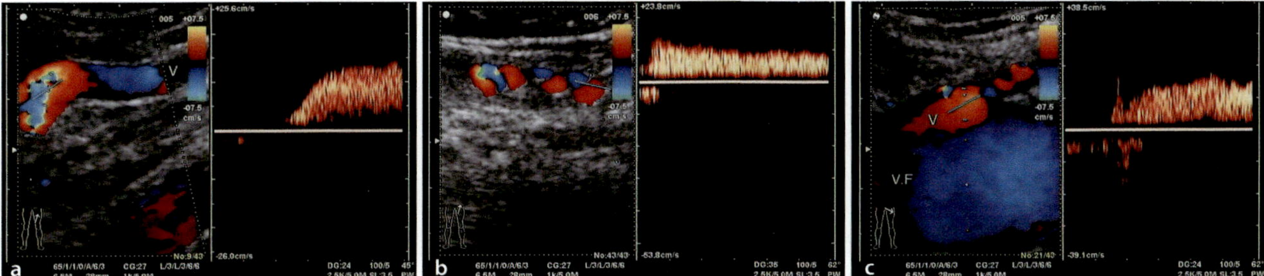

Fig. 3.84a–c (Atlas) Recurrent varicosis.
a If there is visible recurrent varicosis, the course of the affected vein must be evaluated for incompetent valves. This is done using color duplex ultrasound, and the examination begins distally. The example shows a dilated and elongated varix in the medial thigh with peripheral flow (toward transducer) upon Valsalva's maneuver in a patient who underwent stripping of the great saphenous vein.
b A therapeutically relevant diagnostic task is to determine whether a recurrent varix arises from a lateral branch or a perforating vein and whether it communicates with the saphenofemoral junction. A varix communicating with the former saphenofemoral junction (following crossectomy) may have a very thin lumen and show a very tortuous course over a short distance (similar in appearance on color flow image to arterial corkscrew collaterals in thromboangiitis obliterans). Nevertheless, such a varix is clinically relevant and will show reflux upon Valsalva's maneuver; its tortuous course appears on color flow imaging as repeated color reversal due to the changing flow direction relative to the ultrasound beam (and indicates neovascularization).
c A thin vein (V) is seen arising from the femoral vein (V.F) in the area of the former saphenofemoral junction. This vein shows retrograde flow upon Valsalva's maneuver (flow toward transducer indicated by red color; flow above the baseline in the Doppler waveform)

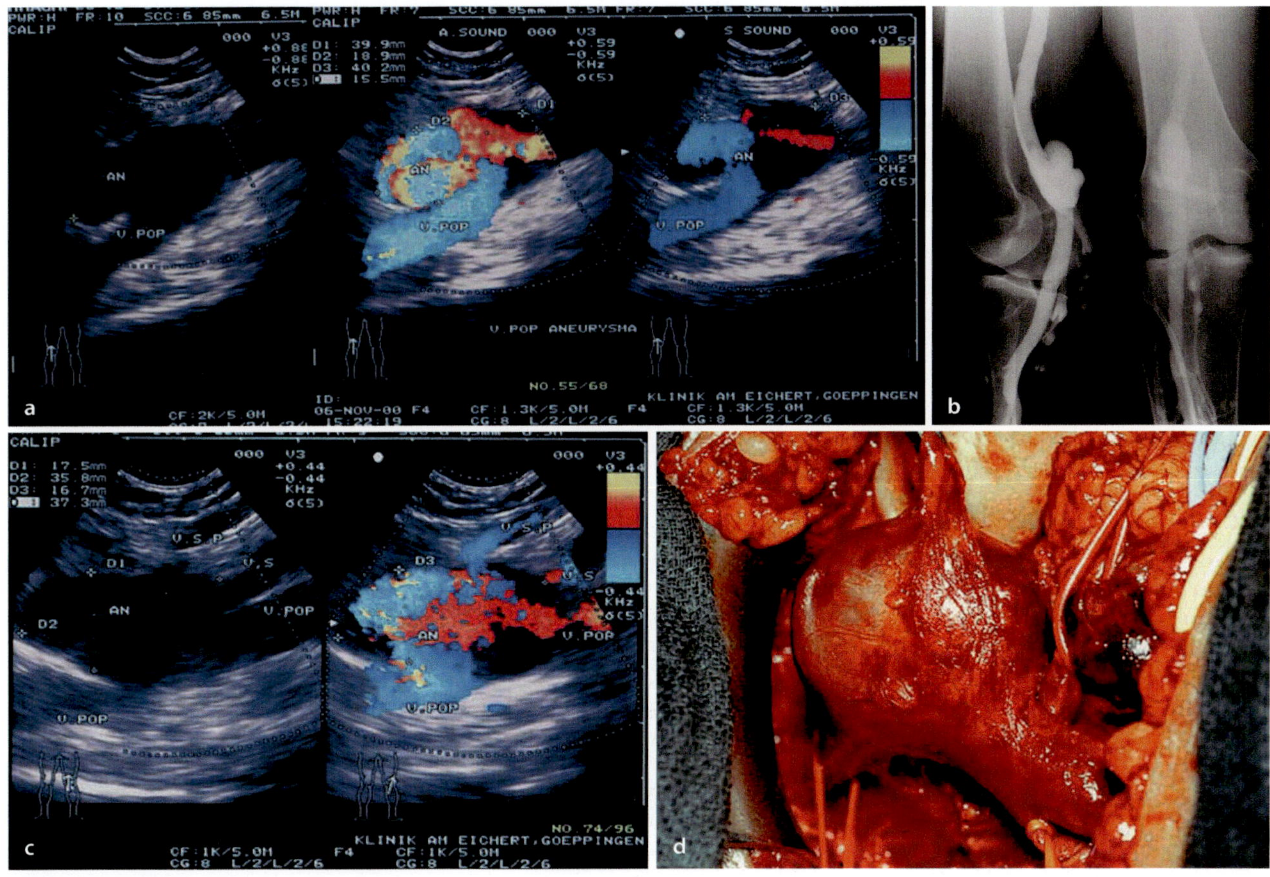

Fig. 3.85a–d (Atlas) Venous aneurysm.
a Gray-scale image depicting a saccular aneurysm (AN) as a distended sac at its preferred site, the popliteal vein (V.POP). The right color flow image (obtained without flow augmentation) reveals zones of nearly complete stasis in the popliteal vein aneurysm. Augmentation of flow (calf compression) induces pronounced eddy currents in the aneurysm (left color flow image).
b Venogram demonstrating saccular aneurysm of the popliteal vein. In a nonthrombosed aneurysm, as in the case shown, opacification corresponds to the sonomorphologic shape of the aneurysm (see gray-scale image in **a**).
c After rotation of the transducer, the small saphenous vein (V.S.P) and a gastrocnemius vein (V.S) entering the aneurysm are depicted. The maximum transverse diameter of the aneurysm is 2.5 cm.
d The intraoperative site confirms the sonomorphologic appearance of the saccular aneurysm. The saccular cranial end is exposed on the left, and the two veins (gastrocnemius vein and small saphenous vein) entering the aneurysm sac are seen in the center. Vascular slings are placed around the popliteal vein (left margin) and a vessel entering the distal popliteal vein (right)

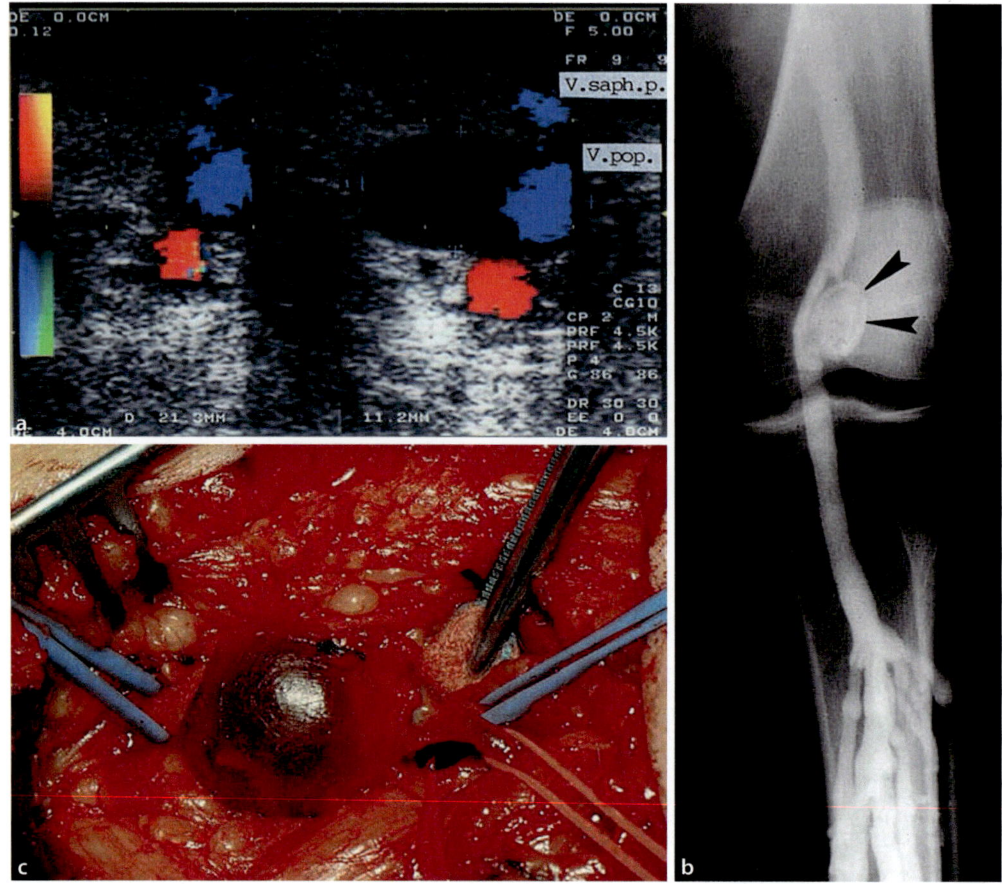

Fig. 3.86a–c (Atlas) Venous aneurysm with thrombus.
58-year-old patient with scintigraphically proven pulmonary embolism. Saccular popliteal vein aneurysm extending to the terminal segment of the sural vein with complete thrombosis sparing only the normal lumen of the popliteal vein.
a The left image depicts the popliteal vein with flow in blue proximal to the aneurysm; the right image shows the dilated segment of the popliteal vein (V.POP) with mural thrombosis.
b Venogram: Mural thrombosis precludes identification of the popliteal vein aneurysm and only aneurysmal dilatation at the entry site of a tributary vein is demonstrated (above knee joint cleft).
c The intraoperative site confirms the ultrasound findings of popliteal vein aneurysm (center) with mural thrombosis of the saccular portion and aneurysmal dilatation of the terminal sural vein. Blue vascular slings are placed around the popliteal vein proximally and distally, and a red sling is placed around the sural vein

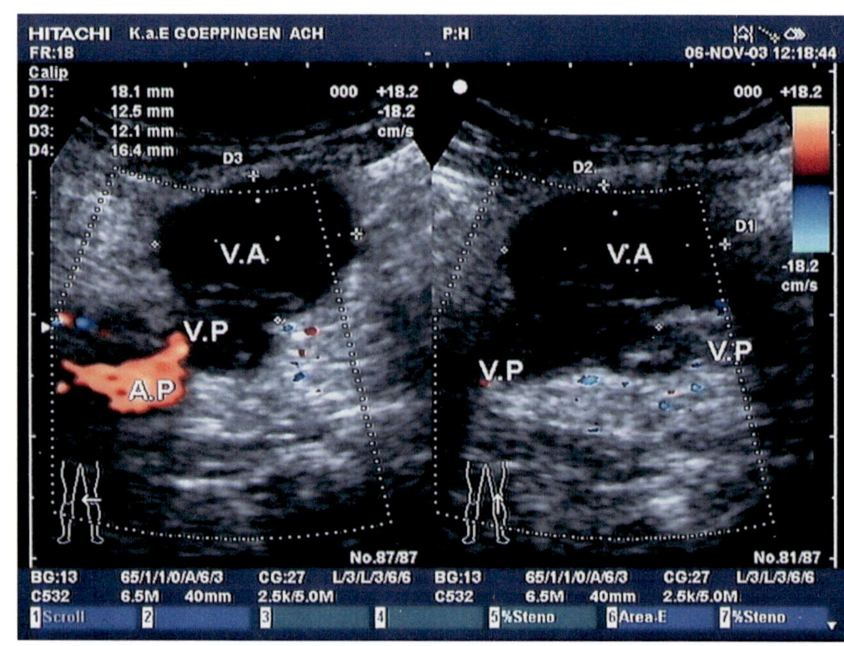

Fig. 3.87 (Atlas) Venous aneurysm and deep vein thrombosis of leg.
There is complete thrombosis of the popliteal vein (V.P). Both the transverse image (left) and the longitudinal image (right) additionally demonstrate a saccular venous aneurysm (VA) with a diameter of nearly 2 cm. The aneurysm is thrombosed as well. This young patient had no other risk factors for venous thrombosis, and it is therefore likely that thrombosis from the venous aneurysm caused secondary popliteal vein thrombosis. Venous aneurysm must be differentiated from an ectatic terminal segment of a varicose small saphenous vein or an ectatic gastrocnemius vein

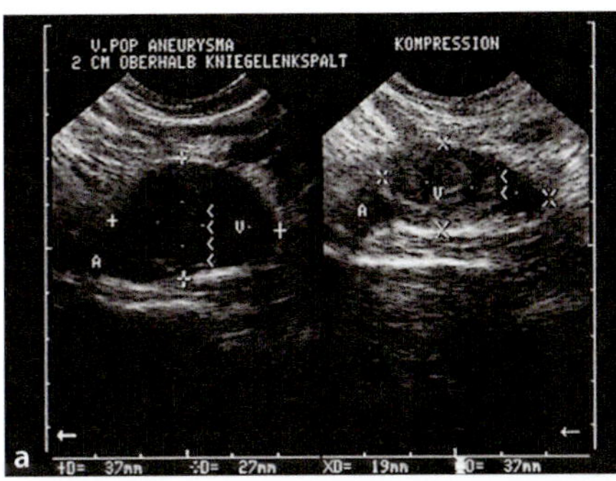

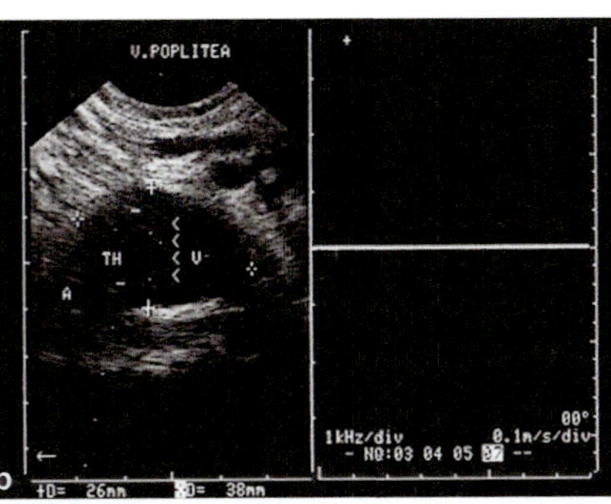

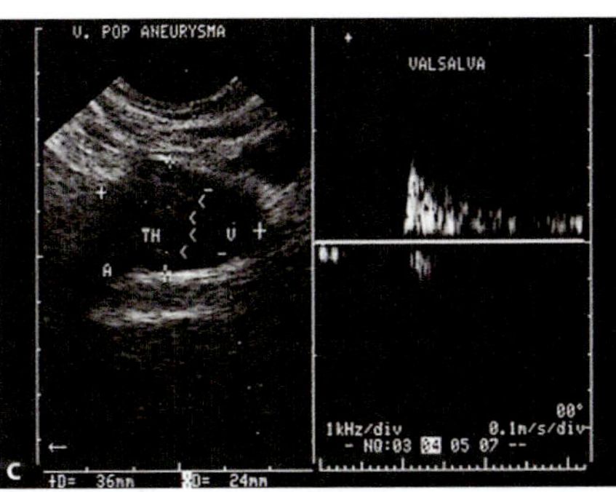

Fig. 3.88a–c (Atlas) Saccular popliteal vein aneurysm.
a 45-year-old patient with recurrent pulmonary embolism; saccular popliteal vein aneurysm with nearly complete thrombosis, leaving only a small residual lumen, demonstrated by sonography and venography.
b,c The aneurysm has a maximum cross-sectional extent of 38 mm. Duplex ultrasound enables differentiation of the thrombotic portion (**b**) from the nonthrombotic residual lumen. Flow is depicted in the patent lumen, and there is reflux during Valsalva's maneuver, indicating valve incompetence (**c**). The patient had concomitant femoral vein incompetence and therefore underwent ligation of the superficial femoral vein to prevent further pulmonary embolism

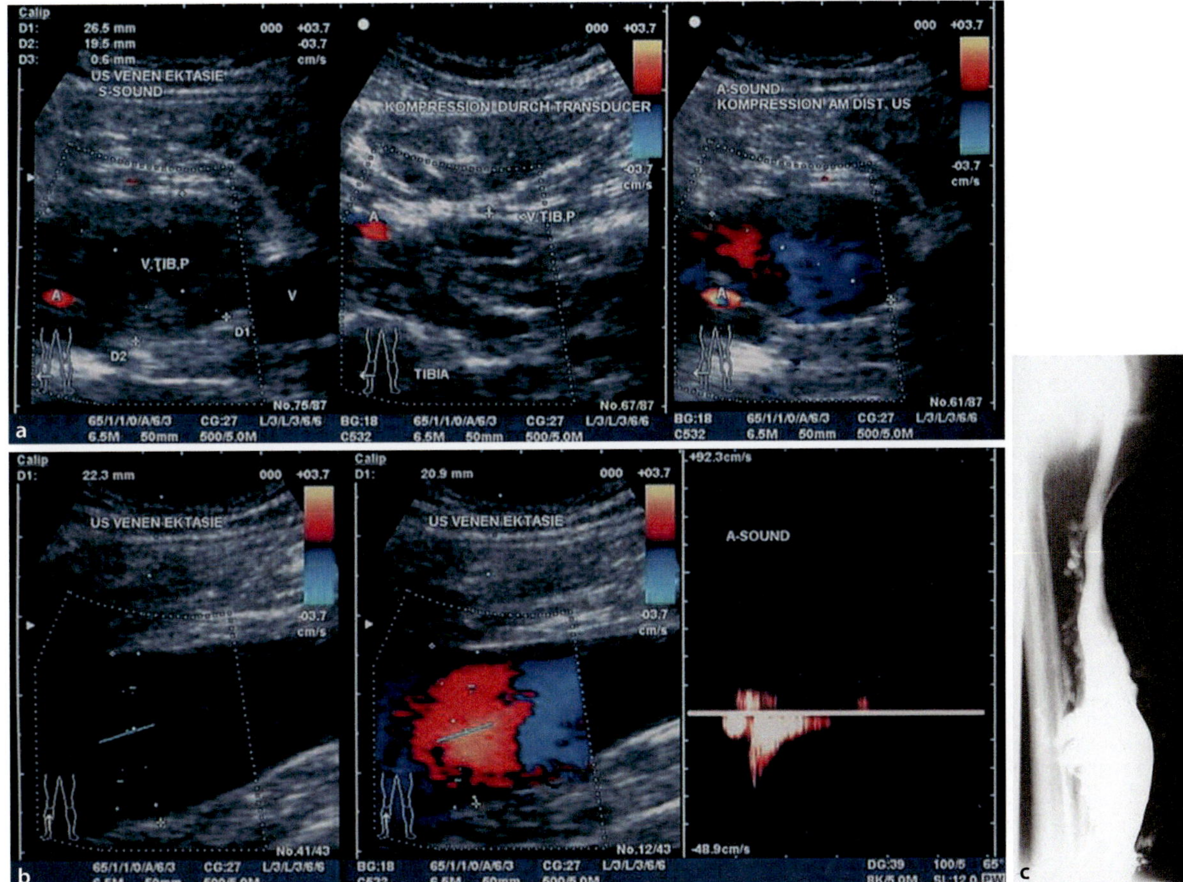

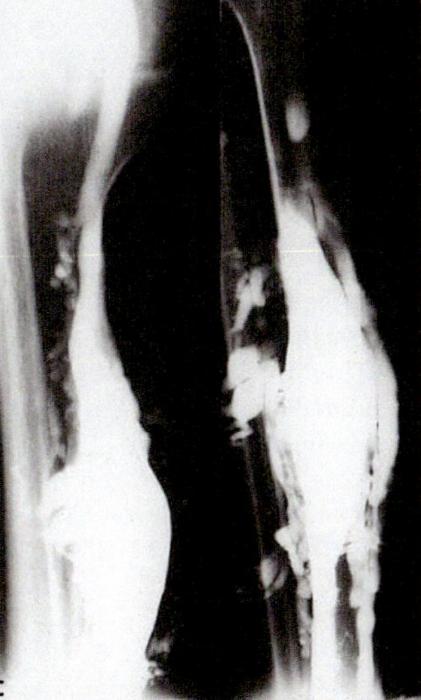

Fig. 3.89a–c (Atlas) Venous ectasia of the calf.
a Ectatic degeneration chiefly involves the muscle veins of the gastrocnemius group, while severe ectasia of the major calf veins is rare. In the 50-year-old patient presented here, spindle-shaped ectatic changes of the posterior tibial vein (V.TIB.P) were the source of scintigraphically proven pulmonary embolism. The B-mode appearance suggests thrombosis. The ectatic veins have a diameter of up to 2.5 cm and can be completely compressed (middle section); the lumen of the posterior tibial vein is indistinguishable (marked). To the left of the vein, the posterior tibial artery is depicted with flow in red. There is no spontaneous flow in the vein (left section), but augmented flow signals can be obtained upon distal compression of the calf (right section).
b The longitudinal image likewise fails to depict spontaneous flow in the spindle-shaped ectatic posterior tibial vein (left). Augmented flow is demonstrated by color duplex scanning and in the Doppler waveform ("A-SOUND") following compression distal to the transducer.
c Venogram: Spindle-shaped ectatic dilatations of muscle veins and major veins in the calf

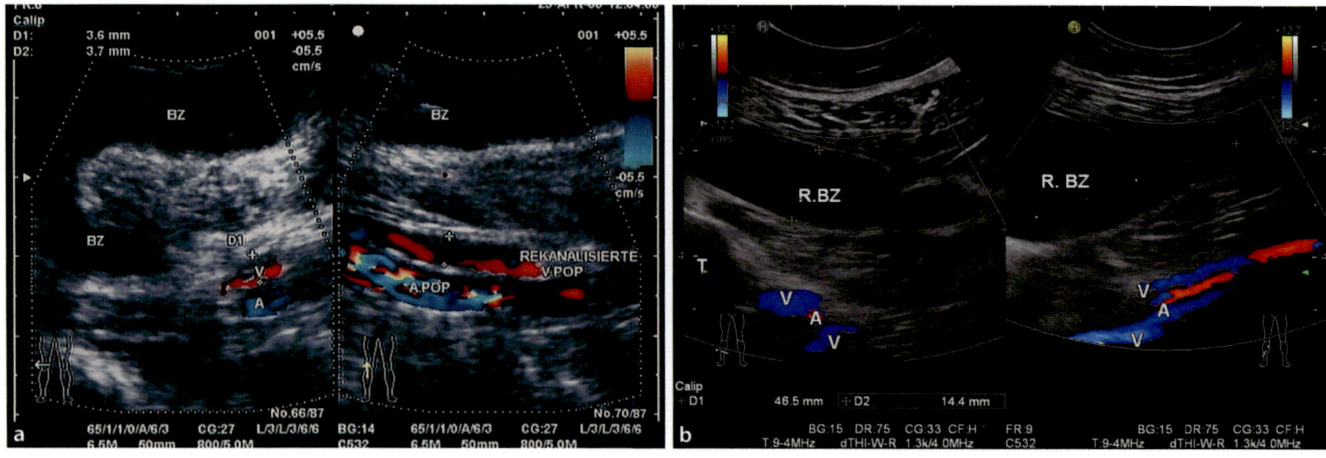

Fig. 3.90a, b (Atlas) Differential diagnosis of venous thrombosis – Baker's cyst.
a Leg pain with acute swelling in this patient is not caused by the postthrombotic changes in the popliteal vein (V) or by recurrent thrombosis, but by a large Baker's cyst (BZ). The transverse view on the left and longitudinal view on the right depict the recanalized vein, but the walls are still markedly thickened. The low PRF adjusted to slow venous flow produces aliasing in the popliteal artery (A.POP).
b Ruptured Baker's cysts present the classic symptoms of calf vein thrombosis. They are typically seen as hypoechoic or anechoic, subfascial leaking structures (in part even between muscle fascia). In the case presented, the leaking fluid extends to the mid-calf level, and there are cystic residues in the popliteal fossa. Baker's cysts can be treated by ultrasound-guided aspiration, resulting in rapid improvement or complete elimination of symptoms. At the same time, ultrasound can confirm patency of calf veins

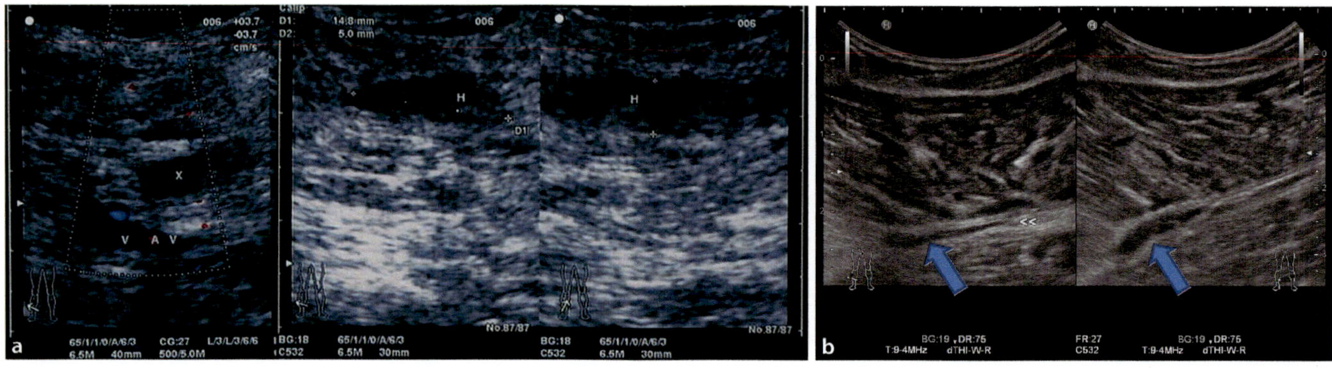

Fig. 3.91a, b (Atlas) Differential diagnosis of calf vein thrombosis – hematoma.
a Another cause of soft tissue swelling and pain to be considered in the differential diagnosis is hematoma, caused, for instance, by a torn muscle. Behind the posterior tibial vein, a hypoechoic structure (X) is depicted in two planes, which explains the local tenderness. A second hematoma is seen in the right image. It is located in the gastrocnemius muscle more distally and closer to the surface.
Calf swelling due to torn muscle.
b Free fluid (blood) secondary to a muscle strain may be very inconspicuous in patients presenting with symptoms of calf vein thrombosis. The examiner must look for bands of low echogenicity at the sites of muscle fasciae, in particular between the gastrocnemius and soleus muscle. The example shows a hematoma (arrow) secondary to a torn muscle with very little free fluid between the gastrocnemius and soleus muscle

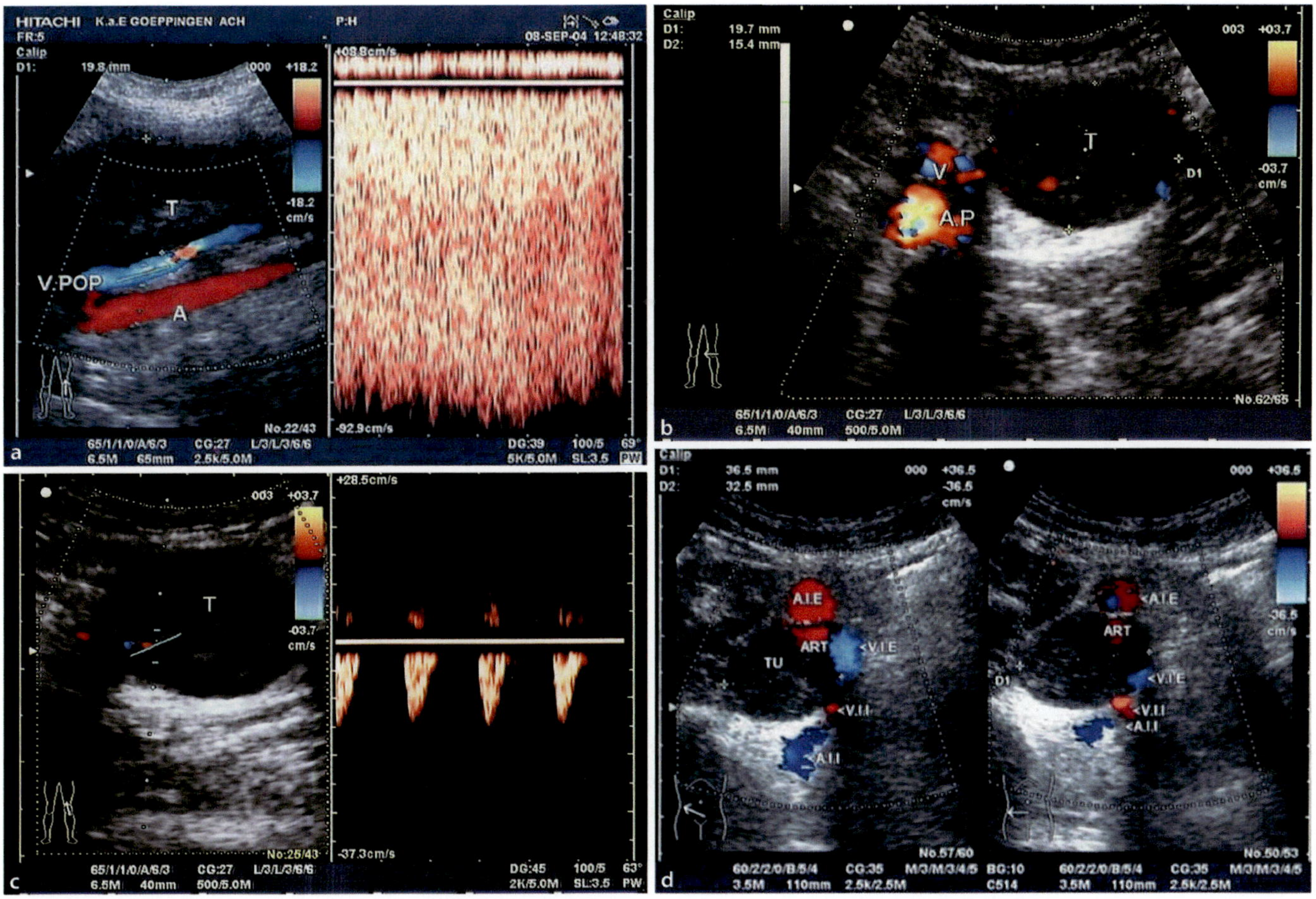

Fig. 3.92a–d (Atlas) Calf swelling due to popliteal fossa tumor.
a External compression of the popliteal vein (V.POP) by a sarcoma (T) in the popliteal fossa, reflected in the Doppler waveform as a high-frequency signal (flow velocity of 90 cm/s, loss of respiratory phasicity).
b 45-year-old woman with calf swelling; differential diagnosis: thrombosis. The detection of flow (low PRF) can help differentiate hypoechoic tumorous lesions from cysts with internal echoes due to intralesional hemorrhage.
c The Doppler waveform shows arterial flow as evidence of a solid tumor (sample volume placed in the area with flow signals in the color duplex image). Schwannoma was diagnosed after removal of the tumor.
d Painful leg swelling caused by a tumor in the iliac bifurcation. Transverse views of the lower abdomen depict the external iliac vein (V.I.E, blue, flow away from transducer) and artery (A.I.E, red, toward transducer) anterior to the tumor and the internal iliac vein (V.I.I, red, toward transducer) and artery (A.I.I, blue, away from transducer) posterior to it. The hypoechoic tumor lies in the bifurcation and primarily compresses the external iliac vein (image on the right obtained slightly more cranially than image on the left). Posterior to the external iliac artery, there is a mirror artifact (ART) due to large acoustic impedance mismatch

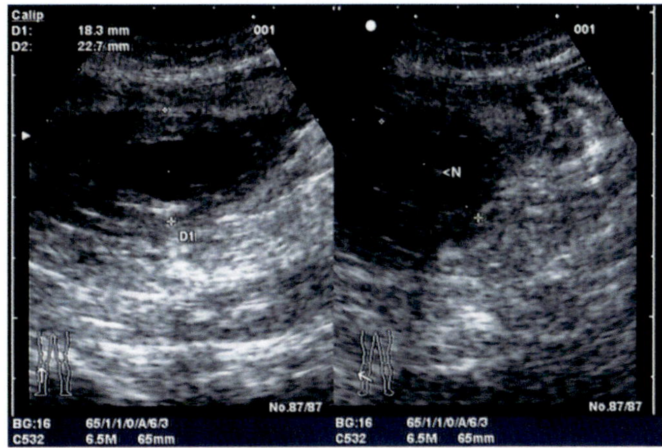

Fig. 3.93 (Atlas) Calf swelling due to subfascial abscess.
An intramuscular abscess is not always associated with inflammation of the skin but may be diagnosed incidentally in patients undergoing ultrasonography for suspected venous thrombosis. It is seen on gray-scale images as a hypoechoic, inhomogeneous structure and is confirmed by ultrasound-guided aspiration (N = needle tip)

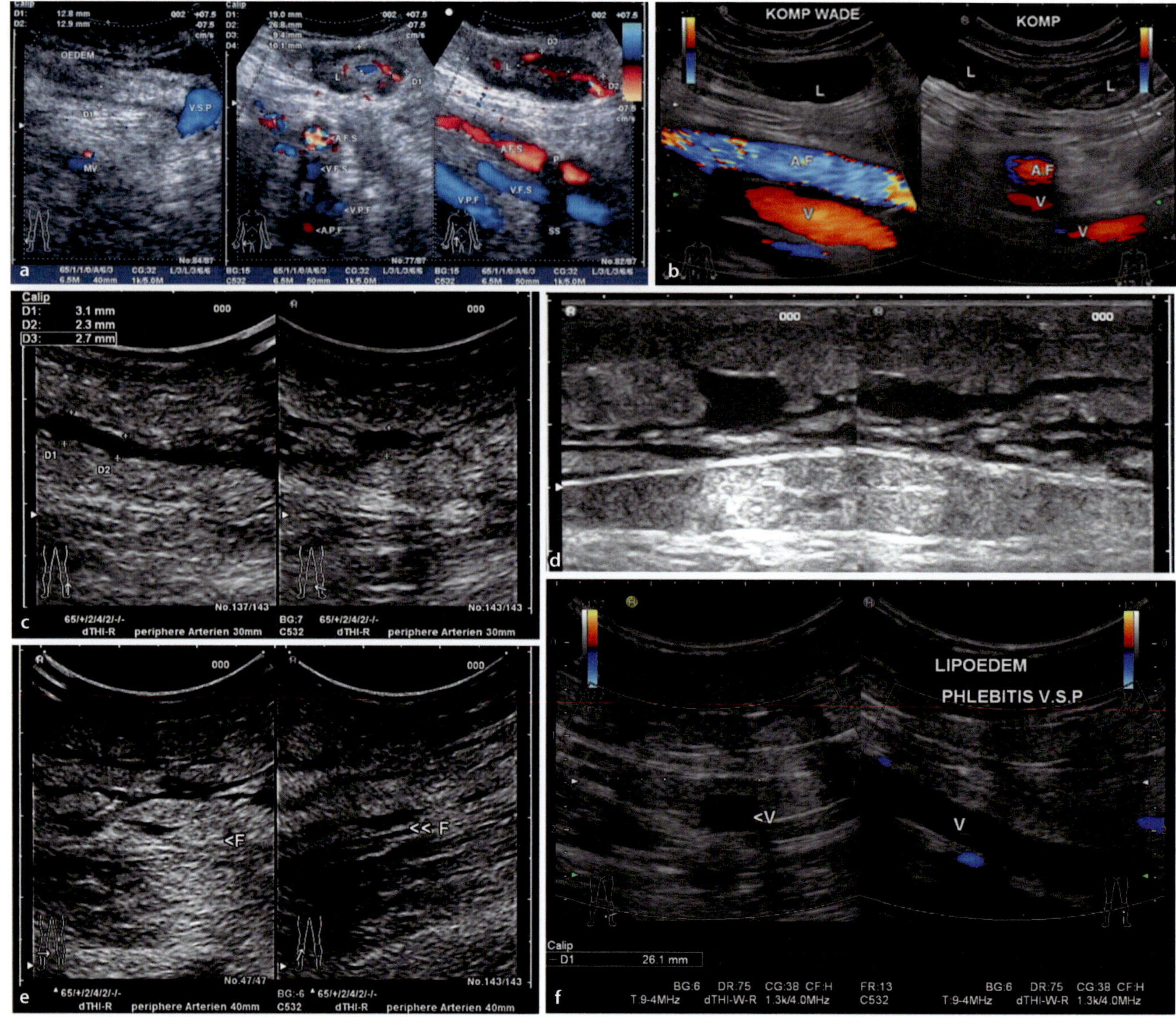

Fig. 3.94a–f (Atlas) Edema of various etiologies, lymphoma, lymphedema, lipedema.
a Apart from thrombosis, leg swelling can be caused by cardiac, inflammatory, or lymphogenic edema with epifascial fluid collections in fatty or connective tissue clefts. Edema causes scattering and thus impairs evaluation of deeper subfascial areas and detection of venous thrombosis below the knee. In the case shown, there is edematous subcutaneous thickening (indicated by calipers, 12 mm). The small saphenous vein (V.S.P) and a gastrocnemius vein (MV) are seen in transverse orientation. Inflammatory edema is associated with reactively enlarged lymph nodes in the groin. They are depicted as hypoechoic, inhomogeneous structures that can be differentiated from thrombophlebitis by gray-scale ultrasound in two planes (round shape). Color duplex imaging with a low PRF depicts the supply and perfusion of the lymph node. Atherosclerosis with wall irregularities and calcified plaque (P) with acoustic shadowing (SS) is seen as an accessory finding.
b Patient presenting with swelling of the calf and thigh as in 4-level thrombosis. Color duplex imaging demonstrates patent deep leg veins. The images show the patent femoral vein with red-coded flow (V). In this patient, leg swelling was due to obstructed lymphatic drainage caused by lymph node metastases from prostate cancer in the true pelvis and groin. Seen here are metastatic lymph nodes (L) in the groin, which are characterized by loss of internal structure, an irregular contour, and low echogenicity.
Calf swelling caused by edema.
c Channel-like structures in the subcutaneous fatty connective tissue (which tend to be near fasciae) on gray-scale images are pathognomonic of lymphedema. For reliable differentiation from edema due to other causes, the dilated lymphatics must be visualized as tubular structures on longitudinal (left) and transverse scans (right). A thin, wall-like structure is occasionally identified by its higher echogenicity between the lumen and connective tissue (left image, adjacent to calipers). Diameter of 2–3 mm.
d Transverse and longitudinal images of lymphedema with markedly dilated lymphatic vessels.
e Edema due to other causes (cardiac, secondary to chronic venous incompetence) has a honeycomb-like appearance on both longitudinal and transverse images, indicating fluid collections in connective tissue clefts of the subcutaneous fatty tissue (F = fascia, underlying muscle tissue without fluid collection).
f Transverse image (left) and longitudinal image (right) showing lipedema (echogenic) in a patient with phlebitis of the small saphenous vein. Like the great saphenous vein, the small saphenous vein courses in a fascial compartment (Cleopatra's eye)

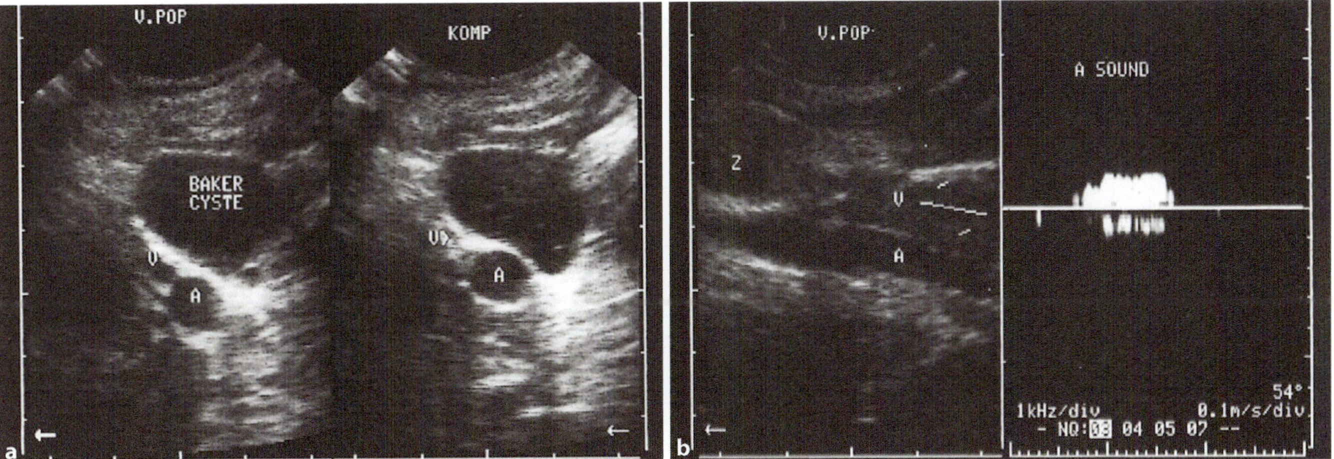

Fig. 3.95 (Atlas) Vein compression by Baker's cyst.
a Patient with calf swelling caused by a large Baker's cyst compressing the vein. The lumen of the vein is still patent but reduced. Pressure applied with the transducer causes complete collapse of the vein as seen on the transverse image (right).
b A month later, the cyst (Z) has increased in size, now compressing the vein and displacing the artery. The Doppler waveform shows no spontaneous flow and only moderate augmented flow upon strong compression of the calf muscles. The sample volume is placed in the vein (longitudinal image)

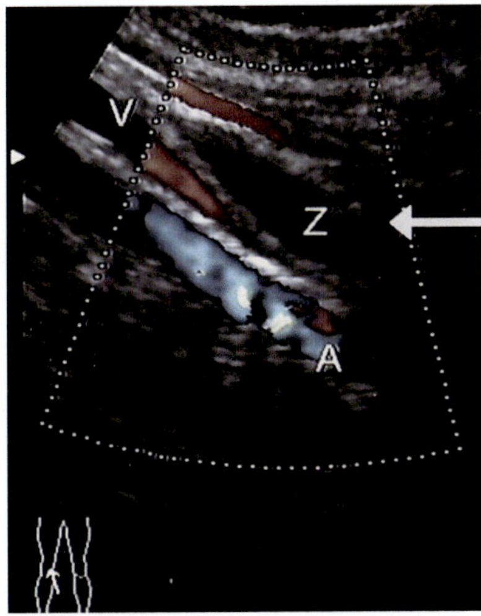

Fig. 3.96 (Atlas) Adventitial cystic disease of the popliteal vein. A cyst (Z) in the wall of the popliteal (V) narrows the lumen distally. Variable filling of the cyst causes intermittent calf swelling with symptom-free intervals. Adventitial cystic disease of the popliteal vein was confirmed intraoperatively

3

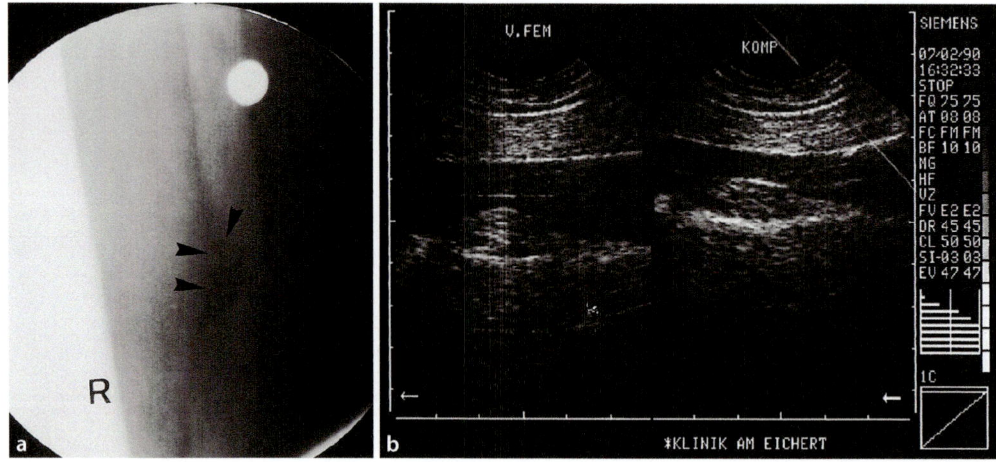

Fig. 3.97a, b (Atlas) Venous wall tumor.
The contrast medium filling defect in the venogram (**a**) is caused by a tumorous lesion of the venous wall depicted by ultrasound (**b**). Ultrasound in longitudinal orientation shows that the wall is not disrupted. Scanning from an anteromedial approach depicts the artery near the transducer and adjacent to the vein, which is compressible (KOMP, right section in **b**). Histologic workup of the surgical specimen yielded the diagnosis of a venous wall fibroma

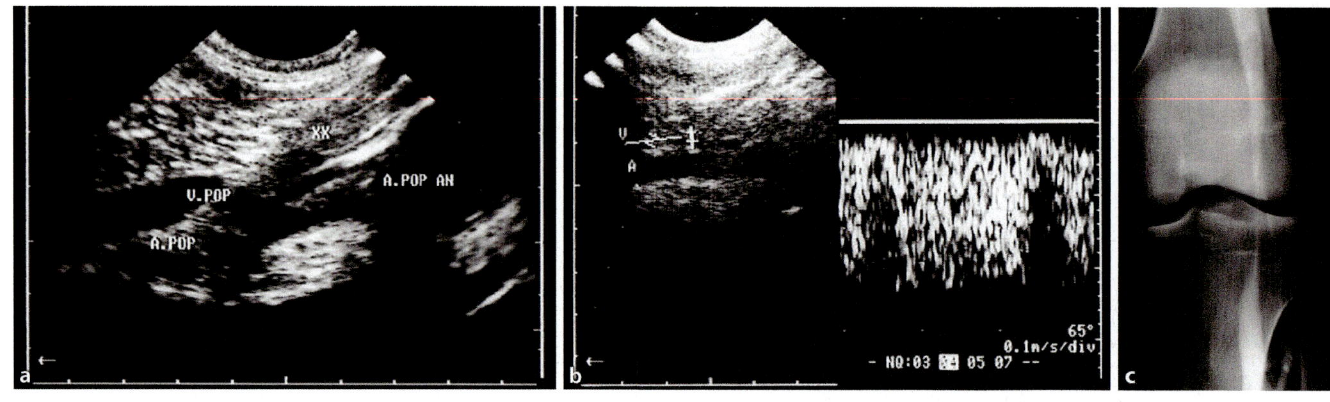

Fig. 3.98a–c (Atlas) Entrapment syndrome.
a An entrapment syndrome of the popliteal artery very rarely involves the popliteal vein as well (see ► Sect. 2.1.6.4.2). In the 45-year-old patient presented here, malformation of the medial head of the gastrocnemius with a lateral extension (XX) to the lateral condyle of the femur (Insua type II) causes stenosis of the popliteal artery with poststenotic, thrombotic dilatation (A.POP AN). The atypical lateral gastrocnemius extension in this case also impairs blood flow in the popliteal vein (V.POP), which is compressed between the dilated artery and the lateral muscle extension (XX).
b In another case – a 35-year-old athletic patient with well-developed calf muscles presenting with calf swelling and exercise-induced pain – ultrasound demonstrates compression of the popliteal vein by a hypertrophied gastrocnemius muscle with two strong heads but normal courses in the popliteal fossa. The Doppler waveform obtained from the compressed popliteal vein with the patient lying in a relaxed position shows a stenosis signal interrupted by arterial pulsation. The vein has a lumen of 2 mm. The angle-corrected flow velocity is over 100 cm/s and respiratory phasicity is lost (same patient as in Fig. 2.95 (Atlas)). In this patient with the rare combination of arterial and venous compression, calf swelling was caused by compression of the popliteal vein at rest and exercise-induced pain by compression of the artery during plantar flexion.
c Venogram: The vein appears compressed. A large popliteal artery aneurysm or a large Baker's cyst may have a similar venographic appearance

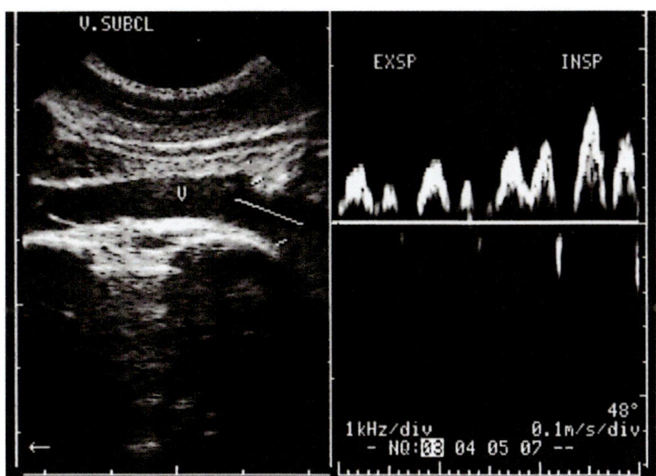

Fig. 3.99 (Atlas) Axillary vein – normal findings.
Junction of axillary and subclavian veins with respiratory phasicity and typical cardiac pulsatility of blood flow. The B-mode image on the left depicts a venous valve

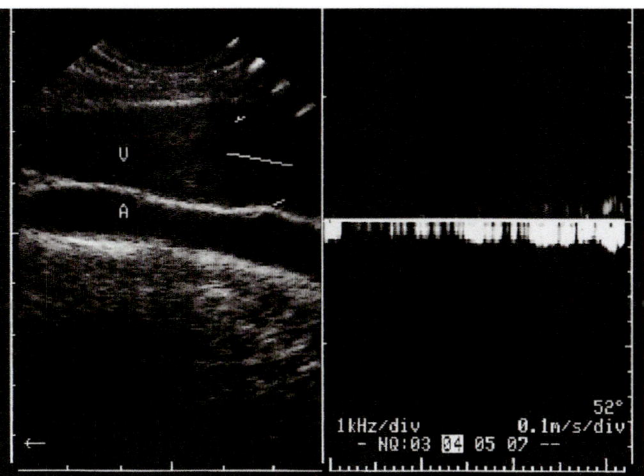

Fig. 3.100 (Atlas) Thoracic outlet obstruction.
Obstruction of venous inflow in the thoracic outlet by a mediastinal tumor is indicated by dilatation of the veins in the B-mode (shown here for the jugular vein). Blood flow is slower and cardiac pulsatility is eliminated

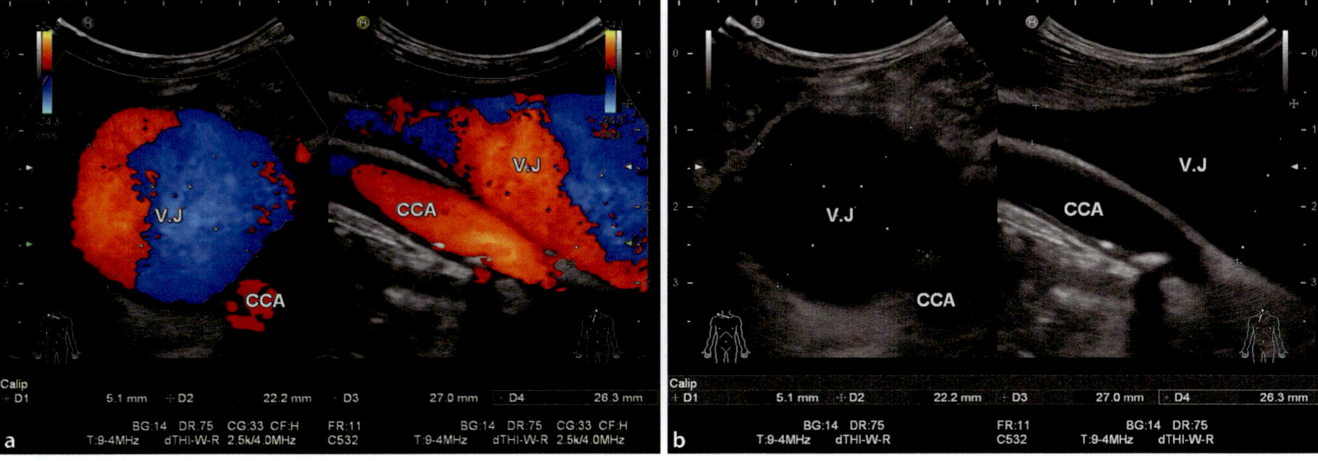

Fig. 3.101a, b (Atlas) Jugular vein aneurysm.
Jugular vein aneurysm (V.J.) measuring 27 mm in size. Aneurysms of the jugular vein can become quite large but thrombosis is very rare, and specific treatment is rarely necessary

3

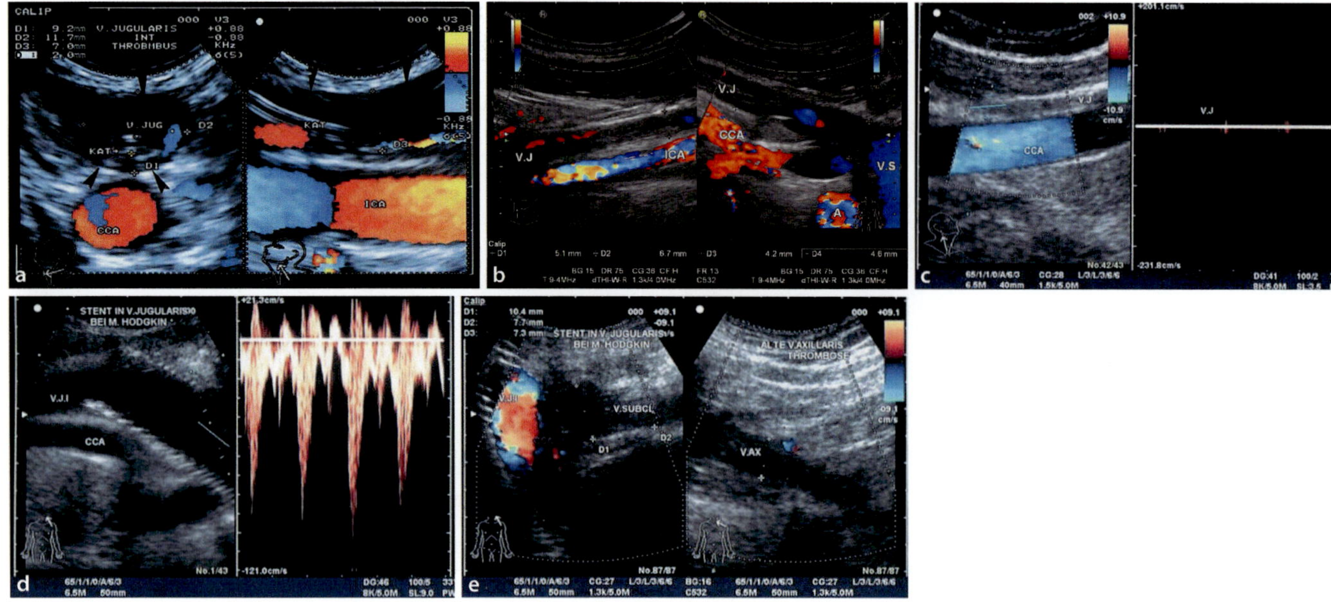

Fig. 3.102a–e (Atlas) Jugular vein thrombosis – central venous catheter.
a Foreign bodies in a vein (pacemaker, central venous catheter) have thrombogenic effects. In the example, the double contour indicates the central venous catheter (KAT) in the thrombosed jugular vein (arrowheads) with residual flow near the wall depicted in blue in transverse orientation (left). The common carotid artery is seen medial to the thrombosed jugular vein (transverse view on the left, longitudinal view on the right). Flow in the artery is in the opposite direction. The color change from red, to black, to blue in the artery is due to a change in flow direction relative to the ultrasound beam.
b Beginning recanalization of the jugular vein (V.J) along its course lateral to the carotid arteries (ICA and CCA) (left image) and proximally, at the site of its junction with the subclavian vein (V.S; right image).
c In older jugular vein thrombosis, there may be partial recanalization or persistent obstruction with depiction of the vein as a connective tissue strand with a rather thin lumen adjacent to the carotid artery. Patients in whom such a condition is identified by ultrasound before implantation of a central venous catheter can be spared an unnecessary puncture.
d In this patient with Hodgkin lymphoma, the mesh-like pattern is a stent placed to maintain patency of the jugular vein obstructed by lymphoma in the thoracic outlet.
e After stenting of the compressed jugular vein (left image), the patient developed thrombosis of the subclavian (V.SUBCL) and axillary veins (V.AX, right image)

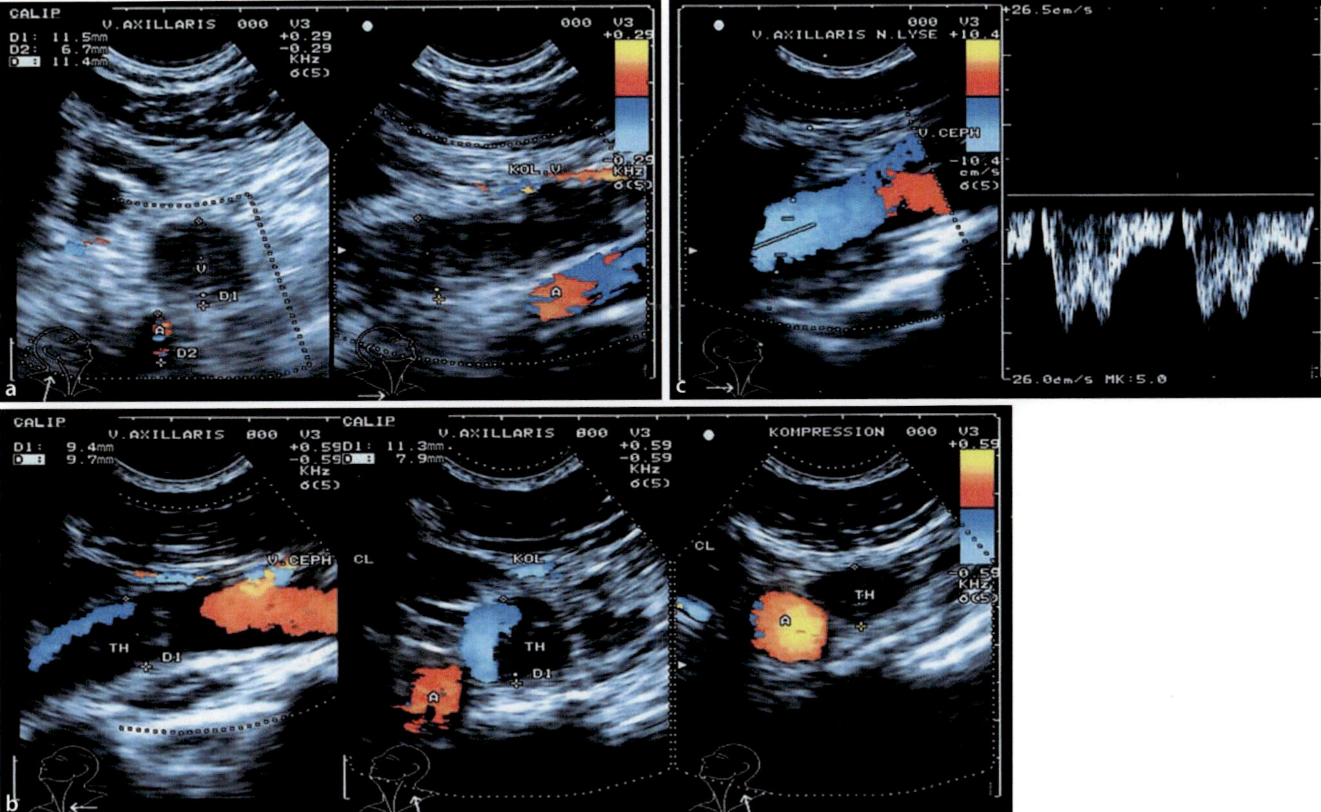

Fig. 3.103a–c (Atlas) Axillary vein thrombosis – thrombolytic therapy.
a Hypoechoic and homogeneous thrombi in the axillary and subclavian veins with clear demarcation from the wall indicate acute thrombosis. The vein is markedly dilated compared to the artery posterior to it. Collateral veins are depicted anteriorly.
b Following two cycles of thrombolytic therapy with ultrahigh-dose streptokinase administration, color duplex imaging demonstrates beginning recanalization. There is complete recanalization of the distal axillary vein (flow depicted in red, toward transducer). In the proximal axillary vein (left section), there is flow along one side of the thrombus (blue, due to change in flow direction relative to transducer). A chest wall collateral is seen anteriorly. The transverse view (middle section) depicts a larger hypoechoic mural thrombus in an otherwise patent axillary vein with flow in blue. The compression test confirms a thrombus and excludes a flow phenomenon due to inadequate instrument settings (right section). The patent lumen is collapsed and only the thrombosed, noncompressible portion is still identifiable as a hypoechoic structure. The transverse scans depict the axillary artery (A) posterocranially (CL = clavicle).
c There is full recanalization of the vein after another cycle of thrombolytic therapy. The Doppler waveform demonstrates respiratory phasicity and cardiac pulsatility of venous blood flow (M-shaped profile). The restoration of cardiac pulsatility indicates that thrombolytic therapy was initiated at an early stage; an older thrombus would have caused inflammatory changes and rigidity of the venous wall

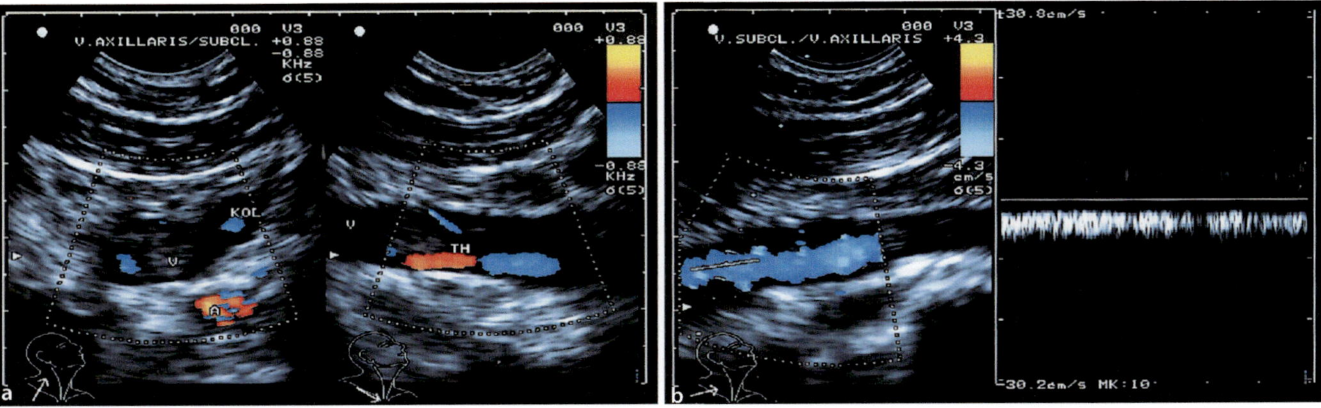

Fig. 3.104a, b (Atlas) Recanalization.
a Thrombosis of the axillary vein as in the case presented in Fig. 3.103 (Atlas); however, five cycles of thrombolytic therapy are necessary before signs of recanalization appear (transverse image on the left, longitudinal image on the right).
b Recanalization of the axillary vein is complete after another three cycles, but the wall is still markedly thickened as indicated by the hypoechoic structure surrounding the patent lumen (blue). The Doppler waveform shows no cardiac modulation of blood flow due to rigidity of the wall resulting from postthrombotic inflammatory changes and possible deposition of thrombotic material. Thrombogenic wall lesions have a high risk of early recurrence. In this patient, recurrent thrombosis of the axillary vein with occlusion was seen 2 days later despite adequate heparinization

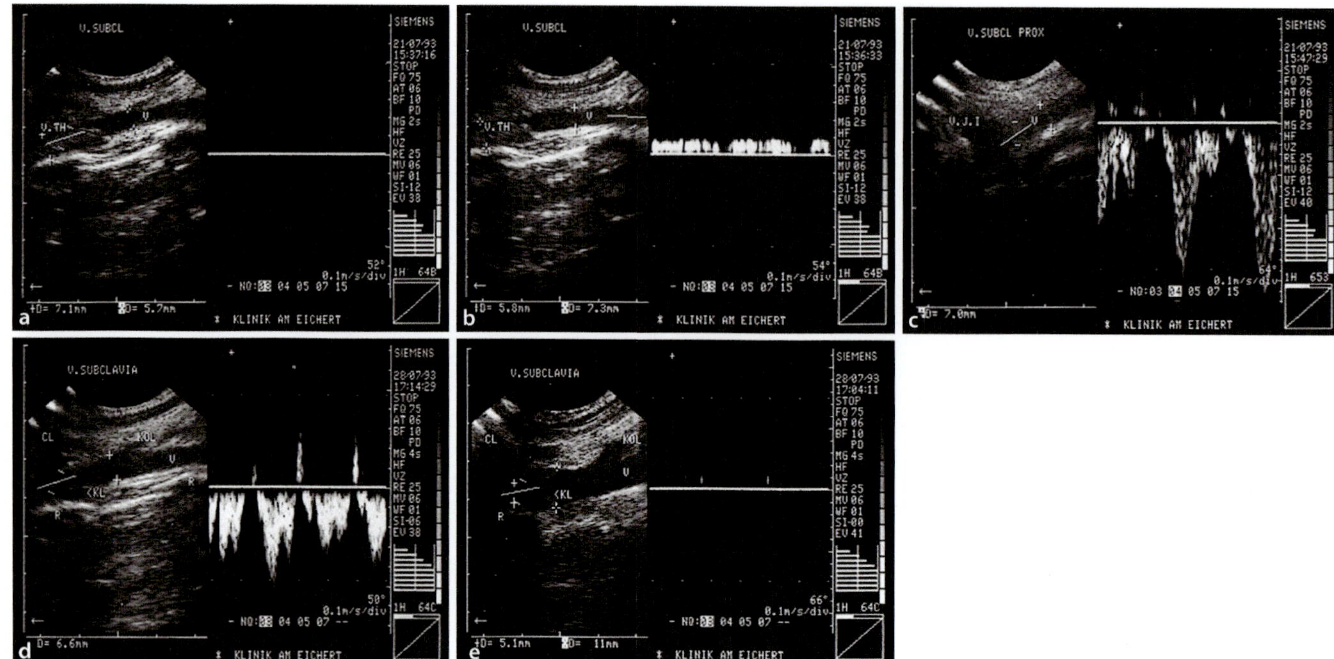

Fig. 3.105a–e (Atlas) Costoclavicular compression syndrome with thrombosis.
a A 17-year-old patient presented with a 5-day history of swelling of the right arm and lividity of the hand and lower arm. She reported recurrent transient but very mild swelling of the arm. Ultrasound identified a short thrombus at the junction of the subclavian vein with the axillary vein immediately distal to the costoclavicular space.
b Upstream of the thrombus, the axillary vein is patent and the Doppler waveform indicates disturbed drainage with loss of respiratory phasicity and cardiac pulsatility.
c Proximal to the clavicle, the subclavian vein is patent and shows normal flow with respiratory and cardiac variation.
d After 3 cycles of ultrahigh-dose streptokinase, recanalization of the vein was observed, and duplex ultrasound confirmed the suspected costoclavicular compression syndrome as the underlying cause of thrombosis. The Doppler waveform from the supine position with the arm relaxed shows a normal flow profile.
e Upon strong pulling of the arm in the posteroinferior direction, the vein becomes dilated distal to the costoclavicular space due to congestion. With the transducer in the infraclavicular fossa, the dilated subclavian and axillary veins as well as collateral veins (KOL) are seen. No flow signal is detected immediately distal to the costoclavicular space, indicating compression-induced occlusion of the subclavian vein. Valves (KL) are seen in the dilated lumen. (CL = clavicle). A Doppler waveform should be obtained to document the costoclavicular compression syndrome because the color duplex findings are difficult to quantify and are more susceptible to artifacts as a result of the maneuvers performed to induce compression

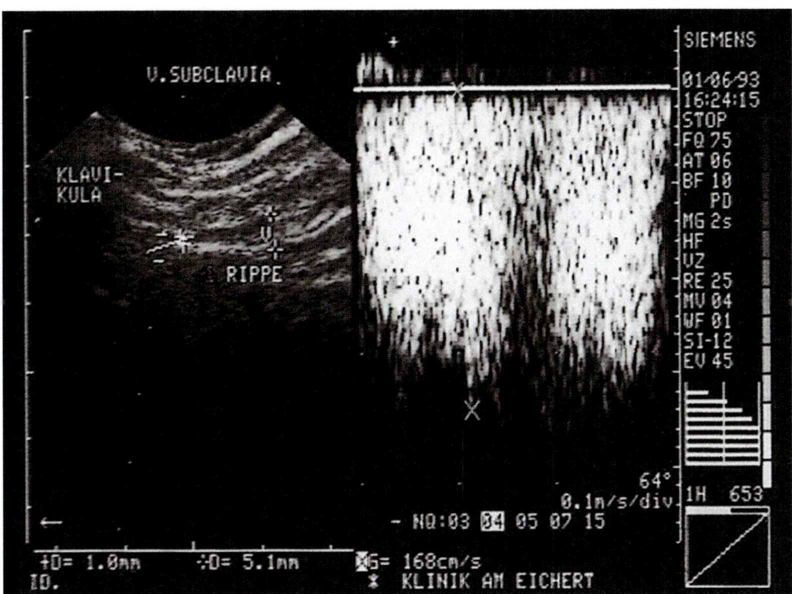

Fig. 3.106 (Atlas) Costoclavicular compression syndrome.
The passage of the vein through the costoclavicular space between the clavicle and the first rib is difficult to depict due to acoustic shadowing. In this area, the vein can only be evaluated if tangential beam orientation is achieved in slender patients. Under these conditions, a continuous high-frequency stenosis signal will be obtained from this vein segment with increasing abduction of the arm. This maneuver may even lead to complete occlusion of the subclavian vein. The findings presented were obtained in a 29-year-old patient with costoclavicular compression syndrome (same patient as in Fig. 3.105 (Atlas), before thrombosis). As in most cases of this syndrome, the subclavian artery was not compressed and showed triphasic flow in the duplex examination. In this patient, the same duplex findings could be elicited when the outwardly rotated arm was pulled in the posteroinferior direction. Extreme hyperabduction can induce compression of the subclavian vein in the costoclavicular space with demonstration of disturbed venous return in the Doppler waveform also in subjects without clinical symptoms of compression syndrome. For this reason, the hyperabduction test must be interpreted with caution. An abnormal Doppler waveform sampled while the outwardly rotated arm is being pulled posteroinferiorly is a more specific sign of the costoclavicular compression syndrome

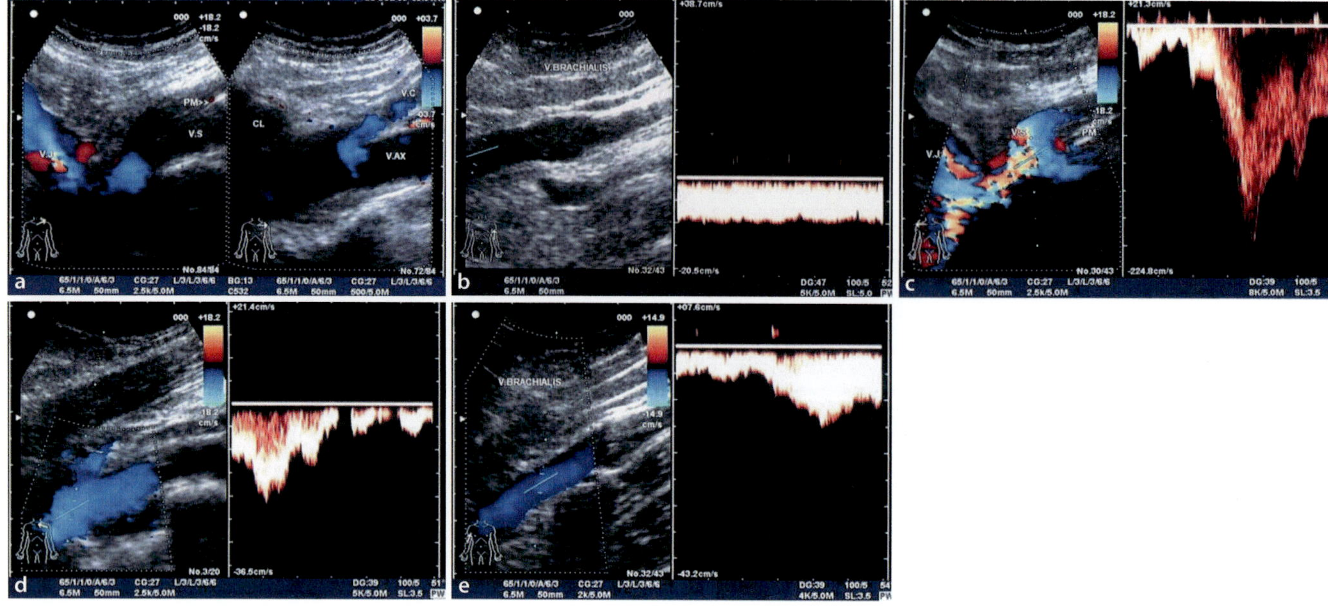

Fig. 3.107a–e (Atlas) Follow-up of subclavian vein thrombosis after pacemaker implantation.
a One week after pacemaker implantation, ultrasound demonstrates thrombosis of the subclavian vein (left) and of the axillary vein (right). Only isolated segments of the partially thrombosed axillary vein show flow signals when scanned with a low PRF. The subclavian vein (V.S) is completely thrombosed to the level of entry of the jugular vein (V.J). The pacemaker probe (PM) is identified by the hyperechoic double reflection in the lumen.
b The Doppler waveform from the brachial vein shows the band-like flow profile with absence of respiratory phasicity typical of upstream flow obstruction (thrombosis).
c After only 2 days of low-molecular heparin (weight-adjusted therapeutic dose), the patient shows surprisingly early spontaneous recanalization. Residual thrombi are seen only around the pacemaker probe (PM). Moreover, there is narrowing of the subclavian vein as it enters the confluence (aliasing, but without demonstration of flow obstruction in the Doppler waveform).
d The axillary vein is completely recanalized with restoration of respiratory phasicity and cardiac pulsatility (confirming absence of a central flow obstruction).
e The brachial vein now exhibits respiratory phasicity of flow with slight cardiac pulsatility, consistent with elimination of the flow obstruction (same sampling site as in **b**)

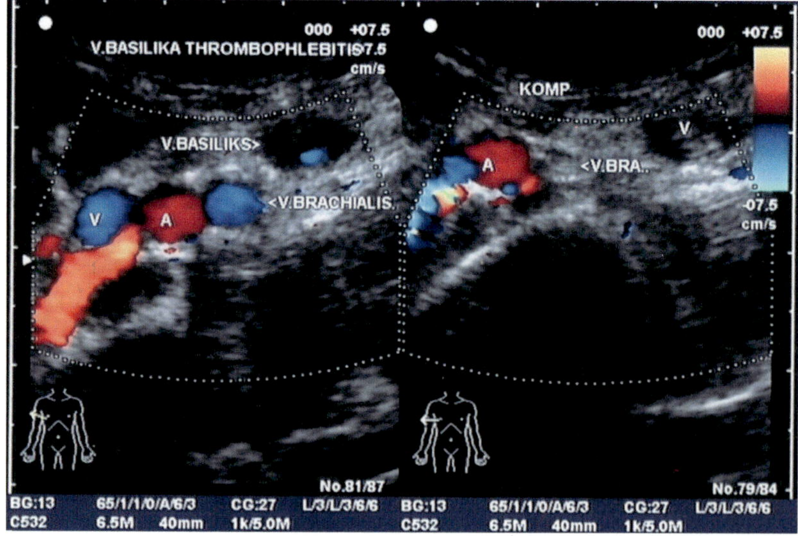

Fig. 3.108 (Atlas) Thrombophlebitis of arm veins. Using the artery as a landmark, the examiner can distinguish deep veins from superficial veins and thus differentiate between thrombosis and thrombophlebitis. In the example, the findings rule out venous thrombosis (brachial vein with flow displayed in blue, compressible as shown on the right) and confirm thrombophlebitis (basilic vein not compressible, superficial course, no accompanying artery)

Arteriovenous Fistulas

W. Schäberle, *Ultrasonography in Vascular Diagnosis*, https://doi.org/10.1007/978-3-319-64997-9_4

4

4.1 Clinical Role of Arteriovenous Fistula Evaluation

4.1.1 Background

Of the 50,000 patients with end-stage renal failure in Germany, each year some 15,000 become candidates for creation of a hemodialysis access. A native arteriovenous (AV) fistula has a better prognosis with longer patency and fewer complications such as infections and is preferred to a synthetic graft (Tordoir et al. 2007). An advantage of a synthetic dialysis access is that it can be used earlier, while a native fistula needs time to mature before it can be used for hemodialysis. A synthetic shunt is the second option in patients whose native vein (typically the cephalic vein) is deemed unsuitable because of a small lumen or because it has undergone thrombotic or fibrotic degeneration as a result of frequent puncture. A minimum flow volume is necessary to ensure adequate dialysis treatment. Protocols in the USA require a flow volume of at least 350 mL/min, while smaller volumes of 200–300 mL/min are still considered acceptable in some European countries including Germany. This requirement informs the preoperative search for a suitable vein for creating an AV fistula and the identification of patients who need a synthetic vascular access. Preoperative vascular mapping contributes important information for selecting the most suitable hemodialysis access for each patient.

4.1.2 Diagnostic Evaluation of Patients with Abnormal and Surgically Created Fistulas

An AV fistula is a direct communication between an artery and a vein that bypasses the capillary bed. **Clinically**, a fistula is recognized by a palpable thrill and a more or less persistent high-frequency bruit that is present throughout the cardiac cycle and varies with fistula flow.

4.1.2.1 Types of AV Fistulas

Congenital, acquired, and therapeutic AV fistulas are distinguished.

A congenital AV fistula can occur in the form of a direct anatomic connection between the arterial and venous system (malformation), the presence of a blood-conducting structure between an artery and a vein (such as an aneurysm), or multiple short circuits in the soft tissue or bone. Congenital fistulas can be part of complex angiodysplastic syndromes. In most patients with an angiodysplastic syndrome, the combination of clinical symptoms usually allows the diagnosis to be made:

- Klippel-Trenaunay syndrome is characterized by unilateral limb hypertrophy with the affected limb showing nevus flammeus and venous anomalies (atypical varicosis and phlebectasia). Sonographically, the dysplastic venous changes are seen as convolutes of varicose veins. AV fistulas, if present, tend to be microfistulas. Such fistulas have no hemodynamic effects and are not apparent on color duplex ultrasound.
- In Parkes Weber syndrome, larger AV fistulas are present (and may be the cause of excessive growth of the affected limb). The feeding arteries and draining veins of these larger fistulas are detectable by duplex ultrasound, which thus allows differentiation of Parkes Weber syndrome from Klippel-Trenaunay syndrome (◘ Fig. 4.2).
- Servelle-Martorell syndrome is characterized by relative undergrowth of the affected limb (typically the arm). The predominant vascular abnormalities are multiple hemangiomas and varicose veins. Demonstration of varicosis by duplex ultrasound may become relevant in the differential diagnosis.

◘ **Table 4.1** Types of arteriovenous (AV) fistulas

Type of fistula	Description
Congenital AV fistula	Direct anatomic connection between the arterial and venous system or indirect communication through short circuits in the soft tissue
Acquired AV fistula	Iatrogenic: complication of arterial catheter examinations or renal transplant biopsy
	Trauma
	Spontaneous
Therapeutic AV fistula	Temporary: after thrombectomy for pelvic vein thrombosis
	Permanent: for hemodialysis access in renal failure

Acquired fistulas usually develop after trauma or iatrogenic vascular injury during invasive procedures such as catheter examinations (◘ Table 4.1).

The third type are **therapeutic fistulas**, which are predominantly created for hemodialysis access. Therapeutic AV fistulas are temporary or permanent and include:

- Temporary AV fistula after thrombectomy for pelvic vein thrombosis
- Fistula to improve patency in patients with a femorocrural bypass graft and poor runoff (controversial)
- AV fistula for hemodialysis access.

4.1.2.2 Creation of a Hemodialysis Access

An AV fistula established for hemodialysis access must:

- have the right size to ensure a minimum flow volume for adequate hemodialysis without inducing arterial steal or cardiac insufficiency,
- have a long enough segment for puncture, and
- be established at a site that causes the least patient discomfort.

The wrist or the bend of the elbow is the best site for a hemodialysis access, both in terms of surgical technique and ease

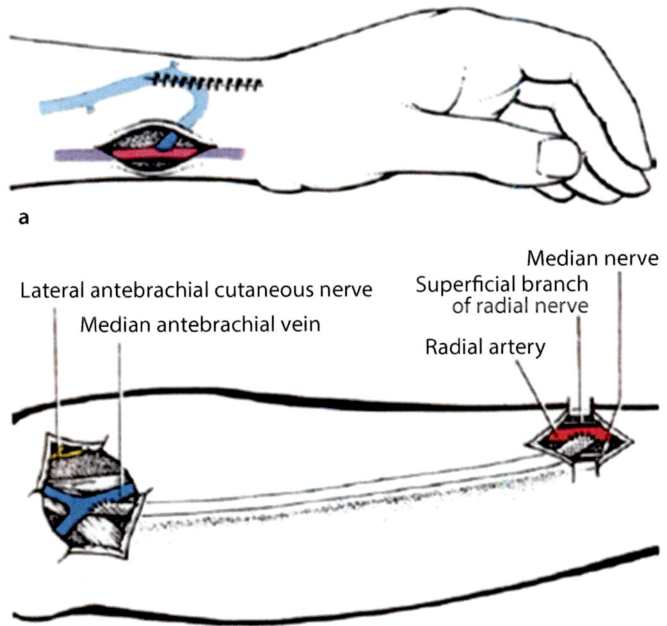

■ **Fig. 4.1** **a** Distal cephalic vein fistula in the forearm: side-to-end anastomosis of the radial artery and distal cephalic vein. **b** Vascular access created with a synthetic conduit: bridge graft connecting the brachial artery and distal cephalic vein (From Heberer and van Dongen 1993)

of access. A minimum fistula flow volume of 300 mL/min is required for dialysis, while a volume exceeding 15–20% of the cardiac output may lead to cardiac insufficiency.

In patients with no adequate vein for creating a direct AV connection, a synthetic graft (polytetrafluoroethylene/PTFE or Gore-Tex) may be interposed.

The classic AV connection for hemodialysis is the Brescia-Cimino fistula, which is an end-to-side anastomosis between the cephalic vein and radial artery at the level of the wrist (■ Fig. 4.1a) or between the cephalic vein and brachial artery in the bend of the elbow. Synthetic accesses are established as loops from the brachial artery at the elbow to the basilic or brachial vein, most commonly as a U-shaped loop implanted subcutaneously in the lower arm. Alternatively, a vascular access can be established with interposition of a straight graft between the brachial artery and the cephalic, axillary, or jugular vein (■ Fig. 4.1b).

The standard diameter of a PTFE prosthesis is 5 or 6 mm. It can be used for hemodialysis immediately after implantation. A direct AV fistula, on the other hand, requires 3–4 weeks to mature before the vein carries enough blood and can be punctured.

Natural AV fistulas have a better prognosis than synthetic accesses, which may be affected by various functional problems requiring repeat revision.

Both the unphysiologically high flow rates and repeat puncture of the access vein induce intimal proliferation, frequently leading to stenosis and occlusion. Published **vascular access patency rates** range widely, depending on the patient population, inclusion criteria, and type of access investigated. The patency rate reported for Brescia-Cimino fistulas is 80–90% after 1 year, 63–87% after 2 years, and approx. 65% after 4 years (Ahmad et al. 1998; Brittinger et al. 1966; Harnoss et al. 1991; Keller et al. 1991, 1988). In contrast, synthetic grafts have patency rates of 62–90% after 1 year, 50–79% after 2 years, and approx. 40% after 4 years (Haimov et al. 1979; Munda et al. 1983; Tellis et al. 1979). Good vascular access function is essential for the quality of life of patients on chronic hemodialysis. To maintain access patency, it is important to ensure timely recognition and proper interpretation of access-related problems. Noninvasive modalities such as color duplex ultrasound are the most suitable diagnostic tests, enabling early identification of the underlying cause of a reduced flow rate through the fistula or other complications and prompt initiation of adequate therapeutic measures.

4.1.2.3 Indications for Color Duplex Ultrasound

Color duplex ultrasound is used in patients with congenital or acquired AV fistulas and patients with a hemodialysis access. The indications include:

- Congenital or acquired nontherapeutic AV fistula:
  - Fistula detection
  - Localization
  - Identification of the feeding artery and draining vein
  - Estimation of fistula flow volume
- Therapeutic AV fistula:
  - Estimation of access flow volume
  - Evaluation of vascular access complications (with search for underlying causes):
    - Fistula flow too low for hemodialysis
    - Peripheral ischemia (hand)/dialysis access steal syndrome (DASS)
    - Arm swelling
    - Fistula occlusion
    - Stenosis (at site of anastomosis or within the fistula)
    - Stenosis of upstream artery or draining vein, peripheral ischemia (arterial steal) due to high fistula flow, and follow-up of outcome after banding
    - Puncture aneurysm
    - Perivascular complications: abscess, hematoma

On color duplex ultrasound, a congenital or acquired (nontherapeutic) AV fistula is characterized by a color Doppler bruit (mosaic of colors) resulting from highly turbulent flow in the fistula and perivascular vibration. Moreover, the higher flow velocity will cause aliasing if the scan parameters are set for depicting normal venous flow.

The Doppler waveform from the feeding artery shows a monophasic flow profile with a large diastolic component, which is due to lower peripheral resistance. The draining vein has an arterialized flow profile with severe turbulence.

The (color) duplex examination allows identification and evaluation of the feeding artery and draining vein.

In patients with an AV fistula for hemodialysis access, ultrasonography enables noninvasive evaluation of access complications and estimation of fistula flow. Measurement of blood flow velocity in the feeding artery has been found to be the most reliable method for determining fistula flow volume, as measurement within the fistula or draining vein is degraded by turbulence and variability of fistula diameter. The measurement in the feeding artery upstream of the venous anastomosis is used to calculate the fistula flow volume by comparing it with the contralateral side or by subtracting blood flow in the artery distal to the fistula. The flow volume is calculated from the time-averaged mean velocity and the cross-sectional area of the vessel.

4.2 Examination Protocol, Technique, and Diagnostic Role

4.2.1 Congenital and Acquired Fistulas

Accurate information on the site of a fistula with its feeding artery and draining vein is helpful for planning the surgical procedure.

When a fistula is suspected on clinical grounds, this information serves to guide the sonographic search (in the color duplex mode) for the abnormal arteriovenous communication, the inflow artery, and the draining vein. The transducer frequency must be adjusted to the required scanning depth. The high flow velocities in a fistula and the occurrence of perivascular vibration artifacts make it necessary to use a high pulse repetition frequency (PRF).

The choice of transducer, patient positioning, and the procedure depend on the body region in which the fistula is clinically suspected (e.g., palpable thrill or limb swelling due to disturbed venous drainage). Perivascular tissue vibration or color bruit is a helpful artifact in color Doppler. It is caused by fast or turbulent flow and can guide the examiner to the site of the abnormal arteriovenous communication.

In spectral Doppler evaluation, the feeding artery is identified by an abnormal, monophasic waveform with a larger diastolic component due to low-resistance flow. Distal to the fistula, the normal triphasic flow profile that characterizes high-resistance flow in peripheral arteries is seen (◻ Fig. 4.2d).

With this in mind, the examiner can identify a large AV fistula with hemodynamically relevant flow by intermittent spectral Doppler interrogation of the artery above and below the site of the suspected arteriovenous communication. The point of transition from monophasic to triphasic flow is where the fistula is located. At the same time, venous return proximal to this point will show pulsatile variation. In addition to precise localization, which is relevant when surgical

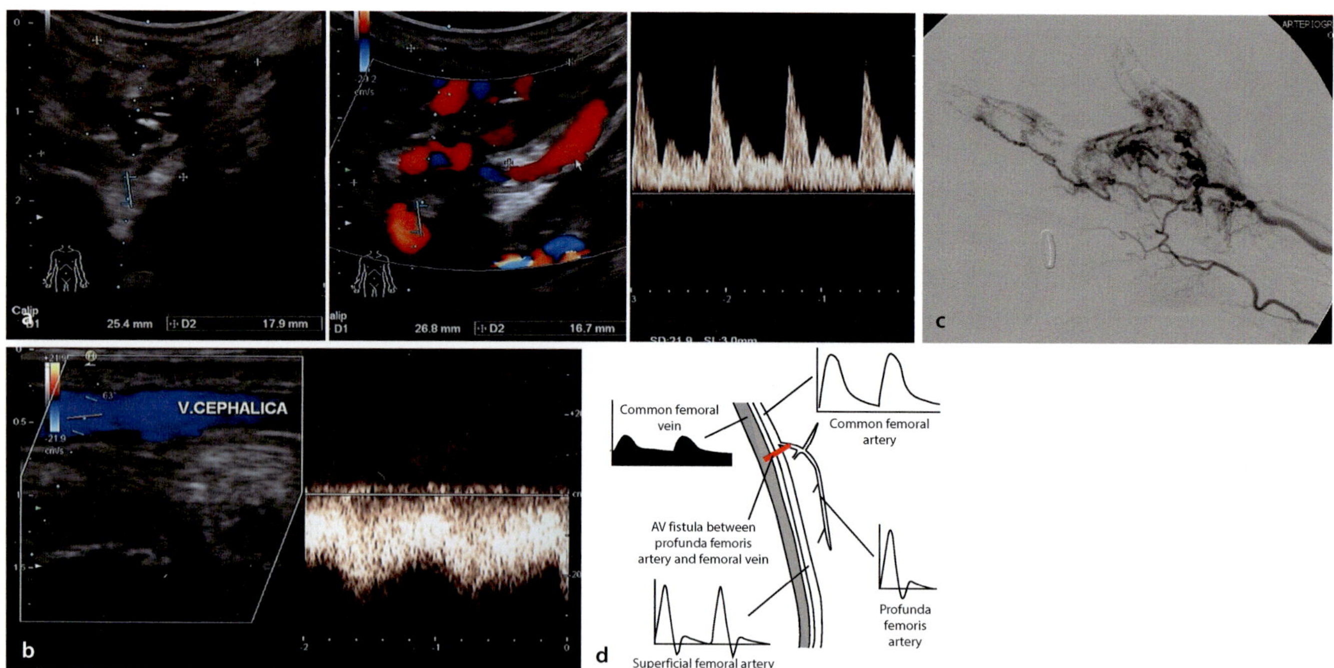

◻ **Fig. 4.2** **a–c** Congenital arteriovenous (AV) fistula. Complex angiodysplasia with a cluster of entangled vessels just distal to the wrist. **a** In the B-mode image (left), the vessels are seen as irregular hypoechoic areas. The color flow image (right) depicts flow signals in an AV macrofistula, where flow is fast enough to be detectable. The Doppler waveform from the feeding artery arising from the radial artery is monophasic with a large diastolic component, which is characteristic of arteries feeding an AV fistula. The arrow indicates the interdigital artery. **b** The Doppler waveform from the cephalic vein draining the fistula shows pulsatile flow. **c** Angiogram showing the cluster of arteriovenous fistulas. **d** A iatrogenic AV fistula commonly develops between the proximal profunda femoris artery and the femoral vein, typically when the puncture is made too far peripherally. The diagrams show the Doppler waveform changes proximal to an AV fistula (common femoral artery, monophasic pattern) and distal to an AV fistula (superficial femoral and profunda femoris arteries, both triphasic). The Doppler waveform from the draining vein proximal to the AV fistula shows pulsatile flow (common femoral vein). The magnitude of the diastolic flow component proximal to the AV fistula reflects the flow volume within the fistula (see ◻ Fig. 4.8 (Atlas))

revision is contemplated, the fistula flow volume may have to be calculated as well. This is done on the basis of the diameter of the feeding artery, determined from the B-mode image, and time-averaged flow velocity (angle-adjusted Doppler measurement), from which the normal blood flow volume of the artery is subtracted. The normal flow volume is determined in the artery of the same name on the contralateral side. Veins draining a fistula are characterized by an arterialized, though often less pulsatile, flow profile.

4.2.2 Hemodialysis AV Fistula

In the sonographic evaluation of therapeutic AV fistulas and their clinical complications, it is not the morphologic or hemodynamic changes as such that are crucial for deciding about the therapeutic consequences, but rather the clinical manifestations they produce. The indication for treatment is chiefly established on the basis of the clinical problems, while the choice of treatment is made on the basis of duplex ultrasound or the results of other imaging modalities (PTA of the existing AV fistula, creation of a new dialysis access, revision, ligation of collateral veins, aneurysm resection, banding, fistula closure).

There is an ongoing controversy about the benefit of regular ultrasound follow-up of hemodialysis access fistulas (see ► Sect. 4.8.2). In general, routine sonographic surveillance is not necessary, while clinical complications and low fistula flow should prompt a timely ultrasound examination to identify the underlying cause. The clinical problems determine the extent of the sonographic examination. In patients presenting with signs of peripheral ischemia or cardiac insufficiency, for instance, it is necessary to quantify the fistula flow volume. If dialysis flow has become insufficient, the examiner must look for stenosis of the feeding artery or draining vein.

A **forearm fistula** is best examined in the sitting patient with the elbow slightly bent and the forearm resting on a support. The superficial course of the arm vessels enables their examination with a high-frequency transducer (7.5–10 MHz). Use of a linear-array transducer has the advantage of providing better contact with the arm. An **upper arm** fistula is examined in the supine patient with the arm comfortably positioned on a support for optimal exposure of the fistula site for transducer maneuvers. A high PRF is necessary to capture the fast blood flow through the fistula, whereas the gain must be downregulated to eliminate vibration artifacts. A lower PRF is necessary to depict slow postocclusive flow. First, the examiner evaluates the fistula in transverse orientation, followed by hemodynamic evaluation in the longitudinal plane with spectral Doppler interrogation of the feeding artery, the access vein or the synthetic graft, and the draining vein. When required, spectral Doppler imaging should include the anastomotic sites.

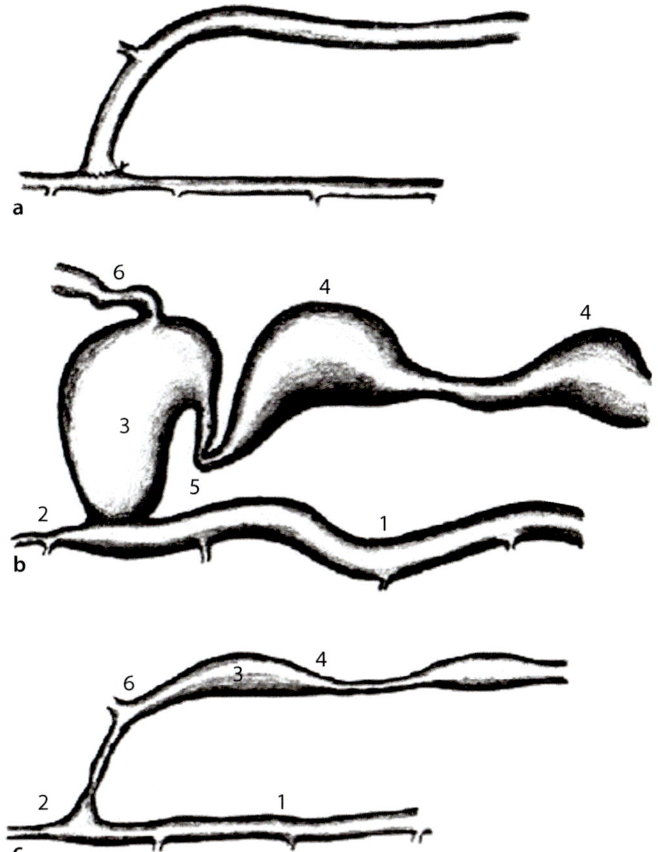

Fig. 4.3a–c Diagram of the morphologic changes that can occur in a hemodialysis access: **a** shortly after creation of the AV fistula; **b** dilatation; **c** stenosis (*1* feeding artery, *2* artery supplying hand distal to access vein, *3* access vein, *4* dilatation and stricture due to scar formation at site of frequent venipuncture, *5* stenosis due to kinking, *6* accessory vein arising from access vein) (From Scholz 1998)

The spectral Doppler findings from these sites, in conjunction with the patient's clinical symptoms, guide the further examination to identify the underlying pathology. In the feeding artery, the indirect stenosis criteria (Fig. 4.12 (Atlas)) can be used when the Doppler waveform is obtained while the access fistula is being compressed to induce high-resistance flow as in a peripheral artery. In inconclusive cases, arterial inflow must be scanned continuously from the subclavian artery to the brachial or radial artery in the longitudinal plane including spectral Doppler sampling.

In patients with a Brescia-Cimino fistula, the access vein and draining veins are evaluated for dilatation or narrowing (Fig. 4.3).

The veins must be examined with very light pressure to avoid compression, which may be misdiagnosed as stenosis. This is achieved by placing several fingers or the edge of the hand holding the transducer on the arm outside the course of the fistula. The transducer can thus be moved with very subtle pressure. Alternatively, undue pressure can be avoided by placing the transducer somewhat lateral to the apex of the

Table 4.2 Structured duplex ultrasound examination of patients with hemodialysis access problems (three-point strategy)

Site of spectral Doppler interrogation	Diagnostic information	Doppler waveform findings (direct/indirect criteria)
Feeding artery proximal to venous anastomosis without and with manual fistula compression	(Central) arterial stenosis, proximal to venous anastomosis	Delayed upstroke, reduced pulsatility (during fistula compression)
	Fistula stenosis	Increasing pulsatility (in proportion to stenosis severity); increased peripheral resistance
Feeding artery distal to venous anastomosis without and with manual fistula compression	Dialysis access steal syndrome (DASS) (symptomatic/asymptomatic)	Reduced PSV, to-and-fro flow, and retrograde flow will be seen in proportion to severity of arterial steal
	Peripheral perfusion reserve	PSV increase (quantitative) with fistula compression
Access vein 2–4 cm from anastomosis	Anastomotic stenosis	Intrastenotic PSV increase (stenosis grading)
	Stenosis of access vein/partial thrombosis	Increasing pulsatility (in proportion to stenosis severity)

vein wall and then tilting it to interrogate the vein. Synthetic grafts are less susceptible to compression.

Apart from palpation, the **course of an AV fistula** is most easily tracked sonographically in transverse orientation. Spectral Doppler measurement is performed in the longitudinal plane at sites suspicious for stenosis. Perivascular vibration artifacts, caused by fast flow, can be eliminated by slightly compressing the area next to the transducer with the flat hand, while at the same time avoiding excessive compression of the vein. Proper positioning is verified in the B-mode by slightly changing the pressure exerted with the transducer. Tortuous veins are better appreciated transversely. In patients with an intricate fistula, an overview of flow directions in the different venous limbs can be obtained in the color duplex mode.

When a narrowing is encountered in the B-mode examination or when aliasing or perivascular tissue vibration (mosaic of colors) appears in the color duplex mode, a Doppler waveform is obtained from that site in longitudinal orientation to confirm stenosis and grade its severity.

While the focus is on vascular assessment, it is also important to pay attention to perivascular structures in longitudinal and transverse planes (and color duplex as needed) to differentiate hematoma, abscess, and AV access aneurysm.

4.2.2.1 Time-Efficient Ultrasound Workup of Hemodialysis Access Problems

Color-coded duplex ultrasound combines two sonographic techniques that enable efficient diagnostic workup of hemodialysis access problems based on the patient's clinical presentation. With gray-scale ultrasound, the examiner can identify the course of the fistula, detect morphologic abnormalities such as aneurysm or luminal narrowing due to scarring, and identify accessory veins diverting blood away from the access vein.

The mainstay of the ultrasound examination is spectral Doppler interrogation for evaluation of fistula flow, arterial perfusion, and stenosis grading. To exploit this unique tool for hemodynamic evaluation of dialysis access problems, the author has developed a time-efficient protocol based on spectral Doppler interrogation of three representative sites (three-point strategy) (Table 4.2) for identification of common, treatable access-related problems.

First, the examiner identifies the brachial artery in the upper arm in transverse orientation and then obtains a waveform in the longitudinal plane. A monophasic waveform with a large diastolic component confirms undisturbed flow through the fistula downstream of the sampling site. A waveform with more pulsatile flow or a triphasic waveform (characteristic of normal high-resistance flow in this artery) indicates obstructed flow in the fistula (occlusion or high-grade stenosis) or in the draining vein (axillary vein thrombosis). Spectral Doppler measurement at this site is then repeated with manual compression of the AV fistula. This should result in a triphasic waveform with a steep systolic upstroke (short acceleration time). Failure to obtain a high-resistance triphasic waveform with absence of a whipping sound during fistula compression suggests an obstructive lesion in the feeding artery upstream of the sampling site (typically the subclavian artery). The examiner then continuously scans the artery up the arm to identify and grade the stenosis.

The second site of spectral Doppler evaluation is the main artery distal to the venous anastomosis. Again, Doppler waveforms are obtained without and with compression of the fistula to assess the steal effect resulting from the hemodialysis access (the finger arteries may be included in the examination in patients with ischemia).

The third site of Doppler interrogation is the access vein approx. 1–3 cm distal from the anastomosis, where fistula flow is assessed and anastomotic stenosis can be identified.

Additional components of the sonographic workup depend on the spectral Doppler findings at these three key sites in conjunction with the patient's clinical symptoms or hemodialysis access problem (inadequate flow volume for hemodialysis, peripheral ischemia (fingers, hand), arm swelling).

4.3 Doppler Waveform Changes Characteristic of AV Fistulas

The low peripheral resistance associated with an AV short circuit results in continuous systolic and diastolic flow and a large diastolic flow component in the feeding artery. This altered flow situation gives rise to a number of specific sonographic findings in patients with an AV fistula:

- Monophasic flow profile due to continuous systolic and diastolic flow with a large diastolic component in the feeding artery
- Pulsatile flow in the arterialized draining vein
- Very turbulent flow across the fistula (along the length of the access vein)
- Perivascular tissue vibration around the fistula
- Dilatation of the inflow artery and draining vein when a hemodynamically relevant AV fistula has been present for many years.

A return to pulsatile flow in the feeding artery of a therapeutic AV fistula indicates low fistula flow due to obstructed venous drainage, fistula stenosis, or fistula occlusion (◘ Figs. 4.15 and 4.18 (both Atlas)).

Perivascular tissue vibration around an AV fistula, especially during systole, is a tissue motion artifact and may be seen in color Doppler as extravascular color (color bruit). The smaller the fistula caliber and the larger the jet, the more pronounced the perivascular vibration artifact. Turbulent flow in the fistula is identified by a mix of colors and by considerable spectral broadening in the Doppler waveform; there may even be retrograde flow components during systole.

The outflow vein is dilated and, due to arterialization, flow is pulsatile and turbulent (resulting in spectral broadening, primarily close to the fistula). Vessel wall and soft tissue vibration artifacts in the color duplex scan can be minimized by slight manual throttling of arterial inflow, which is especially important when performing spectral Doppler measurement for comparison of flow velocities upstream and downstream of a suspected stenosis.

All draining veins have arterialized flow. Accessory venous branches that divert blood away from the access vein, but are unsuitable for hemodialysis, can thus be identified and ligated.

The flow changes in a hemodialysis access that has been used for many years may lead to intricate flow patterns in arteries that are only indirectly, through collaterals, connected to the feeding arteries (e.g., steal phenomena, supply of a radial artery fistula by the palmar arch and ulnar artery). Evaluation of color-coded blood flow directions allows correct interpretation and identification of shunt problems (such as ischemia of the fingers and reduced flow) under such complex flow conditions as well.

The flow velocities derived from spectral Doppler ultrasound vary widely with fistula age and dilatation. Peak systolic velocity (PSV) in the inflow artery may be up to twice as high as in the contralateral counterpart with a large diastolic flow component, resulting in a Pourcelot resistance index of 0.7–0.4. Depending on the diameter, even greater variability in flow velocities of 50–150 cm/s may be seen in the arterialized draining vein. Flow velocity in a synthetic AV access graft varies with arterial inflow and venous outflow resistance. Depending on the graft diameter, systolic velocities range from 100 to 400 cm/s with 60–200 cm/s at end diastole (Lockhart and Robbin 2001).

4.4 Fistula Maturation and Flow Volume Measurement

A decreased flow through the access fistula, due to complications such as stenosis, impairs hemodialysis function. However, only a high-grade fistula stenosis becomes functionally relevant, which, according to Kathrein et al. (1988, 1991), is defined as a decrease in the volume flow rate below 250 mL/min. Although this would seem to be the most obvious thing to do, blood flow is not measured directly in the affected access vein. This is because abrupt changes in diameter, especially in older fistulas, and changes in the lumen shape (elliptical) give rise to errors. Determination of mean velocity within the fistula is also impaired by turbulent flow (spectral broadening). For these reasons, the **flow volume** in an AV hemodialysis access can be **estimated most reliably by determining time-averaged mean flow velocity in the main feeding artery** (typically the brachial artery). Flow volume measurements performed on different ultrasound machines may vary by up to 30%. One reason is the use of different methods for determining the cross-sectional area (direct planimetric measurement or calculation from diameter, leading-edge method). Another is the way in which flow velocity is determined: it may be calculated as the mean velocity across the vessel lumen or as the median velocity. Inadequate receive gain can thus produce measurement errors. Calibration measurements are rarely done before flow volumes are measured. The discrepancies are less relevant as long as serial measurements are performed with the same equipment.

Grosser et al. (1991) compared volume flow measurements performed in the brachial artery, radial artery, and fistula vein and found **the best reproducibility for measurements in the brachial artery**. However, due to blooming effects, the calculation of the cross-sectional area is prone to errors, and the error is larger in smaller vessels such as the radial artery (◘ Fig. 1.28). This is because the error in measuring the vessel diameter is potentiated in the calculated flow volume (because the radius is squared in calculating the cross-sectional area).

Direct flow measurement in the access vein is often unreliable due to the wide luminal variability of Brescia-Cimino fistulas, the oval shape of the cross-sectional area, and turbulent flow, which rarely allows valid determination of mean flow velocity.

Therefore, in patients without any apparent perfusion abnormalities in the arms, bilateral flow measurement has emerged as the more valid method. This is best done in the brachial artery in the mid upper arm, where a good insonation window allows adequate measurement. In patients with adequate, high fistula flow, residual brachial artery contribution to arm perfusion is negligible.

An even more reliable method has been developed by the author and involves two measurements of blood flow velocity in the brachial artery upstream of the arteriovenous anastomosis – one without and one with short manual compression of the fistula. The fistula flow volume is then calculated as the flow volume without compression minus the volume with compression of the fistula (◘ Fig. 4.10e–g). In the author's experience, this method is simple and reliable. It is only limited in individuals with older synthetic loops and in individuals with large arms.

Volume flow is calculated (see ► Sect. 1.1.2.4) by multiplying the cross-sectional area (determined in the B-mode) with the time-averaged mean blood flow velocity (derived from spectral Doppler measurement with an acute angle <50°). This is done automatically when this feature is included in the calculation package. Accurate calculation of the cross-sectional area of the brachial artery is ensured by measuring the diameter using the leading-edge method (to minimize errors due to the blooming effect occurring in gray-scale ultrasound at interfaces of high acoustic impedance such as the vessel wall; ◘ Fig. 1.28) and by taking the variation in arterial diameter through the cardiac cycle into account. To this end, the systolic and diastolic diameters are weighted at a ratio of 1:2 in the equation for cross-sectional area calculation.

Direct determination of flow volume in the access vein is discouraged, especially when a hemodialysis access has been used for a long time. However, when there is complex branching of veins, an attempt can be made to determine the functionally relevant proportion of blood flow through the access vein. To do so, the Doppler sample volume must be placed in a straight segment of the vein with little turbulence and without major caliber variation.

The volume flow rate can also be determined to assess maturity of a newly created hemodialysis access before first use or when maturation appears to be delayed (e.g., low flow). A wide range of volume flow rates from 500 to 1200 mL/min make an AV fistula suitable for hemodialysis.

The predictive value of several ultrasound criteria such as minimum venous diameter for hemodialysis AV fistula maturation was investigated in a retrospective study of 69 patients (Robbin et al. 2002). Fistula adequacy for hemodialysis was 89% in patients with a minimum venous diameter of 4 mm versus 44% for diameters of less than 4 mm. A flow volume of 500 mL/min or greater enabled adequate hemodialysis in 84% of cases versus only 43% if flow volume was less than 500 mL/min. Failure of a fistula to mature should prompt a color duplex ultrasound examination to search for stenosis, focusing on the inflow artery and the anastomosis. Venous outflow obstruction is more likely to induce the formation of a collateral pathway circumventing the access vein, which may cause arm swelling. When too much blood is diverted away from the main vein, the latter may be unsuitable for hemodialysis. Arterial or venous stenosis can be treated by PTA and followed up by serial ultrasonography; however, long-term patency is poor (Clark et al. 2007). An anastomotic stenosis requires surgical revision. Low fistula flow increases the risk of occlusion, which is over 50% when the flow volume drops below 300 mL/min (Lockhart and Robbin 2001; Bay et al. 1998).

4.5 Documentation

The documentation of the ultrasound findings depends on the clinical indication for the examination and the underlying cause of the hemodialysis access complication. Individual images often give only a poor representation of the intricate vascular patterns that may be encountered, especially in hemodialysis patients who have undergone repeat revision of their access. To facilitate serial examinations of hemodialysis access fistulas, images and waveforms from the following sites should be documented routinely:

- A longitudinal view and Doppler waveform from the feeding artery
- A longitudinal view and Doppler waveform from the anastomosis
- A longitudinal view with Doppler waveform from the access vein
- A Doppler waveform from the artery distal to the anastomosis

The documentation of pathology depends on the findings (e.g., stenosis including grading) and the clinical presentation. Prior to surgical revision, all vessel segments involved must be assessed and the findings documented, for example, the axillary or jugular vein if creation of a synthetic graft access is planned. A drawing of the vascular anatomy around the hemodialysis access fistula may be helpful to document complex vascular relationships for subsequent follow-up examinations, to report the findings to colleagues, and to document the sites of measurement (e.g., blood flow velocity without/with fistula compression).

4.6 Vascular Mapping Prior to AV Fistula Creation

Creation of a direct, native arteriovenous fistula for hemodialysis access is always preferable to a synthetic graft. The site should be as distal as possible to minimize ischemic complications and to avoid excessively high flow volumes. Note, though, that a Brescia-Cimino fistula connecting the radial artery and cephalic vein in the forearm has an early failure rate of 15.3% and a 1-year patency rate of only 62.5% (Rooijens et al. 2004). The risk of failure and early occlusion can be lowered by performing preoperative vascular mapping, especially if the creation of a forearm fistula is planned.

Table 4.3 Predictors of adequate AV fistula flow and good hemodialysis access function in preoperative color duplex and spectral Doppler mapping

Preoperative color duplex	Minimum	Doppler waveform
Arterial inflow	>50 cm/s	Triphasic waveform
Arterial diameter	>2.0 mm	–
Venous outflow	–	Venous flow with respiratory phasicity and, toward the center, cardiac pulsatility
Venous diameter (possibly with placement of a tourniquet)	>2.5 mm	–

In most cases, a careful preoperative clinical evaluation will identify the most suitable type of hemodialysis access for the patient (Table 4.3); however, preoperative color duplex imaging has been shown to facilitate the decision and improve the patency rate (Silva et al. 1998; Huber et al. 2002). The radial artery diameter should be at least 2–2.5 mm (Korten et al. 2007); a diameter of <1.5 mm was found to be associated with low flow volumes and an early occlusion rate of up to 45% (Parmar et al. 2007). An atherosclerotic vein may be unsuitable and fail to undergo adequate dilatation. The cephalic vein should be >2.5 mm in diameter to ensure adequate venous drainage. A cephalic vein diameter < 2 mm was reported to result in inadequate fistula maturation in 24% of cases (Mendes et al. 2002). A tourniquet can be placed to estimate the diameter of the vein with maximum filling (Lockhart et al. 2004). The validity of preoperative diameter measurement for predicting AV fistula maturation is confirmed by high intra- and interobserver agreement (Planken et al. 2006). Preoperative color duplex mapping should rule out flow obstruction or sclerosis of the cephalic vein, which may have developed as a result of thrombosis from repeat prior cannulation. Spectral Doppler interrogation should be performed to confirm unobstructed central venous drainage through the axillary vein, seen as normal respiratory phasicity and transmitted pulsatility from the heart.

For ease of cannulation, a superficial vein is preferred for creation of a hemodialysis fistula. Ideally, the candidate vein should not be more than 0.5 cm from the skin surface. If such a vein is not available, e.g., in patients with large arms, the creation of a hemodialysis access may involve mobilization and superficial tunneling of the vein or placement of a synthetic loop.

4.7 Hemodialysis Access Complications

Maintenance of good AV fistula function without complications (arm swelling, peripheral ischemia) is essential for patients on hemodialysis. If clinical evaluation identifies a problem or fistula flow becomes inadequate for dialysis, this should prompt timely workup by color duplex ultrasound. Signs of obstructed venous drainage include edema, swelling of the arm, livid discoloration, prolonged bleeding after removal of the dialysis needles, and increased venous pressure during dialysis. An arterial problem is suggested if there is ischemia with pain and necrosis of the fistula hand (arterial steal) or inadequate flow during dialysis.

Poor fistula flow with inadequate dialysis has many causes. Duplex ultrasound is an excellent tool for workup and identifying the underlying abnormality. The problems include:

- Decreased inflow due to stenosis or occlusion of the feeding arteries
- Decreased drainage due to obstruction of outflow veins (thrombus, stenosis)
- Cardiac insufficiency
- Insufficient blood flow in the access segment due to diversion of blood into venous branches
- AV fistula thrombosis with reduction of patent lumen
- Anastomotic stenosis

In addition, the function and prognosis of a dialysis fistula can be impaired by the following conditions and problems:

- Aneurysm (true or false)
- Local infection, hematoma
- Difficult cannulation due to deep or small vessels

Other hemodialysis access complications are peripheral ischemia (hands, fingers) and arm swelling.

4.7.1 Hemodialysis Access Stenosis

4.7.1.1 Causes of Hemodialysis Access Stenosis

Hemodialysis access stenosis is most commonly caused by neointimal hyperplasia, scarring at puncture sites, and dissection. Intimal proliferation begins 4–8 weeks after creation of the AV fistula, and progression varies widely among individuals. The factors promoting intimal proliferation in an AV fistula include turbulent flow at the anastomosis, intimal damage during cannulation, and increased venous pressure due to high flow rate. The resulting higher shear stress causes chronic damage, triggering repair processes with stimulation of vascular smooth muscle cells. Constriction due to neointimal proliferation tends to occur at valve sites. Finally, the unphysiologically high venous return through the hemodialysis access may be obstructed in the narrow costoclavicular space, which, under normal conditions, presents no clinically relevant flow obstacle.

4.7.1.2 Stenosis Detection and Grading

The clinical presentation and palpation findings as well as problems encountered during hemodialysis (needle clinging – insufficient inflow; increased venous pressure – outflow obstruction) guide the ultrasound examination. Based

Table 4.4 Criteria for identifying relevant hemodialysis access stenosis (Modified from Tordoir et al. 1989; Kathrein 1991; Grosser et al. 1991)

Direct criteria	Indirect criteria
Luminal narrowing (B-mode): diameter < 2 mm indicates high-grade stenosis requiring treatment	Reduced fistula flow volume (<300 mL)
	Prestenotic waveform: return to high-resistance flow (triphasic)
Peak systolic velocity (PSV) ratio cutoffs: - Arterial inflow: >2.0 - Access vein: >3.0 (treatment required for >4–8) - Arteriovenous anastomosis: >3.0	Poststenotic waveform: delayed systolic upstroke

on these clues, the site of the suspected obstruction is evaluated with color duplex imaging and spectral Doppler interrogation using basically the same criteria as for identification of peripheral artery stenosis in patients without an AV fistula. Direct criteria include local flow acceleration, turbulent flow, and perivascular vibration artifacts. Changes in the flow profile (prestenotic versus poststenotic) are of limited value as monophasic flow predominates due to the low resistance resulting from the venous short circuit. Still, a high-grade obstruction will induce increased upstream pulsatility and decreased downstream pulsatility. With a high-resolution transducer, obstructions can be identified in the B-mode. Their hemodynamic significance is then evaluated by spectral Doppler measurement. Moreover, the B-mode information enables differentiation of intramural and extramural causes of luminal narrowing. An example of an intramural process is intimal proliferation. Other steno-occlusive lesions are local thrombotic deposits. These can be differentiated from extramural structures such as hematomas. Early intimal proliferation is seen as a hypoechoic wall deposit or a color filling defect. With further progression, the proliferating intima becomes inhomogeneous and may calcify.

Because normal flow velocity is higher in an AV fistula and the feeding artery, a higher peak systolic velocity (PSV) of 2.5 m/s should be used as a cutoff to identify hemodynamically significant stenosis. Note, though, that most moderate stenoses identified using this higher cutoff do not require treatment unless a patient develops hemodialysis access dysfunction or other complications. Moreover, a doubling of the PSV compared with the prestenotic PSV can serve as a criterion for stenosis in a recently established fistula, but, due to caliber irregularities, is unreliable in older, dilated fistulas. Indirect signs of hemodialysis access stenosis include a return to a triphasic flow profile in the feeding artery and a drop of the fistula flow volume below 250 mL/min (Table 4.4).

Current clinical practice guidelines recommend **duplex ultrasound for quantification of hemodynamically relevant stenosis** (National Kidney Foundation 2006). Compared with the gold standard, DSA, duplex ultrasound was found to have 91% sensitivity and 97% specificity for stenosis detection in a failing hemodialysis access fistula (Doelman et al. 2005).

Stenosis of an AV fistula (e.g., Brescia-Cimino) most commonly affects the anastomosis (55–75%) (Kathrein 1991; Pietura et al. 2005) and the access vein (25%) (Turmel-Rodrigues et al. 2000) (Fig. 4.4). In older AV fistulas, stenotic narrowing may be seen upstream and downstream of dilated segments or occur as a result of scar formation at sites of frequent puncture. Here, a residual lumen <2 mm on B-mode imaging can serve as a predictor of imminent access failure. Otherwise, hemodynamic stenosis grading is more reliable, with flow velocities >300 cm/s suggesting hemodynamically relevant stenosis.

While normal peripheral arteries have high-resistance flow with a triphasic waveform, an artery feeding a hemodynamic access has low-resistance flow with a monophasic waveform. Therefore, as noted above, the indirect criterion of a change from triphasic to monophasic flow cannot be used for stenosis detection unless the waveform is obtained during short manual compression of the AV fistula. With compression, flow should become triphasic, as in a normal native peripheral artery, while persistent monophasic flow indicates stenosis.

The altered hemodynamic situation in and around a hemodialysis access also requires some adjustment of the blood flow velocity cutoffs (absolute values and ratios) identified for stenosis grading in native arteries. Caution is in order when absolute PSV is used because it is affected not only by the known systemic factors such as blood pressure but also by other factors, most notably the fistula flow volume. The effect of the latter is notoriously difficult to quantify. Parameters expressing the stenosis-related increase in blood flow velocity in relation to flow velocity outside the stenosis, e.g., 2 cm upstream, are considered more reliable measures of stenosis severity. In general, it is assumed that a stenosis begins to become hemodynamically relevant when there is doubling of flow velocity or 50% cross-sectional area reduction. This is expressed by a PSV ratio of 2 (intrastenotic PSV divided by prestenotic PSV). In patients with a hemodialysis access, the PSV ratio can also be used to grade stenosis of the venous anastomosis.

As noted, the use of absolute PSV thresholds alone ignores the considerable hemodynamic variability that may be encountered in an artificially created fistula and may lead to false-positive results. Nevertheless, absolute PSV cutoffs of 2.5 ms were used in scientific studies (Kathrein 1991; Grosser et al. 1991; Tordoir et al. 1989). As long as adequate hemodialysis is ensured, flow velocities exceeding 2.5 m/s are acceptable at the anastomosis, and relative stenosis may even be desirable to avoid excessively high fistula flow with ischemia of the hand.

While a PSV ratio cutoff of 2 is assumed to indicate 50% stenosis in the feeding artery, most investigators use a higher ratio of 3 to identify hemodynamically relevant stenosis in the body of the fistula (Fig. 4.4e, f). Even then, the hemodynamic degree alone is no indicator of the therapeutic relevance of the stenosis. In general, treatment is not required unless PSV ratios of 4–8 are measured, and the decision is always made

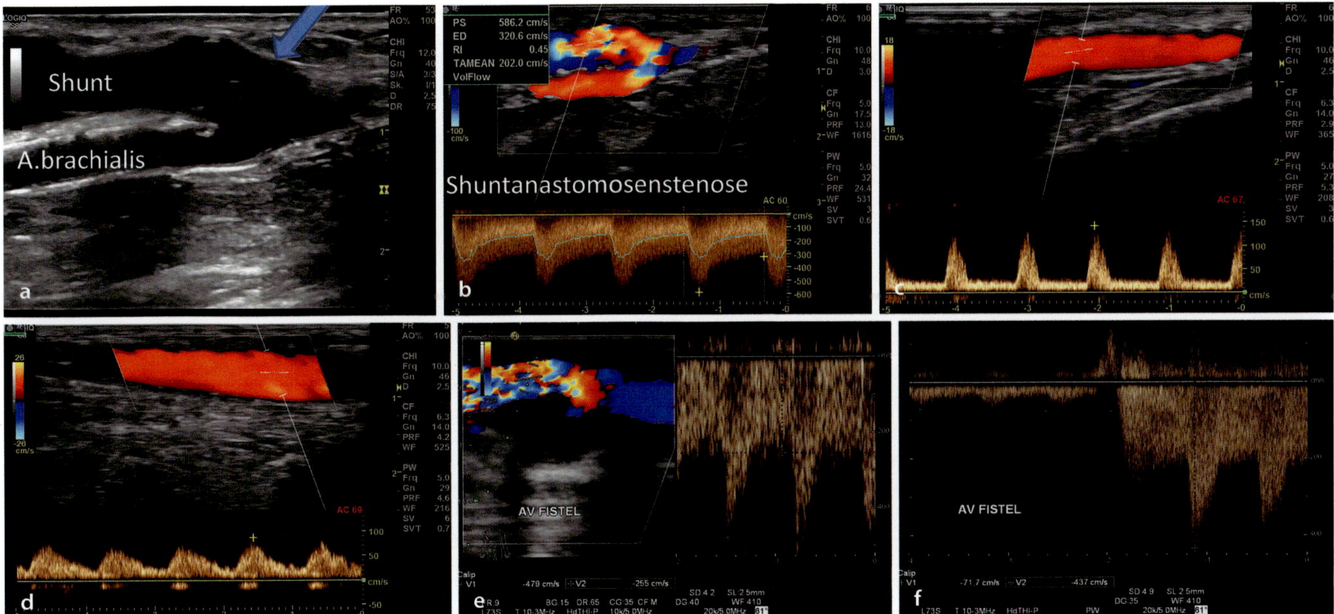

■ **Fig. 4.4a–f** Stenosis of hemodialysis access. **a, b** B-mode image (**a**) demonstrates stenosis at the venous anastomosis of a Brescia-Cimino fistula caused by a flap (arrow) in the access vein (which is seen closer to the transducer than the brachial artery). Peak systolic velocity (PSV) is 6 m/s (**b**), consistent with high-grade stenosis. The automatically calculated time-averaged mean velocity is 202.0 cm/s (TAMEAN in the black inset in the left upper corner in **b**). In the spectral display, mean velocities over time are represented by a green line. A flap as in this patient is often difficult to evaluate by angiography, and the sonographic diameter criterion for therapeutically relevant access vein stenosis (<2 mm in transverse plane) does not apply here. **c** Use of indirect stenosis criteria in the workup of suspected stenosis: The waveform from the brachial artery does not show the expected loss of pulsatility characterizing an artery feeding an AV fistula. Instead, there is slightly pulsatile flow with a small diastolic component, indicating abnormally increased resistance to blood flow through the fistula. **d** The waveform from the access vein distal to the anastomosis shows poststenotic flow with a delayed systolic upstroke and slightly increased PSV. These findings are consistent with an anastomic stenosis. **e, f** Different patient presenting with high-grade AV fistula stenosis with a PSV ratio of 6 (calculated from intrastenotic PSV of 437 cm/s (**f**) and prestenotic PSV of 71 cm/s). The waveform was obtained by continuously moving the transducer across the skin (and includes the sites of prestenotic and intrastenotic PSV measurement). The stenosis is due to an intimal flap and external compression of the fistula by a largely thrombosed, puncture-induced pseudoaneurysm (the vessel wall leak is indicated by residual flow, encoded in blue, within the otherwise thrombosed aneurysm sac). Based on these ultrasound findings, the treatment indicated is surgical revision, not PTA

taking additional parameters such pulsatility of flow in the feeding artery and fistula flow volume into account. The PSV ratio is not reliable unless it can be determined in an access vein segment with a relatively constant diameter. When there is marked widening of the prestenotic segment, the diameter should be used as an alternative diagnostic marker of stenosis.

Flow obstruction in the AV fistula is suggested indirectly by an increase in pulsatility in the feeding artery. High-grade stenosis or occlusion of the AV fistula can even restore the triphasic flow profile characteristic of high-resistance flow in native peripheral arteries. A triphasic waveform obtained in the feeding artery or the vein near the venous anastomosis is thus diagnostic of a relevant flow obstruction downstream of the sampling site (■ Fig. 4.18 (Atlas)).

4.7.1.3 Proximal Feeding Artery Stenosis

When no stenosis has been detected at the anastomosis or in the access vein to explain decreased flow, the search must continue proximally along the inflow (subclavian and axillary arteries). Feeding arteries become susceptible to atherosclerosis after many years of hemodialysis. Since all vessels communicating with the fistula have monophasic flow, a monophasic flow profile cannot be used as a stenosis criterion here. As noted before, the examiner can eliminate the fistula-related modulation of flow in the feeding artery by manually compressing the fistula. During compression, the feeding artery supplies only the arm and hand and the situation is the same as in native peripheral arteries, meaning that both direct and indirect criteria of stenosis apply (■ Fig. 4.12 (Atlas)).

4.7.2 Diagnostic Evaluation for Specific Hemodialysis Access Problems

The following subsections describe the diagnostic workup of common complications in patients with a hemodialysis access and discuss the therapeutic relevance of ultrasound findings in the management of these complications.

4.7.2.1 Peripheral Ischemia

An AV fistula in the arm can lead to critical hypoperfusion of the hand, in particular in patients with pre-existing peripheral arterial occlusive disease (PAOD) or in diabetics with macro- and microangiopathic medial sclerosis and stenotic lesions. In addition to the blood drained through the low-resistance fistula, blood may be diverted from the arteries supplying the

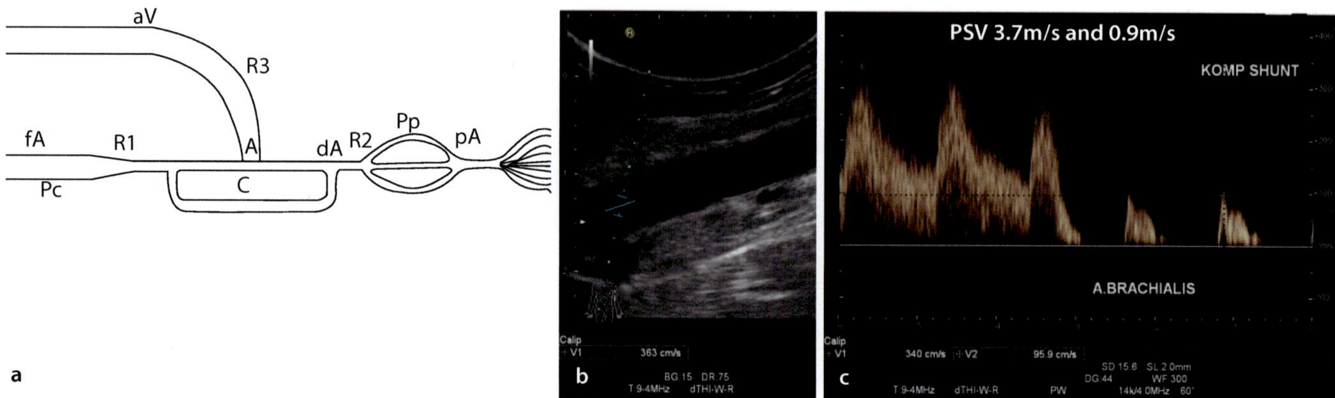

Fig. 4.5 **a** Diagram of factors affecting peripheral perfusion after creation of an AV fistula (for details see text) (*fA* feeding artery, *Pc* central arterial pressure, *dA* draining artery, *Pp* peripheral arterial perfusion pressure, *pA* peripheral arteries, *R1* resistance of feeding artery, *R2* resistance of peripheral vessels, *R3* total resistance of anastomosed vessel, *A* anastomosis, *aV* anastomosed vessel, *C* collateral) (From Scholz 1998). **b, c** High-flow AV fistula with a markedly increased peak systolic velocity (PSV) of >350 cm/s in a long segment of the brachial artery feeding the fistula. The increase is nonfocal, making stenosis unlikely. The Doppler waveform from the brachial artery (**c**) shows flow without manual compression of the AV fistula (left) and with compression (right). During compression, flow in the brachial artery becomes more pulsatile, and a normal PSV of 100 cm/s is measured

forearm and hand. Severe dialysis access steal syndrome (DASS) can cause retrograde flow from the arteries supplying the hand or an increased flow in the ulnar artery if the fistula is supplied by the arteries of the palmar arch. Hypoperfusion of the fingers or even of the whole hand may ensue. The risk of ischemia in the fingers or the hand increases with the severity of PAOD and the magnitude of fistula flow.

A drop in peripheral perfusion pressure below the critical threshold with pain and vital risks to finger areas is dependent on several factors (Fig. 4.5):

- Systemic blood pressure
- Atherosclerosis of peripheral arteries (micro- and macroangiopathy) with increased resistance distal to the venous anastomosis
- Peripheral resistance distal to the venous anastomosis
- Collateralization around the fistula
- Width of anastomosis
- Steal phenomena (DASS)
- Venous outflow resistance
- Proximal stenosis of feeding artery

Macroangiopathic causes of ischemia of the fistula-bearing arm and excessive blood flow through the fistula can be diagnosed by duplex ultrasound. The color duplex examination for peripheral ischemia focuses on identifying sclerotic stenotic lesions of the arm arteries proximal and distal to the arteriovenous anastomosis (with a view to performing PTA or placing a synthetic graft) or on confirming a high-flow fistula with arterial steal (DASS). Once excessive fistula flow has been established as the cause of ischemia, real-time measurement of peripheral flow velocity in response to increasing manual compression of the fistula is performed to estimate the expected effects of different surgical revision techniques (tailoring, banding, or distal revascularization and interval ligation (DRIL)). Duplex ultrasound can also be used for intraoperative monitoring of the effects of flow reduction by cuff placement or plication (Aschwanden et al. 2003; Zanow et al. 2006). Arterial steal results if venous outflow is greater than the capacity of the feeding artery (e.g., due to dilatation). Such a fistula draws blood from areas peripheral to the anastomosis and is characterized by reversed flow in the feeding artery distal to the venous anastomosis.

Peripheral ischemia occurs in 2–8% of all patients with a hemodialysis access. **Identifying the underlying cause** can be complex. Underlying causes include DASS due to excessive fistula flow and a relevant proximal stenosis of the feeding artery presenting with poor hemodialysis flow. Proximal stenosis of the feeding artery can be identified by spectral Doppler interrogation upstream of the venous anastomosis while the fistula is being compressed. During compression of the fistula, the waveform should become triphasic, while a monophasic flow profile and delayed upstroke suggest stenosis of the feeding artery (Fig. 4.12b, c (Atlas)). The stenosis is then localized by mapping the feeding artery upstream of the spectral Doppler sampling site.

The next step is spectral Doppler imaging of the feeding artery just distal to the venous anastomosis, comparing flow in this segment without and with compression of the fistula (Figs. 4.17 and 4.19 (Atlas)). Comprehensive assessment of the **hemodynamic situation** is crucial for deciding about the best therapeutic management (DRIL, banding). If the waveform obtained without compression shows two-and-fro flow (systolic forward flow and diastolic backward flow) or even persistent flow reversal, then this is diagnostic of arterial steal. In a patient with peripheral ischemia, this ultrasound finding is an indication for restricting flow through the vascular access (e.g., banding) or a DRIL procedure (Anaya-Ayala et al. 2012; Scali et al. 2013), and no additional diagnostic tests are necessary. Flow reversal in the distal feeding artery without symptoms of ischemia is observed when there is retrograde filling with backward flow in the brachial artery via the palmar arch, and these patients do not require treatment.

In the absence of steal-related flow changes in the artery distal to the venous anastomosis, manual compression of the fistula will nearly always elicit faster flow (PSV) in this segment and can thus help in estimating a potential beneficial effect of access flow restriction on peripheral perfusion and in deciding which treatment option will restore adequate perfusion of the hand (banding or graft interposition to reduce the lumen; the latter is typically only necessary when a high PSV of >2 m/s is measured in the fistula). The effect of flow-restricting measures can be estimated by pre- and intraoperative determination of flow in the distal feeding artery and the fistula while applying graded compression. Patients in whom high fistula flow has been ruled out as the cause of ischemia are candidates for a DRIL procedure. Before DRIL is performed, it is important, especially in diabetics, to evaluate the distal feeding artery down to the finger arteries for any additional stenotic lesions amenable to treatment (PTA). The search is best performed by levelwise spectral Doppler interrogation of the distal radial artery and the finger arteries with intermittent mapping. The sonographic search for stenosis in this territory is time-consuming and may be limited in diabetics with severe medial calcification. A supplementary angiogram is helpful for detecting stenotic lesions in this territory.

This is the only situation that may require an angiographic examination. Otherwise, the unique hemodynamic information obtained with color duplex imaging is often superior in elucidating underlying vascular access problems in patients with symptoms of ischemia.

When DASS due to excessive fistula flow is suspected, duplex ultrasound can be used to quantify the fistula flow volume (see ► Sect. 4.4). A volume flow rate >1200 mL/min increases the risk of peripheral ischemia and high-output cardiac failure (Bay et al. 1998). In most cases, however, flow quantification is not necessary, and a treatment decision can be made based on the spectral Doppler findings obtained in the feeding artery distal to the venous anastomosis (including the finger arteries) with and without manual compression of the fistula (◘ Fig. 4.17 (Atlas)).

Another cause of peripheral ischemia is flow diversion through competing veins arising from the access vein. Therefore, the access vein should be examined once excessive fistula flow and arterial inflow obstruction have been ruled out as underlying causes of symptomatic ischemia. Accessory veins are marked for subsequent surgical ligation to restore adequate peripheral perfusion.

4.7.2.2 Hemodialysis Access Aneurysm

Because of the superficial location of the hemodialysis access, occlusion or aneurysm can be diagnosed clinically. Duplex ultrasonography may be performed to confirm the clinical diagnosis and to identify the origin and extent of an aneurysm (suture aneurysm, puncture aneurysm) for planning the therapeutic procedure.

Pseudoaneurysm (or false aneurysm) is a typical puncture complication developing when blood escapes through a defect in the arterial wall. The resulting subcutaneous blood collection has a persisting communication with the artery. Color duplex ultrasound identifies a pseudoaneurysm as a perivascular space with pulsatile flow. A pseudoaneurysm of the arterialized access vein is typically associated with obstructed venous drainage (stenosis or partial thrombosis of the access vein or axillary vein). Sonographic demonstration of to-and-fro flow identifies the neck of the pseudoaneurysm. Occasionally, thrombin injection is a treatment option but requires even greater care than in native arteries to avoid thrombin escape into the blood bloodstream and drainage toward the heart. Precautions include complete manual compression of the fistula during thrombin instillation and restriction of arterial inflow by placement of a tourniquet. After these precautions, ultrasound-guided thrombin instillation should begin in the periphery (5000 IU in 5 mL 0.9% NaCl) monitoring clot formation by color duplex ultrasound (◘ Fig. 4.11a, b (Atlas)). A suture aneurysm is a pseudoaneurysm due to suture failure and is commonly associated with infection (◘ Fig. 4.11d (Atlas)).

True vascular access-related aneurysms are focal outpouchings that develop on the basis of degeneration of the wall of the arterialized vein. They are defined as circumscribed increases in diameter to over 15 mm or to twice the diameter of the proximal segment. Fistula dilatation is common due to turbulent flow (especially distal to a narrowed segment) and an increased wall pressure resulting from arterialization of the access vein. Such dilatations may extend over a considerable length of the draining vein when a hemodialysis access has been used for many years (◘ Fig. 4.3).

4.7.2.3 Inadequate or Excessive Fistula Flow

A wide range of fistula flow rates, from 500 to 1200 mL/min, is deemed acceptable for hemodialysis. Rates exceeding 1600 mL/min (Grosser et al. 1991) or 20% of the cardiac output can cause complications such as cardiac insufficiency or ischemia distal to the vascular access. Estimation of the volume flow rate through the fistula may be helpful in various situations such as assessment of the outcome of fistula banding or other flow-restricting measures. As discussed above, various methods exist to quantify fistula flow volume (see ► Sect. 4.4). Theoretically, the most accurate method is to calculate the difference between flow volumes in the feeding artery proximal and distal to the arteriovenous anastomosis. Practically and technically, it is easier and more accurate to calculate fistula flow volume from measurements in the ipsilateral and contralateral brachial artery or from measurements taken without and with compression of the fistula (◘ Fig. 4.10e–g). The latter is the most accurate method. A volume flow rate of less than 300 mL/min is widely assumed to be inadequate for effective hemodialysis, and low flow or a decrease in fistula flow volume over time is regarded as a predictor of hemodialysis access failure.

Poor fistula flow should prompt a search for stenosis, beginning in the feeding artery (for details see ► Sect. 4.7.1). Increased pulsatility in the brachial artery suggests obstruction of the fistula or venous outflow, and the next step is to examine the venous anastomosis (especially in patients with

4

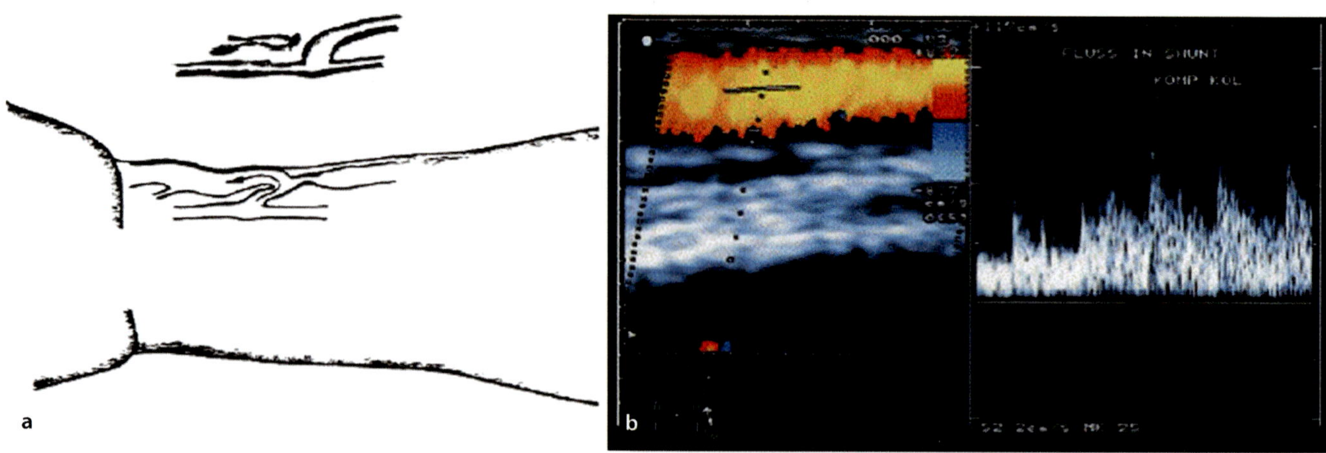

Fig. 4.6 **a** Retrograde arterialization via backward supply to an accessory branch with reduction of fistula flow: such accessory branches can be identified sonographically and marked for ligation (According to Scholz 1998). **b** Brescia-Cimino fistula at the wrist with inadequate flow for hemodialysis. Once stenosis has been ruled out, the examiner must search for accessory branches that divert blood away from the main vein. Such branches need to be ligated to ensure adequate blood flow through the access vein. In the case shown, ultrasound identified an accessory vein with relevant flow. The spectral display shows an increase in PSV within the access vein from 50 cm/s (due to flow diversion) to 75 cm/s (with manual compression of the accessory vein)

a Brescia-Cimino fistula). If there is no flow obstruction at this site, the length of the access segment is scanned, with a focus on stenosis or partial thrombosis. If flow in the fistula is more pulsatile than expected, the examiner should proceed to search for a flow obstruction of the draining veins, especially the axillary and subclavian veins.

Central venous obstruction with impaired venous drainage can lead to congestion and edema. Affected patients may present with arm swelling, especially when there is poor collateralization and fistula flow is high. In these patients, a careful evaluation of the axillary and subclavian veins is warranted to search for venous narrowing. This is accomplished by spectral Doppler evaluation of the axillary vein in the infraclavicular fossa. Normal venous flow in this region should show both respiratory phasicity and atrial pulsatility (W-shaped waveform). Obstructed central venous drainage is suggested when, compared with the contralateral arm, this flow modulation is lost or markedly damped during manual compression of the fistula. Compression is necessary to avoid misinterpretation because phasicity and pulsatility of venous flow may also be modulated by high fistula flow. Also in the infraclavicular fossa, the cephalic vein termination is evaluated for stenosis and the axillary vein for thrombotic deposits.

Luminal narrowing of the draining vein is seen in up to 40% of hemodialysis patients but may be asymptomatic if collaterals are present (Hecking et al. 2006; Neville et al. 2004). Venous obstruction often occurs secondary to a central venous intervention or placement of a central venous catheter. With 93% sensitivity and 94% specificity, color duplex ultrasonograpy has replaced venography in diagnosing obstructed venous drainage (Grogan et al. 2005). Color duplex imaging is also the method of choice for post-interventional evaluation of the access vein and central venous outflow. The primary patency rate after PTA alone is only 7–43% versus 11–70% for PTA with stenting (Mickley 2006). In patients with a synthetic dialysis access, narrowing primarily occurs at the site of the venous (distal) anastomosis and is due to intimal hyperplasia (Gaanterman et al. 1995; Roy-Chaudhury et al. 2001). In a study of 38 patients with clinically suspected hemodialysis access graft stenosis examined by Doppler ultrasound and angiography, Robbin et al. (1998) found ultrasound to reliably depict stenoses of access grafts and draining veins using PSV criteria. A focal two- to three-fold PSV increase was associated with 75% or greater stenosis.

Vascular access thrombosis can progress to partial or even complete occlusion. It has many causes including pre-existing stenosis, puncture complications (dissection, wall hematoma), fistula infection, and local compression, and the risk is higher in patients with episodes of hypovolemia or hypotension.

Another cause of **low fistula flow** (once stenosis has been ruled out) is **diversion of blood through collateral veins** coursing parallel to the access vein. Dilated accessory veins with large flow volumes can cause arm swelling. If the branches arise close to the venous anastomosis, patients may develop symptomatic arterial steal. Inadequate dialysis flow, new-onset steal-related symptoms (especially if they develop some time after creation of the dialysis fistula) (Fig. 4.19a-d (Atlas)), and arm swelling should prompt a color duplex examination to search for branching veins along the length of the access vein (in transverse orientation). Flow velocity and diameter of the branch vein are measured to determine the amount of blood diverted from the hemodialysis access vein. In addition, a branch vein can be compressed to estimate the flow increase likely to occur in the access segment after ligation. A relevant branch vein identified sonographically can then be marked for ligation (Fig. 4.6). The presence of branch veins may also be the reason that an AV fistula fails to mature. In this case, ligation will lead to maturation within a short time.

Flow volumes of over 1500–2000 mL/min may occur in patients with a more proximal hemodialysis access (bend of the elbow) if the cephalic vein is dilated and the anastomosis is too wide. Such high flow rates can lead to high-output cardiac insufficiency, especially in patients with compensated cardiac insufficiency or pre-existing cardiac damage. Quantification of the fistula flow volume by duplex ultrasound (the most reliable method for this purpose) can help avoid this complication, allowing identification of candidates for banding and assessment of the adequacy of flow reduction after treatment.

4.7.2.4 Arm Swelling

Venous outflow obstruction in patients with a hemodialysis access may be due to (partial) central vein thrombosis or terminal stenosis of the cephalic vein (◘ Figs. 4.15 and 4.18 (both Atlas)) and can present with arm swelling. Obstructed central venous drainage is suggested when there is increased pulsatility of flow in the access near the anastomosis and is confirmed by compression ultrasound or duplex ultrasound with the transducer in the infraclavicular fossa (incomplete compressibility of the vein with marginal flow around the clot). In patients with a loop graft, venous outflow obstruction may also be due to a stenosis upstream of the venous anastomosis. If no outflow obstruction is identified, the examiner proceeds to scan the length of the fistula in the transverse plane beginning at the venous anastomasosis to look for large-caliber accessory veins arising from the access vein. (◘ Figs. 4.16 and 4.19 (both Atlas)). When pressure in an accessory vein is high, it not only drains blood to the heart but also diverts blood to the forearm and hand. Venous flow reversal is identified sonographically, and these veins are then marked for surgical ligation.

Other complications cause circumscribed swelling. An example is pseudoaneurysm at puncture sites, which is identified on color flow images by the characteristic to-and-fro flow through a persisting communication with the parent vessel. Like a pseudoaneurysm developing as a complication of femoral artery puncture, a hemodialysis-access-related pseudoaneurysm can be treated by ultrasound-guided thrombin instillation. However, to prevent drainage of thrombin toward the center, even greater precautions should be taken including short manual compression of the access segment downstream of the aneurysm during instillation (◘ Fig. 4.11a, b (Atlas)).

4.8 Diagnostic Role of Duplex Ultrasound Compared with Other Modalities

Gray-scale ultrasound identifies both morphologic vascular changes of a hemodialysis access (dilatation, aneurysm, narrowing, thrombosis) and perivascular lesions (hematoma, abscess). (Color) duplex imaging provides quantitative information on fistula flow and identifies stenoses of the access vein and inflow artery. Ultrasonography thus enables more comprehensive evaluation of suspected hemodialysis access complications and their differential diagnosis than the mere visualization of vascular morphology by angiography. Angiography has the advantage of providing a better overview of the vascular anatomy around an AV fistula, but evaluation of complex vascular patterns may be impaired by overlying vessels. Sonographically detected pathology such as stenosis, length of dilated segment, or venous short circuits can be directly marked on the skin for surgical management. Ultrasound has 91–98% sensitivity and specificity in identifying arterial and venous stenosis, and provides unique information on the complex hemodynamic situation around an AV hemodialysis access and its pathology. This information is more relevant for deciding about the best treatment strategy in patients with hemodialysis access problems or complications (e.g., low flow, peripheral ischemia, arm swelling) than the morphologic information provided by angiography.

4.8.1 Therapeutic Decision-Making

Color duplex ultrasound is an excellent tool for the pretherapeutic evaluation of patients with an occluded Brescia-Cimino fistula, providing valuable information for deciding between surgical and interventional management. Over time, a hemodialysis access may degenerate with alternating widening and constriction. These changes are detectable by ultrasound, also in patients with large arms. Luminal narrowing due to scar formation at puncture sites is sonographically characterized by a thin lumen and thickened walls, which may additionally appear more echogenic. The ultrasound findings thus guide the treatment decision, allowing identification of patients whose vascular access problems can be managed by an endovascular procedure with thrombectomy and those requiring surgical revision with placement of a synthetic graft (narrowing due to scar formation). Surgical revision is also necessary in patients with ectatic/aneurysmal dilatation and thrombotic deposits on the walls in conjunction with thromboembolic occlusion. Hemodynamic assessment with differentiation of excessive versus normal fistula flow is the basis for selecting the best therapeutic strategy when patients present with peripheral ischemia (▶ Sect. 4.7.2.1).

The decision as to when a stenosis should be treated may be difficult, especially in patients with a Brescia-Cimino fistula that has been used for many years. Because of the degenerative changes of such fistulas, characterized by the alternation of narrowed and widened segments, higher cutoffs (absolute PSV or PSV ratio) than in native arteries are required to identify therapeutically relevant stenosis. Blood flow velocity alone is no reliable measure in a natural fistula and should always be interpreted in conjunction with fistula adequacy. Conversely, in a synthetic graft with its invariable diameter, the PSV ratio allows reliable stenosis grading.

At the anastomosis of both native fistulas and synthetic grafts, the PSV ratio is an unreliable parameter. Here, an absolute PSV of 2.5 m/s suggests stenosis with beginning hemodynamic relevance. Again, this says nothing about the therapeutic relevance of the stenosis. On the contrary, as long as there is adequate flow for hemodialysis, a relative stenosis may even be desirable to prevent dialysis access steal syndrome (DASS) with symptomatic peripheral ischemia. In these patients, elimination of the stenosis may even be contraindicated and can inadvertently induce ischemia, especially if preinterventional spectral Doppler interrogation already shows to-and-fro-flow in the feeding artery distal to the arteriovenous anastomosis. Therefore, to make the right therapeutic decision, it is crucial to always interpret the hemodynamic sonographic findings in conjunction with the patient's clinical presentation or hemodialysis access problems.

The results of a recent study (Schäberle and Leyerer 2014) in 51 patients with common hemodialysis access problems (37% peripheral ischemia, 53% poor fistula flow, 10% arm swelling) confirm that the three-point ultrasound protocol presented above (► Sect. 4.2.2.1) allows reliable pretherapeutic identification of underlying causes and initiation of appropriate treatment. In 47 of the 51 patients (92%), this protocol resulted in adequate management of the underlying problems without a need for revision of the therapeutic approach. This study also showed the structured protocol to be time-efficient, requiring on average 8 minutes for diagnostic workup of hemodialysis access problems.

4.8.2 Surveillance Programs?

There is an ongoing controversy about the benefit of routine duplex ultrasound surveillance in preventing thrombosis and prolonging vascular access survival in hemodialysis patients (Vachharajani 2012). It is undisputed, though, that duplex ultrasound is highly accurate in detecting vascular access stenosis (Finlay et al. 1993; Older et al. 1998; Doelman et al. 2005), and there is published evidence showing the benefit of early revision for imminent access failure diagnosed on the basis of sonographic flow measurement (Bay et al. 1998) or stenosis detection and grading (Older et al. 1998). This position is confirmed by a recent study showing that, while surveillance programs result in a 2.6% higher rate of fistula interventions, they also reduce the fistula thrombosis rate by 8.4% (Jiang et al. 2013). Despite the high diagnostic accuracy of ultrasound in identifying the etiologies of vascular access problems (aneurysm, stenosis, partial thrombosis) (Pietura et al. 2005; Doelman et al. 2005), the authors of a large meta-analysis (Tonelli et al. 2008) and a recent review (Paulson et al. 2013) conclude that surveillance programs are not justified because they do not lower the risk of access loss.

Nevertheless, there are proponents of surveillance programs for native fistulas, while it is undisputed that regular monitoring of synthetic access grafts does not significantly improve outcome. This conclusion is not based on scientific studies but on experience and data obtained in the follow-up of synthetic bypass grafts for steno-occlusive disease in peripheral arteries of the leg.

Another issue is whether the more or less aggressive reintervention policy is justified in all patients in whom routine surveillance reveals relevant hemodialysis-access-related stenosis. As discussed above, it is not always necessary or even desirable to treat a stenosis as long as there is adequate fistula flow for hemodialysis. In certain scenarios, the elimination of a stenosis might even cause a steal effect with symptomic peripheral ischemia. While the controversy about routine surveillance remains to be solved, it is undisputed, though, that signs of hemodialysis access problems such as reduced blood flow should prompt timely sonographic evaluation tailored to the clinical situation.

Timely workup is the basis for adequate and individualized management. The following listing summarizes the hemodialysis access problems and underlying causes that are amenable to sonographic workup and differentiation (with figure references in brackets):

- **Inadequate or low fistula flow**
  - Decreased inflow due to stenosis of the feeding artery (◘ Fig. 4.12 (Atlas))
  - Stenosis of the anastomosis or access vein (◘ Figs. 4.13 and 4.15 (Atlas), ◘ Fig. 4.4)
  - Decreased drainage due to proximal venous outflow obstruction (stenosis or (partial) thrombosis) (◘ Figs. 4.15 and 4.18 (Atlas))
  - Partial thrombosis of access vein with reduction of patent lumen
  - Has fistula maturation occurred? (◘ Fig. 4.21 (Atlas))
  - Inadequate fistula flow due to diversion of blood flow into (parallel) accessory veins (◘ Figs. 4.6 and 4.16 (Atlas))
- **Peripheral ischemia**
  - Hyperfunctioning fistula (DASS) (◘ Fig. 4.5; ◘ Figs. 4.10, 4.14, 4.17, and 4.20 (Atlas))
  - Arterial stenosis (◘ Fig. 4.12 (Atlas))
  - (Prominent accessory vein (◘ Figs. 4.6, 4.16 and 4.20 (Atlas)))
- **Arm swelling**
  - Stenosis/Thrombus of draining vein (◘ Figs. 4.15, 4.18, 4.19, and 4.20 (Atlas))
  - Prominent accessory vein with blood flow (retrograde) parallel to fistula flow (◘ Figs. 4.16, 4.19, and 4.20 (Atlas))
- **Degenerative dilatation** (◘ Fig. 4.11 (Atlas)), **pseudoaneurysm** (◘ Fig. 4.11 (Atlas)), **infection**

Hemodialysis patients may present with complex clinical problems as a result of the intricate hemodynamic patterns that may develop in and around their vascular access over time. Such cases require an individual sonographic approach to obtain a comprehensive overview of the vascular situation including possible differential diagnoses, which is essential for identifying the best therapeutic strategy.

4.9 Atlas: Arteriovenous Fistulas

◘ Table 4.5 lists the figures presented in the Atlas. The figures illustrate normal findings, methodology, and vascular abnormalities in patients with an arteriovenous fistula.

◘ **Table 4.5** Arteriovenous fistulas – figures

Entity/Pathology	Figure
Spontaneous AV fistula	◘ Fig. 4.7 (Atlas), page 280
Iatrogenic AV fistula	◘ Fig. 4.8 (Atlas), page 280
Hemodialysis access – normal findings and volume flow measurement	◘ Fig. 4.9 (Atlas), page 281
Hemodyalisis access complications – high-flow fistula, peripheral ischemia; volume flow measurement	◘ Fig. 4.10 (Atlas), page 282
Fistula flow volume calculation from measurement in the feeding artery (brachial artery) without and with fistula compression	◘ Fig. 4.10 (Atlas), page 283
Aneurysm of hemodialysis access – puncture aneurysm, suture aneurysm, degenerative dilatation	◘ Fig. 4.11 (Atlas), page 284
Stenosis of proximal feeding artery	◘ Fig. 4.12 (Atlas), page 285
Anastomotic stenosis	◘ Fig. 4.13 (Atlas), page 285
Hemodialysis access complication – peripheral ischemia, arterial steal	◘ Fig. 4.14 (Atlas), page 286
Hemodialysis access complication – reduced fistula flow, terminal cephalic vein stenosis	◘ Fig. 4.15 (Atlas), page 286
Hemodialysis access complication – peripheral ischemia	◘ Fig. 4.16 (Atlas), page 287
Peripheral ischemia after creation of hemodialysis access – accessory vein ligation	◘ Fig. 4.16 (Atlas), page 287
Peripheral ischemia – arterial steal with retrograde flow in palmar arch	◘ Fig. 4.17 (Atlas), page 288
Outflow obstruction – central vein thrombosis downstream of hemodialysis access	◘ Fig. 4.18 (Atlas), page 288
Peripheral ischemia – to-and-fro flow, anastomotic stenosis, accessory vein	◘ Fig. 4.19 (Atlas), page 289
Hemodialysis access complication – progressive swelling of forearm and hand	◘ Fig. 4.20 (Atlas), page 290
Failure of fistula maturation due to stenosis close to anastomosis	◘ Fig. 4.21 (Atlas), page 290

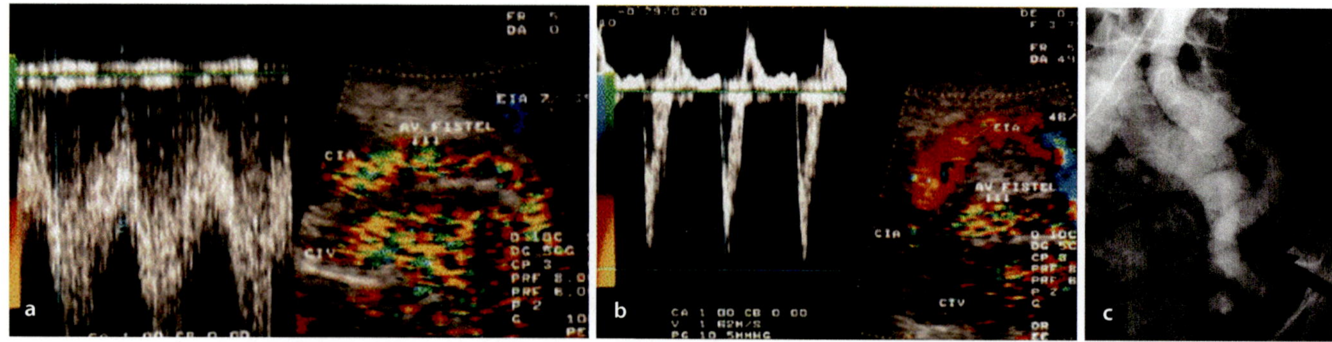

Fig. 4.7a–c (Atlas) Spontaneous AV fistula.
a Ultrasound examination to rule out thrombosis in a patient with leg swelling. The color flow image obtained while scanning the veins at the pelvic level shows a color bruit in the surrounding tissue, consistent with perivascular tissue vibration caused by an AV fistula. There is highly turbulent flow in the feeding common iliac artery (CIA) and in the internal iliac artery. The Doppler waveform from the internal iliac artery near the fistula shows the high diastolic flow typical of a short circuit between the arterial and venous system. The arched internal iliac artery is depicted with turbulent flow to the level of the fistula (mosaic of colors). Turbulent flow is also depicted in the common iliac vein (CIV) posterior to it. The elongated external iliac artery (EIA) is seen anteriorly.
b Unlike the internal iliac artery supplying the fistula, the external iliac artery (EIA) shows pulsatile, triphasic flow on color duplex and in the Doppler waveform. Using intermittent spectral Doppler interrogation along the internal iliac artery and vein, the examiner can gradually approach the site of the fistula, which is identified by an abrupt increase in peak systolic and especially diastolic velocities.
c Contrast medium flow in angiography reveals the AV short circuit in the pelvis. Ultrasonography is superior to angiography in precisely localizing the fistula. The arrows indicate the iliac artery and vein

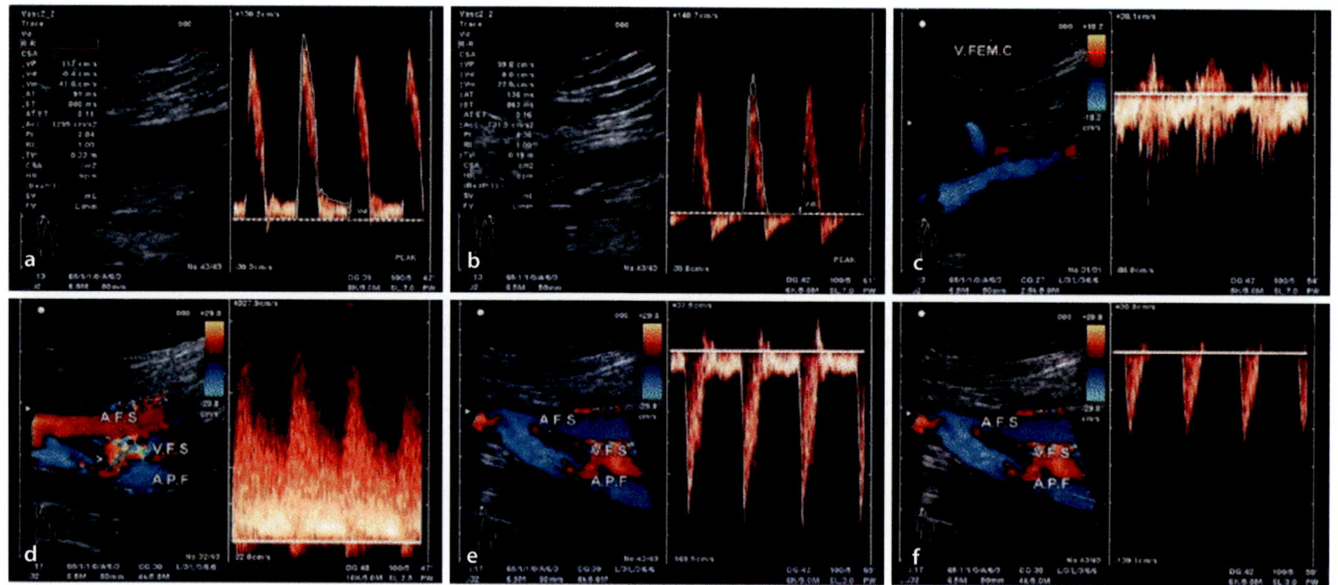

Fig. 4.8a–f (Atlas) Iatrogenic AV fistula.
a There is continuous diastolic flow in the common femoral artery on the right compared to the contralateral side. The time-averaged velocity (TAV) is 47.6 cm/s with a peak systolic velocity (PSV) of 117 cm/s and an end-diastolic velocity (EDV) of 10 cm/s.
b Comparison with the unaffected side shows flow in the left common femoral artery to be triphasic with a PSV of 99.8 cm/s and a TAV of 22.9 cm/s. The common femoral artery diameter is the same on both sides.
c The common femoral vein on the right has a pulsatile flow profile (with flow toward the center displayed in blue) characteristic of an arterialized vein draining an AV fistula (Fig. 4.2d).
d The case presented is a typical example of a iatrogenic AV fistula as a complication of cardiac catheterization. This type of iatrogenic fistula nearly always develops between the superficial femoral vein and the profunda femoris artery and typically occurs when the access site in the groin is chosen too low. The search for the fistula reveals the connection between the profunda femoris artery (A.P.F; blue flow away from transducer) to the superficial femoral vein (V.F.S) with a high-frequency flow signal (aliasing, red) and a flow velocity of over 3.5 m/s. Anteriorly, the superficial femoral artery is depicted (A.F.S; red, toward transducer).
e The Doppler waveform from the profunda femoris artery (A.P.F) proximal to the AV fistula shows a large diastolic flow component and the same flow profile as the common femoral artery.
f Distal to the AV fistula (see **d**), the profunda femoris artery (A.P.F; coded in blue) shows a triphasic profile without end-diastolic flow. This change in flow pattern proves that the AV fistula is located between the two sampling sites (in **e** and **f**)

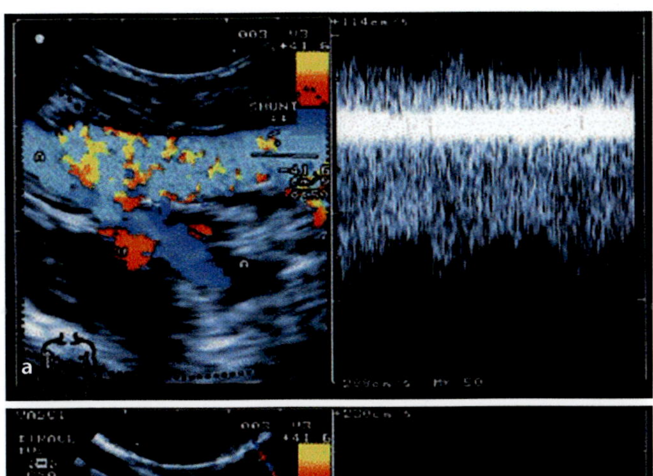

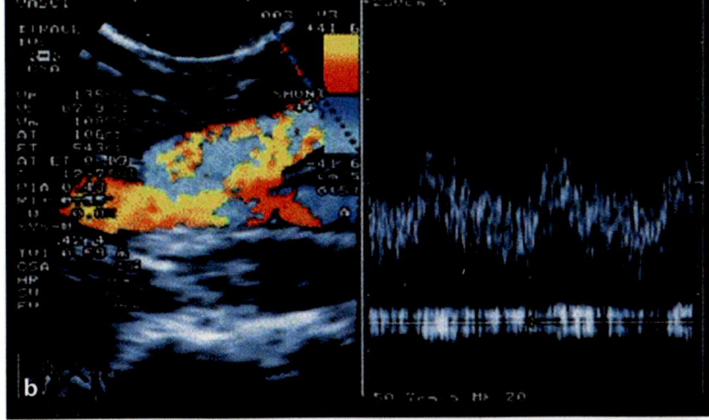

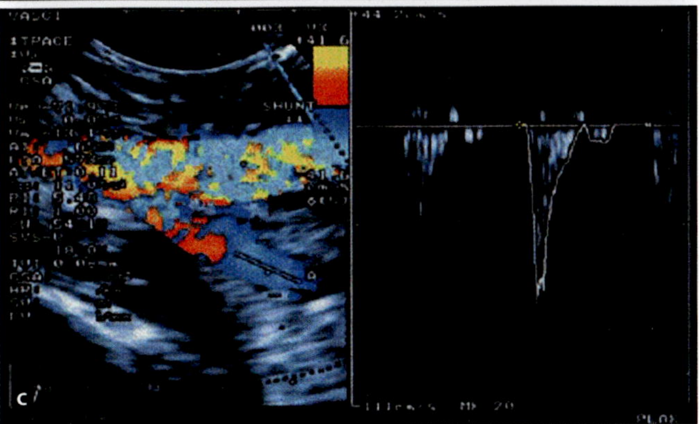

Fig. 4.9a–c (Atlas) Hemodialysis access – normal findings and volume flow measurement.
a Oblique image of the anastomosis of a Brescia-Cimino fistula (end-of-vein-to-side-of-artery anastomosis) in the bend of the elbow with marked turbulence at the anastomosis. Stretched brachial artery coursing posterior to the anastomosis.
b The color flow image (left) shows the proximal brachial artery with flow coded in red and mild aliasing on the left and the distal brachial artery on the right (coded blue). The sharp transition from red to blue appears to indicate flow reversal but is due to a change in flow direction relative to the transducer. In the color flow image, faster blood flow in the feeding artery is indicated by brighter colors. The Doppler waveform from the feeding artery (right) shows a large diastolic flow component (end-diastolic velocity (EDV) of 95 cm/s). With a calculated average flow velocity of 108 cm/s and a brachial artery diameter of 4.8 mm, the flow volume in the feeding artery is 1170 mL/min.
c The brachial artery segment distal to the AV fistula has the typical flow profile of arm arteries: triphasic waveform without an end-diastolic component. The flow volume calculated for the brachial artery segment just distal to the venous anastomosis is 129 mL/min ($0.16\ cm^2 \times 60 \times 13$ cm/s). The fistula flow volume, calculated as the difference in flow volumes between the brachial artery upstream and downstream of the venous anastomosis, is 1040 mL/min

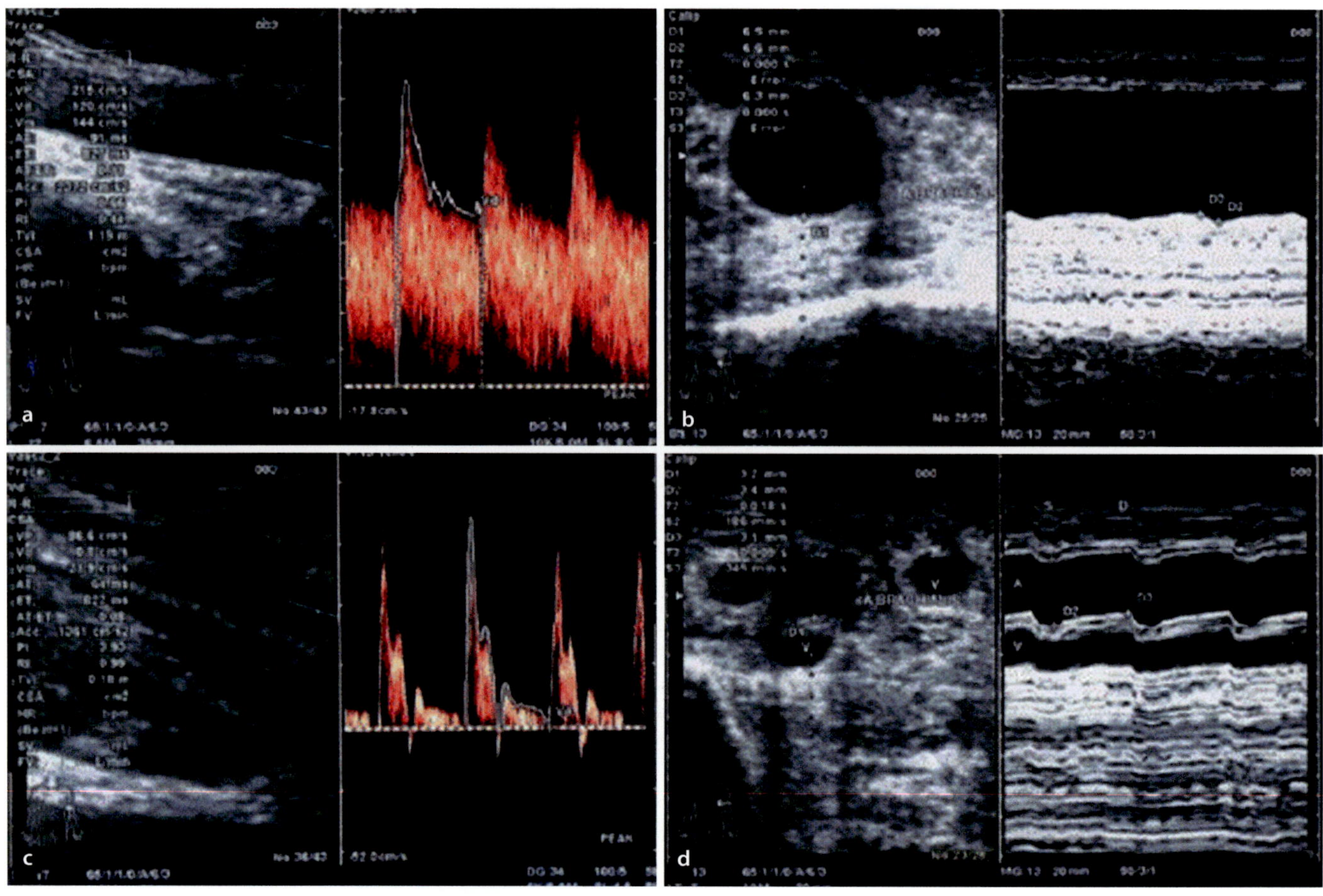

Fig. 4.10a–j (Atlas) Hemodyalisis access complications – high-flow fistula, peripheral ischemia; volume flow measurement. Excessive fistula flow can lead to dialysis access steal syndrome (DASS) with ischemia of the hand or cardiac insufficiency. Since hemodialysis patients often have considerable comorbidity, the fistula must be examined as a possible cause of newly occurring signs of cardiac insufficiency. Duplex ultrasound is the simplest and most reliable method for estimating the flow volume in the AV fistula. A more reliable method for determining fistula flow volume (compared with the method illustrated in Fig. 4.9b, c) is measurement of the flow volume in the brachial artery in both arms with calculation of the fistula flow volume as the difference between the fistula-bearing arm and the non-fistula-bearing arm.
a When this feature is available, the system's software calculates the mean time-averaged velocity (TAV) from the Doppler waveform recorded with an angle of less than 60° (144 cm/s in this case).
b At the same site, the vessel diameter is measured in the B-mode scan (6.5 mm). For accurate calculation of the vascular cross-sectional area, the systolic and diastolic diameters have to be measured (using the leading-edge method, Fig. 1.28) and weighted at a ratio of 1:2. This is done in the time-motion mode with an angle of insonation perpendicular to the vessel (i.e., as close to 90° as possible). In the example, a flow volume of 2778 mL/min is calculated from the mean TAV and cross-sectional area.
c The same measurements are performed in the brachial artery of the non-fistula-bearing arm, where the flow profile is triphasic with a mean TAV of 21.9 cm/s.
d After calculation of the mean cross-sectional area from the systolic and diastolic diameters, a mean flow volume of 108 mL/min is calculated. The example also illustrates the flow-induced dilatation of the arterial vessels as a cause of increased flow in long-standing AV fistulas (the diameter differences between the views with spectral Doppler displays (**a**, **c**) and those with time-motion displays (**b**, **d**) are due to the use of different scales).
e–j Fistula flow volume calculation from measurement in the feeding artery (brachial artery) without and with fistula compression.
e Patient presenting with peripheral ischemia and clinical dilation of the access vein 11 years after establishment of an AV fistula in the bend of the elbow. Sonographic measurement reveals dilatation of the feeding brachial artery with a systolic diameter of 6.8 mm and diastolic diameter of 6.4 mm, from which a vascular cross-sectional area of 0.34 cm^2 is calculated (with 1:2 weighting of systolic and diastolic diameters).
f Without compression of the fistula, the brachial artery upstream of the AV anastomosis has a time-averaged velocity (TAV) of 120 cm/s with a flow profile characteristic of an artery feeding an AV fistula.
g With manual compression of the fistula, TAV determined at the same site in the brachial artery is 10 cm/s, and the waveform is triphasic (which is the pattern characteristic of high-resistance flow in peripheral arteries). The fistula flow volume calculated from these measurements is high and is diagnostic of a hyperfunctioning AV fistula: $0.34 \times (120-10) = 37.4$ cm^3/s or 2.24 l/min (cross-sectional area multiplied by (TAV without fistula compression minus TAV with fistula compression)).
h Distal to the AV anastomosis, the brachial artery shows retrograde flow with a monophasic waveform, consistent with arterial steal.
i With manual compression of the AV fistula, there is normal flow to the periphery with a triphasic waveform in the distal brachial artery.
j Dilated access vein with large caliber variation (in part with oval vessel cross-section) and turbulent flow, which precludes reliable direct flow volume determination in the access vein

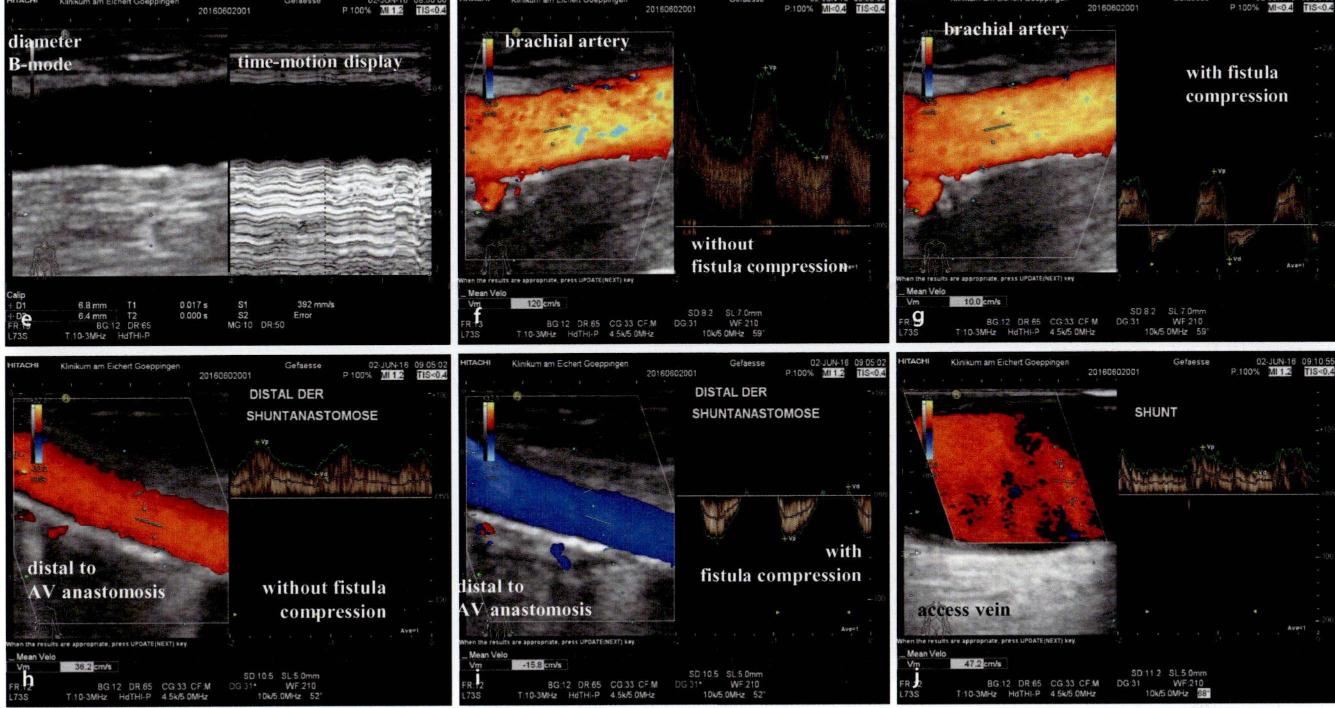

■ **Fig. 4.10** (continued)

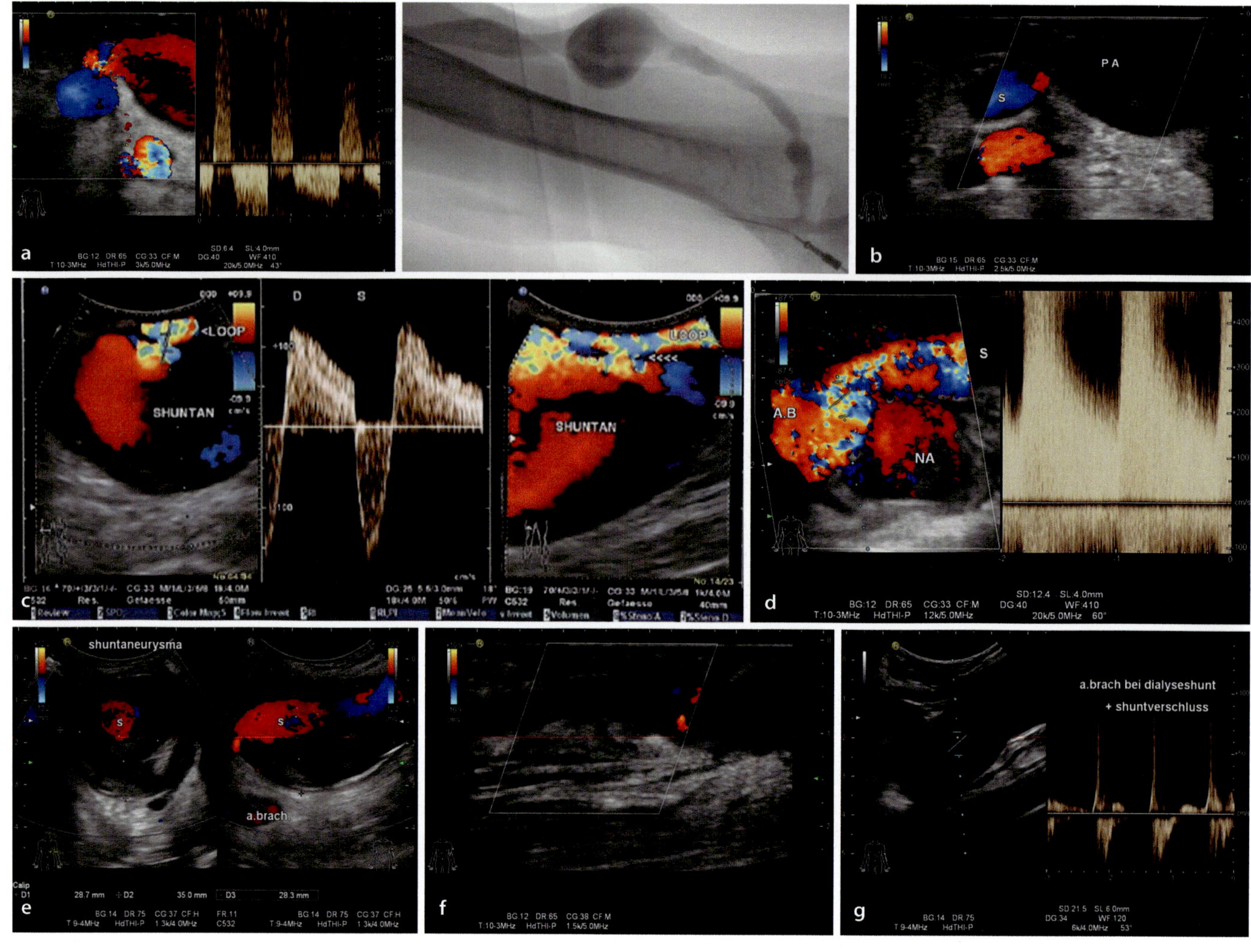

◘ Fig. 4.11a–g (Atlas) Aneurysm of hemodialysis access – puncture aneurysm, suture aneurysm, degenerative dilatation.
a A puncture aneurysm is a pseudoaneurysm with little tendency to thrombose spontaneously. It is frequently due to obstructed venous outflow (see ◘ Figs. 4.15 and 4.20 (Atlas)). In the case presented here, puncture aneurysm developed 6 years after creation of an AV fistula in the bend of the elbow. Color duplex and spectral Doppler show the typical features of a pseudoaneurysm: systolic inflow through the aneurysm neck and outflow from the sac throughout diastole. The standard treatment is surgical repair. In rare cases, it is possible to treat a fistula-related pseudoaneurysm by thrombin instillation. This requires very confident identification of the aneurysm neck and very strict precautions to minimize the risk of thrombin spillage. The measures to be taken include temporary complete manual compression of the fistula (blue) (confirmed by ultrasound) downstream of the aneurysm (red) to prevent escape into the outflow vein and throttling of inflow by placement of a tourniquet upstream of the aneurysm. With these precautions, thrombin instillation begins near the wall in the portion away from the neck using ultrasound to monitor correct needle placement. To avoid thrombosis, compression of the fistula must be released immediately after clotting of the aneurysm sac has occurred.
b Following thrombin injection, ultrasound confirms complete thrombosis of the puncture aneurysm (PA) with some residual pulsation in the aneurysm neck (red). The hemodialysis access (S, blue) is patent.
c Woman with a long history of hemodialysis and a loop in the thigh following loss of hemodialysis fistulas in both arms due to multiple complications. A posterior puncture aneurysm was suspected, due to iatrogenic piercing of the far wall of the access segment (SHUNTAN). The Doppler waveform obtained with the sample volume placed in the leak between the loop and the aneurysm shows the changes characteristic of a pseudoaneurysm: flow into the aneurysm (below the baseline, away from transducer) during systole (S) and back into the loop as a result of the changed pressure during diastole (above the baseline, toward transducer). In inconclusive cases, a spectral Doppler measurement can thus help differentiate between severe ectasia of the fistula (only in a direct AV fistula without an interposed conduit) and puncture aneurysm (pseudoaneurysm).
d Suture aneurysm and anastomotic stenosis in a patient with an AV fistula in the bend of the elbow (A.B = brachial artery, S = fistula vein). The sonographic findings include a PSV > 500 cm/s, aliasing, and turbulent flow.
e–g Brescia-Cimino fistula (> 10 years) with aneurysmal dilatation and partial thrombosis (**e**). The longitudinal image (**f**) shows that, due to thrombosis, the patent lumen of the dilated portion is of the same diameter as the adjacent normal segment (which is why this aneurysm would escape detection by angiography). There is a patent accessory branch vessel, and downstream of its origin, the access vein is occluded. At sites of frequent needle puncture, the access vein is narrowed due to scarring (left part of **f**). As a result of the long use of the fistula for hemodialysis, the feeding brachial artery is also dilated (**g**) and shows triphasic flow due to partial obstruction of the access vein. Based on these findings, the indication for creation of a new hemodialysis access can be established without additional diagnostic tests or prior attempts to revise the existing fistula

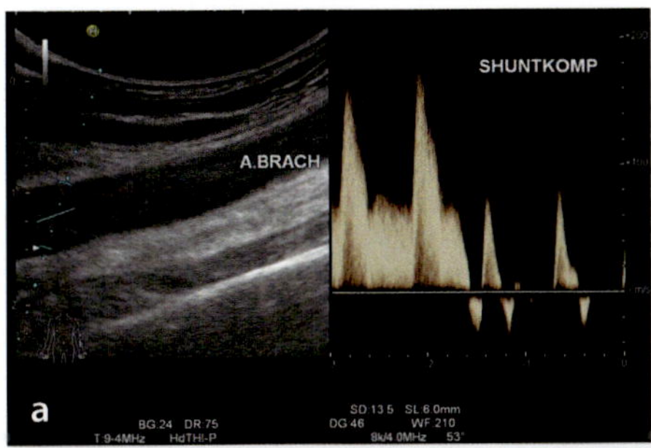

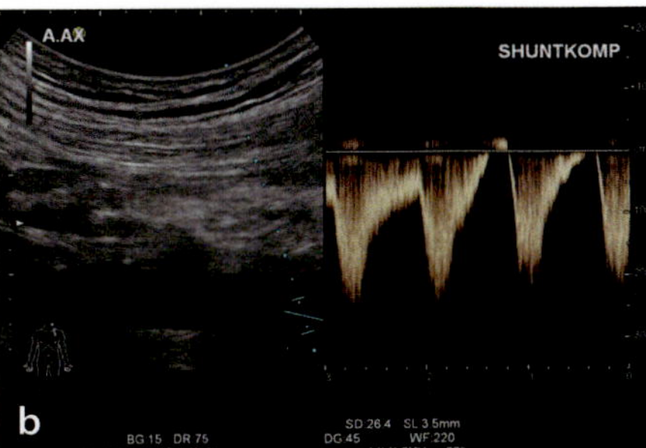

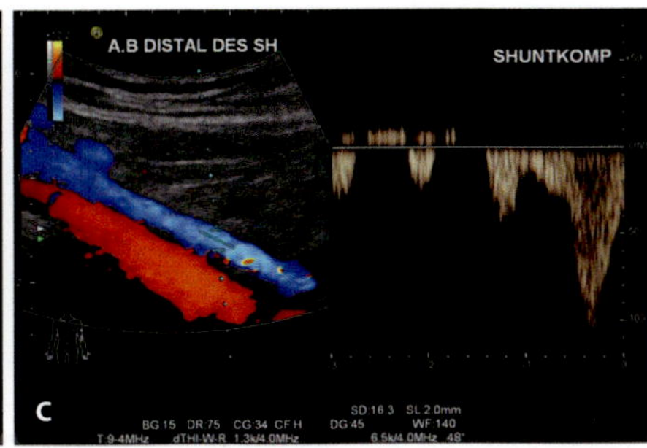

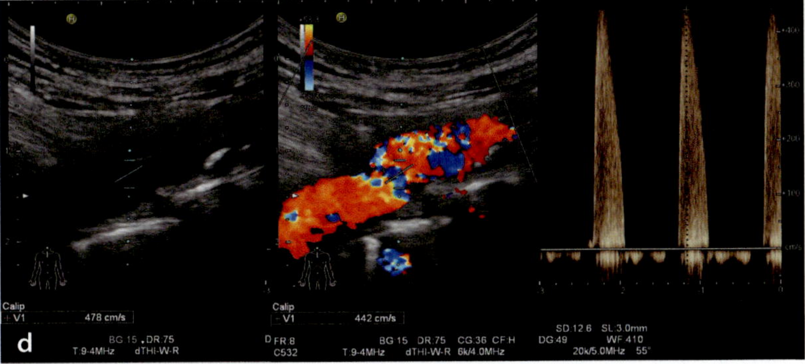

Fig. 4.12a–d (Atlas) Stenosis of proximal feeding artery.
a Brachial artery with the typical, monophasic flow profile of an artery feeding an AV fistula (left portion of waveform). With manual fistula compression (right portion of waveform, SHUNTKOMP), flow becomes triphasic (as in a peripheral artery without an AV fistula), and the indirect criteria can be used to rule out upstream (proximal) stenosis. (Without manual fistula compression, a triphasic waveform in the feeding artery of a hemodialysis access indicates occlusion of the access vein or high-grade venous outflow obstruction.)
b Patient with ischemic finger pad necrosis and higher-grade subclavian artery stenosis. Manual compression of the fistula results in decreased flow velocity in the axillary artery, and the spectral Doppler display (right portion of waveform, SHUNTKOMP) shows the indirect signs of upstream stenosis: delayed systolic upstroke (prolonged rise time) and monophasic flow profile.
c The Doppler waveform from the brachial artery distal to the venous anastomosis shows to-and-fro flow due to arterial steal; manual fistula compression elicits increase in flow (right portion of Doppler waveform, SHUNTKOMP) and features of poststenotic flow (monophasic profile with delayed systolic upstroke).
d The subclavian artery stenosis, the underlying cause of ischemia in this patient, can only be graded while the fistula is being compressed. During compression, a PSV of 450 cm/s is measured, indicating >75% stenosis. (Fistula compression allows the examiner to use both the direct and indirect criteria for peripheral artery stenosis grading also in individuals with an AV fistula)

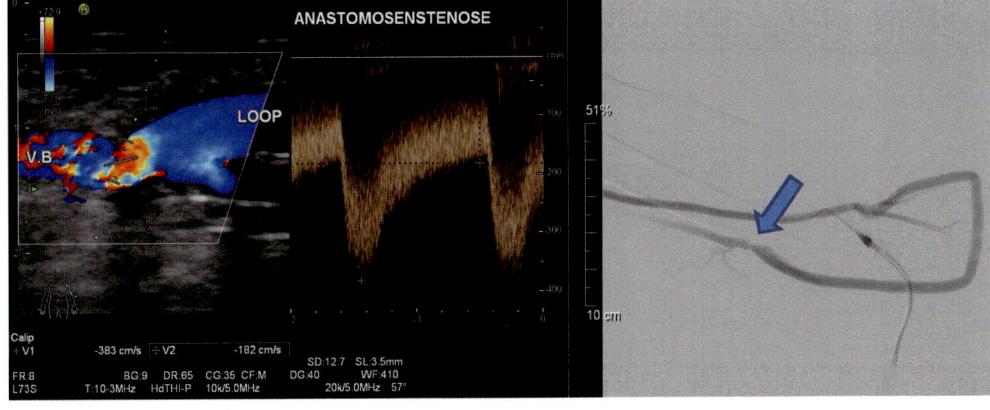

Fig. 4.13 (Atlas) Anastomotic stenosis.
Forearm loop AV graft with higher-grade stenosis at the venous anastomosis (PSV of 5 m/s). The stenosis (indicated by arrow in the angiogram) is difficult to evaluate or grade in a single angiographic projection

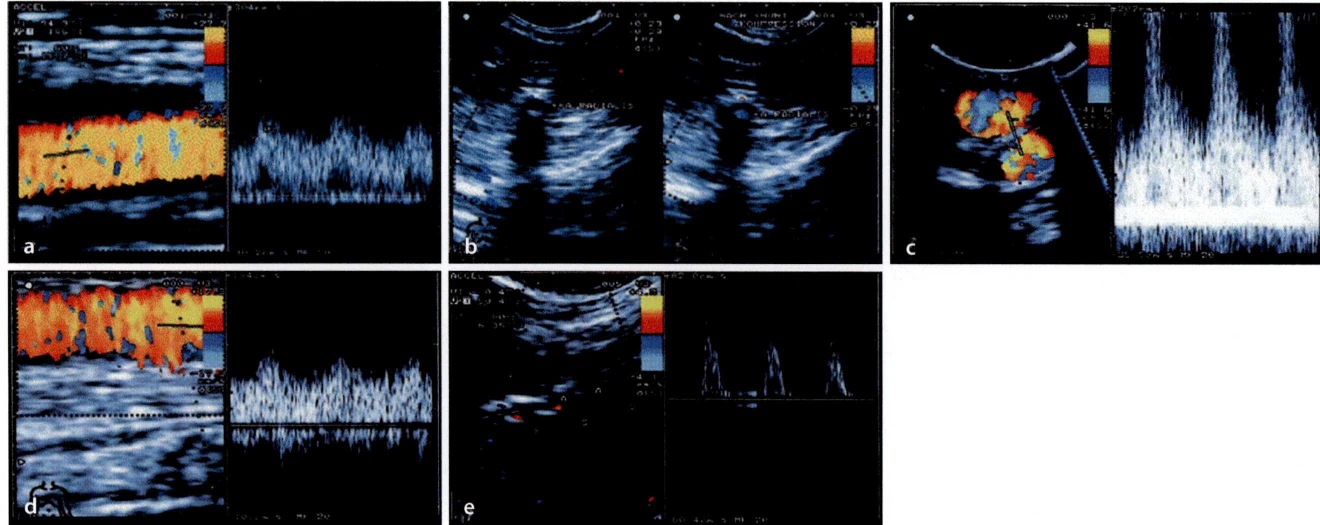

Fig. 4.14a–e (Atlas) Hemodialysis access complication – peripheral ischemia, arterial steal.
a A patient with a hemodialysis access in the bend of the elbow which functioned for many years developed ischemic necrosis of the finger pads. The AV fistula was found to be patent and showed a high flow rate with a peak systolic velocity (PSV) of 186 cm/s and end-diastolic velocity (EDV) of 94 cm/s.
b Without compression of the fistula, no flow is detected in the radial artery by color duplex or spectral Doppler. The transverse view of the radial artery on the left demonstrates marked medial sclerosis with posterior acoustic shadowing obscuring flow. The image on the right shows blood flow coded in blue in the radial artery upon compression of the fistula. Angiography also requires compression of the fistula to visualize the distal radial artery (not shown).
c Banding of the fistula causes stenosis in this area with a PSV of 280 cm/s and EDV of 100 cm/s.
d As a result of banding, there is a decrease in blood flow in the fistula (PSV of 95 cm/s and EDV of 60 cm/s).
e Although visualization is impaired by medial sclerosis, flow with a PSV of 50 cm/s is detectable in the radial artery (A) after banding. However, only isolated spot-like flow signals are depicted in the radial artery despite a high gain (indicated by posterior artifacts due to overmodulation) and a low PRF. The calcified plaques and medial sclerosis cause acoustic scattering and shadowing (S)

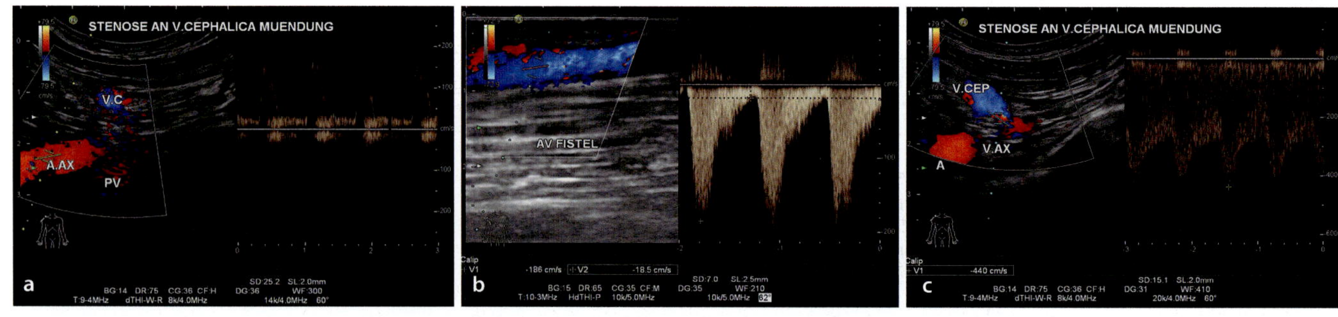

Fig. 4.15a–c (Atlas) Hemodialysis access complication – reduced fistula flow, terminal cephalic vein stenosis.
a In a patient with a long-standing Brescia-Cimino fistula, there is increased pulsatility of arterial inflow, shown here in the axillary artery. Color bruit (PV, perivascular vibration) is seen in the tissue adjacent to a high-grade stenosis at the termination of the cephalic vein (VC) (see **c**).
b The hemodialysis access is patent and shows normal flow, but pulsatility is increased as well (reduced diastolic flow velocity), consistent with increased venous drainage resistance more centrally.
c In this patient, reduced flow with increased pulsatility in the fistula is due to a high-grade stenosis of the terminal cephalic vein (V.CEP) (which takes an arched course and is difficult to image in a single plane) with a PSV >420 cm/s. This hemodialysis access problem can present with arm swelling (V.ax = axillary vein)

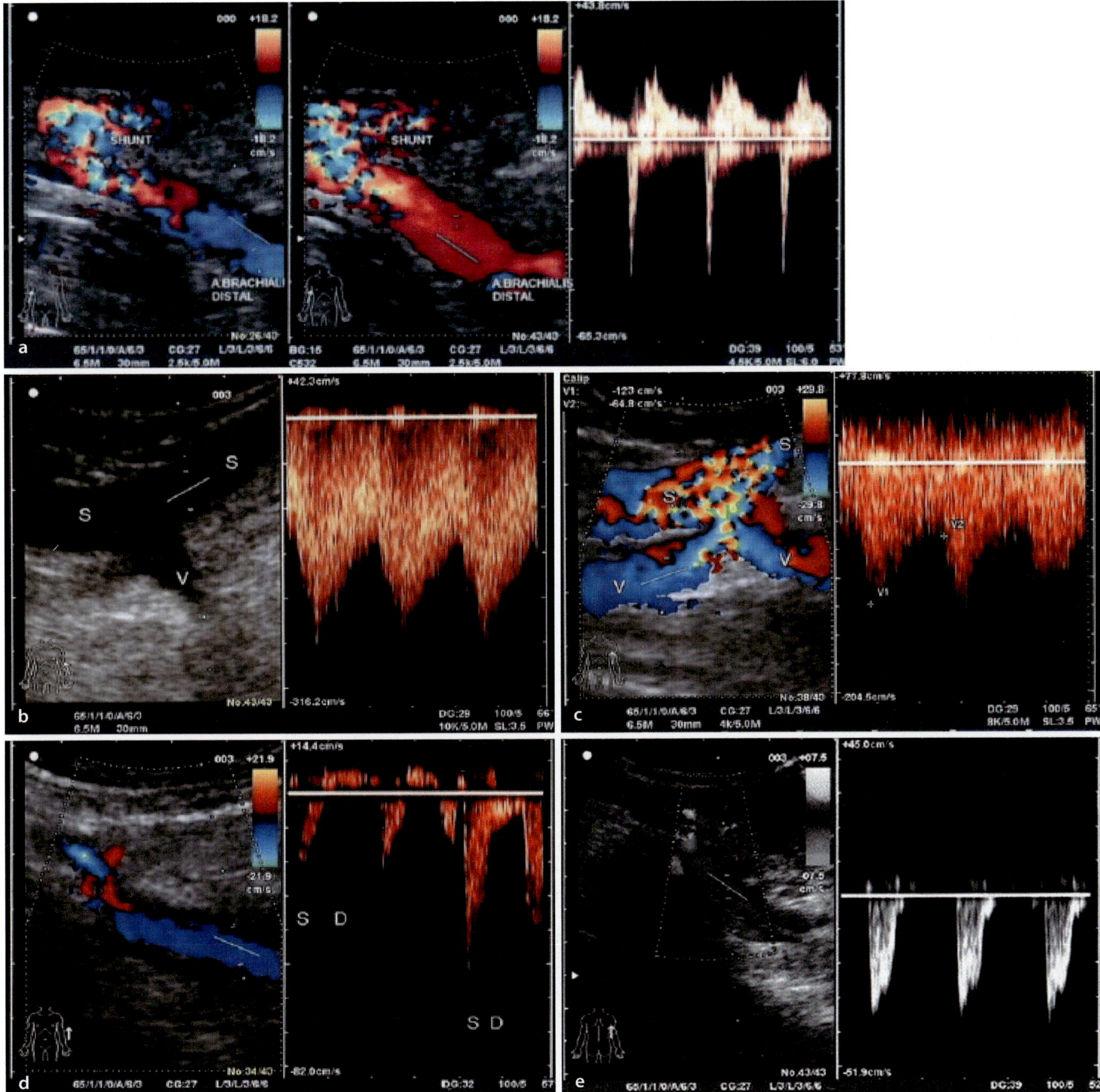

Fig. 4.16a–e (Atlas) Hemodialysis access complication – peripheral ischemia.
a Patient with hemodialysis access in the bend of the elbow presenting with peripheral ischemia and hand pain. High flow through the fistula causes to-and-fro flow in the brachial artery distal to the venous anastomosis. The alternating forward and backward flow is demonstrated both by color duplex (systolic flow away from transducer depicted in blue and diastolic flow toward transducer and fistula depicted in red) and spectral Doppler. To-and-fro flow in the distal feeding artery in conjunction with a high-flow fistula does not cause peripheral ischemia when perfusion is maintained via collaterals.
b–e Peripheral ischemia after creation of hemodialysis access – accessory vein ligation.
b When banding or any other type of fistula revision including closure is contemplated, the course of the fistula vein should be evaluated to search for accessory branches or communications with deeper veins. If flow in such an accessory vein is high, it can divert blood away from the access vein. In the example shown, the cephalic vein, which is the access vein (S), is only slightly dilated with a diameter of 1.2 cm, but flow is high with a peak systolic velocity (PSV) of approximately 2.5 m/s (upstream of the origin of the accessory vein).
c There are two dilated accessory veins (V) with diameters of 8 and 7 mm. The Doppler waveform from one of the veins shows a PSV of 123 cm/s and an end-diastolic velocity (EDV) of 60 cm/s with similar velocities in the second vein (waveform not shown).
d There is to-and-fro flow in the proximal radial artery shortly after its origin from the brachial artery: slow orthograde flow during systole with a PSV of 20 cm/s and diastolic backward flow (D) with an EDV of 8 cm/s. Compression of the fistula (right) results in systolic and diastolic forward flow (into the periphery, away from transducer) with a postischemic increase in the diastolic component (PSV of 40 cm/s and EDV of 10 cm/s).
e The accessory veins described in **c** were sonographically marked and exposed for ligation to improve hand perfusion and salvage the dialysis access. Following revision, the improved hemodynamic situation is demonstrated by repeat spectral Doppler measurement at the same site as in **d**: orthograde flow is restored (without backward flow), and the PSV is 35 cm/s (compare the waveform in **d**). The patient's symptoms resolved after the intervention

Fig. 4.17a–c (Atlas) Peripheral ischemia – arterial steal with retrograde flow in palmar arch.
a Patient with a dilated Brescia-Cimino fistula in the wrist (12 mm diameter) and ischemic pain in the finger pads but with an otherwise well-functioning access (fistula not shown). There is high flow in the proximal radial artery (not shown) with retrograde flow in the distal segment (coded in red, toward transducer). The Doppler waveform confirms retrograde flow with reduced systolic flow velocity (S) and a high end-diastolic flow velocity (EDV) of 75 cm/s (D). Compression of the fistula elicits flow reversal (KOMP SHUNT) with an orthograde flow direction (away from transducer) and a large diastolic flow component (postischemic) in the radial artery.
b The ulnar artery shows high orthograde flow (aliasing in the color flow image) toward the periphery (coded in blue, away from transducer; below the baseline in the waveform). The Doppler waveform is that of an artery supplying an AV fistula with a large diastolic component (EDV of 44 cm/s) and a high PSV of 100 cm/s. Upon compression of the fistula (KOMP SHUNT), the flow pattern normalizes (triphasic flow characteristic of peripheral arteries) with a PSV of 45 cm/s. These findings are consistent with arterial steal due to a high-flow fistula; arterial blood flow is insufficient, and the ulnar artery is recruited to also supply the fistula via the palmar arch, which explains the retrograde flow in the radial artery distal to the fistula. Based on these sonographic findings, the patient underwent ligation of the radial artery distal to the fistula. This measure eliminated arterial steal and restored adequate blood supply to the hand through the ulnar artery.
c Drawing illustrating blood flow in this situation (arrows indicate flow direction)

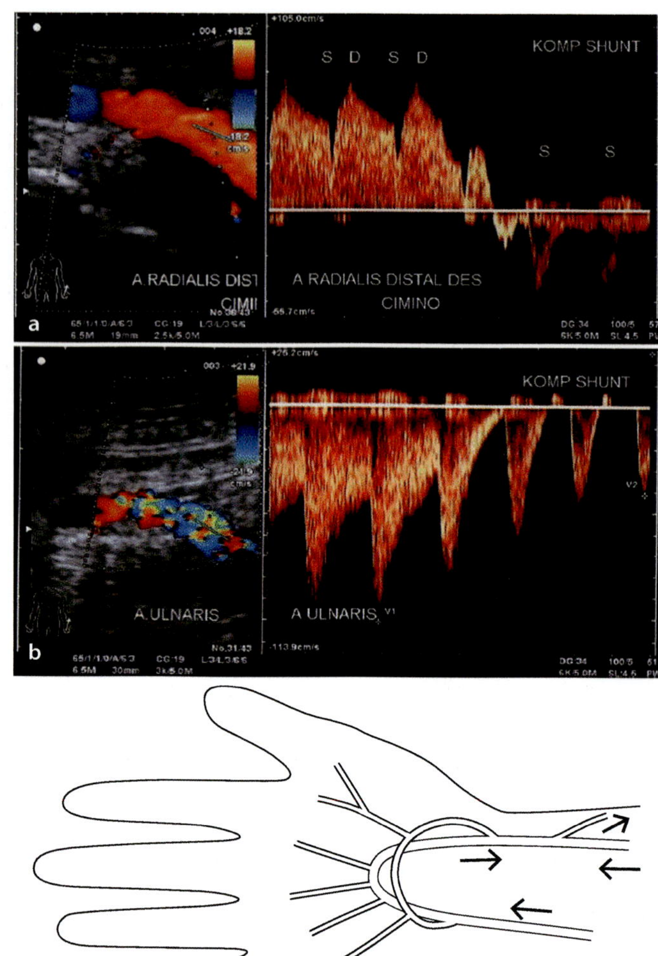

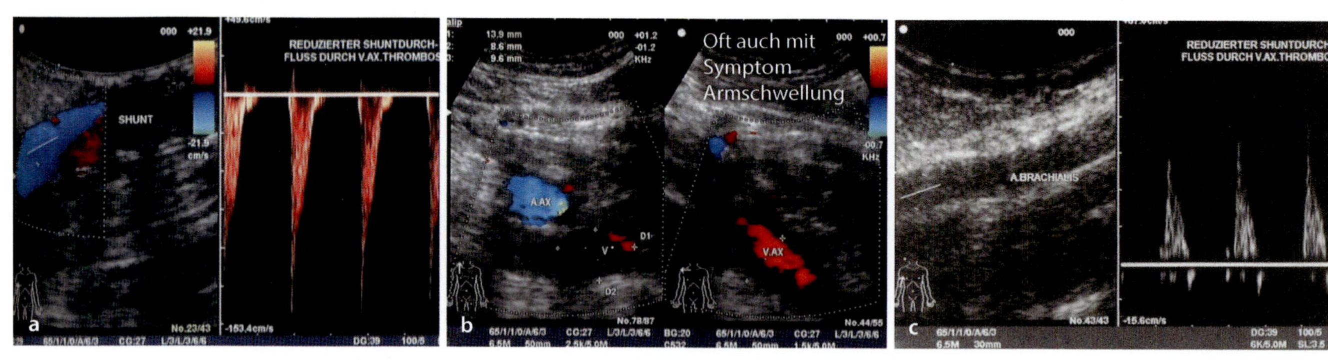

Fig. 4.18a–c (Atlas) Outflow obstruction – central vein thrombosis downstream of hemodialysis access.
In patients with a stenotic lesion upstream of a hemodialysis access, the Doppler waveform from the fistula is less pulsatile with a delayed systolic upstroke and an increased diastolic flow component (resembling venous flow). Conversely, impaired venous drainage (thrombosis, stenosis, compression) results in a more pulsatile flow profile.
a The Doppler waveform from the hemodialysis access lacks a diastolic component, suggesting an increased flow resistance (flow obstruction) downstream of the site of sampling.
b Color duplex imaging demonstrates thrombosis of the axillary vein with some residual flow near the walls coded in red. The lumen of the vein (V) is nearly completely filled by the thrombus.
c The outflow obstruction leads to high-resistance flow in the brachial artery feeding the hemodialysis fistula, which is indicated by a return to a triphasic waveform (i.e., the flow profile characteristic of normal peripheral arteries). When inadequate blood flow during hemodialysis is due to impaired venous drainage, this is suggested by spectral Doppler interrogation of the feeding artery or of the access vein and then confirmed by continuous evaluation of venous outflow to identify the site of obstruction. In the case presented here, thrombosis of the axillary vein was revealed. In patients with a synthetic loop graft, the differential diagnosis of a triphasic waveform includes stenosis of the venous anastomosis

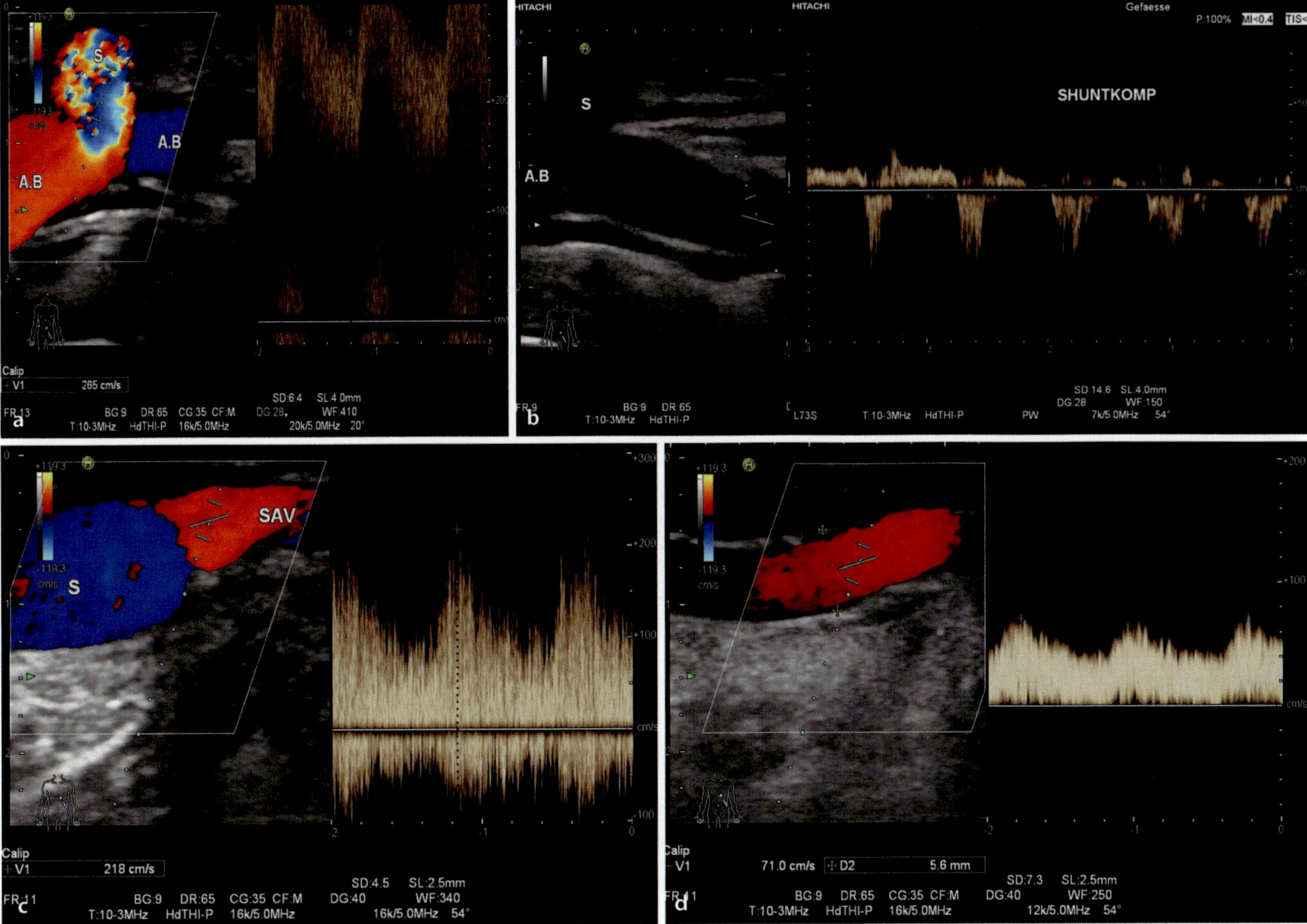

Fig. 4.19a–d (Atlas) Peripheral ischemia – to-and-fro flow, anastomotic stenosis, accessory vein.
a Patient with AV fistula (S) in the bend of the elbow (A.B = brachial artery) presenting with peripheral ischemia and mild swelling of the hand. The ultrasound examination reveals high-grade anastomotic stenosis (aliasing, peak systolic velocity (PSV) of >6 m/s, peak end-diastolic velocity (EDV) of 2.5 m/s).
b Despite the high-grade anastomotic stenosis, there is to-and-fro flow in the brachial artery distal to the venous anastomosis. During manual fistula compression, forward flow is restored in this segment.
c Close evaluation of the fistula vein (displayed in blue; S) identifies a large accessory vein (red; SAV) with blood flow into the hand.
d Color flow imaging and spectral Doppler interrogation demonstrate a large flow volume in the accessory vein (PSV of 80 cm/s, diameter of 1 cm) with blood flow to the periphery (red). The accessory vein was marked, and subsequent ligation led to resolution of peripheral pain and hand swelling. The anastomotic stenosis was left untreated

4

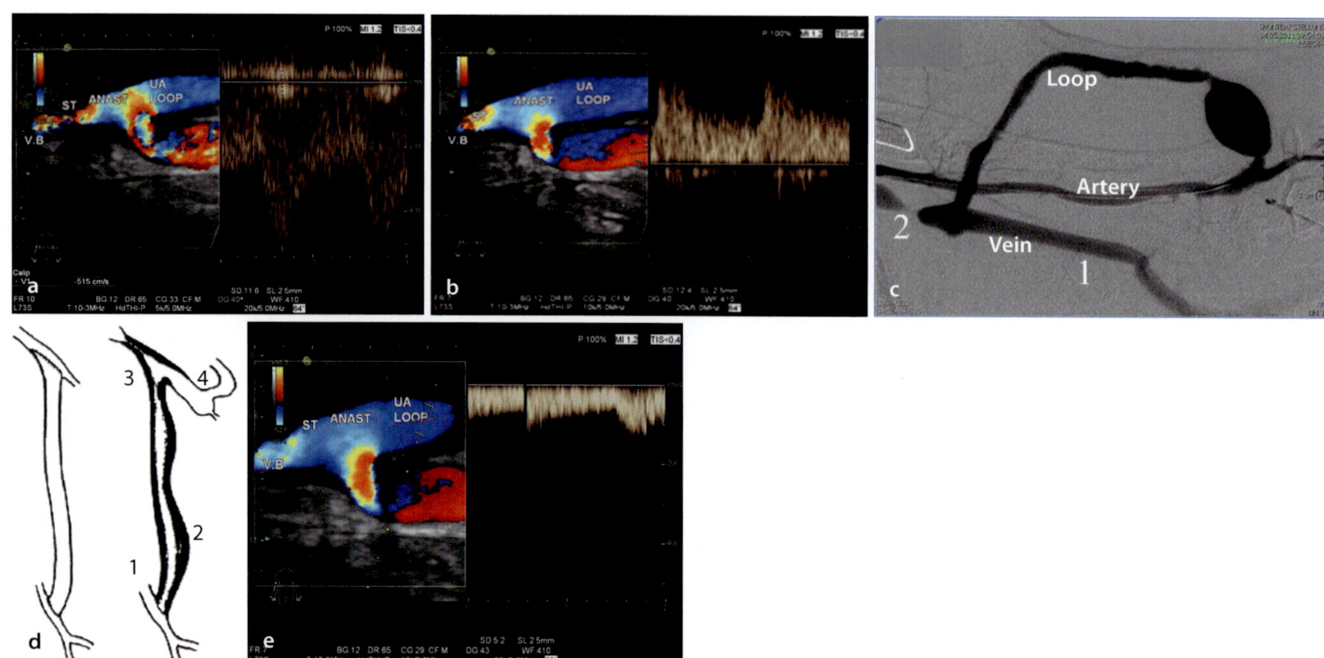

Fig. 4.20a–e (Atlas) a–c Hemodialysis access complication – progressive swelling of forearm and hand. Patient with a history of interposition of a synthetic graft (onto basilic vein) to replace a failing AV fistula 1 year before presenting with progressive swelling of the forearm and hand.

a Duplex ultrasound with a peak systolic velocity (PSV) of up to 5.5 m/s indicates high-grade stenosis (ST) of the basilic vein (V.B) just central to the venous anastomosis (ANAST).

b The stenosis causes flow toward the hand in the dilated basilic vein distal to the anastomosis (red, flow toward transducer). Venous drainage to the hand is the cause of hand swelling in this patient. As a result of this reversed venous drainage, the more central stenosis (see Fig. 4.15) causes neither increased pulsatility in the access segment nor a drop in blood flow below the limit required for adequate hemodialysis function. However, the stenosis may cause dilatation, prolonged bleeding after hemodialysis, and puncture aneurysm.

c The PTA angiogram obtained on the basis of the ultrasound findings provides an overview of the complex flow situation with central stenosis of venous drainage and dilatation of the vein peripheral to the anastomosis (right).

d Diagram of late morphologic changes in an AV fistula for hemodialysis (right drawing): stenosis at venous anastomosis (3); dilatation of access vein and scarring due to frequent puncture (2); dilatation of distal draining vein (4); stenotic changes of feeding artery due to progressive atherosclerosis (1) (From Scholz 1998).

e Normal hemodialysis flow despite high-grade stenosis of the access vein central to the anastomosis (**a**). Normal flow is ensured due to venous drainage via retrograde flow in forearm veins. Aliasing in the center of the image (yellow and red colors at the origin of the draining vein, which shows red-coded, retrograde flow) is due to a very small Doppler angle at this site (with the beam tangential to the direction of blood flow) (see Figs. 1.18b and 1.50b)

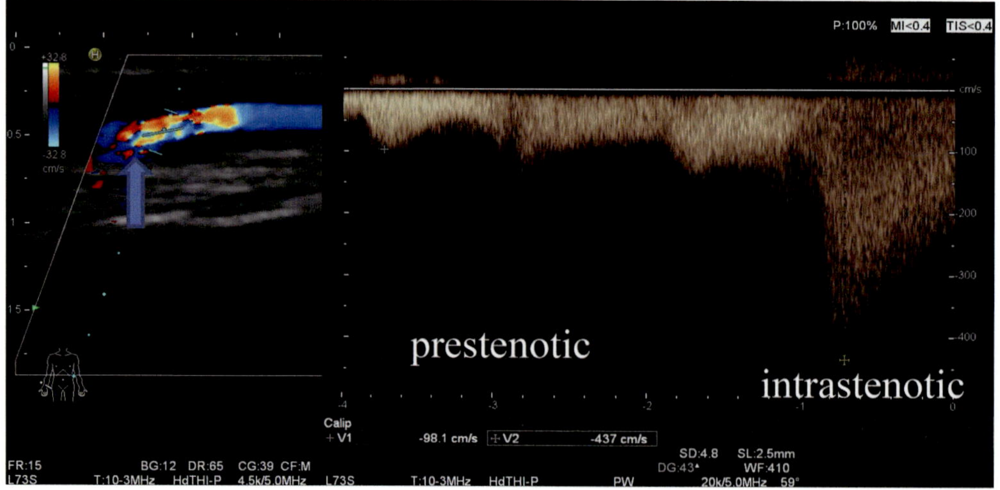

Fig. 4.21 (Atlas) Failure of fistula maturation due to stenosis close to anastomosis. Patient with a persistent thin access vein (2 mm) 5 weeks after creation of an AV hemodialysis access. Ultrasound identifies high-grade stenosis as the underlying cause (arrow; with a peak systolic velocity (PSV) ratio > 4; calculated from an intrastenotic PSV of 437 cm/s and a prestenotic PSV of 98 cm/s). The stenosis is not apparent morphologically (B-mode image), only in the waveform. The possible cause is an intimal flap or intraoperative trauma (for intimal flap see Fig. 4.4)

Extracranial Cerebral Arteries

W. Schäberle, *Ultrasonography in Vascular Diagnosis*, https://doi.org/10.1007/978-3-319-64997-9_5

Cardiovascular disease is the most common cause of death in Western industrialized countries. The most serious cerebrovascular manifestation is stroke with its complications, which is fatal in one third of cases. Patients who survive cerebral infarction often suffer from irreversible damage and paralysis and require permanent care. With atherosclerosis of the carotid artery circulation becoming more common with age, cerebral infarction gains relevance as the population ages (Fabres et al. 1994; Mannami et al. 2000; Roederer et al. 1984). Over 60–70% of all ischemic cerebral infarctions are caused by arterial embolism, typically arising from the carotid artery (Bock et al. 1993; Evans 1999; Roederer et al. 1984).

Carotid endarterectomy (CEA), first performed by De Bakey in 1953, is a highly effective surgical procedure for reducing the risk of stroke in patients with atherosclerosis of the carotid system. This has been confirmed in several large trials in individuals with symptomatic carotid artery stenosis performed in Europe (European Carotid Surgery Trial (ECST)) and the USA (North American Symptomatic Carotid Endarterectomy Trial (NASCET)) as well as in an asymptomatic population (Asymptomatic Carotid Atherosclerosis Study (ACAS)) (◘ Table 5.1). These studies compared the natural history with the morbidity and mortality after carotid surgery stratified by clinical stage and degree of carotid artery stenosis. The results of all three studies suggest that carotid reconstruction is beneficial in individuals with symptomatic high-grade stenosis (>70%) and in selected cases of 60–70% symptomatic stenosis. In high-grade asymptomatic stenosis, however, surgical repair is beneficial only in individuals with a low risk of perioperative morbidity and plaque morphology predictive of a high risk of embolism.

Suitable diagnostic tests are necessary for identifying those patients who will benefit from the therapeutic measures confirmed in these large trials to be advantageous. More specifically, this involves identifying individuals with carotid stenosis who are at a high risk of embolism and will benefit from CEA. Color duplex ultrasound is a noninvasive method that can be repeated at any time and has evolved into a highly accurate method for quantifying the degree of carotid stenosis (the risk of embolism increases with the degree of stenosis). Moreover, sonography also provides information on plaque morphology, the second major factor affecting the risk of embolism. Another feature associated with the risk of embolism and inflammatory activity is plaque neovascularization, which can be evaluated by contrast-enhanced ultrasound (CEUS).

The superficial course of the carotid arteries, without interfering structures, enables detailed sonographic evaluation of the arterial segment accounting for the majority of cerebral infarctions. Given these ideal scanning conditions and the fact that the vast majority of carotid stenoses occur at the origin of the internal carotid artery (ICA), continuous wave (CW) Doppler ultrasound alone is already highly accurate in detecting higher-grade carotid stenosis.

(Color) duplex ultrasound provides both morphologic and blood flow information, thus enabling precise evaluation of arterial lesions and their locations in conjunction with determination of their hemodynamic relevance based on the measurement of angle-corrected spectral Doppler velocities. Sonographic assessment of plaque morphology contributes further information for estimating the risk of embolism. Taken together, the sonographic findings are sufficient to identify candidates for surgery or medical management of carotid artery stenosis without the need for additional invasive tests.

◘ Table 5.1 Results of randomized multicenter trials comparing surgical versus medical treatment of symptomatic (NASCET, ECST) and asymptomatic carotid artery stenosis (ACAS)

Parameter	NASCET	ECST	ACAS
No. of patients	659	778	1659
- Surgical management	328	455	825
- Medical management	331	323	834
Perioperative stroke rate	2.1%	6.6%	1.4%
Morbidity/mortality rate (natural history)	5.8%	7.5%	2.3%
Risk reduction (relative)	65%	43%	53%
- Men			66%
- Women			17%

NASCET North American Symptomatic Carotid Endarterectomy Trial, *ECST* European Carotid Surgery Trial, *ACAS* Asymptomatic Carotid Atherosclerosis Study

5.1 Normal Vascular Anatomy and Important Variants

5.1.1 Carotid Arteries

The brain derives its blood supply from the two carotid arteries and the two vertebral arteries. The latter unite at the inferior border of the pons to form the basilar artery. In over 70% of individuals, the left common carotid artery (CCA) arises directly from the aortic arch before the origin of the subclavian artery (◘ Fig. 5.1a). The right CCA originates from the brachiocephalic trunk or artery (innominate artery), which arises from the aortic arch and additionally gives off the subclavian artery. The most important variants of the supra-aortic arteries, which originally developed from the branchial arches, are:

- Common origin of the brachiocephalic trunk and left CCA from the aortic arch (13%)
- Persisting communicating trunk arising from the aortic arch and giving off first the left CCA and then the brachiocephalic trunk (9%)
- Bilateral brachiocephalic trunk dividing into the CCA and the subclavian artery (1%)
- Situs inversus (very rare).

5

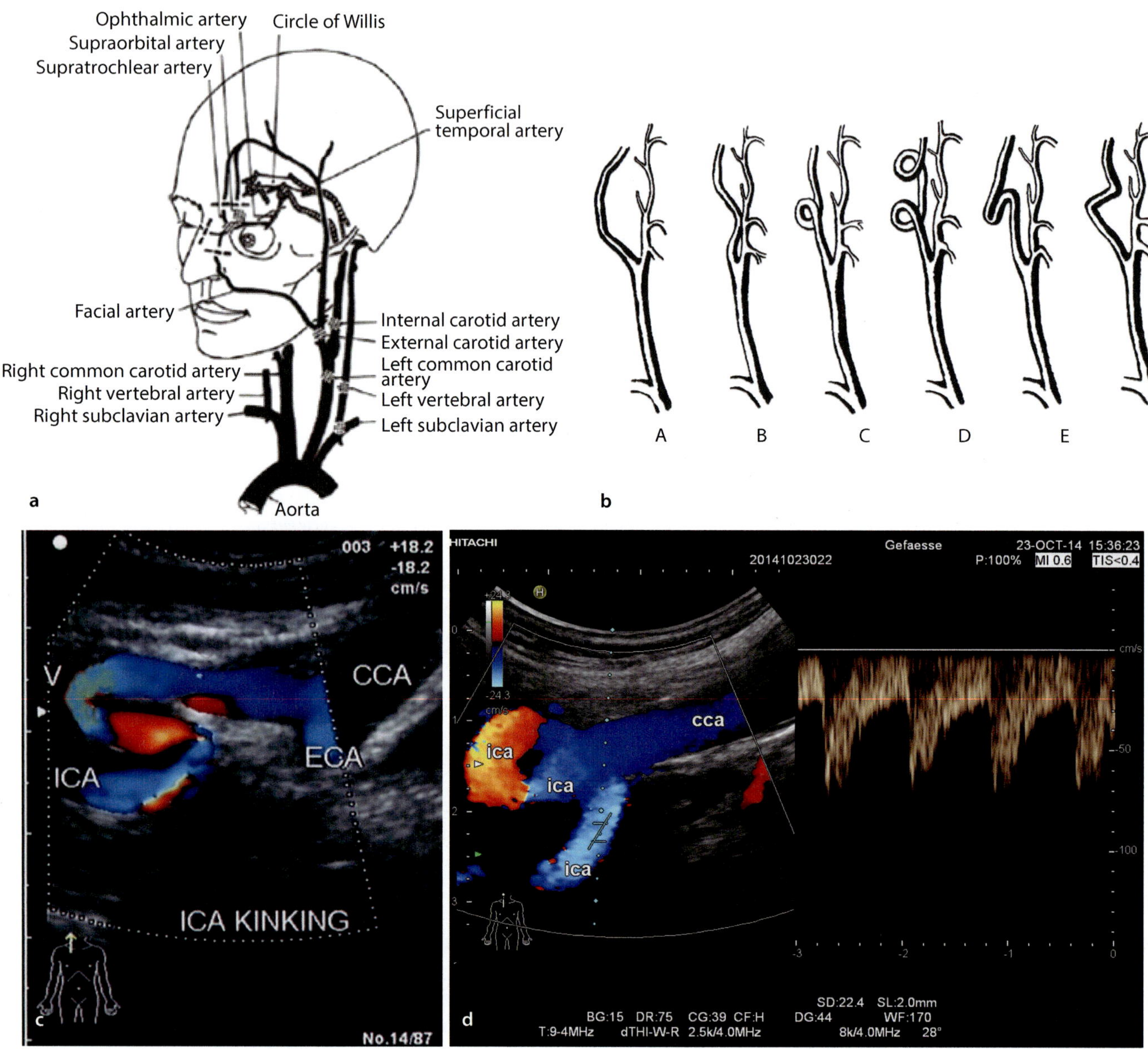

Fig. 5.1 **a** Diagram of the arteries supplying the brain (marked are the sites for taking representative measurements and documenting results). **b** Variants resulting from elongation of the internal carotid artery (ICA) (shown for the left artery): **A** C-shaped course, **B** S-shaped course, **C** coiling, **D** double coiling, **E** kinking, **F** double kinking. **c** Color flow image showing severe kinking of the ICA (corresponding to **E** in **b**), indicated by a change in blood flow direction relative to the transducer (change from blue to red color coding). **d** Color flow image showing coiling of the ICA (corresponding to **C** in **b**), indicated by a change in color coding due to a change in flow direction relative to the transducer (blue – away from transducer/toward the heart; red – toward transducer)

The normal brachiocephalic trunk on the right has a length of 4–5 cm. It crosses under the brachiocephalic vein and, behind the right sternoclavicular joint, divides into the right subclavian artery and the right CCA.

The two CCAs course cranially accompanied by the vagus nerve and the internal jugular vein, which runs anterolateral to the carotids. The carotid bifurcation is usually located at the C4–C5 level, which roughly corresponds to the level of the thyroid cartilage, but there is wide interindividual variation (Fig. 5.2). Typically, the larger ICA arises from the posterolateral aspect. It has a widened portion at its origin, called the carotid bulb. Unlike the external carotid artery (ECA), the ICA does not give off branches along its extracranial course.

Elongation of the ICA is associated with **kinking** (90° angle between adjacent segments) or **coiling** (360° loop) (Fig. 5.1b–d). Carotid elongation develops with age. Arterial hypertension is considered a predisposing factor. Kinking or coiling results from the limited space available between the two points of fixation, the bifurcation and the base of skull, but even severe kinking rarely causes hemodynamically significant stenosis (see Fig. 5.51 (Atlas)).

The ECA arises from the anteromedial aspect of the ICA; in approx. 10% of individuals its point of origin is lateral or posterolateral. On its course, it first gives off the superior thyroid artery (STA) and then branches to supply the skin and extracranial organs (facial and temporal arteries).

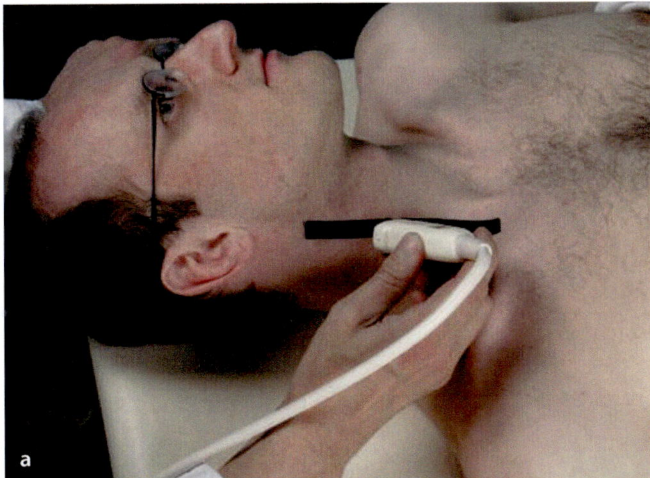

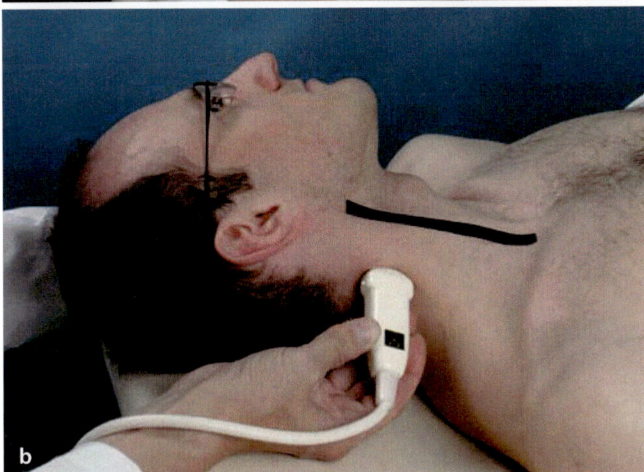

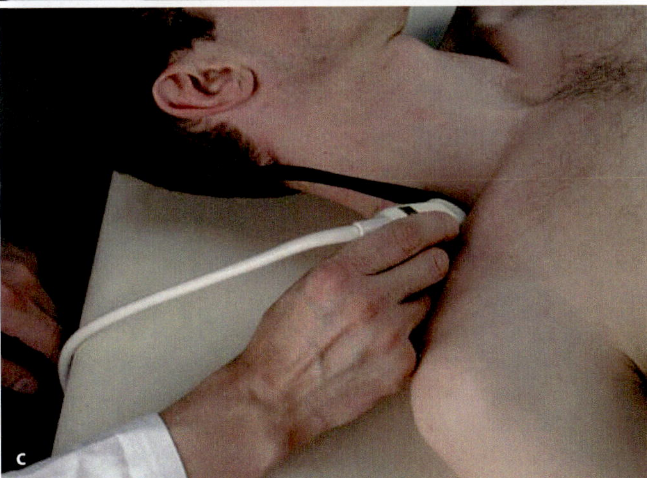

Fig. 5.2 Transducer positions for examination of the extracranial carotid artery and vertebral artery (courses indicted by thick black lines). **a** Anterolateral transducer position (in front of sternocleidomastoid muscle) for scanning the carotid artery. **b** Posterolateral position (behind sternocleidomastoid muscle) for scanning the carotid artery. **c** Transducer position for scanning the origin of the vertebral artery

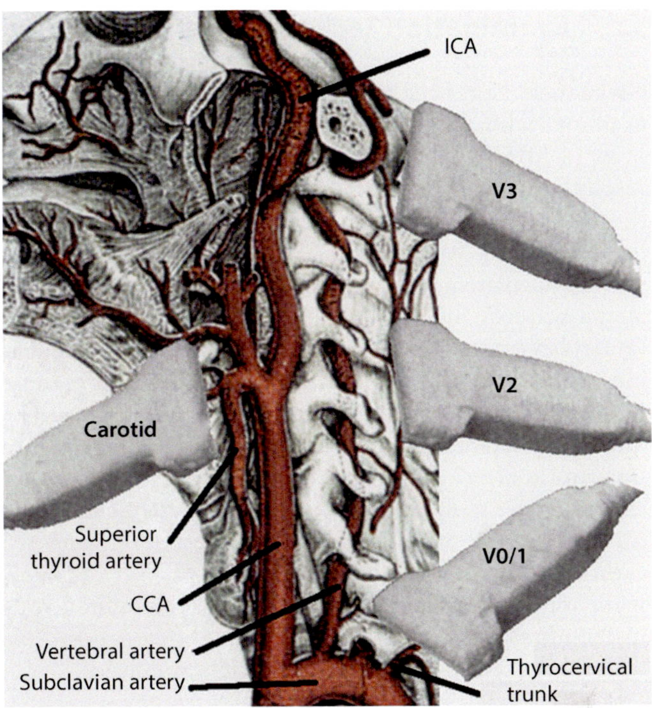

Fig. 5.3 Vascular anatomy of the extracranial cerebral arteries. Transducer positions for imaging the carotid bifurcation and the extracranial vertebral artery segments (V0/1, V2, and V3)

5.1.2 Vertebral Arteries

The two vertebral arteries originate from the ipsilateral subclavian arteries at the C6 level and then pass through the transverse foramina of the corresponding vertebrae, thus taking a partially intraosseous course on their way to the skull base. They often differ in caliber and may exhibit unilateral hypoplasia or aplasia, which is compensated for by contralateral hypertrophy. The left vertebral artery typically has a larger caliber and, in up to 4% of the population, arises directly from the aortic arch.

Somewhat distal to the vertebral artery, the thyrocervical trunk arises from the subclavian artery. The differentiation is significant in the duplex ultrasound examination. For a precise description of the site of lesions, the vertebral artery is divided into five segments (Fig. 5.3):

- The V0 segment, which is the origin of the vertebral artery from the subclavian artery
- The V1 segment, which extends from the origin to the C6 transverse process
- The V2 segment, which is the part coursing through the cervical vertebral foramina
- The V3 segment, which takes an arched course around the atlas and is therefore also referred to as the atlas loop
- The V4 segment, which is the intracranial part of the vertebral artery.

The V2 segment of the vertebral artery communicates with branches of the thyrocervical trunk and the V3 segment with the occipital artery (ECA branch).

Anatomic variants of the vertebral artery render the diagnosis more difficult. These include unilateral hypoplasia, an origin directly from the aortic arch (5% for the left vertebral artery, no risk of subclavian steal syndrome), and an abnormal course (entry into the cervical spine below or sometimes above the C6 level in 10% of individuals).

5.2 Examination Technique and Protocol

Given their superficial location, the cerebral arteries can be examined with a high-frequency transducer (5–7.5 MHz or even 10 MHz), yielding B-mode images with high spatial resolution. The ultrasound examination is performed with the patient in the supine position and the head slightly hyperextended. While some examiners prefer to sit to the right of the patient, it is recommended that the examiner sit at the patient's head, from were all transducer positions (anterolateral, posterolateral) can be reached with little movement and without exerting undue pressure because his or her elbow can rest on the edge of the couch (◘ Fig. 5.2). This is important for continuously evaluating the course of the carotid artery and for performing the temporal artery tap maneuver to identify the ECA and differentiate it from the ICA (◘ Fig. 5.6). The course of the arteries and the carotid bifurcation are identified in the transverse plane, while the Doppler waveform is sampled longitudinally. As in the ultrasound examination of other body regions, the left of the screen is superior and the right is inferior.

5.2.1 Carotid Arteries

The examination begins by obtaining a survey of the carotid bifurcation in transverse orientation to determine the location and course of the internal carotid artery (ICA) and external carotid artery (ECA) in relation to each other. The following variants may be encountered:

- In approx. 90% of the population, the ICA courses posterolateral to the ECA.
- In approx. 10% of individuals, the ICA is seen at the same level and medial to the ECA.
- In rare cases, the ICA is located anterior to the ECA.

For Doppler angle correction and precise identification of stenosis or plaque, the examiner must move the transducer around to obtain a view depicting the carotid bifurcation as a tuning fork. There are three standardized approaches for longitudinal imaging:

- Positioning of the transducer between the larynx and sternocleidomastoid muscle for sagittal anteroposterior sections (◘ Fig. 5.2a)
- Lateral approach through the sternocleidomastoid muscle
- Posterolateral approach with the transducer posterior to the sternocleidomastoid muscle (◘ Fig. 5.2b)

The posterolateral transducer position will enable good visualization of the bifurcation in most patients whose ICA follows a normal course. In this position the ICA is depicted near the transducer.

B-mode ultrasound is used for preliminary exploration of carotid artery anatomy and for obtaining initial information on the vessel wall in transverse orientation and in the longitudinal views presented above (◘ Fig. 5.4).

Sonomorphologically, the normal arterial wall is composed of three layers: an inner layer depicted as a hyperechoic line next to the lumen; a middle zone seen as a somewhat broader, hypoechoic layer; and an outer layer of slightly higher echogenicity, which is poorly demarcated from the perivascular fatty tissue. Since ultrasound does not visualize tissues or tissue layers directly but rather the echoes reflected by interfaces between zones of different acoustic impedance, the three layers seen do not exactly match the three anatomic wall layers – the intima, media, and adventitia. The intima and media are sonographically indistinguishable, which is why it is not possible to evaluate the intima alone. It is therefore common practice to measure the thickness of the intima–media complex instead.

The sonographic **thickness of the intima–media complex** is used as an early indicator of subclinical atherosclerosis and a measure of therapeutic outcome in interventional studies (e.g., to monitor statin therapy). It is therefore desirable that a standardized method for measuring carotid intima–media thickness (IMT) be used to minimize interobserver variability. A perpendicular angle of incidence ensures optimal evaluation of the vessel wall, which is the case if the target vessel courses parallel to the skin surface. If the angle is smaller, the examiner should move the transducer back and forth or rotate it slightly to ensure that the wall is evaluated in a plane showing the maximum vessel diameter. IMT is measured in the far wall of the CCA to exploit the blood-filled lumen as an acoustic window for optimal visualization of the two echogenic lines demarcating the intimal and medial layers. The leading-edge method (see ► Sect. 1.1.2.4 and ◘ Fig. 5.5) is recommended to minimize blooming artifacts (which appear at boundaries with a large mismatch in acoustic impedance). Serial IMT measurements should always be performed at the same site; most investigators prefer the far wall 2–3 cm proximal to the carotid bifurcation. Use of a high-frequency transducer (> 10 MHz) is recommended for evaluation of the wall as axial resolution and measurement accuracy increase with transducer frequency (see ◘ Table 1.2). Note, however, that although it is technically feasible, differentiation of structures smaller than 0.01 mm is beyond the resolution capacity of the human eye (and may introduce measurement errors, blooming, etc.). Finally, it is recommended that the measurement of IMT be performed at end diastole to minimize variations through the cardiac cycle (Meyer and Strobel 2008).

No agreement exists regarding the need for detailed sonomorphologic characterization of plaque in routine clinical examination. While most patients with over 70% stenosis (according to ECST criteria, which corresponds to 50% stenosis according to NASCET criteria) are candidates for surgery based on this degree of stenosis alone, plaque morphology becomes relevant for therapeutic decisions in patients with 60–70% stenosis and in patients with asymptomatic high-grade stenosis.

The morphologic evaluation of the vessel wall and plaque is followed by spectral Doppler measurement in the longitudinal plane. Color duplex imaging can provide clues regarding steno-occlusive lesions: stenosis is suggested by aliasing and an occlusion by the absence of color filling in the lumen.

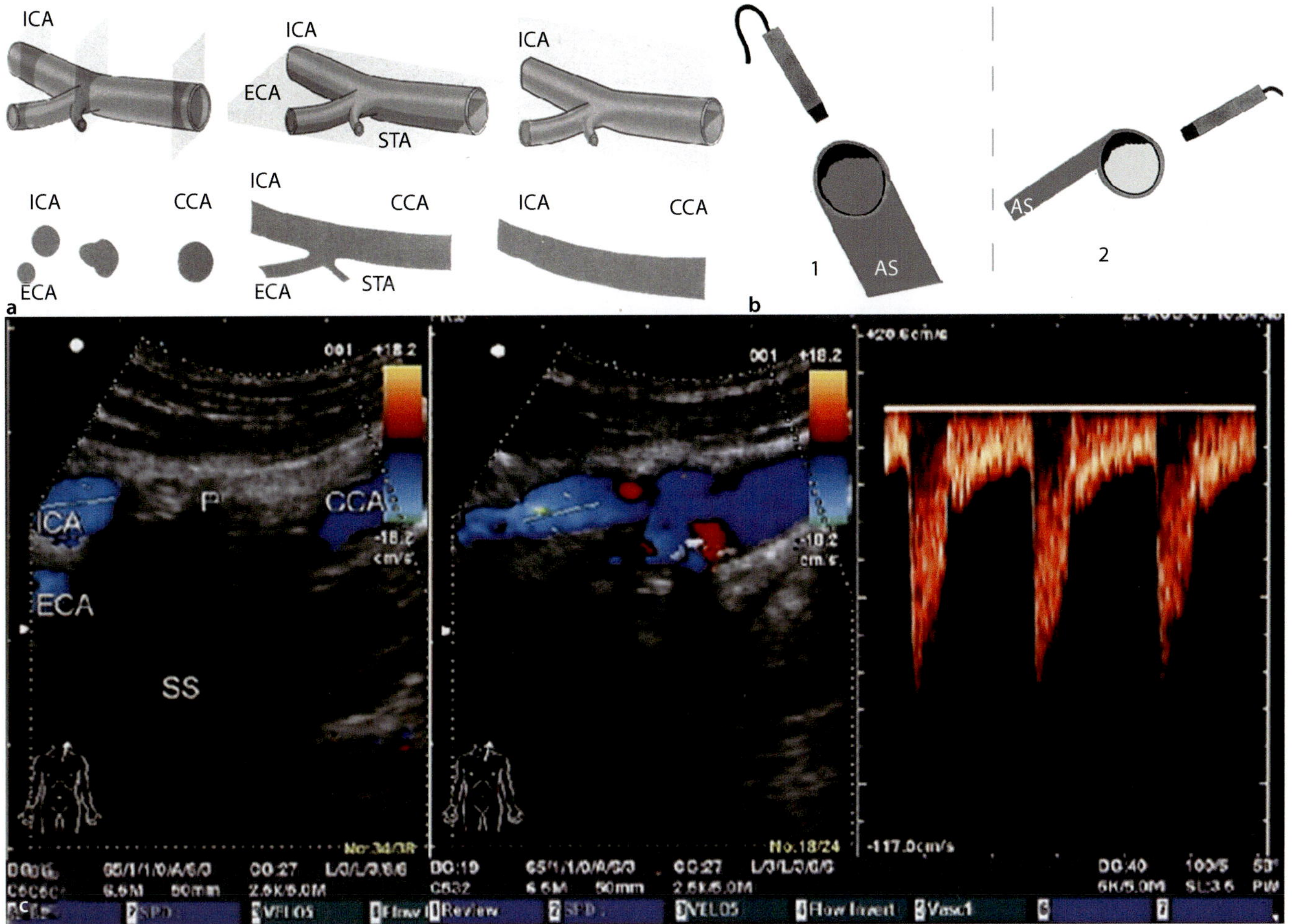

Fig. 5.4 **a** Diagrams illustrating the ultrasound examination of the carotid bifurcation. The leftmost drawing illustrates the sites of transverse examination for an overview and identification of the carotid arteries. The second drawing illustrates the posterolateral transducer position, which usually depicts the carotid bifurcation as a tuning fork with the internal carotid artery (ICA), which runs posteriorly, appearing closer to the transducer and the external carotid artery (ECA) appearing farther away from it. Often, this transducer position allows sonoanatomic identification of the ICA by demonstrating its wider bulb and also of the ECA by visualizing the superior thyroid artery (STA) arising from it; this position also enables evaluation of plaque morphology. The third drawing illustrates the anterior transducer position, which is used for plaque evaluation or spectral Doppler interrogation in cases where acoustic shadowing due to calcified plaque impairs imaging in the posterolateral position. **b** Diagram illustrating how posterior acoustic shadowing (AS) obscuring the lumen can be circumvented by rotating the transducer from position 1 (e.g., posterolateral position) to position 2 (e.g., anterior position) to enable evaluation of plaque morphology/surface and assessment of stenosis in the presence of calcified plaque. Position 2, unlike position 1, will also allow spectral Doppler imaging. The drawings illustrate how even a small, calcified plaque can impair evaluation of the vascular lumen if the vessel is examined in only one plane. **c** The left image (obtained with the transducer in a posterolateral position) illustrates how acoustic shadowing from calcified plaque in the carotid bulb completely eliminates flow signals from the ICA and ECA and obscures vascular structures in the B-mode. The second image, obtained after changing the transducer position to circumvent the sickle-shaped calcified plaque, allows evaluation of both the bulb and the ICA. There are no signs of hemodynamically relevant luminal narrowing. No flow acceleration is demonstrated by color duplex or spectral Doppler, ruling out relevant stenosis caused by the plaque

Moreover, the color duplex mode can facilitate identification of the course of a kinked or coiled ICA.

While color duplex imaging is optional for initial orientation, angle-corrected **Doppler waveforms** in the longitudinal plane must be obtained for quantification of blood flow velocity in the CCA, ICA, and ECA (Table 5.2). Spectral Doppler sampling should be performed in the ICA at short intervals. Use of a larger sample volume will often enable continuous examination of the CCA and ICA in the duplex mode, especially from the posterolateral approach. In this way, a continuous spectrum can be obtained and analyzed throughout the CCA and ICA, similar as with CW Doppler ultrasound. The ECA is scanned only at its origin for differentiation from the ICA and for the identification of possible stenosis.

The posterolateral transducer position is usually superior to the anterior position for spectral Doppler interrogation. From this transducer position, the bifurcation appears as a tuning fork with the ICA close to the transducer, and the CCA, the bulb, and long segments of the ICA and ECA can be evaluated in a single view. This facilitates angle correction, and the intervening soft tissue improves visualization. However, when the ICA is kinked or coiled, different scanning planes are necessary to identify a long enough straight segment of the artery for angle correction.

5

To **minimize errors in flow velocity measurement in the ICA**, the examiner should try to achieve a **Doppler angle of < 60°** (see Fig. 1.23 and ► Sect. 1.1.4.6). This requires selection of an adequate transducer. When a linear transducer with beam steering is used, even maximum cranial deflection (technically limited to 20°) gives an angle of insonation no smaller than 70° for an artery coursing parallel to the skin surface (90°–20° = 70°). While a linear transducer provides the best resolution for morphologic assessment of the vessel wall in the B-mode, a curved-array transducer with a small footprint affords greater flexibility in achieving an adequate angle for spectral Doppler interrogation along the tortuous course of the ICA. Curved-array transducers are also superior to linear transducers in patients with short necks and in interrogating vessel segments near the base of the skull. The view is optimal when the artery is depicted with parallel walls along the entire width of the monitor. In the 10% of individuals with a medial origin of the ICA, the tuning fork view of the bifurcation is occasionally obtained when an anterior approach is used. If this is not possible, the transducer is first tilted for selective visualization of the origin of the ECA and then tilted laterally for visualization of the origin of the ICA.

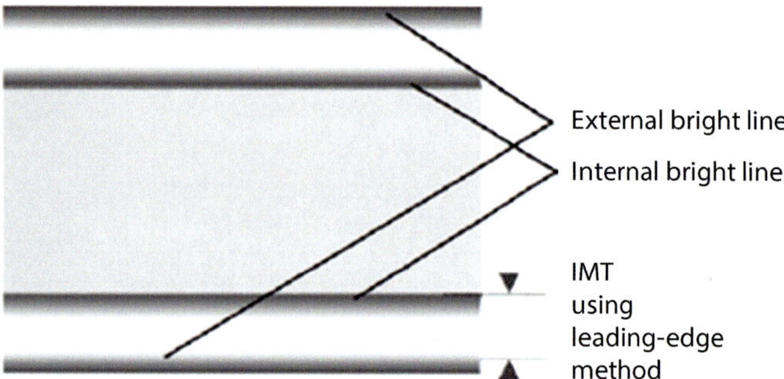

Fig. 5.5 Measurement of intima–media thickness (IMT). The intima and media cannot be distinguished sonographically. The first bright echo is the interface between the blood and the intima (interface between tissues of different acoustic impedance) with the second bright echo representing the border between the adventitia and the perivascular connective tissue. The wall layer between these two reflections is the intima–media complex. Its thickness is measured using the leading-edge method (see Figs. 1.28 and 5.52 (Atlas))

Longitudinally, the **ICA** is continuously followed to the base of the skull, for which the **posterolateral transducer position** works best in most patients. Different approaches may be required to follow a coiled or kinked ICA and to identify concomitant stenosis. Whenever the duplex findings are inconclusive, a Doppler waveform should be obtained.

A lower-frequency (5 MHz) curved-array transducer (with a small footprint) should be used in patients with poor insonation conditions or for evaluation of the deeper portions of the extracranial ICA near the base of the skull.

When **color-coded duplex ultrasound** is used, the gain and pulse repetition frequency (PRF) must be chosen so as to ensure good color filling of the vessel lumen without aliasing (color reversal from red to blue or vice versa). Transverse views are obtained with the transducer slightly tilted to achieve an adequate Doppler angle. With adequate instrument settings, changes in the color flow pattern suggest pathology, which must then be confirmed by spectral Doppler analysis.

Calcified plaques completely reflect the ultrasound pulse and thus cast acoustic shadows, impairing both color duplex and conventional duplex as well as B-mode imaging. Color coding is most severely affected by acoustic shadow-

Table 5.2 Ultrasound examination of the carotid arteries (sequence of steps)

Ultrasound method	Purpose
B-mode: transverse plane	Course, possibly differentiation of ICA/ECA (STA origin, vessel diameter)
B-mode: longitudinal plane (anterior and posterolateral transducer positions)	Search for plaque, plaque characterization, differentiation of nonatherosclerotic vascular disease
Color duplex (optional): posterolateral transducer position, anterior approach as needed	Course (kinking, coiling), initial clues regarding the presence of stenosis (aliasing). Supplementary information when ICA/ECA differentiation is difficult (STA origin)
Spectral Doppler (PW Doppler): in longitudinal orientation (never transverse plane); posterolateral or anterior transducer position (angle <60°). Adequate Doppler angle may be easier to achieve using a curved array transducer with a small radius (can be tilted)	Confirmation of stenosis, stenosis grading Differentiation of ICA and ECA (temporal artery tap) Indication for surgery (CEA)
Additional B-mode examination with high-resolution transducer (linear array) for evaluation of plaque morphology: patients with 60–70% ICA stenosis by ECST criteria/local degree (equivalent to 40–50% NASCET stenosis)/stage II or 60–80% stenosis/stage I	Plaque morphology: echolucent/echogenic, homogeneous/inhomogeneous, smooth/irregular surface; standardized analysis of echogenicity, e.g., GSM, may be used (indication for repair and type of repair)
Power mode, B-flow mode, or CEUS in selected patients	Plaque ulcer, detailed evaluation of plaque surface

CEA carotid endarterectomy, *CEUS* contrast-enhanced ultrasound, *ECA* external carotid artery, *ECST* European Carotid Surgery Trial, *GSM* gray-scale median, *ICA* internal carotid artery, *NASCET* North American Symptomatic Carotid Endarterectomy Trial, *STA* superior thyroid artery, *PW* pulsed wave

Table 5.3 Criteria for differentiating the ICA and ECA

Criterion	Reliability
ICA posterolateral to ECA	This is the case in only 90% of individuals, while 10% have a medial ICA origin
Less pulsatile flow (large diastolic flow component) in ICA compared to ECA	Reliable under normal conditions; patients with ECA stenosis will also have a large diastolic flow component in the ECA waveform
Larger lumen of ICA, especially of bulb	Fairly reliable under normal conditions but not valid in the presence of multiple (calcified) plaques
Doppler waveform from ECA shows pulsation transmitted upon intermittent tapping of temporal artery	Reliable
ECA gives off arterial branches (1st branch: STA) and ICA does not	Reliable if origins can be identified but often impaired by multiple plaques with acoustic scattering and shadowing

ECA external carotid artery, *ICA* internal carotid artery, *STA* superior thyroid artery

ing. In such situations, the pulsed Doppler, enabling focused application of a higher beam intensity with a high gain, will usually provide a Doppler waveform with a weak amplitude that still allows assessment of blood flow. If the calcification does not involve the entire inner circumference, the examiner can try and improve flow evaluation in the residual lumen by insonating the vessel from a different direction to obtain a view that depicts the calcified plaque on the wall away from the transducer (Fig. 5.4).

Under normal conditions, **the ICA and ECA are easily differentiated** on the basis of their sonoanatomic relationship, the demonstration of branches arising from the external but not from the internal carotid artery, and the widened bulb at the origin of the ICA. Compared with the ICA, the ECA has more pulsatile flow with a smaller diastolic component in the Doppler waveform. However, in patients with high-grade stenosis of the carotid bifurcation, acoustic scattering and shadowing may impair B-mode evaluation, and the stenosis-related hemodynamic changes also affect the flow profile in the ECA in that diastolic flow increases and the waveform becomes less distinct from the ICA waveform. Internalization is also observed when the ECA is recruited as a collateral for an occluded ICA. In such cases, the examiner can use the temporal tap sign to identify the ECA. The temporal tap maneuver involves rhythmical tapping of the temporal artery (anterior to the ear). The oscillations will be transmitted to the ECA and appear in the Doppler waveform from the ECA origin, especially in diastole (Table 5.3), regardless of whether the artery is normal or whether stenosis is present (Fig. 5.6). Weaker transmission will still be noted in the CCA, while the tap maneuver has no effect on the ICA waveform.

5.2.2 Vertebral Arteries

The vertebral artery can be examined by ultrasound from its origin to just before the atlas loop in the longitudinal plane from a lateral approach in the supine patient. It is not possible to scan the entire length of the vertebral artery because segments of it are obscured by the transverse processes of the cervical vertebrae. The origin from the subclavian artery is best appreciated using a curved-array transducer with a small radius, while the remainder can also be scanned with a linear probe, ideally with a frequency of 5–7.5 MHz. The **V2 segment** with its accompanying vein is easiest to identify between the acoustic shadows from the transverse processes. Because the paired vertebral arteries are linked via several pathways, steno-occlusive disease in one branch has different hemodynamic effects than an obstruction in an unpaired, organ-supplying artery. In terms of flow physiology, the vertebral circulation constitutes a parallel circuit of vascular resistances. Kirchhoff's second law states that, in a parallel circuit, current is inversely proportional to resistance. According to the Hagen-Poiseuille law, a small change in vascular diameter (hyperplastic vertebral artery, atherosclerotic stenosis, or luminal narrowing caused by dissection) will markedly reduce flow in the artery because the effect that vascular diameter has on flow in the equation is raised to the fourth power. Because the vertebral arteries are paired, 60–70% stenosis will reduce blood flow by 90–95%, and the contralateral artery largely maintains blood supply to the posterior circulation, spontaneous thrombosis of the vertebral artery is quite common when higher-grade stenosis is present.

Stenosis at the origin of the vertebral artery may be difficult to identify and evaluate, especially in obese patients with a short neck. In addition, marked tortuosity of the vertebral artery at its origin from the subclavian artery can impair Doppler angle correction. Tortuosity may further contribute to poor flow, but this is not uncommon at the origin of the vertebral artery and does not necessarily mean that stenosis is present. Identification of vertebral stenosis by color duplex imaging is easier and more reliable in the V2 segment, but higher-grade stenosis of the V2 segment is rare, and luminal narrowing of this segment is more commonly caused by dissection. The technically less challenging examination of the V2 segment is sufficient in patients with suspected subclavian steal syndrome. In general, however, the V0/V1 segment

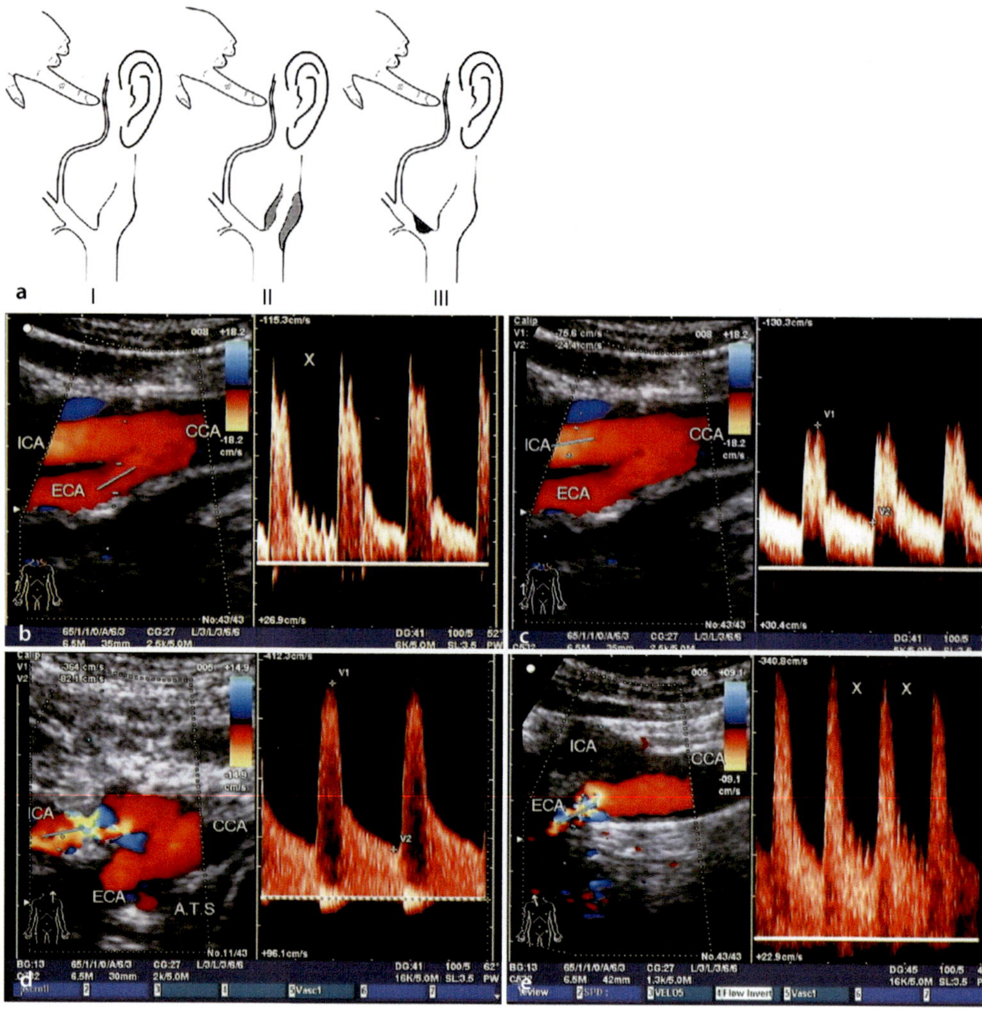

Fig. 5.6 Duplex ultrasound examination of the carotid bifurcation and differentiation of the internal carotid artery (ICA) and external carotid artery (ECA). Flow in the ECA is more pulsatile and is modulated by the signal transmitted upon rhythmical tapping of the temporal artery (**a I** and **b**), especially during diastole (X). The oscillations resulting from the temporal tap do not affect the waveform from the ICA (**a I** and **c**). When stenosis is present, differentiation between the ICA and ECA on the basis of pulsatility is difficult, and plaque may impair identification of the superior thyroid artery (A.T.S) arising from the ECA or of the wider bulb of the ICA. The temporal artery tap, however, still provides a clearcut differentiation, as the oscillation is not transmitted into a stenotic ICA (**a II** and **d**). The Doppler waveform from a stenotic ECA (**a III** and **e**) shows similar pulsatility of flow as the waveform from a stenotic ICA, and transmission of the oscillations produced by temporal tapping (X) into the ECA allows differentiation of the two arteries in this situation

should be examined because it is the preferred site of vertebral artery pathology (curved-array transducers are more suitable than linear transducers).

To evaluate the vertebral arteries, the examiner can proceed in **one of two ways: in slender patients with good insonation conditions, the vertebral artery is identified at its origin from the subclavian artery** (Figs. 5.2c and 5.3), where stenosis can be ruled out by obtaining a Doppler waveform in **longitudinal orientation**. In patients with a poor acoustic window or complex sonoanatomy, the examiner first locates the CCA longitudinally to then identify the vertebral artery between the transverse processes of the cervical vertebrae; this is accomplished by slight posterolateral movement and medial angulation of the transducer (see Fig. 5.87 (Atlas)). Acoustic shadowing from the transverse processes at regular intervals precludes complete evaluation of the V2 segment (Fig. 5.7). From the V2 segment, the examiner can then follow the artery downward to identify its origin. The atlas loop will come into view when the transducer is moved cranially and angled (Fig. 5.87 (Atlas)).

In the color duplex mode, the examiner follows the length of the vertebral artery to its origin, looking for luminal narrowing or aliasing. Any luminal narrowing should be quantified by obtaining a Doppler waveform.

A full evaluation includes measurement of the vertebral artery diameter and comparison with its counterpart in order to differentiate a **hypoplastic artery** from other vascular pathology. Arterial diameters are determined in the V2 segment (B-mode).

When a patient with trauma and **suspected vertebral artery dissection** is examined, the focus of the ultrasound examination should be on the segment running through the cervical vertebral foramina (V2 segment). When looking for **atherosclerotic vertebral artery stenosis**, on the other hand, it is the origin from the subclavian artery which requires close attention. To locate the origin, it may be necessary to first identify the subclavian artery in the cervical triangle and then use the color mode to identify the vertebral origin (V0/V1) at the cranial edge of the subclavian artery. Because of its tortuous course at the origin, the vertebral artery may easily move out of the scan plane. The vertebral artery origin must not be confused with the thyrocervical trunk, which arises more distally and is easier to visualize. The two can be distinguished from one another by rhythmically tapping the vertebral artery below the mastoid (atlas loop); this signal is transmitted to the vertebral artery and modulates the Doppler waveform from the vertebral artery origin (see procedure described for identification of the ECA using the temporal tap at the end of ▶ Sect. 5.2.1 and Fig. 5.7b).

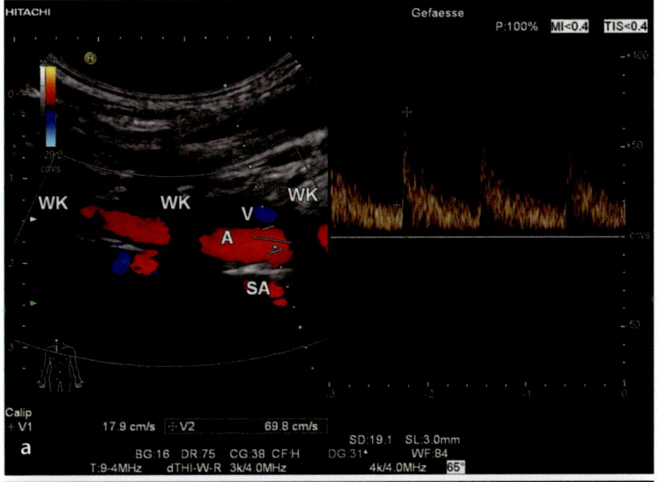

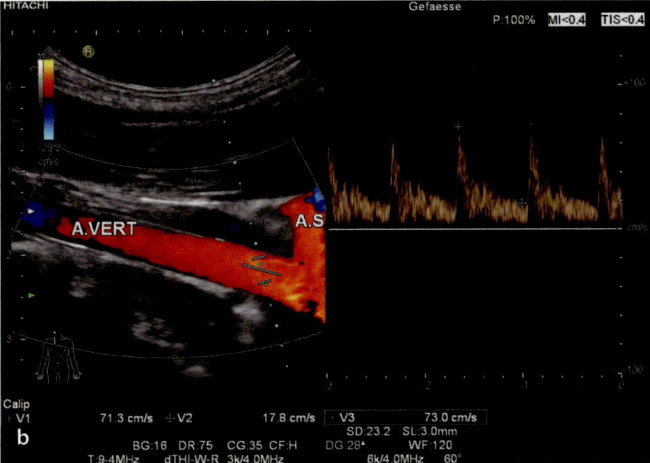

◘ **Fig. 5.7** **a** Image showing the V2 segment of the vertebral artery (A) between the vertebral processes (WK, acoustic shadowing). A segment of the vertebral vein (blue) is also seen (SA = mirror artifact). **b** Vertebral artery (A.VERT) at its origin (V0/V1 segment) from the subclavian artery (A.S.) with a monophasic waveform typical of low-resistance flow. The peak systolic velocity (PSV) is 72 cm/s, and the end-diastolic velocity (EDV) is 18 cm/s. Oscillations generated by tapping the vertebral artery below the mastoid are transmitted to the vertebral artery and appear in the waveform (left portion)

In the vertebral artery, spectral Doppler evaluation is also important to determine the direction of blood flow. In patients with normal vertebral artery flow at rest and suspected **exercise-induced subclavian steal syndrome** due to subclavian artery stenosis or occlusion, the increased demand during muscle activity can be reproduced during the examination. With continuous spectral Doppler recording in the vertebral artery, a blood pressure cuff around the upper arm is inflated to over 250 mmHg and then released after 3–5 min to induce reactive hyperemia in the arm. If high-grade stenosis or occlusion of the proximal subclavian artery with subclavian steal and vertebrovertebral crossover is present, this maneuver will induce flow reversal in the ipsilateral vertebral artery and an increase in flow velocity in the contralateral vertebral artery.

5.3 Documentation

Normal findings should be documented in longitudinal views (B-mode) of both CCAs, ICAs, and ECAs, vertebral arteries (V1 or V2 segment), and subclavian arteries with the corresponding Doppler waveforms (including angle-corrected flow velocity measurements) (see sites for taking representative measurements in ◘ Fig. 5.1a). Abnormal findings are documented in additional B-mode images and the corresponding Doppler waveforms obtained from the sites of pathology in longitudinal orientation. Systolic and end-diastolic flow velocities obtained with angle correction must reflect the degree of stenosis. Finally, the report should contain information on the localization of stenotic and nonstenotic plaques (B-mode images for documentation) and a description of plaque morphology.

5.4 Normal Findings

5.4.1 Carotid Arteries

The common carotid artery (CCA) has a constant luminal diameter of approx. 7 mm. Flow is pulsatile with a large diastolic component. The internal carotid artery (ICA) has a peak systolic velocity (PSV) ranging from 60 to 100 cm/s (◘ Table 5.4). At its origin, the wider lumen (bulb) and vessel branching lead to eddy currents even under normal conditions. PSV is lower in the bulb, and flow separation may lead to retrograde flow on the side opposite the external carotid artery (ECA), seen as color reversal in color duplex images (see ◘ Figs. 5.49 (Atlas) and ◘ 1.45b).

The normal thickness of the **intima–media complex** measured in the B-mode (from the lumen–intima interface, the first bright line, to the media-adventitia interface, the second bright line) is **0.5–0.6 mm** and increases somewhat with age.

Supplying the brain, the ICA has low-resistance flow with a **Doppler waveform** that is characterized by a steep systolic upslope followed by monophasic flow with a fairly large dia-

◘ **Table 5.4** Average blood flow velocities and diameters of the extracranial cerebral arteries (meta-analysis)

Artery	PSV (cm/s)	EDV (cm/s)	D (mm)
CCA	50–80	15–30	6.0–7.5
ICA	60–90	20–40	4–6
ECA	60–100	10–20	3.5–4.5
Vertebral artery	20–70	5–35	3–5

CCA common carotid artery, *D* diameter, *ECA* external carotid artery, *EDV* end-diastolic velocity, *ICA* internal carotid artery, *PSV* peak systolic velocity

5

Table 5.5 Causes of abnormal pulsatility (Doppler waveform) in the extracranial cerebral arteries

Change	Cause
Reduced pulsatility	High-grade proximal flow obstruction AV fistula or angioma in distal segment Hyperperfusion (e.g., in hyperthyroidism) Aortic stenosis
Increased pulsatility	High-grade distal flow obstruction Increased intracranial pressure Severe cerebral microangiopathy Aortic insufficiency Low heart rate

AV arteriovenous

stolic component. Conversely, flow in the ECA is more pulsatile with a smaller diastolic component. The common carotid artery, supplying both territories, has a mixed waveform. As in all other vascular territories, pulsatility in the carotid system is determined by peripheral resistance and vessel elasticity and therefore increases with age (Table 5.5).

5.4.2 Vertebral Arteries

Published data on blood flow velocities in the vertebral arteries vary widely from 19 to 98 cm/s for peak systolic velocity (PSV) and from 6 to 30 cm/s for end-diastolic velocity (EDV). The resistance index (RI) ranges from 0.62 to 0.75 (Tratting et al. 1992). Assessment of the vertebral artery, especially at its origin, is impaired by **caliber variation** and the occurrence of congenital hypoplasia. At the same time, evaluation of the origin is important because it is the most common site of stenosis.

The normal diameter of the vertebral artery is 3–5 mm but it is common for one vertebral artery to be larger than the other, resulting in right–left diameter differences of over 2 mm.

In case of **lateral differences in flow velocity** and poor visualization of the origin, the examiner must differentiate a proximal stenosis from hypoplasia.

The following **criteria suggest hypoplasia**:

- Unilateral caliber reduction (luminal diameter typically <2 cm)
- Contralateral hyperplasia (luminal diameter typically >3.5) and side difference typically >2 mm
- Flow velocity (PSV) lower than on the contralateral side
- Unchanged waveform; however, flow is often more pulsatile with a reduced diastolic flow component (see Figs. 5.87 (Atlas), 5.39, and 5.40).

In contrast, stenosis is indicated by less pulsatile flow, a smaller systolic component, and more pronounced diastolic flow in the waveform obtained downstream of the lesion.

5.5 Clinical Role of Duplex Ultrasound

5.5.1 Carotid Arteries

The carotid bifurcation is the preferred site of carotid artery stenosis. An important underlying mechanism is turbulent flow with increased wall tension resulting from the abrupt change in diameter in the bulb and flow division in the bifurcation. This mechanism and shear forces cause higher intimal stress in the carotid bulb. As a result, carotid plaque tends to develop along the outer wall opposite the flow divider (Fig. 5.10). This stressful hemodynamic situation with flow division is also visible on color duplex ultrasound (Figs. 1.44b and 5.49 (Atlas)).

The aim of sonographic assessment of the extracranial cerebral arteries is to **prevent cerebral infarction** with its harmful sequelae and permanent deficits (Fig. 5.8).

Several duplex ultrasound parameters can contribute to estimating a patient's **cardiovascular risk**. Besides intima-media thickness (IMT) measured in the common carotid artery (CCA), the **resistive index** (**Pourcelot index**) determined in the internal carotid artery (ICA) is gaining significance in the assessment of early stages of atherosclerosis and as a predictor of cardiovascular morbidity and mortality. A study investigating RI progression from a baseline RI of 0.66 ± 0.08 found a continuous increase in cardiovascular events as the RI increased (Uthoff et al. 2008).

While diagnostic ultrasound and treatment of peripheral vessels are symptom-oriented, the purpose of carotid artery evaluation is prognosis-oriented in that it aims at identifying patients at risk for stroke and initiating adequate preventive measures in these high-risk patients (Tables 5.6 and 5.7). Duplex ultrasound examinations of the extracranial cerebral arteries are performed for the following reasons:

- Identification of the underlying cause in patients with a transient ischemic attack (TIA), prolonged reversible ischemic neurologic deficit (PRIND), or stroke (additional CT and echocardiography)
- Workup of asymptomatic carotid artery stenosis suspected on clinical grounds (auscultation, risk factors, atherosclerosis with coronary heart disease or pelvic artery stenosis)
- Indication for operative treatment of carotid stenosis: plaque morphology, hemodynamic stenosis grading
- Workup of a pulsatile neck mass (aneurysm, transmission of pulsation through extravascular tumor)
- Workup of traumatic intimal dissection
- Diagnostic evaluation for inflammatory disease (Takayasu's arteritis, temporal arteritis)
- Workup of disturbed perfusion in the posterior circulation (vertebral artery stenosis, subclavian steal syndrome due to subclavian artery occlusion)
- Diagnosis of brain death
- Follow-up after surgical repair (carotid endarterectomy) or PTA with stenting (immediately after intervention, then at 6-month intervals).

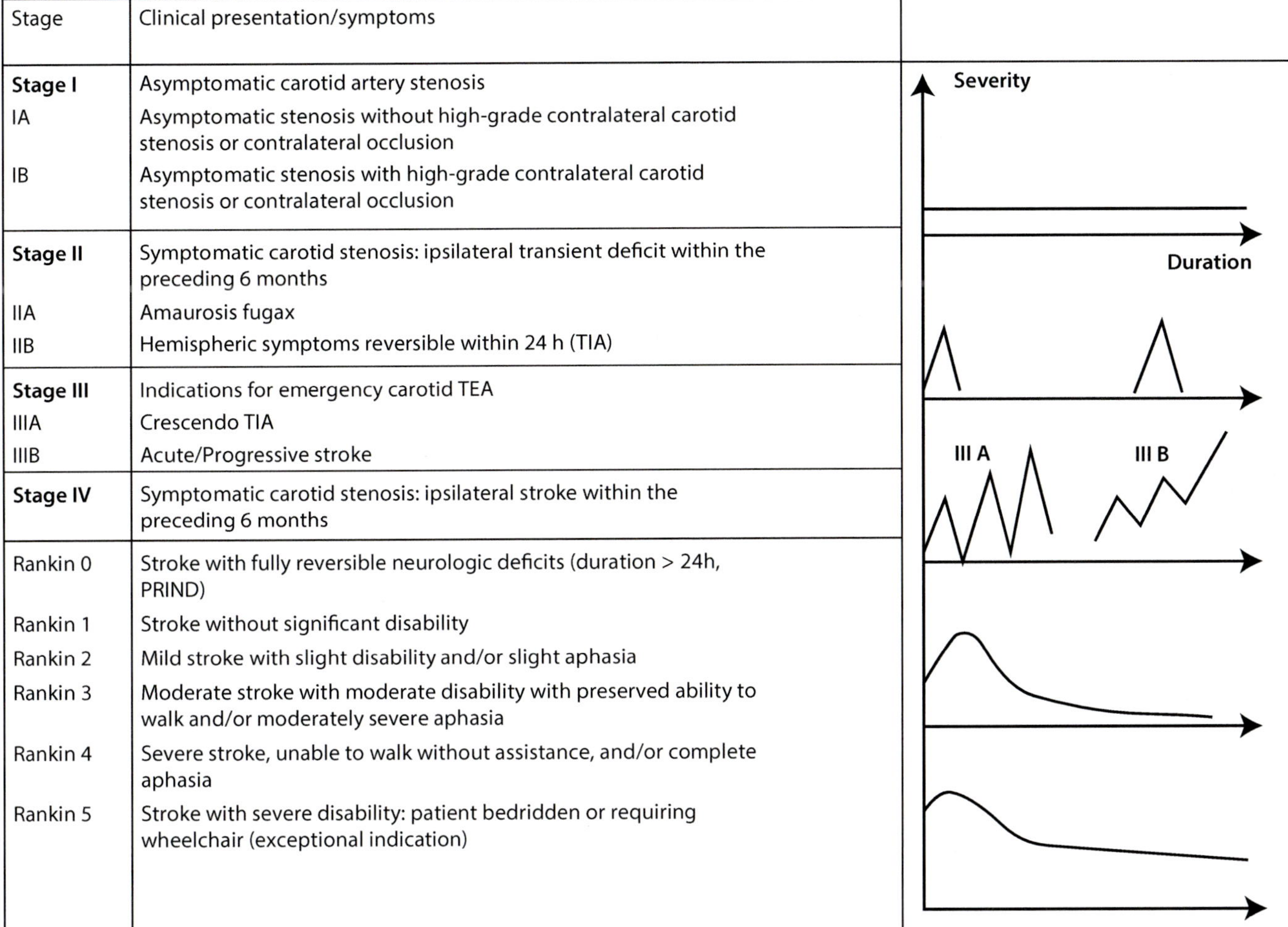

Stage	Clinical presentation/symptoms
Stage I	Asymptomatic carotid artery stenosis
IA	Asymptomatic stenosis without high-grade contralateral carotid stenosis or contralateral occlusion
IB	Asymptomatic stenosis with high-grade contralateral carotid stenosis or contralateral occlusion
Stage II	Symptomatic carotid stenosis: ipsilateral transient deficit within the preceding 6 months
IIA	Amaurosis fugax
IIB	Hemispheric symptoms reversible within 24 h (TIA)
Stage III	Indications for emergency carotid TEA
IIIA	Crescendo TIA
IIIB	Acute/Progressive stroke
Stage IV	Symptomatic carotid stenosis: ipsilateral stroke within the preceding 6 months
Rankin 0	Stroke with fully reversible neurologic deficits (duration > 24h, PRIND)
Rankin 1	Stroke without significant disability
Rankin 2	Mild stroke with slight disability and/or slight aphasia
Rankin 3	Moderate stroke with moderate disability with preserved ability to walk and/or moderately severe aphasia
Rankin 4	Severe stroke, unable to walk without assistance, and/or complete aphasia
Rankin 5	Stroke with severe disability: patient bedridden or requiring wheelchair (exceptional indication)

Fig. 5.8 Classification of extracranial carotid artery stenosis. Higher-grade carotid stenosis ≥50% (by NASCET criteria) or ≥70% (by ECST criteria) based on angiography or ultrasound. Graphic representation of the duration (horizontal axis) and severity (vertical axis) of the respective neurologic deficits. *PRIND* prolonged reversible ischemic neurologic deficit, *TEA* thromboendarterectomy, *TIA* transient ischemic attack

Table 5.6 Risk of stroke in surgically versus medically managed patients with carotid artery stenosis. Perioperative risk (stroke/death) and absolute risk reduction (ARR) of ipsilateral stroke over a 5-year period in patients with symptomatic carotid artery stenosis[a]

Degree of carotid stenosis (%)	Operative risk[b] (%)	Risk of stroke		ARR[c] (%)	P	NNT
		Surgical (%)	Medical (%)			
< 30	6.7	12	10.0	2.2	0.05	–
30–49	8.4	15	18.2	3.2	0.6	31
50–69	8.4	14	18.6	4.6	0.04	22
70–99	6.2	10	26.0	15.9	< 0.001	6

ECST European Carotid Surgery Trial, *NASCET* North American Symptomatic Carotid Endarterectomy Trial, *NNT* number needed to treat
[a]Summary of results obtained in 6029 randomized patients from the ECST (n = 3018), the VA (Veterans Affairs) trial 309 (n = 189), and the NASCET (n = 2885)
[b]All strokes/deaths occurring within 30 days; a total of 3248 patients were operated on
[c]Including perioperative stroke/death

Table 5.7 Extracranial cerebral arteries – duplex ultrasound findings and therapeutic consequences

Diagnosis	Ultrasound findings, clinical presentation, and stenosis degree by ECST criteria (with equivalent NASCET degrees in brackets; see Tables 5.8 and 5.9)	Therapy
Plaques	No hemodynamic stenosis, asymptomatic or symptomatic	Medical management
ICA stenosis	Hemodynamically significant stenosis <70% (<50% NASCET), asymptomatic	Medical management
	Stenosis >70% (>50% NASCET), asymptomatic Evaluation of plaque (vulnerable?) using B-mode, CEUS	Surgical reconstruction (CEA) acceptable but only proven if perioperative risk is low (according to ACAS study): Weighing of best medical treatment ← → CEA, CAS: – If perioperative morbidity/mortality rate < 3% – Annual stroke rate of 2% in medical care group versus 1% in surgical group – Surgery only if life expectancy >5 years
	50–70% stenosis (30–50% NASCET), symptomatic B-mode: plaque morphology	Surgical reconstruction (CEA): – Acceptable; however, not proven in patients with TIA <6 months and plaque morphology suggesting high risk of embolism (ulceration, hypoechogenicity, irregular surface)
	> 70% stenosis (>50% NASCET), symptomatic	Proven indication for surgery (CEA): Risk reduction relative to natural history increases as the perioperative morbidity and mortality rate decreases (target: < 5%)
	> 70% stenosis (>50% NASCET), stage IV	Surgery only after nearly complete resolution of symptoms approx. 2–6 weeks after acute event Prophylactic surgery of asymptomatic side may be indicated if there is stenosis on this side as well
ICA occlusion	Stage IV	Usually no operation, emergency operation may be contemplated only immediately after the event (mortality of up to 9%); otherwise medical management; repair may be indicated in patients with multiple-vessel disease
Subclavian artery stenosis/occlusion	Steal syndrome, symptomatic	PTA, extrathoracic bypass procedure or transposition
ECA stenosis	High-grade	External carotid angioplasty indicated only in multiple-vessel disease (occlusion of ICA) with borderzone ischemias and proven extracranial and intracranial collateralization
Carotid artery dissection	Mostly due to trauma, asymptomatic, patent or thrombosed false lumen	Medical management, anticoagulation (intimal flap becomes attached or false lumen undergoes obliteration or thrombosis in most cases). Fixation or resection of intimal flaps only in exceptional cases with pronounced neurologic deficits and floating flaps
Kinking or coiling	Asymptomatic, no stenosis	Medical management
	Symptomatic if associated with stenosis	Resection
Inflammatory vessel disease (Takayasu's arteritis, temporal arteritis)	Wall thickening (macaroni sign) with or without hemodynamically significant stenosis	Cortisone therapy, no surgical reconstruction
Carotid body tumor	Well-perfused tumor in the carotid bifurcation (color duplex)	Complete tumor resection; embolization only in patients with a high risk of morbidity
Vertebral artery stenosis	High-grade stenosis, asymptomatic	Medical management
	High-grade stenosis, symptomatic	Chiefly located at origin, surgical reconstruction or PTA

ACAS Asymptomatic Carotid Atherosclerosis Study, *CAS* carotid artery stenting, *CCA* common carotid artery, *CEA* carotid endarterectomy, *CEUS* contrast-enhanced ultrasound, *ECA* external carotid artery, *ECST* European Carotid Surgery Trial, *ICA* internal carotid artery, *NASCET* North American Symptomatic Carotid Endarterectomy Trial, *PTA* percutaneous transluminal angioplasty, *TIA* transient ischemic attack

Over the last decades, **carotid endarterectomy (CEA)** has evolved into a suitable method for treating high-grade ICA stenosis – the major underlying cause of cerebral infarction. The main drawback of CEA, and of carotid artery stenting (CAS), is that it may cause what it is supposed to prevent, namely TIA or stroke. This is why the surgical risk must be weighed against the risk of untreated stenosis. Numerous prospective randomized multicenter studies compared the natural history and the surgical risk for symptomatic and asymptomatic carotid stenoses of different degrees (see ◘ Table 5.1). Endarterectomy in symptomatic carotid stenosis aims at eliminating the vascular source of emboli and/or residual flow obstruction in individuals with a history of cerebral infarction.

The **European Carotid Surgery Trial** (**ECST**) and the **North American Symptomatic Carotid Endarterectomy Trial** (**NASCET**) compared antiplatelet therapy versus endarterectomy in patients with symptomatic carotid artery stenosis. Re-analysis of the pooled data suggests that CEA statistically highly significantly reduces the risk of ipsilateral stroke by 16% after 5 years in individuals with 70–99% stenoses (by ECST criteria, which is equivalent to >50% stenosis by NASCET criteria). In other words, six operations have to be performed to prevent one ipsilateral stroke over a 5-year period (number needed to treat (NNT)). In individuals with 50–69% stenosis, absolute risk reduction (ARR) drops to 4.6%. CEA has no advantage in individuals with stenoses <50% and is harmful in those with <30% stenosis compared to the natural history of the disease. The rate of severe perioperative complications (stroke, death) was found to be 6.2% for patients with stenosis greater than 70% versus 8.4% for those with 50–69% stenosis (◘ Table 5.6).

The wider use of validated noninvasive diagnostic modalities such as Doppler and duplex ultrasound and the known relationship between coronary heart disease and carotid stenosis and their associated risk of stroke make it more and more important to establish reliable criteria for identifying patients with subclinical carotid artery stenosis who would benefit from prophylactic surgery. However, in this population with a lower risk of spontaneous stroke (annual rate of less than 1% in stenosis <70% versus approx. 2.5% in those with >70% stenoses, depending on other findings and comorbidity), it is more difficult to demonstrate a statistical benefit of therapeutic measures. While other studies revealed no benefit of operative treatment in this population, the **Asymptomatic Carotid Atherosclerosis Study** (**ACAS**) demonstrated an advantage for the patients operated on for carotid stenoses of 60–99% compared to patients undergoing medical treatment (ACAS 1995). The 5-year stroke risk was 5.1% in the surgical group versus 11% in the medical care group. The perioperative risk of stroke and death was 2.3% including the rate of 1.2% of preoperative angiography. The American Heart Association (AHA) recommends surgery for asymptomatic carotid artery stenosis >60% if the center performing the intervention has a perioperative risk of less than 3%.

In clinical practice, patient management is primarily based on the sonographic degree of stenosis (which determines the risk of embolism) and the patient's clinical stage (◘ Table 5.7).

Apart from the degree of stenosis (◘ Fig. 5.11), **plaque morphology** is another major determinant of stroke risk. Ulcerated plaques with superimposed thrombi, intraplaque hemorrhage, and atheromatous plaques are associated with a higher risk of stroke compared to smooth, fibrous plaques. However, no imaging modality exists that enables a satisfactory estimate of the risk of embolism on the basis of plaque morphology.

Yet, in certain cases, the sonomorphologic appearance may be useful in estimating the risk of embolism. Some studies suggest that hypoechoic plaques have a two to five times greater tendency to embolize than hyperechoic ones.

Arterial emboli from atherosclerotic plaques in carotid stenosis account for 55–60% of all strokes (territorial infarction; ◘ Fig. 5.9a). Another 30–35% are due to cardiogenic embolism, and less than 5% are due to hemodynamically reduced perfusion, especially in multiple-vessel disease (borderzone infarction). Other rare causes accounting for less than 5% of cases are inflammatory vessel disease, microangiopathy, and dissection.

5.5.1.1 Stenosis Grading

Despite the clinical relevance of internal carotid artery (ICA) stenosis, there is no agreement about how it should be quantified, and various methods have been proposed. The **difficulty in grading ICA stenosis** is chiefly attributable to the greater width of the carotid bulb, the preferred site of ICA stenosis. Patients with thick plaques in this slightly dilated portion of the carotid artery may have a considerable risk of embolism, while the degree of narrowing has little or no hemodynamic effect (◘ Fig. 5.10).

Basically, two methods exist for grading and reporting ICA stenosis:

- The ECST (European Carotid Surgery Trial) method: local degree of stenosis
- The NASCET (North American Symptomatic Carotid Endarterectomy Trial) method: distal degree of stenosis

The **local degree of stenosis** is defined as the ratio of the patent residual lumen to the local vessel lumen without the plaque and gives the best estimate of plaque thickness (which is relevant for the ensuing risk of embolism) and the true extent of vascular obstruction. However, angiography enables only a rough and indirect estimate of the local degree of a stenosis because, unlike duplex ultrasound, it does not depict the original vessel diameter.

The **distal degree of stenosis** is calculated from the diameter of the residual lumen of the stenosed segment and that of the distal ICA (which is fairly constant up to the base of the skull). This method allows accurate assessment of the reduction in blood supply to the brain caused by a stenosis and classifies mild to moderate stenosis of the carotid bulb as hemodynamically nonsignificant (◘ Figs. 5.9b and 5.10).

5

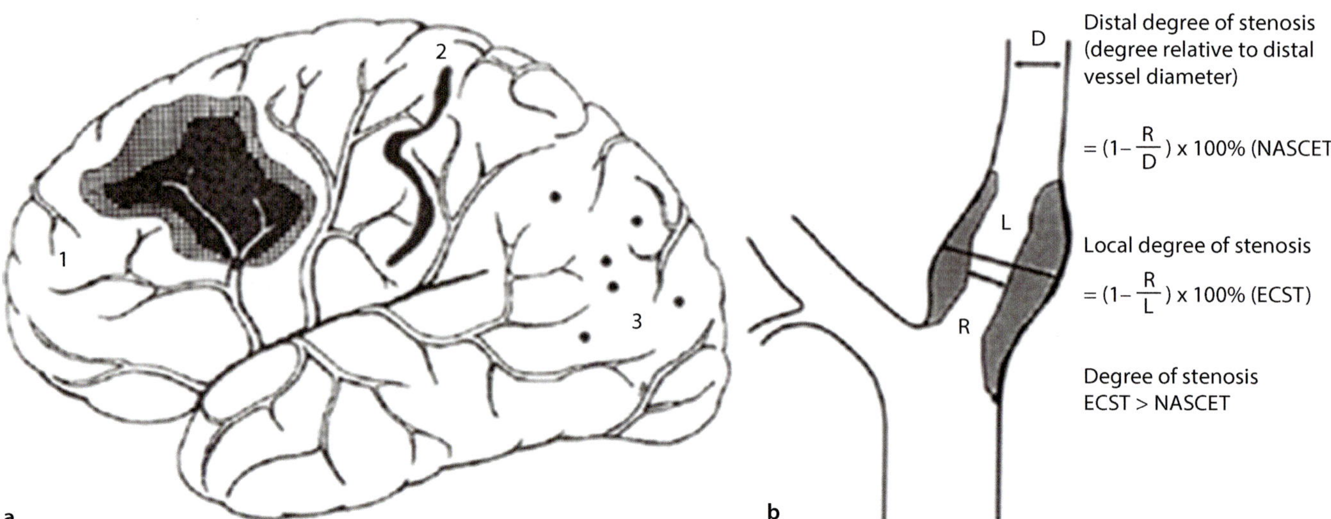

Fig. 5.9 **a** Types of cerebral infarction. **1** Territorial infarction: caused by arterioarterial embolism (carotid, cardiac). **2** Borderzone infarction: hemodynamic origin, reduced perfusion in terminal vascular bed, chiefly in patients with multiple-vessel disease. **3** Lacunar infarction: microangiopathy. **b** Methods of stenosis grading (local versus distal degree of stenosis). Due to the larger vessel diameter in the bulb, a stenosis classified as mild to moderate using the local grading method may not be classified as a stenosis when the distal grading method is used. Since the stenosis-related decrease in perfusion only has a minor role in the development of cerebral ischemia, whereas plaque thickness is crucial for the associated risk of embolism, the local degree of stenosis is clinically more relevant. For instance, eccentric plaques causing only moderate stenosis of the bulb may already carry a considerable risk of embolism based on their thickness

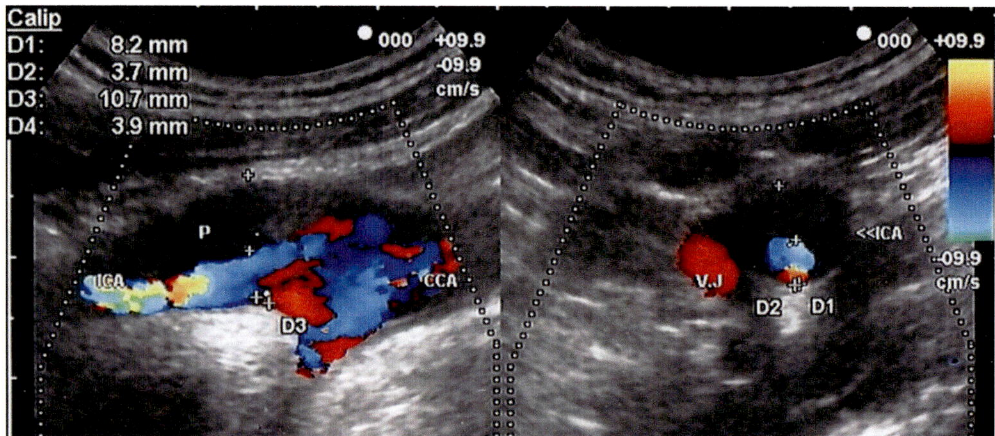

Fig. 5.10 Color duplex ultrasound (longitudinal image on the left and transverse image on the right) demonstrating hypoechoic eccentric plaque of the carotid bulb. Calculation using the local grading method yields a 65% diameter reduction (60–70% stenosis). According to the distal stenosis grading method (NASCET) (diameter of the distal ICA in the longitudinal image: almost 5 mm), this is a 20–30% stenosis and surgery is not indicated. Conversely, the local degree of stenosis (ECST) establishes an indication for surgery, especially when additionally considering plaque morphology (hypoechoic) and configuration (very eccentric and thickness >5 mm: high shear stress). The final decision for surgery also depends on the patient's age and concomitant diseases. The example illustrates how the method used for stenosis grading (local versus distal) might lead to different therapeutic consequences (see Fig. 5.15)

The confusion about carotid artery stenosis grading, both in scientific publications and in routine clinical practice, is mainly attributable to the fact that the distal grading method is primarily used in the USA, while determination of the local degree, which is also favored in Germany, is more common in Europe. Hence the NASCET used the former and the ECST the latter. To overcome this confusion, a consensus conference in 2010 issued the recommendation that the distal degree of ICA stenosis (NASCET criteria) should be used in reports. In other words, authors using the local degree of stenosis, which is a better predictor of the risk of embolism, should explicitly say so. Before this consensus was reached, the local grading method was favored by the German Society of Ultrasound in Medicine (Deutsche Gesellschaft für Ultraschall in der Medizin, DEGUM) (Widder et al. 1986).

Table 5.8 Correspondences between distal (NASCET) and local (ECST) degrees of internal carotid artery (ICA) stenosis

Grading method	Degree of stenosis								Study
Distal (%)	0	50	60	67	70	75	85	90	NASCET
Local (%)	40	70	75	80	82	85	90	95	ECST

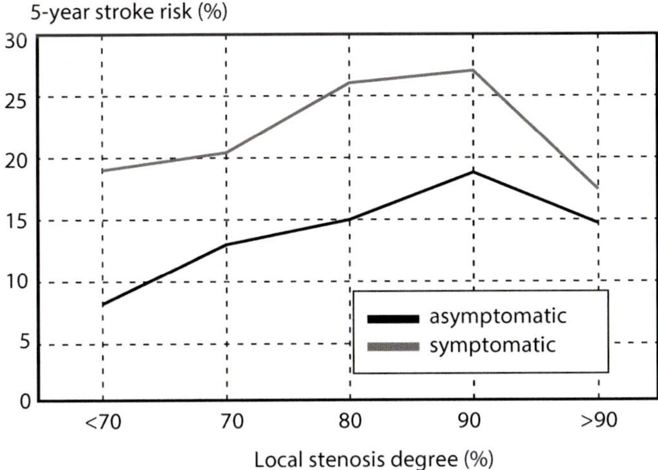

Fig. 5.11 Risk of ipsilateral cerebral infarction by degree of internal carotid artery (ICA) stenosis in symptomatic and asymptomatic individuals (According to Widder 2004)

As the relation between the diameter of the carotid bulb and that of the distant internal carotid is fairly constant, the degrees of ICA stenosis by NASCET and ECST criteria can be easily **converted into each other** using the following equations:

- Local (ECST) degree of stenosis (%) = 0.6 × distal (NASCET) degree (%) + 40%
- Distal (NASCET) degree of stenosis (%) = local (ECST) degree of stenosis (%) – 40%/0.6

The resulting correspondences between the distal and local degrees of ICA stenosis are presented in Table 5.8.

Plaque causing luminal narrowing of up to 40% in the carotid bulb is classified as a nonstenotic lesion using the distal quantification method because stenosis with a local degree of up to 30% reduces the bulbous lumen only to the diameter of the distal carotid artery (Fig. 5.11). Note, however, that hemodynamic alterations are less relevant for the risk of cerebral infarction than the **risk of embolism**, which **increases with plaque thickness**. Therefore, eccentric plaque in the bulb may already pose a considerable risk of embolism before it causes hemodynamic effects.

Angiography, the traditional gold standard for carotid artery assessment, has methodological limitations as it grades a stenosis on the basis of purely morphologic criteria. It is an invasive procedure that involves radiation exposure and contrast-medium-related side effects as well as the risk of minor stroke in 1.3–4.5% of cases and major stroke in 0.6–1.3% (Davies and Humphrey 1993; Dion et al. 1987; Hankey et al. 1990; Moore 2003). The risk of angiography is higher in symptomatic stenoses than in asymptomatic ones, and the risk of inducing stroke may be as high as 12.5% in patients with bilateral high-grade carotid stenosis (Theodotou et al. 1987). The ACAS provides the most detailed analysis. According to this study, angiography performed at radiologic centers is associated with a combined neurologic morbidity and mortality of 1.2% in asymptomatic patients, which is only slightly lower than the 1.52% risk associated with carotid endarterectomy (CEA) in the same patient population. In light of these findings, it was recommended to perform CEA without prior diagnostic angiography (Chervu et al. 1994) (Fig. 5.12). This is made possible in part by the use of high-resolution ultrasound, which has been shown in comparative studies with histologic workup to be superior to angiography in assessing plaque morphology and the ensuing risk of embolism (Ten Kate et al. 2010; Honda et al. 2004).

5.5.1.2 Plaque Morphology

Ultrasound measurement of carotid **intima-media thickness (IMT)** has become an established technique for estimating the risk of cardiovascular morbidity and mortality. IMT is used as a surrogate marker for pre- or subclinical atherosclerosis and for monitoring the outcome of treatment (e.g., statins) in interventional studies.

Risk factors such as long-standing hypertension or hyperlipoproteinemia damage the intima, first becoming manifest as thickening of the intima-media complex. Thickening above 1 mm is considered abnormal and a thickness of 2 mm or more is defined as plaque (Li et al. 1996).

However, thickening of the intima–media complex is also an age-related phenomenon. While IMT is below 0.6 mm in young healthy individuals (Rubbia et al. 1994), an average increase of 0.1 mm per decade of life is regarded as normal after the age of 40 (Homma et al. 2000). **Serious arterial wall changes** should be expected when the **increase in thickness exceeds 1.5 mm**. Individuals with an IMT > 1.5 mm or small focal plaques often have aortic plaques, which have been implicated as a cause of embolic cerebral infarction. Measurement of IMT therefore provides a general estimate of the total atherosclerotic burden, and patients with marked thickening of the intima-media complex have an increased embolic risk arising from atherosclerotic plaques in the aortic arch.

Intimal lipid accumulation is a crucial mechanism in **plaque development**. Macrophages infiltrate the atherosclerotic lesions and phagocytose cholesterol, giving rise to foam cells. Following recruitment of muscle cells and fibroblasts, a

5

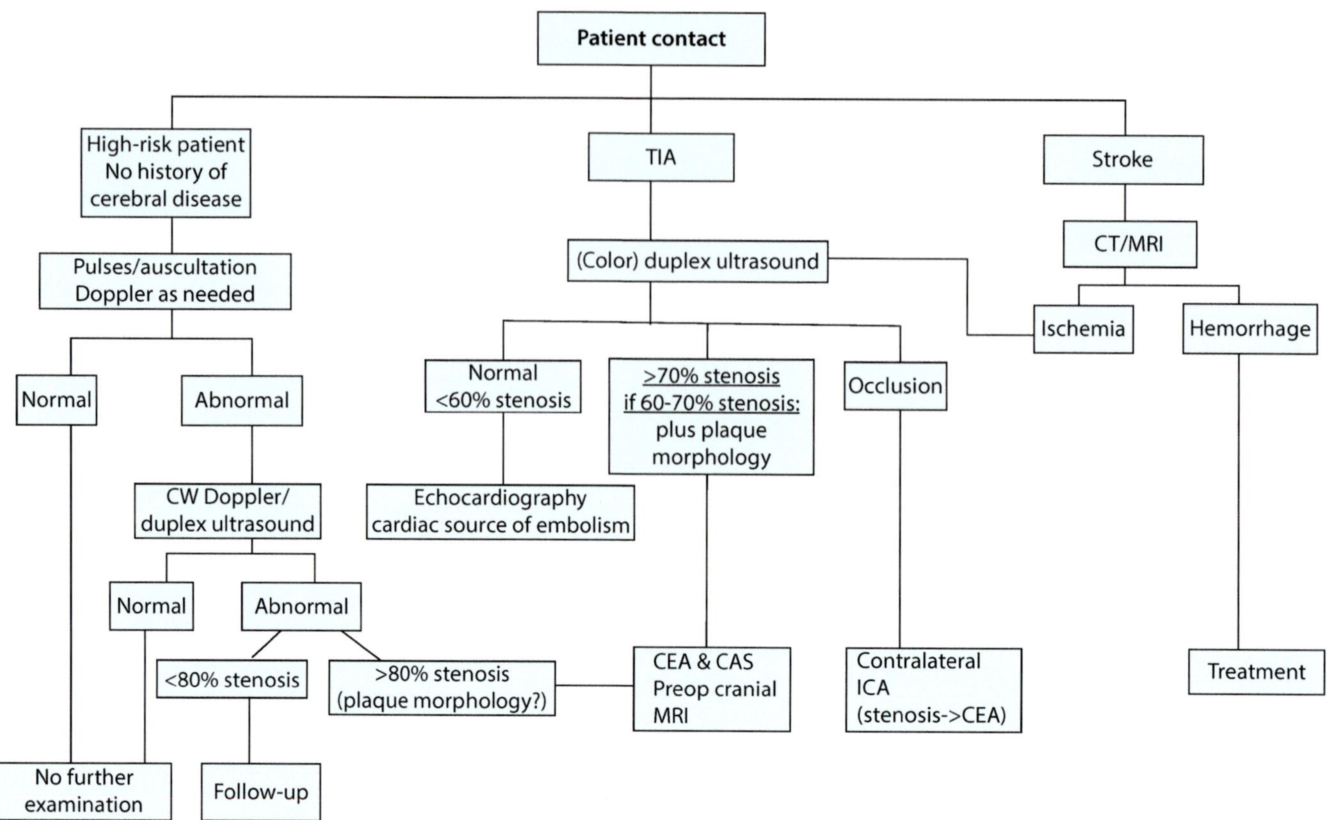

Fig. 5.12 Diagnostic algorithm in patients with suspected internal carotid artery (ICA) stenosis. Degrees of stenosis in the algorithm are ECST degrees (with 70% stenosis by ECST criteria being equivalent to 50% stenosis by NASCET criteria). If >70% ECST stenosis (>50% NASCET) has been diagnosed by duplex ultrasound, the patient can proceed to surgery without further preoperative imaging of the carotid arteries. In patients with 60–70% ECST stenosis (40–50% NASCET), plaque morphology on B-mode imaging is considered as an additional criterion in identifying those for whom carotid endarterectomy (CEA) is recommended (see Figs. 5.9b and 5.10 and Table 5.9)

collagen matrix is formed, and advanced lesions may develop a fibrous cap. Inflammatory processes appear to play an important role in the further development and also in rendering a plaque vulnerable. Mechanisms such as intimal stress and damage in conjunction with slow flow but high wall pressure contribute to plaque development opposite a flow divider in vessel bifurcations (► Sect. 1.2.1 and Fig. 1.44).

Once a plaque has reached a certain thickness, it disturbs the nutrition of the intima, which is not supplied by vessels of its own but through diffusion from the vessel lumen. The initial plaque continues to grow through the accumulation of lipids, lipoproteins, and cholesterol. The interruption of the nutrient supply can lead to central necrosis (Fig. 5.13) with formation of an atheroma, which may become organized through fibroblast invasion and thus develop into a stable lesion. Alternatively, there may be rupture of the covering intimal layer with discharge of degenerative atheromatous debris into the bloodstream and embolization to the brain. Neovascularization and inflammatory processes appear to contribute to plaque vulnerability (Fig. 5.14). As a result of lipid inclusion and central necrosis, a plaque can increase in size to such an extent that it represents a considerable obstacle to pulsatile blood flow. Sonographically, such a plaque is identified by **pulsatile longitudinal movement with the blood flow**. Fibroblast invasion leads to sclerosis, ultimately resulting in calcification of the plaque.

A rapid **increase in plaque size** may also be due to internal hemorrhage, which is attributed to very minute, vulnerable vessels growing in from the adventitia. Exposure to flowing blood can lead to rupture of the thin plaque cap (intima) with embolization to the brain of necrotic or thrombotic plaque components (Fig. 5.13). Plaque rupture triggers repair processes with re-endothelization of the former plaque area, resulting in a rather smoothly covered niche that poses no risk of embolization. Unfortunately, this fairly harmless state may be difficult to differentiate from ulceration by angiography and ultrasound alike.

Less harmless sequelae are ulcerative defects with incomplete re-endothelialization that may still release thrombotic material into the bloodstream.

The turbulent flow occurring in stenotic segments can induce the deposition of thrombotic material, especially at the distal end of a plaque, with ultimate progression to occlusion of the ICA.

The risk of embolism is determined not only by the degree of stenosis but also by plaque morphology as such. The following types of plaques can be distinguished in the carotid system on the basis of their macroscopic appearance:

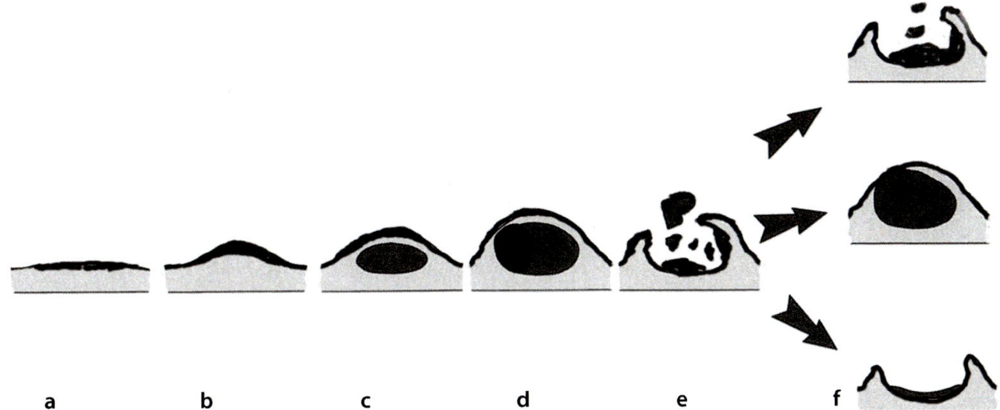

Fig. 5.13a–f Stages of plaque development. **a** Initial atherosclerotic wall thickening (intima-media complex thickening). **b** Further increase in wall thickness. **c** Plaque increases in size through lipid accumulation and may undergo central necrosis (atheroma); disturbed nutrition of the plaque. **d** Intramural hemorrhage through rupture of ingrowing vessels. **e** Rupture of the plaque cap induced by pulsatile blood flow (longitudinal pulsation) with ulceration mainly of proximal portions. **f** Re-endothelialization of the ulcer with formation of a washed-out niche as a fairly stable residue (bottom); re-endothelialization of the vulnerable plaque (middle); or persisting ulcerative plaque with recurrent embolism and only partial repair of the vulnerable surface (top)

- Flat, fibrous plaque
- Atheromatous or soft plaque
- Calcified or hard plaque
- Ulcerative plaque
- Hemorrhagic plaque

In a large series of 1252 consecutive patients, Park et al. (1998) correlated plaque morphology in carotid endarterectomy specimens with clinical symptoms. The incidence of plaque ulceration was 77% in patients with transient ischemic attacks (TIAs) and 79% in those with prior stroke, which was significantly higher than in asymptomatic patients (60%). The incidence of intraplaque hemorrhage did not differ significantly between symptomatic and asymptomatic patients but was significantly higher in patients with greater than 90% carotid stenosis.

For estimation of the risk of embolism, it would be desirable to have an imaging modality (like ultrasound or contrast-enhanced ultrasound (CEUS)) that provides reliable information on plaque morphology. This is difficult, however, since most atherosclerotic lesions are chiefly composed of variable amounts of atheromatous material with high lipid content and fibrous material rich in collagen. The inhomogeneous composition of plaques is reflected in their ultrasound appearance, but it is not possible to identify individual plaque components on the basis of their echogenicity and to exploit this information for predicting the risk of embolism. Specifically, ulcerated plaques are difficult to differentiate from washed-out cavities that have become re-endothelialized.

5.5.2 Vertebral Arteries

Transient ischemic attacks (TIAs) or strokes due to pathology of the vertebrobasilar system are much less common than those arising from the carotid territory. Stenosis at the origin of the vertebral artery rarely requires surgical or interventional treatment, in particular because the risk of embolism is lower. In patients with multiple-vessel disease and a global reduction in cerebral perfusion, repair is mainly done in the carotid territory.

While lesions in the carotid system present with highly specific hemispheric symptoms, the clinical manifestation is much less specific when the vertebrobasilar system is involved. Dizziness is the chief symptom, but may also be caused by numerous nonvascular conditions. Apart from atherosclerotic lesions, acute symptoms of vertebrobasilar insufficiency may be due to dissection, typically occurring after trauma.

In patients with subclavian artery occlusion, the vertebral artery is scanned to evaluate its collateral function in subclavian steal syndrome (complete vs. incomplete).

Ultrasound is the method of choice for morphologic assessment as well as demonstration of atherosclerotic lesions and dissection. Published data suggest that the vertebral artery is amenable to sonographic assessment in over 80–90% of cases, depending on the segments included in the analysis.

5.6 Ultrasound Criteria, Measurement Parameters, and Diagnostic Role

5.6.1 Carotid Arteries

5.6.1.1 Plaque Evaluation and Morphology

5.6.1.1.1 Intima-Media Thickness

There has been a long controversy regarding the role of B-mode plaque evaluation in estimating the risk of embolism, and even more recent studies have not clarified this issue. What is undisputed is that B-mode sonomorphologic criteria allow a detailed description and classification of

5

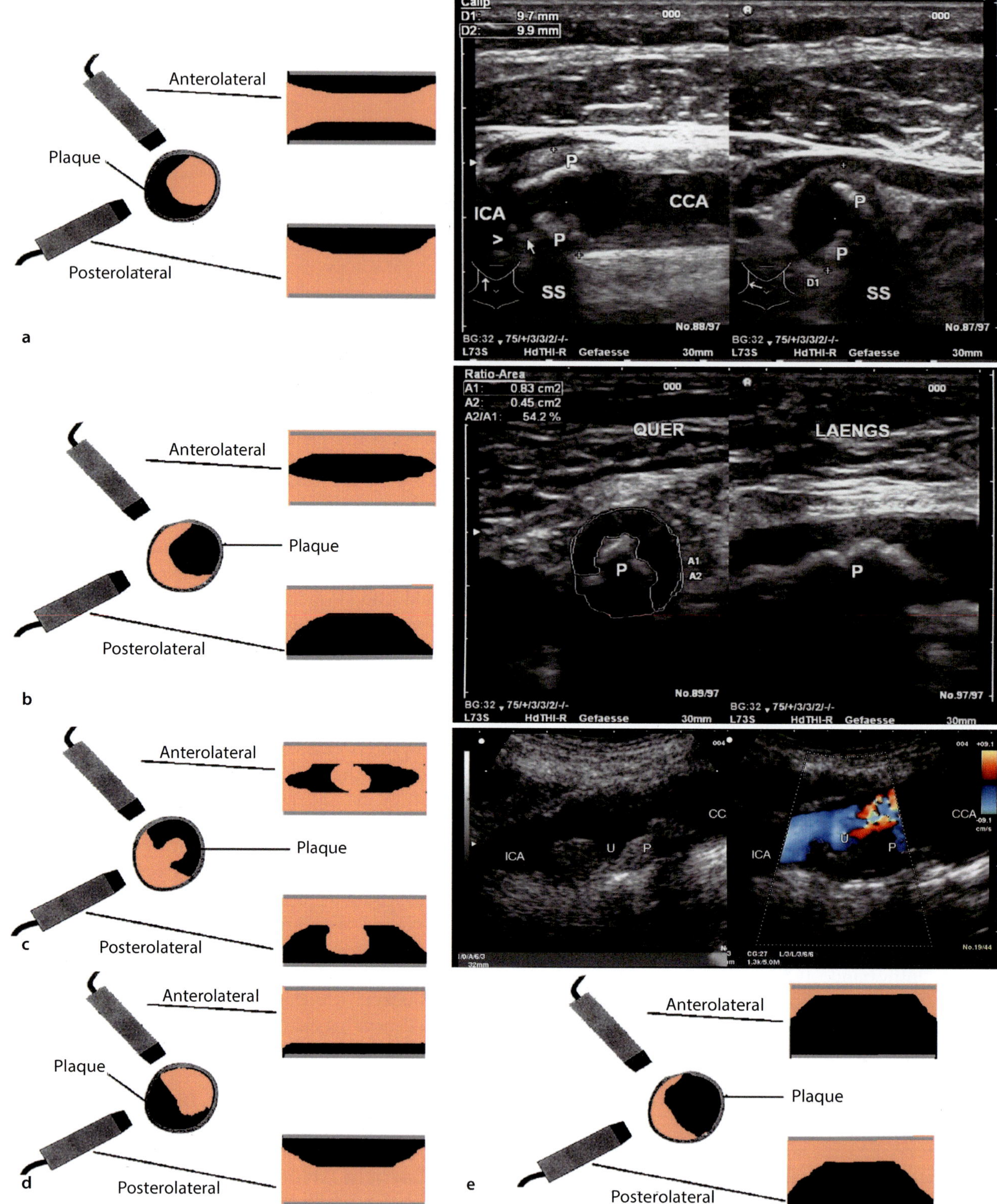

Fig. 5.14a–e Scanning in at least two planes (as in angiography) is required for sonographic plaque characterization (thickness, morphology) (anterior and posterolateral transducer positions). If, for instance, a small bowl-shaped plaque is imaged in only one plane, the degree of stenosis can be overestimated or underestimated (see Fig. 5.27). Diagrams **a–e** illustrate different sonomorphologic plaque shapes (transverse plane on the left and anterolateral and posterolateral longitudinal sections on the right). The drawings show eccentric concave (**a, d**) and convex (**b, e**) plaques and ulceration (**c**) and illustrate how eccentric plaques convexly protruding into the lumen can be overestimated in certain scan planes, while concave eccentric plaques may be underestimated. The plaques in **a** and **b** (diagrams and corresponding ultrasound images) cause roughly the same cross-sectional area reduction (approx. 50%) but differ in thickness and in the amount of diameter reduction they cause (how these parameters are evaluated depends on the scan plane). With the transducer in the posterolateral position, the degree of stenosis caused by a large eccentric plaque (examples **b** and **e**) may be overestimated; with an anterior approach, it may be slightly underestimated. **c** Ulcer in a large eccentric plaque. In this example, only the posterolateral transducer position allows adequate evaluation (as illustrated by the diagrams)

plaques with good interobserver and intraobserver agreement. Technical developments and the use of high-resolution transducers (>10 MHz) have improved the detection and evaluation of small plaques as well as the measurement of intima-media thickness (IMT). The latter is therefore increasingly being used to identify individuals with an increased cardiovascular risk.

The thickness of the intimal and medial layers can be most reliably measured in longitudinal orientation using the leading-edge method (see ◘ Figs. 5.52 and 5.53 (both Atlas) and ► Sect. 5.2.1). This method allows measurement of the intima-media complex with good interobserver agreement and was used to determine age-related IMT reference values. The normal IMT is <0.7 mm, with a thickness > 1 mm being abnormal and >2 mm representing plaque. Homma et al. (1997, 1999, 2000) found a linear increase in IMT from a mean of 0.49 mm before age 40 to 1.02 mm in subjects older than 100 and proposed the following formula for calculating age-related normal IMT: (0.009 × age) + 0.116.

The intima and media cannot be differentiated sonographically, and this is why the intima-media complex is measured to identify atherosclerotic thickening of the intima. The media is thickened in patients with inflammatory vascular conditions.

Interventional studies (e.g., of statin treatment; Hedblad et al. 2001; Kang et al. 2004) used serial sonographic IMT measurement to monitor treatment outcome, assuming a measurement accuracy with an error of less than 0.1 mm (Reley et al. 1992; Meyer and Strobel 2008). This accuracy requires an axial resolution that only a transducer with a very high frequency of >15 MHz can offer. Such transducers in turn may not provide the penetration necessary for imaging the CCA in all patients. Transducers with a frequency of 10 MHz or less have a maximum axial resolution of approx. 0.2 mm and are unlikely to detect changes of less than 0.1 mm in serial measurements. In addition, deviations of 0.1–0.2 mm result from interobserver variability and the use of different ultrasound systems (Baldassarre et al. 2000; Kanters et al. 1997). Despite these limitations, high-resolution transducers provide a good option for monitoring IMT.

Various sites in the CCA and ICA have been explored to measure IMT, and the **distal CCA** 2–3 cm proximal to the bifurcation has emerged as the **best site for IMT measurement**. Areas of plaque should be excluded, but once plaque has been demonstrated, IMT measurement is no longer required to estimate the cardiovascular risk (Poli et al. 1988; Bond et al. 1989; Ebrahim et al. 1999; Sun et al. 2002; Homma et al. 2001; Sakaguchi et al. 2003; Sutton-Tyrrell et al. 1992; Meyer and Strobel 2008).

Long circumferential thickening of the arterial wall, especially when homogeneous and hypoechoic, could point to early vasculitis. Suspected vasculitis should be ruled out or confirmed by additional clinical and laboratory examinations and sonographic evaluation of the vascular territories most susceptible to this condition (subclavian artery).

Small plaques in the ICA become more frequent in the normal population after age 50 with a prevalence of up to 80% in those over 80. Because they are so common and their natural history is unclear, the significance of small ICA plaques and their therapeutic relevance remain unclear.

5.6.1.1.2 Plaque Features

Carotid plaque and stenosis mainly occur in the bifurcation and the first 2 cm of the ICA and ECA. This is because the local reduction in blood flow velocity occurring in zones of separation (with local eddy currents) (see ◘ Fig. 1.44b) increases pressure on the arterial wall, which can cause local intimal damage. Carotid bulb plaque therefore tends to arise in the separation zone of the bifurcation and hence opposite the ECA origin (◘ Figs. 5.18 and 5.16). The natural dilatation of the bulb additionally contributes to the higher pressure (Bernoulli equation). The superficial location of these carotid segments enables imaging with a high-resolution, high-frequency transducer that also allows evaluation of plaque morphology. The **morphologic description** of a plaque comprises the following **features**:

- Localization:
  - Anterior/posterior wall
  - Proximal/distal
- Extent:
  - Circular/semicircular
  - Plaque diameter
- Plaque configuration:
  - Concentric
  - Eccentric
- Plaque surface:
  - Clearly delineated/poorly delineated/not delineated
  - Smooth/irregular (0.4–2.0 mm fissures); ulcer (> 2.0 mm deep)
- Plaque composition:
  - Homogeneous/inhomogeneous
- Echogenicity:
  - Echogenic (with or without acoustic shadowing)/ echolucent/cannot be visualized

The great flexibility in positioning the transducer facilitates plaque evaluation in different planes in a way not afforded by other cross-sectional imaging modalities. Nevertheless, the individual ultrasound scan reduces the three-dimensional (3D) plaque to a two-dimensional (2D) representation (◘ Fig. 5.14). Serial measurement of plaque thickness over time – an important predictor of the risk of embolism – thus becomes unreliable using B-mode ultrasound alone. Therefore, it is recommended to insonate the plaque from different directions and measure its greatest thickness instead of using standardized planes for measurement. Plaque configuration also contributes to the risk of embolism and must not be neglected. The **risk is higher for an eccentric plaque** because it is thicker on one side and the shear forces acting on this thicker plaque portion protruding into the lumen are greater than those acting on a concentric plaque – even when the two are causing the same degree of stenosis (◘ Fig. 5.15).

Using a high-resolution transducer, the examiner should first obtain an unbiased impression of plaque morphology

5

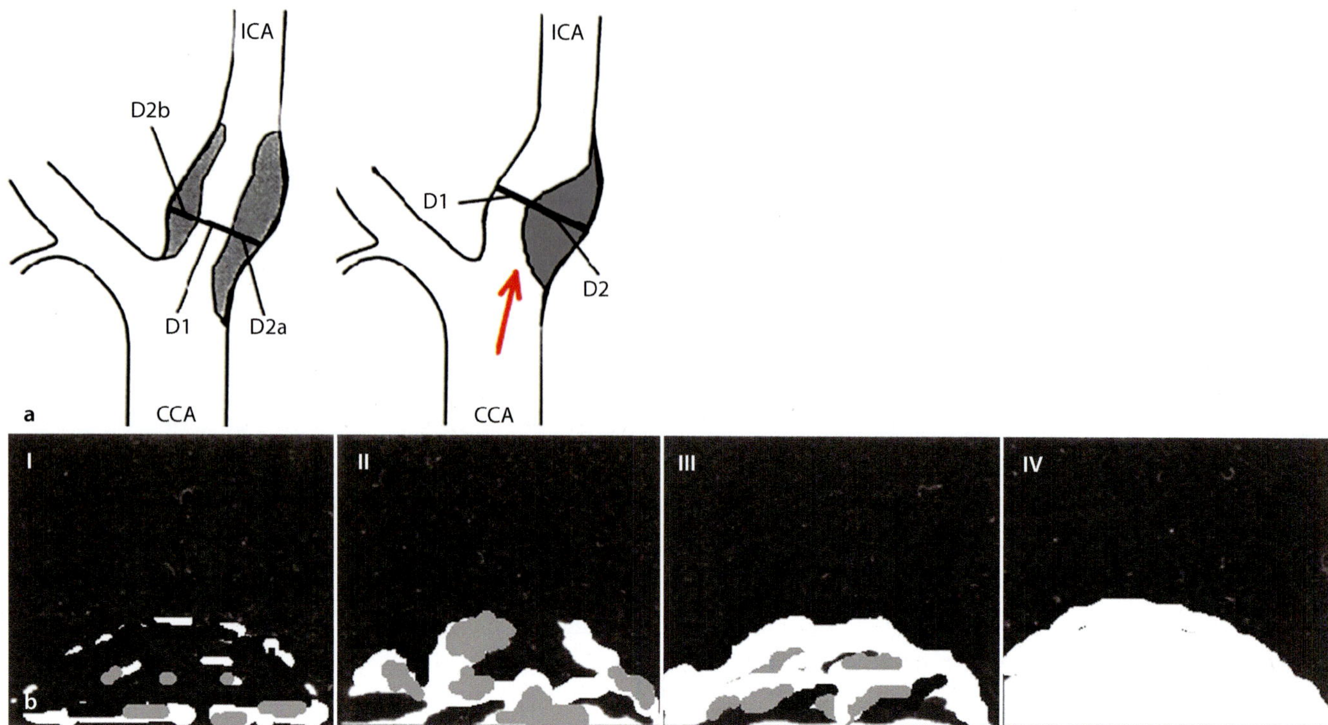

Fig. 5.15 **a** Diagrams illustrating internal carotid artery (ICA) stenosis caused by concentric (left drawing) versus eccentric plaque (right drawing). Although the degree of stenosis is the same (approx. 65% based on the local grading method/ECST ceriteria), an eccentric plaque is thicker (twice as thick in the example) and therefore poses a higher risk of embolism: the shear forces acting on it (red arrow) are greater, and the plaque is therefore more likely to rupture. **b** Sonomorphologic types of carotid artery plaque (based on the Gray-Weale classification; see Figs. 5.57, 5.58, and 5.59 (Atlas)): Type I – predominantly echolucent lesions with a low gray-scale value, similar to that of the lumen; the surface is interrupted and not consistently visible. Type II – mixed, substantially echolucent lesions with small areas of echogenicity and interrupted, irregular surfaces. Type III – mixed, substantially echogenic lesions with mostly regular and clearly delineated surfaces. Type IV – predominantly echogenic lesions of uniform density with mostly smooth and clearly delineated surfaces

without any gross pathologic criteria or prognostic factors in mind. Plaque appearance on gray-scale images provides no direct information whatsoever about plaque composition – whether fibrous, atheromatous, stable, unstable, or ulcerated. Instead, the examiner must always bear in mind that the ultrasound image is a display of differences in acoustic impedance between tissues and does not reflect tissue properties directly.

The **plaque surface**, which is the boundary between flowing blood and the plaque components, is described in terms of visibility and irregularity or disruption. Note, however, that the visibility of a reflecting structure such as the plaque boundary is primarily determined by the angle of incidence of the ultrasound beam (i.e., the intensity with which the boundary is depicted depends on whether the returning echoes have been reflected or scattered by the interface; see Figs. 1.2 and 1.3).

5.6.1.1.3 Plaque Differentiation

The way in which a gray-scale ultrasound image is formed also plays a role when evaluating plaque makeup and echotexture. Echodensity is described in shades of gray ranging from very dark to very bright (echolucent to echogenic). The reference values used are those of the hypoechoic flowing blood (lowest gray-scale value) and the hyperechoic boundary (high gray-scale value) between the adventitia and surrounding connective tissue in the far wall. The echotexture can be described as homogeneous (uniform appearance) or inhomogeneous (irregular distribution of bright pixels or absence of echoes). In a heterogeneous plaque, echolucent areas near the surface are most relevant for estimating the risk of embolism. Acoustic shadowing is the only ultrasound phenomenon that provides direct information on a histopathologic tissue feature, as it indicates total reflection of the incident ultrasound beam by a calcified structure. It is a sign of a calcified plaque, which is more stable. The Gray-Weale classification was proposed to provide a unified description on the basis of the many criteria of plaque morphology used in the literature and distinguishes four types of plaques based on echogenicity (Gray-Weale et al. 1988; Fig. 5.15b).

Supplementing this classification with other important criteria including plaque surface characteristics (Geroulakos et al. 1994; Langsfeld et al. 1989; Lusby 1993; Widder 1995), one can **distinguish the following types of plaques** on ultrasound (Figs. 5.16, 5.57 (Atlas), and 5.58 (Atlas)):

- Type IV: echogenic and homogeneous plaque with a clearly delineated, smooth surface
- Type III: plaque of mixed echogenicity with predominantly echogenic portions and an irregular surface

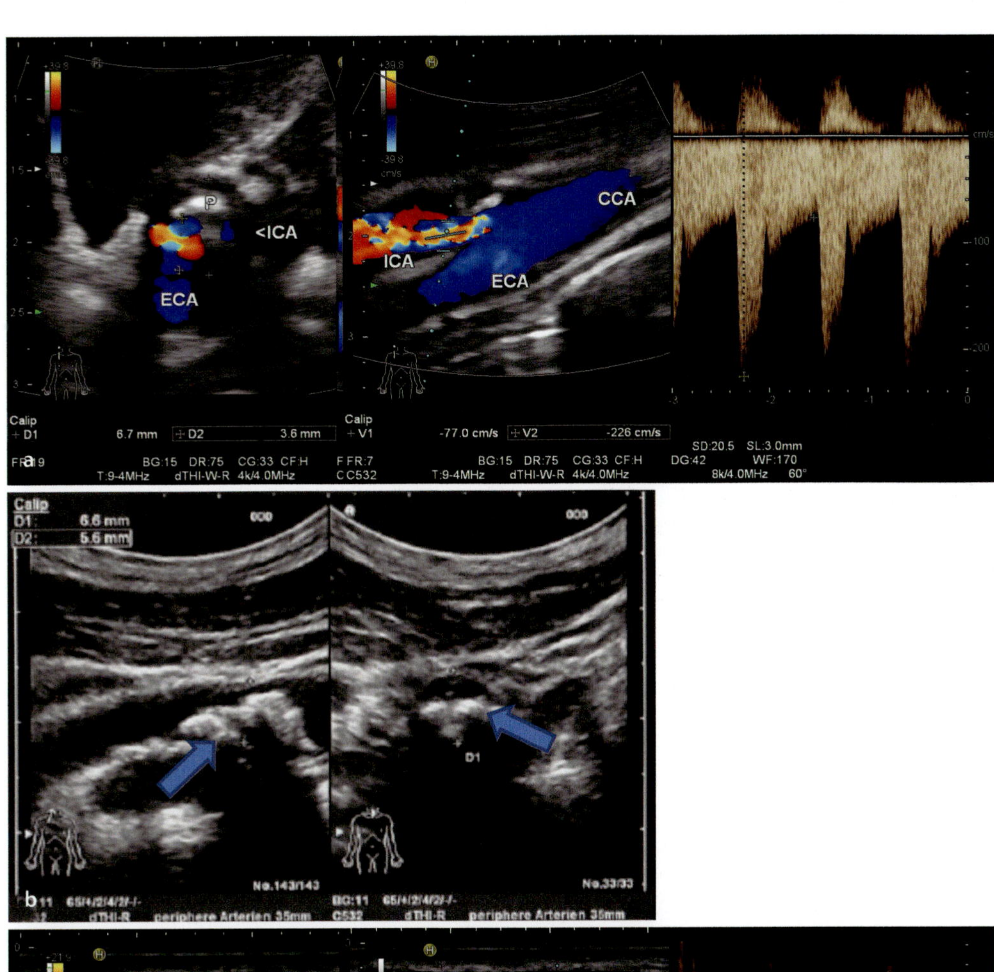

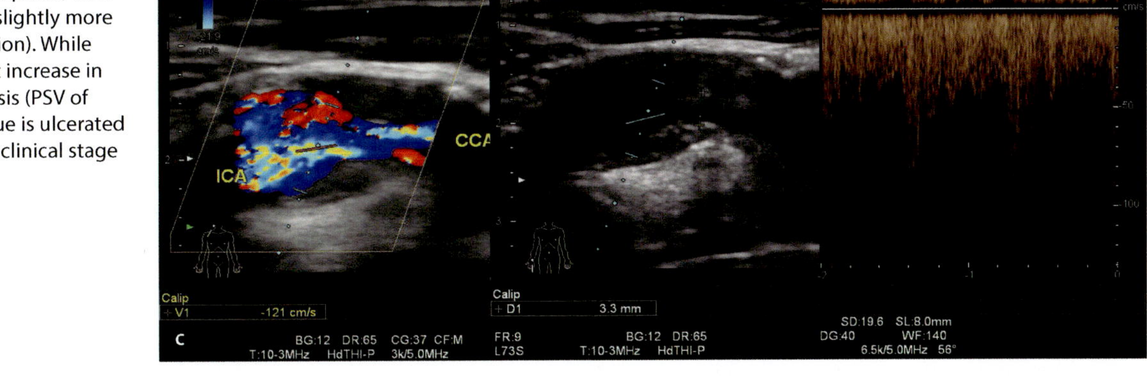

Fig. 5.16a–c Evaluation of plaque morphology. **a** Relatively hyperechoic, partially inhomogeneous, noncalcified plaque (type III) with a smooth surface (indicated by P in the left image) causing higher-grade stenosis with a peak systolic velocity (PSV) of 230 cm/s (>70% ECST stenosis/>50% NASCET stenosis). Overall, the morphologic features suggest a stable lesion, except that it is eccentric and thus exposed to greater shear stress (compared with a concentric plaque). **b** Echogenic, calcified (acoustic shadowing), and very eccentric plaque with a rather regular surface (longitudinal image on the left and transverse image on the right). The small indentation in the center of the lesion suggests an irregularity rather than ulceration. The longitudinal image (different perspective) suggests a higher-grade stenosis compared with the transverse image (70% diameter reduction). **c** Very hypoechoic, concentric plaque, almost indistinct from flowing blood, with hemodynamically moderate stenosis (PSV of 130 cm/s; 50–60% ECST stenosis/40% NASCET stenosis). Figure 5.19 shows the same plaque 6 months later (CEUS; different plane, with the transducer in a slightly more posterolateral position). While there is only a slight increase in the degree of stenosis (PSV of 150 cm/s), the plaque is ulcerated and the patient has clinical stage II disease

- Type II: predominantly echolucent or heterogeneous plaque with a poorly delineated surface
- Type I: plaque not visualized or suggested only by isolated echogenic spots in an otherwise echolucent lesion; the color flow mode is required to estimate plaque size based on the extent of the color filling defect

Assigning a plaque to one of these four categories faces two fundamental problems. First, most plaques are very heterogeneous, with components belonging to different categories, while other portions are not visualized at all and simply cannot be categorized. And one must also bear in mind that the echoes used to form the image are affected by the interaction of ultrasound with structures in the body and are not a direct representation of the target tissue (see ▶ Sect. 1.1.1.4). Second, an intraoperative analysis has shown that echolucent plaques are fibrous or atheromatous with surprisingly similar frequency (Widder et al. 1990).

Despite these discouraging remarks, the following assumptions are valid regarding the modified Gray-Weale classification of plaques.

Some studies suggest that **predominantly echolucent** plaque with isolated bright spots (type I) corresponds to atheroma with lipid inclusions and intraplaque hemorrhage, which make the plaque unstable and have been shown to be associated with a significantly increased risk of stroke.

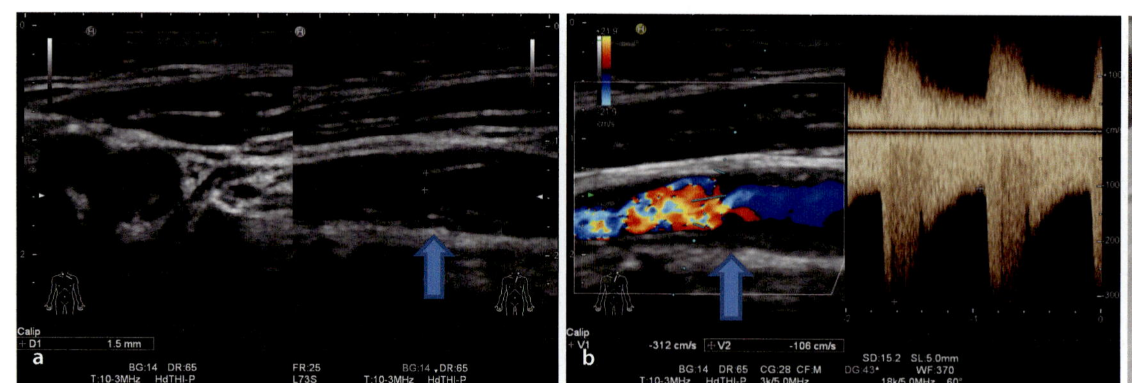

Fig. 5.17a–c Long, high-grade internal carotid artery (ICA) stenosis caused by a substantially echolucent plaque (type II) with an irregular surface. **a** The B-mode image reveals a predominantly concentric plaque with a conspicuous, tooth-like protrusion (arrow). **b** The color duplex examination shows that the eccentric component of the plaque causes high-grade stenosis with a peak systolic velocity (PSV) of 312 cm/s and an end-diastolic velocity (EDV) of 108 cm/s. The stenosis jet is seen distally. This plaque configuration is associated with an increased risk of triggering a cerebral event during an endovascular intervention, and patients should therefore undergo carotid endarterectomy (CEA) instead. **c** Nevertheless, the patient opted for coronary artery stenting (CAS). Angiographically, the subtotal occlusion caused by the protruding portion of the plaque is not seen due to poor spatial resolution of contrast filling

Echogenic and **homogeneous plaques** with a smooth surface (type IV), on the other hand, are associated with a low risk of embolization (see Figs. 5.16, 5.17, 5.58 (Atlas), 5.59 (Atlas), and 5.60 (Atlas)). Unfortunately, the **most common plaques (types II and III)** are difficult to assess in terms of prognosis, and sonomorphologic risk assessment has a disappointingly low accuracy of 50–70%. Despite its rather disappointing overall accuracy, under certain circumstances, sonographic plaque classification can provide useful information for selecting patients for surgery. These include in particular patients with asymptomatic high-grade stenosis or symptomatic 50–70% stenosis and type I or IV plaque.

5.6.1.1.4 Plaque Thickness

A thicker plaque protruding into the lumen on one side is exposed to greater shear stresses (seen sonographically as longitudinal pulsatile movement of the plaque), which may cause rupture of the vulnerable cap with discharge of embolic material into the bloodstream. This is why an eccentric plaque poses a greater risk of embolism compared with a concentric plaque (which is flatter because it occupies the entire inner circumference of the lumen) causing the same degree of stenosis (Figs. 5.10, 5.15a, 5.16, and 5.57 (Atlas)).

Progressive luminal narrowing due to plaque thickening leads to higher flow velocities in the stenotic segment (>350 cm/s), which in turn increases the risk of ulceration and embolism (Beach 1992). The risk of central necrosis and subsequent ulceration also increases with plaque length. This is due to nutritional disturbance, which additionally increases with plaque thickness (diffusion).

A **rapid increase in overall plaque size** with formation of large, echolucent areas, e.g., due to hemorrhage, in serial examinations indicates a **markedly increased risk of embolism** and is an indication for surgery.

Ulceration following **rupture of the plaque cap** is characterized on B-mode images by a heterogeneous echotexture with disruption of the surface or a crater-like defect.

The results of a large prospective multicenter study of 1121 patients with medically treated higher-grade carotid artery stenosis followed up for up to 7 years suggest that the cerebrovascular risk increases considerably with the plaque area, regardless of stenosis severity (Nicolaides 1995).

Several other studies, including investigations using 3D ultrasound, confirm that complications such as ulceration may become more common as the plaque volume increases (Schminke et al. 2000; AbuRahma et al. 2002; Pedro et al. 2002).

5.6.1.1.5 Plaque Morphology: Plaque Surface

Prediction of the risk of embolism on the basis of the sonomorphologic appearance of carotid plaque is confronted with a general problem, namely that **studies already fail to yield consistent results** regarding the correlation between **pathomorphologic features of plaques** such as ulceration, soft atheromatous deposits, and hemorrhage and the clinical stage (symptomatic vs. asymptomatic patients). While some investigators (Park et al. 1998; Sterpetti et al. 1991) demonstrated a statistically significant correlation between plaque ulceration and the occurrence of transient or persistent neurologic deficits, others did not find such a correlation (Hill et al. 1994; Van Damme et al. 1992). This explains the highly discrepant results regarding the accuracy of predicting embolism on the basis of the sonographic evaluation of plaque morphology.

Another issue is that published data are often difficult to compare. Studies correlating morphologic features of plaques with clinical stages (and the ensuing risk of embolism associated with the plaque) use different designs and subjective criteria for defining what constitutes echolucency/echogenicity or an irregular surface. Therefore, suggestions to **standardize the description of plaques** were made as early as the 1990s. De Bray et al. (1997) recommended using the echo levels of the following structures as reference values in describing plaque echogenicity: an echolucent plaque corresponds to the

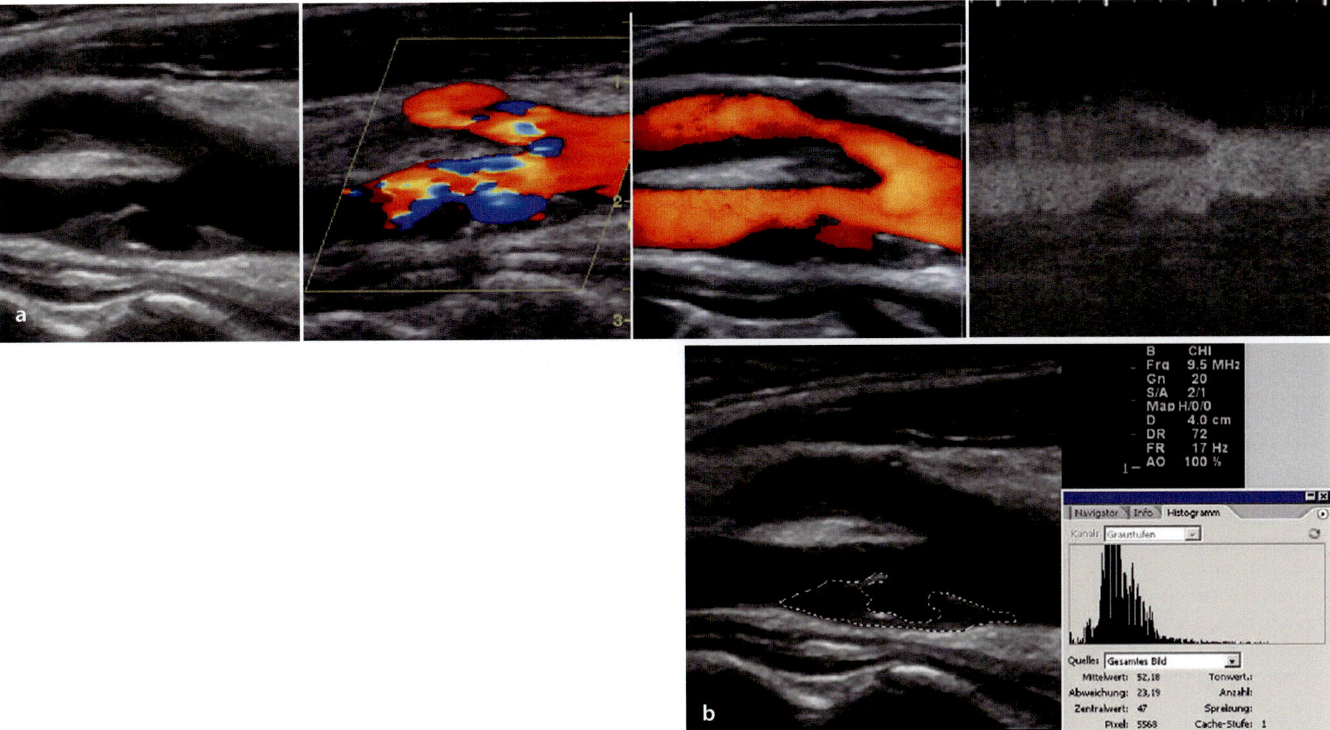

Fig. 5.18a, b Echolucent eccentric plaque at the origin of the internal carotid artery (ICA) with deep ulcer (> 2 mm). **a** Images from left to right: B-mode, color duplex, power Doppler, and B-flow mode. While the ulcerated portion is clearly differentiated from the patent lumen in the B-mode image, the power mode and B-flow mode allow the most accurate evaluation of the ulcer contour and delineation from flowing blood. Sonographic plaque morphology (echogenicity and plaque configuration) is used as an additional criterion in identifying candidates for surgery or in deciding about the best reconstructive approach (carotid artery stenting versus carotid endarterectomy). Different ultrasound techniques are used to improve morphologic plaque characterization, and both B-flow and contrast-enhanced ultrasound (CEUS) allow more accurate evaluation of plaque configuration and better identification of bowl-shaped defects. However, even with these techniques, it remains difficult to differentiate a plaque ulcer with a high risk of embolism from a washed-out niche, which, in terms of embolism risk, is considered rather harmless (see Fig. 5.13). **b** Computation of the gray-scale median (GSM) of the echolucent carotid plaque shown in **a**. The plaque is outlined in a normalized B-mode image (linear scaling using input and output values of two reference points: blood, 0–5; adventitia, 185–195), and the computer program (Adobe Photoshop CS) generates a histogram representing its composition and a median value (GSM of 47 in this case) (Figure courtesy of Werner Lang)

echogenicity of flowing blood, a less echolucent plaque to that of the sternocleidomastoid muscle, and a hyperechoic plaque to that of bone. For the plaque surface, they propose a distinction between smooth and irregular, with an irregular surface being defined as the presence of fissures 0.4–2.0 mm deep, while ulceration is assumed when craters with a depth of more than 2 mm are present (Fig. 5.18).

Ultrasound was reported to have 97% sensitivity and 81% specificity for detecting surface irregularities of lesions (Kagawa et al. 1996). An angiographic study found a correlation between an irregular surface and microscopic plaque rupture and hemorrhage in histologic examinations (Lovett et al. 2004). Both angiographic studies (Rothwell and Warlow 1999) and sonographic studies reported an increased risk of embolism for plaques with an irregular surface (Prabhakaran et al. 2006). Other investigators found a high correlation between plaques with an irregular surface and carotid artery stenosis with neurologic symptoms (Eliasziw et al. 1995; AbuRahma et al. 1999; Kessler et al. 1995; Steinke et al. 1992); however, only a few studies used a prospective design (Handa et al. 1995; Kitamura et al. 2004; Rothwell et al. 2000).

Sonographic demonstration of plaque ulceration was reported to be associated with an increased risk of ipsilateral cerebrovascular ischemia (Sitzer et al. 1995; De Bray et al. 1997; AbuRahma et al. 1998; Pedro et al. 2002). Other investigators deny such an association (Meairs and Hennerici 1999), failing to identify significant differences in plaque surface between symptomatic and asymptomatic patients.

An **irregular plaque surface**, **plaque ulceration**, or poststenotic **dead-water zones** can lead to local platelet aggregation with release of small thrombi into the bloodstream. While it is possible, in principle, to depict ulcerated areas as crater-like defects within hyperechoic plaques (Fig. 5.18), plaques are frequently heterogeneous and a fresh ulcer (Fig. 5.57 (Atlas)) is difficult to differentiate from a washed-out niche (with any imaging modality) (Fig. 5.13). Six studies investigating the validity of color duplex ultrasound in the detection of plaque ulceration yielded a wide range of accuracies with a mean sensitivity of 60% (38–94%) and mean specificity of 74% (33–92%) (Widder et al. 1990; Comerota et al. 1990; Sitzer et al. 1996; Kardoulas et al. 1996; Banafsche et al. 1998; Saba et al. 2007). The European Carotid Plaque Study (1995) found 47% sensitivity and 63% specificity for B-mode ultrasound alone.

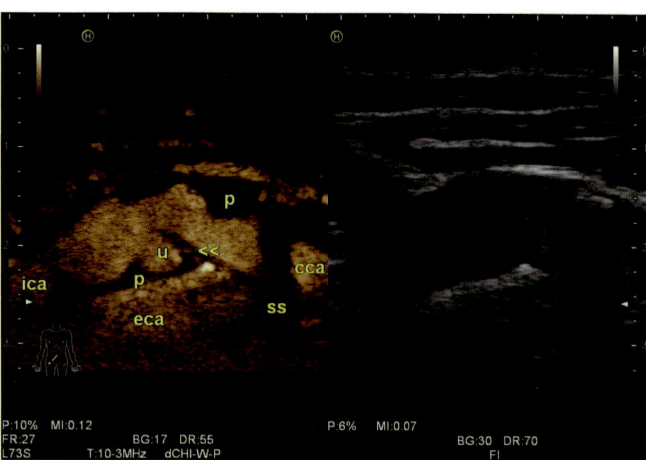

Fig. 5.19 Internal carotid artery stenosis (stage II) caused by a very echolucent plaque (60% ECST stenosis as estimated by color duplex). The contrast-enhanced ultrasound (CEUS) image (left) allows excellent evaluation of the plaque contour (p) including ulceration (u) and demonstrates neovascularization (<<) in the ulcerated portion. No neovascularization is detected in the plaque portion close to the transducer (p). CEUS suffers from the same artifacts as other ultrasound techniques. In the example shown, there is acoustic shadowing (ss) due to calcification. The bright spots in this portion of the plaque are also visible in the corresponding gray-scale image (right) and therefore do not represent neovascularization but echogenic components of the plaque. This example nicely illustrates the importance of interpreting CEUS in conjunction with the corresponding B-mode image in order to avoid misdiagnosis of bright spots

In the large cohort study of 1939 patients without a history of stroke already cited above (Prabhakaran et al. 2006), an irregular plaque surface was identified as a major risk factor with a three times higher cumulative 5-year risk of ischemic stroke compared to a regular plaque surface (8% vs. <3%).

On the other hand, **ulceration tends to be overestimated** because a very irregular plaque surface (Fig. 5.17) or a normal vessel segment between two adjacent plaques may be mistaken for ulceration. The B-mode criterion for ulceration is a deep crater (>2 mm) with a smaller diameter on the luminal side (bowl-shaped). If the B-mode findings are inconclusive, additional color duplex ultrasound, B-flow imaging, or contrast-enhanced ultrasound (CEUS) (Figs. 5.13 and 5.19) should be used to improve evaluation of the defect shape and to identify echolucent areas in an otherwise more echogenic plaque (Figs. 5.14, 5.17, and 5.18). Overall, though, differentiation of ulcerated plaque from a harmless washed-out niche remains difficult with any method (Fig. 5.13).

Subintimal intraplaque hemorrhage depicted on B-mode ultrasound as echolucent and heterogeneous areas can lead to rupture of the plaque cap (ulceration) and is therefore associated with an increased risk of stroke. Hemorrhage was found to be six times more common in surgical specimens from symptomatic patients than in specimens from asymptomatic patients. Recent hemorrhage is demonstrated by ultrasonography with a sensitivity of 72–91% and a specificity of 65–88% (Bluth et al. 1986; Widder et al. 1990).

5.6.1.1.6 Plaque Echogenicity: Influencing Factors

The difficulties just discussed have not discouraged attempts to differentiate vulnerable and stable plaques in terms of the risk of embolism they pose (Fig. 5.18). Uncomplicated or stable plaques are assumed to be homogeneously fibrous or partially calcified and to have an intact fibrous cap. Conversely, unstable plaques predominantly consist of atheromatous material (Fig. 5.17) and may contain necrotic areas and blood: a plaque cap is either absent or appears thinned or visibly interrupted. Several investigators assume that degenerative processes induced by inflammation or bacterial infection (which may lead to necrotic zones and intralesional hemorrhage) play an important role in the development of high-risk lesions (Libby 2002; O'Leary et al. 1991; O'Donnell et al. 1985; Bassiouny et al. 1977).

A number of studies (European Carotid Plaque Study Group 1995; Kardoulas et al. 1996; AbuRahma et al. 1998; Gronholdt et al. 1997, 2002; Droste et al. 1997) agree that echolucency indicates high lipid content or intralesional hemorrhage – features known to be associated with an increased risk of embolism. This is also the explanation given for the four-fold higher risk of ischemic cerebrovascular events in patients with echolucent plaques found in the Tromsø study (Figs. 5.16, 5.17, and 5.57 (Atlas)) (Mathiesen et al. 2001). Widder et al. report low sensitivity of 34% and specificity of 36% for intraplaque hemorrhage (with histologic correlation) and 51% sensitivity and 68% specificity for atheromatous plaque makeup (Widder et al. 1990). Inflammatory processes, which are known to trigger plaque growth, may also contribute to the echolucency of vulnerable plaques. This would explain the higher cardiovascular risk of patients with echolucent carotid artery plaques.

Overall, sonographic evaluation of echogenicity is very subjective and also depends on the instrument settings used. In general, a plaque is classified as echolucent if it is less echogenic than the adjacent sternocleidomastoid muscle (see Fig. 5.57 (Atlas)). Very echolucent plaques are indistinguishable from flowing blood on B-mode ultrasound. Bright spots within the lesion may be the only sign that an atheromatous plaque is present (Figs. 5.57 and 5.58 (both Atlas)). In these cases, color duplex imaging is required to indirectly reveal the plaque border as a filling defect. Increasing deposition of collagen and cellular matrix is believed to be associated with higher echogenicity. Very bright echoes are characteristic of dense fibrous or calcified areas and, in conjunction with acoustic shadowing, indicate a calcified plaque. Calcification in a plaque may be focal or diffuse. If acoustic shadowing obscures the vessel wall or precludes spectral Doppler interrogation, the transducer can be moved to avoid the intervening structure (Fig. 5.4).

A **heterogeneous ultrasound appearance** suggests a mixed plaque, and inhomogeneous components in a predominantly echolucent lesion appear to be associated with a higher risk of embolism. AbuRahma et al. (1998) found an improved detection of intraplaque hemorrhage when evaluation of echogenicity was supplemented by evaluation of plaque heterogeneity with an increase in sensitivity to 76% and specificity to 85%.

Plaques with areas of lower echogenicity near the luminal surface appear to carry a higher risk of embolism. Published studies, however, provide no clear answer as to whether the risk is higher for homogeneous versus heterogeneous plaques (Sztajzel et al. 2006; El-Barghouty et al. 1994; Wijeyaratne et al. 2003).

For these reasons, caution is advised when applying histologic terms to the description of ultrasound appearances of carotid plaques, and it is emphasized again that a gray-scale image is a display not of tissues but of interfaces between areas of different acoustic impedance. In terms of physics, higher echogenicity in a gray-scale image, therefore, merely means that a tissue contains more such interfaces. To stay on the safe side, as long as the correlation between the sonographic appearance and histologic makeup of a plaque is still vague, it is recommended that the examiner simply describe the plaque (Woodcock et al. 1992).

In summary, though, a number of prognostic features associated with a low versus high risk of embolism can be derived from the sonographic appearance of a carotid plaque:

- Low risk:
  - Predominantly echogenic and homogeneous plaque
  - Plaque surface smooth and clearly delineated
  - Calcification
  - Short plaque (<1 cm)
  - Thin plaque (<4 mm)
- High risk:
  - Predominantly echolucent lesion with isolated bright spots, difficult to delineate from surrounding blood
  - Ulceration
  - Long plaque (>1 cm)
  - Plaque diameter >4 mm
  - Longitudinal pulsatile movement of the plaque in the direction of blood flow

5.6.1.1.7 Gray-Scale Analysis: Potential and Limitations

As already mentioned, apart from plaque surface, echogenicity is the most important prognostic criterion. Although atheromatous material and lipid inclusions are widely assumed to correspond to echolucent plaque areas when scanned with a high-frequency transducer, a controversy exists as to the value of gray-scale ultrasound for plaque analysis. The assumption that inhomogeneous and hypoechoic plaques are unstable (Bräsen et al. 1997) is confirmed by a number of prospective studies showing that plaques with these features and predominantly heterogeneous portions are associated with a significantly higher risk of ipsilateral cerebrovascular ischemia than echogenic, homogeneous plaques (El-Barghouty et al. 1996; Geroulakos et al. 1994; Bock et al. 1993; Langsfeld et al. 1989). Other studies (Meairs and Hennerici 1999; Hill and Donato 1994), including the Asymptomatic Carotid Stenosis Trial (Halliday et al. 2010), failed to establish a statistically significant association between clinical symptoms and the sonographic appearance of carotid plaque.

To overcome the inherent limitations of subjective assessment of both plaque echogenicity and homogeneity and the dependence of these features on the equipment and instrument settings used, various methods of standardization have been proposed. The most common quantitative ultrasound measure of plaque echogenicity is the so-called **gray-scale median (GSM)**, which involves the computation of normalized images in which the darkest and brightest areas (blood and adventitia) are invariably assigned values of 0–5 (echolucent) and 180–200 (hyperechoic) (▫ Fig. 5.18b).

The GSM of the plaque in the normalized image allows objective differentiation of echolucent lesions with a GSM of <35 from echogenic lesions with a GSM of >65. While a GSM >65 was found to correlate well with fibrocalcified plaques, a GSM <35 correlated poorly with the presence of a lipid core (40–60% sensitivity) or atheromatous plaque (El-Barghouty et al. 1996; Gronholdt et al. 1998, 2001; Aly and Bishop 2000; Tegos et al. 2000; Ciulla et al. 2002). Another study reported 84% sensitivity and 75% specificity for identifying intralesional lipid cores using stratified GSM analysis rather than whole-plaque analysis (Sztajzel 2005).

The authors of a large prospective multicenter study with follow-up of 1121 patients with carotid artery stenosis (Nicolaides 1995) conducted a detailed analysis of associations between plaque echogenicity (using different GSM ranges) and cerebrovascular events and found good interobserver agreement (correlation of 0.93) for GSM determination. Compared with echogenic plaques (GSM >30), the risk of cerebrovascular events was more than five times higher for very echolucent plaques with a GSM <15 and more than three times higher for plaques with a GSM of 15–29.

Standardized determination of echogenicity to estimate plaque vulnerability might also help in deciding between carotid artery stenting (CAS) and carotid endarterectomy (CEA). The Imaging in Carotid Angioplasty and Risk of Stroke (ICAROS) study shows that carotid plaque echolucency (GSM ≤25) increases the risk of stroke during CAS. This study found a 7.1% risk of cerebrovascular events during CAS for echolucent plaques with a GSM of ≤25 versus 1.5% for hyperechoic plaques ($p = 0.01$) (Biasi et al. 2004).

Technically, gray-scale analysis and characterization of the plaque surface from sonographic images are less reliable for plaques causing high-grade stenosis versus those causing mild to moderate stenosis. Sonographic evaluation is also limited when a plaque is inhomogeneous or calcified.

While several studies (El-Barghouty et al. 1995, 1996; Pedro et al. 2000; Kakkos et al. 2007) investigating plaque echolucency using GSM analysis (see ▫ Fig. 5.18b) show that echolucent plaques are associated with an increased risk of stroke (Pollak et al. 1998), there is another study that suggests that computer-assisted texture analysis of carotid plaque in ultrasound images predicts embolism more accurately than GSM analysis (Kakkos et al. 2007).

In yet another study, standardized gray-scale analysis of plaque morphology showed good interobserver agreement, while plaque sonomorphology correlated poorly with the histopathologic findings in the surgical specimens from patients having undergone eversion endarterectomy (Denzel 2003).

Attempts have also been made at improving the evaluation of plaque echogenicity by means of **3D ultrasound**; however, a study using a standardized protocol did not find 3D ultrasound to be superior to 2D ultrasound in evaluating the echogenicity of ICA plaque (Denzel et al. 2009). Neither ultrasound nor any other imaging modality can consistently differentiate a fresh plaque ulcer from a harmless cavity.

As an ultrasound image is created from echoes reflected at interfaces of different acoustic impedance, a **heterogeneous tissue containing more interfaces has higher echogenicity**. This is why hemangiomas in the liver are echogenic. Inhomogeneous tissue is more echogenic than homogeneous tissue regardless of its stiffness (hard–soft). Applied to plaques with their variable pathomorphologic composition, this means that the echogenicity of plaques with a high risk of embolism resulting from a high lipid content or intraplaque hemorrhage (as such predominantly echolucent) is not uniform but is instead dependent on how the lipid and blood are integrated into the plaque matrix and on the resulting plaque structure. Hence, these plaques may also appear echogenic. Conversely, a stable, fibrous plaque (based on pathomorphologic criteria) can have low echogenicity when the plaque matrix contains fewer interfaces. This is an inherent limitation of the sonographic evaluation of plaque morphology.

It follows that it is not possible to derive carotid plaque makeup from echogenicity although scientific evidence suggests that echolucency predicts a three to five times higher risk of embolism. This lack of correlation between plaque composition and sonographic appearance was impressively confirmed in a study using GSM values to classify ICA plaques as echolucent (GSM <32) and echogenic (GSM ≥32) (Gonçalves et al. 2004). Surgical specimens were prepared for biochemical and chromatographic analysis to determine the elastin, calcium, collagen (by measuring hydroxyproline), and lipid (chromatography) content of the plaques. The analysis revealed that calcium hydrocarbonate content was significantly higher in echogenic plaques and elastin content in echolucent plaques. No significant differences between echolucent and echogenic plaques were found for collagen, cholesterol, or triglycerides. Detailed analysis of plaque lipids by linear regression also failed to reveal differences between the two types of plaques. These findings are in disagreement with numerous other studies and also contradict the widely held assumption that echolucent plaques have a high lipid content and therefore pose a greater risk of embolism than echogenic plaques, which are assumed to be fibrous. Thus, we are confronted with the **paradoxical situation** that, while echolucent plaques tend to be associated with a higher risk of embolism (symptomatic carotid artery stenosis), there is no histologic basis for this observation as no significant correlation has been found between echogenicity and a histologically vulnerable plaque (e.g., high lipid content).

New techniques of sonographic image processing may provide new insights into plaque morphology and thus improve the differentiation of vulnerable and stable plaques. While conventional B-mode ultrasonography processes the amplitude of the reflected echoes, an alternative technique using high-resolution transducers as in intravascular ultrasound (IVUS) differentiates the reflected echo pulses by frequency. This technique is based on the assumption that different tissues (necrosis, fibrosis, lipid-rich tissue) reflect the ultrasound with different frequencies. The authors concluded that sonographic evaluation of plaque morphology using this technique might have the potential to improve tissue differentiation and to thus help discriminate vulnerable plaques with necrotic portions and a high lipid content from more stable, fibrotic plaques (Reid et al. 2005).

Virtual histology IVUS is another technique that was introduced to characterize carotid plaque composition. The frequencies reflected by different plaque components (fibrous, necrosis, calcification, and lipid core) are collated and coded with different colors, and this information is then superimposed on the original IVUS image as a color map of plaque composition. For example, red can be used to indicate plaques considered to be vulnerable (e.g., plaques with hemorrhagic or necrotic components, lipid-rich plaques). While this technique was primarily expected to influence coronary interventions, virtual histology IVUS might also have a role in the pretherapeutic assessment of other vascular territories that are amenable to interventional dilatation with stenting, most notably the carotid and renal arteries. A worldwide registry to define the clinical role of virtual histology IVUS was planned when this technique was introduced.

5.6.1.1.8 Carotid Plaque Characterization Using Contrast-Enhanced Ultrasound

Contrast-enhanced ultrasound (CEUS) improves the differentiation of the hypoechoic intima-media complex and of atherosclerotic plaques from flowing blood. The adventitia in turn is also characterized by higher echogenicity. CEUS thus allows good evaluation of the plaque contour and plaque surface (irregularities, ulceration) (◘ Fig. 5.19) and is especially useful for the detection of echolucent plaques, which may be difficult to differentiate from flowing blood when conventional gray-scale imaging is used (van der Oord 2013). CEUS with enhancement of flowing blood is thus useful for the diagnosis of subclinical atherosclerosis and can help in detecting very low flow, which distinguishes very severe stenosis or pseudo-occlusion from true occlusion.

Ultrasound microbubbles increase the intensity of Doppler signals from blood, improving evaluation of irregular plaque surfaces and ulceration and identification of echolucent plaques (Kono et al. 2004). Despite these advantages, CEUS does not solve the notorious problem of differentiating a harmless residual defect from plaque ulceration (◘ Fig. 5.13).

The microbubbles also enter smaller vessels such as intraplaque neovessels and proliferating vasa vasorum, seen as bright reflections within the plaque (◘ Fig. 5.19). **Neovascularization** identified by CEUS can thus serve as an additional marker of carotid plaque vulnerability. Several studies have shown a significant correlation between plaque neovascularization demonstrated by CEUS and histopathology (Hoogi et al. 2011; Staub et al. 2013), symptomatic carotid artery plaque (Xiong et al. 2009), and echolucency (Staub et al. 2011). The accuracy of semiquantitative evaluation of plaque neovascularization by CEUS has been confirmed in studies with histologic correlation and in an animal model (Coli et al. 2008; Shah et al. 2007; Hoogi et al. 2011; Vavuranakis et al. 2013).

Histopathologic studies show that plaque neovascularization through **vasa vasorum proliferation** from the adventitia (fragile vessels) correlates with plaque vulnerability (Pelisek 2012) and with increasing thickness of the plaque (Sluimer et al. 2009). Plaque growth is also triggered by hypoxia and inflammatory processes.

Providing a semiquantitative measure of plaque neovascularization, **CEUS can make an important contribution** to the differentiation of vulnerable and stable carotid plaques and to the prediction of a patient's cardiovascular risk.

Several retrospective studies (Staub et al. 2010; Faggioli et al. 2011; Yiong et al. 2009) confirm an association between increased plaque neovascularization as identified by CEUS and a higher incidence of cerebrovascular events (stroke, TIA). Thicker plaques, especially echolucent ones, have higher neovascularization on CEUS (Staub et al. 2011). However, the examiner should be aware that neovascularization is more difficult to identify in echogenic plaques and that not all bright spots indicate neovascularization. To avoid misinterpretation of such spots, it is important to exactly match CEUS images with the corresponding real-time gray-scale images (◘ Figs. 5.19 and 5.57 (Atlas)).

Inflammation is an another factor contributing to plaque vulnerability. Higher levels of C-reactive protein (CRP) are associated with faster plaque progression and have been shown to predict cardiovascular events (Hermus et al. 2010). A recent study reports an association between elevated CRP levels and more extensive plaque neovascularization, as assessed by CEUS (Staub 2015). In a rabbit model of atherosclerosis, CEUS was found to have the potential for monitoring the response to statin treatment, showing regression of plaque vascularization in serial examinations (Tian et al. 2013).

In summary, available evidence suggests that CEUS can improve evaluation of morphologic plaque features and allows semiquantitative determination of plaque neovascularization. Therefore, CEUS has the potential to improve risk stratification of carotid plaque compared with the prediction of cerebrovascular events based on stenosis severity alone (Eyding et al. 2011). This in turn can contribute to a better selection of candidates for invasive prophylactic treatment. Moreover, the demonstration of vulnerable carotid artery plaque based on neovascularization allows identification of patients at an increased risk of cardiovascular events (Hellings et al. 2010) who may benefit from optimization of their medical treatment.

5.6.1.2 Stenosis Quantification/Grading

In the prophylactic approach to carotid artery stenosis (prevention of worst case), the severity of stenosis is the basis for patient management and the choice between best medical treatment and invasive options (surgery or intervention). The foremost diagnostic task in these patients, therefore, is to ensure reliable stenosis grading.

The indirect criteria used in the assessment of peripheral artery stenosis, such as changes in peristenotic pulsatility, are of little use in the carotid territory. Pulsatility of blood flow varies with peripheral resistance and vessel wall elasticity. Several factors can lead to increased carotid artery pulsatility including reduced wall elasticity (e.g., in medial sclerosis), increased intracranial pressure, aortic insufficiency, and bradycardia (◘ Table 5.5). A decrease in pulsatility is observed in the presence of an AV fistula with hyperperfusion or in tachycardia.

As in the peripheral arteries, higher-grade carotid artery stenosis is associated with increased pulsatility in the prestenotic segment and decreased pulsatility in the poststenotic segment. The effect on pre- and poststenotic pulsatility correlates with the severity of stenosis (indirect stenosis criterion).

Sonographically, intrastenotic flow velocity (peak systolic velocity (PSV) and end-diastolic velocity (EDV)), which increases according to the continuity equation, is the most important direct criterion of a flow-limiting stenosis caused by carotid plaque. In addition, the stenosis disturbs blood flow, especially when caused by an eccentric plaque. Laminar flow becomes unstable with features ranging from the presence in the Doppler waveform of slow flow components in an otherwise clear window to turbulent flow with a retrograde component. For grading, the site of stenosis is identified in the longitudinal plane, and a Doppler waveform is obtained with the sample volume placed in the stenotic jet (the distal plaque end when the stenosis is short). A measurable increase in flow velocity does not occur until a plaque causes a diameter reduction of at least 30–40% (by NASCET criteria/distal degree of stenosis, which is equivalent to 50% ECST stenosis/local degree). This is the threshold above which a stenosis becomes hemodynamically significant and can be quantified by spectral Doppler. However, the inability to quantify lower-grade stenosis has no therapeutic consequences. Instead, if the plaque is clearly seen, the planimetric method can be used to roughly estimate the degree of mild to moderate stenosis from transverse and longitudinal gray-scale images. The planimetric method is prone to errors for stenoses caused by echolucent plaques.

Therefore, the planimetric method should not be used to quantify hemodynamically relevant, higher-grade stenosis even if the patent lumen appears to be clearly delineated on color flow images. Measurement of the cross-sectional area requires a 90° angle of insonation relative to the vessel axis, which is the worst angle for Doppler imaging and results in inaccurate visualization of the patent lumen. A higher color gain does not overcome this problem because the resulting color spillover obscures the boundary between flowing blood and the plaque, making the lumen appear larger than it actually is. Another inherent drawback of color flow imaging is that the images are generated by interpolation, which also

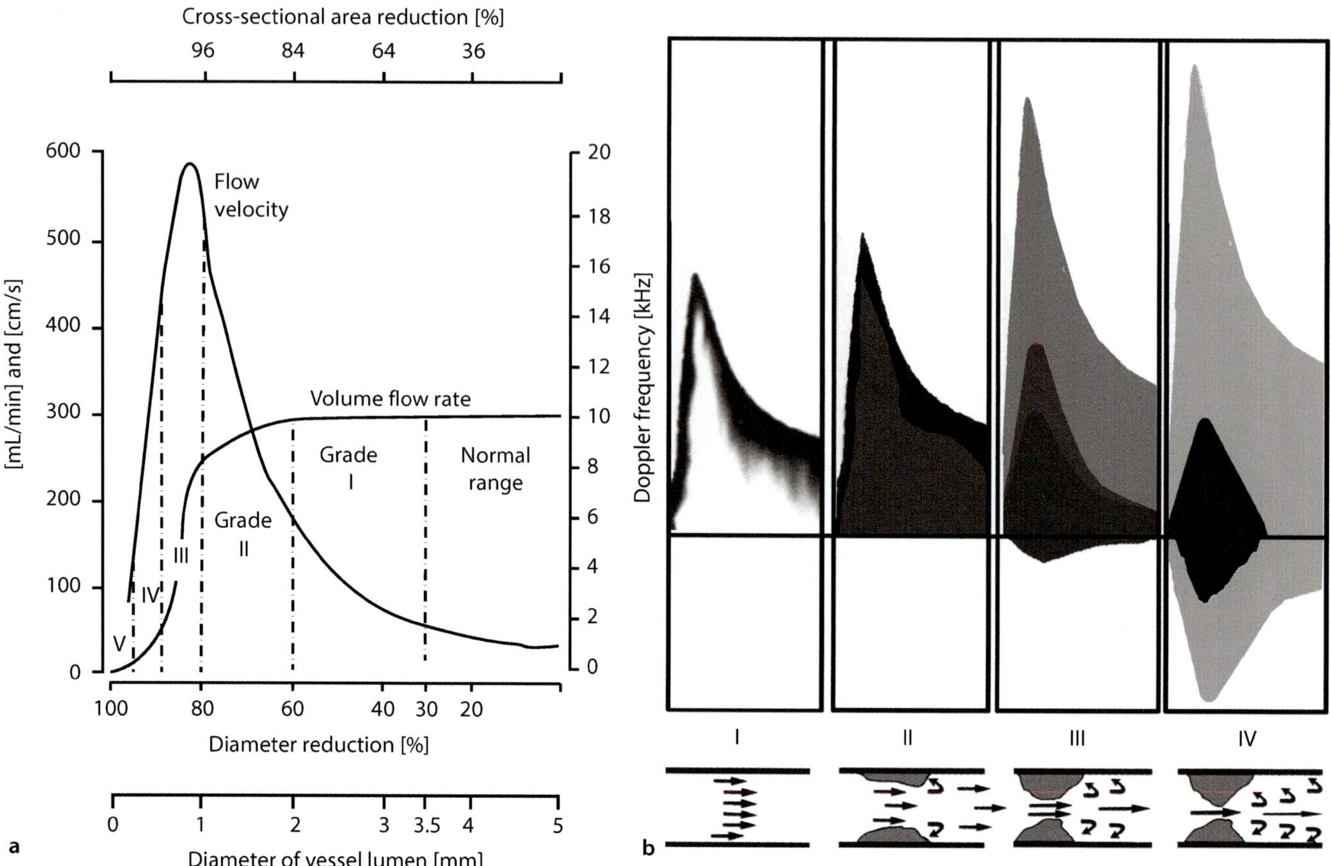

Fig. 5.20 **a** Flow in the carotid artery under idealized conditions: changes in peak systolic velocity (PSV) (given as Doppler shift frequency in KHz) and volume flow rate (in mL/min) with progressive stenosis of the internal carotid artery (expressed as percentage diameter and cross-sectional area reduction). Relevant flow acceleration occurs at diameter reductions >50%. **b** Flow disturbance and PSV increase with the degree of luminal narrowing caused by a stenosis. **I** Normal Doppler waveform with a so-called clear window (laminar flow). **II** Mild flow disturbance results in increasing filling of the clear window (flow disturbance caused by eccentric plaque) and beginning increase in PSV; mild to moderate stenosis. **III** Further PSV increase with onset of turbulent flow (low-frequency components) in moderate to severe stenosis. **IV** PSV increase and marked turbulence, reflected in the predominance of low-frequency flow with retrograde components. When very high-grade stenosis is present, excessive gain is frequently necessary to visualize the high-frequency systolic flow components (low amplitude)

contributes to overestimation of the patent lumen. For these reasons, the hemodynamic method of stenosis quantification is superior and should be used in all cases of clinically relevant stenosis (≥50%).

In view of these limitations in the assessment of plaque size by both B-mode and color duplex ultrasound, hemodynamic stenosis quantification by spectral Doppler analysis is clearly the best method for estimating the severity of higher-grade carotid artery stenosis. It is based on the continuity equation and calculates the diameter reduction from the angle-corrected flow velocity measured in the stenosis.

Luminal narrowing between 50% and 70% is compensated for by autoregulatory mechanisms, which maintain relatively constant blood supply by recruiting collateral pathways and reducing peripheral resistance. Although a <50% diameter reduction causes a slight increase in flow velocity, the increase is not clinically relevant and cannot be measured reliably (as flow velocity is also influenced by systemic effects, which are difficult to account for) (Fig. 5.20). Nevertheless, <50% stenosis may become apparent by signs of disturbed or turbulent flow, seen as spectral broadening and increasing loss of the clear window or as retrograde flow during systole. These indirect signs are more pronounced when the stenosis is caused by an eccentric plaque compared with a concentric plaque.

In summary, all carotid artery stenoses causing at least 50% luminal narrowing are graded on the basis of the Doppler frequency or angle-corrected flow velocity. Thus, it cannot be emphasized enough that **great care must be taken in setting the Doppler angle correction cursor.** This is an absolute prerequisite for accurate stenosis grading and is especially important when the degree of carotid artery stenosis is used to identify candidates for surgery. Normally, the Doppler cursor is aligned with the vessel wall, assuming that the blood flows parallel to the wall. When an eccentric plaque is present, however, the blood flow direction within the stenosis changes since the jet is redirected by the plaque protruding into the bloodstream (Fig. 5.21). Aligning the angle correction cursor with the actual flow direction visualized in the duplex mode will give a more accurate Doppler

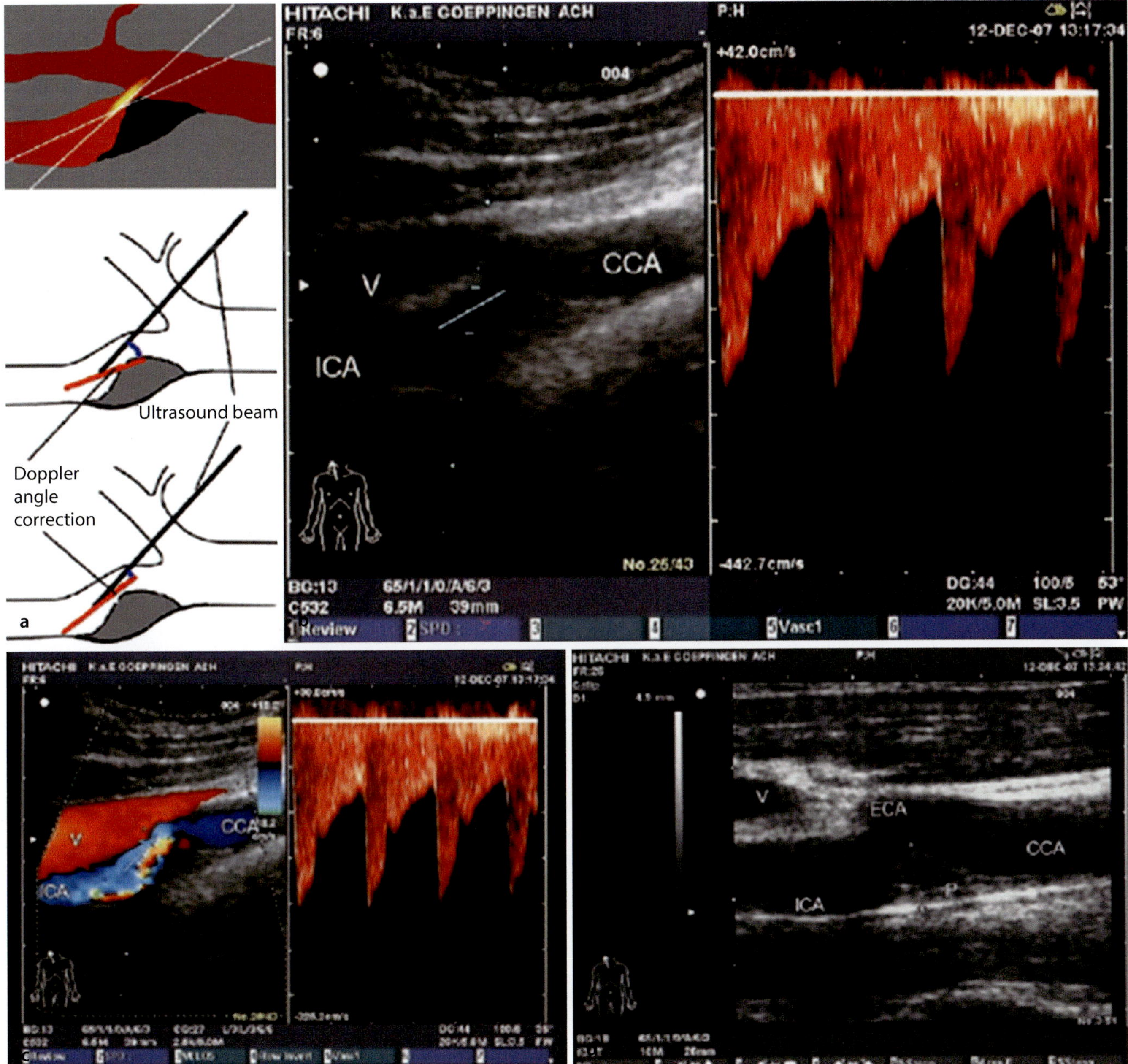

Fig. 5.21 **a** The Doppler angle correction cursor (red) is usually aligned parallel to the vessel wall (middle diagram) because it is assumed that blood flow is parallel to the wall (black line represents the ultrasound beam and blue the Doppler angle). When an eccentric plaque is present, the flow jet visualized by color duplex imaging is frequently not parallel to the wall but is deviated toward the plaque (yellow in the top diagram). Alignment of the Doppler angle correction cursor parallel to the stenosis jet depicted in the duplex scan can result in a discrepancy of 5–10%, when compared with correction parallel to the vessel wall (bottom diagram). **b** Eccentric stenosis at the origin of the internal carotid artery (ICA): measured with Doppler angle correction parallel to the vessel wall, a peak systolic velocity (PSV) of 280 cm/s is calculated, corresponding to >70% stenosis (by ECST criteria) (53° Doppler angle relative to arterial wall). **c** The flow jet depicted in the color duplex image (aliasing indicated by yellow color coding) is at a smaller angle to the ultrasound beam (see **a**). With the corrected Doppler angle of 35° (relative to stenosis jet), a PSV of 210 cm/s is calculated from the (same) Doppler shift frequency, corresponding to <70% stenosis by ECST criteria). The divergent results with regard to PSV and degree of stenosis illustrate that the standard method of Doppler angle correction does not yield adequate results when the assumption on which it is based does not hold. **d** Sonomorphologically, the plaque has two features of vulnerability: low echogenicity and marked eccentricity with longitudinal pulsation in the real-time B-mode (high shear stress acting on the plaque, see Fig. 5.15a; plaque thickness of 4.9 mm). These plaque features justify an indication for surgery, even in patients with stage I disease. Note the clearer definition of the plaque (P) in **d** compared with **b**. Plaque conspicuity decreases with the angle between the ultrasound beam and the wall (due to increased scatter)

angle measurement than alignment with the vessel wall; the discrepancy may be up to 5–10°. When the angle is small (30–50°), a 5° error in aligning the cursor results in a negligible error in calculating blood flow velocity. An angle of less than 50° is difficult to obtain in the carotid bifurcation, but one should always try for an angle smaller than 60°. In a curved segment such as the origin of the ICA, setting the angle correction cursor is limited and even a 60° Doppler angle is difficult to achieve (see ◘ Fig. 1.23). Setting the angle may be easier using a convex transducer instead of a linear array.

Bulky plaque with an irregular surface disrupts blood flow, causing eddy currents, turbulence, and reversed flow. This is reflected in the Doppler waveform as progressive spectral broadening with loss of the clear window and reversed systolic flow.

Eddy currents with retrograde flow may lead to confusion in interpreting the spectral Doppler information when the **size and site of the sample volume** are not carefully chosen. A small sample volume near the vessel wall will primarily capture the reversed flow components, while a narrow volume in the center of the flow jet will only register the high velocities, missing the turbulent flow components (supplementary direct stenosis criteria). For adequate hemodynamic evaluation, the sample volume must encompass the entire vessel lumen to register both the high velocities in the jet and turbulent flow near the wall (◘ Fig. 5.22). Nevertheless, PSV measured in the stenotic jet remains the most relevant criterion for stenosis grading. In general, the increase in flow velocity is greatest just distal to the point of maximal stenotic narrowing seen in the B-mode image, especially when the stenosis is short. According to the continuity equation, intrastenotic flow acceleration does not occur until there is a diameter reduction of at least 50% or an area reduction of 75% (see ◘ Fig. 5.53 (Atlas)).

Intrastenotic flow velocity increases in proportion to the degree of stenosis (◘ Table 5.9, ◘ Fig. 5.20) and is highest in subtotal occlusion. At the same time, friction occurring at the high velocities associated with subtotal occlusion acts as a decelerating force (decreasing the velocity of most reflecting blood components). Nevertheless, a high gain will depict isolated high-frequency signals in the flow jet as an indicator of the high degree of the stenosis. Distal to a high-grade stenosis (measured in the ICA close to the skull base), the systolic flow velocity decreases with the degree of stenosis (postocclusive flow reduction).

5.6.1.2.1 Primary and Secondary Criteria for Carotid Stenosis Grading

A set of primary and secondary stenosis criteria have been evaluated for grading carotid stenosis (◘ Fig. 5.23 and ◘ Tables 5.9 and 5.10).

Although peak systolic velocity (PSV) is the central measure of the severity of luminal narrowing according to the continuity equation, a number of additional criteria have emerged and can contribute to an accurate assessment of carotid stenosis severity, especially in inconclusive cases or patients with intricate plaque configuration. This multiparametric sonographic approach to the diagnostic evaluation of carotid stenosis enables both adequate preoperative workup (without additional diagnostic tests) and provides a basis for follow-up (and not merely reduces the evaluation to the separation of <70% stenosis versus >70% stenosis). Establishing an accurate baseline status is important because rapid progression of asymptomatic carotid stenosis is the most important marker of increased stroke risk.

▪ Primary Stenosis Criteria (◘ Table 5.9)

Maximum peak systolic velocity (PSV) is the highest flow velocity derived from the angle-corrected Doppler waveform obtained by continuous interrogation of the stenotic segment. PSV increases in proportion to the degree of stenosis. When stenosis is caused by irregular or eccentric plaque, Doppler angle correction (<60%) is most reliably accomplished by placing the sample volume in the stenotic jet identified by color duplex imaging (◘ Fig. 5.21). Jet flow velocity is typically highest just distal to the stenotic plaque, which is why acoustic shadowing by a short calcified plaque usually does not interfere with Doppler interrogation. When subtotal occlusion is present, friction loss can lead to a lower PSV than expected from the degree of luminal narrowing alone (◘ Fig. 5.24c). The examiner needs to be aware of this pitfall to avoid underestimating carotid stenosis severity. Other factors influencing PSV are:

- Stenosis length: due to friction, PSV is lower in a long high-grade stenosis (◘ Fig. 5.24d) compared with a short stenosis
- Collateral function: intrastenotic PSV is increased in a carotid artery collateralizing its occluded contralateral counterpart (◘ Fig. 5.50 (Atlas)), as is PSV in the common carotid artery (CCA).

In all of these situations, carotid stenosis grading based on PSV alone becomes unreliable.

B-mode ultrasound: Before carotid artery stenosis becomes hemodynamically relevant (<30% NASCET/<50% ECST stenosis), it is only detectable with B-mode imaging. When the plaque is clearly demarcated based on its echogenicity, diameter reduction and possibly luminal reduction (planimetry) can be determined from B-mode images. Accurate quantification of mild stenosis is not required clinically. Instead, the plaque should be characterized in terms of surface properties, echogenicity, homogeneity, and shape in transverse and longitudinal orientation (◘ Fig. 5.14).

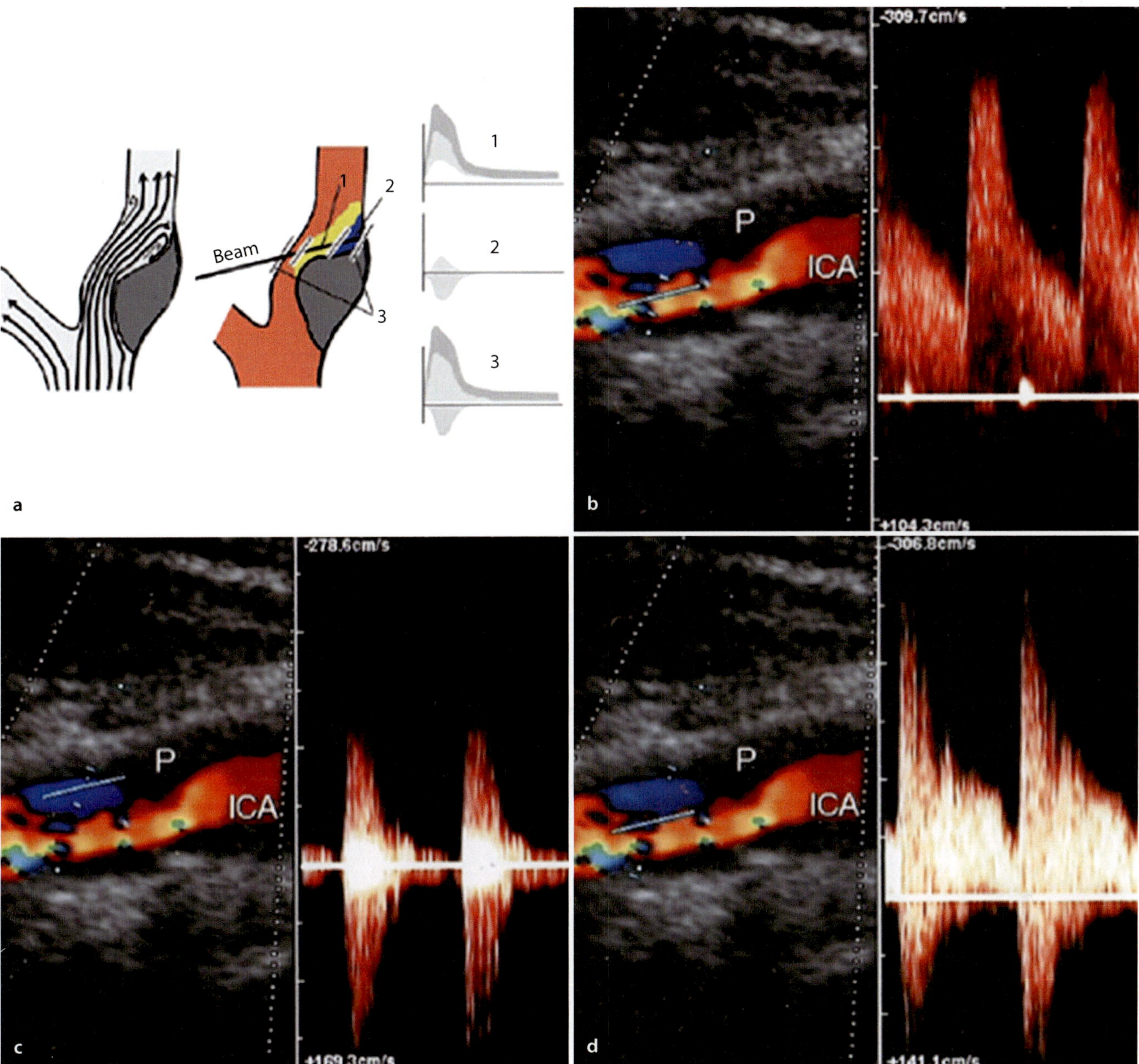

Fig. 5.22 **a** The left drawing shows the course of flow in a high-grade stenosis caused by eccentric plaque in the internal carotid artery (ICA) with eddy currents and retrograde flow components directly behind the plaque. The middle drawing shows the duplex color coding (based on mean velocity) of blood flow velocity and direction in a stenosis. Flow velocity is highest in the flow jet, which is indicated by aliasing (color change from red to yellow); flow reversals at sites of eddy currents are indicated by red and blue color. The Doppler waveforms (diagrams on the right) represent blood flow velocity and direction at different sampling sites in the area of a carotid stenosis (indicated by the numbers 1–3). The waveform from the center of the stenosis (1) selectively represents the high flow velocity in the stenotic jet. The waveform measured in a small sample volume placed directly behind the plaque (2) represents blood flow in the area of eddy currents, seen as predominantly retrograde flow (displayed below the baseline in the waveform). Adequate selection of a sample volume covering the entire width of the arterial lumen (3) depicts both maximum peak systolic velocity (PSV) and the eddy currents distal to the plaque. **b** Color duplex image and Doppler waveform from a sample volume placed in the stenotic jet (aliasing with color change from red to yellow to light blue) in an eccentric ICA plaque. **c** The waveform obtained with the sample volume placed close to the wall directly behind the plaque predominantly represents eddy currents (color change from red to black to blue), which appear predominantly as retrograde flow (below the baseline in the waveform). **d** With a sample volume covering the entire width of the lumen, the waveform reflects both the high PSV and the eddy currents with retrograde flow components

Table 5.9 Multiparametric approach using a set of primary and secondary criteria for grading the severity of internal carotid artery (ICA) stenosis using duplex ultrasound (Modified according to Neale et al. 1994; Faught et al. 1994; Moneta et al. 1995; AbuRahma et al. 1998; Grant et al. 2003; and Arning et al. 2010). Later Investigators using the NASCET criteria for grading ICA stenosis propose lower threshold velocities: PSV of 130 cm/s for 50% stenosis and 230 cm/s for 70% stenosis (AbuRahma et al. 2011; Jahromi et al. 2005)

Distal degree (NASCET) (%)		10	20–40	50	60	70	80	90	Occlusion
Local degree (ECST) (%)		45	50–60	70	75	80	90	95	Occlusion
Primary criteria	1. B-mode image	+++	+						
	2. Color duplex image	+	+++	+	+	+	+	+	+++
	3. PSV at the site of maximum stenosis (cm/s)	<100	120–160	>200	>250	>300	>350–400	200–500	No flow signal
	4. PSV in the poststenotic segment (cm/s)					>50	<50	<30	No flow signal
	5. (Beginning) collateralization (periorbital arteries/ACA)					(+)	++	+++	+++
Secondary criteria	6. Decrease in diastolic velocity in the prestenotic segment (CCA)					(+)	++	+++	+++
	7. Abnormal flow in the poststenotic segment			+	+	++	+++	(+)	
	8. EDV at the site of maximum stenosis (cm/s)		<50	<90	<100	>100	>100		
	9. Confetti sign				(+)	++	++		
	10. Carotid stenosis index (ICA/CCA PSV ratio)			≥2	≥3	≥4	≥4.5		

Number of plus signs indicates diagnostic relevance (compared with other criteria)
ACA anterior cerebral artery, *CCA* common carotid artery, *EDV* end-diastolic velocity, *ICA* internal carotid artery, *PSV* peak systolic velocity

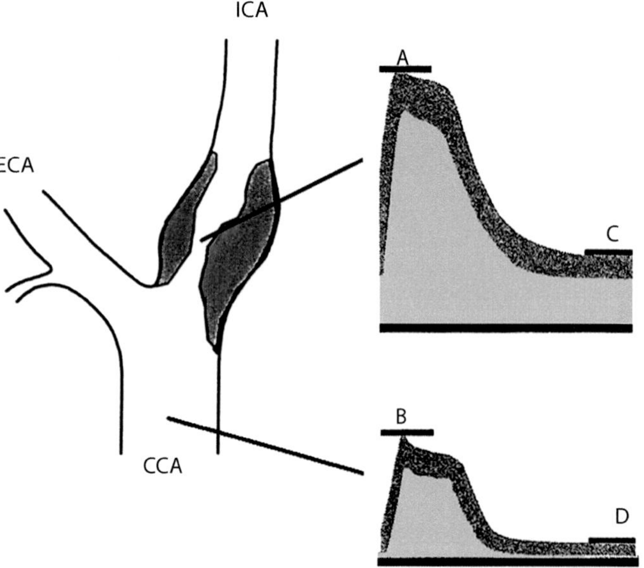

Fig. 5.23 Stenosis criteria for grading internal carotid artery (ICA) stenosis. A = peak systolic velocity (PSV) within the stenosis (the most reliable parameter based on scientific evidence); C = peak end-diastolic velocity (EDV) in the stenosis; A/B = ratio of intrastenotic PSV in the ICA and PSV in the common carotid artery (CCA); C/D = ratio of peak EDV in the stenosis and peak EDV in the CCA

Table 5.10 Pitfalls in carotid stenosis grading due to other factors affecting peak systolic velocity (PSV)

Stenosis grading	Factor/Source of error
Underestimation of stenosis (of risk of embolism)	Episode of low blood pressure Proximal stenosis, e.g., aortic stenosis Very-high-grade stenosis, subtotal occlusion Long stenosis Tandem stenosis (additional distal/intracranial stenosis) Very eccentric stenosis
Overestimation of stenosis	High blood pressure at time of examination Hyperperfusion (contralateral carotid occlusion or very-high-grade stenosis) Very pulsatile flow (medial sclerosis in diabetes mellitus) Small or contracted vessels Very short stenosis

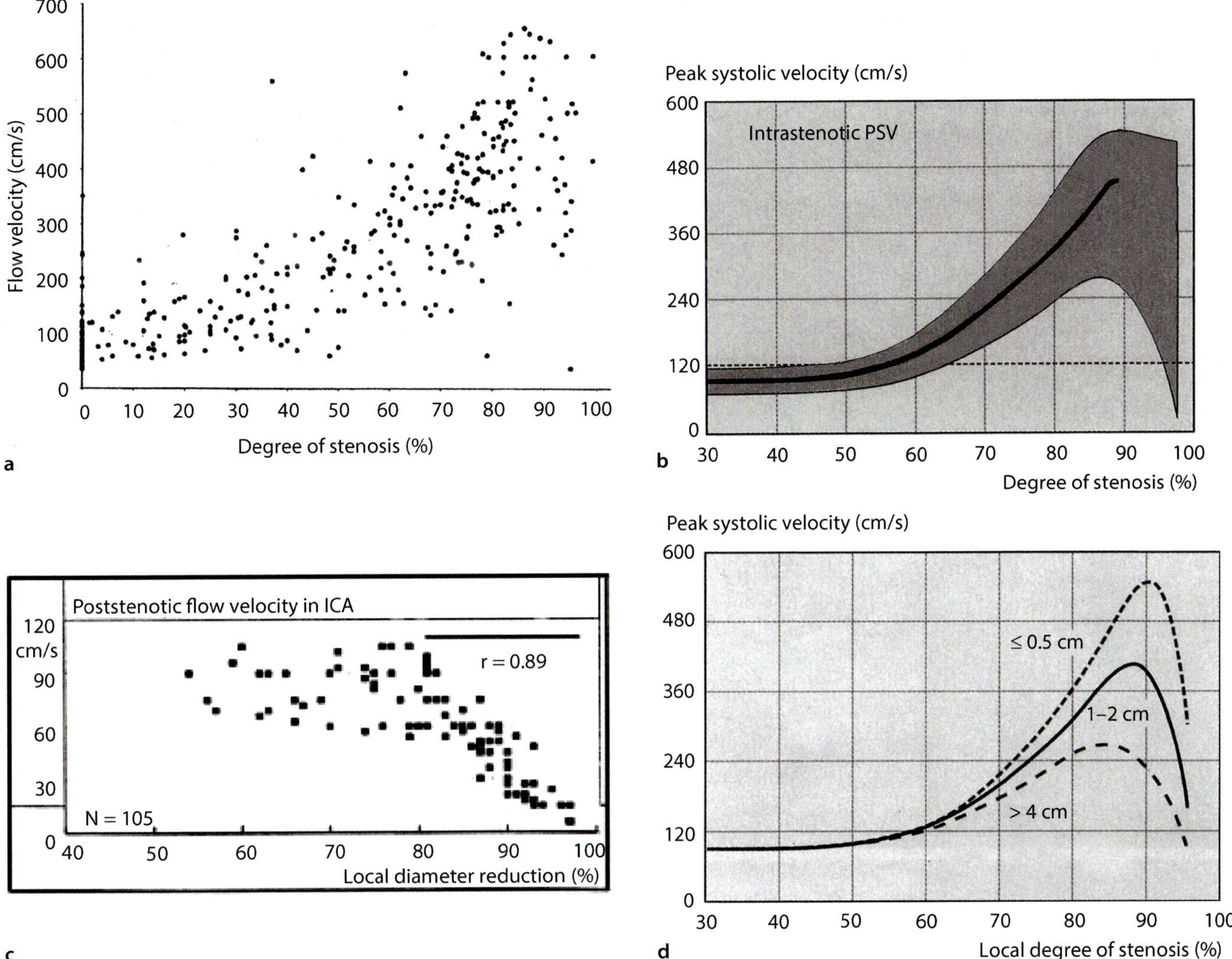

Fig. 5.24 **a** Internal carotid artery (ICA) stenosis: relationship between angiographic stenosis and intrastenotic peak systolic velocity (PSV) for calculating the distal degree of stenosis (Fig. 5.7b) (From Moneta et al. 1995); differences in plaque morphology are one factor contributing to scatter (see Fig. 5.27). **b** Flow velocity (PSV) as a function of stenosis severity (local degree). Intrastenotic PSV increases continuously with luminal diameter reduction (according to the continuity equation) and degreases again in very-high-grade stenosis/subtotal occlusion due to friction loss, especially when a long carotid segment is stenosed. **c** Distribution of poststenotic PSV as a function of local diameter reduction. Poststenotic PSV tends to decrease when the degree of stenosis is at least approx. 85% (According to Görtler et al. 1994). **d** Relationship between the length of stenotic plaque (length of stenosis) and expected maximum PSV as a function of stenosis severity. When a long high-grade stenosis is present, friction loss may lead to a lower PSV in the stenotic jet than would be expected from the degree of stenosis. This association is especially important when luminal narrowing is due to dissection. However, the actual decrease in PSV to be expected also depends on plaque configuration and has not been investigated systematically (According to Widder 2004)

Color duplex ultrasound performed with properly adjusted settings (gain, PRF) allows qualitative evaluation but no grading of carotid artery stenosis. The color mode may help in differentiating plaque from flowing blood in the patent lumen but reliable determination of the degree of luminal narrowing is not possible due to inherent methodological limitations, especially in transverse orientation (see ► Sect. 1.2.3). Color flow images may also facilitate differentiation of subtotal and total occlusion.

Poststenotic PSV should be measured as far cranially as possible (distal to the stenosis jet). It is decreased in high-grade stenosis (poststenotic PSV >50 cm/s in <70% stenosis (NASCET) versus <30 cm/s in >90% stenosis) (see Table 5.9). Comparison of poststenotic PSV with the contralateral side is advisable.

Presence of collateral circulation can point to carotid stenosis. Abnormal flow (reversed flow direction, reduced flow) in the supratrochlear artery is a sign of high-grade ICA stenosis. Collateralization is more reliably detected intracranially using transcranial duplex ultrasound. A variety of arteries can be recruited to bridge a stenosed carotid artery; therefore, identification of a single collateral with increased flow taken alone is not a reliable indicator of carotid stenosis. In most examinations, searching for collaterals is not necessary or helpful for estimating stenosis severity.

5

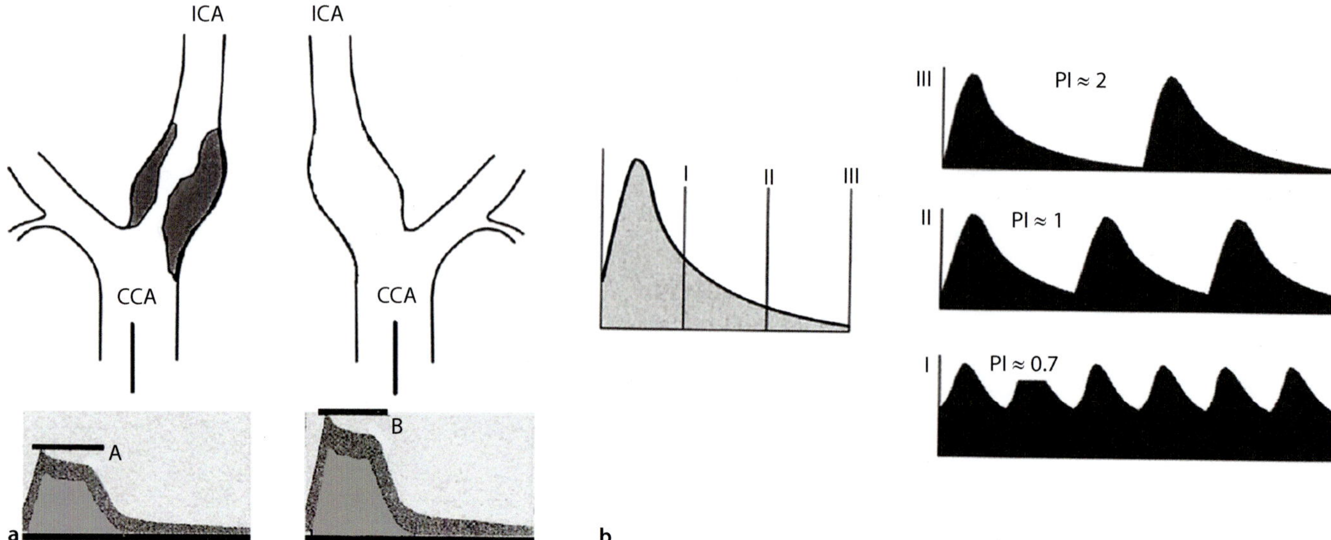

Fig. 5.25 **a** Unilateral high-grade internal carotid artery (ICA) stenosis or occlusion (left diagram) leads to an increase in flow velocity in the contralateral common and internal carotid arteries if they function as the primary collateral pathway; this must be borne in mind in stenosis grading (diagrams from Widder and Görtler 2004). **b** Because end-diastolic velocity (EDV) decreases with the duration of diastole, stenosis grading on the basis of EDV is dependent on a patient's heart rate (as well as other systemic factors such as blood pressure at the time of measurement, contralateral occlusion, wall elasticity). As a consequence, resistance indices, which incorporate EDV, also vary with heart rate (see Fig. 1.28c, d)

Secondary Stenosis Criteria (Table 5.9)

Reduced diastolic flow velocity in the common carotid artery (CCA): Flow velocity in the CCA, particularly during diastole, decreases when higher-grade ICA stenosis is present. Pulsatility increases prestenotically, and the CCA flow profile becomes more like that of the ECA (externalization). The increase in pulsatility is determined not only by the degree of ICA stenosis but also by the number of ECA branches recruited as collaterals: the stenosis-related increase in pulsatility is damped more markedly when more ECA branches provide collateral flow. The ECA waveform thus becomes less pulsatile, i.e., more like that of the ICA (internalization), which in turn affects the flow pattern in the CCA.

Turbulent flow is often more conspicuous acoustically (like foodsteps on gravel) than visually in the waveform. Transition from normal laminar to turbulent flow occurs at sites of stenotic narrowing when the Reynolds number exceeds 2000 and in the poststenotic segment (sudden widening of the lumen with flow separation). The occurrence of turbulent flow depends not only on stenosis severity but also strongly on plaque configuration and surface.

Intrastenotic end-diastolic velocity (EDV) increases with the severity of carotid stenosis. An EDV of >50 cm/s suggests that at least 50% stenosis is present with velocities >80–100 cm/s suggesting high-grade stenosis (>70%). This parameter is especially useful for quantifying subtotal occlusion, in which PSV is more difficult to determine (Carpenter et al. 1996). Note, though, that EDV increases with the patient's heart rate because a higher heart rate means a shorter end-diastolic phase (Fig. 5.25b).

Perivascular tissue vibration occurs in the soft tissues around higher-grade carotid stenosis. This phenomenon can cause what is known as the confetti sign in color duplex imaging (adequate gain and PRF) or can be auscultated because the tissues vibrate at audible frequencies.

Carotid stenosis index or ratio of PSV in the ICA to that in the ipsilateral CCA (ICA/CCA PSV ratio): Absolute flow velocities are influenced by physiologic and abnormal systemic factors (hypertension, aortic valve stenosis, medial sclerosis, contralateral occlusion, intracranial collateralization). The effect of these factors can be reduced by calculating the ratio of PSV in the stenosis to PSV in the prestenotic segment of the same vascular territory (Moneta et al. 1993; Howton et al. 2008; Carpenter et al. 1995). However, as the ECA also arises from the CCA, the ratio will be altered if the ECA is stenosed or acts as a collateral in the presence of ICA stenosis (Figs. 5.23 and 5.25).

Ratio of intrastenotic to poststenotic systolic velocity (PSV) in the ICA (see ► Sect. 1.2.3 and Fig. 1.48): Identical degrees of stenosis (risk of embolism) can be associated with different intrastenotic and above all poststenotic velocities, depending on the length of the stenosis (Fig. 5.24d). In a long (high-grade) stenosis, friction losses result in a lower intrastenotic PSV. To account for the resulting error in stenosis grading, it has been proposed to calculate the ratio of intrastenotic to poststenotic velocity, preferably using intensity-weighted mean flow velocities rather than PSV. A cutoff of 5 is assumed to indicate higher-grade carotid stenosis (Ranke et al. 1999; Table 5.11). This parameter is considered unreliable and is used very rarely.

Table 5.11 Sensitivity, specificity, and accuracy of duplex ultrasound in internal carotid artery (ICA) stenosis grading using different sonographic criteria (angiography as reference standard). Some studies report local (ECST) degrees of carotid stenosis, while others report distal (NASCET) degrees of stenosis (see Fig. 5.9b). Some authors provide no information on the method of stenosis grading used

Author	Year	N	Method (parameter)				Results				
			Degree of stenosis (%)	PSV (cm/s)	EDV (cm/s)	PSV ratio	Sensitivity (%)	Specificity (%)	PPV (%)	NPV (%)	Accuracy (%)
Faught et al.	1994		70		130						93
Polak et al.	1992		50	125							83
Huston et al.	2000	915	50	130	70	1.6	92	90	90	91	91
		915	70	230		3.2	86	90	83	92	89
Soulez et al.	1999		70				94	81	62	98	
			60			2.9	94	80	72	96	
AbuRahma et al.	1998		50	140			92	95	97	89	93
			60	150	65		82	97	96	86	90
			70	180	96		85	95	91	92	92
Grant et al.	2000		70	225							90
Carpenter et al.	1996	110	70	210			94	77	68	96	83
		110	70		70		92	60	73	86	77
		110	70			3.3	100	65	65	100	79
Hood et al.	1996	457	70	230	100		78	97	88	94	93
Carpenter et al.	1995		60	230			98	87	88	98	92
			60		40		97	52	86	86	86
			60			2.0	97	73	78	96	76
			60	230	40	2.0	100	100	100	100	100
Browman et al.	1995	75	70	175			91	60			
Moneta et al.	1995	176	60	260	70	3.2–3.5	84	94	92	88	90
Neale et al.	1994	60	70	270	110		96	91			93
Moneta et al.	1993		70	325	130	4	83	90	80	92	88
Eckstein et al.	2001	68	70 (ECST)	180			92	42	82	67	79
Finkenzeller et al.	2008	21	50	120	50	1.5	Correlation with IADSA, r = 0.852 (Pearson)				
			70	200	100	2.0					

EDV end-diastolic velocity, *IADSA* intra-arterial digital subtraction angiography, *NPV* negative predictive value, *PPV* positive predictive value, *PSV* peak systolic velocity

Stenosis Grading Using the Primary and Secondary Criteria

Degrees of Carotid Stenosis (Table 5.9, Figs. 5.20, 5.21, 5.22, 5.23, and 5.24):

- Low-grade stenosis (<20–40% by NASCET criteria) and plaque morphology are evaluated by B-mode ultrasound. While a slight increase in intrastenotic flow velocity may be apparent in the Doppler waveform or color duplex images, the increase is not hemodynamically relevant and precludes quantification.
- Moderate stenosis (50% NASCET/70% ECST) is associated with a PSV of up to 200 cm/s. Whether turbulent

flow occurs depends on plaque configuration. The carotid stenosis index may be increased above 2, while the other parameters are unaffected or the changes are not diagnostically meaningful.

- Moderate to high-grade stenosis (60% NASCET) causes local flow acceleration with color aliasing and a PSV of up to 250 cm/s. There may be turbulent flow and beginning signs of perivascular tissue vibration.
- High-grade stenosis (70% NASCET) is associated with aliasing, a PSV of up to 300 cm/s, and beginning effects on secondary criteria (collateral flow, supratrochlear artery). Turbulent flow is apparent, the confetti sign may be seen, and intrastenotic EDV is increased (>100 cm/s).
- High- to very-high-grade stenosis (80%) leads to even more marked changes compared with high-grade stenosis (PSV of 350–400 cm/s, carotid stenosis index of >4). Poststenotic velocity is decreased.
- Subtotal occlusion (90%) is associated with a further increase in intrastenotic PSV; on the other hand, intrastenotic PSV may be lower due to greater friction loss (PSV range of 200–500 cm/s). With very high receive gain, it is often possible to capture the low-amplitude, high-frequency jet components. The diagnosis of subtotal ICA occlusion is corroborated by a decrease in poststenotic flow velocity (<30 cm/s) and an increase in CCA pulsatility.
- Occlusion of the ICA is characterized by the absence of flow signals (color duplex and waveform) throughout the extracranial ICA. Sonographic evaluation should extend to the skull base in order not to miss pseudo-occlusion (see, however, persistent primitive hypoglossal artery (PPHA), ► Sect. 5.6.1.3.1). In addition, flow in the CCA is decreased and becomes more pulsatile; and collateral circulation can be demonstrated.

▪ Critical Appraisal of PSV: The Main Criterion of Carotid Stenosis

The parameters for grading internal carotid artery (ICA) stenosis outlined above have accuracies of 83–97% using intra-arterial angiography as the gold standard. Several studies found good interobserver agreement both for grading ICA stenosis (kappa = 0.7) and for identifying candidates for surgery (kappa = 0.72; Griffiths et al. 2001). When the degree of carotid stenosis determined using absolute parameters provides no definitive basis for recommending surgery, effects of systemic conditions such as hypertension or hypercirculation (fever, hyperthyroidism) should be considered (◘ Table 5.10). Medial sclerosis in long-standing diabetes mellitus leads to pulsatile flow with a larger systolic component and a smaller diastolic component. Contralateral carotid artery occlusion (◘ Fig. 5.25) or high-grade stenosis and multiple-vessel disease with vertebral artery involvement may also lead to artificially elevated flow velocities (Busuttil et al. 1996) in the carotid system; another factor to be considered in interpreting carotid blood flow velocities is collateralization (see ◘ Figs. 5.68 and 5.69 (both Atlas)). To avoid overestimation in these situations, a higher PSV cutoff of 140–150 cm/s should be used to discriminate between low-grade and hemodynamically significant (>20–40%) carotid artery stenosis (modified according to AbuRahma et al. 1995). Not taking these factors into account will lead to false-positive results and overestimation of carotid stenosis (Horrow et al. 2000; Busuttil et al. 1996).

In the study of Busuttil et al. (1996), duplex ultrasound overestimated the degree of carotid stenosis in patients with severe contralateral disease, falsely suggesting high-grade stenosis in 27% of cases (using angiography as the reference). Following unilateral carotid endarterectomy (CEA), PSV on the unoperated side decreased on average by 36 cm/s. Other investigators reported a 20–40% higher PSV due to compensatory flow in patients with over 90% contralateral stenosis (Henderson et al. 2000).

The compensatory increase in PSV is determined not only by the severity of contralateral stenosis but also by the contribution of the ICA to collateral circulation and by the recruitment of other collaterals (ipsilateral ECA and supratrochlear artery, posterior circulation).

In another study including 107 patients with asymptomatic 50–99% contralateral carotid artery stenosis (PSV >125 cm/s), a postoperative duplex examination showed a mean decrease in PSV of 48 cm/s (10%) and a mean decrease in EDV of 36 cm/s (19%) (Abou-Zamzam et al. 2000). The authors concluded that patients with severe bilateral carotid stenosis **should be restudied with duplex scanning after the first operation before undergoing CEA of the contralateral side.**

Pitfalls in carotid stenosis grading (◘ Table 5.10) include:

- Acoustic shadowing due to long calcified plaque (>2 cm) precludes measurement of intrastenotic PSV (rotation of transducer to avoid areas of acoustic shadowing, see ◘ Fig. 5.4)
- Plaque configuration: very eccentric plaque with little hemodynamic effect (relatively low PSV) but high risk of embolism due to plaque thickness (◘ Figs. 5.15, 5.27, and 5.57e (Atlas))
- Presence of bilateral higher-grade stenosis (PSV overestimates stenosis because collateral function results in higher PSV than expected on the basis of the degree of stenosis alone; ◘ Figs. 5.68 and 5.69 (both Atlas)) or presence of tandem stenosis (PSV underestimates ICA stenosis, even if the second stenosis is in the aorta)
- PSV underestimates the degree of long stenosis (◘ Fig. 5.24d)
- High bifurcation: carotid bulb and proximal ICA cannot be insonated adequately (switching to a curved-array transducer with small footprint may help)
- Mistaking occlusion for pseudo-occlusion in individuals with refilling of the ICA through a PPHA (◘ Fig. 5.31)
- Recanalization of ICA occlusion (◘ Fig. 5.30)
- Carotid aneurysm with thrombosis as source of embolism (◘ Fig. 5.72 (Atlas))
- Carotid dissection (◘ Figs. 5.44 and 5.45)
- Vasculitis (◘ Fig. 5.46)

Normal blood flow velocity is higher in the thinner vessels of slim patients or arteries narrowed by other factors such as temporary vascular contraction compared with the velocities determined in a general population. This will then translate into higher PSV in a stenotic segment (◘ Fig. 5.49 (Atlas)).

As already mentioned, a long high-grade stenosis (in particular a stenosis of >3 cm) will cause a less pronounced increase in PSV than a shorter stenosis of the same degree (◘ Fig. 5.24d). The thresholds defined in investigations using angiography as the gold standard are usually based on the most common stenosis length of 1–2 cm. According to the Hagen-Poiseuille law, flow resistance also depends on the **length of the narrowed segment.** A very short stenosis will cause a more marked increase in PSV, and this is why the length of the stenosis has to be considered in stenosis grading as well (although no detailed study-based data exist).

An intracranial stenosis of the carotid territory occurring **in tandem** with an extracranial **ICA stenosis** reduces extracranial flow velocity, resulting in a less marked increase in PSV across the extracranial stenosis (stenosis mismatch). A tandem lesion with high-grade intracranial stenosis may be suggested:

- if flow velocity in the distal extracranial ICA is markedly lower than would be expected from the degree of upstream stenosis and
- if flow is more pulsatile than expected (◘ Table 5.10).

Some authors prefer measurement of end-diastolic velocity for stenosis grading, arguing that this parameter is less affected by the patient's blood pressure at the time of the examination. Nevertheless, data from comparative studies still show PSV to be the most reliable velocity parameter for stenosis grading since EDV varies with the patient's heart rate and other systemic factors (◘ Fig. 5.25b). Repeated measurement of constant blood flow in the same vessel at increasing heart rates would yield increasingly higher EDVs due to shortening of the cardiac cycle, resulting in an artificially lower resistive index (RI).

The **effects of systemic factors** such as hypertensive episodes or greater pulsatility due to reduced wall elasticity can be minimized by calculating the ratio of PSV in the ICA to that in the ipsilateral CCA (ICA/CCA PSV ratio or carotid stenosis index) for stenosis grading. This ratio can be determined as a supplementary parameter whenever absolute PSV suggests a borderline stenosis and it is assumed that the measurement was influenced by systemic factors.

The compilation of studies in ◘ Table 5.11 shows that accuracy rates of over 90% can be achieved in stenosis grading on the basis of the hemodynamic parameters derived from duplex ultrasound (using angiography as the gold standard). Hence, the accuracy of duplex imaging is comparable to the interobserver variability between two radiologists evaluating the same angiograms (◘ Tables 5.12 and 5.13). Taken together, published data indicate that ultrasound achieves consistently good results with sensitivities and specificities of approximately 90% in detecting greater than 70% carotid artery stenosis (relevant for identifying surgical candidates). For carotid stenoses of 50–70%, several studies and a meta-analysis of 41 studies investigating different imaging modalities in comparison with intra-arterial digital subtraction angiography (IADSA) found sensitivities for duplex sonography that were 5–30% lower but specificities of over 90% (Wardlaw et al. 2006). An explanation for these results is not apparent from the meta-analysis, but the use of different criteria (threshold velocities) for defining hemodynamically relevant stenosis (50% stenosis or greater), systemic factors (blood pressure, wall elasticity), and different hemodynamic effects of eccentric versus concentric plaques (◘ Fig. 5.27b) appear to be contributing factors.

◘ **Table 5.12** Agreement between two independent radiologists in identifying and classifying hemodynamically significant carotid artery stenosis on angiography

Author/year	Agreement between two independent radiologists (%)
Croft et al. 1980	88
Moneta et al. 1993	93

◘ **Table 5.13** Accuracy of angiography in comparison with pathologic workup of surgical specimens

Author/year	Accuracy of angiography compared with pathology (%)
Croft et al. 1980	79

The question regarding the most valid velocity parameter for the grading of carotid artery stenosis – PSV, EDV, or ICA/CCA PSV ratio – still remains open. Published data yield no uniform picture and the heterogeneity of study designs makes results difficult to compare.

A study of the **ICA PSV/CCA PSV ratio** determined by duplex ultrasound in more than 300 carotid artery examinations with receiver operating characteristic (ROC) analysis found good accuracy for the detection of 70–99% NASCET stenosis using a cutoff of 4 (Moneta et al. 1993). Other investigators achieved good accuracies with different cutoffs (◘ Table 5.11).

Nevertheless, **PSV** has turned out to be the most reliable velocity parameter in detecting and quantifying high-grade carotid artery stenosis, showing consistently high accuracy in many studies (Arning et al. 2003; Lal et al. 2004; Lewis and Wardlaw 2002) (◘ Table 5.11). If the ultrasound examination is technically adequate, patients in whom higher-grade stenosis is diagnosed can be scheduled for surgery without additional imaging tests for stenosis grading (Grant et al. 2003; Lewis and Wardlaw 2002). The decision to recommend carotid endarterectomy (CEA) always involves weighing the predicted risk of future vascular events against perioperative and postoperative morbidity/mortality. Various attempts at defining the best PSV cutoff for identifying

5

hemodynamically relevant stenosis (>50%) by means of ROC curve analysis in studies using angiography as the reference standard show that a higher PSV improves specificity, albeit at the cost of sensitivity; conversely, a lower cutoff velocity improves sensitivity but lowers the specificity of the method (see ◘ Fig. 6.9: ROC analysis for determining the cutoff velocity for renal artery stenosis; ◘ Fig. 2.19: for profunda femoris stenosis). This situation is impressively illustrated by a study of Moneta et al. (1995), who investigated different PSV cutoffs for identifying 60–99% carotid artery stenosis in a larger patient population. A PSV cutoff of 200 cm/s yielded high sensitivity of 93% but poor specificity of 76% (84% accuracy), while a cutoff of 300 cm/s resulted in low sensitivity of 78% and high specificity of 95% (87% accuracy). The best compromise was to use a PSV cutoff of 260 cm/s, which yielded the highest accuracy of 88% with 86% sensitivity and 91% specificity.

Using a combination of PSV >260 cm/s and EDV >70 cm/s, Moneta et al. achieved 84% sensitivity, 94% specificity, 92% positive predictive value, and 90% accuracy in discriminating 60–99% stenosis. Similar results were obtained with an ICA/CCA PSV ratio > 3.2 (◘ Table 5.11). In asymptomatic patients, the statistical benefit of prophylactic CEA is smaller, and the number needed to treat to prevent one stroke is higher than is the case for patients with symptomatic carotid stenosis. For this reason it has been proposed that velocity thresholds with a higher positive predictive value be used in asymptomatic patients. For an intrastenotic PSV cutoff of 290 cm/s combined with an EDV of 80 cm/s, the authors reported a 95% positive predictive value for 60–99% asymptomatic ICA stenosis (angiography).

Technical advances and the advent of high-resolution transducers led to improved **sensitivities and specificities of 90–95%** in correctly identifying hemodynamically significant carotid artery stenosis. The correlation of intra-arterial angiography and color-coded duplex imaging is 0.8–0.9 (Faught et al. 1994; Sitzer et al. 1993).

Despite these good results, some caution is in order in view of the range of PSV cutoffs proposed for defining hemodynamically relevant stenosis (Elgersma et al. 1998) and the scatter apparent in ◘ Fig. 5.24a. In one study, PSV values ranging from 50 to 530 cm/s were measured for 70% angiographic stenosis (Hunink et al. 1993). This variation cannot be fully explained by measurement errors and failure to take the hemodynamic effects of different plaque configurations (◘ Fig. 5.27) into account.

Because carotid stenosis grading based on PSV cutoffs alone is prone to errors, the German Society of Ultrasound in Medicine (Deutsche Gesellschaft für Ultraschall in der Medizin, DEGUM) advocates a multiparmatric approach using the set of primary and secondary criteria discussed above (► Sect. 5.6.1.2.1 and ◘ Table 5.9). Several decades of sonographic and vascular surgical experience from the clinician's perspective confirm that this sonographic approach allows reliable preoperative carotid stenosis grading (Khaw 1997). The practice is different in North America, where carotid ultrasound examinations are performed by sonographers

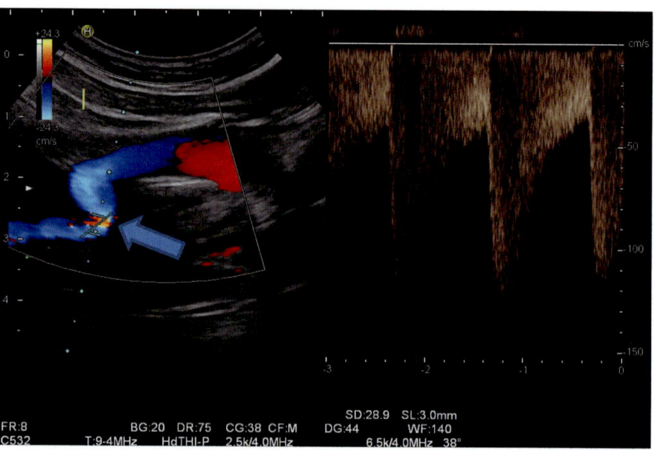

◘ **Fig. 5.26** Severe kinking (acute angle) of the internal carotid artery (ICA) can cause stenosis. However, in a kinked segment, stenosis grading is limited because Doppler angle correction is difficult to accomplish, and additional parameters such as turbulent flow need to be used to corroborate the diagnosis. In the example, a PSV of 135 cm/s is measured in the kinked distal ICA. This PSV suggests 30–40% stenosis (by NASCET criteria, equivalent to 50–60% ECST stenosis)

and PSV alone is used for stenosis grading. The different philosophies necessarily result in different recommendations regarding PSV cutoffs: while the Radiological Society of North America (RSNA) recommends one standardized PSV cutoff to detect all carotid stenoses >70%, the DEGUM advocates a more flexible approach based on PSV measurement in conjunction with additional parameters (◘ Fig. 5.24b).

Despite the variation in flow velocities measured for a given angiographic degree of stenosis and despite the pitfalls in determining PSV discussed above, it is safe to conclude that there is good overall agreement between hemodynamic stenosis quantification by duplex ultrasound and angiographic stenosis grading (◘ Tables 5.10, 5.11, 5.12, and 5.13).

Another aspect worth mentioning here is that a study investigating ultrasound machines from different manufacturers in a phantom model of predefined flow velocities found differences in flow velocity measurements on the order of 5–10% (Fillinger et al. 1996). This is another issue that tends to be overlooked when discussing differences in reported scientific data.

Atherosclerotic elongation of the ICA leads to tortuosity, kinking, and coiling due to the limited space available between the carotid bulb and the base of the skull. Such changes typically do not require treatment and are often incidental findings that impair duplex ultrasound evaluation. Only kinking stenosis, especially when symptomatic, should be operated on (see ◘ Fig. 5.51 (Atlas)).

Even severe **kinks or coils will produce a stenosis** only if the artery takes a sharp turn; they may however impair flow velocity measurements due to the difficulty of achieving an adequate Doppler angle. Therefore, **indirect criteria such as turbulent flow** must be considered as well (◘ Fig. 5.26). In severe ICA kinking, the degree of luminal narrowing may vary with different functional positions of the cervical spine.

Most stenoses at the origin of the ICA (bulb), the most common site of carotid stenosis, are due to atherosclerosis. Distal carotid stenosis is rare and typically has other underlying causes such as fibromuscular dysplasia, wall dissection (usually due to trauma), or kinking.

Collateralization also affects the risk of embolism in steno-occlusive carotid disease. Intrastenotic PSV in an 80–90% stenosis is lower when there is good collateralization as opposed to the same degree of stenosis in a patient with poor collateral pathways. Lower intrastenotic velocities reduce the risk of embolism because wall shear stress is lower.

The **poststenotic ICA diameter** is another **prognostic factor**. When a high-grade ICA stenosis develops slowly, the decrease in blood supply is compensated for by the recruitment of collaterals. As a result, carotid blood flow on the side of stenosis is decreased. A subgroup analysis of the ECST shows that a reduced poststenotic ICA lumen has important prognostic implications for patients with high-grade stenosis (Rothwell et al. 2000). In this analysis, patients with poststenotic narrowing of the ICA defined as an ICA/CCA ratio of <0.42 (which usually means <3 mm) had a two thirds lower stroke rate than patients with similar stenosis severity but without narrowing at 5-year follow-up. The authors assume that poststenotic narrowing may be protective as blood flow distal to the stenosis is insufficient to carry emboli to the brain.

For the reasons outlined before, color flow imaging (color duplex or power mode) is inaccurate for stenosis quantification (diameter reduction in longitudinal plane or **cross-sectional area reduction in transverse plane**) on the basis of the width of color-coded flow relative to the lumen diameter at the site of maximum stenosis. The inherent methodological limitations (angle dependence of the flow signal) can be overcome by using the B-flow technique, which allows better differentiation of flowing blood from the vessel wall or plaque because of its superior discrimination of echoes from mobile and stationary reflectors. A small study (21 patients) evaluated the performance of different imaging techniques in discriminating 50–95% stenosis (by NASCET criteria) compared with intra-arterial DSA, which served as the gold standard. In this study, **B-flow imaging** (see ◘ Fig. 5.86) showed the highest correlation (Pearson) with DSA (R = 0.94), followed by contrast-enhanced MRI (1.5 Tesla, standard coil; R = 0.9117), color duplex ultrasound, and reconstructed contrast-enhanced CT (both R = 0.85) (Finkenzeller et al. 2008). Note, however, that plaque evaluability in both B-mode and B-flow imaging crucially depends on plaque morphology, in particular on the presence of calcification. The accuracy of stenosis grading with B-flow imaging decreases with the severity of calcification.

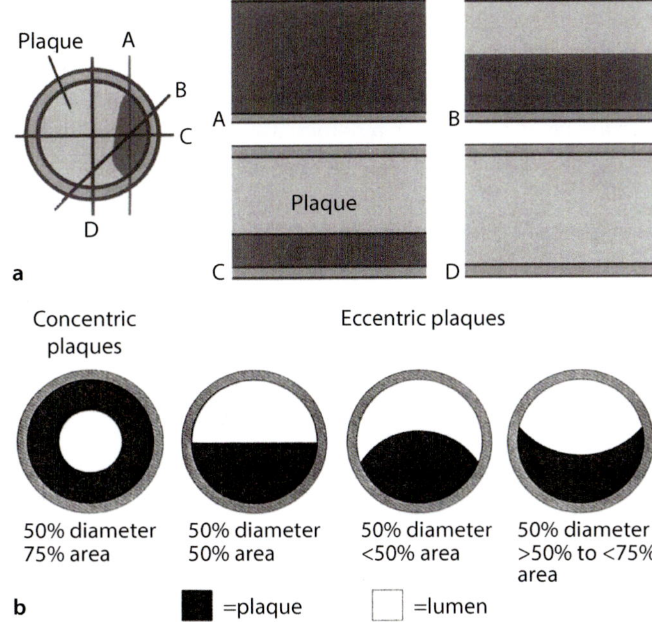

◘ **Fig. 5.27** **a** Eccentric luminal narrowing can vary widely in appearance and suggest different degrees of stenosis, depending on the imaging plane (angiography and B-mode ultrasound). The diagrams illustrate how the same plaque can lead to different estimates of the degree of stenosis caused by it: A: 0%, B: approx. 50%, C: approx. 70%, D: 100%. This source of misinterpretation results from the reduction of the three-dimensional vascular lesion to the two-dimensional imaging plane. Color duplex facilitates evaluation of eccentric plaques, which, if possible, should be assessed in transverse and longitudinal orientation. **b** Plaque morphology (concentric–eccentric) can lead to variable degrees of cross-sectional area reduction despite identical diameter reduction. Eccentric plaques are thicker than concentric ones, even when they cause the same degree of stenosis. Because they protrude into the lumen, eccentric plaques are exposed to greater shear stress (longitudinal pulsation) and are thus more susceptible to rupture and embolism. These two factors (reduction to two planes and differences in plaque configuration) explain the discrepancies in stenosis quantification between duplex ultrasound and angiography when eccentric plaques are present. Differences in plaque configuration lead to problems when stenosis grading on the basis of hemodynamic criteria with duplex ultrasound is compared with angiography using diameter reduction as a morphologic criterion. For instance, a 50% diameter reduction measured angiographically and indicating a 50% stenosis corresponds to a 50% stenosis based on hemodynamic grading (expressed in terms of cross-sectional area reduction) when the plaque is eccentric, but to a 75% stenosis when the plaque is concentric. With duplex ultrasound, stenosis grading is based on hemodynamic criteria derived from the Doppler waveform. A cross-sectional area reduction of 75% results in a PSV (local grading method) of approx. 240 cm/s (PSV ratio of 4) versus 120 cm/s (PSV ratio of 2) for 50% area reduction (in peripheral arteries)), while the angiographic diameter reduction is 50% in both cases (local degree of stenosis). PSV ratio = prestenotic PSV/intrastenotic PSV; degree of stenosis = (1–1/PSV ratio) × 100. The degree of stenosis determined hemodynamically is a more adequate marker of the severity of blood flow reduction (in relation to cross-area reduction). This is also relevant in evaluating peripheral or renal artery stenosis (see ◘ Fig. 2.17)

▪ Inherent Methodological Differences Between Ultrasound and Angiography

The gold standard, angiography, also has pitfalls – even when the stenosis is evaluated in different projections and quantification is done in the plane with the most severe luminal narrowing. Independent interpretations of the same angiograms by two radiologists show variation in accuracy ranging from 80% to 93%. **Errors in angiographic stenosis grading** arise from the fact that the 3D plaque is projected onto the 2D film, where the resulting degree of narrowing varies with the imaging plane (◘ Fig. 5.27a). In DSA, stenosis grading is also influenced by the concentration of contrast medium. Moreover, plaques of different configuration which produce the same diameter reduction produce different reductions in the cross-sectional area. Hence, they differ in hemodynamic relevance, giving rise to different increases in PSV (◘ Fig. 5.27b).

Angiography is based on the distal method of carotid stenosis grading. With this method, luminal narrowing of the ICA bulb on the order of 30% merely means that the lumen of the bulb is reduced to the width of the distal ICA, and no stenosis is diagnosed (◘ Fig. 5.10).

In an analysis of 1001 angiograms of the ICA, 34% of stenoses were classified as 70–99% stenoses by ESCT criteria versus only 16% by NASCET criteria (distal grading method) (Rothwell et al. 1994).

▪ Stenoses of the Common Carotid Artery (CCA) and External Carotid Artery (ECA)

Compared with the ICA, the ECA has a more pulsatile flow profile with a smaller diastolic component. Stenosis typically occurs at the ECA origin but becomes clinically relevant only in the presence of concomitant ICA occlusion and maintenance of brain perfusion via extracranial branches such as the supratrochlear artery or, very rarely, in patients with multiple-vessel disease and globally reduced perfusion of the brain with collateral pathways involving ECA branches. Due to the higher pulsatility of blood flow in the ECA, the PSV cutoff should be higher than for the same degree of stenosis in the ICA; therefore, we may safely assume that a PSV of 250–300 cm/s suggests higher-grade ECA stenosis. Consequently, there is no need for ROC analysis to determine cutoffs for grading ECA stenosis.

Stenosis of the CCA is rare. The most common sites of CCA stenosis are the origin of the artery from the aortic arch or from the brachiocephalic trunk and the distal CCA segment just below the bifurcation. Between these two sites, CCA stenosis can be graded using the intrastenotic-to-prestenotic PSV ratio (see ◘ Fig. 5.38a). In patients with subtotal or total CCA occlusion, branches of the ECA (such as the superior thyroid artery) can be recruited to ensure blood flow to the ICA. Depending on the course of the collateral pathways, the ECA will show variable retrograde filling. The hemodynamic stenosis criteria for the CCA are the same as for the ICA.

5.6.1.3 Occlusion

Occlusions of the carotid territory are chiefly due to local thrombus formation secondary to stenosing atherosclerosis at the origin of the ICA. As there are no arteries emptying into or arising from the extracranial portion of the ICA (except in individuals with a persistent primitive hypoglossal artery (PPHA); see ► Sect. 5.6.1.3.1 and ◘ Fig. 5.31), an occlusion will extend to the level of the next branching in the petrous bone or intracranially into the ophthalmic artery. Embolic carotid occlusion mainly affects the distal, intracranial segments of the internal carotid system. In the most severe form, there will be to-and-fro flow in the Doppler waveform (thump pattern), and the thrombus may extend cranially to the level of the bifurcation. Differentiation between subtotal and total ICA occlusion is important as surgery is usually only recommended for subtotal occlusion. Unfortunately, the ingrowth of vessels into the connective tissue of an organized occlusion makes it difficult to distinguish the two. Thus, the depiction of color-coded flow signals in the ICA segment near the skull base indicating a patent lumen is the decisive criterion for establishing the differential diagnosis. Contrast-enhanced ultrasound (CEUS) may be helpful in differentiating subtotal or pseudo-occlusion from true occlusion of the ICA.

Adjusting the scanner settings (low wall filter, low pulse repetition frequency, high gain) is important for detecting slow flow and small blood volumes in **pseudo-occlusion.** With adequate settings, the absence of flow distal to the atherosclerotic lesion is the most reliable evidence of ICA occlusion. Since no vessels arise from the ICA extracranially, the Doppler waveform sampled far distal to the bulb (near skull base) provides the most reliable information for differentiation, especially since there are no structures interfering with the Doppler signal (such as calcified plaques). Blood flow distal to a subtotal occlusion often assumes a venous character with a slow systolic velocity in spectral Doppler analysis. Using these criteria, color duplex ultrasound has a positive predictive value of 92.5–96.7% (Kirsch et al. 1994).

B-mode imaging is not very reliable in detecting ICA occlusions, especially recent ones, when intraluminal structures are still absent. Once transformation of the thrombus has occurred, occlusion may be identified in the B-mode by the presence of internal echoes from connective tissue in the shrunken lumen. However, an occluded artery is often difficult to distinguish from surrounding tissue.

When the ICA is occluded, even greater care is required so as **not to confuse the ICA and the ECA**. In ICA occlusion, the ECA supplies the brain (◘ Fig. 5.61 (Atlas)) through the supratrochlear artery, resulting in a less pulsatile Doppler waveform with a larger diastolic component (◘ Figs. 5.28 and 5.29). In this setting, the identity of the ECA must be confirmed by rhythmically tapping the temporal artery and looking for the transmitted pulsation (◘ Fig. 5.28). This is important to avoid making a mistake and localizing the occlusion to the ECA. Moreover, the examiner should be aware that, because ECA occlusion is typically short, the distal ECA tends to be refilled via collaterals. In this situation, the waveform from the postocclusive ECA segment becomes more like the ICA waveform (◘ Fig. 5.30).

Recanalization following ICA occlusion is very rare, and, if it occurs, it is generally associated with thromboembolic occlusion. It is characterized by flow signals in a tortuous and thin artery. Often, hypoechoic areas are seen near the wall of the shrunken lumen throughout the extracranial ICA (◘ Fig. 5.30). Spectral Doppler analysis will not reveal a stenosis jet but typically only slow flow and greater pulsatility compared with the normal ICA.

In the rare cases of CCA occlusion, the ICA may be refilled by branches of the ECA recruited as collaterals (e.g., superior thyroid artery; see ◘ Fig. 5.63 (Atlas)). The corre-

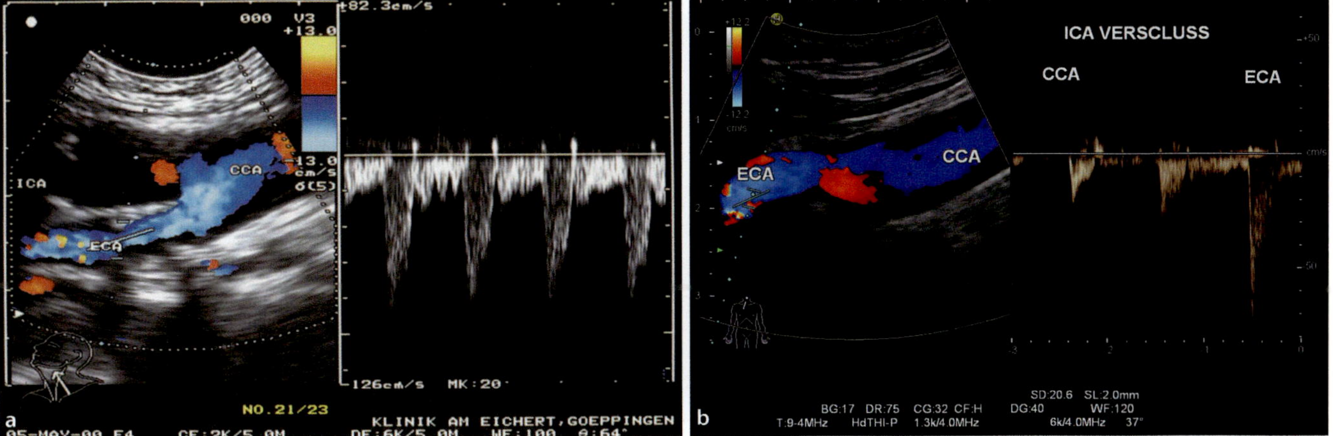

Fig. 5.28 **a** Image of the carotid bifurcation showing occlusion of the internal carotid artery (ICA) (absence of flow in the color flow image and Doppler waveform). The Doppler waveform from the external carotid artery (ECA) shows a rather large diastolic flow component and pulsatility as in the ICA, indicating that the ECA supplies the brain. Tapping of the temporal artery with transmission of this effect into the waveform proves that the waveform is actually from the ECA. **b** The normal common carotid artery (CCA) has a mixed waveform (combining features of ICA and ECA blood flow). When the ICA is occluded, as in the example shown, pulsatility in the CCA becomes more like that in the ECA (left part of waveform) and flow velocity is reduced. The Doppler tracing was obtained by moving the transducer from the CCA to the ECA (while maintaining a constant Doppler angle). In this patient, the contribution of the ECA to collateral flow is small

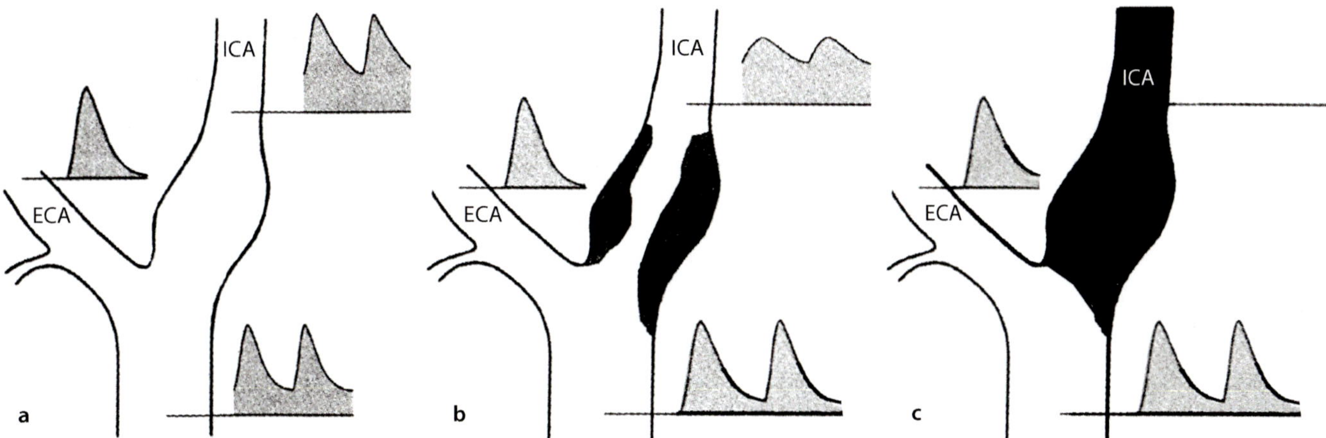

Fig. 5.29a–c Diagrams of Doppler waveforms illustrating normal and abnormal findings in the carotid territory. **a** Normal flow patterns – internal carotid artery (ICA): low-resistance flow with little pulsatility and large diastolic flow component; external carotid artery (ECA): pulsatility higher than in the ICA (the ECA mainly supplies skin and muscles and therefore faces a higher peripheral resistance) but lower than in the extremity arteries, due to the ECA's supply to the glands; common carotid artery (CCA): mixed type, pulsatility intermediate between that of the ICA and ECA, which it supplies. **b** High-grade stenosis or occlusion of the ICA – flow in the CCA becomes increasingly pulsatile, approaching the flow pattern of the ECA (as the influence of the ICA on the CCA waveform recedes or disappears). If the ECA additionally assumes collateral function and supplies the brain via the supratrochlear artery, the ECA waveform will become less pulsatile (low peripheral resistance). ICA waveform distal to high-grade ICA stenosis: characteristic postocclusive flow with delayed systolic upslope and decreased pulsatility, i.e., larger diastolic flow component and reduced peak systolic velocity (PSV). The difference is less striking than the change from triphasic to monophasic flow in extremity arteries because the ICA is a low-resistance artery and already has a monophasic flow profile under normal conditions. **c** ICA occlusion – with the CCA exclusively supplying the ECA, its flow increases in pulsatility and the waveform becomes similar to that of the ECA. The ECA may partially supply the brain (e.g., via the supratrochlear artery), reflected in a less pulsatile flow pattern with a larger diastolic component

sponding Doppler waveform will show retrograde flow in the proximal ECA with reversal to forward flow, but with a highly postocclusive character, in the ICA.

Bypass grafting is indicated only in multi-vessel disease with reduced global cerebral perfusion, which may manifest as borderzone infarction.

5.6.1.3.1 Persistent Primitive Hypoglossal Artery

A persistent primitive hypoglossal artery (PPHA) is an embryonic communication between the anterior and posterior cerebral circulations, which normally resolves and obliterates during early embryonic development. PPHA is rare and is typically detected incidentally by angiography. The

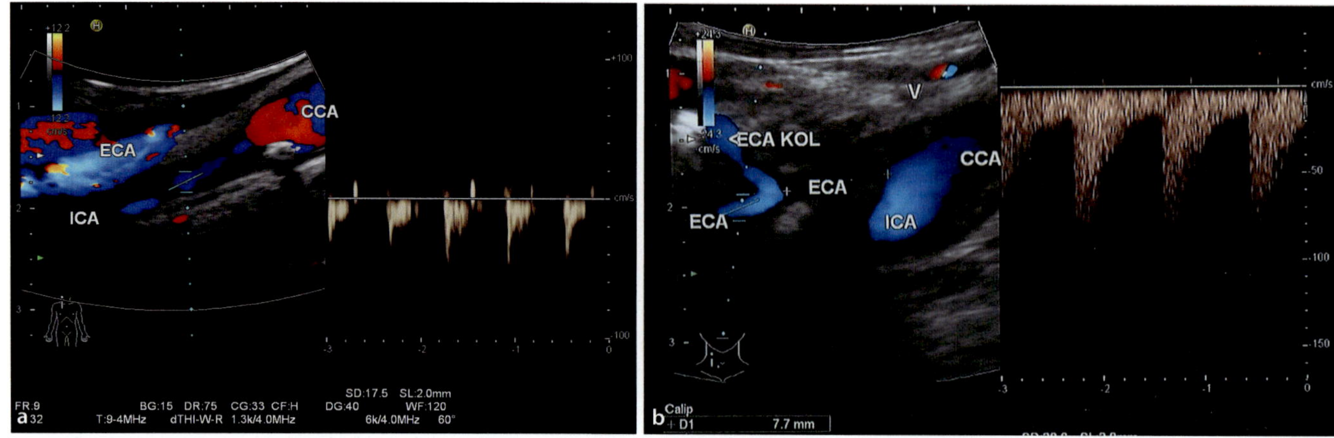

Fig. 5.30 **a** Recanalization after internal carotid artery (ICA) occlusion (thin patent lumen with slow, pulsatile flow). The external carotid artery (ECA) takes a more superficial course. **b** When insonation conditions are poor and acoustic shadowing from calcified plaques prevents thorough evaluation, ECA occlusion may be mistaken for ICA occlusion. To avoid this error, it is important to follow the occluded artery cranially: in the example, the distal portion of the occluded ECA is refilled by a collateral (ECA KOL). When the ICA is occluded, distal refilling only occurs in individuals with a persistent primitive hypoglossal artery (PPHA). Another pitfall to be borne in mind is that the postocclusive ECA waveform becomes more like that from the ICA (internalization; **b**). In this situation, the temporal tap maneuver can help confirm the identity of the ECA (Fig. 5.6)

reported incidence is 0.027–0.26% (Yilmaz et al. 1995). Autopsy data suggest that patients with a PPHA typically have other variants of vascular anatomy (Vasovic et al. 2008). A common association is a hypoplastic or aplastic vertebral artery with the main supply to the posterior circulation coming from the ICA via the PPHA (Elhammady et al. 2007). This is why patients with high-grade carotid stenosis may show disturbed perfusion of the posterior circulation (Kanazawa et al. 2008; Yuasa et al. 2005). In very rare cases of total or subtotal ICA occlusion, a PPHA supplies blood to the distal ICA (Fig. 5.31). In 2007, Ehammady et al. published what they claimed to be the first report of a PPHA with retrograde flow in a patient with high-grade proximal ICA stenosis. Much earlier, however, in 1992, Widmann and Sumpio reported a patient with flow in the distal ICA and absence of flow proximally, which was initially misdiagnosed as pseudo-occlusion. Intraoperatively, they found proximal ICA occlusion and distal refilling via a PPHA. Published data on the frequency of PPHAs (incidentally) detected during carotid artery ultrasound examinations are not available. In a retrospective analysis of 6300 patients who underwent carotid duplex ultrasound for suspected carotid stenosis or other indications, the author identified PPHA in 0.08% of cases. More than half of the PPHAs (0.05%) showed retrograde flow because they functioned as collaterals in proximal ICA occlusion. It is expected that, with awareness of this collateral pathway, more PPHAs will be identified by color duplex ultrasound in the future (Schäberle 2013). However, the sonographic detectability of PPHA strongly depends on the insonation conditions and is impaired in severe atherosclerosis with calcified plaques. Therefore, the frequency is likely to vary with the composition of the patient population investigated.

A PPHA with normal flow typically has a thin caliber (Fig. 5.31d, e) and is more difficult to detect and differentiate from ECA branches than a dilated PPHA recruited as a collateral in high-grade ICA stenosis or occlusion (Fig. 5.64b–d (Atlas)).

Sonoanatomically, a PPHA arises from the ICA slightly cranial to the bulb and runs to the skull base dorsomedial to the ICA. It courses through the hypoglossal canal to join the vertebrobasilar system, where aneurysmal dilatation may occur.

In addition, there may be compression of the hypoglossal nerve, and iatrogenic injury of the PPHA during carotid endarterectomy (CEA), like high-grade carotid stenosis, can cause disturbed perfusion of the posterior circulation in patients with a hypoplastic vertebral artery.

5.6.1.4 Postoperative Follow-Up

5.6.1.4.1 Carotid Endarterectomy (CEA)

Three operative techniques are available for carotid endarterectomy (CEA) in patients with carotid artery stenosis (Fig. 5.32).

In patients with a wide carotid bulb, CEA can be performed with direct closure of the arteriotomy. A possible complication of this procedure is the inadvertent creation of a relative stenosis compared with the distal ICA lumen by pulling the vessel wall too tight.

This complication can be prevented by **interposing a synthetic or venous patch** after CEA to compensate for the relative narrowing that may be created by primary closure. Too wide a patch, on the other hand, will lead to ectasia or even aneurysm with development of turbulent flow.

In **eversion CEA**, the ICA is transected at its origin, and the outer layer over the stenosing plaque-intima cylinder is everted and dissected along the vessel until the intima appears fairly normal again. At this point the cylinder is transected, and the outer wall layer is re-inserted into the common carotid artery (CCA).

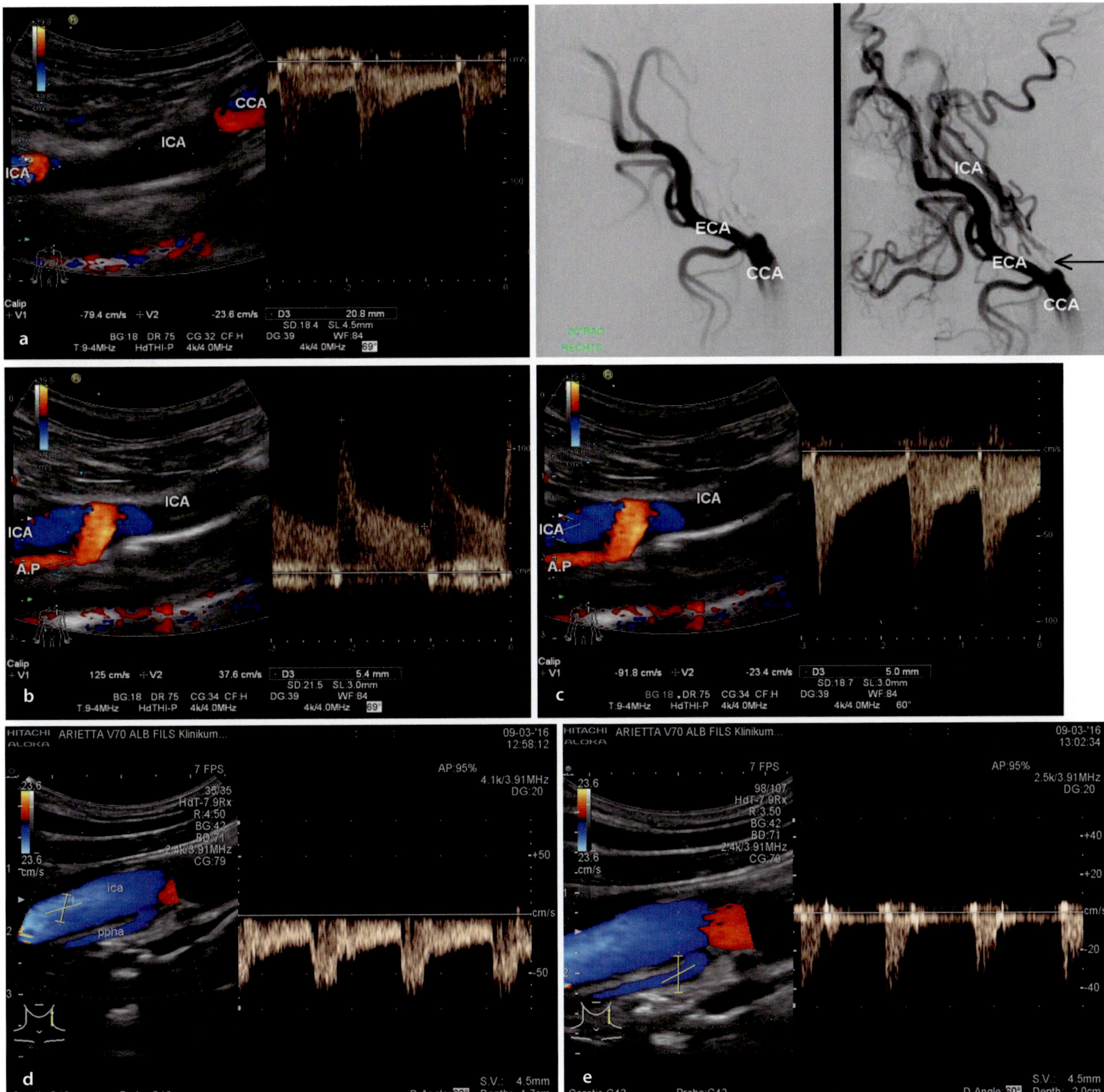

Fig. 5.31 Persistent primitive hypoglossal artery (PPHA) **a** Patient with atrial fibrillation and absolute arrhythmia and sonomorphologic findings pointing to embolic internal carotid artery (ICA) occlusion. Sonographic evaluation shows a normal common carotid artery (CCA) and bifurcation, while no flow is detectable in the ICA just distal to the bifurcation. The distal extracranial ICA segment has monphasic flow and normal ICA pulsatility (PSV of 90 cm/s). The patient subsequently underwent angiography. The first angiogram confirms ICA occlusion with distal refilling via a PPHA, which ensures adequate blood flow in the affected ICA territory. In this situation, the contralateral ICA or posterior cerebral circulation is not required to provide compensatory blood flow to the brain. The second angiogram shows the late phase of refilling of the distal ICA via the PPHA. **b** Dilated PPHA with retrograde flow (red, toward transducer, A.P) with a PSV of 125 cm/s (the occluded segment of the ICA is seen in the right half of the image). **c** The patent distal ICA has a normal-diameter lumen and a flow volume similar to an unobstructed ICA (PSV of 95 cm/s and normal pulsatility). These findings confirm good perfusion via the dilated PPHA. Delayed systolic upslope (acceleration time), compared with the unaffected contralateral side, is the only sign of postocclusive flow in the waveform from the distal ICA. Based on these ultrasound findings, surgery is unnecessary or even harmful. In addition, duplex ultrasound identified a compensatory increase in blood flow in the vertebral artery (PSV of 110 cm/s; not shown). **d, e** Normal ICA with PPHA. The example illustrates the incidendal detection of a PPHA, seen as a thin artery arising from the unobstruced extracranial ICA (**d**, with ICA waveform). The flow direction is orthograde (blue), as in the ICA (**e**, with PPHA waveform). Normally, the ICA does not give off extracranial branches. Color reversal (from red to blue) is due to a change in flow direction relative to the transducer (curved array)

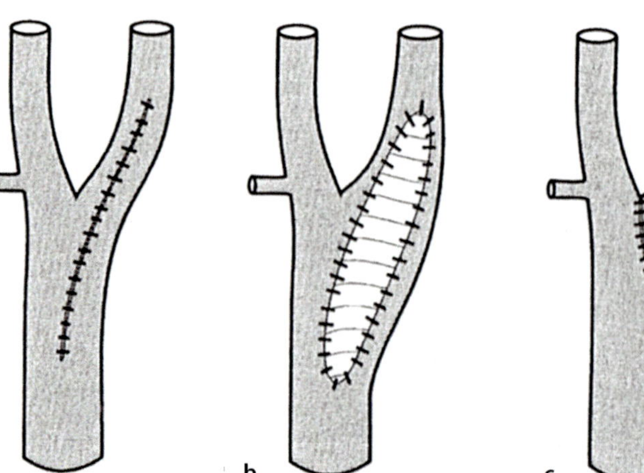

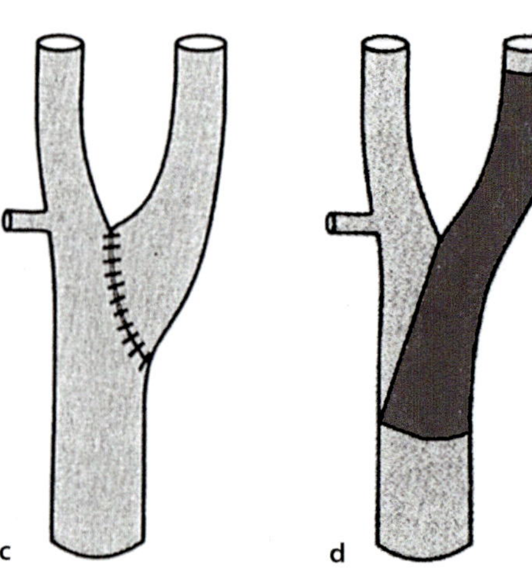

Fig. 5.32a–d Surgical and interventional restoration of patency in internal carotid artery (ICA) stenosis. **a** Carotid endarterectomy (CEA) with direct closure. **b** CEA with patch angioplasty. **c** Eversion CEA. **d** Percutaneous transluminal angioplasty (PTA) with carotid artery stenting (CAS)

Each CEA technique alters postoperative carotid bulb anatomy in a specific way: while CEA with patch insertion leads to an unphysiologically wide carotid bulb, the other two CEA techniques reduce bulb width to the normal ICA diameter. As a result of the loss of normal bulb anatomy, the correlations that exist in the native ICA no longer apply, and the two methods of carotid stenosis grading (local versus distal) yield the same results. The PSV ratio (intrastenotic to prestenotic PSV in the ICA) therefore often allows reliable grading of recurrent stenosis after CEA (which tends to involve the segment distal to the bifurcation or the distal end of the segment operated on). However, in the follow-up of patients after CEA with patch insertion, the hemodynamic effects of the caliber variation at the distal patch end must be taken into account in interpreting the sonographic findings.

Moreover, each CEA technique is **prone to specific complications** that must be carefully ruled out by postoperative ultrasonography. The complications of the primary closure technique, apart from relative narrowing as an early complication, include an intimal step or an intimal flap. Elongation of the ICA can lead to kinking with development of a stenosis unless the excessive segment is resected.

Patch angioplasty is susceptible to thrombotic deposits, but these may resolve, even after days, following treatment with heparin and platelet aggregation inhibitors (see Fig. 5.78 (Atlas)). However, such thrombotic deposits can also induce transient ischemic attacks (TIAs) or early occlusion. Aneurysmal dilatation due to excessive correction gives rise to turbulent flow. Suture aneurysms primarily occur in association with infection and after insertion of a synthetic patch. At the junction of the patch with the distal ICA, detachment of the intima can lead to the same complications as direct closure. Use of a venous patch can give rise to the formation of a true aneurysm due to the physiologically weaker venous wall. Over time, patients may develop recurrent stenosis. Hence, in the follow-up examination, special attention must be paid to intimal hyperplasia in the suture area.

Suture line complications are rare in eversion CEA, while step formation at the transition to the native intima is somewhat more common (Table 5.14).

Table 5.14 Sonographic evaluation for postoperative complications after carotid endarterectomy (CEA)

CEA technique	Evaluation of operative site	Evaluation of distal ICA
CEA with direct closure	Relative stenosis, recurrent or residual stenosis	Intimal step, intimal flap, intimal dissection, kinking, intimal hyperplasia
CEA with patch angioplasty	Thrombotic deposits in the patch area without/with hemodynamically significant stenosis, suture aneurysm, ectasia, infection, recurrent stenosis	Intimal step, intimal flap, intimal dissection, kinking, intimal hyperplasia
Eversion CEA	Retraction of suture line, suture aneurysm, recurrent stenosis	Intimal flap, intimal step, intimal dissection, intimal hyperplasia

The specific complications of the different CEA techniques must be borne in mind when performing the mandatory postoperative duplex scan. Postoperative sonography is impaired by scattering through edema, which may affect both B-mode and spectral Doppler imaging. The use of a lower-frequency transducer (5 or even 3.5 MHz) yields B-mode images with a poorer resolution but often facilitates both the identification of the target artery within the edematous tissue and spectral Doppler measurement for exclusion of early occlusion, residual stenosis, or thrombotic deposits.

The **development of recurrent stenosis** has been investigated in numerous studies with postoperative follow-up by duplex ultrasound (Fig. 5.33). However, the studies do not address the problem of the diagnostic accuracy of ultrasound in detecting the above-described early complications under the poorer postoperative insonation conditions (Figs. 5.78 and 5.79 (Atlas)). Clinical experience indicates that patients with transient ischemic attacks (TIAs) after CEA with patch

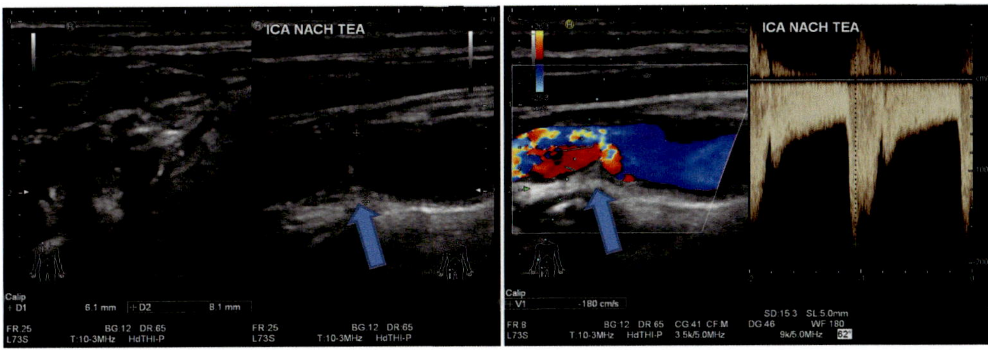

Fig. 5.33 Moderate recurrent carotid stenosis in transverse and longitudinal orientation (caused by a flap-like, floating structure, indicated by arrow in the 2 longitudinal views) after carotid endarterectomy (CEA) with patch angioplasty (seen in the near wall). The PSV is 180 cm/s

closure often have thrombotic deposits on the synthetic patch, even if no hemodynamic effect is apparent in the Doppler waveform. The deposits may completely resolve within days to weeks under heparin and antiplatelet therapy. No studies have investigated these complications in terms of their possible impact on patch selection. Color duplex ultrasound allows differentiation of intimal dissection and intimal flaps, which are often seen as hyperechoic floating structures in the bloodstream.

The flow pattern in a suture aneurysm is the same as in a pseudoaneurysm. To-and-fro flow can be demonstrated by color duplex or spectral Doppler (see ▶ Sect. 2.1.6.3 and Figs. 5.70 and 5.71 (both Atlas)).

If semiclosed endarterectomy of the external carotid artery (ECA) is performed, intimal flaps or dissection may give rise to stenosis or occlusion. They rarely have functional or clinical significance but must be considered in the differential diagnosis when examining the ICA.

The intimal step at the proximal end of the operated on segment in the CCA is often highly conspicuous in the B-mode image but has no clinical or functional relevance as the step flattens out in the direction of the flowing blood.

Recurrent stenosis within the first 12 months of surgery is due to neointimal proliferation (unless the operation has been technically inadequate). Recurrence seen after 2 years is attributable to the progression of atherosclerosis. Based on the follow-up data from more than 160 studies including over 62,000 patients, the average restenosis rate is 6% (range, 0–50%) (Kallmayer et al. 2014). Plaque echogenicity (mean GSM) is lower than in primary ICA stenosis (Fig. 5.35e) without this indicating a higher stroke risk (Pavela et al. 2014). The incidence of symptomatic recurrent carotid stenosis is 2% with the recurrence rate being markedly higher after CEA with direct closure than after patch angioplasty (12% versus 5%). Overall, approx. 20% of all stenoses seen after CEA are accounted for by residual stenoses, 50% develop within 2 years, and 30% occur later. Long-term follow-up of 380 patients for 16 years revealed restenosis rates of 5.8%, 9.9%, 13.9%, and 23.4% after 1, 3, 5, and 10 years, respectively; however, only 2.1% of patients were found to have high-grade recurrent stenosis (> 80%) (Mattos et al. 1993; Roth et al. 1999). In the follow-up after CEA, sonographic evaluation of the unoperated side with identification of progressive atherosclerosis appears to be more relevant than imaging of the side where CEA was performed. It has been proposed that routine duplex surveillance in the first 6 months is not required when an intraoperative completion study has confirmed the technical adequacy of the repair (Pross et al. 2001; Fig. 5.34). However, experience seems to indicate that it is common to detect thrombotic deposits in patients with postoperative TIAs despite normal intraoperative findings, especially when a synthetic patch has been used. Such deposits respond well to heparin treatment (follow-up within 4 weeks is recommended).

5.6.1.4.2 Carotid Artery Stenting (CAS)

Following percutaneous transluminal angioplasty (PTA) with carotid artery stenting (CAS), ultrasound depicts the stent as a mesh-like structure. A diagnostic Doppler waveform is difficult to obtain from the stented carotid segment during the first days, presumably because the stent is not yet incorporated. After this initial period, the scanning conditions are the same as before stent placement. Stents are also prone to thrombotic deposits, which may cause stenosis but will recede after initiation of treatment with heparin and platelet antiaggregators. The distal stent end is especially prone to recurrent stenosis (Figs. 5.35, 5.82 (Atlas), and 5.83 (Atlas)).

Scientific evidence suggests that higher blood flow velocity cutoffs are needed for postinterventional surveillance of patients after CAS (Stanziale et al. 2005). **Loss of compliance of the arterial wall** after stent insertion results in higher normal velocities; thus, it has been proposed that a PSV of up to 150 or 180 cm/s should be considered normal in a stented carotid artery segment (Chahwan et al. 2007; Lal et al. 2004).

5.6.1.4.3 Scientific Discrepancies Regarding Restenosis Grading After CAS

Several studies investigating restenosis after carotid artery stenting (CAS) proposed peak systolic velocity (PSV) thresholds of 150–240 cm/s for >50% stenosis and 300–450 cm/s for >70% (to 80%) stenosis (Alexander et al. 2007; AbuRahma et al. 2008; Lal et al. 2008; Stanziale et al. 2005; Kwon et al. 2007; Zhou et al. 2008; Chi et al. 2007). Most of these studies assessed stenosis severity using North American Symptomatic Carotid Endarterectomy Trial (NASCET) methodology. When European Carotid Surgery Trial (ECST) methodology is used, the PSV cutoffs for identifying equivalent degrees of

5

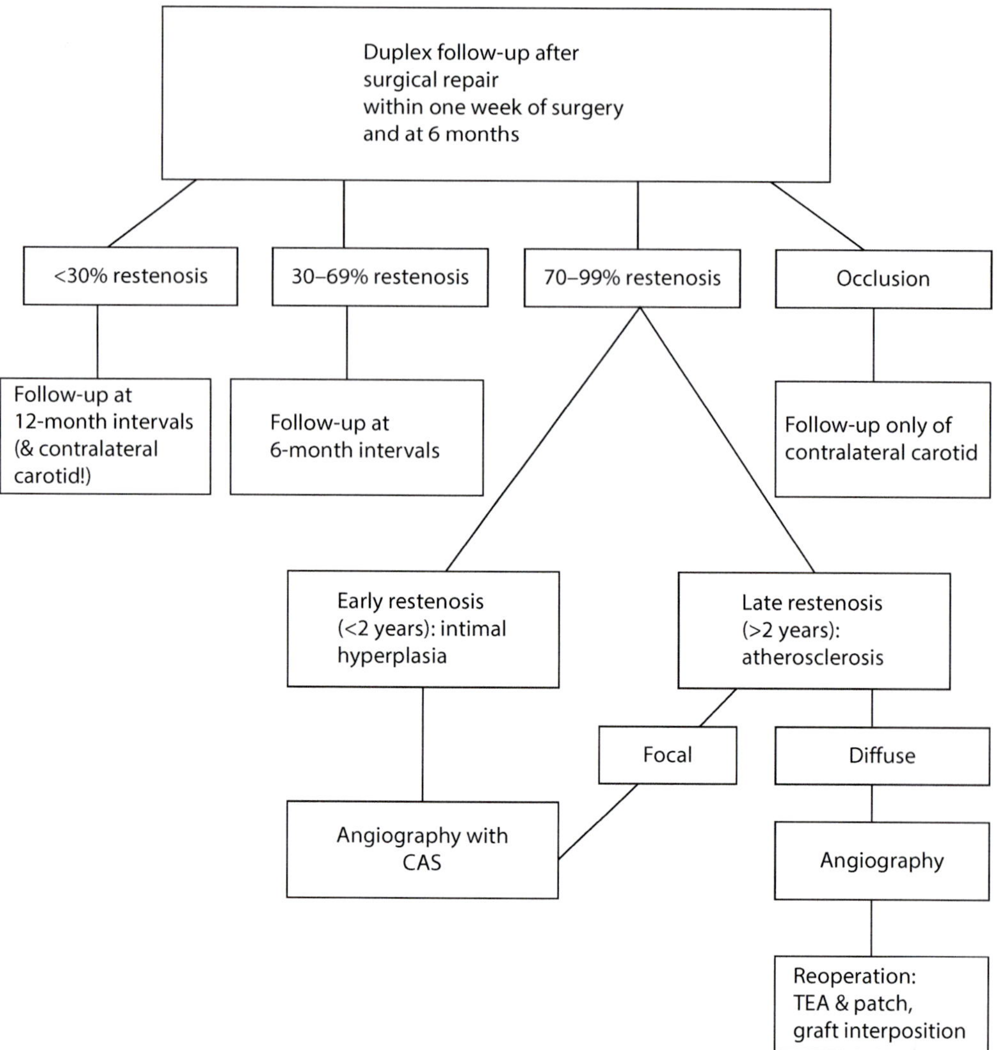

Fig. 5.34 Diagnostic algorithm for the follow-up of patients after carotid endarterectomy (CEA) based on NASCET grading of restenosis. *CAS* carotid artery stenting, *TEA* thromboendarterectomy

stenosis should be approx. one third lower because a given PSV indicates a higher-grade local stenosis (ECST) compared with the distal degree (NASCET). The second issue to be considered is that different velocity criteria apply when grading in-stent restenosis compared with restenosis in a nonstented carotid artery. Two studies investigating carotid restenosis proposed cutoffs of 180 and 200 cm/s for >50% restenosis (NASCET criteria) in unstented carotid arteries versus 220 and 240 cm/s for in-stent restenosis (Lal et al. 2008; Chi et al. 2007). According to these studies, the cutoff for in-stent restenosis is only approx. 10–20% higher than for restenosis in native carotid arteries.

The need for modified velocity criteria in stented carotid arteries was also confirmed by AbuRahma et al. (2008), who conducted a ROC analysis to determine cutoffs for different degrees of in-stent carotid restenosis. In this study, a PSV threshold of 154 cm/s for >30% stenosis (by NASCET criteria) showed 99% sensitivity and 89% specificity. The optimal PSV cutoff for >50% stenosis was 224 cm/s, which had 99% sensitivity, 90% specificity, 99% positive predictive value, 90% negative predictive value, and 98% overall accuracy. The ideal cutoff for >80% stenosis was 325 cm/s with 100% sensitivity, 99% specificity, and 99% accuracy. The diagnostic accuracy of absolute PSV was compared with end-diastolic velocity (EDV) and also with the ratio of PSV in the stented ICA to the PSV in the CCA. This comparison showed that PSV provided the most reliable criterion for sonographic stenosis grading in 144 patients in whom the results were compared with angiography. Nineteen of the patients had >50% in-stent restenosis. Large PSV ranges were found for different categories of stenosis (defined by angiography, NASCET criteria): range of 142–256 cm/s with a mean PSV of 178/s for 30–50% stenosis (n = 38); 201–408 cm/s with a mean PSV of 278 cm/s for 50–80% stenosis (n = 11); and 58–613 cm/s with a mean of 403 cm/s for 80–99% stenosis (n = 8).

A minor limitation of published ultrasound studies of carotid in-stent restenosis is the small number of cases investigated. Although some study populations include more than 100 patients with duplex ultrasound after CAS (Table 5.15), ROC analysis was usually performed in subsets of 10–20 patients who underwent angiography because they had restenosis of at least 50% and were candidates for possible reintervention.

Moreover, most studies use CT angiography (or magnetic resonance imaging) as the method of reference for color duplex imaging rather than the gold standard of angiography in two or three planes, neglecting the inherent methodological limitations of CT angiography, especially in the carotid bifurcation. This introduces an additional inaccuracy into the ROC analysis of sonographic velocity thresholds. Most investigators use catheter-based angiography only in patients undergoing repeat PTA for higher-grade stenosis; as a result, the gold standard is available only for these cases.

In the discussion of velocity thresholds for quantifying carotid in-stent restenosis compared with restenosis of nonstented arteries, it was initially overlooked that the approximately one third higher cutoffs proposed in studies using NASCET methodology could not simply be converted to equivalent cutoffs for in-stent restenosis grading using ECST methodology. Instead, it turned out that PSV cutoffs for diagnosing in-stent restenosis based on ECST methodology should only be slightly higher than cutoffs for nonstented arteries (see ◘ Table 5.9). Higher blood flow velocities in stented carotid segments may be attributable to several factors. One is rigidity of the stented arterial wall, which results in higher PSV within the stent; however, it has also been shown that pulsatility varies with the stent device used. At the same time, it is hard to believe that the difference in rigidity between a stented segment and an atherosclerotic, calcified ICA with higher-grade stenosis is so large as to explain a 30% difference in PSV or to justify a 30% higher PSV cutoff for in-stent restenosis. The lumen reduction by the stent does not explain this difference either.

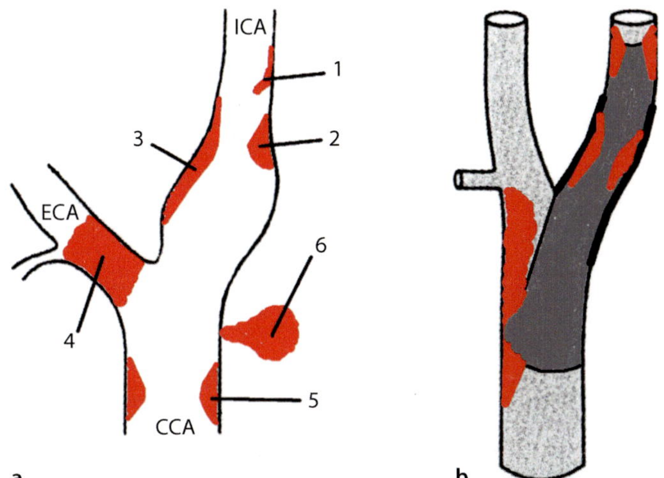

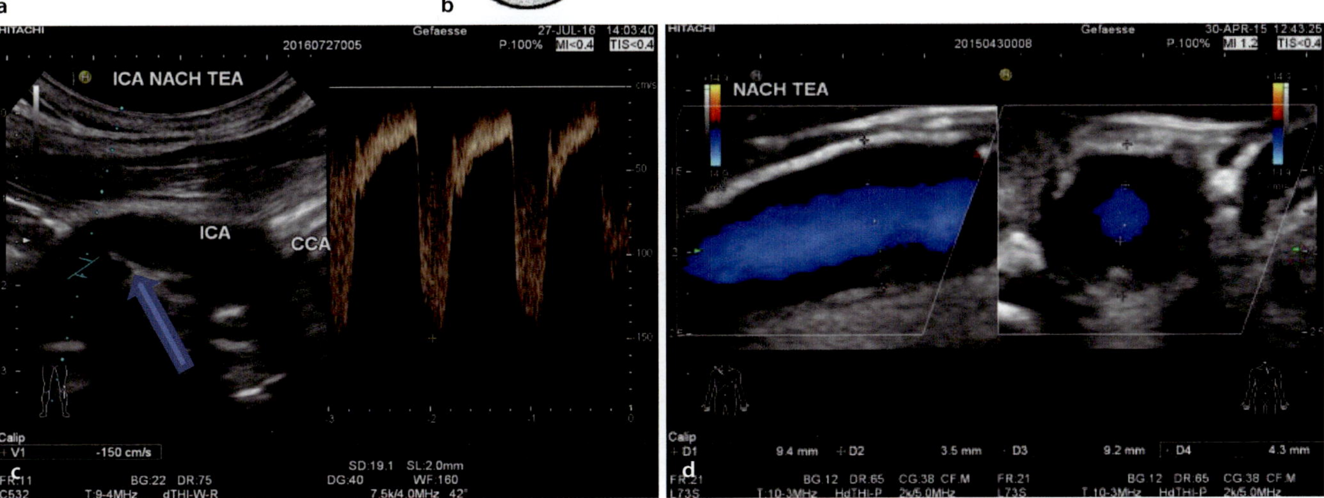

◘ **Fig. 5.35** **a** Common sites of early and late complications and progressive atherosclerosis after carotid endarterectomy (CEA): **1** intimal flap; **2** recurrent stenosis due to plaque; **3** neointimal proliferation with recurrent stenosis; **4** postoperative external carotid artery (ECA) occlusion; **5** damage from clamping, step, plaque progression at proximal end of CEA; **6** suture aneurysm. **b** Early and late complications after carotid artery stenting (CAS): neointimal hyperplasia; recurrent plaque with stenosis; ECA stenosis, when ICA stent crosses the ECA origin. (For stent dislocation, see ◘ Fig. 5.85 (Atlas)). **c** Moderate recurrent stensosis caused by intimal flap (arrow) seen at follow-up 1 week after CEA (PSV of 150 cm/s). **d** Recurrent stenosis caused by neointimal proliferation 8 months after CEA. **e** Recurrent stenosis caused by plaque (P) due to progressive atherosclerosis is often identified by echolucency without this indicating an increased risk of embolism (images obtained 6 years after CEA). The Doppler waveform confirms high-grade recurrent stenosis with a PSV of 350 cm/c. **f** Suture aneurysm. This patient presented with local swelling due to a large hematoma after CEA. The ultrasound examination reveals to-and-fro flow (with systolic (s) inflow and diastolic outflow (d) in the waveform from the site of suture line rupture identified by color duplex ultrasound. A suture line rupture should always alert the examiner to the possibility of infection as an underlying cause

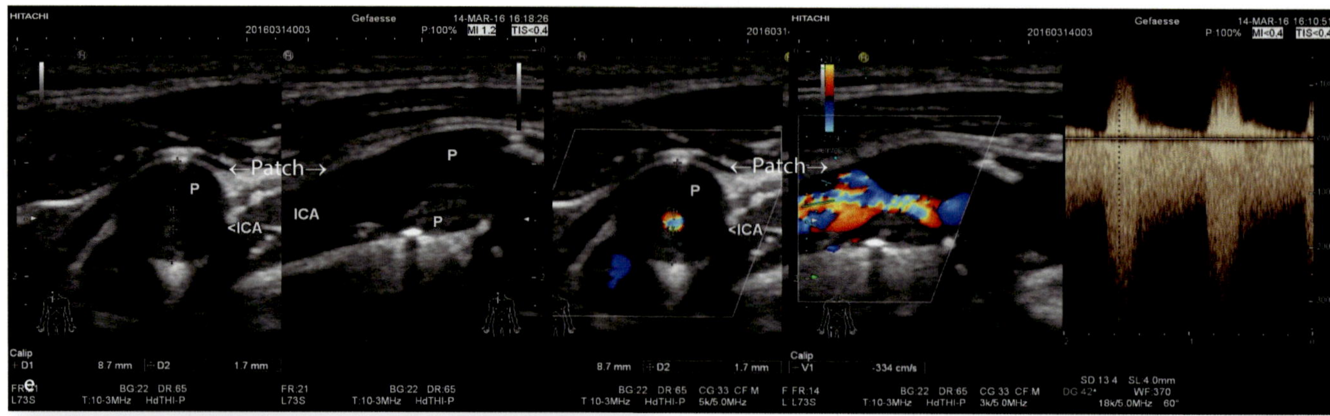

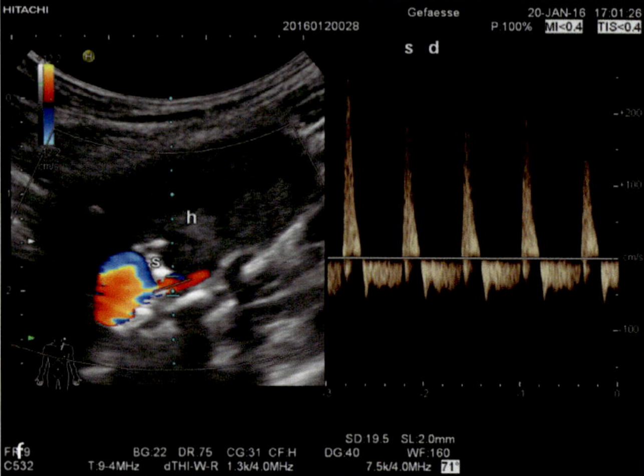

Fig. 5.35 (continued)

Table 5.15 Dzsound criteria for in-stent restenosis after carotid artery stenting (CAS)

Author, year	No.	PSV (cm/s)			ICA/CCA ratio		
		> 50%	> 70%	> 80%	> 50%	> 70%	> 80%
AbuRahma 2008	144/19	224		325	3.4		4.5
Lal 2008	189/29	220		340	2.7		4.1
Stanziale 2005	118/19	225	350		2.5	4.75	
Peterson 2005			170				
Chi 2007	13	240	450		2.45	4.3	
Wei Zhou 2008	237/22		300			4	
Kwon 2007		200			2.5		

No.: total number of patients with CAS examined with duplex ultrasound/number of patients who underwent angiography or CT angiography
CCA common carotid artery, *ICA* internal carotid artery, *PSV* peak systolic velocity

5.6.1.4.4 Stenosis Grading Based on the Continuity Equation

As recurrent stenosis at the proximal stent end (i.e., the junction between the common carotid artery (CCA) and the stent) is less common than in-stent restenosis or stenosis at the distal stent end (Fig. 5.37b), **abrupt doubling of peak systolic velocity (PSV)** in a continuous Doppler measurement – which is well established for diagnosing stenosis in peripheral arteries – can be used for the diagnosis of hemodynamically relevant in-stent restenosis (50% stenosis) in the carotid system as well (Figs. 5.36, 5.37, and 5.38). When the increase in intrastenotic PSV is determined using the

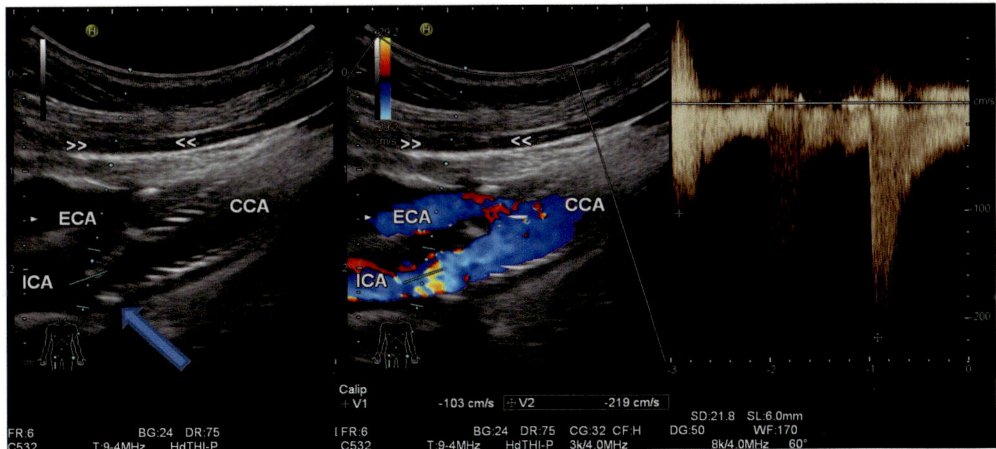

Fig. 5.36 Patient with restenosis after carotid artery stenting (CAS). Continuous spectral Doppler imaging revealed a focal increase in peak systolic velocity (PSV) in the stent from 100 cm/s in the prestenotic segment to 210 cm/s in the stenosis. For this measurement, the spectral Doppler waveform was recorded by moving the transducer along the artery in a cranial direction in order to continuously shift the sample volume from the prestenotic to the intrastenotic segment of the stent, while maintaining a constant Doppler angle (the segment along which the Doppler tracing was recorded is indicated by > > … < < in the B-mode image). The pre- and intrastenotic PSVs give a PSV ratio of 2, consistent with 50% in-stent restenosis. Restenosis in this case is not caused by stent dislocation but by the rigidity of the snugly fitting stent: elastic recoil of the short, stenotic, brace-like plaque at the origin of the ICA (identified by hyperechogenicity) results in conical tapering of the stent. The example illustrates how PSV increases as the cross-sectional area decreases along the tapering stent. Although the stent is patent, increasing flow resistance in the narrowing portion of the stent causes hemodynamically relevant stenosis. This type of stenosis is more difficult to identify by angiography

PSV ratio, this velocity should be related to PSV just upstream of the in-stent restenosis rather than to PSV in the common CCA. However, in some studies (AbuRahma et al. 2008; Lal et al. 2008; Stanziale et al. 2005; Peterson et al. 2005; Chi et al. 2007), investigators determined the CCA/ICA PSV ratio for diagnosing ICA in-stent restenosis, proposing cutoff ratios of 2.5–3.4 for >50% stenosis and 4–4.5 for >70% or >80% stenosis. While calculation of the intrastenotic PSV increase in relation to the PSV in the CCA accounts for systemic effects on PSV as well as compensatory flow increases in patients with contralateral steno-occlusive ICA lesions, in-stent restenosis grading using the CCA/ICA PSV ratio is subject to the same pitfalls as in the native arteries: PSV in the CCA varies with the volume flow rate in the external carotid artery (ECA), which increases when the ECA is recruited as a collateral. This problem can be avoided by measuring the prestenotic PSV for calculation of the velocity ratio in the proximal ICA, which is often possible, as in-stent restenosis in the carotid territory tends to occur upstream of the origin of the ECA. Using the PSV from the proximal ICA is more reliable because it is not influenced by other factors such as hemodynamic effects of branching arteries, diameter variations, or differences in vessel wall rigidity. Ideally, the prestenotic PSV for calculation of the velocity ratio should be measured within the stent to eliminate possible effects of the stent on vessel lumen width or wall rigidity. Use of the PSV ratio also avoids the well-established problems that arise from the wide variation in absolute PSVs measured for a given angiographic degree of stenosis and the fact that this parameter is affected by a variety of other factors (AbuRahma et al. 2008). In a compilation and analysis of an as yet small number of patients, the author identified nine patients with higher-grade carotid in-stent restenosis, classified as >75% stenosis based on the continuity equation and a cutoff ratio of intra- to prestenotic PSV in the ICA of >4. Absolute intrastenotic PSV in these nine patients ranged from 230–455 cm/s (Figs. 5.36, 5.37, and 5.38 and Figs. 5.81, 5.82, and 5.83 (Atlas)). All nine cases were confirmed by subsequent angiography. Stenosis grading using this PSV ratio is different from both ESCT and NASCET methodology (local versus distal carotid stenosis grading) but is methodologically closer to the latter. Differences in diameter between the carotid bulb and the distal ICA are eliminated when a stent is in place. In this artificial situation of a relatively constant ICA diameter, it follows from the continuity equation that a PSV ratio of 2 or doubling of PSV indicates 50% cross-sectional area reduction, while a ratio of 4 corresponds to 75% area reduction in the stent. A 75% cross-sectional area reduction corresponds to 50% diameter reduction when caused by circumferential stenosis. Conversely, 50% diameter reduction caused by an eccentric plaque results in a smaller cross-sectional area reduction, and therefore the resulting stenosis has a less severe hemodynamic effect and causes a smaller increase in PSV (Fig. 5.27). While causing less severe stenosis, an eccentric plaque is thicker and exposed to greater shear stress, which increases the risk of embolism (Fig. 5.15a). This risk must be taken into consideration as well when assessing the therapeutic relevance of carotid in-stent restenosis.

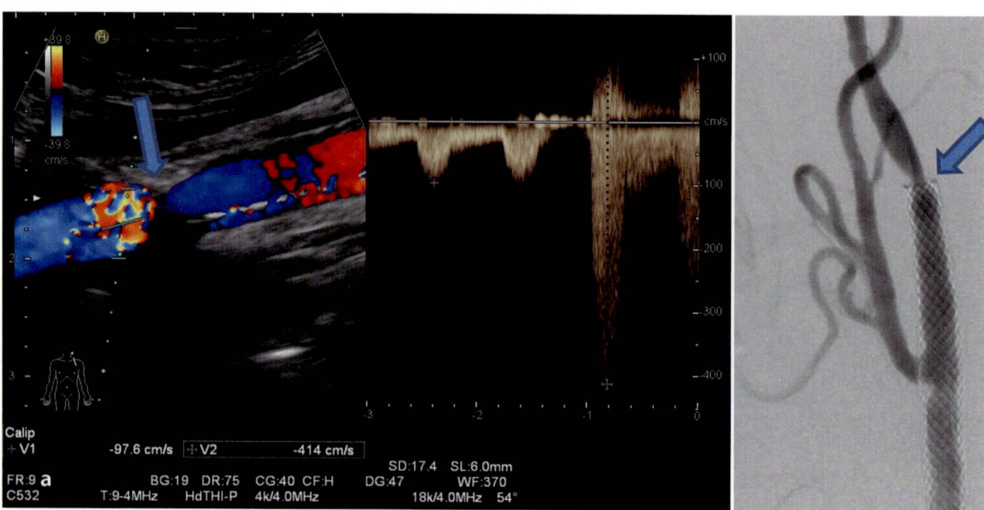

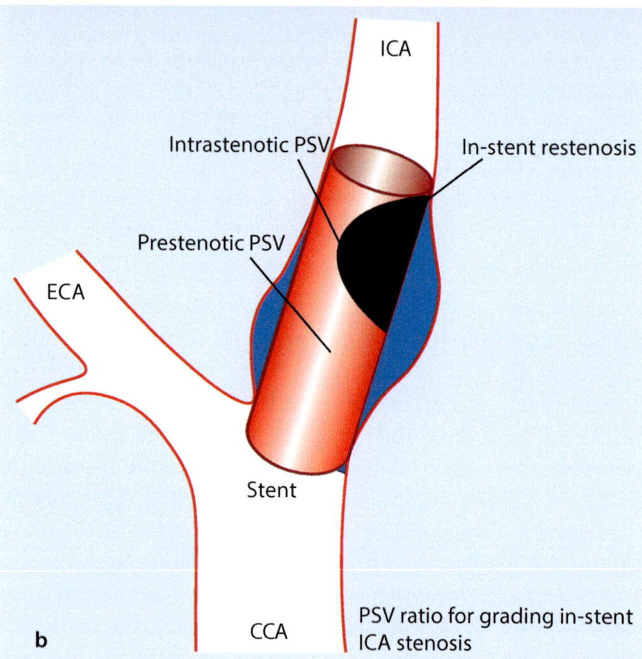

Fig. 5.37 **a** High-grade carotid in-stent restenosis at the distal stent end with an intrastenotic-to-prestenotic PSV ratio of >4 (calculated from intrastenotic PSV of 414 cm/s and prestenotic PSV of 97.6 cm/s – the latter measured in the stent just distal to the ECA origin). The site of PSV increase is identified by moving the transducer cranially while obtaining a continuous spectral tracing at a constant Doppler angle (curved-array transducer, tilted to achieve good Doppler angle, 54° in the example) (see Fig. 5.83b (Atlas) for another example of high-grade in-stent restenosis with a PSV ratio > 4 but with an absolute intrastenotic PSV of only 268 cm/s). The angiogram (right) shows high-grade ICA in-stent restenosis (projection plane). **b** Diagram illustrating the author's approach to grading carotid in-stent restenosis based on the continuity equation (see Fig. 1.44 and ► Sect. 1.2.3). This approach avoids the confusion regarding distal versus local stenosis grading (NASCET versus ECST) and exploits the fact that a stented carotid artery segment has a fairly constant diameter and that most in-stent restenoses occur within the stent farther away from the ECA origin or even at the distal stent end. The drawing shows the sites where prestenotic and intrastenotic PSV for calculation of the PSV ratio should be measured. This is the most accurate method for grading in-stent restenosis of the ICA (see Figs. 5.81, 5.82, and 5.83 (all Atlas))

B-flow ultrasound (see Fig. 5.86 (Atlas)) and contrast-enhanced ultrasound (CEUS) (Clevert et al. 2011) (see ► Sect. 5.6.1.1.8) allow very accurate morphologic grading of carotid in-stent stenosis. The diagnostic performance is comparable to angiography, while B-flow imaging affords higher spatial resolution.

5.6.1.4.5 Stent Dislocation

While ultrasound provides no valid diagnostic information in patients with dislocation of an aortic stent, it is well suited to evaluate patients with suspected dislocation of an ICA stent. In the carotid territory, duplex ultrasound with a high-frequency transducer provides highly resolved information

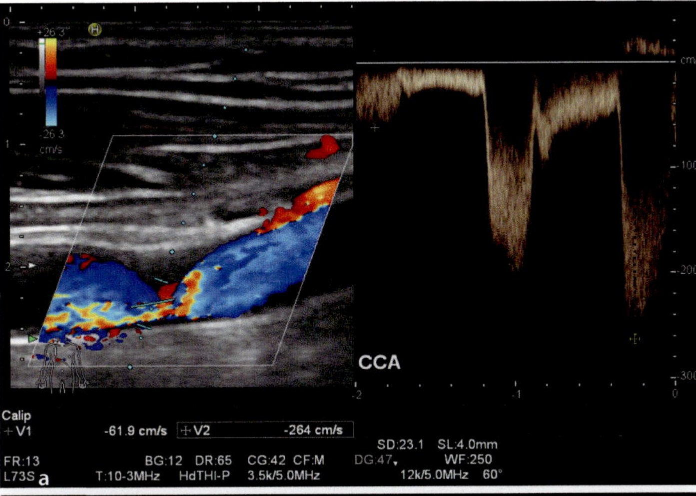

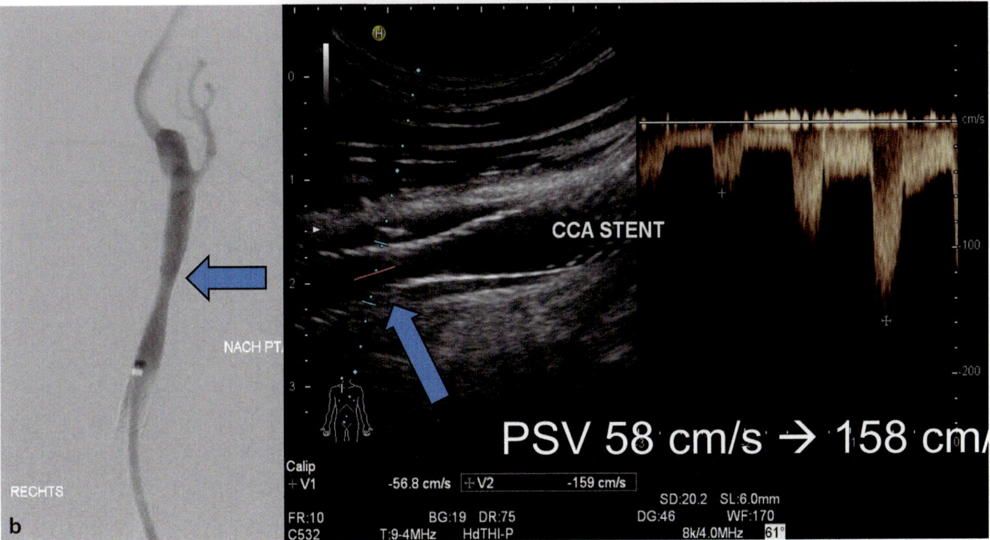

Fig. 5.38a, b Illustration of stenosis grading in a native common carotid artery (CCA) and stented CCA using the continuity equation. Study-based velocity cutoffs have not been defined for grading CCA stenosis. **a** In this patient, >75% stenosis is diagnosed based on a peak systolic velocity (PSV) ratio > 4 (calculated from PSVs of 264 and 61 cm/s). **b** Following stent implantation, the patient developed in-stent restenosis due to elastic recoil of the plaque; restenosis is classified as moderate based on a PSV ratio of 2.7 (PSVs: 158/58 cm/s) (see Figs. 5.36 and 5.37 for how to obtain a continuous spectral Doppler tracing for PSV measurement along the stented arterial segment). The angiogram confirms in-stent restenosis (arrow) of the CCA

on blood flow within the stent or between the stent and the wall of the native artery (see Fig. 5.85 (Atlas)). The findings can be corroborated by contrast-enhanced ultrasound (CEUS), and the time-motion mode provides additional information on pressure-related stent movement within the arterial lumen. A diameter mismatch between the artery and an uncoated stent can result in blood flow between the stent and the native arterial wall. Here, ultrasound is superior to angiography because, following opacification, the thin bloodstream outside the stent lumen is difficult to differentiate from flow within the lumen.

Straightening of an elongated and tortuous ICA by a rigid stent can lead to **kinking** distally. Color duplex imaging allows identification of kinks and associated stenosis as well as any (postural) reduction in cerebral perfusion, which may occur in patients with bilateral carotid stents.

5.6.2 Vertebral Arteries

5.6.2.1 Stenosis

The origin of the vertebral artery may be difficult to evaluate by color duplex imaging when a kink or loop is present. Arising at a right angle from the subclavian artery, the vertebral artery exhibits disturbed flow at its origin, which must not be mistaken for stenosis. The curved course at the origin may lead to Doppler angle uncertainty and an unreliable flow velocity calculation for stenosis grading.

Virtually all **atherosclerotic stenoses** of the vertebral artery occur at its origin. Since there is wide variation in peak systolic velocities and in the flow volume of the vertebral arteries and there may be marked differences in caliber between the two vertebral arteries (hyperplasia, hypoplasia), no absolute cutoff value (as for the carotid arteries) can be defined to discriminate between low-grade and hemodynamically significant stenosis (Figs. 5.39 and 5.40). Therefore, indirect criteria such as turbulent flow at the origin or markedly reduced pulsatility compared with the contralateral artery can be considered but should be interpreted with caution. Vertebral artery stenosis is suggested when PSV at the origin is at least 50% higher than in more distal segments. Grading of stenosis at the vertebral artery origin is difficult for several reasons:

- Absolute PSV cutoff: unreliable due to interindividual variation and variable perfusion
- Comparison with contralateral side: precluded due to variability or possible hypoplasia

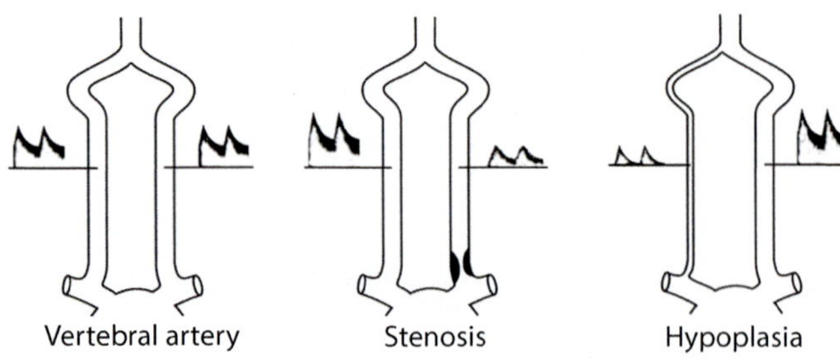

Fig. 5.39 Diagrams of Doppler waveforms illustrating normal and abnormal findings in the vertebral arteries (▶ Sect. 5.4.2). The first drawing presents normal waveforms from the right and left vertebral arteries. The second drawing illustrates the situation when the left vertebral artery is stenosed. The postocclusive waveform is characterized by a delayed systolic upstroke, decreased peak systolic velocity (PSV), and a relatively large diastolic component. The third drawing shows one hypoplastic and one hyperplastic vertebral artery. The waveform from the hypoplastic artery differs from a poststenotic waveform in that diastolic velocity is decreased as well (Modified according to Widder 1995)

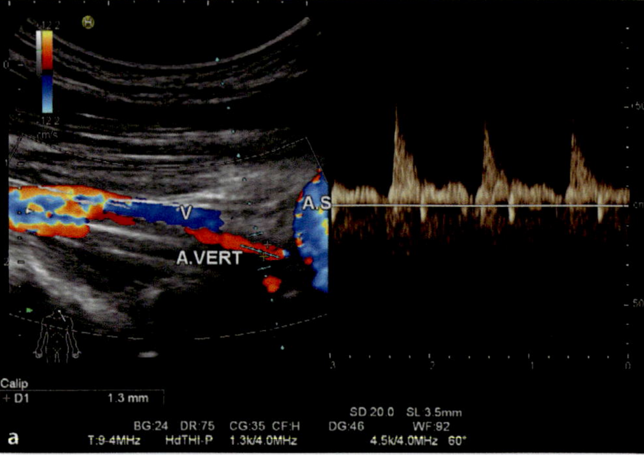

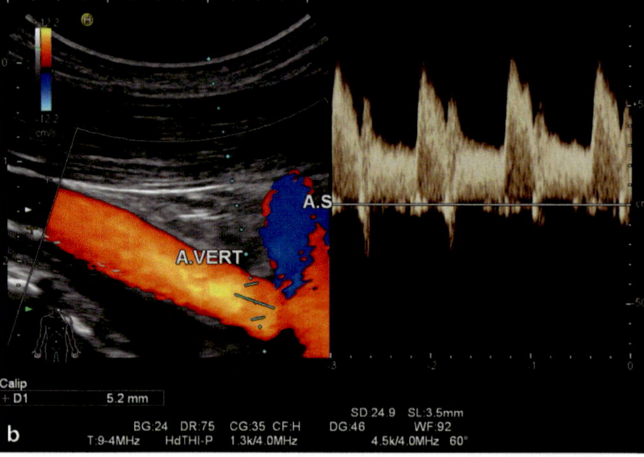

Fig. 5.40 **a** Severe hypoplasia of the vertebral artery (A.VERT) at its origin from the subclavian artery (A.S). The hypoplastic artery has a diameter of 1.3 mm with a peak systolic velocity (PSV) of 45 cm/s and relatively pulsatile flow in the waveform. The vertebral vein (V) is seen along the artery, and there is aliasing in the left half of the image. **b** The diameter of the contralateral vertebral artery shows a compensatory increase to 5.2 mm with a PSV of 80 cm/s

- Intrastenotic-to-prestenotic PSV ratio: not meaningful due to completely different hemodynamic situation in the subclavian artery.

In view of these difficulties, an **exception** is made here and the **intrastenotic-to-poststenotic PSV ratio** is accepted for stenosis grading (see nomogram in Fig. 1.48). High-grade stenosis is diagnosed when there is a marked increase in PSV (>160 cm/s; see Fig. 5.88 (Atlas)).

More distal vertebral artery stenosis (involving the prevertebral V1 segment or intertransverse V2 portion) is rare, and luminal narrowing of these segments is virtually always due to dissection or inflammatory vascular disease.

5.6.2.2 Occlusion

A vertebral artery can become occluded if it is affected by progressive atherosclerosis or atherosclerosis extending from the subclavian artery. These occlusions are limited to the prevertebral portion (V0 and V1 segments), and since collateralization via the spinal arteries and contralateral vertebral artery is good, they are typically detected incidentally and rarely cause brain stem infarction. Occlusion of the proximal vertebral artery is diagnosed by the absence of flow signals from these segments after scan parameters have been adjusted to slow flow. A Doppler waveform recorded distal to an occluded vertebral artery segment reflects the complex hemodynamic situation arising from variable collateralization but will typically show signs of abnormal flow (reduced or otherwise altered pulsatility) (see Fig. 5.90 (Atlas)). While contrast-enhanced ultrasound (CEUS) usually allows good differentiation of an occluded vertebral artery from a patent or refilled artery, differentiation from a very hypoplastic vertebral artery (which is notoriously difficult to identify) can pose a problem. This applies especially if the occlusion extends to the intertransverse portion (V2 and V3 segments); however, this portion will only be involved if occlusion is due to dissection. Intracranial occlusion downstream of the origins of the first intracranial branches leads to a markedly higher pulsatility in the upstream segment and slower diastolic blood flow. Higher pulsatility (or even to-and-fro flow) may point to basilar artery occlusion.

5.6.2.3 Dissection

Dissection of the vertebral artery may occur after trauma or spontaneously and affects the intertransverse portion (V2 segment). Even a very long dissection will typically spare the first few centimeters of the artery. CEUS can help in visualizing the true and false lumen. A diagnostic problem may arise if there is long dissection with thrombosis of the false lumen, which may be mistaken for a hypoplastic vertebral artery. In case of dissection, an eccentric tubular structure of low echogenicity, often taking a spiral-like course, is visualized along a long portion of the patent vertebral artery lumen (depiction of flow by color duplex). The differential diagnosis includes vasculitis, which is a rare condition causing circumferential arterial wall thickening.

5.6.2.4 Subclavian Steal Syndrome

The vertebral artery system is of special significance in the subclavian steal syndrome. Proximal stenosis or occlusion of the subclavian artery diverts blood away from the basilar territory when the ipsilateral arm is used. Clinically, the steal phenomenon is characterized by symptoms of intermittent brain stem and cerebellar ischemia including dizziness, ataxia, and drop attacks. Flow reversal in the ipsilateral vertebral artery is typically triggered by exercise but can also occur at rest. In this situation, blood is supplied to the affected arm by other cerebral arteries, in particular the contralateral vertebral artery.

The subclavian steal syndrome is diagnosed by the demonstration of reversed flow in the vertebral artery at rest or upon provoked hyperemia in the ipsilateral arm (see ◘ Figs. 5.91, 5.92, and 5.93 (all Atlas)).

The severity of the subclavian steal syndrome varies with the extent of the occlusive process in the subclavian artery and the role of the vertebral artery in collateral flow to the arm. The increasing significance of the ipsilateral vertebral artery as a collateral is reflected in the Doppler waveform, which shows changes ranging from increasing systolic deceleration, to to-and-fro flow with retrograde systolic flow and antegrade diastolic flow (incomplete steal), to complete retrograde flow (complete steal) (◘ Fig. 5.41).

In the most common situation, known as vertebrovertebral crossover, a steal effect chiefly occurs in the contralateral vertebral artery as the feeding vessel and chiefly manifests as an increase in diastolic flow in response to a provocative maneuver (◘ Figs. 5.42 and 5.93 (Atlas)). Other collateral pathways include the thyrocervical trunk, chest wall vessels, and cervical vessels supplying soft tissue. The better the collateral circulation, the less severe the steal effect in the ipsilateral vertebral artery and the less severe the patient's symptoms.

The **provocative test** for eliciting a **steal effect** in patients with less collateral flow through the vertebral artery is performed by applying an upper arm cuff inflated to over 200 mmHg for 3–5 min to induce ischemia in the ipsilateral arm. Subsequent deflation will lead to a postischemic increase in flow velocity in the arm arteries, resulting in an increase of the steal effect in the vertebral artery. This is reflected in the waveform by an increase in retrograde flow or even complete flow reversal despite a predominance of antegrade flow at rest.

Duplex ultrasound is the method of choice for evaluating patients with subclavian occlusion and symptoms of subclavian steal. It enables detailed evaluation of the steal effect in the vertebral artery and differentiation of the stages of

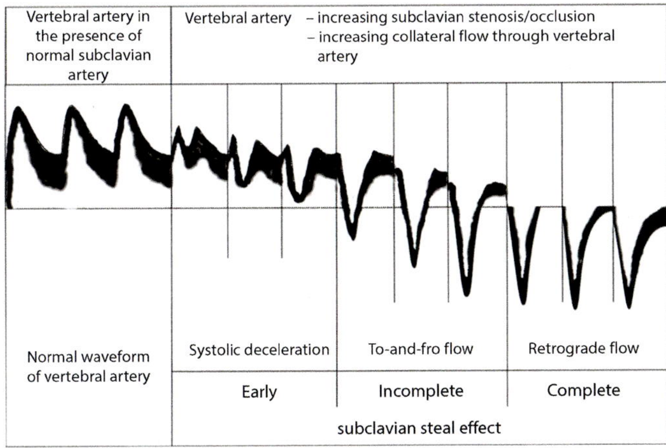

◘ **Fig. 5.41** Changes in the Doppler waveform from the ipsilateral vertebral artery in subclavian artery occlusion with subclavian steal. Depending on collateralization and the hemodynamic role of the vertebral artery as a collateral pathway, changes already occurring without provocative maneuvers may include systolic deceleration, to-and-fro flow, and retrograde flow (in patients with marked vertebrovertebral crossover). Provocation may elicit more severe changes in the postischemic phase, e.g., an increase in the retrograde flow component or transition from systolic deceleration to retrograde flow (see ◘ Figs. 5.91, 5.92, and 5.93 (Atlas))

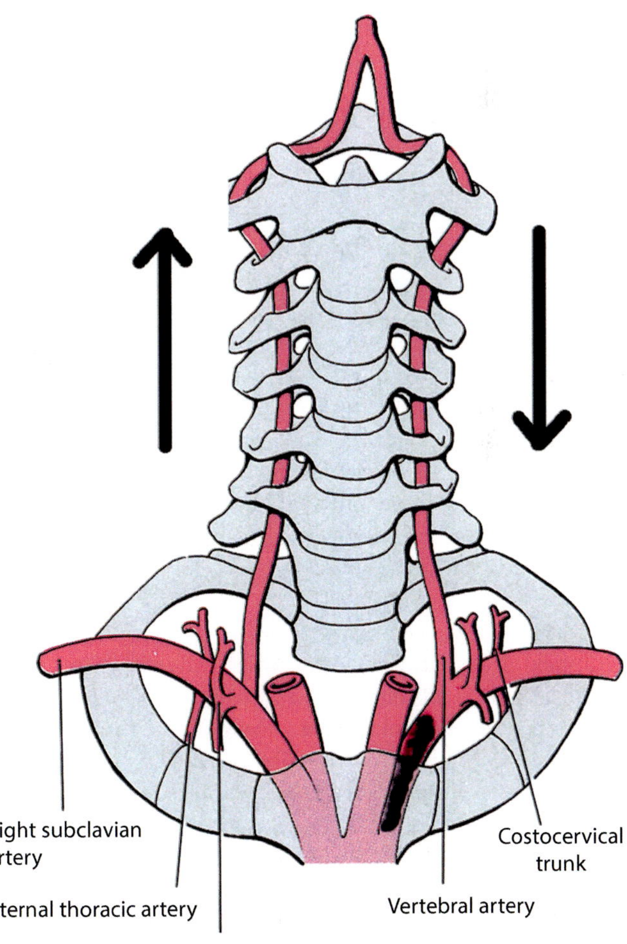

◘ **Fig. 5.42** Diagram of the course of the vertebral arteries and blood flow direction (arrows) in occlusion of the left subclavian artery (marked in black). Flow in the ipsilateral vertebral artery is reversed. Other collateral pathways are the internal thoracic artery, thyrocervical trunk, and costocervical trunk (Modified according to Heberer and van Dongen 1993)

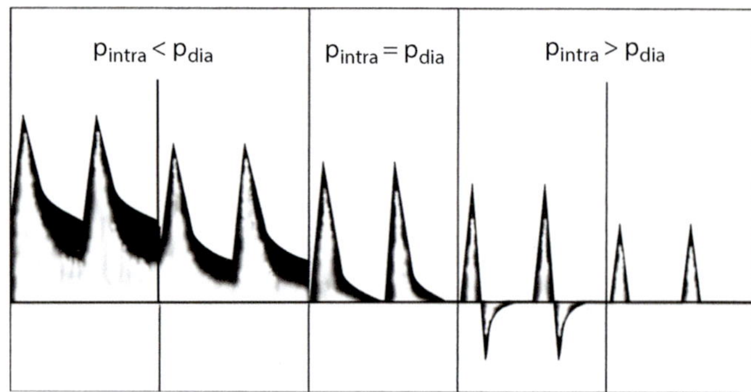

Fig. 5.43 Effects of increasing intracranial pressure on pulsatility in the extracranial cerebral arteries. The diagrams of the Doppler waveforms from left to right reflect the decreasing diastolic component (P_{dia} = diastolic blood pressure) with increasing intracranial pressure (P_{intra}) (According to Widder 1995)

incomplete steal. However, occlusion of the subclavian artery, just as of the carotid artery, may have no therapeutic relevance in patients without neurologic symptoms or clinical complaints.

5.7 Diagnosis of Brain Death

An elevated intracranial pressure associated with trauma, hemorrhage, or edema is reflected in signs of increased peripheral resistance in proximal arterial segments. In the Doppler waveform from the internal carotid artery (ICA), increasing intracranial pressure is indicated by a corresponding decrease in the diastolic flow component or even to-and-fro flow with a systolic forward and diastolic backward component (Figs. 5.43 and 5.95 (Atlas)). However, the correlation between intracranial pressure and the pulsatility index varies as it is affected by individual factors and autoregulatory processes as well as the underlying disease. Therefore, no reproducible absolute values of intracranial pressure can be derived from the Doppler waveform or the pulsatility index.

Nevertheless, interpretation of the **Doppler waveform** will yield information on relevant elevations of intracranial pressure. When intracranial pressure exceeds diastolic blood pressure, the diastolic flow component disappears or becomes retrograde (to-and-fro flow) (see Fig. 5.95 (Atlas)), suggesting cessation of cerebral blood flow (Hassler et al. 1991). Transcranial Doppler sonography has been an accepted diagnostic modality for shortening the waiting time for diagnosing cerebral circulatory arrest in Germany since the early 1990s. If, for technical reasons, the typical changes in the Doppler waveform cannot be demonstrated in the basal cerebral arteries, cerebral circulatory arrest can be diagnosed by using duplex sonography to demonstrate these changes in the flow profile (Fig. 5.43) of the extracranial ICA or in the vertebral arteries. In this situation, care must be taken to clearly identify the arteries supplying the brain and to differentiate them from other segments such as the ECA.

5.8 Rare (Nonatherosclerotic) Vascular Diseases of the Carotid Territory

5.8.1 Dissection

Arterial dissection is the spontaneous or traumatic separation of the arterial wall layers caused by blood surging in through a tear in the intima. Alternatively, blood leaking from the vasa vasorum can enter the vessel wall; in this case there is no communication with the lumen. The extravasated blood elevates the intima, resulting in the creation of a false lumen alongside the true arterial lumen. If blood dissects between the media and adventitia, the latter is elevated, giving rise to a pseudoaneurysm. A blind-ending false lumen becomes thrombosed and compresses the true lumen, causing high-grade stenosis or occlusion in severe cases. When there is a second tear at the distal end, the blood can re-enter the true lumen and flow through both lumina.

Dissection may cause various complications with manifestations ranging from headache to hemisymptoms. Seventy percent of patients with dissection of the internal carotid artery (ICA) have no or only mild neurologic deficits, while 25% present with severe neurologic symptoms. Spontaneous resolution is common when the false lumen becomes thrombosed and subsequent shrinkage of the thrombus causes the compression of the true lumen to recede.

There are three underlying **causes** of carotid dissection with different symptoms, treatments, and prognoses:

- Spontaneous dissection
- Traumatic dissection (blunt trauma or iatrogenic after puncture) (Fig. 5.75 (Atlas))
- Aortic dissection (Stanford type A) with subaortic extension (Fig. 5.73 (Atlas))

Common carotid artery (CCA) dissection resulting from aortic dissection begins in the proximal portion, from where it can progress into the carotid bifurcation. In patients with suspected CCA dissection, the artery is examined in the transverse plane, starting as far anteriorly as possible using a convex or curved array transducer. Spontaneous dissection of the CCA is very rare but may occur in patients with Marfan's syndrome (Harrer et al. 2006).

Traumatic and spontaneous **carotid dissection** typically affects the ICA including the portion near the skull base, which is why the ultrasound examination must focus on these segments.

Cerebral infarction due to dissection is primarily seen in adolescents, and dissection accounts for approx. 20% of strokes in younger patients. It is typically due to trauma and rarely occurs spontaneously, commonly affecting arterial segments prone to injury from bony structures such as the skull base (carotid arteries) or the transverse foramina (vertebral arteries). Following an acute phase with a relatively high risk of embolization and occlusion, dissection has a good prognosis due to spontaneous recanalization over time.

The location and superficial course of the carotid arteries allow good B-mode evaluation of the **sonomorphologic**

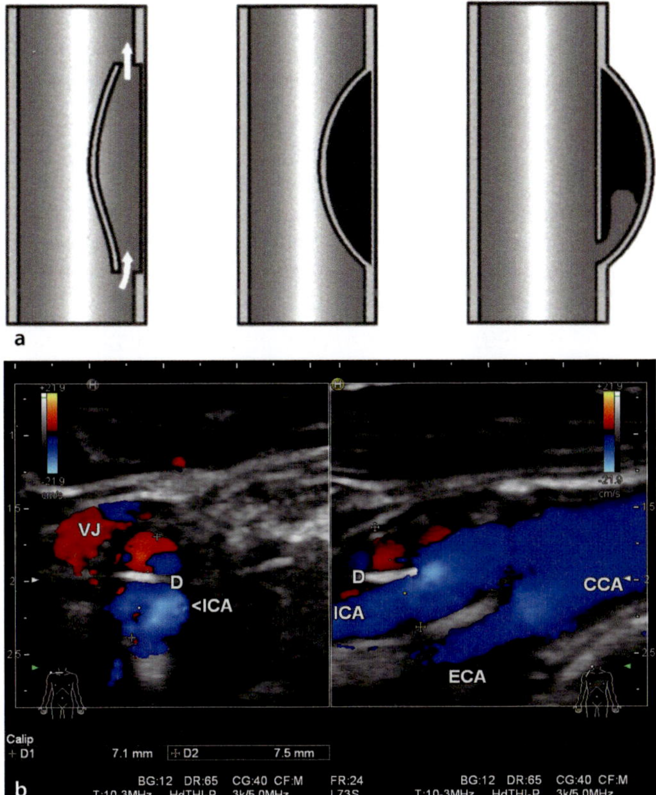

■ **Fig. 5.44** **a** Diagrams of the sonomorphologic findings in different forms of dissection. The first drawing shows intimal dissection with entry and re-entry. The second drawing illustrates the situation in internal dissection with narrowing of the true lumen due to thrombosis of the false lumen. The third drawing presents the situation in external dissection, which is characterized by intramural hemorrhage between the media and adventitia with spindle-shaped or saccular dilatation but with little or no compression of the true lumen; this may lead to the formation of a pseudoaneurysm. **b** Ultrasound findings in older posttraumatic dissection of the internal carotid artery (ICA) with a relatively hyperechoic dissection membrane (D) in transverse and longitudinal orientation. The dissection begins in the carotid bulb and extends 4 cm cranially (ECA = external carotic artery, CCA = common carotid artery). To-and-fro flow in the false lumen is common, especially when there is distal thrombosis in external dissection (see **a**)

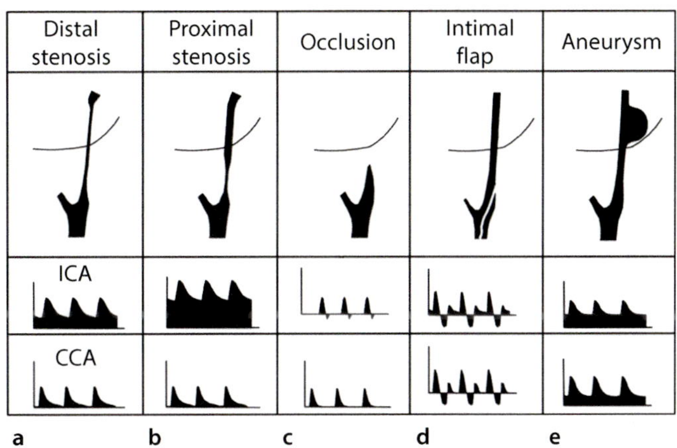

■ **Fig. 5.45** Diagrams of different flow profiles in dissection of the internal carotid artery (ICA). The waveform changes depend on the location and extent of dissection, presence of thrombosis, and sites of entry and re-entry (From Widder 1995). **a** Long ICA dissection with varying flow velocities due to caliber irregularities of the patent segment. **b** Short dissection with circumscribed flow acceleration at the site of luminal narrowing, which may be difficult to differentiate from atherosclerotic stenosis or fibromuscular dysplasia. **c** Dissection-induced occlusion of the ICA with thump pattern (to-and-fro sign) in the patent segment and externalization of the common carotid artery (CCA). **d** If the true and false dissection lumina are patent, flow profiles vary widely with the sites of entry and re-entry. The waveform from the true lumen depends on the degree of flow obstruction caused by the dissection. Fluttering of the intimal flap leads to a multiphasic waveform. **e** Distal formation of a pseudoaneurysm (typically beneath base of skull) cannot be detected by ultrasound because proximal flow is normal

features of carotid dissection with a high-resolution transducer (■ Fig. 5.44):

- An **intraluminal intimal flap** separating the true and false lumen; the flap can often be seen flapping back and forth with pulsation (see ■ Figs. 5.73 and 5.75 (both Atlas)).
- In **internal dissection** (intimal tear) with **thrombosis of the false lumen**, the thrombotic material will appear as a hypoechoic eccentric structure narrowing the true lumen over a variable length. The thrombosed false lumen typically has a somewhat higher echogenicity than the adjacent patent lumen (see ■ Fig. 5.74 (Atlas)).
- In **external dissection**, intramural hemorrhage with thrombosis will result in aneurysmal dilatation with low echogenicity of content and a visibly elevated adventitia.
- In patients with an **intimal tear**, the intima will be visualized as a flapping structure of higher echogenicity within the arterial lumen. In older dissection, the intimal flap may assume the appearance of a circumscribed wall deposit in an otherwise normal-appearing artery. Short dissection can be iatrogenic – the result of inadvertent injury to the opposite arterial wall with the needle during catheterization and may cause short stenosis due to a structure protruding into the lumen and difficult to distinguish from plaque-like deposits.

Spectral Doppler findings obtained in a patent false lumen are highly variable, depending on the individual constellation and the site of sampling relative to the entry and re-entry points. There may be to-and-fro flow or even retrograde flow. The flow signal from the true carotid artery lumen may be obscured by the more intense signal from the moving intimal flap.

Thrombosis of the false lumen is usually identified by a slightly higher echo level compared with the patent lumen. The Doppler waveform varies widely with the extent and type of dissection (see ■ Fig. 5.73 (Atlas)). In patients with dissection-induced occlusion distal to the ICA origin, a knocking waveform (thump pattern) is obtained, and there is externalization of the CCA. Dissection with luminal narrowing is characterized by a waveform with a higher Doppler shift frequency and an increased angle-corrected flow velocity in the residual lumen over a long stretch of the ICA. With only minimal luminal narrowing, the spectral Doppler tracing from the ICA and CCA appears fairly normal (■ Fig. 5.45).

Carotid dissection can be caused by blunt trauma to the neck or hyperextension of the cervical spine. Additionally, it may be iatrogenic, the result of puncture of a cervical vein, or secondary, the result of an aortic dissection extending into the CCA (type I according to De Bakey) (◘ Fig. 5.73 (Atlas)). Rarely, CCA dissection extends into the ICA with patency of long stretches of the true and false lumen. In this form there may be forward flow in both lumina or, depending on the site of re-entry, to-and-fro flow or retrograde flow in the false lumen (see ◘ Fig. 5.74 (Atlas)).

A study evaluating the usefulness of different **duplex criteria** in 23 patients with ICA dissection confirmed by MRI/MR angiography or conventional angiography revealed a detection rate of only 47.8% when morphologic criteria alone were used (intramural hematoma, double lumen). Additional use of hemodynamic criteria (hemodynamic evidence of distal stenosis or occlusion) increased the detection rate to 73.9%. Sonographic follow-up after 3–6 weeks established a correct diagnosis in 91.3% of cases (hemodynamic signs of distal stenosis or occlusion with signs of resolution). Using **both morphologic and hemodynamic criteria**, duplex ultrasound is highly sensitive in detecting dissection; however, in some cases a sonographic follow-up examination is necessary for a definitive diagnosis (Arning 2005).

Dissection causing high-grade stenosis of the patent lumen can be diagnosed with 96% sensitivity using ultrasound with determination of hemodynamic parameters (Benninger et al. 2006).

5.8.2 Vasculitis

Primary and secondary forms of vascular inflammation are distinguished. Secondary vasculitis is associated with autoimmune diseases (collagen disease, systemic rheumatic disease), infections, and malignancies. These typically affect smaller vessels, and therefore rarely involve the large arteries supplying the brain.

Three categories are distinguished according to the size of the vessels affected: small-cell vasculitis (Wegener's granulomatosis, Churg-Strauss syndrome, hypersensitivity vasculitis), which is not amenable to diagnosis by ultrasound; vasculitis of medium-sized vessels (Kawasaki's disease, polyarteritis nodosa – often with dilatative changes), which is amenable to diagnosis by ultrasound; and vasculitis of large vessels (giant cell arteritis with two subtypes: Takayasu's arteritis and Horton's disease/temporal arteritis).

Takayasu's arteritis, occasionally called pulseless disease, can affect the large arteries supplying the brain. It is a primary vasculitis and typically occurs before age 40. It is a giant cell arteritis, predominantly of the aorta and its major branches, with the common carotid artery (CCA) and the subclavian artery as the extracranial cerebral arteries most frequently affected. The mesenteric, renal, and iliac arteries may also be affected. As with all other forms of vasculitis, inflammatory thickening of the arterial wall (media) causes various degrees of luminal narrowing. The external carotid artery (ECA) can be involved in Takayasu's arteritis (with occlusion being quite common) but not the internal carotid artery (ICA). Involvement of the latter suggests Horton's disease.

Horton's disease of the extracranial cerebral arteries has a prevalence of 0.75% in individuals older than 50, and continues to become more prevalent with age. This form of giant cell arteritis also affects medium-sized and large arteries, predominantly the arteries of the abdomen and extremities as well as the supra-aortic arteries.

The **etiology** is unknown but an immunologic basis is likely. Takayasu's arteritis predominantly occurs in younger women, while Horton's giant cell arteritis is more common after age 60. General symptoms include weakness, headache, fever, and weight loss. These symptoms as well as unspecific signs of inflammation are present before vascular stenosis or occlusion occurs, and an ultrasound examination of the preferred sites of these conditions – the subclavian artery and the CCA – should be performed whenever either of these two diseases is suspected. If the suspicion is confirmed by sonography, cortisone therapy is initiated to prevent vascular complications. In patients with suspected Horton's arteritis, the ultrasound examination should include not only the subclavian and axillary arteries but also the temporal artery (which may be tender and firm on palpation).

5.8.2.1 Ultrasound Findings in Takayasu's Arteritis

The B-mode ultrasound appearance of Takayasu's arteritis is characterized by circumferential, homogeneous, and hypoechoic thickening of a long arterial wall segment, which primarily affects the media but may also extend to the intima (the so-called macaroni sign). In color duplex ultrasound, a hypoechoic halo is seen around the patent lumen. With progression, the thickening wall can cause stenosis, and even secondary thrombotic occlusion may occur. When repair of an occluded subclavian or common carotid artery is contemplated, it is pivotal to carefully differentiate thromboembolic from atherosclerotic occlusion and to establish whether occlusion is attributable to inflammatory wall thickening. The latter requires initial immunosuppressive treatment before any attempt at repair can be made.

Concentric wall thickening distinguishes vasculitis from dissection with thrombosis of the false lumen, which instead causes eccentric narrowing of the true lumen (see ◘ Fig. 5.76 (Atlas)). The appearance is also distinct from that of **atherosclerotic lesions**, which primarily involve the intima, exhibit focal variation, are more hyperechoic, and have irregular surfaces. While atherosclerosis can cause concentric luminal narrowing in patients with lipid metabolism disorders or diabetes mellitus, atherosclerotic lesions are primarily seen in the carotid bulb and the ICA. Conversely, Takayasu's arteritis affects the CCA and very rarely extends beyond the carotid bifurcation. Arteritis may also cause dilatation of the proximal aortic branches.

Ultrasonography allows early diagnosis of the disease (Taniguchi et al. 1997) and is the method of choice for

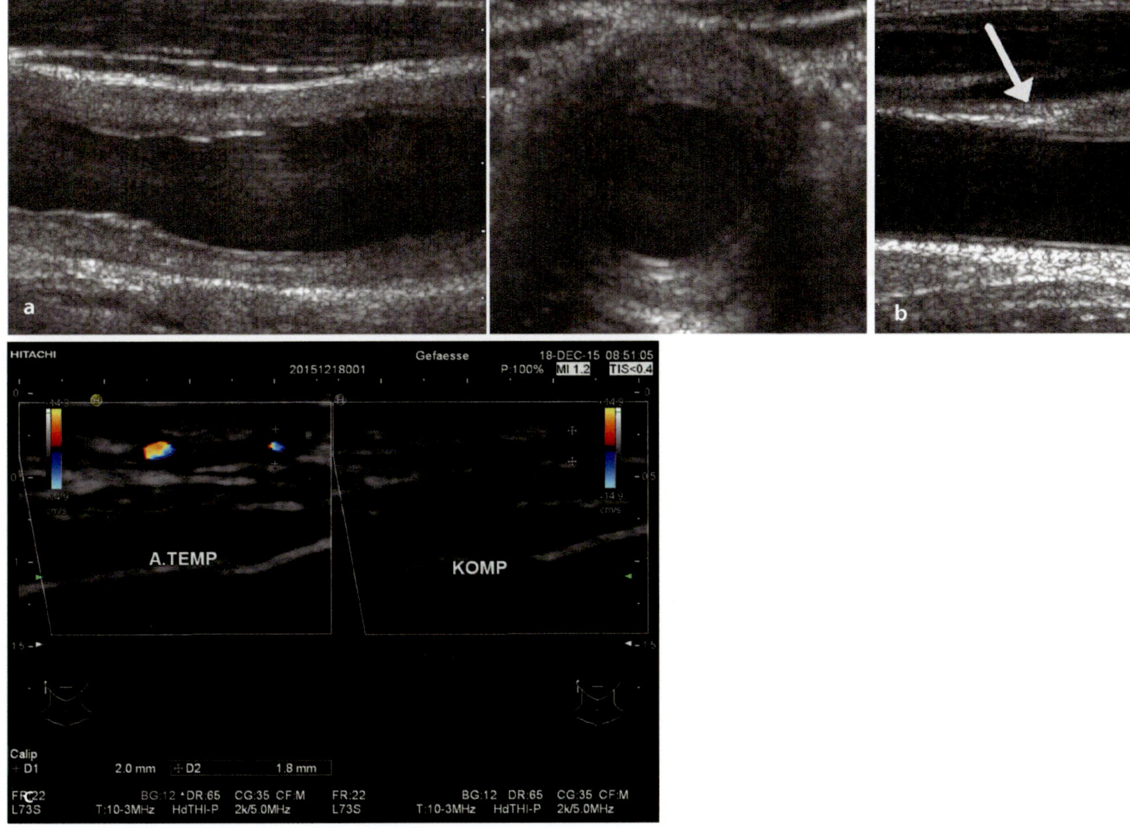

Fig. 5.46 **a** Longitudinal and transverse images of circumferential wall thickening in Takayasu's arteritis. The longitudinal view (left) nicely illustrates that hypoechoic inflammatory wall thickening predominantly involves the media. In this patient the innermost layer, or intima, is additionally thickened by atherosclerosis. **b** Inflammatory wall lesions in Takayasu's arteritis predominantly involve arterial segments close to the aorta, in particular the subclavian artery and the common carotid artery (CCA), while the internal carotid artery (ICA) is not involved. The image shows the transition from the thickened wall of the CCA to the carotid bifurcation, which is free of arteritis (arrow). In the left part of the image, the thickness of the artery wall is normal (Courtesy of K. Amendt). **c** Patient with arterial wall thickening due to arteritis of the posterior branch of the temporal artery (A.TEMP). The affected branch has a thin residual lumen, while the anterior branch appears normal without relevant wall thickening. The right image shows the situation during compression (KOMP): the thickened wall of the affected branch prevents compression, indicated by a lumen diameter of 1.8 mm while pressure is being applied with the transducer (versus 2.0 mm without compression). The unaffected anterior branch is fully compressible (no flow signals, no wall thickening)

follow-up (Park et al. 2001; Fukudome et al. 1998), especially for documenting the regression of inflammatory wall thickening in patients on immunosuppressive treatment. The Doppler waveform will show a continuously but only moderately increased flow velocity, depending on the degree of concentric narrowing. Ultrasound has a markedly higher accuracy than angiography, in particular in early disease. Severe inflammatory wall thickening can cause vascular occlusion (Fig. 5.46). Medical therapy with the administration of anti-inflammatory and immunosuppressive agents is the **treatment of choice**. Bypass surgery is discouraged, even in occlusion, as the patency rate is poor.

In Takayasu's arteritis (and other inflammatory vascular conditions such as Horton's disease), **contrast-enhanced ultrasound (CEUS)** allows good differentiation of the thickened media (hypoechoic, thickened intima-media complex) from the hyperechoic, patent lumen and from the adventitia and also allows evaluation of vasa vasorum proliferation. This information is useful for estimating inflammatory activity and monitoring the response to immunosuppressive treatment. A study of Takayasu's arteritis using CEUS demonstrated microbubble accumulation in the concentrically thickened carotid wall as a sign of neovascularization in acute disease and a strong decrease in enhancement during immunosuppressive treatment (Schinkel et al. 2014).

5.8.2.2 Ultrasound Findings in Horton's Disease

Although historically referred to as temporal arteritis, Horton's giant cell arteritis can also involve the extracranial cerebral arteries (like Takayasu's arteritis) as well as the subclavian and axillary arteries. Involvement of the ophthalmic artery is dreaded as it can lead to blindness. Horton's disease is an immunovasculitis of individuals beyond age 50. Thickening of the temporal artery, if involved, points to the diagnosis. Histologic workup of a segment of the diseased temporal artery was long considered the diagnostic gold standard. In the sonographic examination, the main branch of the superficial temporal artery is identified in transverse orientation at the level of the jaw and traced upward until it divides into frontal and parietal branches, which are also examined. Thickening of the temporal artery may be segmental rather than continuous, which is why the entire temporal artery must be imaged and evaluated in longitudinal and transverse planes in the B-mode (◘ Fig. 2.103d). Care must be taken to use a low PRF and sensitive receive gain. Temporal arteritis, like any form of vasculitis, causes circumferential wall thickening (halo or macaroni sign) with a wall thickness of 0.5–1.5 mm (Schmidt et al. 1997, 1993; Stammler et al. 2000). Blood flow velocity is decreased, and wall pulsation is absent or lower in the diseased temporal artery than on the contralateral side. These parameters have a high positive predictive value (Schmidt and Gromnica-Ihle 2002; Schmidt 2006), but normal findings in the temporal artery do not rule out Horton's disease as the temporal artery is involved in only approx. 60% of patients. The axillary artery is involved in approx. 50% of patients (Schmidt et al. 2008) and should be examined as well (see ◘ Figs. 2.46 and 2.49). Inflammatory wall thickening recedes under immunosuppressive treatment, which correlates with a drop in laboratory inflammatory parameters.

High-resolution ultrasound of the temporal artery (if involved) has 97% specificity (Schmidt and Blockmans 2005), and if the sonographic examination provides definitive evidence of vasculitis, treatment can be started without obtaining a biopsy (guidelines of the German Association of Scientific Medical Societies, AWMF guidelines). A biopsy is only required when ultrasound findings are inconclusive or normal but clinical signs suggest arteritis. A biopsy should be obtained from a sonographically suspicious wall segment to preclude false-negative results (as involvement is segmental). Since demonstration of flow in small vessels crucially relies on adequate instrument settings (gain, PRF), the diagnosis can be corroborated by testing for compressibility. The temporal artery can be compressed against the skull, and incompressibility of the residual lumen confirms inflammatory wall thickening (Aschwanden et al. 2013).

5.8.3 Fibromuscular Dysplasia

Fibromuscular dysplasia is a rare nonatheromatous and noninflammatory vascular disease of unknown etiology that typically involves the renal arteries (hypertension). It is a disease of medium-sized arteries and can therefore also affect the extracranial carotid territory, causing TIAs or even stroke. Approx. 30% of patients with fibromuscular dysplasia have intracranial aneurysm. In the vast majority of cases, steno-occlusive disease is due to hyperplasia of smooth muscle cells and must be differentiated from degenerative and inflammatory vascular conditions.

Fibromuscular dysplasia is characterized by multiple stenoses alternating with normal or dilated arterial segments, producing a beaded appearance on angiograms and **high-resolution ultrasound images** (the so-called string-of-beads sign). Color duplex or power Doppler imaging will detect flow in the residual lumen, allowing differentiation of the patent lumen from the dysplastic arterial wall. The sonomorphologic appearance allows differentiation from atherosclerotic lesions, aided by the fact that fibromuscular dysplasia typically occurs in young women without atherosclerotic lesions in other vascular territories.

The **duplex ultrasound appearance** is characterized by multiple stenoses, which may alternate with dilated segments. Depending on the severity of steno-occlusive lesions, direct and indirect signs of stenosis may be present. Carotid fibromuscular dysplasia is rarely diagnosed with duplex ultrasound as the first imaging test because the lesions causing the string-of-beads appearance usually spare the proximal 3–5 cm of the ICA. When fibromuscular dysplasia is suspected, the examiner must follow the ICA as far cranially as possible using a curved array transducer and lowering both the transmit frequency and the pulse repetition frequency toward the skull base. In general, ultrasound can only detect advanced disease with hemodynamically relevant stenosis located not too far cranially. Ultrasound studies report a prevalence of 0.05–0.14% (Labropoulos et al. 2007; Arning 2004) compared with 0.61% in a catheter angiography study (Sandok 1983).

5.8.4 Aneurysm

Aneurysm of the ICA is rare and may occur secondary to atherosclerotic or inflammatory vascular disease (◘ Figs. 5.70, 5.71, and 5.72 (Atlas)).

A **true aneurysm** is an aneurysm involving all three arterial wall layers and can be congenital, typically in patients with connective tissue disease, or it can be acquired. Mycotic or inflammatory aneurysm is caused by a localized infection of the arterial wall in the setting of inflammatory conditions of the head or neck region or in individuals in whom hematogenous spread has occurred, for example, in endocarditis. True aneurysms of the carotid territory must be distinguished from pseudoaneurysms, which typically develop after surgery or trauma.

True aneurysms of the extracranial cerebral arteries are very rare with reported rates of 0.4% (Painter et al. 1985) to 5.5% (Liapis et al. 1994). They are accounted for by atherosclerosis in 32% of cases, thrombosis in 17%, and dissection in 37% (Moreau et al. 1994). Before the era of antibiotic treatment, most true aneurysms were mycotic aneurysms developing secondary to tuberculosis and syphilis (Konstantinidis et al. 1998). Only 5% of mycotic aneurysms were reported to involve the extracranial carotid arteries (Brown et al. 1995). Mycotic aneurysms have become very rare and are usually caused by staphylococci or streptococci, or less commonly by salmonella infections.

An aneurysm of the extracranial cerebral arteries becomes apparent as a pulsating neck mass. B-mode ultrasound depicts the focal dilatation of the artery (saccular or spindle-shaped), and color duplex imaging allows evaluation of the patent lumen and demonstration of thrombotic deposits.

The definition of aneurysm that applies to the extracranial carotid and vertebral arteries (abrupt doubling of the lumen diameter) cannot readily be applied to the wider carotid bulb. Here, normal diameter variation must be differentiated from true aneurysmal dilatation, which is usually assumed when the external diameter reaches 14–15 mm. Clinically, however, it is more relevant to identify thrombotic deposits in saccular, dilated arterial segments, which can give rise to embolism and cause cerebral infarction.

A spontaneous stroke rate of up to 50% has been reported for untreated carotid aneurysm (Valentine 2003), suggesting that even smaller aneurysms should be operated on. Other complications may result from local compression of adjacent structures such as the internal jugular vein, the trachea, the esophagus on the left side, and occasionally of a cerebral nerve (Numenthaler 1986). Rupture of carotid aneurysm is rare.

Color duplex ultrasound (or MR angiography) is the method of choice, enabling precise evaluation of the diameter and extent of the aneurysm as well as differentiation of thrombotic deposits (which is not possible with angiography) (see ◘ Fig. 5.72 (Atlas)).

Suture aneurysm is a pseudoaneurysm that may be noted as a pulsatile mass of the neck or may be detected at sonographic follow-up after carotid endarterectomy. Color duplex ultrasound differentiates flow within the aneurysm from thrombotic material, and the characteristic "steam engine sound", caused by a high-frequency systolic signal and retrograde flow throughout diastole, can be heard in the aneurysm neck when Doppler interrogation is performed (see ◘ Fig. 5.71 (Atlas)). The indication for surgical revision can be established without preoperative angiography.

5.8.5 Arteriovenous Fistula

An arteriovenous (AV) fistula is usually a sequela of trauma or iatrogenic manipulation (puncture, central venous catheter) and is conspicuous as a mosaic of colors due to perivascular tissue vibration. Spectral Doppler interrogation will not always demonstrate the fistula directly, which is why the diagnosis relies on the demonstration of high flow velocity in the feeding artery, especially during diastole, and arterialized flow in the vein. The Doppler waveform obtained within the fistula depends on the flow volume but resembles the pattern in a stenosis with high systolic and diastolic flow velocities. AV fistulas in the carotid system primarily involve the common carotid artery (CCA) and the internal jugular vein because they lie close together. The fistula flow volume can be estimated by calculating the flow volume on the ipsilateral side by multiplying the mean flow velocity with the cross-sectional area of the CCA proximal to the fistula and then subtracting the CCA flow volume of the contralateral side.

When a dural AV fistula is suspected (typically presenting with pulse-synchronous tinnitus), sonographic evaluation of the occipital artery in the retroauricular area directly in front of the mastoid can confirm the fistula by demonstration of a characteristic high-frequency signal. A fistula with a large blood flow volume is identified by a unilateral increase in flow velocity in the ECA (and CCA). The increase in PSV is apparent in a long ECA segment, distinguishing fistula from stenosis (short focal PSV increase).

5.8.6 Idiopathic Carotidynia

Idiopathic carotidynia was first mentioned in 1927 and has been recognized as a distinct clinical entity by the International Headache Society (IHS) since 1988. It is a neck pain syndrome presenting with severe unilateral pain of the upper neck region and responding well to treatment with nonsteroidal anti-inflammatory drugs. Ultrasound demonstrates echolucent, often eccentric thickening of the vessel wall, usually causing only moderate luminal narrowing (◘ Fig. 5.47) because the main part of the thickening extends outward. While the findings resemble the appearance in dissection or vasculitis, carotidynia differs from dissection (with thrombosed false lumen) in that it involves the bifurcation with the distal CCA and proximal ICA and presents with local pain, while dissection tends to involve more cranial segments of the ICA and causes headache. Magnetic resonance imaging (MRI) was reported to show no evidence of intramural hematoma but enhancement after administration of contrast medium, suggesting an inflammatory wall lesion

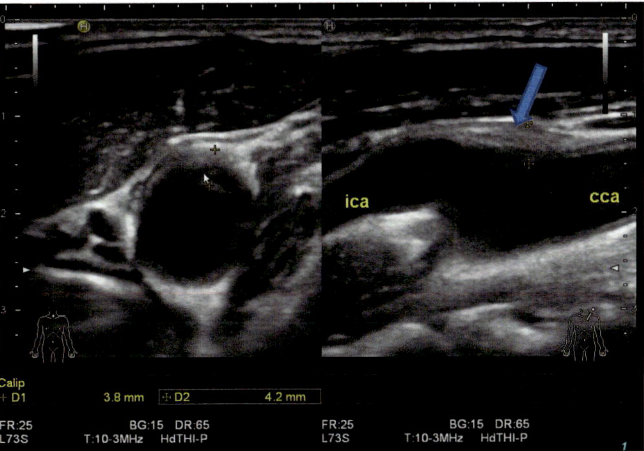

◘ **Fig. 5.47** Idiopathic carotidynia with wall thickening at the origin of the internal carotid artery (ICA). Thickening primarily involves the outer wall layer (two-layered appearance of the arterial wall)

(Burton et al. 2000; Arning 2004). As the thickened wall does not constrict the lumen, no hemodynamic signs of stenosis can be detected. Carotidynia is an example of a well-established clinical entity that required the advent of state-of-the-art imaging to identify underlying morphologic changes (high-resolution ultrasound and MRI). The symptoms resolve spontaneously with follow-up imaging after 4 weeks demonstrating a return to almost normal wall thickness.

5

5.8.7 Vasospasm

Vasospasms can be induced by mechanical manipulation or medications taken to treat vasculitis, or they can occur during episodes of migraine. They can cause cerebral or ocular ischemia, but the stenosis caused by spasm is usually of such short duration that only a few reports describe it being visualized by ultrasound (Janzarik et al. 2007; Mosso et al. 2007). It is assumed that most instances of vasospasms go undetected. Treatment is with calcium antagonists. Color duplex imaging will show a narrow lumen with stenotic flow, returning to normal within hours. No morphologic wall changes are apparent; recurrent vasospasms usually affect the same arterial segment.

5.8.8 Compression by Tumor, Carotid Body Tumor

Compression of a carotid segment by cervical tumors or lymph node metastases is rare and more commonly affects the internal jugular vein. Carotid body tumors are highly vascularized masses located at the carotid bifurcation, where they cause the typical saddle deformity (splaying of the internal and external carotid branches by the tumor mass) on ultrasound. In the color duplex mode, multiple small tumor vessels are demonstrated.

The tumor arises from the 3–4 mm carotid body, a structure in the bifurcation that functions as a chemoreceptor and regulates PO_2, PCO_2, and the pH value. Carotid body tumors are primarily supplied with blood from external carotid branches and rarely also from the thyrocervical trunk. They are assumed to develop from paraganglial tissue, probably a residue of the neural crest. Hence, there may be multiple tumors and rarely also parajugular or paravagal tumors as well as tumors at the aortic arch.

Histologically, adenomatous and angiomatous subtypes can be distinguished. The latter is very highly vascularized with an impressive appearance on color duplex imaging. Tumor growth in the area of the carotid bifurcation can encase or compress the arteries (◘ Fig. 5.48). Color duplex evaluation of the localization and vascularization of the tumor contributes to the preoperative differentiation, and the information on tumor extension facilitates radical surgical removal.

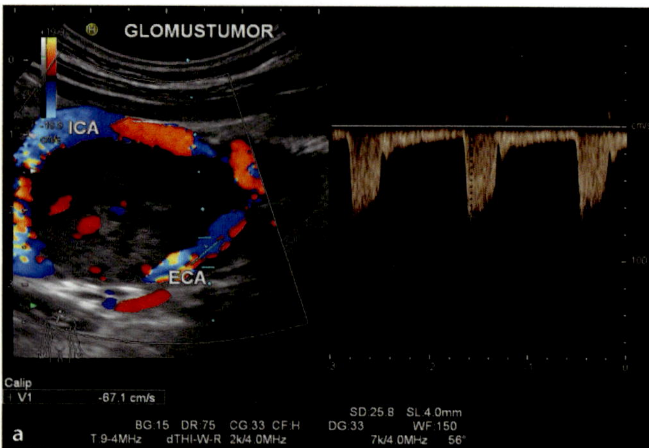

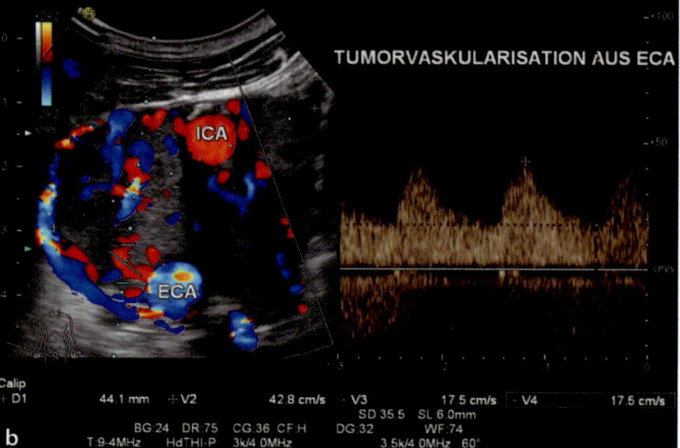

◘ Fig. 5.48 **a** Longitudinal view of a carotid body tumor in the bifurcation splaying the internal carotid artery (ICA) and external carotid artery (ECA) in a 57-year-old patient. The tumor receives its blood supply from ECA branches; tumor vascularization is relatively low. The sample volume is placed in the ECA. **b** 64-year-old patient with a palpable, pulsatile neck mass on the right side. The transverse color duplex image shows a highly vascularized carotid body tumor measuring 4–5 cm and encasing segments of the ICA and ECA. The Doppler waveform from a tumor-feeding artery arising from the ECA shows a very large diastolic flow component

Color duplex imaging is also the method of choice for monitoring the outcome of tumor embolization in elderly or multimorbid patients (◘ Fig. 5.95 (Atlas)) in whom surgical resection should be avoided. Serial ultrasound allows evaluation of tumor growth and tumor vascularization.

5.9 Diagnostic Role of Duplex Ultrasound in Evaluating the Extracranial Cerebral Arteries

As a noninvasive diagnostic test, duplex ultrasound is the method of choice for confirming or ruling out suspected steno-occlusive lesions of the carotid system. In the stepwise diagnostic workup, it follows after the patient's history has been obtained and a physical examination performed. The

Table 5.16 Role of duplex ultrasound in carotid artery surgery and stenting

Decision to be made	Duplex criteria
Indication for surgery	Degree of stenosis Plaque morphology Nonatherosclerotic vascular narrowing/disease Tandem stenosis
Timing of operation	Early surgery, risk of occlusion/reischemia
Type of surgery/anesthesia	Kinking: shortening of ICA Site of plaque/plaque length: general versus local anesthesia Plaque morphology: surgery versus stenting (CEA – CAS)
Technical success	Degree of residual/recurrent stenosis following surgery/stenting Complications of surgery
Outcome	Recurrent stenosis, follow-up

CAS carotid artery stenting, *CEA* carotid endarterectomy, *ICA* internal carotid artery

formerly widely used CW Doppler technique is less expensive, easy to perform, and has an accuracy of over 90% in detecting therapeutically relevant higher-grade carotid stenosis (Keller et al. 1988; Neuerburg-Heusler 1984). It is a suitable screening modality for patients with a reasonable suspicion of carotid stenosis if abnormal findings are subsequently verified by duplex imaging. However, anatomic anomalies and sudden changes in the angle of insonation due to kinking or coiling of the carotid artery may give rise to false-positive findings, and low-grade stenosis escapes detection by CW Doppler.

Duplex ultrasonography is **noninvasive** and has a sensitivity and specificity of over 90% in quantifying internal carotid artery (ICA) stenosis, making it the **diagnostic test of choice** (Table 5.16). This is all the more so since angiography, the traditional gold standard, has its limitations as well. Its accuracy, determined by comparing the image interpretations performed by two independent radiologists, is 88–93%, which is similar to the comparison of duplex ultrasound and angiography. This agreement is surprising since duplex ultrasound is based on hemodynamic evaluation while angiography is a morphologic method. Angiography is limited by the fact that 3D plaques protruding into the vessel lumen are reduced to the two film dimensions, which impairs the reliability of stenosis measurement – despite mandatory assessment in two or three planes.

Duplex sonography is also the method of choice in all patients with nonatherosclerotic vascular conditions (inflammatory disease, dissection, aneurysm) because B-mode scanning depicts not only the luminal narrowing but wall changes and perivascular structures as well.

The complications of angiography include a stroke rate of 1–3% (Waugh and Sacharias 1992), which is almost as high as the rate of complications experienced centers achieve with surgical management by carotid endarterectomy (CEA). For this reason, the indication for CEA is increasingly based on duplex ultrasound alone. In addition to the preoperative localization and quantification of carotid stenosis, sonography is also preferred for follow-up after CEA or carotid artery stenting (CAS).

In patients with high-grade internal carotid artery (ICA) stenosis (70% ECST stenosis/50% NASCET stenosis; see Fig. 5.9b and Table 5.9), the stenosis degree alone establishes the indication for surgery and, if the sonographic examination allows confident grading, no further stenosis quantification or B-mode evaluation of plaque morphology is necessary. Sonomorphologic evaluation of plaque vulnerability only has a role in stage II disease and moderate stenosis of 60–70% or in stage I disease with high-grade stenosis, where a decision needs to be made between best medical treatment and surgery.

Many studies have been performed to investigate sonographic properties of plaques (e.g., echogenicity, surface, and contour) and to identify features that might allow prediction of the risk of embolism, but no consistent picture has emerged, and results are even contradictory. Furthermore, published data are not easily comparable because investigators use different study designs, descriptive criteria, and classification systems. Nevertheless, a few general conclusions regarding plaque morphology and echogenicity appear to be generally accepted. For one, the risk of stroke increases with plaque thickness, which is why the same degree of stenosis is associated with a greater risk of embolism when caused by an eccentric plaque than when caused by a concentric plaque. This is because an eccentric plaque protruding into the blood stream is more susceptible to rupture of its cap. Such a plaque is often identified by characteristic longitudinal pulsation in the direction of blood flow in real-time B-mode ultrasound. An irregular surface seen on B-mode scans suggests atheromatous rather than fibrous plaque. Plaque with high lipid content is assumed to be echolucent and has an up to four times higher risk of embolism. In evaluating plaque echogenicity, however, the examiner must always bear in mind the **inherent technical limitations** of ultrasound resulting from the fact that a sonographic B-mode image is generated from echoes reflected off boundaries between tissues of different acoustic impedance. This means that low echogenicity merely indicates that a tissue is homogeneous but allows no conclusions to be drawn regarding other tissue properties such as elasticity. Moreover, evaluation of echogenicity is subjective and also depends on the equipment and settings used. To overcome these limitations, a standardized measure of plaque echogenicity, the gray-scale median (GSM), has been proposed. While this standardized analysis shows good interobserver correlation, agreement between sonomorphologic plaque classification and histopathologic examination of eversion CEA specimens is poor. Again, no consistent picture emerges from scientific studies with some authors describing high correlation between histopathologic results and sonomorphologic appearance and others reporting poor or no correlation (Ratiff et al. 1985; Droste et al. 1997; Biasi et al. 1999; Widder et al. 1990; Schulte-Altedorneburg et al. 2000; Denzel et al. 2003; Gonçalves et al. 2004).

Despite these limitations, **sonographic plaque analysis** can contribute additional information for **estimating the risk of stroke**. Rapidly progressive stenosis is four times more likely to cause TIAs and cerebral infarction than less progressive stenosis of a similar degree (Widder et al. 1992). Heterogeneous, mostly echolucent plaque is more likely to progress. Moreover, one also has to be aware that similar plaques may develop differently. Plaques considered harmless on the basis of their sonomorphologic and macroscopic appearance may rapidly turn into vulnerable, high-risk plaques, when intralesional hemorrhage occurs, for instance.

Overall, though, caution must be exercised in predicting the risk of embolism from the sonomorphologic appearance of plaque.

Neovascularization of plaques has received increasing attention as a major culprit in plaque vulnerability. **Contrast-enhanced ultrasound (CEUS)** allows semiquantitative assessment of plaque neovascularization, which is why it has a growing role in identifying plaques with an increased risk of embolism. Moreover, CEUS allows very good delineation of the plaque contour and plaque surface.

Initial CW Doppler imaging, as it used to be advocated by some investigators, is no longer necessary since a color duplex examination performed with adequate instrument settings enables continuous hemodynamic evaluation. Supplementary transcranial ultrasonography, on the other hand, provides useful additional information on intracranial arterial anomalies and stenosis.

Duplex or color duplex ultrasound is highly reliable in evaluating the carotid bifurcation, the preferred site of carotid stenosis. Angiography does not yield any additional information in this area. The hemodynamic assessment by duplex ultrasound is superior in grading ICA stenosis compared with angiography, which merely depicts the perfused lumen in relation to the adjacent vessel segment. Only ultrasound provides information on plaque morphology (see ▶ Sect. 5.6.1.1 and ◘ Fig. 5.27). In the NASCET study, there was poor agreement between angiography and intraoperative findings with regard to the evaluation of plaque surface properties such as ulceration.

Angiography has the advantage of providing a good overview of the target vascular anatomy and allows better documentation of the findings. Another advantage of angiography is the detection of **stenosis near the aortic arch and the base of the skull as well as intracranially**. If the sonographic findings in these carotid segments are inconclusive, angiography should be performed.

If no angiography is performed prior to CEA, the ultrasound examination must be performed with great care, especially with regard to establishing the identity of the ICA and ECA. High gain is required to differentiate between subtotal and total occlusion. In particular if the examination is impaired by calcified plaques, the examiner must attempt to depict flow signals in the artery up to the base of the skull. However, a control angiography should be done in such cases and also if stenosis grading is impaired by heavy calcification.

Angiography or intra-arterial digital subtraction angiography (DSA) is indicated only in those cases where the sonographic examination is inconclusive or the examination of the extracranial cerebral arteries reveals indirect evidence of intracranial vascular pathology. Alternatively, a transcranial duplex examination can be performed.

In addition to angiography and color duplex ultrasound, the extracranial and intracranial cerebral arteries can be examined by **CT angiography** or **MR angiography**. Unlike conventional angiography, which is a 2D projection technique, CT and MR angiography yield 3D datasets of blood flow in a specific body region, which can then be reconstructed in multiple planes for vascular evaluation.

A helical CT angiogram depicts the target vessels in relation to surrounding structures and is obtained after injection of iodine-based X-ray contrast medium. Arterial evaluation may be limited by adjacent structures of similar attenuation or bones and by premature opacification of veins. Bones may degrade the visualization of the carotid siphon, while superimposed veins and calcified plaques may limit adequate arterial evaluation in the area of the carotid bifurcation. Time-consuming image postprocessing is required to ensure adequate evaluation in these cases. Overall, CT angiography tends to underestimate the degree of ICA stenosis (Clevert et al. 2005; Patel et al. 2002; Zhang et al. 2005). CT angiograms have high spatial resolution and are highly sensitive in detecting small flow volumes and slow flow, for example, distal to subtotal occlusion, but provide little information on blood flow direction or other hemodynamic parameters.

As with CT angiography, MRI also allows 3D reconstruction for the depiction of target vessels in relation to surrounding structures. Nearby bones do not limit evaluation and a contrast agent is not generally required but will markedly improve image quality and depiction of vessels with slow-flowing blood.

The **signal intensity of blood on MR images** is determined by various factors including the MR pulse sequence or slice thickness used, the course of the vessel relative to the imaging plane, and blood flow velocity and flow profile. The depiction of flowing blood by MRI is complex. Two basic phenomena are time-of-flight and phase-contrast effects, which are exploited by different MR techniques to highlight arteries and/or veins. Time-of-flight MR angiography can be manipulated to selectively image either the arteries or veins. To selectively highlight the arteries, the venous signal is suppressed. This is accomplished by application of a saturation band to flip longitudinal magnetization into the transverse plane, thereby suppressing venous enhancement in the imaging volume that would result from the inflow effect. The phase-contrast technique obtains information on the vascular system from deliberately induced flow-related phase shifts. These phase shifts depend on the speed of flowing protons and can be measured to calculate blood flow velocity. In-flow and phase-contrast MR angiography only use flow effects for vascular imaging. Contrast-agent-based MR techniques exploit the selective shortening of the T1 relaxation time of flowing blood (from 1200 to 50 ms) during intravascular passage of the contrast agent to generate image contrast between vessels and stationary tissues. The use of special phased-array coils markedly improves the signal-to-noise ratio while at the same time shortening image acquisition time and increasing spatial resolution, thereby improving the differentiation of peripheral arteries and veins.

MR angiography differs from CT angiography in that blood flow itself rather than the contrast-enhanced blood is visualized in the image, and arteries and veins are differentiated using different pulse sequences and imaging techniques. Vessels are most accurately depicted on MR angiograms when blood flow is laminar. Vortexing and turbulent flow in a stenotic segment may impair quantitative assessment and lead to overestimation of the degree of stenosis, especially when the time-of-flight technique is used (Clevert et al. 2006; Patel et al. 2002, 1995). These flow phenomena may also lead to misinterpretation in bifurcations and at the origins of branches. Use of a contrast agent is necessary to visualize very slow flow. The combination of conventional MRI with MR angiography is an ideal imaging tool for a comprehensive evaluation of intracranial perfusion and parenchymal changes, providing diagnostic information to supplement color duplex ultrasound (extracranial cerebral arteries and stenosis quantification in the carotid bifurcation) in patients considered for CEA.

With the methodological limitations outlined above, CT angiography is most beneficial in evaluating the anterior and posterior arteries near the base of the skull as well as the origins of arteries arising from the aortic arch. MR angiography, on the other hand, enables good evaluation of the entire intracranial arterial territory including the carotid siphon. **Color duplex imaging**, however, performed with a high-frequency transducer remains the most suitable imaging tool for assessing the extracranial arteries supplying the brain, including the detection of pathology and stenosis grading. This is suggested by studies comparing different imaging modalities with the traditional gold standard (i.e., angiography performed in two or three planes).

Several studies show that the gold standard, DSA, underestimates ICA stenosis compared with histology (Pan et al. 1995; Schenk et al. 1988; Alexandrov et al. 1993), while a more recent in vitro study reports significant overestimation for higher-grade stenosis ($p = 0.0007$) (Smith et al. 2012). The authors conclude that the accuracy of DSA is affected by plaque configuration (mountain-shaped lesions, irregular surface). Another source of error is the contrast medium concentration, which determines plaque conspicuity. The same study shows that CT angiography and, surprisingly, MR angiophy also underestimate stenosis severity.

With 92% sensitivity and 74% specificity, contrast-enhanced MR angiography is less accurate in identifying stenosis requiring surgical management than duplex ultrasound, and it is also inferior in stenosis grading. The two modalities are supplementary, with duplex ultrasound enabling adequate evaluation of the extracranial carotid system and MR angiography providing information on the intracranial vessels as well as on the supra-aortic origins of arterial branches. Together, the two modalities enable comprehensive diagnostic evaluation prior to surgical repair of ICA stenosis.

The indication for surgical management or PTA in patients with subclavian steal syndrome due to subclavian artery obstruction can be established if the clinical suspicion is confirmed by duplex imaging, but only angiography will enable exact identification of collateral pathways.

If initial management of ICA stenosis is conservative (e.g., antiplatelet or statin treatment), follow-up ultrasonography should focus on identifying changes in plaque morphology and progression of stenosis. Rapid progression of stenosis and changes in plaque morphology are two important criteria for switching to surgery. In patients treated by CEA, a follow-up ultrasound examination is performed immediately after surgery and then at 6-month to 1-year intervals, depending on the findings. A focus of follow-up is on identification of recurrent stenosis and complications such as suture aneurysm.

5.10 Atlas: Extracranial Cerebral Arteries

◘ Table 5.17 lists the figures presented in the Atlas. The figures illustrate normal findings, methodology, and vascular diseases of the extracranial cerebral arteries.

◘ **Table 5.17** Extracranial cerebral arteries – figures

Entity/Pathology	Figure
Carotid bifurcation – ICA/ECA differentiation	◘ Fig. 5.49 (Atlas), page 358
ECA stenosis	◘ Fig. 5.49 (Atlas), page 358
PSV dependence on systemic factors – blood pressure	◘ Fig. 5.50 (Atlas), page 358
Kinking without/with stenosis	◘ Fig. 5.51 (Atlas), page 359
Coiling	◘ Fig. 5.51 (Atlas), page 359
Measurement of intima-media thickness (IMT)	◘ Fig. 5.52 (Atlas), page 360
Measurement of intima-media thickness (IMT) – plaque	◘ Fig. 5.52 (Atlas), page 360
Stenosis with beginning hemodynamic effects	◘ Fig. 5.53 (Atlas), page 361
Moderate ICA origin stenosis	◘ Fig. 5.54 (Atlas), page 361
Distal ICA stenosis	◘ Fig. 5.55 (Atlas), page 362
High-grade ICA origin stenosis	◘ Fig. 5.56 (Atlas), page 362
Evaluation of plaque morphology	◘ Fig. 5.57 (Atlas), page 363, 364
Plaque morphology – surface structure	◘ Fig. 5.58 (Atlas), page 364
Plaque morphology – long concentric carotid stenosis (smooth, regular surface)	◘ Fig. 5.59 (Atlas), page 365
Plaque morphology – high-grade stenosis with ulceration	◘ Fig. 5.60 (Atlas), page 366
ICA occlusion	◘ Fig. 5.61 (Atlas), page 367
Signs of recanalization in ICA occlusion	◘ Fig. 5.62 (Atlas), page 367
CCA occlusion – collaterals	◘ Fig. 5.63 (Atlas), page 368
Complete extracranial carotid territory occlusion	◘ Fig. 5.64 (Atlas), page 369
PPHA as collateral in ICA occlusion	◘ Fig. 5.64 (Atlas), page 369
Occlusion of the brachiocephalic trunk – collateral pathways	◘ Fig. 5.65 (Atlas), page 370
CCA stenosis	◘ Fig. 5.66 (Atlas), page 370
High-grade stenosis of the brachiocephalic trunk	◘ Fig. 5.67 (Atlas), page 371
ICA occlusion – compensatory flow increase in collateral pathways	◘ Fig. 5.68 (Atlas), page 371
Pitfall of PSV-based ICA stenosis grading in contralateral ICA occlusion	◘ Fig. 5.69 (Atlas), page 371
Suture aneurysm	◘ Fig. 5.70 (Atlas), page 372
Complications after carotid endarterectomy – suture aneurysm	◘ Fig. 5.71 (Atlas), page 372
True ICA aneurysm	◘ Fig. 5.72 (Atlas), page 373
Mycotic ICA aneurysm	◘ Fig. 5.72 (Atlas), page 373
Dissection of CCA	◘ Fig. 5.73 (Atlas), page 374

Table 5.17 (continued)

5

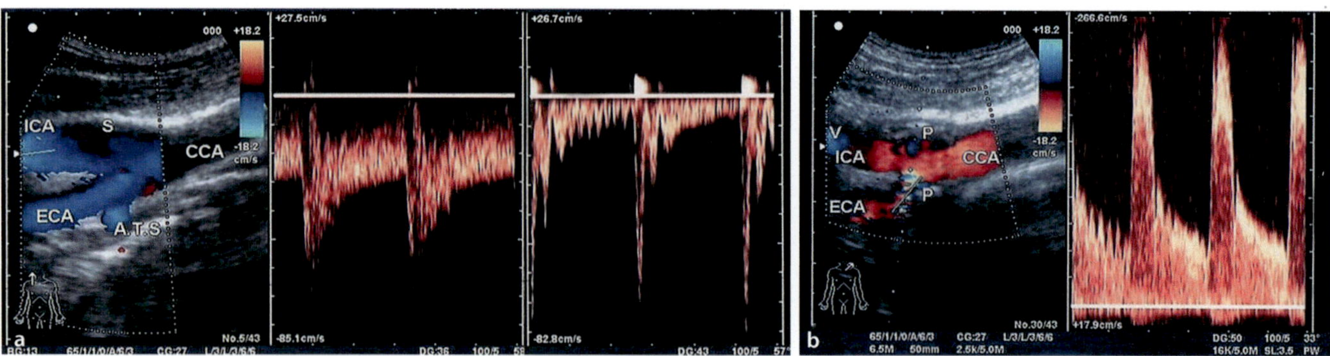

Fig. 5.49a, b (Atlas) **Carotid bifurcation – ICA/ECA differentiation.**
a Longitudinal view of the carotid bifurcation obtained with the transducer in the posterolateral position. The internal carotid artery (ICA) is closer to the transducer. The color change in the bulb indicates retrograde flow components due to flow separation (S) (see Fig. 1.44b). The Doppler waveform of the ICA is characterized by a fairly large end-diastolic flow component. The external carotid artery (ECA) is identified further away from the transducer with flow separation at its origin (red) and the superior thyroid artery (A.T.S) arising from it. The Doppler waveform on the left is from the ICA, the waveform on the right from the ECA. The ECA waveform is more pulsatile compared with the ICA waveform and reflects the oscillations caused by tapping of the temporal artery anterior to the ear (left portion of waveform).
ECA stenosis.
b Stenosis of the ECA reduces pulsatility in the stenotic segment, which may make it difficult to correctly assign the stenosis to the ICA or ECA. When the ECA waveform is altered by stenosis and becomes internalized, the temporal tap sign enables reliable differentiation of the two arteries. (Inverted color encoding of flow direction compared to **a**)

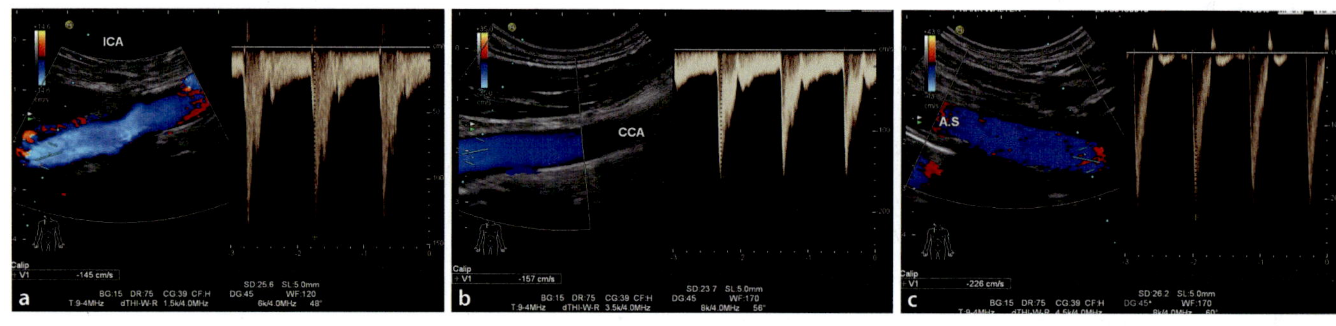

Fig. 5.50a–c (Atlas) **PSV dependence on systemic factors – blood pressure.**
Peak systolic velocity (PSV) is higher in hypertension. This patient with a blood pressure of 205/100 mmHg during the ultrasound examination had a PSV of 145 cm/s in the ICA (**a**), a PSV of 157 cm/s in the CCA (**b**), and a PSV of 230 cm/s in the axillary artery (**c**) without signs of stenosis in gray-scale or color duplex images. These PSVs were present in long segments of the arteries and also in the contralateral arteries. In a patient with normal blood pressure, these PSVs would suggest 50–60% stenosis

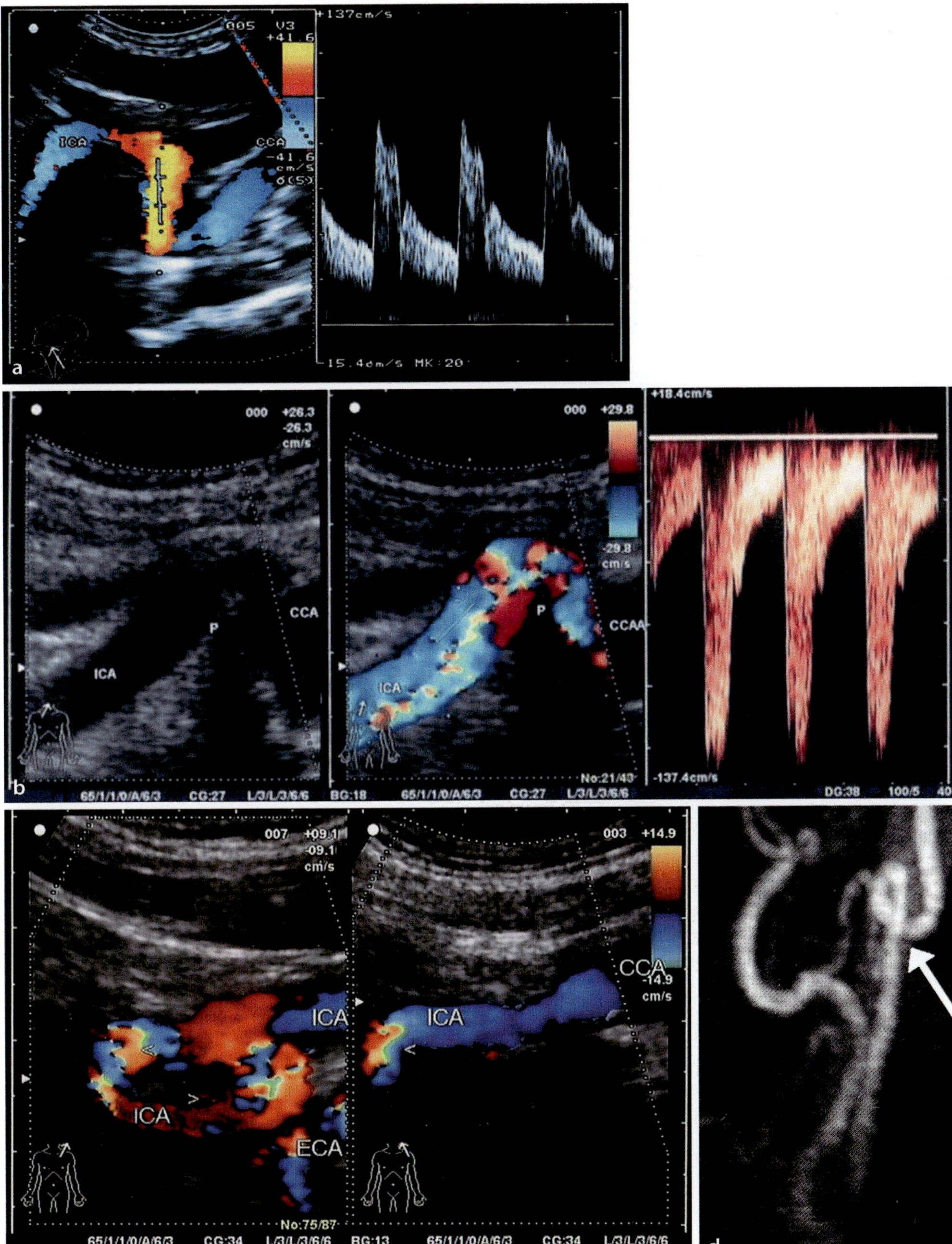

Fig. 5.51a–d (Atlas) Kinking without/with stenosis.
a Elongation of the internal carotid artery (ICA) may lead to kinks or coils (see Fig. 5.1). The resulting tortuosity of the ICA can lead to different angles of insonation with localized increases in the Doppler shift frequency, which must not be misinterpreted as evidence of stenosis. The corresponding color duplex image will show color aliasing in vessel segments insonated at a small angle. Depending on the insonation angle used, kinks or coils in the course of the ICA may be depicted as flow reversal (change in color coding). The color flow image (left) depicts the junction of the common carotid artery (CCA) with the ICA on the right and the distal ICA on the left. The Doppler waveform obtained after angle correction shows laminar flow with a PSV of 95 cm/s, confirming that aliasing in the color mode is due to a small insonation angle. The color change from red to blue is caused by the change in flow direction relative to the transducer.
b Stenosis due to ICA kinking is rare. Such a stenosis may be caused by sclerotic wall changes with plaque (P) at the site of the kink. Here, a PSV of 145 cm/s indicates a stenosis of approximately 60% (by ECST criteria; see Fig. 5.9b and Table 5.9).
Coiling.
c Coiling of the tortuous ICA is seen on color duplex images as a change in color coding, which indicates a change in flow direction relative to the transducer. The right section shows the proximal, straight segment of the ICA (first 2.5 cm) with the arrowhead indicating the transition to the coiled segment. The left section depicts the coiled segment and the transition from the straight portion (change from blue, flow away from transducer, to red, flow toward transducer). A coiled ICA segment is often not visualized in a single plane, but in most cases flexible transducer positioning will allow full evaluation. In the example, one segment is imaged at a 90° Doppler angle, resulting in the artifactual absence of flow. Color aliasing is due to use of a low pulse repetition frequency.
d Angiogram showing the loop (arrow) in the distal extracranial ICA

5

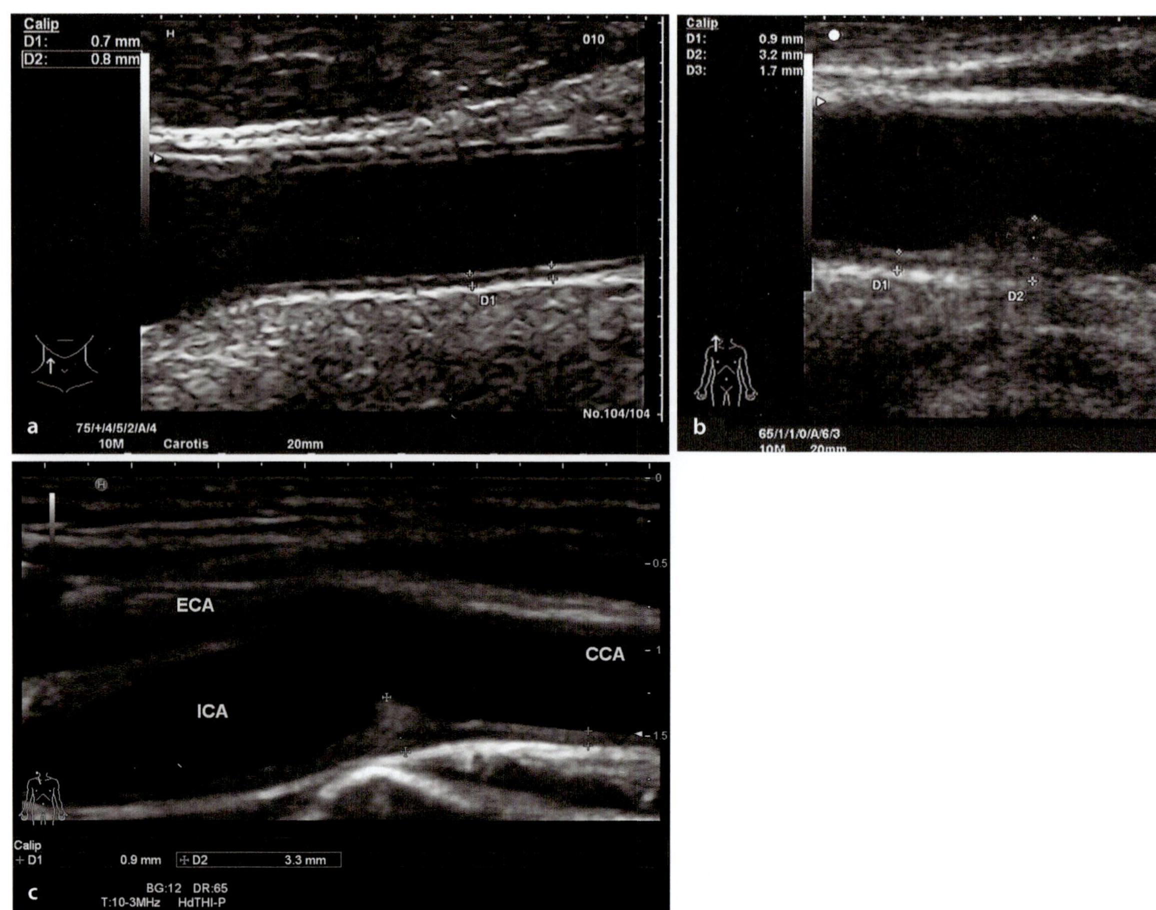

Fig. 5.52a–c (Atlas) Measurement of intima-media thickness (IMT).
a 38-year-old man with a history of hyperlipidemia, in whom an intima-media thickness (IMT) of 0.8 mm was measured in the far wall 2 cm proximal to the bifurcation (indicated by calipers). An IMT of 0.8 mm is abnormal for the patient's age but would be normal for an individual over 60 (see Fig. 5.5).
b In another patient, measurement in the far wall of the common carotid artery (CCA) just before the bifurcation shows thickening of the intima-media complex to 0.9 mm and a plaque with a maximum thickness of 3.2 mm and an irregular surface to the right of it.
Measurement of intima-media thickness (IMT) – plaque.
c The thickness of the intima-media complex is measured in the wall away from the transducer, where the interface between the perfused lumen and the intima produces a sharp reflection due to the intervening flowing blood. The intima and media are indistinct with the second bright reflection occurring at the boundary between the adventitia and the surrounding connective tissue. The layer between these two reflections, which is measured, is the intima-media complex. The IMT of 0.9 mm measured in this case is abnormal in a 50-year-old individual. A plaque is defined as an IMT >2 mm. In the example, an eccentric plaque measuring 3.3 mm in thickness is seen in the center of the image

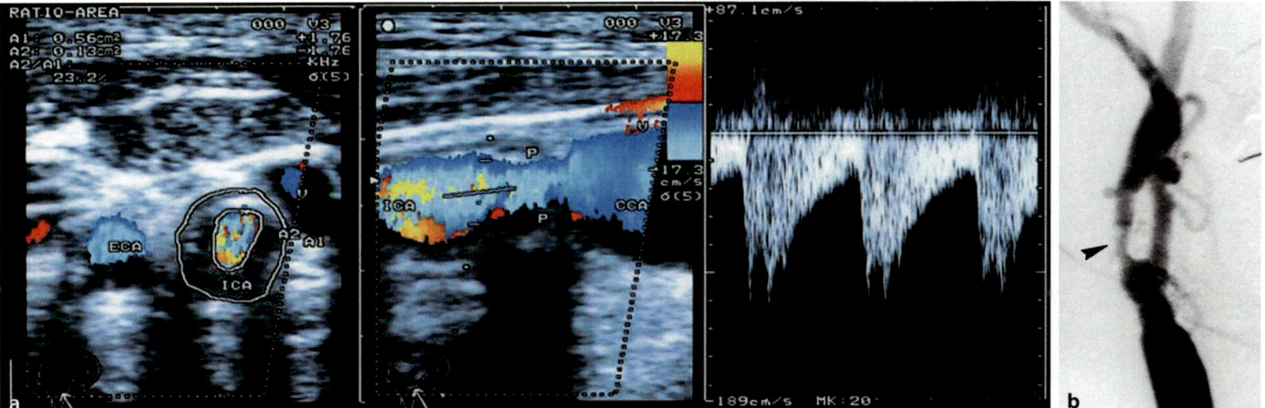

■ **Fig. 5.53a, b (Atlas) Stenosis with beginning hemodynamic effects.**
a A circular plaque in the internal carotid artery (ICA) reduces the cross-sectional area by 75% (left image). To achieve complete color filling of the perfused lumen in the transverse plane, a low pulse repetition frequency (PRF) is employed, which produces aliasing. In the right image, faster blood flow in the center of the artery is indicated by brighter blue and yellow and eddy currents as a change in color coding (red) (see ► Sect. 1.2.3). The hemodynamic stenosis severity with a peak systolic velocity (PSV) of 128 cm/s and spectral broadening correlates with the cross-sectional area reduction. A 65–83% cross-sectional area reduction corresponds to a 40–60% diameter reduction (by ECST criteria; see ■ Fig. 5.9b and ■ Table 5.9), suggesting a stenosis which is just becoming hemodynamically significant. This is shown here for illustration only, and measurement of the cross-sectional area reduction from a transverse image should not be used for stenosis grading (perpendicular angle of insonation results in lower Doppler shift frequencies, and turning up the gain for color imaging can result in blooming artifacts). All relevant stenoses are graded hemodynamically from angle-corrected spectral Doppler measurement in longitudinal orientation.
b Angiogram: Moderate stenosis of the ICA origin

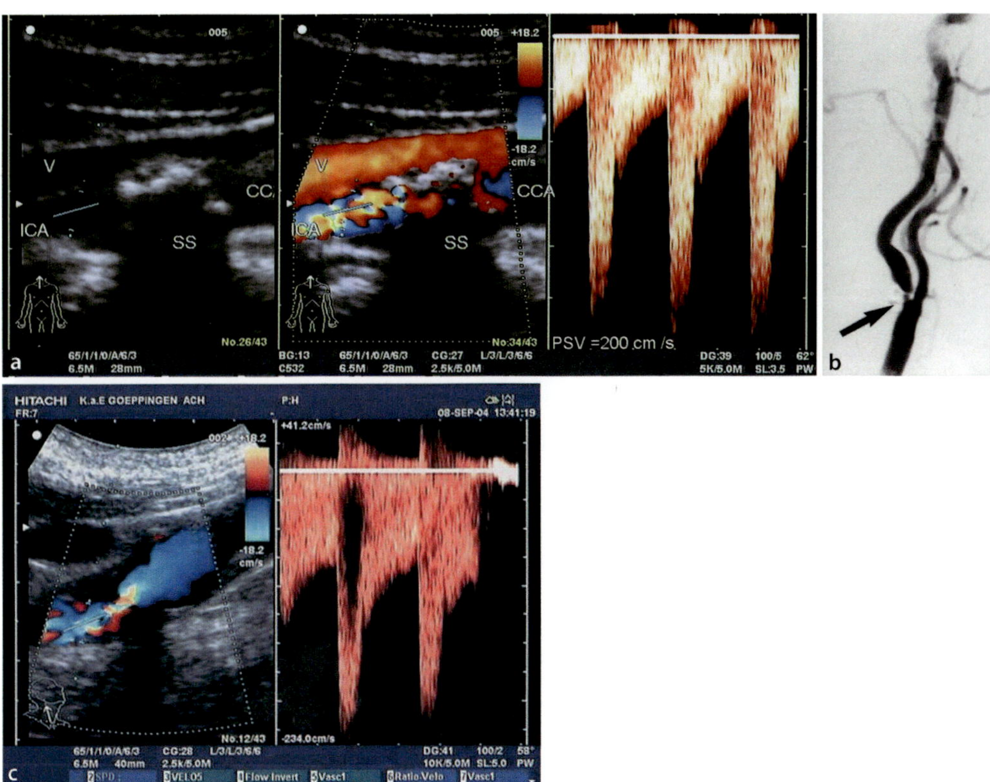

■ **Fig. 5.54a–c (Atlas) Moderate ICA origin stenosis.**
a The severity of luminal narrowing caused by plaque at the internal carotid artery (ICA) origin cannot be evaluated in the gray-scale mode due to calcification with posterior acoustic shadowing (SS). Color flow imaging is also impaired. Distal to the acoustic shadow, there is an eccentric jet with aliasing (yellow) and turbulent flow. Peak systolic velocity (PSV) is increased to 200 cm/s and end-diastolic velocity (EDV) to 70 cm/s, consistent with approx. 70% stenosis by ECST criteria (equivalent to 50% NASCET stenosis; see ■ Fig. 5.9b and ■ Table 5.9). In this case, it was not possible to depict flow by moving the transducer and thus avoiding the calcification. Instead, a high gain was used to obtain a Doppler waveform from the area of acoustic shadowing for hemodynamic quantification of the stenosis by measuring PSV at the site of the plaque.
b Angiogram: 60–80% diameter reduction.
c Example of a plaque causing a similar degree of stenosis as in **a** but with better visualization of the stenosis because the plaque is not calcified. Echolucency suggests a vulnerable plaque, but the surface is smooth. The plaque causes moderate to severe stenosis of the carotid bulb (aliasing, PSV of 225 cm/s and EDV of 80 cm/s). The B-mode image (left) depicts the common carotid artery (CCA) on the right and the ICA on the left, both with flow coded in blue

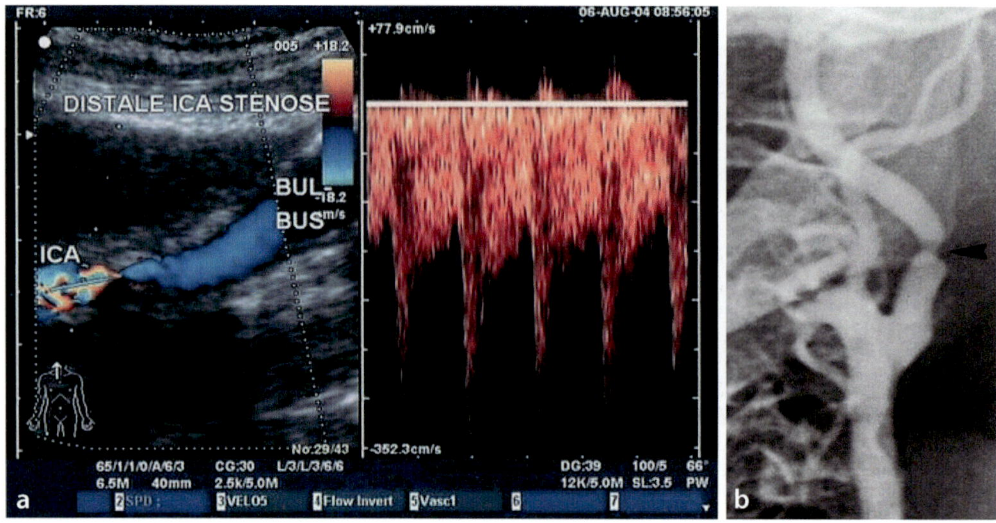

◘ Fig. 5.55a, b (Atlas) Distal ICA stenosis.

a From a posterolateral transducer position, stenosis is depicted in the internal carotid artery (ICA) approx. 2.5 cm upstream of the origin of the external carotid artery (ECA). In the color duplex image, stenosis is suggested by aliasing; the plaque is echolucent. A peak systolic velocity (PSV) of 380 cm/s suggests a diameter reduction of >80%. More distal evaluation of the ICA is precluded by acoustic shadowing and scattering produced by connective tissue structures at the base of the skull. In the postoperative evaluation after carotid endarterectomy (CEA), it is important to exclude stenosis at the distal patch end.

b Angiogram: Filling defect (arrowhead) just below the skull base and normal origin of the ICA

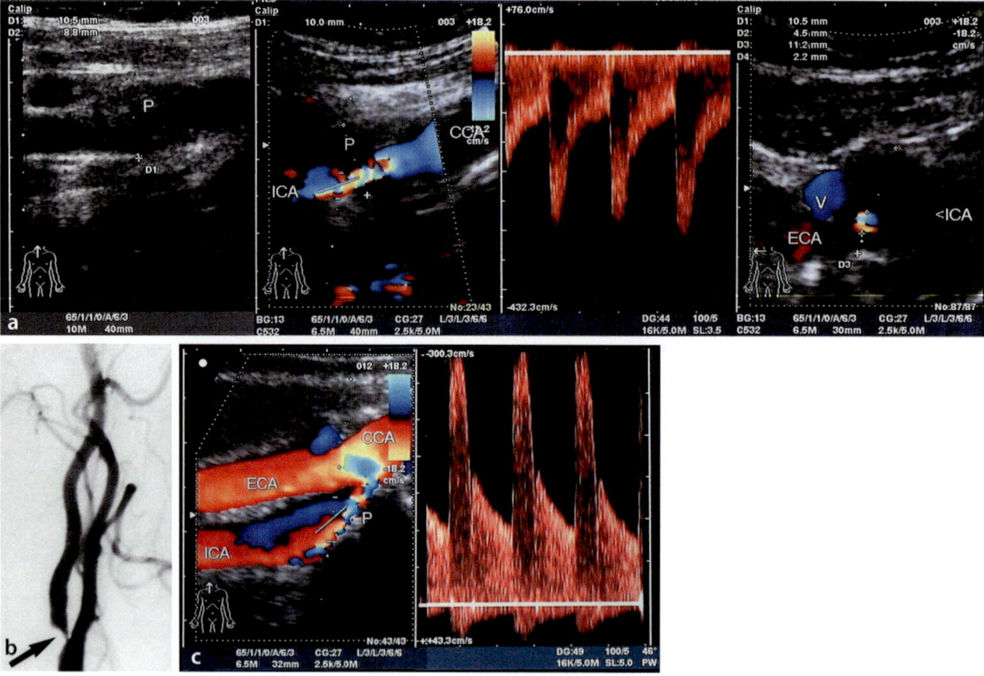

◘ Fig. 5.56a–c (Atlas) High-grade ICA origin stenosis.

a Echolucent, smooth plaque (P) at the origin of the internal carotid artery (ICA) is difficult to delineate from flowing blood (leftmost image). There is aliasing in the longitudinal color flow image with a peak systolic velocity (PSV) of 3 m/s, indicating high-grade stenosis. Blue indicates normal flow direction toward the brain (away from transducer); red indicates turbulent flow with retrograde components. The transverse view (rightmost image) displays the sonomorphologic appearance of the echolucent, eccentric plaque in the carotid bulb (ICA, indicated by calipers) and the resulting high-grade luminal narrowing. The external carotid artery (ECA) and jugular vein (V) are seen lateral to the ICA. Accurate stenosis grading is not possible from transverse views (see ◘ Fig. 5.53 (Atlas) and ► Sect. 1.2.3); a rough estimate is that the diameter reduction is >80%.

b Angiogram: High-grade stenosis (arrow) of the ICA caused by eccentric plaque.

c Eccentric high-grade ICA stenosis, which, unlike the stenosis in **a**, is caused by a calcified plaque (P) with acoustic shadowing (PSV of 380 cm/s). In this example, the color coding follows the convention adopted in some textbooks on vascular ultrasound to invariably depict arteries in red and veins in blue. Therefore, the arteries are displayed in red although the blood flow direction is away from the transducer. Also seen are turbulent flow components (see ◘ Fig. 5.22a)

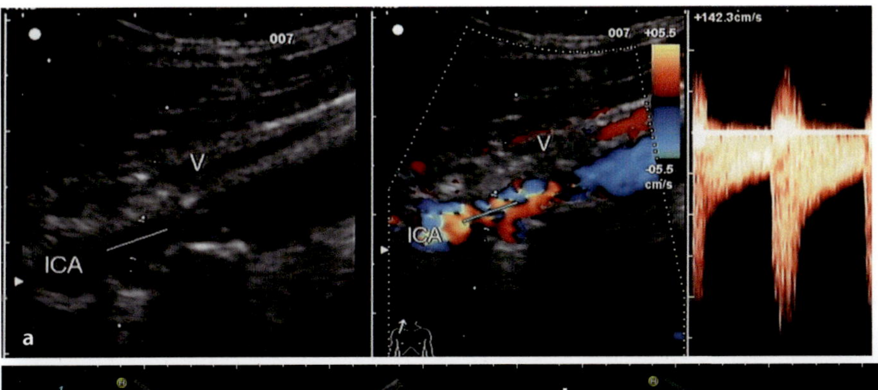

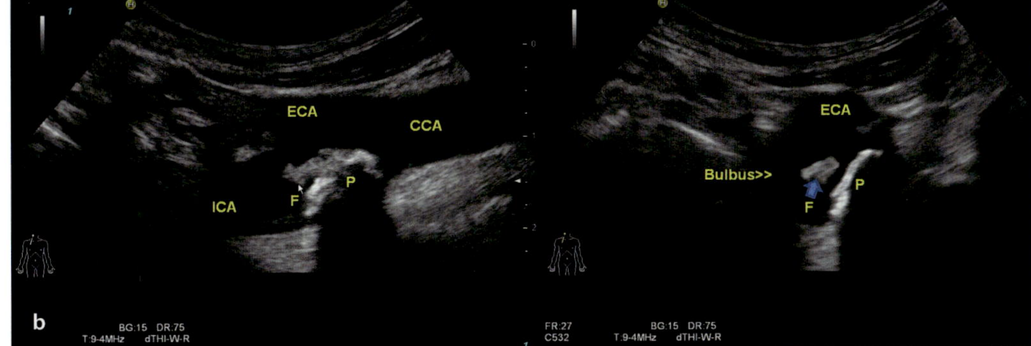

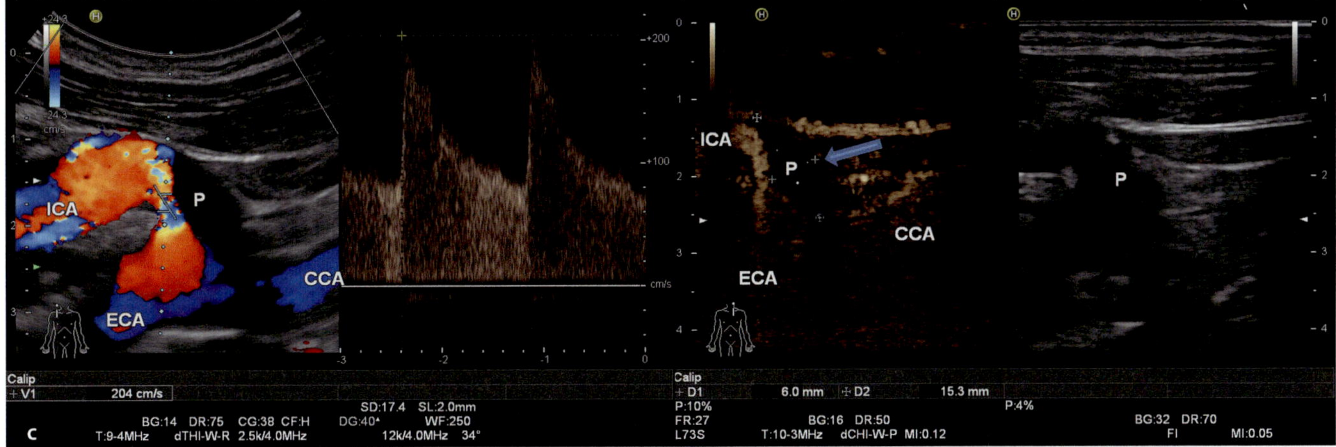

◘ Fig. 5.57a–e (Atlas) Evaluation of plaque morphology (◘ Figs. 5.14, 5.15, and 5.18).

a Example of a partially calcified plaque with echolucent noncalcified portions and a bowl-shaped defect at the distal end. The sharp demarcation of the defect with a bright boundary is more in keeping with a harmless defect niche rather than fresh ulceration (and was confirmed intraoperatively). The peak systolic velocity (PSV) of 2.5 m/s indicates >70% stenosis by ECST criteria (equivalent to >50% stenosis by NASCET criteria; see ◘ Fig. 5.9b and ◘ Table 5.9). Mix of red and blue within the defect indicates eddy currents (see ◘ Fig. 5.18a, e).

b Echogenic plaque (P) protruding into the lumen at the internal carotid artery (ICA) origin (longitudinal image on the left, transverse image on the right). Acoustic shadowing indicates calcification of the plaque. The stenosis has no hemodynamic relevance and does not explain the patient's symptoms (TIAs), which are attributable to a floating portion (F) identified by real-time ultrasound. (In unclear cases, the time-motion mode can be used to demonstrate plaque motion, see ◘ Fig. 2.57 (Atlas).)

c Color duplex (left) and contrast-enhanced ultrasound (CEUS) (right) of echolucent eccentric plaque (P) causing high-grade stenois at the ICA origin. The fact that no contrast microbubbles enter the plaque in the CEUS examination indicates absence of neovascularization and hence a less vulnerable plaque. However, this very eccentric plaque may be highly vulnerable because it is prone to intralesional hemorrhage. The echolucent plaque is difficult to differentiate from surrounding blood in B-mode ultrasound (rightmost image), and color duplex is necessary to delineate the eccentric plaque from flowing blood (leftmost image). If no gray-scale median (GSM) analysis is performed, the echogenicity of the plaque can be evaluated by comparing it with that of the sternocleidomastoid muscle anterior to the artery (closer to the transducer). The low echogenicity of the plaque in this example corresponds to a GSM < 20.

d Echolucent, eccentric plaque (P) causing moderate stenosis (Doppler waveform) at the ICA origin (color duplex on the left, CEUS on the right). CEUS clearly shows signs of (mild) plaque neovascularization (arrows; grade 2). This example also illustrates the discrepancy between the risk of embolism resulting from plaque thickness (arrow in transverse view on the left; 5.5 mm versus 8 mm bulb diameter) and the hemodynamic relevance of the stenosis (PSV of 160 cm/s, consistent with approx. 60% ECST stenosis and 40% NASCET stenosis).

e Six months later, color duplex ultrasound reveals nearly unchanged plaque thickness (not shown), while CEUS shows increased neovascularization (grade 3) of the proximal plaque portion (site of high shear stress) but little neovascularization in the distal portion (grade 1). This plaque is homogenenous in terms of echogenicity but inhomogeneous in terms of neovascularization

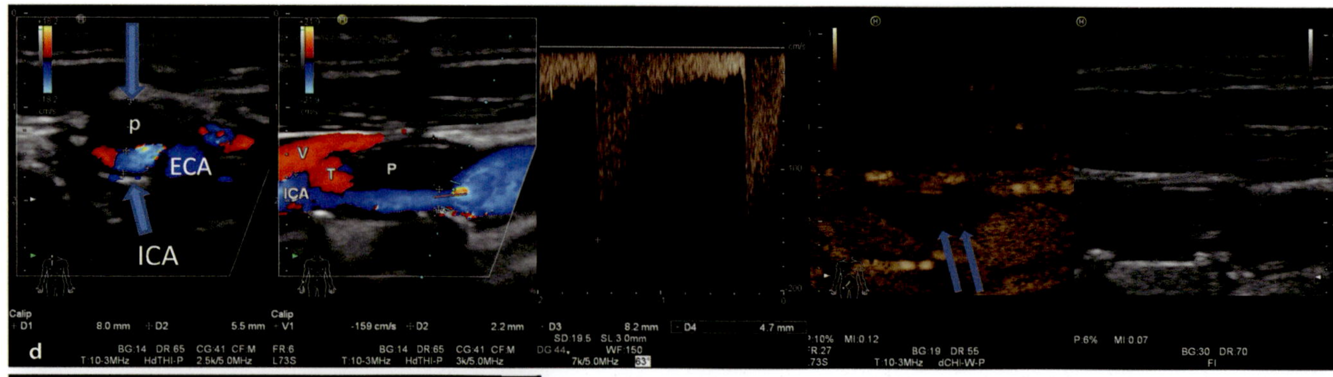

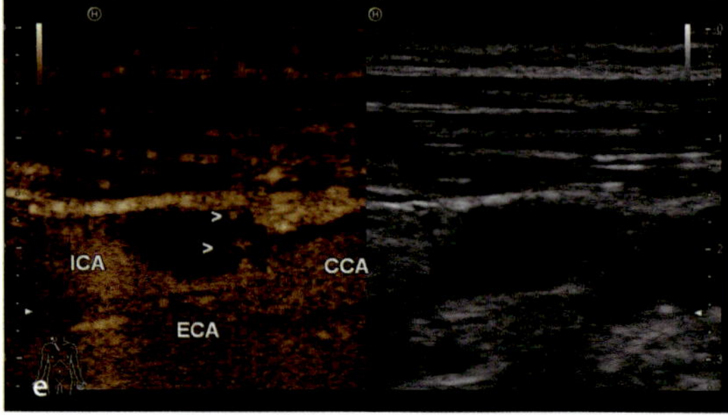

◘ **Fig. 5.57** (continued)

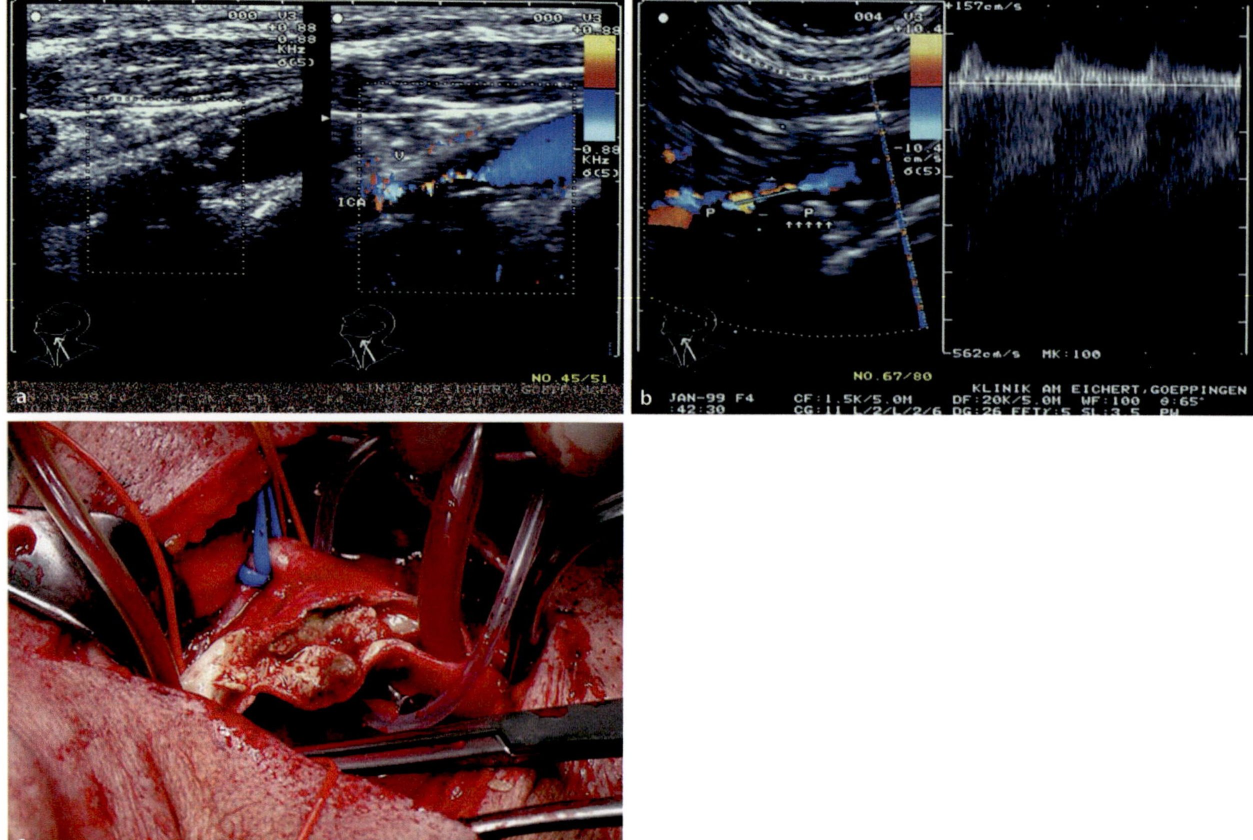

◘ **Fig. 5.58a–c (Atlas) Plaque morphology – surface structure** (see ◘ Fig. 5.15, ► Sect. 5.6.1).
a Sagittal B-mode image showing inhomogeneous plaques with ill-defined contours. Bright spots suggest that the plaque extends almost to the center of the artery. Color duplex imaging is necessary for adequate evaluation, showing a very small residual lumen between the two plaques on the far and near wall. Flow acceleration is indicated by aliasing. Type IV plaque: echolucent, inhomogeneous, surface not delineated from vessel lumen.
b Spectral Doppler measurement with the sample volume placed in the stenotic jet confirms high-grade stenosis with a peak systolic velocity (PSV) > 4 m/s.
c Intraoperative confirmation of high-grade stenosis with a long plaque, predominantly of the atheromatous type (consistent with the ultrasound findings)

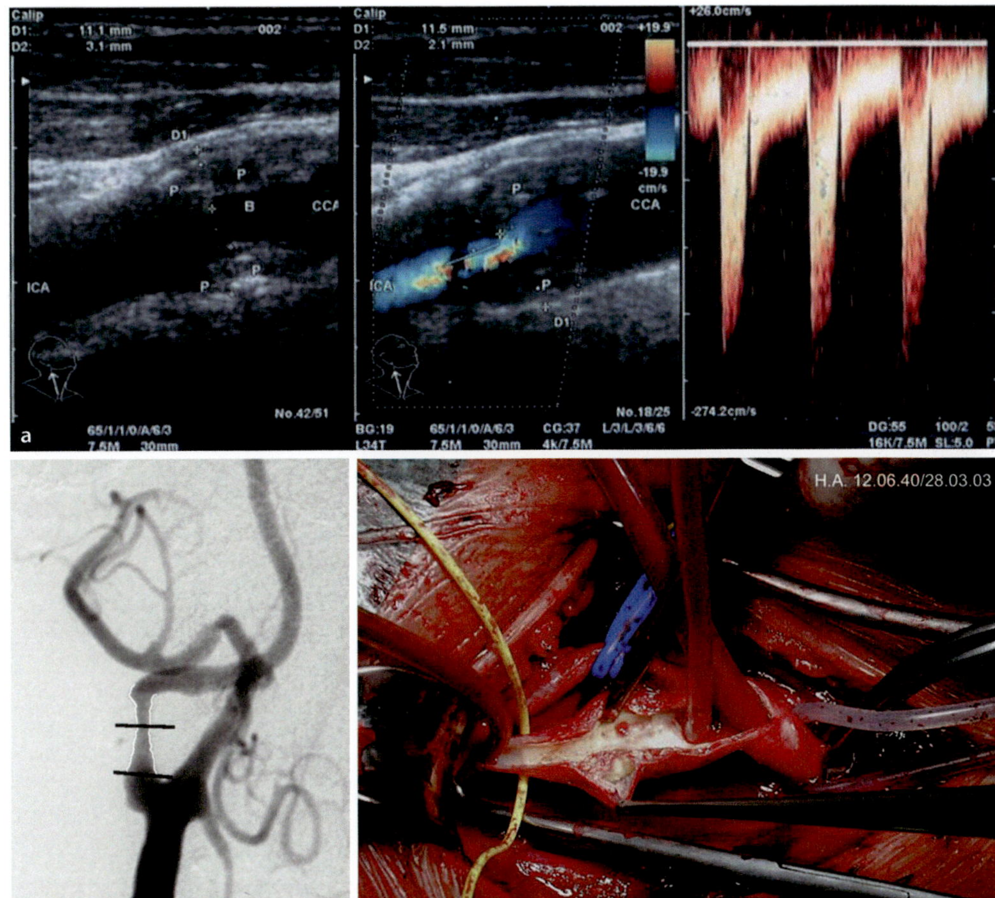

Fig. 5.59a–c (Atlas) Plaque morphology – long concentric carotid stenosis (smooth, regular surface).
a Gray-scale image depicting a concentric, fairly homogeneous and smoothly marginated plaque in the center with a just barely visible, extremely echolucent portion extending cranially. Only the color duplex image enables differentiation of the echolucent distal plaque portion and perfused lumen. The peak systolic velocity (PSV) determined by spectral Doppler measurement is 230 cm/s.
b Angiogram confirming a long concentric, smooth stenosis.
c Intraoperative photograph showing mostly fibrous plaque with a smooth surface (for this plaque composition, a higher echogenicity would have been expected in the preceding ultrasound examination)

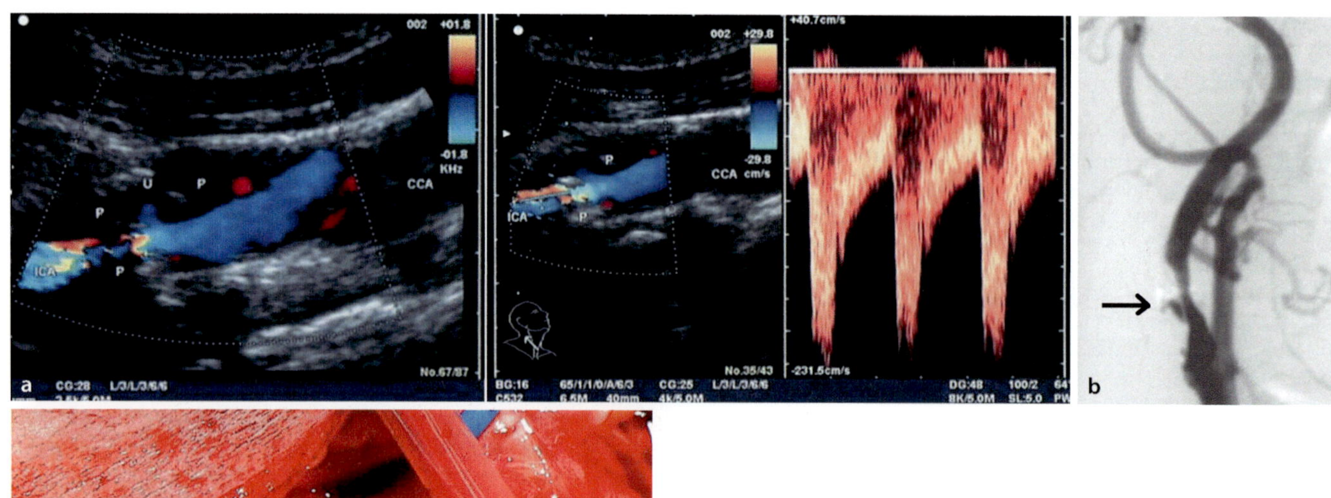

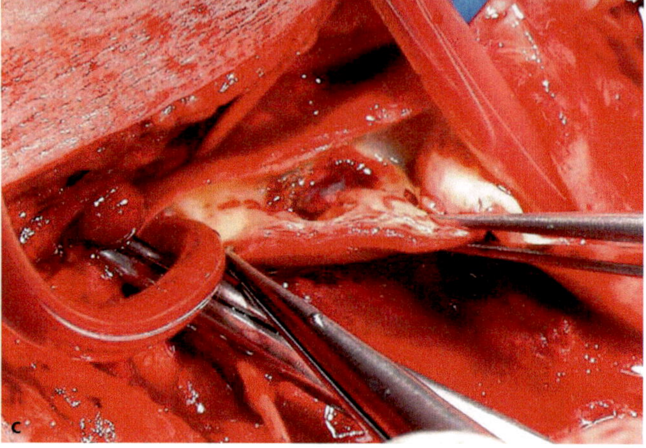

Fig. 5.60a–c (Atlas) Plaque morphology – high-grade stenosis with ulceration.
a Echolucent plaque (P) with ulceration (U) at the internal carotid artery (ICA) origin. The concentric plaque causing high-grade stenosis begins directly distal to the ulceration. Ulceration often occurs in the proximal portion of a highly stenotic plaque protruding far into the lumen. The arriving pulse wave (often depicted as longitudinal pulsatile plaque movement by gray-scale imaging) may cause rupture of the vulnerable plaque cap. In the example, the peak systolic velocity (PSV) in the stenotic jet (indicated by aliasing) is 220 cm/s.
b Angiography with a filling defect confirming the plaque contour demonstrated by ultrasound and also the ulceration.
c Intraoperatively, the atheromatous plaque and adjacent ulceration are confirmed at the sites already identified by ultrasonography and angiography

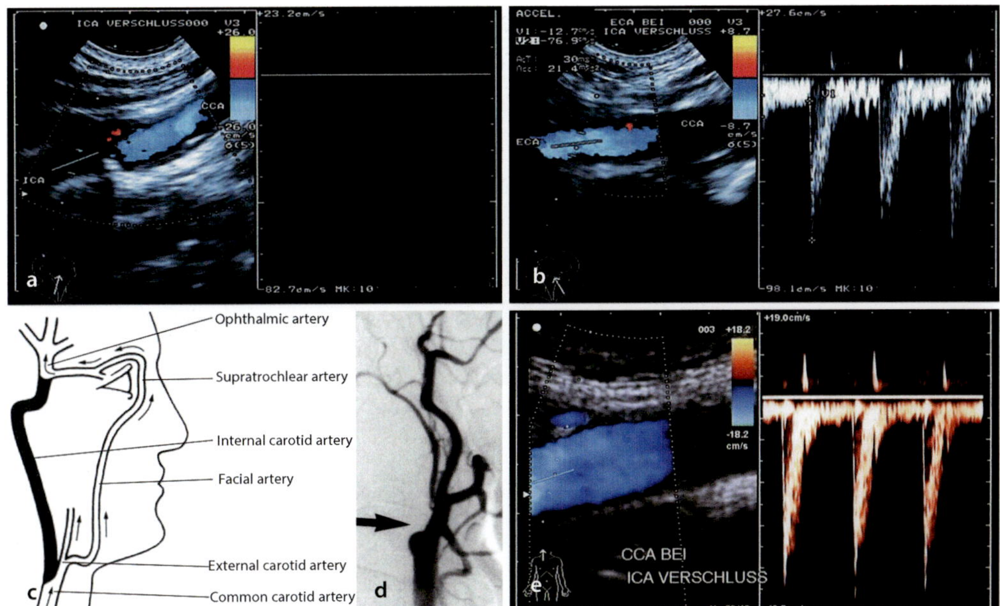

Fig. 5.61a–e (Atlas) ICA occlusion.

a Patient with occlusion of the internal carotid artery (ICA) indicated by the absence of flow signals both in the color flow image and in the Doppler waveform. There is a calcified plaque with acoustic shadowing at the ICA origin. The common carotid artery (CCA) is patent (right part of color flow image). To differentiate occlusion from subtotal occlusion, the ICA must be scanned to the level of the mandibular angle using high gain to detect low flow.

b In this patient, the external carotid artery (ECA) provides collateral flow via the supratrochlear artery, resulting in a larger diastolic flow component in the ECA waveform. To avoid confusion with the ICA in this situation, the identity of the ECA should be confirmed using the temporal tap maneuver. Rhythmical tapping of the temporal artery (branch of ECA) causes oscillation in the ECA waveform (as shown here) but not in the ICA waveform.

c Diagram of collateralization of ICA occlusion via the ECA and supratrochlear artery (CW Doppler).

d Angiogram: ICA occlusion (arrow).

e In ICA occlusion, flow in the CCA becomes more pulsatile with a Doppler waveform becoming more like that of the ECA, the only artery supplied by the CCA in this situation (known as externalization of the CCA)

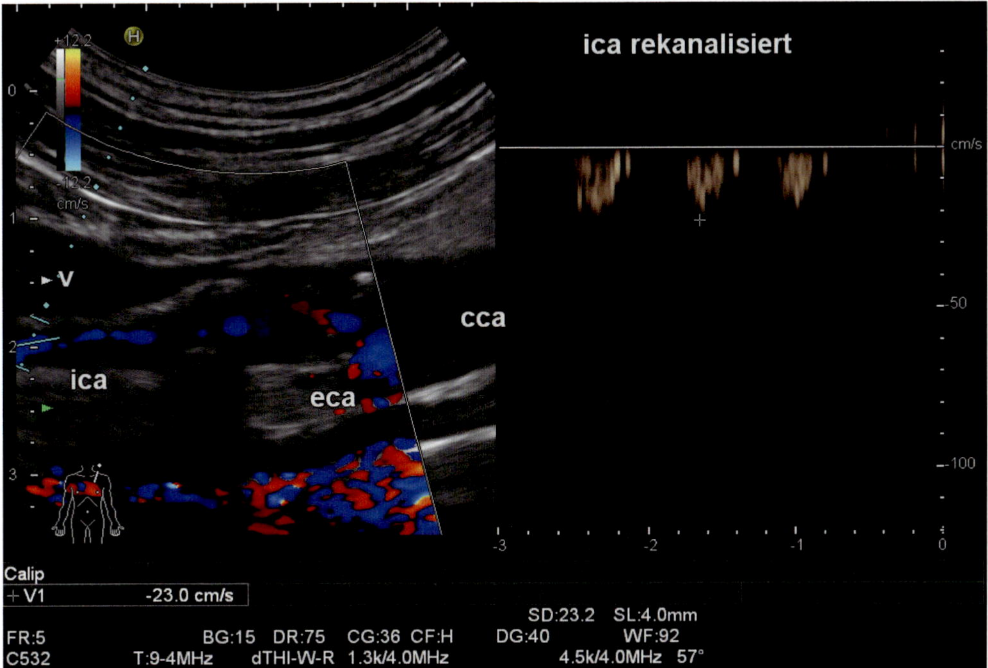

Fig. 5.62 (Atlas) Signs of recanalization in ICA occlusion.

When examining a patient with suspected internal carotid artery (ICA) occlusion, the examiner must search for flow signals using a low pulse repetition frequency (PRF). Recanalization is uncommon and must be differentiated from pseudo-occlusion. The latter is characterized by a patent poststenotic segment of normal width with very slow flow filling most of the lumen, while isolated high-frequency flow signals may be identified in the subtotally occluded segment when high gain is used. In occlusion with recanalization (as in the case presented here), flow signals indicating a thin, meandering current are depicted centrally in the otherwise occluded and shrunken extracranial ICA, which is often filled with more hypoechoic residues marginally. Unlike stenotic narrowing, recanalization is characterized by slow flow (23 cm/s in the example with atypical ICA flow signal due to changed resistance). The meandering recanalization channels can disappear from the scan plane, which should not be misinterpreted as absence of blood flow in the color flow image (artifact farther away from transducer due to low PRF)

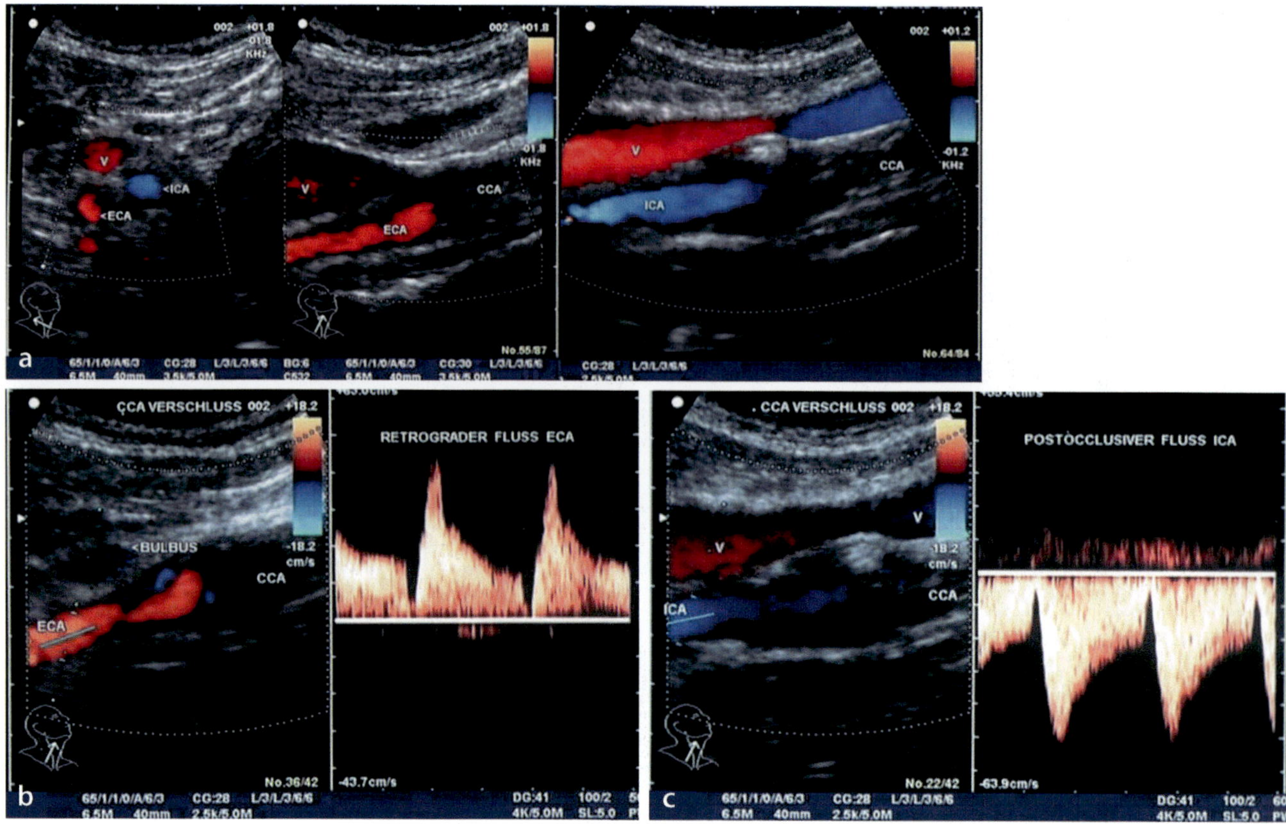

Fig. 5.63a–c (Atlas) CCA occlusion – collaterals.
a In patients with occlusion of the common carotid artery (CCA) and a patent bifurcation, the internal carotid artery (ICA) is refilled via branches of the external carotid artery (ECA), primarily the superior thyroid artery, which in turn is supplied by branches of the thyrocervical trunk.
b Distal ECA branches may likewise contribute to the supply of the ICA. It is therefore common to see retrograde flow in a long segment of the ECA (displayed in red, toward the heart, same flow direction as in the accompanying internal jugular vein).
c ICA with forward flow (displayed in blue, away from transducer). The ICA waveform (like the waveform from the ECA) shows postocclusive flow with damping and a delayed systolic upstroke

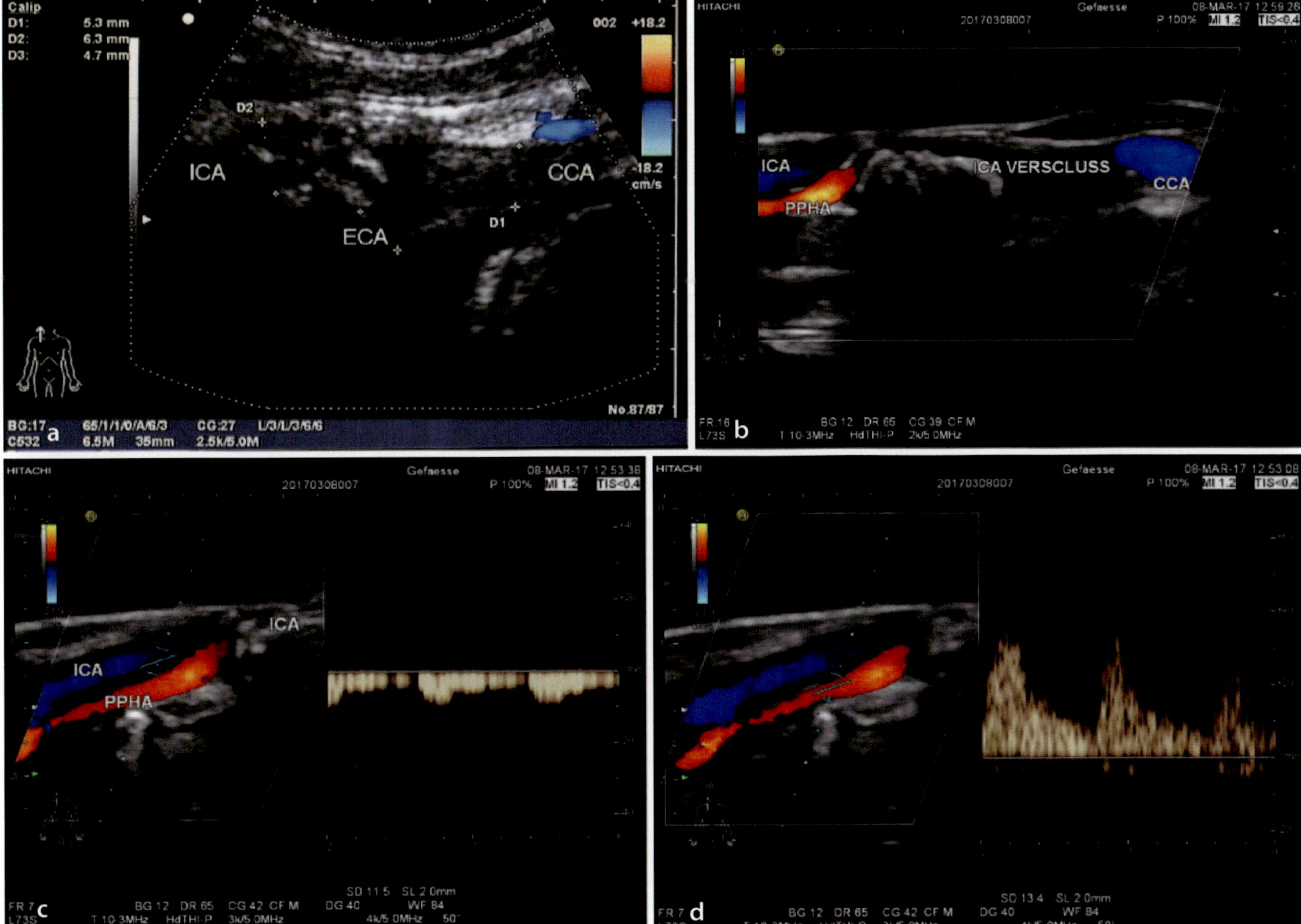

Fig. 5.64a–d (Atlas) Complete extracranial carotid territory occlusion.
a When the common carotid artery (CCA) is occluded, the examiner should begin by identifying the bifurcation and then try to detect flow in the internal carotid artery (ICA) and external carotid artery (ECA). Evaluation is limited when large plaques with acoustic shadowing are present. An occluded segment appears very heterogeneous and contains areas of higher echogenicity, making it difficult to delineate the arterial lumen from the surrounding connective tissue. The arteries are indicated by calipers (CCA: D1; ICA: D2; ECA: D3). The only patent vessel with flow (blue) is a vein in the top right corner of the image.
PPHA as collateral in ICA occlusion.
b Atherosclerotic occlusion (2 cm in length) of the mid-segment of the ICA. The distal ICA receives blood supply via a persistent primitive hypoglossal artery (PPHA).
c Flow velocity in the postocclusive segment of the ICA is markedly reduced (peak systolic velocity (PSV) of 10 cm/s).
d The PPHA with red-coded flow toward the heart (PSV of 40 cm/s) refills the proximally occluded ICA

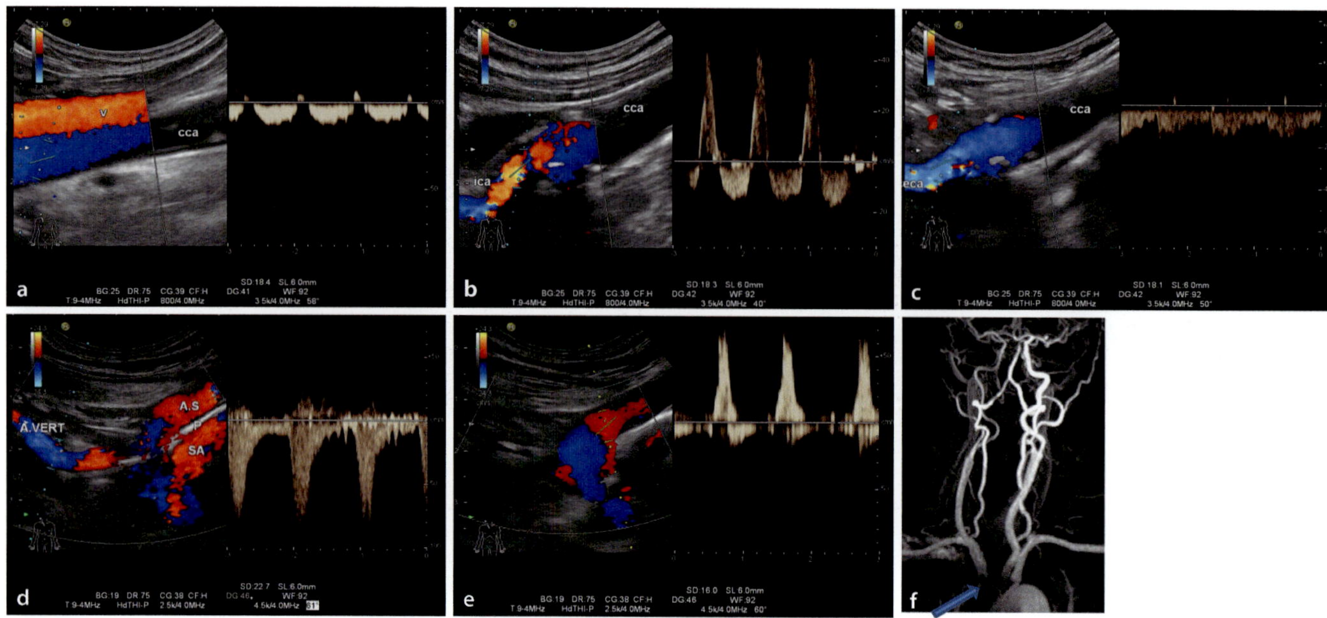

Fig. 5.65a-f (Atlas) Occlusion of the brachiocephalic trunk – collateral pathways. Duplex ultrasound allows excellent hemodynamic evaluation of collateral channels.
a There is alternating forward and backward flow in the common carotid artery (CCA) with predominantly orthograde diastolic flow and slow retrograde systolic flow (blue-coded flow toward the brain in the CCA, red-coded flow in the jugular vein).
b Alternating flow directions (red/blue) in the internal carotid artery (ICA) with orthograde flow during diastole and rather high retrograde flow during systole (red, toward transducer; peak systolic velocity (PSV) of 50 cm/s) indicate that the ICA has been recruited as a collateral and supplies the ECA territory via the intracranial circulation during systole.
c The retrograde systolic flow in the ICA refills the ECA, where the flow direction is normal and the waveform shows postocclusive flow.
d There is retrograde flow in the vertebral artery (A.VERT), which supplies the subclavian artery (A.S) (SA = mirror artifact; oscillations from temporal tap in the waveform during diastole).
e The resupplied subclavian artery shows postocclusive flow.
f The MR angiogram shows occlusion of the brachiocephalic trunk and provides a (morphologic) overview of collateral pathways but – unlike spectral Doppler – no information on the relative flow contributions of the individual collaterals

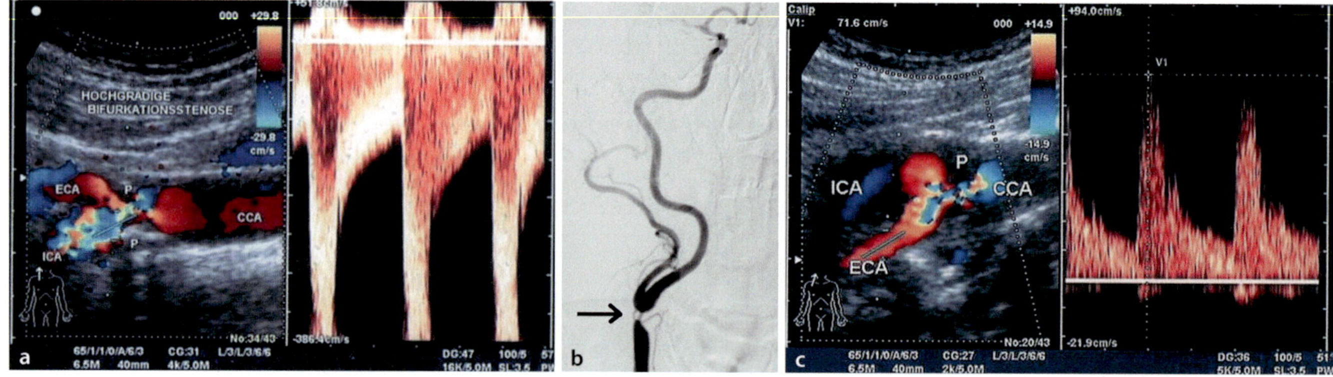

Fig. 5.66a–c (Atlas) CCA stenosis.
a Preferred sites of common carotid artery (CCA) stenoses are the origin proximally and the area of the bifurcation distally. In the example, concentric plaques (P) cause high-grade stenosis just before the CCA divides into the internal carotid artery (ICA) and external carotid artery (ECA). The stenosis is indicated by aliasing in the color flow image and confirmed by spectral Doppler analysis with a peak systolic velocity (PSV) of more than 4 m/s.
b Angiogram confirms the high-grade stenosis of the distal CCA just before the bifurcation.
c With increasing stenosis of the distal CCA, communicating vessels entering the ECA, e.g., via the superior thyroid artery, are recruited as collaterals. In the case shown here, high-grade stenosis of the CCA (P) is suggested by aliasing. There is retrograde flow in the ECA (displayed in red, toward transducer) with refilling of the ICA. The Doppler waveform from the ECA shows backward flow to the heart (toward transducer). The large diastolic component reflects the fact that the ECA supplies the brain indirectly via the ICA. (Posterior transducer position as opposed to anterior position in **a**)

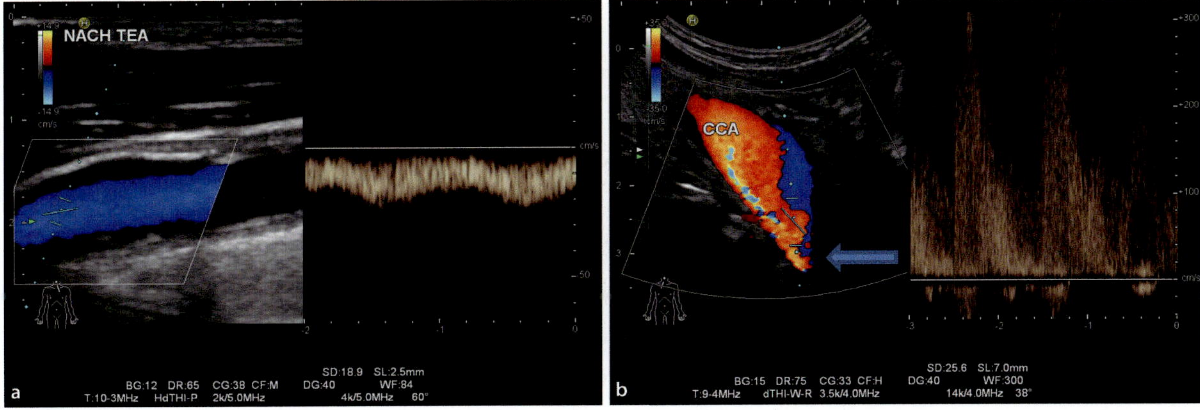

Fig. 5.67a, b (Atlas) High-grade stenosis of the brachiocephalic trunk.
a In a patient after carotid endarterectomy (CEA), the waveform from the internal carotid artery (ICA) shows the typical features of poststenotic flow (low PSV, delayed systolic rise). Neointimal proliferation is apparent (identified by low echogenicity). These findings should prompt a search for stenosis proximally.
b High-grade stenosis of the brachiocephalic trunk with a PSV > 3 m/s (aliasing technically not avoidable due to high Doppler shift frequency with acute insonation angle). The sample volume is placed in the stenosis jet (indicated by turbulent flow, encoded in blue). Only a short portion of the stenotic segment is evaluable because the artery leaves the scanning plane

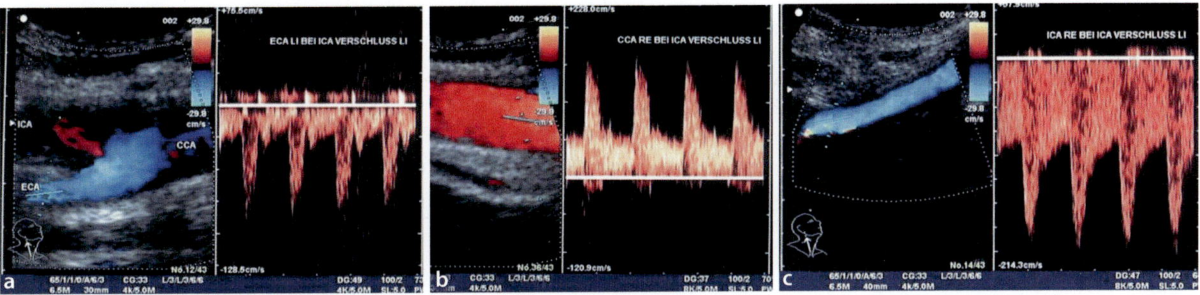

Fig. 5.68a–c (Atlas) ICA occlusion – compensatory flow increase in collateral pathways.
Occlusion of the internal carotid artery (ICA) is compensated for by larger flow volumes in the collateral arteries. The resulting higher flow velocities must not be misinterpreted as indicating stenosis. Faster flow is detectable in long segments of the collaterals, while no stenosing structures are identified.
a The ipsilateral external carotid artery (ECA) can become a collateral, seen as internalization of the ECA waveform (to-and-fro flow – knocking waveform in the bulb).
b Occasionally, there may be an increased compensatory flow in the contralateral common carotid artery (CCA) as well (150 cm/s in the case shown).
c PSV of 200 cm/s in a long segment of the contralateral ICA. The increase is rarely as impressive as in this case and varies with the contributions of other collaterals

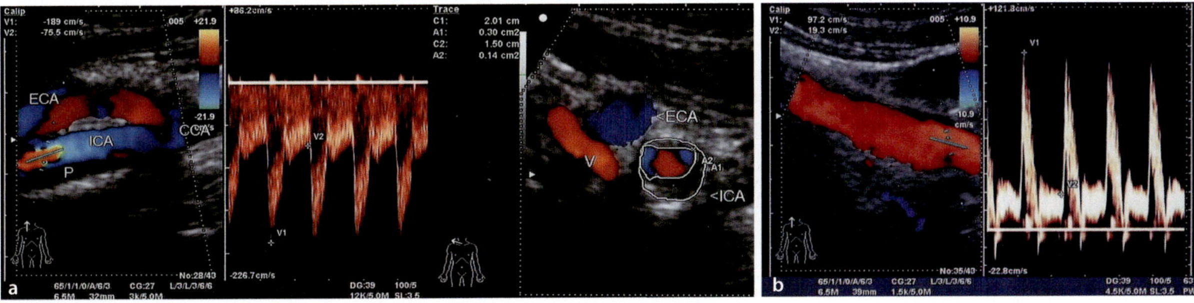

Fig. 5.69a, b (Atlas) Pitfall of PSV-based ICA stenosis grading in contralateral ICA occlusion.
a Long echolucent plaque (P; longitudinal image on the left) of the internal carotid artery (ICA) causing <50% luminal narrowing, while the peak systolic velocity (PSV) of 189 cm/s suggests 60–70% stenosis (by ECST criteria). The maximum diameter reduction determined in the ICA in the transverse plane (right image) is just below 50% (beware of inherent limitations using this method), corresponding to a 50% cross-sectional area reduction (as the plaque is predominantly eccentric), which is not hemodynamically relevant. Cross-sectional area of patent lumen: 0.14 cm^2; total cross-sectional area of ICA: 0.3 cm^2.
b To determine whether the increased PSV in the ICA is due to an increased blood flow volume to compensate for contralateral ICA occlusion, flow velocity in the common carotid artery (CCA) is measured. In the example, a high PSV of 97.2 cm/s in the CCA indicates that at least part of the PSV increase in the ICA is attributable to collateral flow. Consequently, the PSV in the ICA overestimates stenosis severity and, to arrive at a correct estimate, allowance must be made for the contribution due to collateral flow

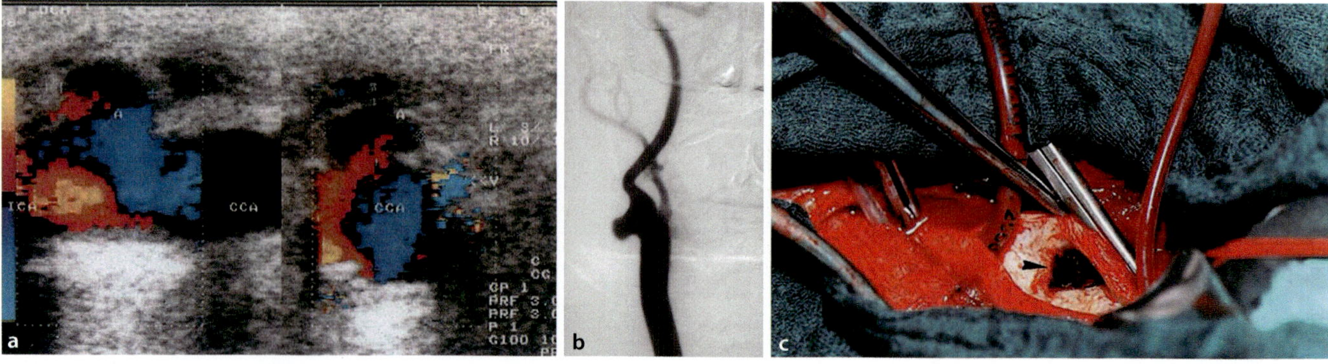

Fig. 5.70a–c (Atlas) Suture aneurysm.
a Pulsatile mass of the neck 3 years after carotid endarterectomy (CEA). Color duplex sonography identifies a circumscribed outpouching with flow signals in the patch area at the origin of the internal carotid artery (ICA). Incomplete color filling of the pouch suggests partial thrombosis. No demonstration of stenosis.
b Angiogram confirms saccular aneurysm of the ICA bulb.
c Intraoperatively, a suture aneurysm covered by connective tissue structures is seen with thrombotic deposits in the aneurysmal sac (arrowhead)

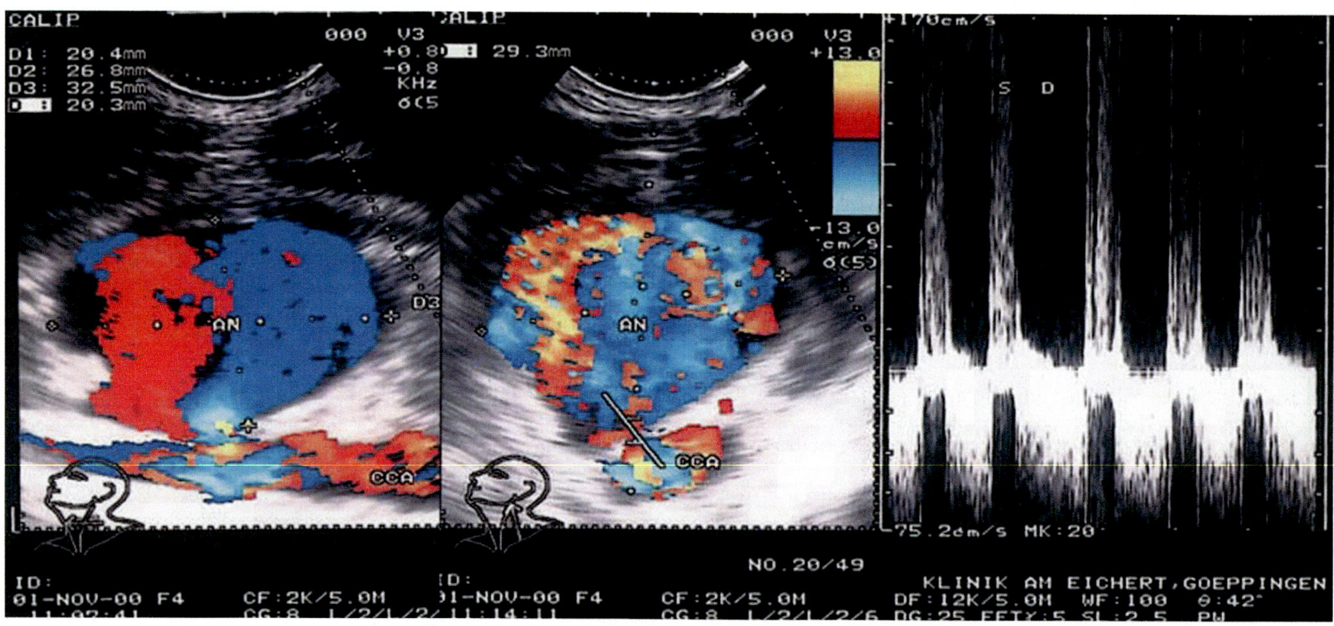

Fig. 5.71 (Atlas) Complications after carotid endarterectomy – suture aneurysm.
Virtually all pseudoaneurysms of the carotid system are due to trauma or occur in the form of suture aneurysms after carotid endarterectomy (CEA), particularly in patients who have undergone synthetic patch angioplasty. Suture aneuryms often indicate infection of the patch. The longitudinal (left) and transverse color flow images (right) show a conspicuous mushroom-like structure protruding from the vessel, which can be palpated as a pulsating mass in most cases. The color coding varies with the presence and extent of thrombosis. The spectral waveform from the aneurysmal neck shows the typical to-and-fro sign indicating high-frequency systolic flow into the aneurysm and flow into the carotid lumen throughout diastole

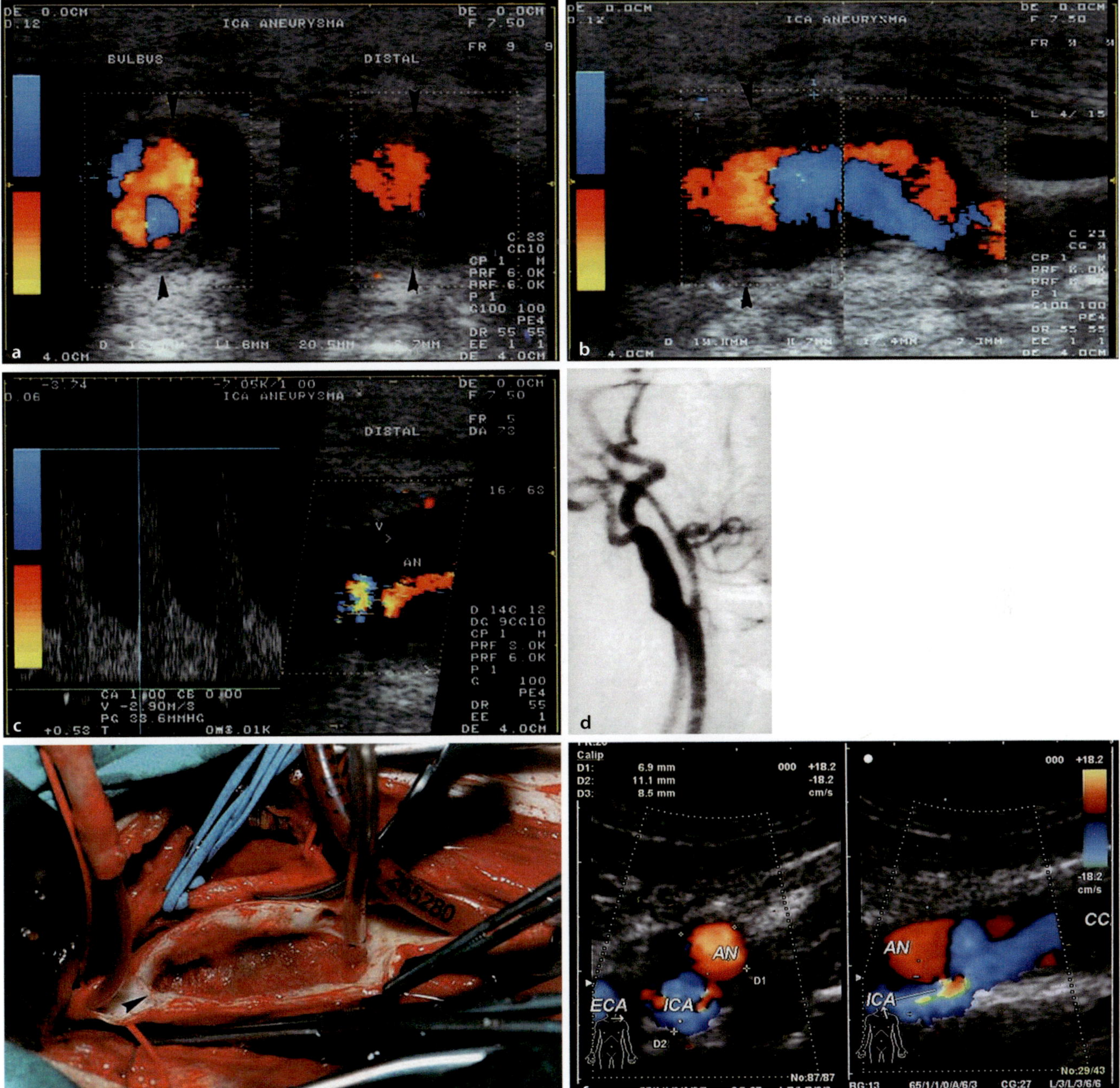

Fig. 5.72a–f (Atlas) **True ICA aneurysm.**

a Transverse image showing the patent lumen of the internal carotid artery (ICA) surrounded by hypoechoic aneurysmal thrombotic deposits (arrowheads) both in the bulb area (left) and in the distal segment (right). The aneurysm has a diameter of 2 cm.

b The longitudinal image allows evaluation of the shape of the ICA aneurysm (common carotid artery (CCA) on the right and ICA on the left). The image impressively shows the total extent of the aneurysm (arrowheads) and the size of the hypoechoic thrombotic portion in relation to the color-coded patent lumen. The color change indicates eddy currents.

c At the distal end of the aneurysm there is flow acceleration with turbulence and aliasing (inverted display). Flow velocity is increased to 2.9 m/s (inverted waveform depicting flow away from transducer above the baseline).

d Angiogram: Ectasia of the ICA. The mural thrombi make the aneurysm appear smaller than it actually is, and angiography does not provide information on the hemodynamic significance of the stenosis at the distal end of the aneurysm; all that is seen is less pronounced opacification due to luminal narrowing in the anteroposterior projection.

e Intraoperative site confirming the spindle-shaped aneurysm of the proximal ICA with mural thrombosis and fibrotic stenosis at its distal end (arrowhead). CCA with shunt on the right and distal ICA on the left with the aneurysm of the proximal ICA in between. The aneurysm is thrombosed and shows fibrous luminal narrowing at its distal end. A blue vascular sling is placed around the ECA.

Mycotic ICA aneurysm.

f Transverse (left) and longitudinal (right) images of a saccular aneurysmal dilatation (AN) of the proximal ICA. The transverse view nicely depicts the aneurysm with flow toward the transducer (red). Flow direction in the ECA is normal (blue, toward the head)

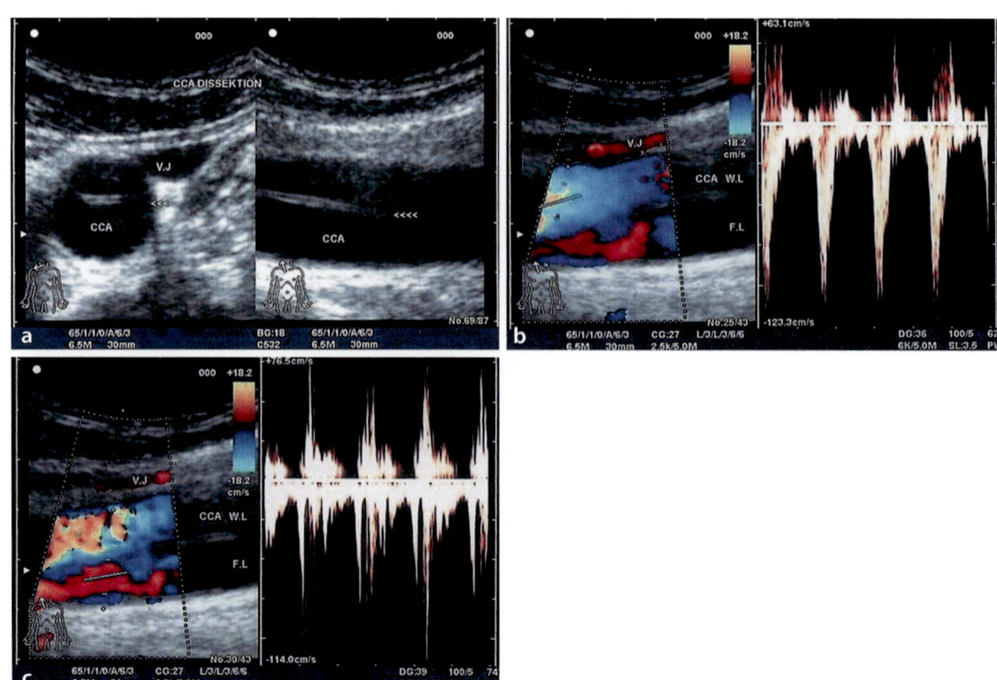

Fig. 5.73a–c (Atlas) Dissection of CCA.
In De Bakey type I aortic dissection, the dissection extends into the common carotid artery (CCA).
a The B-mode image depicts the dissection in longitudinal and transverse planes as an intraluminal flap oscillating during the cardiac cycle.
b Color flow imaging differentiates the true lumen of the CCA (CCA W.L) with antegrade flow toward the brain from the false lumen (F.L) (V.J, jugular vein).
c The flow direction demonstrated in the false lumen depends on the placement of the sample volume relative to the re-entry site. Forward flow is demonstrated if the re-entry is distal to the sample volume and to-and-fro flow, as in the example, if it is proximal. The image shows flow in the true lumen displayed in blue (toward the periphery, away from transducer) and aliasing, while there is to-and-fro flow in the false lumen (here displayed in red, toward transducer)

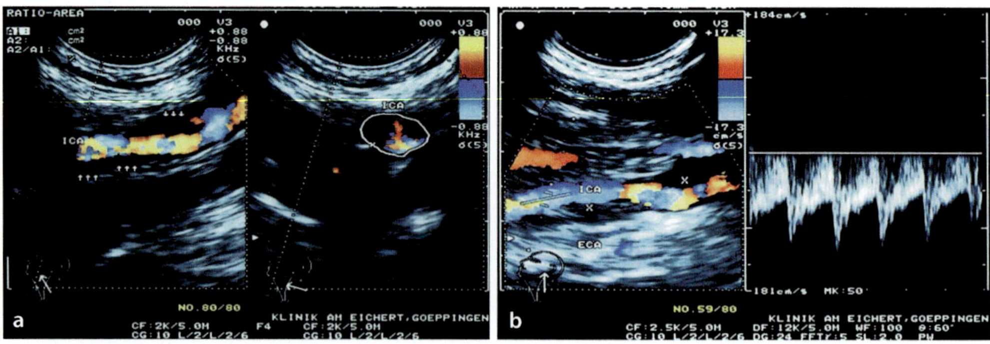

Fig. 5.74a, b (Atlas) Posttraumatic ICA dissection.
a Long posttraumatic dissection of the internal carotid artery (ICA) extending from the bifurcation to the base of the skull with thrombosis of the false lumen. Unlike atherosclerotic changes, thrombotic dissection is characterized by a homogeneous and hypoechoic sonomorphologic appearance. The thrombosed false lumen is long and tortuous and partly attaches to the vessel wall. Occasionally, as in this example, the entry site can be identified by the depiction of pulsatile flow signals in the color duplex mode (right image).
b The blood flow velocity measured by spectral Doppler indicates that the luminal narrowing due to the dissection does not yet cause higher-grade stenosis (PSV of 120 cm/s)

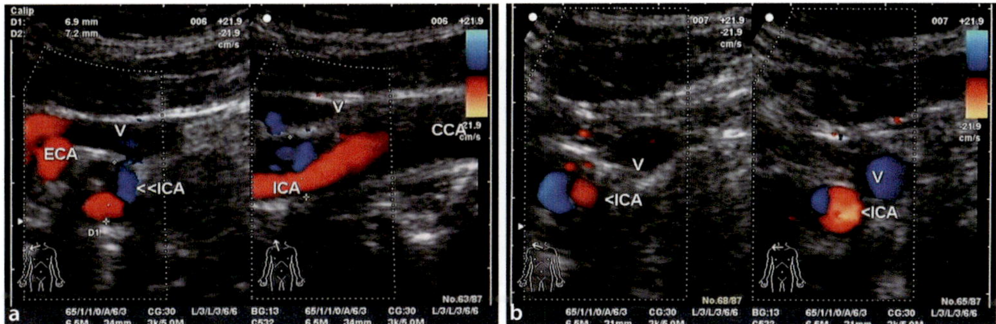

Fig. 5.75a, b (Atlas) Posttraumatic ICA dissection with patent true and false lumen.
a Posttraumatic ICA dissection extending from the carotid bulb to the skull base. The longitudinal image on the right (inverted display) shows the true lumen coded in red and the false lumen coded in blue. The transverse image (left) shows 50% diameter reduction of the true lumen and partial thrombosis (hypoechoic portion) of the false lumen (coded in blue) (V = internal jugular vein; ECA = external carotid artery).
b Following the course of the ICA cranially in transverse orientation reveals that the false lumen extends to the skull base. The image shows the proximal ICA on the left and its distal portion on the right. The true lumen is coded in red (inverted display)

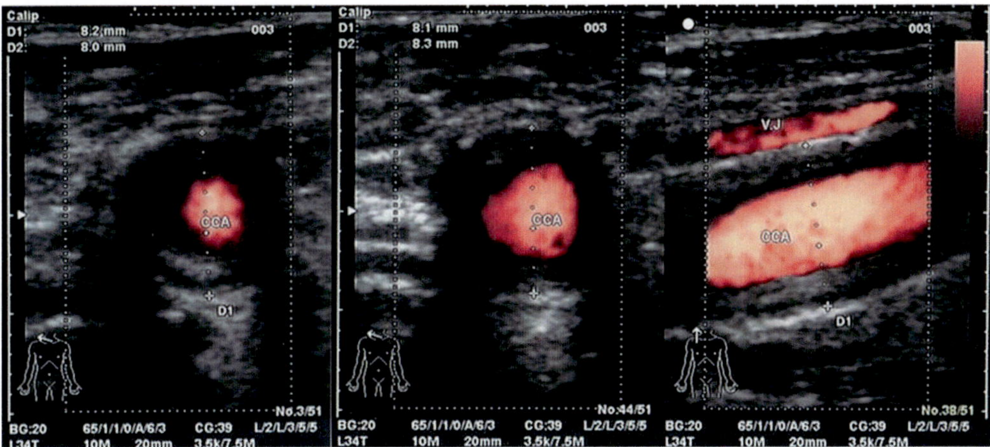

Fig. 5.76 (Atlas) Takayasu's arteritis.
Concentric wall thickening is pathognomonic of arteritis. Takayasu's arteritis predominantly affects the subclavian artery and common carotid artery (CCA). The example shows the CCA in the power Doppler mode. The transverse image (leftmost section) demonstrates concentric diameter reduction (>50%), which involves a long vessel segment. The transverse image in the middle and the longitudinal image on the right obtained after 2 weeks of cortisone treatment show slightly reduced but persistent concentric wall thickening of the CCA

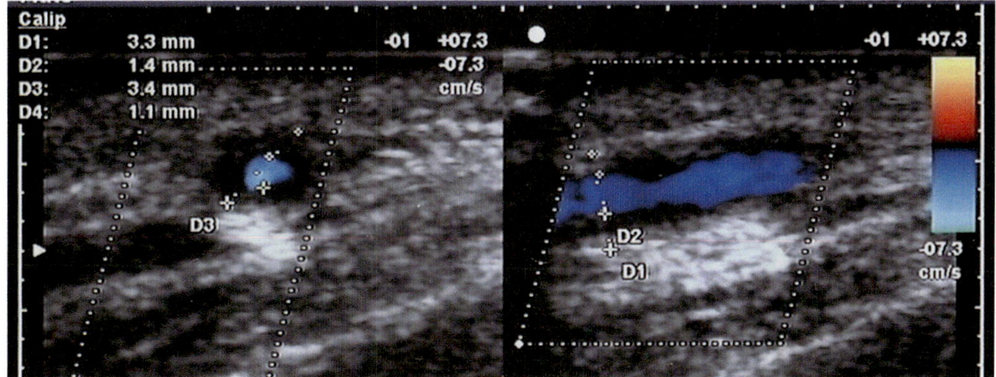

Fig. 5.77 (Atlas) Temporal arteritis.
Transverse (left) and longitudinal (right) images of the temporal artery showing luminal narrowing (size reduction from 3 to 1 mm; calipers) due to inflammatory concentric wall thickening

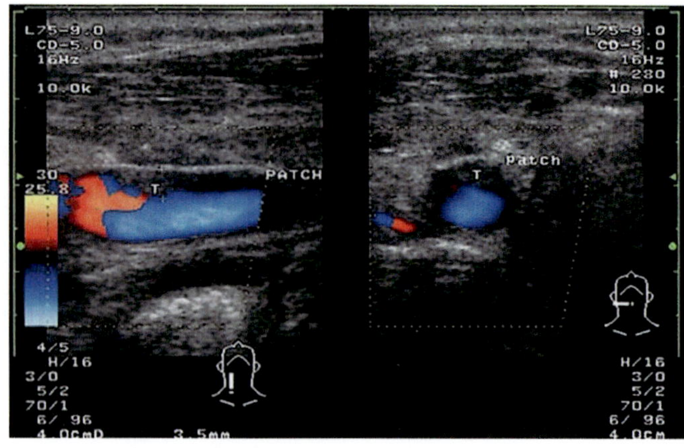

Fig. 5.78 (Atlas) Postoperative follow-up after carotid endarterectomy (CEA).
Postoperatively, there may be luminal narrowing due to thrombotic deposits, in particular when a synthetic patch has been interposed. Thrombotic deposits protruding far into the lumen and causing hemodynamically relevant narrowing are a source of embolism. The patch itself is seen as a bright line (wall near transducer) with a hypoechoic deposit on the luminal side (T)

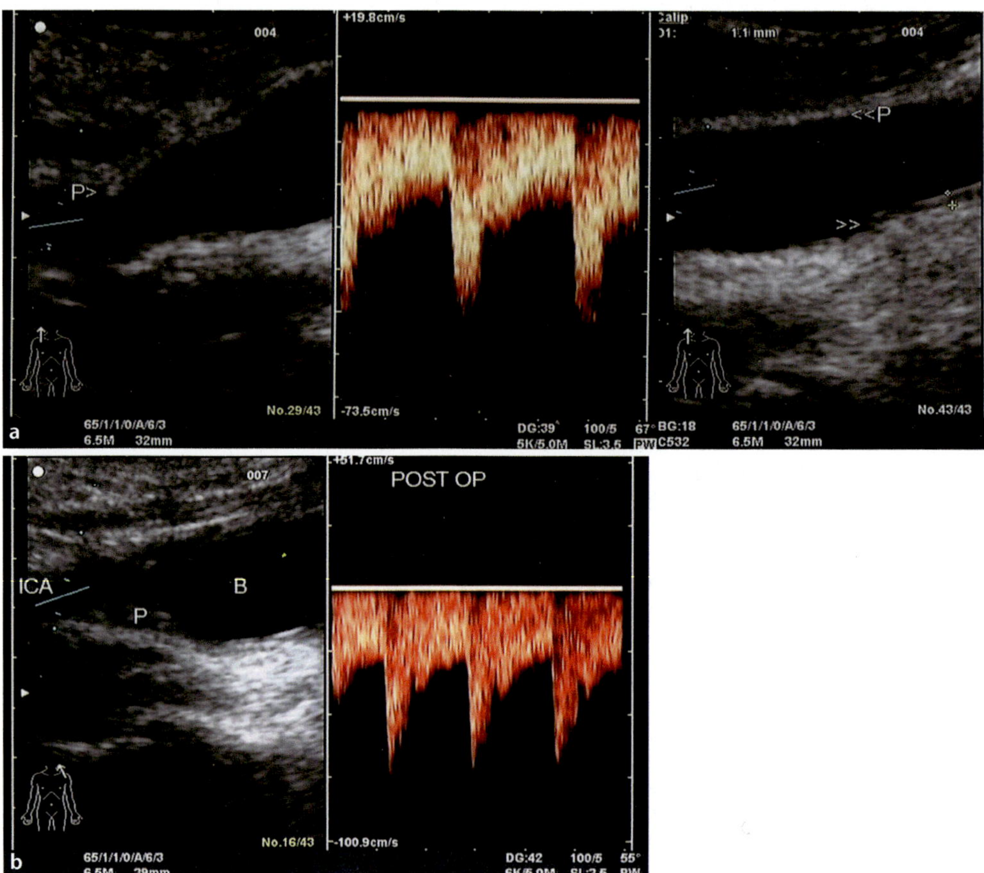

Fig. 5.79a, b (Atlas) Carotid endarterectomy with patch closure.
a Early postoperative sonomorphologic appearance of the vessel wall after carotid endarterectomy (CEA) with patch angioplasty (Dacron patch). The image on the left depicts the transition from the patch (P) to the native internal carotid artery (ICA) with the sample volume for Doppler measurement. The corresponding Doppler waveform indicates normal flow velocities. The image on the right shows the proximal end of CEA and the patch (P) with a step in the far wall at the transition (indicated by double arrowheads). The caliber mismatch is unproblematic, causing no flow obstruction because the larger diameter is downstream. Intima–media thickness (IMT) in the common carotid artery (CCA) is increased to 1.1 mm (calipers).
b At 6-month follow-up after CEA with patch closure, there is evidence of early neointimal formation at the transition from the patched segment to the distal ICA. There is good evaluation of this segment (P) using gray-scale imaging, which shows no hemodynamiclly relevant luminal narrowing (PSV of 90 cm/s)

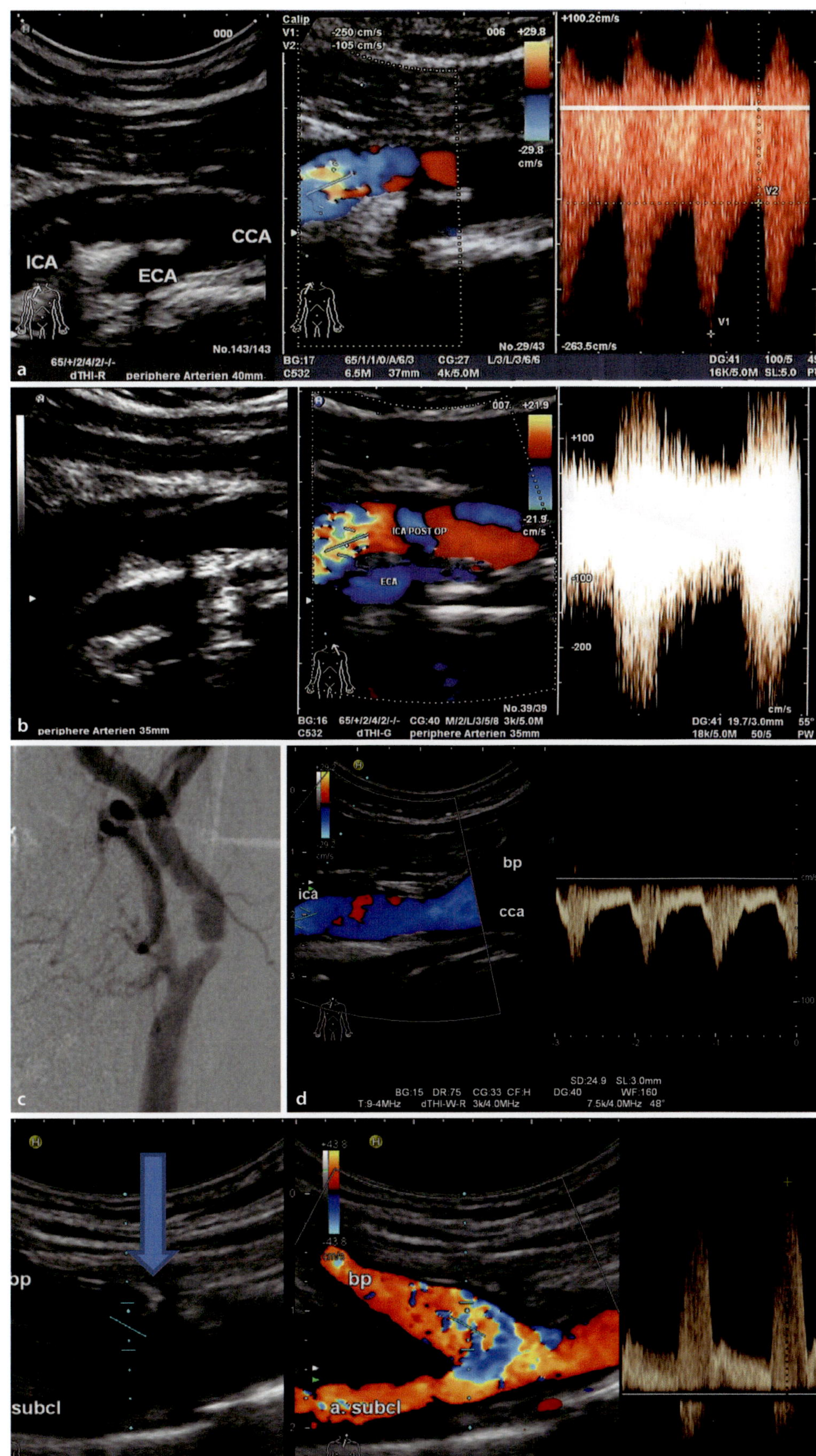

Fig. 5.80a–e (Atlas) Recurrent stenosis after carotid endarterectomy (CEA)

a Postoperative B-mode image (left) after carotid endarterectomy (eversion) shows an intimal flap within the lumen (to the right of the "ICA" label) with aliasing in the color duplex mode (color spillover obscuring the flap). The peak systolic velocity (PSV) of 250 cm/s indicates >70% stenosis (by ECST criteria; see Fig. 5.9b and Table 5.9).

b Thrombosis progressed due to thrombotic deposits and neointimal proliferation within a few weeks (PSV >300 cm/s with very turbulent flow in the stenotic segment).

c Angiogram confirming high-grade stenosis after CEA due to intimal flap and thrombotic deposits.

Anastomotic stenosis after bypass procedure between subclavian artery and ICA for CCA occlusion.

d Doppler waveform from the internal carotid artery (ica) distal to the bypass graft anastomosis shows typical signs of poststenotic flow (delayed systolic rise and slightly reduced PSV of 70 cm/s).

e These findings are attributable to proximal stenosis at the site of anastomosis of the bypass graft (bp) with the subclavian artery (a.subcl). There is aliasing in the color duplex image, and Doppler interrogation demonstrates >70% stenosis (PSV of 350 cm/s). The B-mode image (left) reveals a flap (arrow). This flap is obscured by color spillover in the color duplex mode and was not adequately seen in the angiogram (not shown)

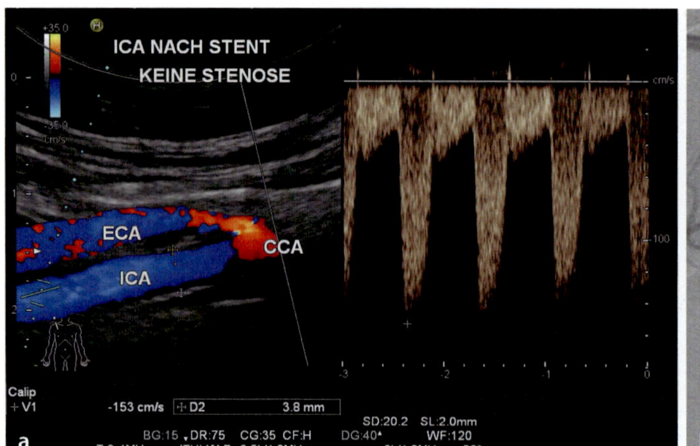

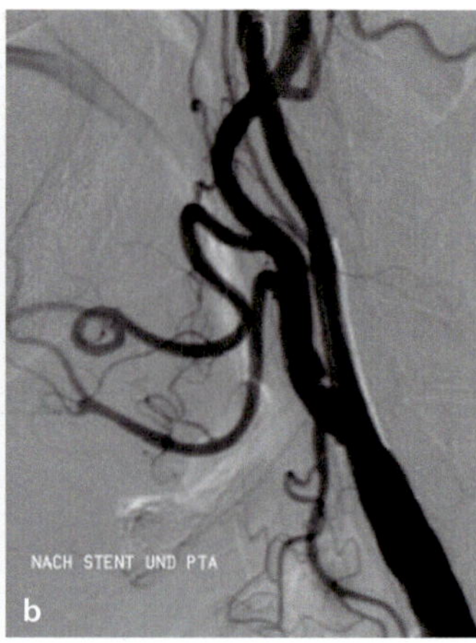

Fig. 5.81a, b (Atlas) Change in pulsatility after carotid artery stenting (CAS).
a Changes in the Doppler waveform after carotid artery stenting (CAS). A long segment of the internal carotid artery (ICA) exhibits an increased peak systolic velocity (PSV) of 153 cm/s and slightly increased pulsatility without evidence of stenosis (3.8 mm stent diameter). The PSV measured in the stented segment would indicate 40% NASCET stenosis and 50–60% ECST stenosis in the native ICA. Here, the higher PSV and greater pulsatility are due to the smaller lumen and rigidity of the stented segment, respectively.
b Angiogram without signs of residual or recurrent stenosis in the stented ICA. The patent lumen within the stent is smaller than that of the native artery

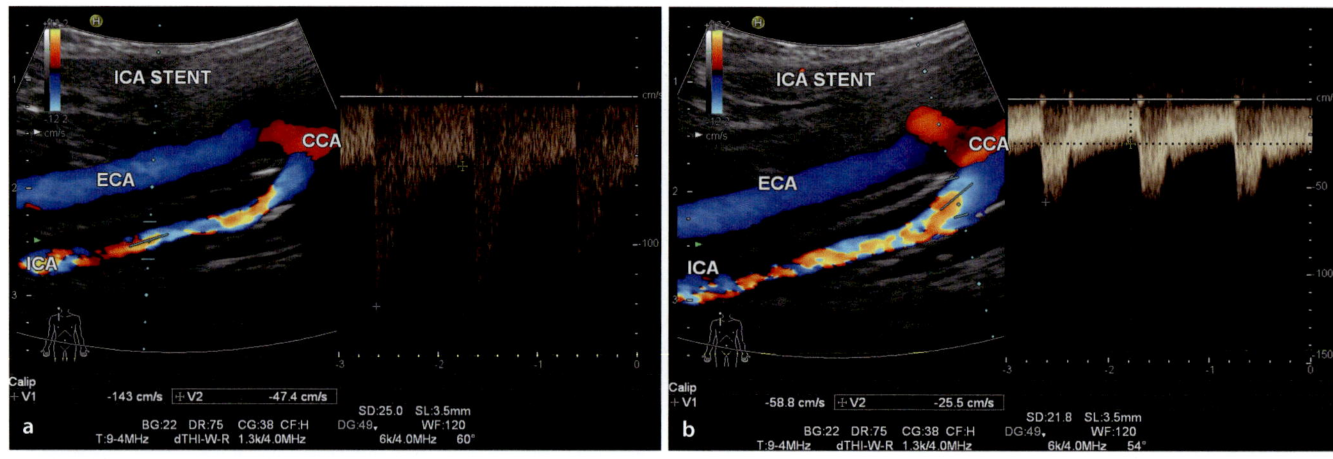

Fig. 5.82a, b (Atlas) ICA in-stent restenosis – neointimal proliferation.
Examination of the internal carotid artery (ICA) after stenting shows long-stretched narrowing of the stented lumen due to neointimal proliferation. The morphologic appearance suggests 50% lumen reduction
a. The peak systolic velocity (PSV) measured in this segment is 143 cm/s (which is similar to the PSV measured in the nonstenotic stented ICA, see Fig. 5.81a). However, a PSV ratio of 2 is calculated from this PSV and the PSV of 58 cm/s measured in the proximal stented segment (bulb)
b. A ratio of 2 corresponds to approx. 50% stenosis according to the continuity equation. The PSV ratio allows reliable grading of in-stent restenosis because the stent creates a straight channel of uniform caliber, and there a no hemodynamic effects of arteries arising from the stented segment. This example illustrates that the PSV ratio is a more reliable parameter than absolute intrastenotic PSV for grading carotid in-stent restenosis

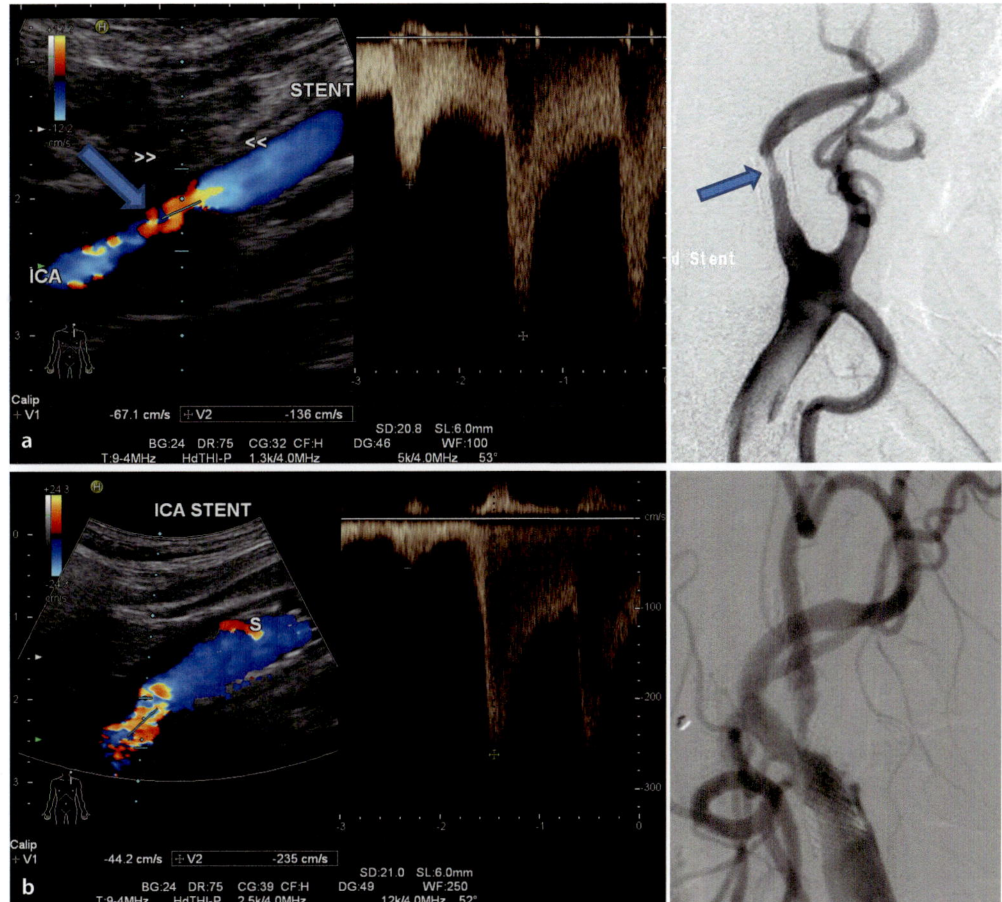

◻ Fig. 5.83a, b (Atlas) Grading of in-stent restenosis – PSV ratio.
a In-stent restenosis of the internal carotid artery (ICA) can be identified and graded sonographically by obtaining a continuous spectral Doppler tracing of the stented arterial segment. Because a stented segment has a rather constant diameter, determination of the peak systolic velocity (PSV) ratio in the stented portion allows reliable identification and grading of in-stent restenosis. In the case presented, the Doppler tracing shows a focal increase in PSV from 67.1 to 138 cm/s in the stented segment, indicating >50% stenosis. Conversely, the absolute intrastenotic PSV of 138 cm/s is still below the PSV cutoff for hemodynamically relevant in-stent restenosis identified by ROC curve analysis. The Doppler waveform shown was obtained by continuous spectral Doppler recording from the proximal to the distal stented ICA segment (indicated by ">> <<" in the color duplex image). The left portion of the waveform reflects the hemodynamic situation upstream of the stenosis, while the right portion shows the abrupt increase in PSV at the site of in-stent stenosis. The corresponding angiogram shows in-stent restenosis at the distal stent end (arrow).
b High-grade in-stent restenosis 1.5 cm upstream of the origin of the external carotid artery with a PSV ratio of 5 (calculated from an intrastenotic PSV of 268 cm/s and a prestenotic PSV of 44 cm/s). The abrupt increase in PSV was identified by continuous spectral Doppler recording moving the tilted transducer (at an angle of 52°) along the artery in a cranial direction. The angiogram shows 80% ICA in-stent restenosis (projection plane)

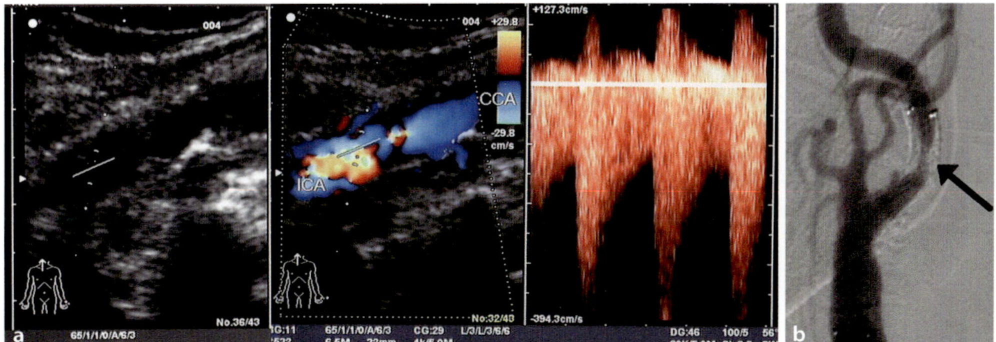

◻ Fig. 5.84a, b (Atlas) High-grade in-stent restenosis after carotid artery stenting (CAS).
a High-grade in-stent restenosis 2 years after carotid artery stenting (CAS). Mixed echogenic and echolucent plaque with an intrastenotic peak systolic velocity (PSV) of almost 4 m/s.
b Angiogram: High-grade in-stent restenosis of the ICA, confirming the ultrasound findings presented in **a**

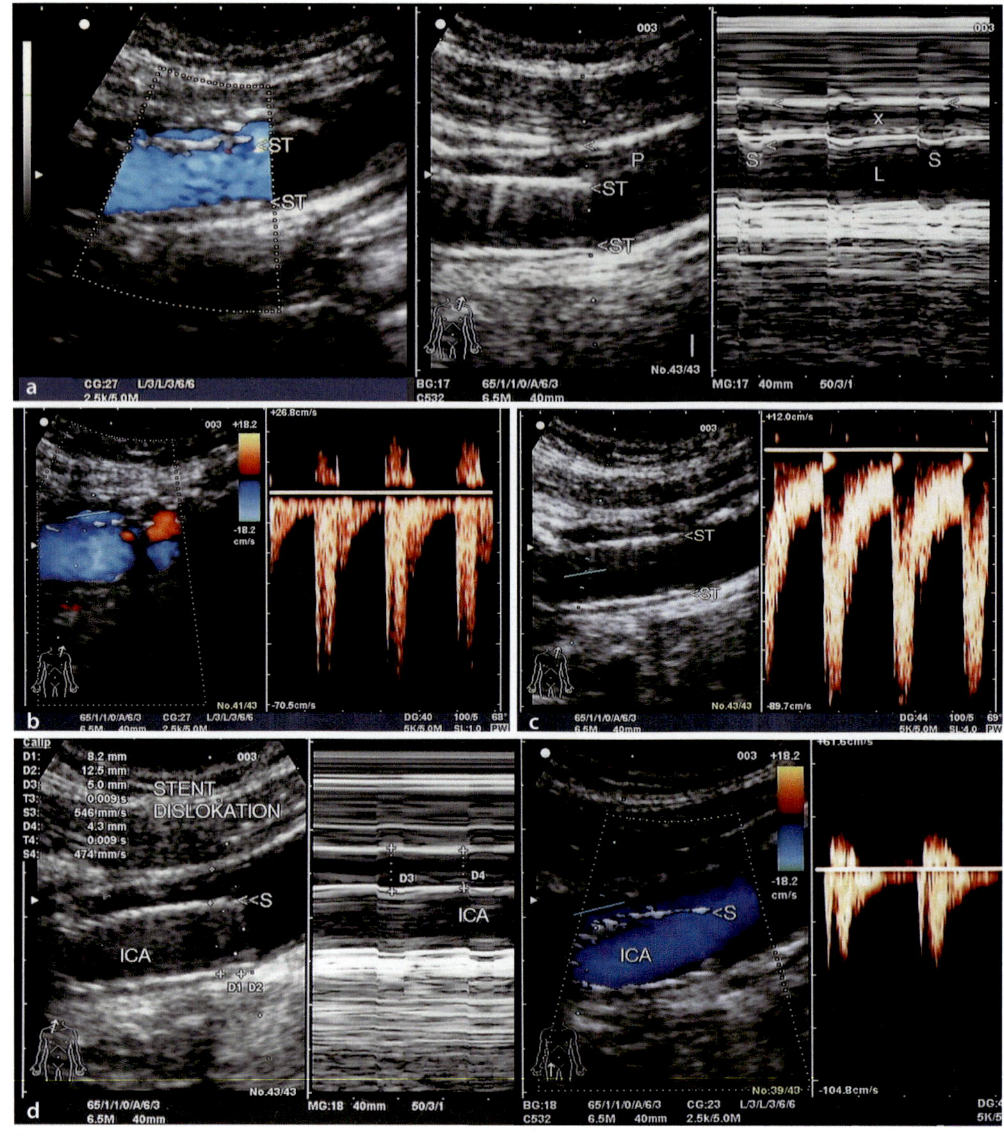

Fig. 5.85a–d (Atlas) Stent dislocation.
a Longitudinal image (left) and time-motion image (right) showing dislocated stent (ST) in the internal carotid artery (ICA). There appears to be a lumen with blood flow between the stent and the vessel wall, as indicated by flow signals. Note that the stent is subject to pulsatility effects (in the time–motion display), showing paradoxical stent motion as the stent is compressed by the flowing blood and pressure in the false lumen (X) during systole (S).
b The Doppler waveform from the false lumen between the stent and the arterial wall demonstrates flow along the stent toward the head with a peak systolic velocity (PSV) of 60 cm/s.
c The stent lumen is not compromised (PSV of 90 cm/s).
d The patient initially refused a repeat intervention and the stent became even more dislodged with an increase in the size of the lumen between the stent and the arterial wall. In the gray-scale image (leftmost image), a long segment of the stent including its end is seen to be detached from the arterial wall closer to the transducer, while it tightly adheres to the opposite wall. The color flow image and spectral Doppler show flow between the detached stent and the native arterial wall. The time-motion mode (which displays movement of structures over time) shows pulsatile movement of the detached stent, resulting in a variable distance between the stent and the native arterial wall of 5 mm (D3) during systole and 4.2 mm in late diastole (D4). The Doppler waveform shows more pulsatile flow in the lumen between the stent and the native arterial wall than within the stent

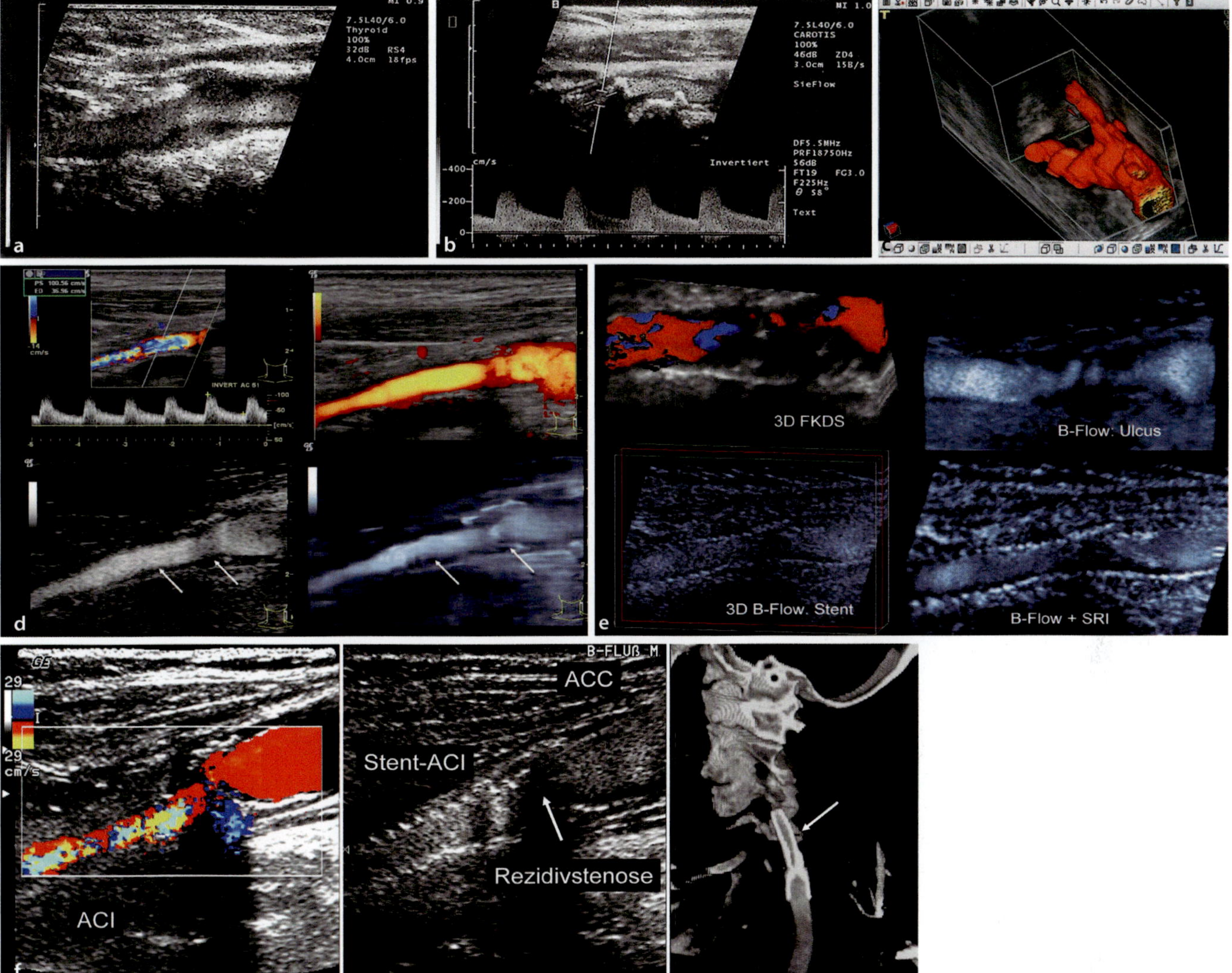

Fig. 5.86a–f (Atlas) Alternative ultrasound techniques: B-flow mode, 3D ultrasound.
a B-mode flow imaging analyzes the amplitude signal of the reflecting particles in the interval between two pulses. The movement of reflecting particles is encoded in terms of flow direction, velocity, and number. A narrowed vessel segment is depicted with higher signal intensity as a result of the larger number of reflecting particles and faster flow due to the reduced cross-sectional area. In addition to hemodynamic parameters, the B-flow mode also provides morphologic images with high resolution of plaques and the vessel wall, enabling good differentiation of the plaque surface and surface irregularities (ulceration) from the patent lumen. The image presented shows plaque on the near and far walls of the carotid bulb. The luminal narrowing resulting from these plaques is indicated by the higher signal intensity of the perfused lumen in this segment.
b Advantages of B-flow imaging are its little angle dependence and the good morphologic discrimination between vessel wall and patent lumen. Its major drawback is its susceptibility to artifacts induced by the highly pulsatile wall motion that occurs in the presence of high-grade stenosis caused by plaque. Like all ultrasound techniques, the B-flow mode is impaired by signal scattering and acoustic shadowing due to calcified structures. This is why B-flow imaging has not replaced the hemodynamic spectral Doppler technique in detecting and characterizing vascular pathology. The example illustrates how the B-flow image is degraded by acoustic shadowing from calcified plaque. The higher signal in the vessel lumen indicates the stenotic jet. Still, spectral Doppler interrogation continues to be the most reliable method for quantifying high-grade stenosis.
c Three-dimensional displays can provide a good overview of vascular anatomy and relationships in the presence of atypical variants or elongation. At its current state of development, however, this technique contributes little to stenosis grading and evaluation of plaque morphology (see **e**). Due to artifacts caused by vessel pulsation and atherosclerotic plaques, 3D displays have no advantage over 2D displays in answering relevant angiologic and vascular surgical questions. The example depicts the CCA on the right with the superior thyroid artery above and the ICA (bottom) and ECA (top) on the left.
d–f B-flow imaging for evaluation of in-stent restenosis (Images **d–f** courtesy of M. Jung, from Schäberle 2011).
d Color duplex with spectral Doppler analysis (top left) and power Doppler mode (top right) shows normal findings after carotid artery stenting (CAS). The B-flow mode (bottom left) and B-flow with speckle reduction imaging (SRI) (bottom right) confirm that there is no relevant luminal narrowing but the images do not depict wall deposits or neointimal proliferation within the stent.
e High-grade ICA stenosis before (top) and after (bottom) CAS. B-flow imaging (top right) is superior in visualizing the plaque surface and ulcer compared with the color duplex mode (top left: 3D reconstruction). The images after CAS were obtained using the B-flow mode (bottom left) and the B-flow mode with SRI (bottom right); the B-flow mode is comparable to contrast-enhanced ultrasound (CEUS) in terms of stent delineation and allows morphologic stenosis grading.
f Color duplex image, B-flow image, and CT angiogram of high-grade ICA in-stent restenosis. Like all ultrasound techniques, B-flow imaging is degraded by artifacts such as acoustic shadowing, which limits morphologic stenosis grading using this technique

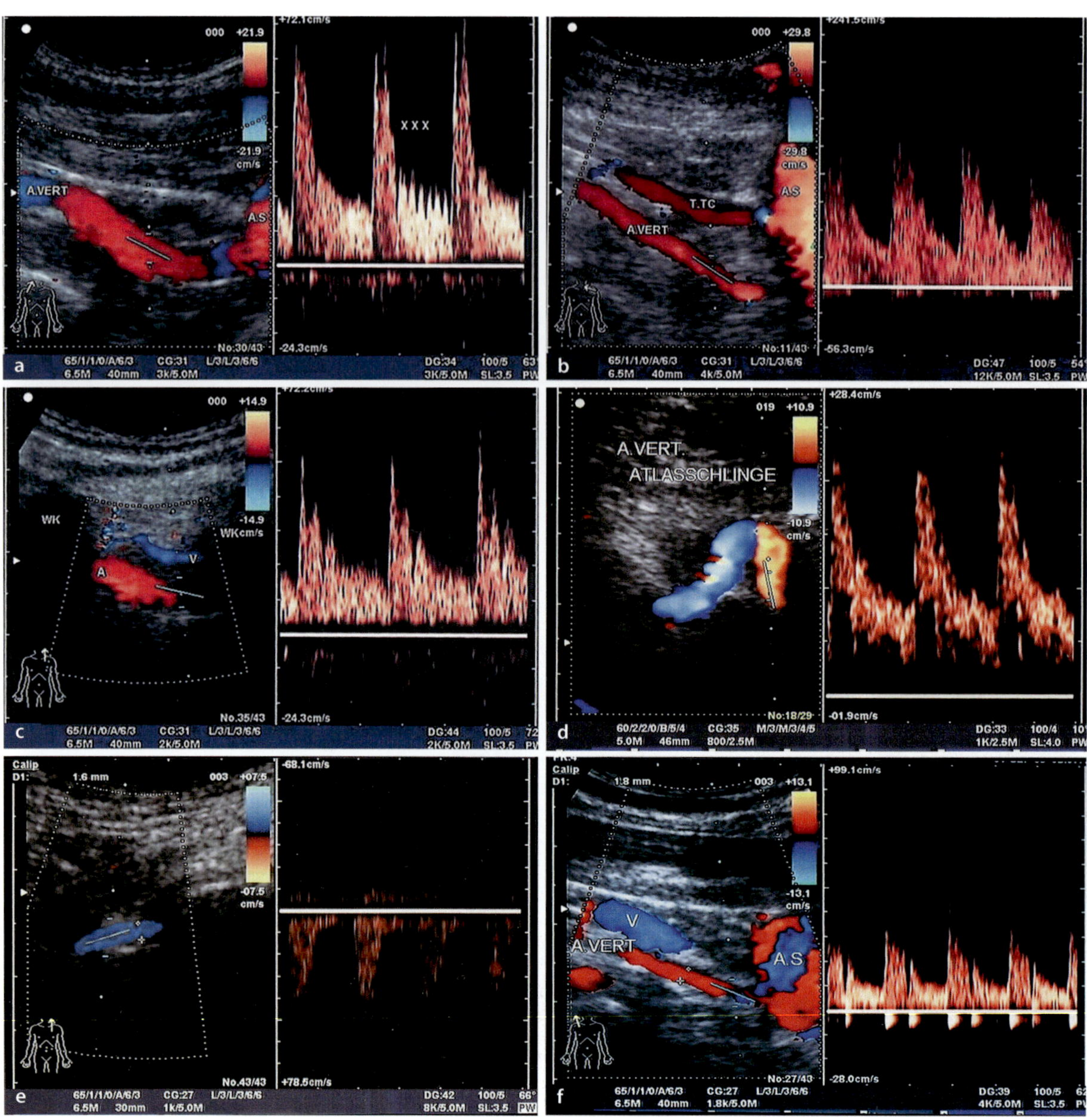

Fig. 5.87a–g (Atlas) Vertebral artery.

a Origin of the vertebral artery from the subclavian artery interrogated with the transducer in the supraclavicular position. The flow profile is similar to that of the internal carotid artery (ICA). The identity of the vertebral artery is confirmed by transmission of the oscillations elicited by tapping the mastoid area (as illustrated in the waveform shown).

b Care must also be taken not to confuse the thyrocervical trunk (T.TC) with the vertebral artery (A.VERT). It supplies the thyroid and therefore has a similar waveform and comes more easily into view, in particular when the insonation conditions are poor, because its origin from the subclavian artery is closer to the transducer than the origin of the vertebral artery.

c Vertebral artery coded in red between two transverse processes (WK). The vein (V) is depicted closer to the transducer with flow in blue.

d Spectral Doppler imaging of the vertebral artery by interrogation of the atlas loop (transducer placed below the mastoid and directed toward the contralateral eye) stems from the era of CW Doppler ultrasound and has become less important with the advent of duplex ultrasound. However, this approach is useful to sample the vertebral artery Doppler spectrum during functional testing performed to diagnose postural compression of the vertebral artery by a vertebral body. In this setting, evaluation of the atlas loop enables follow-up of postocclusive waveform changes in a fairly fixed position during movements of the neck. As with CW Doppler, changes in flow direction are reflected in the Doppler waveform. In the example, there is flow toward the transducer in the proximal portion of the atlas loop. In the distal atlas loop, flow is away from the transducer.

Hypoplastic vertebral artery.

e Hypoplastic vertebral artery with a diameter of 1.6 mm and reduced flow velocity, in particular during diastole (PSV of <40 cm/s and EDV of <5 cm/s). A compensatory increase in flow is measured in the contralateral vertebral artery (PSV of 90 cm/s and diameter of 4 mm; not shown).

f, g Vertebral artery hypoplasia.

f Hypoplastic vertebral artery (A. VERT) with a diameter of 1.9 mm depicted at the origin from the subclavian artery (A.S).

g The contralateral vertebral artery, also shown at the origin from the subclavian artery (A.S), is hyperplastic (diameter of 4.7 mm). The Doppler waveform from the hypoplastic vertebral artery shows more pulsatile flow. Individuals with a very hypoplastic vertebral artery have an increased risk of brain stem infarction. Moreover, as in the patient shown, certain rotational movements of the head can cause transient brain stem syndrome resulting from intermittent compression of the contralateral hyperplastic artery on its course through the foramina. This can cause reproducible episodes of vertigo with certain head positions, which will disappear after a few seconds when the head is returned to its normal position

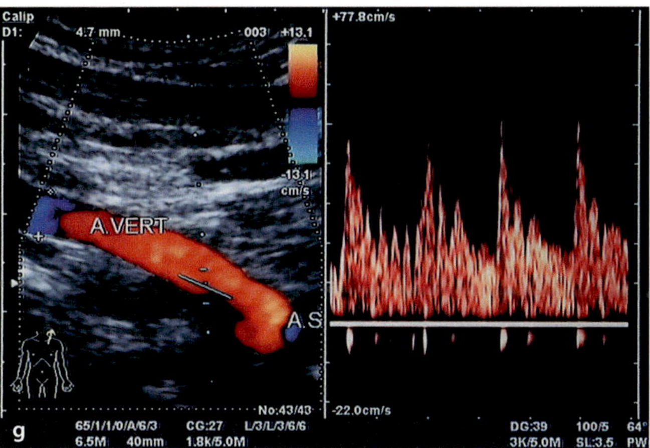

Fig. 5.87 (continued)

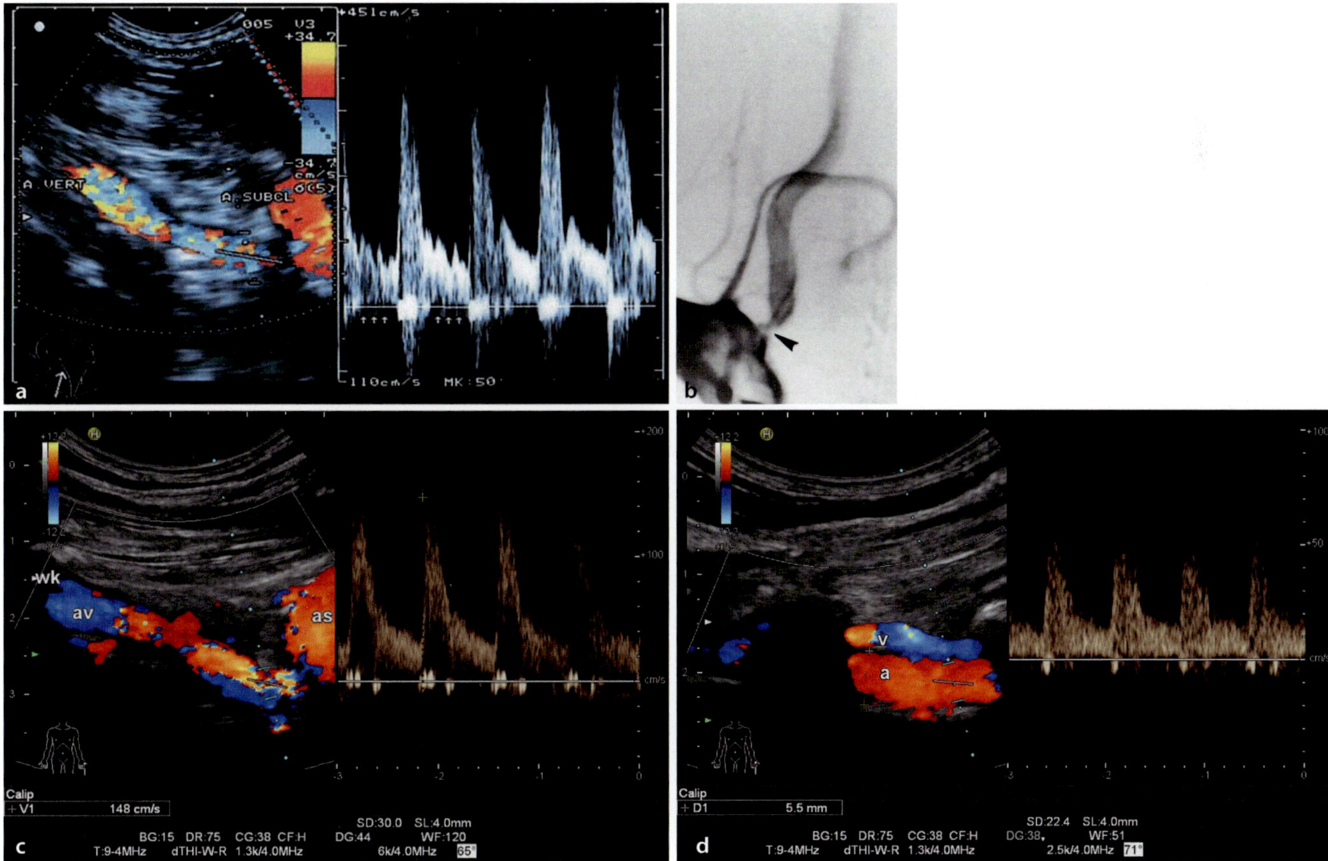

Fig. 5.88a–d (Atlas) Vertebral artery origin stenosis.
a Color duplex imaging shows aliasing due to turbulence at the origin of the vertebral artery (coursing leftward in the display) from the subclavian artery (A.SUBCL). At the origin, color coding is absent from the lumen due to plaque with acoustic shadowing. The spectral waveform documents the stenosis with a peak systolic velocity (PSV) of 320 cm/s and an end-diastolic velocity (EDV) of 80 cm/s. The vertebral artery is distinguished from the thyrocervical trunk, which has a similar flow profile, by the transmission of the oscillations from rhythmical tapping of the distal vertebral artery below the mastoid (indicated by arrows in the waveform).
b Angiogram: Stenosis (arrowhead) at origin of vertebral artery.
Grading of vertebral artery stenosis.
c Grading of vertebral artery stenosis based on absolute PSV cutoffs (as used for grading ICA stenosis) is unreliable due to the wide normal PSV variation in the vertebral arteries. In the case presented, there is borderline stenosis with a PSV of 150 cm/s. This case also illustrates the difficulties in achieving adequate Doppler angle correction in the arched course of the vertebral artery. The ratio of intrastenotic to poststenotic PSV allows reliable grading of mild to moderate stenosis but not of high-grade stenosis.
d A rather high poststenotic PSV of 60 cm/s with a slightly delayed systolic rise is measured in the V2 segment, and the resulting PSV ratio indicates approx. 60% stenosis

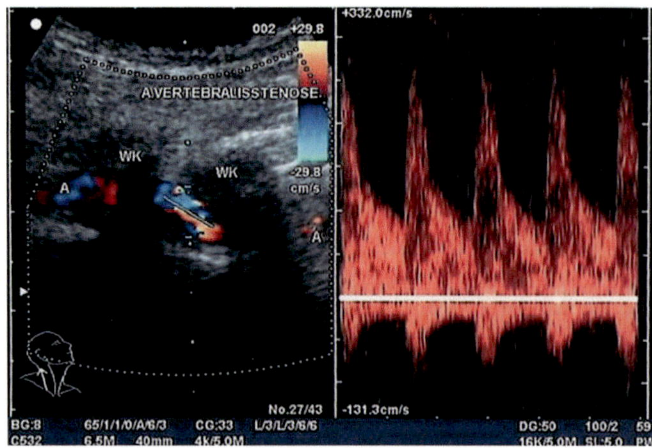

Fig. 5.89 (Atlas) Distal vertebral artery stenosis.
Atherosclerotic vertebral artery stenosis typically occurs at the origin from the subclavian artery. A more distal stenosis (in the V2 segment between C4 and C5, as in the example presented) often has other causes such as constriction of the passageway through the transverse processes by exostosis or dissection. An increase in flow velocity (here 250 cm/s) indicates stenosis only if it is localized. Increased flow throughout the vertebral artery suggests a compensatory increase in perfusion due to hypoplasia of the contralateral branch or atherosclerotic occlusion of other arteries supplying the brain

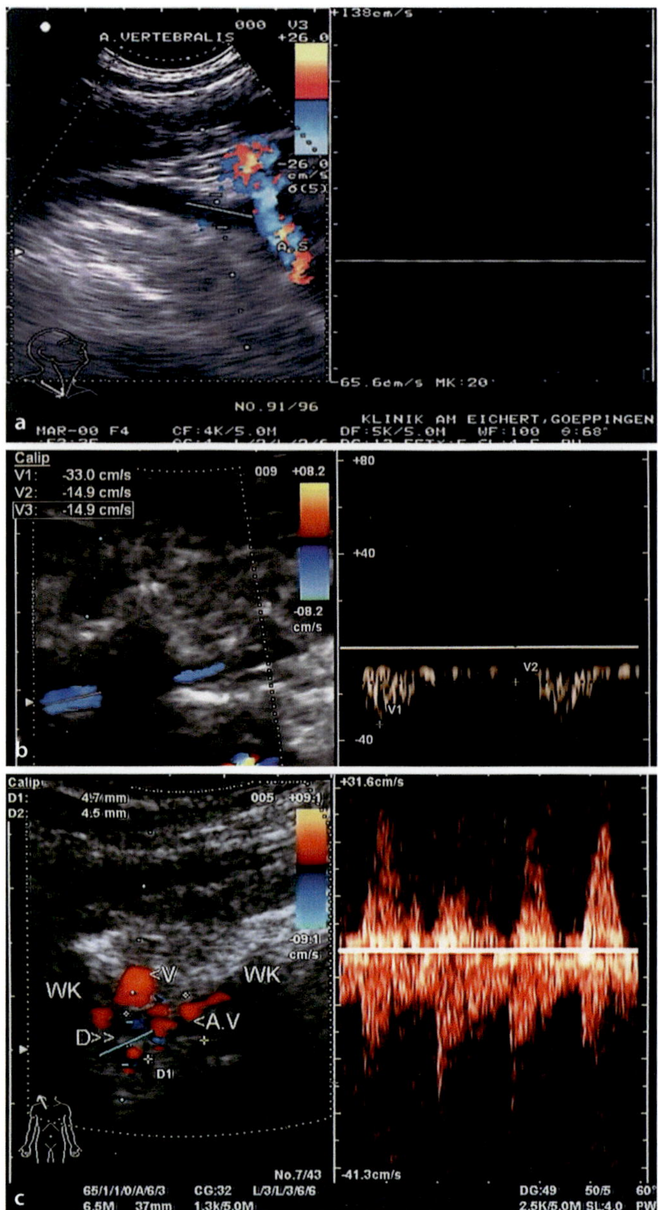

Fig. 5.90a–c (Atlas) Vertebral artery occlusion.
a Both color duplex and spectral Doppler fail to depict flow signals in a tubular structure arising from the subclavian artery. The course of the structure corresponds to that of the vertebral artery, and the findings are consistent with vertebral artery occlusion.
b Thin vertebral artery (2.2 mm) with refilling through spinal vessels just before the atlas loop and postocclusive flow (delayed systolic rise and slow flow with a PSV of 32 cm/s).
Vertebral artery dissection.
c Following a failed endovascular intervention, an intimal flap (D) is visible in the vertebral artery between the transverse processes. At the site of sampling, flow in the true and false lumina is in opposite directions (coded in red and blue; above and below the baseline in the Doppler waveform; V = vertebral vein). The vertebral artery lumen is indicated by calipers; the false lumen is patent in the left part of the image and thrombosed in the right part

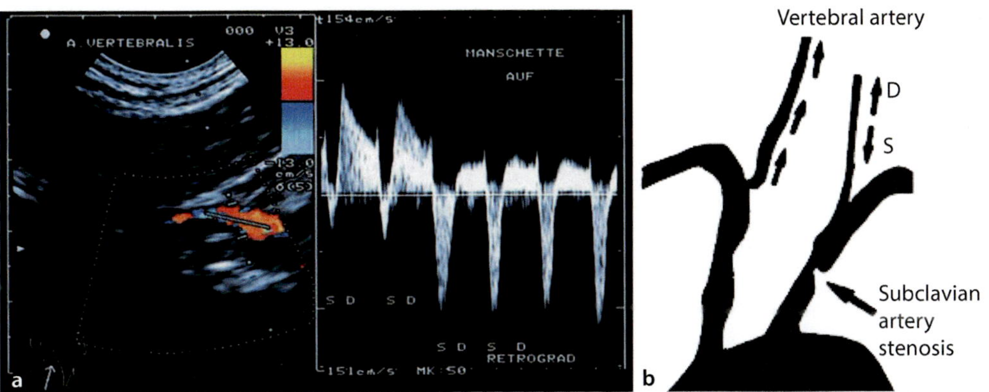

Fig. 5.91a, b (Atlas) Subclavian steal syndrome with to-and-fro flow in the vertebral artery.
a The steal phenomenon in the vertebral artery varies with the severity of subclavian artery stenosis. The respective changes can be reproduced during the examination using an arm cuff to induce and release ischemia while recording a Doppler waveform. To-and-fro flow may be preserved and only change from primarily cranial flow to primarily central flow (toward subclavian artery. In the case shown, compression of the ipsilateral arm results in high diastolic flow in the cranial direction with only little retrograde flow in systole. Upon deflation of the arm cuff, there is a change in to-and-fro flow with a large retrograde systolic flow component (S) and only little antegrade flow in diastole (D).
b Diagram of to-and-fro flow in the vertebral artery in ipsilateral subclavian artery stenosis

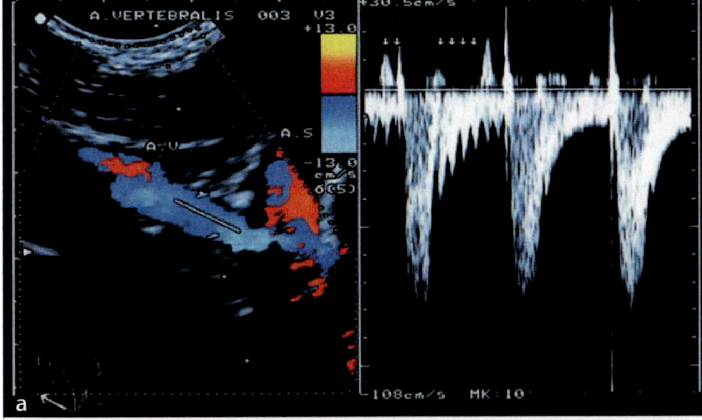

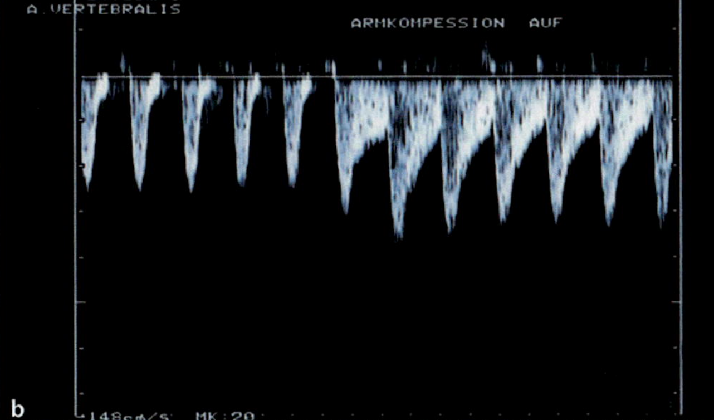

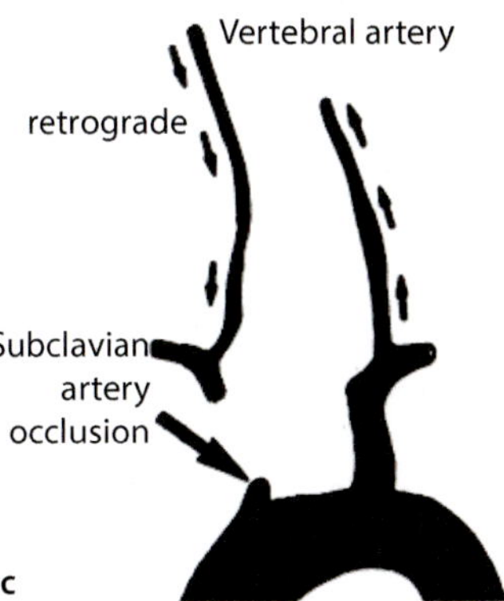

Fig. 5.92a–c (Atlas) Subclavian steal syndrome with retrograde flow in the vertebral artery.
a In this patient with severe subclavian steal syndrome, retrograde flow from the ipsilateral vertebral artery (A.V) into the subclavian artery (A.S) is already seen at rest (displayed in blue). This is verified by the spectral Doppler tracing with confirmation of the identity of the vertebral artery by transmission of oscillations from tapping in the mastoid region. The subclavian artery is occluded proximal to the site of entry of the vertebral artery.
b Following ischemia upon release of the arm cuff, the Doppler waveform shows a marked increase in retrograde flow, in particular in diastole.
c Diagram of retrograde flow in the vertebral artery in ipsilateral subclavian artery occlusion with complete subclavian steal syndrome

5

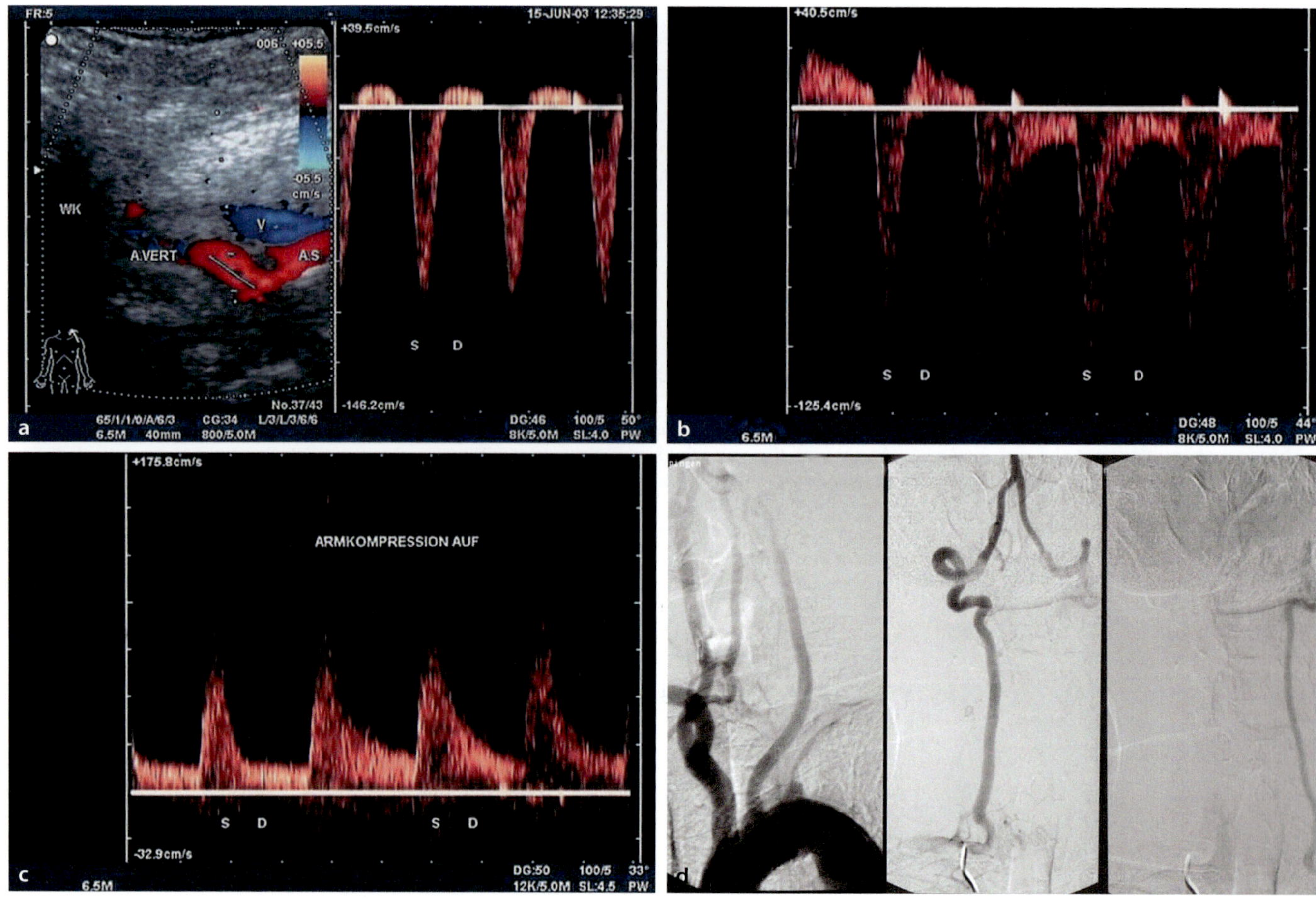

Fig. 5.93a–d (Atlas) Subclavian steal syndrome with vertebrovertebral crossover.
a Image showing the origin of the vertebral artery in central subclavian artery occlusion. The spectral waveform recorded at the origin of the vertebral artery (A.VERT) from the subclavian artery (A.S) demonstrates to-and-fro flow with a retrograde systolic component (away from transducer, toward heart) and an antegrade diastolic component (toward transducer, toward brain). The passage of the artery through the transverse process (WK) is shown at the left margin of the image.
b In the provocative test, compression of the ipsilateral brachial artery with reduction of blood flow into the arm arteries leads to an increase in antegrade diastolic flow in the ipsilateral vertebral artery compared to rest (see **a**). Ischemia induced by release of the cuff (mid-portion of the waveform) results in a change from to-and-fro flow to a constant reversed flow from the vertebral artery into the subclavian artery (away from transducer).
c An increase in systolic and diastolic flow velocity (S = systole, D = diastole) in the contralateral vertebral upon release of the cuff around the brachial artery on the side of the occluded subclavian artery proves vertebrovertebral crossover in subclavian steal syndrome. In the example shown, the increase in velocity is not very pronounced, suggesting that there are other collateral routes to bypass the occluded subclavian artery.
d Angiogram with depiction of contrast medium crossover in occlusion of the left subclavian artery. The temporal course of the contrast medium passage shows flow from the right subclavian artery (left) into the right vertebral artery (middle) and into the left vertebral artery (right)

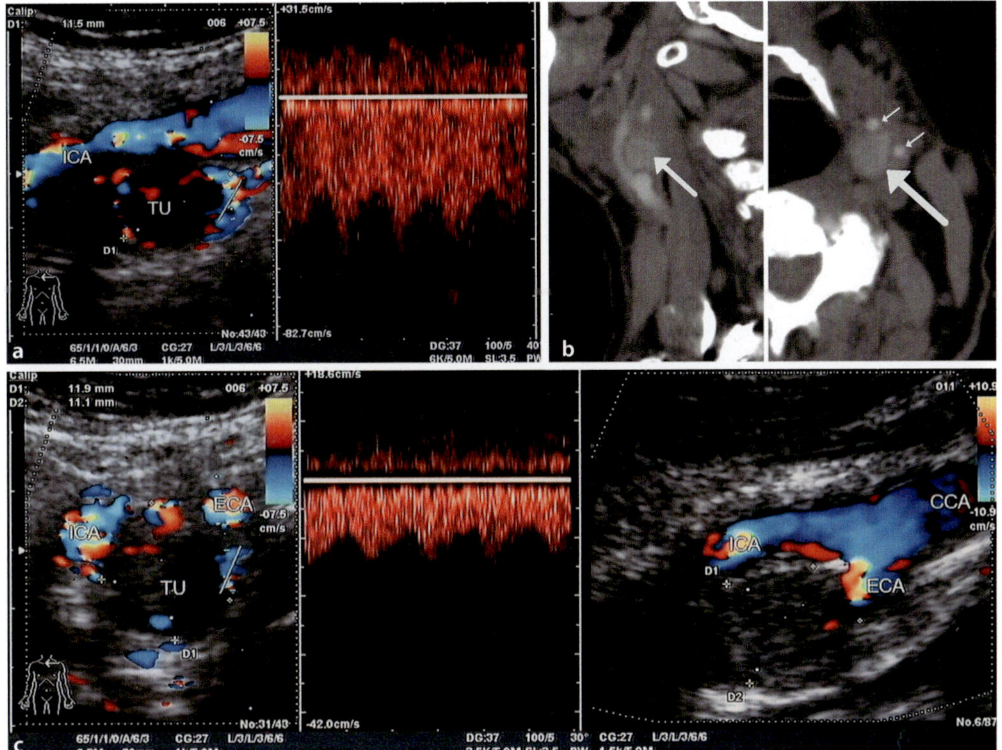

Fig. 5.94a–c (Atlas) Carotid body tumor.
a Ultrasound shows a rather well vascularized carotid body tumor (TU) supplied by the external carotid artery (ECA). There is relatively high flow in the feeding artery with a peak systolic velocity (PSV) of >80 cm/s. The tumor is hypoechoic and measures 11 × 18 mm.
b Longitudinal and axial computed tomography images of the glomus tumor (large arrow); small arrows indicate the internal carotid artery (ICA) and ECA.
c Following transarterial tumor embolization in this 82-year-old patient, perfusion in the tumor is markedly reduced (TU) and a patent feeder arising from the ECA has a PSV of only 15 cm/s. A growing carotid body tumor typically splays the carotid bifurcation. Lateral growth, as in this patient, is less common. Even less common are carotid body tumors encasing the vessels or developing in the back of the neck. A carotid body tumor in atypical location, as in the case presented here, must be differentiated from lymphoma (which is more common). The primary criterion on duplex ultrasound is good vascularization (transverse view on the left, longitudinal view on the right)

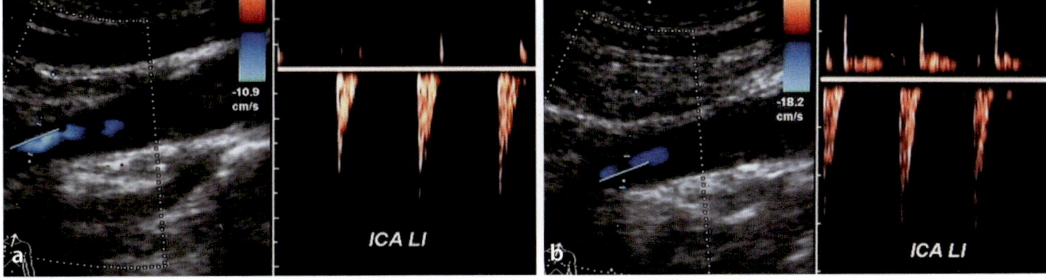

Fig. 5.95a, b (Atlas) Diagnosis of brain death.
Diastolic flow velocity determines the pulsatility of blood flow, and this in turn is governed by vessel wall elasticity and especially by the degree of peripheral resistance. In the carotid territory, peripheral resistance can increase when there is an increase in intracranial pressure, and diastolic flow velocity reflects diastolic blood pressure as a function of intracranial pressure. An increase in intracranial pressure therefore causes a decrease in diastolic flow velocity, and the end-diastolic flow component is eliminated when intracranial pressure matches diastolic pressure. This can result in a flow signal resembling postocclusive flow (as shown in **a**): high pulsatility, no diastolic flow, and markedly reduced peak systolic velocity (PSV) (20 cm/s in the example, knocking waveform). The pressure situation can lead to to-and-fro flow with markedly reduced orthograde flow velocity (PSV of 30 cm/s in **b**) and retrograde diastolic flow. To-and-fro flow or a waveform showing only early diastolic peaks indicates cerebral circulatory arrest

Visceral and Retroperitoneal Vessels

W. Schäberle, *Ultrasonography in Vascular Diagnosis*, https://doi.org/10.1007/978-3-319-64997-9_6

6.1 Abdominal Aorta, Visceral and Renal Arteries

6.1.1 Vascular Anatomy

6.1.1.1 Aorta

The abdominal aorta begins at the level of the diaphragm, crossing it via the aortic hiatus at the T12 vertebral level, and descends in front of or slightly to the left of the vertebral column. The diameter of the aorta decreases on its downward course from 25 to 20 mm. A diameter of up to 30 mm as a result of age-related dilatation is considered normal. An abrupt increase in diameter to more than 1.5 times that of the normal proximal segment is regarded as evidence of an aneurysm. The abdominal aorta divides into the two common iliac arteries at the L4/L5 level. The three major sources of intestinal blood supply are the celiac trunk, the superior mesenteric artery, and the inferior mesenteric artery. These visceral branches arise from the anterior aspect of the aorta. Their pattern of supply is complex and has numerous variants. The lumbar arteries originate from the lateral aspect, and the two renal arteries course in a retroperitoneal direction. The arteries arising from the aorta, from superior to inferior, are described in detail below (◘ Fig. 6.1).

6.1.1.2 Visceral Arteries

Just below the aortic aperture of the diaphragm, the aorta gives off the celiac trunk, or celiac artery, which, after 2–3 cm, divides into its two main branches, the common hepatic and splenic arteries. The common hepatic artery courses between the head of the pancreas and the lower edge of the liver into the hepatoduodenal ligament, where it gives off the right gastric artery and gastroduodenal artery, two important collaterals that connect to the superior mesenteric artery. It then continues to the liver as the proper hepatic artery. The splenic artery is in part very tortuous as it courses along the upper border of the pancreas to the splenic hilum and supplies not only the spleen but also the body and tail of the pancreas as well as the greater curvature of the stomach.

Approx. 0.5–2 cm below the celiac trunk lies the origin of the superior mesenteric artery at the L1/L2 level. It arises anteriorly at an acute angle of 15–30° relative to the aorta, and its proximal segment runs parallel to the aorta between the pancreas and renal vein. After approx. 4–5 cm, it gives off the inferior pancreaticoduodenal and middle colic arteries, which supply the proximal two-thirds of the transverse colon. The distal superior mesenteric artery divides into the jejunal, ileal, and ileocolic arteries supplying the small intestine.

Many anatomic variants exist. In 55% of the population, the celiac trunk gives off the hepatic artery and splenic artery (type I according to Michel's classification). In type II (10%), the replaced left hepatic artery arises from the left gastric artery. In type III (11%), the replaced right hepatic artery, which supplies the right hepatic lobe, arises from the superior mesenteric artery (see ◘ Figs. 6.3e and 6.52b (Atlas)). These two common variants lead to altered hemodynamics at the origin of the superior mesenteric artery (larger diastolic

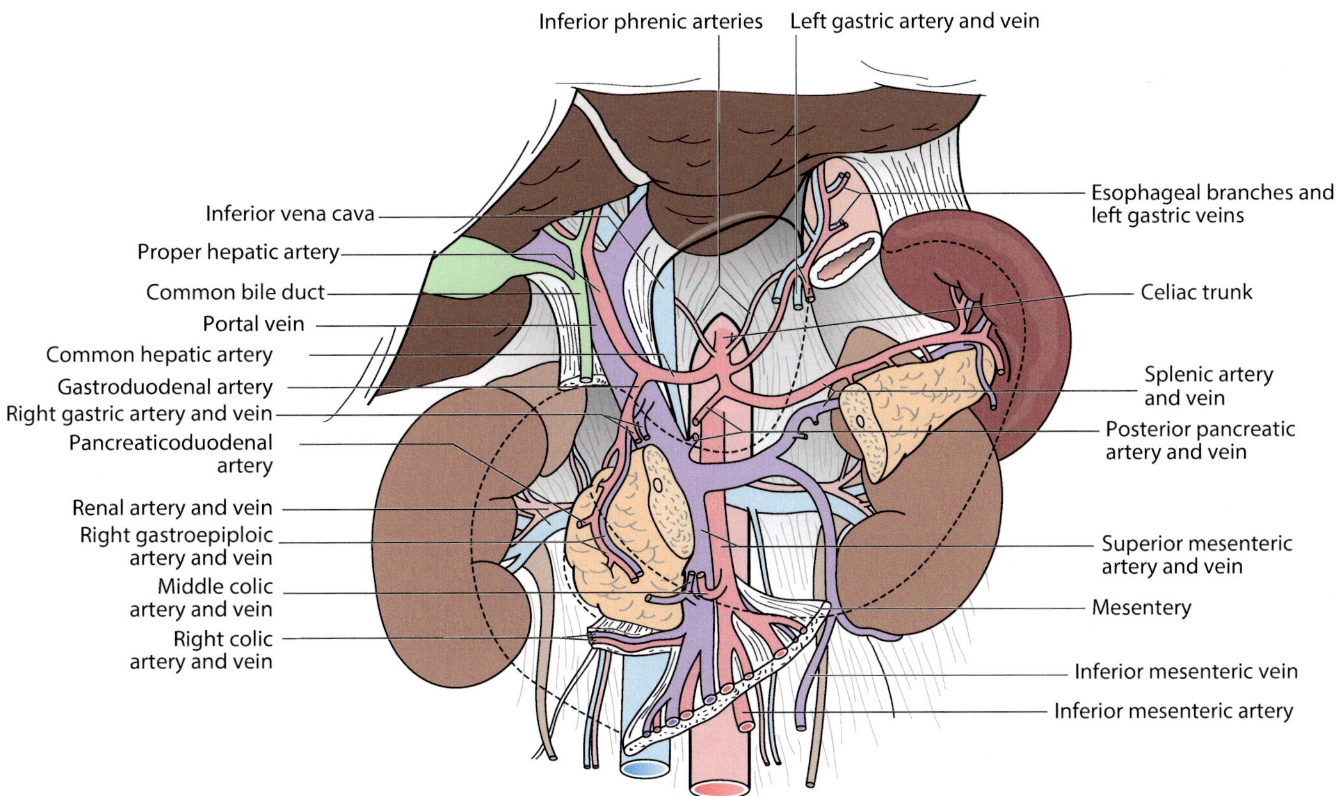

◘ **Fig. 6.1** Vascular anatomy of the upper abdomen (From Luther 2014)

component). Another variant is the presence of accessory hepatic arteries, for example, arising from the superior mesenteric artery (7%). A rare variant is a common origin of the hepatic, splenic, and superior mesenteric arteries from the aorta (4.5%). There is good collateralization of the visceral arteries, which is why chronic proximal occlusion of a single visceral artery usually has no adverse effect.

The inferior mesenteric artery originates at the L3 level, approx. 4–5 cm above the aortic bifurcation, and descends anterior to and somewhat to the left of the aorta. It is not visualized consistently due to its small caliber of approx. 2–4 mm.

6.1.1.3 Renal Arteries

The renal arteries arise from the aorta at right angles at the L2 level approx. 1–2 cm below the mesenteric artery. The right renal artery often arises somewhat higher than the left renal artery and crosses under the inferior vena cava, while the left renal artery takes an almost horizontal course to the left renal hilum. Two or more renal arteries are present in approx. 25% of the population. The renal arteries divide into the segmental arteries just before the hilum. The segmental arteries successively split into interlobar, arcuate, and interlobular arteries.

6.1.2 Examination Protocol and Technique

With a scanning depth of up to 20 cm, a valid and diagnostic duplex scan of the intra-abdominal and retroperitoneal arteries can only be obtained using a low-frequency transducer with a higher receive gain and a high enough frame rate. Slender patients can be examined with a 5 MHz transducer, but 3.5–2 MHz transducers will be necessary in most cases. Sector scanners or curved-array transducers with a small footprint make it easier to achieve a suitable Doppler angle (<70°, ideally <60°). Spectral Doppler sampling is impaired by the longer pulse delay with increasing depth of the vessel of interest.

The examiner is confronted with a dilemma here since a high pulse repetition frequency (PRF) is required to detect fast flow, while the depth of the target vessels necessitates the use of a low PRF, making aliasing a more common problem when evaluating stenosis of an abdominal vessel. This problem can be overcome by reducing the transmit frequency and scanning at a smaller insonation angle. To achieve an adequate frame rate in the color mode, a small color box just large enough to cover the area of interest must be chosen (as the frame rate is lower when more scan lines are processed).

The patient is positioned supine with the arms along the side of the body and a relaxed abdominal wall. Other preparations are usually not necessary. To reduce artifacts, the examiner can apply gentle pressure with the transducer and push interfering gas-filled bowel loops out of the way or compress them. Exerting pressure with the transducer additionally reduces the scanning depth (skin level – aorta). However, exerting pressure may be painful and should be done gently in patients with a history of abdominal surgery and extensive adhesions.

The examination of the abdominal and retroperitoneal vessels begins with the identification of the aorta just below the diaphragm. The examiner then follows the aorta in transverse orientation down to the division into the iliac arteries, localizing the origins of the visceral and renal arteries on the way.

6.1.2.1 Aorta

6.1.2.1.1 Protocol for Ultrasound Examination of the Abdominal Aorta and Aortic Aneurysm

The sonographic evaluation of the abdominal aorta begins by following its course in transverse orientation from the diaphragm to the bifurcation. Adequate characterization of dilated aortic segments and their extent includes the common and internal iliac arteries in longitudinal and transverse planes. **An abdominal aortic aneurysm (AAA)** is defined as a focal increase in diameter to twice that of the proximal segment or a diameter > 3 cm. The length of an aneurysm is not relevant for the decision when to operate and only adds to the confusion in the numbers game. What is relevant though is whether an aneurysm begins above or below the renal artery origins and how close an infrarenal aneurysm extends to the renal artery origins. The peripheral extent of an AAA is of interest in terms of involvement of the common iliac artery and possibly of the internal iliac artery. The iliac arteries are evaluated in transverse and longitudinal orientation (oblique abdominal view). This information is important for therapeutic decision making and preoperative planning.

To **measure an AAA**, the examiner first localizes the largest diameter and then moves the transducer around to identify a plane depicting a circular structure with a small diameter. This maneuver will avoid overestimation of the aneurysm, which would result from measuring the size in oblique orientation and which is a common pitfall, especially in the presence of dilatative atherosclerotic processes with elongation and arching of the aorta. With its flexible selection of scan planes, ultrasound is superior to computed tomography, which relies on the acquisition of standardized axial slices.

In the **diagnostic evaluation** of patients with suspected **stenosis**, a spectral Doppler tracing of the aorta is obtained in longitudinal orientation. Occlusion of the aorta is most easily identified by the absence of flow in the duplex mode and then confirmed by acquisition of a Doppler waveform. The vena cava to the right of the aorta can serve as a landmark.

6.1.2.1.2 Protocol for Ultrasound Follow-Up After Endovascular Aneurysm Repair (EVAR)

Color duplex ultrasound (CDUS) (◘ Figs. 6.77, 6.78, 6.79, 6.80, 6.81, and 6.82 (Atlas)) and **contrast-enhanced ultrasound (CEUS)** (◘ Fig. 6.36 and ◘ Figs. 6.82 and 6.38 (Atlas)) rely on different mechanisms to detect flowing blood. Endoleaks are a common complication of endovascular aneurysm repair (EVAR) for abdominal aortic aneurysm (AAA). CDUS requires a minimum Doppler shift frequency to detect flowing blood and thus fails to detct very slow flow or flow in anatomic areas where a sufficiently small Doppler angle cannot be accomplished. Recall that, according to the Doppler equation, a smaller angle of insonation results in a higher Doppler shift frequency. Hence, a small angle improves the detection of slow flow.

Following intravenous injection, ultrasound microbubbles enhance the signal from flowing blood, rendering CEUS more sensitive to low flow and slow flow within a stent graft and in the extravascular space following escape through an endoleak compared with conventional color duplex imaging. When CDUS is used for endoleak detection, it is important to use a lower PRF (as for the sonographic examination of veins), possibly in conjunction with a longer persistence and higher gain. For hemodynamic characterization of an endoleak, flow should be characterized by spectral Doppler interrogation at the site of entry into the residual aneurysm sac. When the B-mode image shows inhomogeneous echogenicity, hypoechoic areas should be scrutinized closely in the color duplex mode.

CEUS for endoleak detection is performed after bolus injection of 1.2–2.4 mL SonoVue. The abdominal aorta including the stent graft and its limbs is examined in transverse orientation. Following arrival of the contrast microbubbles, the examiner first scrutinizes the proximal and distal anchorage of the stent graft to identify a possible type I endoleak using a low mechanical index (MI) to avoid rapid destruction of the microbubbles (transmit power reduced to 10–20% of the output power). Type II endoleaks (patent lumbar arteries, inferior mesenteric artery) will typically become apparent after a short delay (late arterial to venous phase) following arrival of the contrast agent in the stent graft. For identification of a type II endoleak, the entire residual aneurysm sac is first imaged in transverse orientation, which may be supplemented by longitudinal and oblique planes as required (video). To avoid misinterpretation of the CEUS scan, it is important to compare the findings with the corresponding B-mode image (special software). Especially in patients with a complex stent graft, the final step is to examine the renal artery origins and mesenteric arteries for patency and stenosis.

The microbubble contrast solution is supplied along with large-lumen cannulas and glass syringes to minimize microbubble destruction (shear stress and wall adherence) during handling. The dynamic examination of the target anatomy begins immediately after administration of the microbubble bolus and saline flush. The arterial phase begins 10–20 s after injection; after 30 s, the venous phase begins.

6.1.2.2 Visceral Arteries

The short celiac trunk with the division into the hepatic and splenic arteries is often identified in the transverse view as a conspicuous palm-leaf-shaped structure. Slight angulation of the transducer may be necessary to identify and visualize the origins of these arteries. The proper hepatic artery can be followed along its course anterosuperior to the portal vein in the hepatoduodenal ligament.

Also in transverse orientation, the course of the **splenic artery** to the spleen can be followed. The hepatic and splenic arteries are characterized by rather large diastolic flow components as they supply parenchymal organs. From a clinical point of view, sonographic examination of these arteries is performed for two reasons only: to evaluate patients with suspected iatrogenic vascular complications after major abdominal surgery and to search for aneurysm. Visceral artery aneurysms are rare and most commonly occur in the splenic artery, followed by the hepatic artery.

The **superior mesenteric artery** is identified at its origin in longitudinal orientation and tracked as far as possible along its course parallel to the aorta. In inflammatory bowel disease, B-mode imaging enables evaluation of intestinal wall thickening, while blood flow velocity in the superior mesenteric artery provides a measure of inflammatory activity. Inflammatory bowel disease is associated with an increased peak systolic velocity (PSV) and above all with an increased diastolic velocity.

The superior mesenteric artery arises at the level of the celiac trunk or as far as 2 cm below it. It descends parallel to the aorta and is thus seen as a round structure with a smaller diameter anterior to the aorta in transverse images. Doppler spectra are sampled in transverse planes in the celiac trunk and the hepatic and splenic arteries and longitudinally in the superior mesenteric artery. A better Doppler angle is achieved when the transducer is moved downward and tilted (◘ Figs. 6.2 and 6.3). Patients with an elongated and arched proximal segment of the superior mesenteric artery should be asked to breathe in slightly, which will shift the mesentery downward, thereby stretching the proximal segment for improved Doppler angle correction.

An atypical origin of the **hepatic artery** from the superior mesenteric artery affects the hemodynamics of the superior mesenteric artery (larger diastolic component). Therefore, the celiac trunk must always be included in an examination

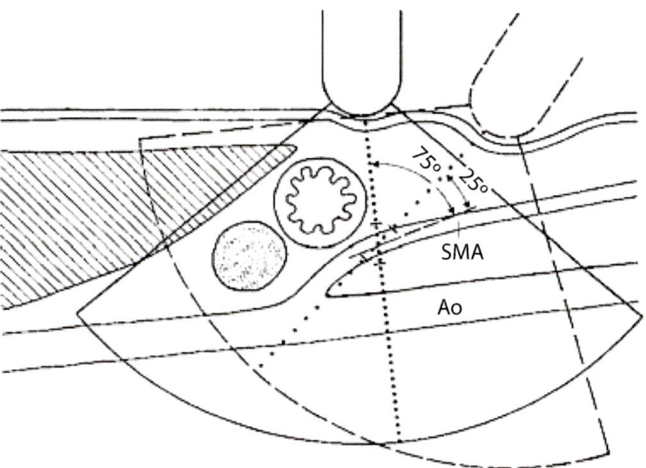

◘ **Fig. 6.2** Diagram of the origin of the superior mesenteric artery (SMA) from the aorta (Ao), illustrating how the Doppler angle can be improved from 75° to 25° by moving the transducer distally and then tilting it cranially

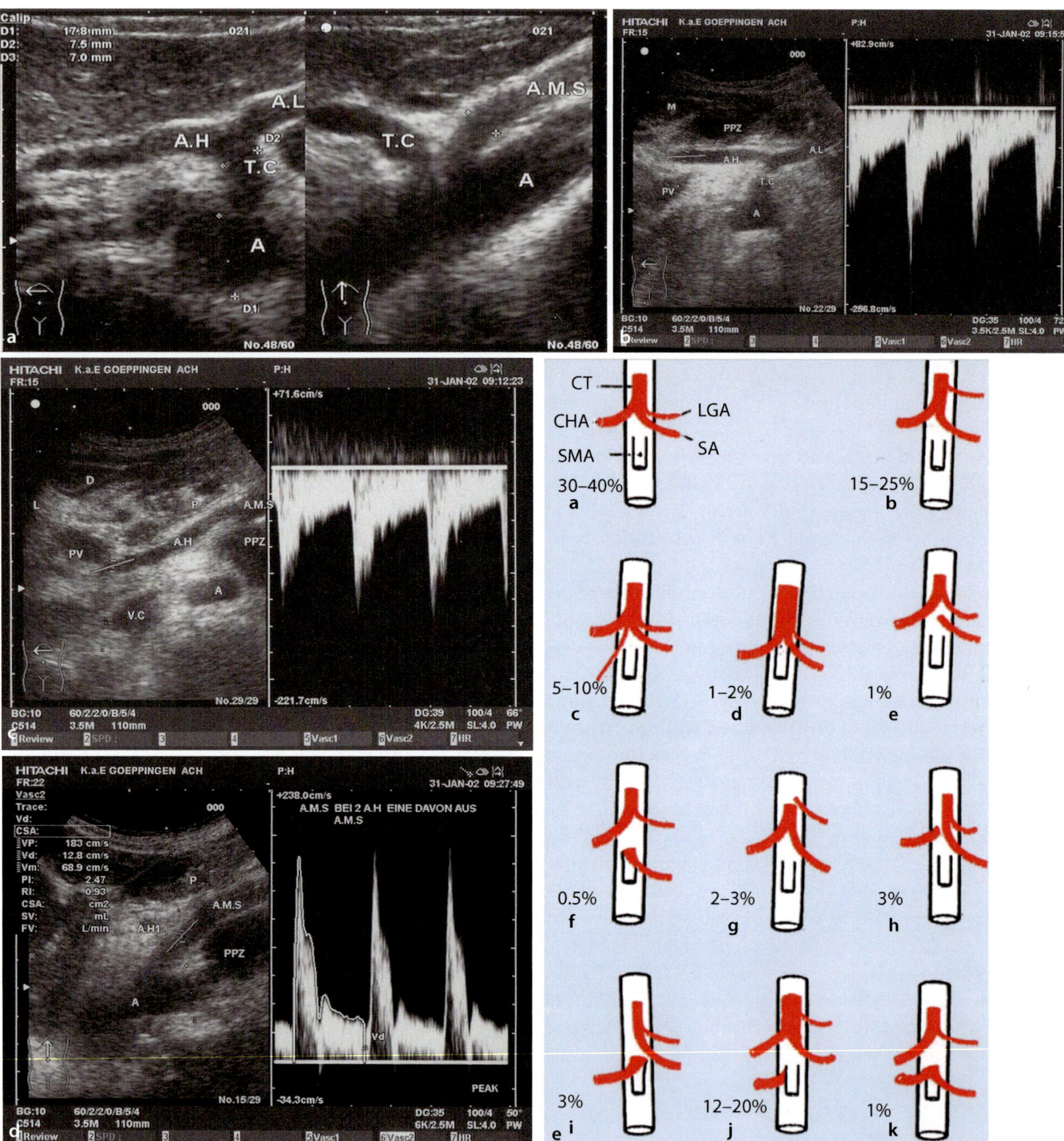

Fig. 6.3 **a** Sonoanatomy of the celiac trunk and superior mesenteric artery. The left image shows the origin of the celiac trunk (T.C) from the aorta (A) in transverse orientation. The celiac trunk varies in length from 1 to 4 cm and divides into the hepatic artery (A.H) and splenic artery (A.L). The hepatic artery is contained within the hepatoduodenal ligament, coursing beneath the liver to the liver hilum. The right image shows the origins of the celiac trunk (T.C) and superior mesenteric artery (A.M.S) from the aorta in longitudinal orientation. The mesenteric artery descends in front of the aorta (sometimes slightly to the left or to the right of the aorta). The celiac trunk divides early, leaving the scan plane, so that only a short segment is typically seen on longitudinal abdominal scans. **b–d** Variants of hepatic artery (A.H) anatomy. The example shows an individual with two hepatic arteries: one hepatic artery arising from the celiac trunk (T.C) and supplying the left hepatic lobe (**b**) and a second hepatic artery arising from the superior mesenteric artery (A.M.S) and supplying the right hepatic lobe (**c**). The hepatic artery arising from the superior mesenteric artery affects the pulsatility of blood flow in the latter (larger diastolic component, see waveform in **d**). PPZ = pancreatic pseudocyst, P = pancreas, PV = portal vein, V.C = vena cava, A = aorta. **e** Diagram illustrating variants of visceral artery origins from the abdominal aorta. CT, celiac trunk; SMA, superior mesenteric artery; CHA, common hepatic artery; SA, splenic artery; LGA, left gastric artery

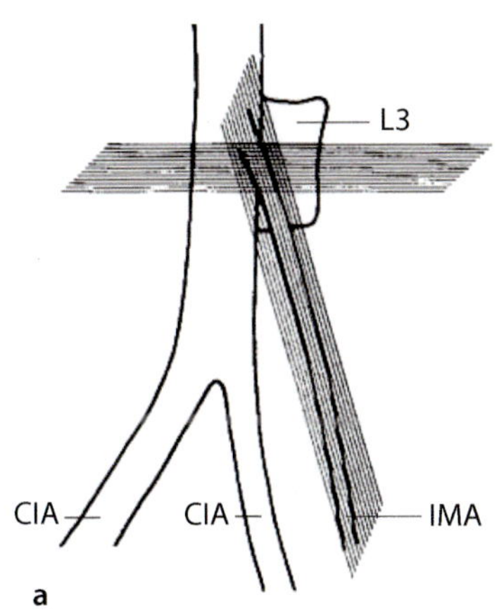

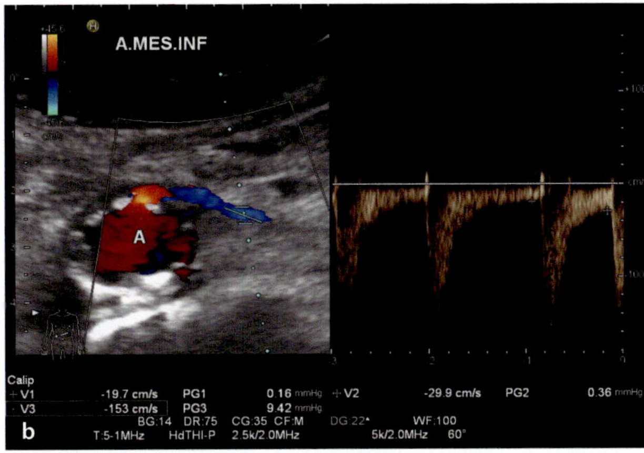

Fig. 6.4 a Diagram of the origin of the inferior mesenteric artery (IMA) about 3 cm above the aortic bifurcation. The IMA arises from the left anterolateral aspect of the aorta and is identified with the transducer in transverse orientation and applying slight pressure while moving it upward from the bifurcation until the proximal IMA comes into view. In most individuals, the IMA can then be scanned over a length of 2–5 cm, but will not be visualized when the acoustic window is poor (CIA, common iliac artery). **b** Oblique mid-abdominal view for identifying the inferior mesenteric artery at its origin from the abdominal aorta (A), from where it can be followed downward (blue-coded flow). The waveform illustrates the dependence of end-diastolic velocity (EDV) and the resistive index (RI) on heart rate (patient with absolute arrhythmia). For a heartbeat with long diastole, the EDV of 19 cm/s gives an RI of 0.87, while the EDV of 29 cm/s from a heartbeat with a short diastole gives an RI of 0.81 (see Figs. 1.28d and 5.25)

of the mesenteric arteries to identify the hepatic artery origin. If the artery does not arise from the celiac trunk, the mesenteric artery must be searched for a replaced hepatic artery. In the evaluation of suspected acute mesenteric occlusion, the main trunk is evaluated, including spectral Doppler sampling, and subsequently the artery is tracked downward into its branches, the jejunal, middle colic, ileocolic, and right colic arteries. After adequate instrument adjustment with a high but artifact-free gain and low PRF, the origins of these vessels are located in the mesentery to then confirm or rule out embolic occlusion of these branches. Occlusion suggested by absence of flow in the color duplex mode should be confirmed by spectral Doppler.

The **inferior mesenteric artery** is less relevant clinically and is most easily depicted roughly halfway between the origin of the renal artery and the aortic bifurcation in the transverse plane or in an oblique orientation with the transducer face directed toward the left lower abdomen (Fig. 6.4). If involvement of multiple visceral arteries is suspected, Doppler spectra are obtained from their origins to identify stenosis or occlusion.

To obtain reproducible measurements, the visceral arteries, just like the extremity arteries, should not be scanned during periods of hyperemia. This means that the examination should be performed **after a period of fasting** since blood flow velocity is markedly increased after a meal.

Scatterers such as bowel gas can be pushed aside by applying pressure with the transducer. A small Doppler angle is achieved by moving and tilting the transducer, so that the sample volume in the target vessel comes to lie at the lateral edge of the B-mode scanning field displayed on the monitor.

The respiratory mobility of the intra-abdominal organs including the intra-abdominal and retroperitoneal vessels makes it necessary to scan the vessels during maximum inspiratory breath-holding or during shallow breathing with little respiratory motion. Proper breathing must be practiced with the patient before the examination.

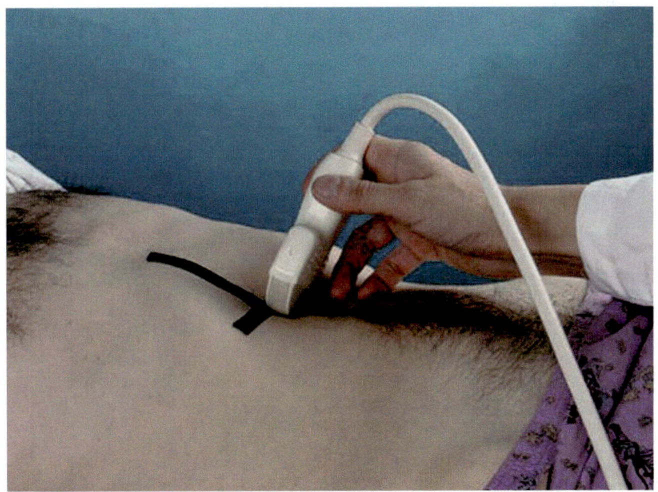

Fig. 6.5 Epigastric transducer position (transverse upper abdominal view) for evaluation of the renal arteries

6.1.2.3 Renal Arteries

One way of identifying the renal arteries at their origins just below the easily visualized superior mesenteric artery is to localize the latter in transverse orientation and to then move the transducer 1–2 cm downward and look for the renal arteries as they arise from the aorta to the left and right (Fig. 6.5). A second landmark is the left renal vein (hypoechoic, broader band), which overcrosses the aorta, coursing between the aorta and the superior mesentering artery, before entering the vena cava. The left renal artery typically arises some millimeters below the right renal artery

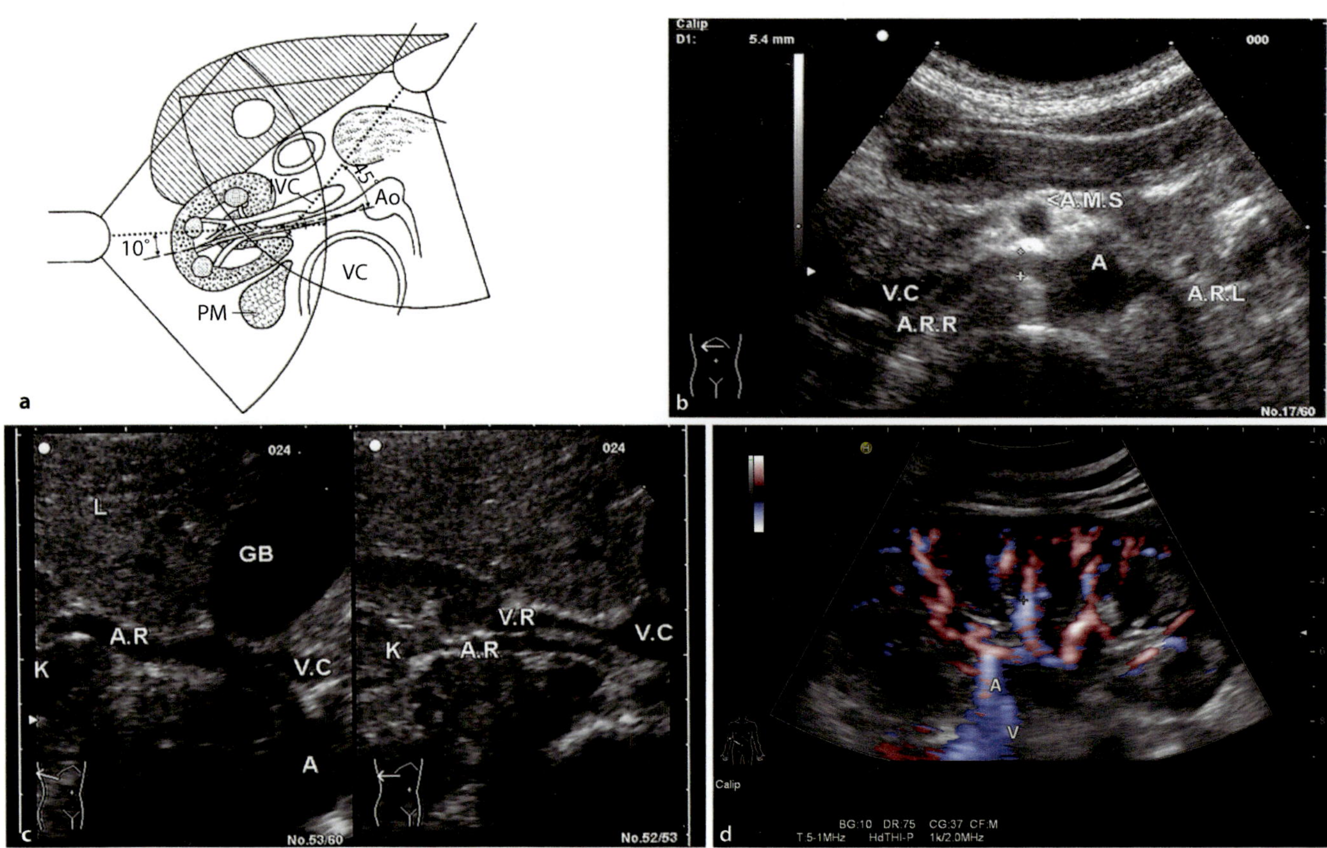

◘ Fig. 6.6 **a** Diagram of the right renal artery as it arises from the aorta (Ao) and of the renal vein entering the inferior vena cava (IVC). Anterior transducer position with a Doppler angle of 45°; lateral position with a Doppler angle of 10° (VC, vertebral column; PM, psoas muscle). **b** Sonoanatomy of the renal arteries (epigastric view). The renal artery origins from the aorta at the L1 level are seen in the epigastrium 1–2 cm below the superior mesenteric artery (A.M.S) orgin. It is rare, but when both arteries are visualized in the same plane, from the aorta to the renal hilum, the appearance suggests spread wings. Often, however, it is necessary to direct the transducer face toward the respective side in order to visualize a long segment of the renal artery; this is because the vascular bundle suspending the kidney is pulled slightly downward at its distal end. The right renal artery (A.R.R) passes under the vena cava (V.C) on its way to the renal hilum, while the left renal artery (A.R.L) courses posteroinferior to the pancreatic head in the retroperitoneum to reach the left renal hilum. **c** Visualization of the left renal artery is often impaired by air in the colon. On the right side, the liver and vena cava can be used as an acoustic window to achieve complete evaluation of the renal artery from its origin to the renal hilum. The left section (paramedian view) shows the right renal artery (A.R) from the renal hilum (K) to the aorta (A), deep to the liver (L), gallbladder (GB), and vena cava (V.C). **d** Flank view of the kidney and hilum with the renal vein (V) and renal artery (A): branches from segmental to interlobar arteries are visible (red indicates arteries, blue indicates veins)

and both do not usually take a strictly horizontal course but move slightly downward. The right renal artery first courses anteriorly in a slightly curved fashion and then arches underneath the vena cava (◘ Fig. 6.6a–c). Up to 20% of individuals have an accessory renal artery (coursing to the lower pole), which should be searched for downstream of the origin of the main renal artery.

The origins and proximal 3 cm of the renal arteries can be visualized and evaluated in over 90% of cases, while visualization of the middle third is often incomplete due to overlying bowel gas, especially on the left. The middle segment of the renal artery is easier to scan on the right, where the vena cava can be used as an acoustic window. Interfering bowel gas can be displaced by pressing the transducer against the bowel until the target segment is seen. The transducer is then moved to the right or left to achieve an optimal angle for spectral Doppler recording (as illustrated for the superior mesenteric artery in ◘ Fig. 6.2).

For **stenosis identification using indirect criteria** (acceleration time, resistive index with side comparison), both renal arteries can be examined from the flank, identifying the artery in the renal hilum. In slender to moderately obese patients, the right paramedian approach can be used to follow the renal artery to its origin using the liver as an acoustic window (coronal view or banana peel view).

The distal third of the renal artery can be scanned continuously from the flank starting at the renal hilum and following the course of the artery proximally (◘ Fig. 6.6). This transducer position also allows good Doppler measurement with a relatively small angle. The individual segmental arteries are identified in the color mode and evaluated for origin stenosis by having the patient exhale or hold his or her breath in inspiration. If **renal artery infarction** is suspected, the renal parenchyma is evaluated for perfusion defects seen on color duplex scans as wedge-shaped areas without flow signals (high but artifact-free gain, low PRF). Moving the transducer around, the examiner must also try and image arteries supplying the renal parenchyma in the upper and lower pole. A small Doppler angle is important in order not to mistake absence of flow signals due to a large Doppler angle for infarction (the problem is illustrated for upper pole arteries in ◘ Fig. 1.30b).

6.1.2.3.1 Ultrasound Technique

Over the last 25 years, a total of four different methodological approaches for diagnosing renal artery stenosis (RAS) using color duplex ultrasound (CDUS) have been evaluated. Two approaches use direct criteria and two use indirect criteria for RAS grading.

- **Direct Criteria**

RAS grading based on direct criteria uses either absolute peak systolic velocity (PSV) or the renal-aortic ratio (RAR). Grading from maximum PSV is based on the continuity equation (which states that PSV is inversely proportional to stenotic cross-sectional area reduction).

The RAR relates the PSV measured in the stenotic renal artery to PSV in the aorta, which thus serves as an individual standard of comparison. The RAR was proposed to eliminate systemic effects (such as blood pressure during the examination) on PSV. However, even the RAR has limitations as there are other factors that influence hemodynamics in the aorta and these are difficult to account for.

- **Indirect Criteria**

Indirect criteria for identifying RAS are derived from Doppler waveforms obtained at the renal hilum. One criterion of ipsilateral RAS is a decrease in the resistive index (RI) of >0.05.

The second indirect criterion is a longer acceleration time distal to higher-grade RAS. Acceleration time is the interval from end-diastole to maximum PSV.

Some authors prefer PSV measurement at the hilum as an indirect criterion to circumvent the difficulties that may be encountered in measuring PSV in the proximal renal artery. However, it is known from other vascular territories that indirect criteria are not reliable unless higher-grade stenosis is present. While their specificity is adequate for 50–70% stenosis, sensitivity is poor (typically ≤70%).

As a general rule, any accessory arteries must be included in the evaluation when indirect criteria are used because renal hypertension can also be induced by steno-occlusive disease in an accessory artery.

A **transplant kidney** can often be imaged with a higher frequency than the abdomen in general, in particular when examining slender patients (4–7 MHz). Both the transplant renal artery and the vein should be continuously imaged by color duplex sonography with spectral Doppler sampling for stenosis quantification at the arterial and venous anastomoses. Additional Doppler measurements are obtained at sites of aliasing along the length of the transplant vessels (unless aliasing is due to the use of an inadequate PRF). As for all Doppler measurements, it is important to achieve an angle of insonation of less than 60° for measuring flow velocity, which may be difficult because the vessels are often tortuous. In the B-mode, the examiner assesses the echogenicity and contour of the parenchyma and looks for perirenal fluid collections, which can compress the vein or obstruct the flow of urine from the transplant, causing dilatation of the renal pelvis and calyces.

6.1.3 Normal Findings

6.1.3.1 Aorta

The aorta changes in diameter and pulsatility from proximal to distal. The flow profile shows continuous diastolic flow immediately below the diaphragm and becomes triphasic, as in peripheral arteries, below the origins of the renal arteries. The diameter of the aorta decreases from a mean of 25 mm to 15–20 mm just above the bifurcation. Progressive age-related dilatation with diameters of up to 30 mm of the infrarenal portion is considered normal, in particular in individuals with atherosclerotic vascular lesions (Rieger and Schoop 1998). An aneurysm is diagnosed when aortic enlargement exceeds 3 cm.

6.1.3.2 Visceral Arteries

Supplying parenchymal organs (liver and spleen) with a low peripheral resistance, the celiac trunk and hepatic and splenic arteries have Doppler waveforms with a monophasic flow profile and a relatively large diastolic component, resulting in a low pulsatility index of 0.6–0.8. Studies demonstrate wide interindividual variation in peak systolic velocity (PSV) and end-diastolic velocity (EDV) and in vessel diameters (◘ Table 6.1). This situation makes it difficult to define cutoff values for identifying hemodynamically significant stenosis.

The **Doppler waveform of the superior mesenteric artery** reflects a mixed type combining the high pulsatility of peripheral arteries and the low pulsatility of arteries supplying parenchymal organs. At the same time, the superior mesenteric artery waveform is a good example of demand-adjusted changes in pulsatility. After a meal, there is an increase in PSV, but above all in EDV, due to the reduced peripheral resistance, which is the main factor responsible for a lower postprandial pulsatility index.

In a study of normal vessels in 30 volunteers performed by the author as early as 1987, measurements in the superior mesenteric artery yielded a PSV of 134 ± 22.8 cm/s and an EDV of 20.8 ± 4.4 cm/s. Mean flow velocity was 23.4 ± 5.6 cm/s. During digestion-related hyperemia 1 h after eating, PSV was increased to 196 ± 25 cm/s and EDV to 47.5 ± 8.3 cm/s. Mean postprandial flow velocity was 46 ± 7.4 cm/s. In the time-motion display, the diameter of the superior mesenteric artery varied on average between 8.04 mm during systole and 7.4 mm during diastole (◘ Fig. 6.7). Based on these values, mean blood volume increased by 126%, from 639 mL/min preprandially to 1447 mL/min postprandially.

Table 6.1 Normal values for the visceral arteries

Artery (studies)	PSV (cm/s)	EDV (cm/s)	Mean (cm/s)	RI	Diameter (mm)
Celiac trunk (Bowersox et al. 1991; Jäger et al. 1992; Moneta et al. 1988)	100–237	23–58	45–55	0.66–0.82	6–10
Splenic artery (Nakamura et al. 1989; Sato et al. 1987)	70–110		15–40		4–8
Hepatic artery (Jäger et al. 1992; Nakamura et al. 1989; Sato et al. 1987)	70–120		20–40		4–10
Superior mesenteric artery[a] (Jäger et al. 1986; Sato et al. 1988; Sabba et al. 1991; Bowersox et al. 1991; Schäberle and Seitz 1991)	124–218	5–30	15–35	0.75–0.9	5–8

Duplex parameters: *PSV* peak systolic velocity, *EDV* end-diastolic velocity, *mean* mean blood flow velocity, *RI* resistive index
[a]Values including preprandial and postprandial measurements

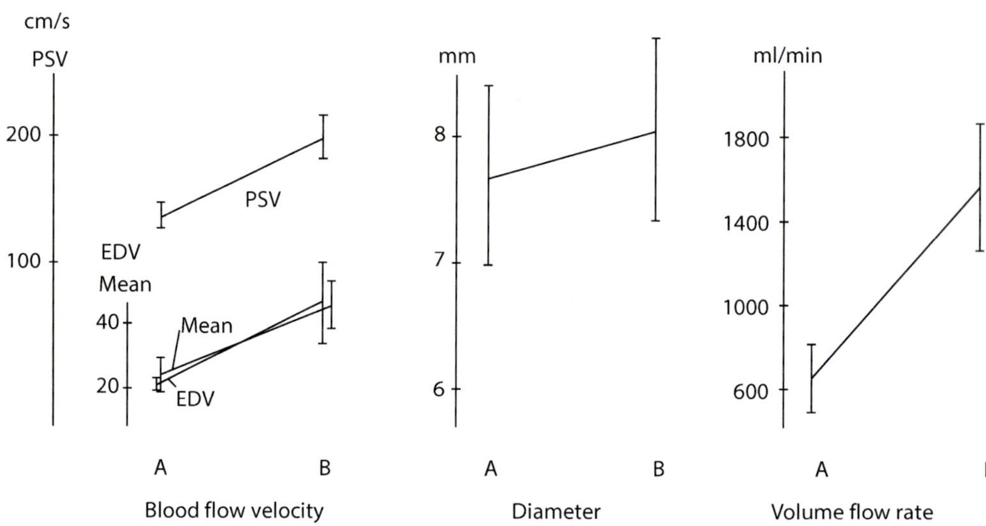

Fig. 6.7 Preprandial (A) and postprandial (B) mean values (±15) of peak systolic velocity (PSV), end-diastolic velocity (EDV), and mean blood flow velocity (Mean) in the superior mesenteric artery in 30 healthy subjects. Also shown are the corresponding preprandial and postprandial vessel diameters and volume flow rates

Apart from mechanical, metabolic, and neural mechanisms, mesenteric artery perfusion is affected by **vasoactive substances**, in particular gastrointestinal hormones like gastrin, secretin, and glucagon as well as other vasoactive hormones like catecholamines, histamine, and bradykinin. The effect on mesenteric perfusion of drugs like nitrates, ergotamine, narcotic agents, or calcium antagonists can be demonstrated by flow measurements performed with duplex ultrasound. In the above-quoted study, it was also shown that mean blood flow velocity after nifedipine administration increased from 23.9 to 41.8 cm/s, corresponding to a 75% increase. The Pourcelot index decreased from 0.84 to 0.77, which is comparable to the postprandial decrease. These observations show that increased mesenteric perfusion is primarily attributable to a reduced peripheral resistance in the mesenteric territory (see Fig. 6.51 (Atlas)).

In patients with anatomic variants (hepatic artery arising from the superior mesenteric artery), higher threshold velocities must be defined (see Fig. 6.52 (Atlas)). Moreover, blood flow in the superior mesenteric artery is also altered when the artery is recruited as a collateral in steno-occlusive disease of the celiac trunk.

Diagnostic evaluation of the inferior mesenteric artery is of little clinical significance. Systolic and diastolic flow velocities are comparable to those in the superior mesenteric artery but flow tends to be somewhat more pulsatile. Angle-corrected measurements in 20 subjects performed by our group yielded an average PSV of 109 cm/s and EDV of 10 cm/s with wide interindividual variation. The flow profile was found to resemble that of the superior mesenteric artery but typically with a small diastolic component.

6.1.3.3 Renal Arteries

The renal arteries supply low-resistance parenchymal organs and therefore have a flow profile with little pulsatility and a large diastolic component. Measurements performed in 102 renal arteries without abnormalities on control angiography yielded a mean PSV of 84.7 ± 13.9 cm/s and EDV of 31.2 ± 7.8 cm/s. The Pourcelot index was 0.66 ± 0.07 (findings by our group, 1988). Evaluation of the renal arteries for exclusion of stenosis by duplex imaging is possible in 85–90% of cases; the proximal third as the preferred site of atherosclerotic stenoses can be evaluated in over 90% of cases. The flow velocities reported in the literature not only vary widely from one study to the next but also within the studies. The range is <60–140 cm/s for PSV and 20–65 cm/s for EDV with a Pourcelot index of 0.6–0.8. Reported diameters range from 5 to 8 mm (Karasch et al. 1993; Hoffmann et al. 1991; Schäberle et al. 1992).

PSV, EDV, and the Pourcelot index are affected by vessel elasticity and peripheral resistance. Moreover, they are influenced by systemic blood pressure. In diabetics, medial sclerosis with reduced wall compliance and parenchymal changes result in lower diastolic flow and a higher Pourcelot index. PSV is slightly higher than in subjects with normal vessels.

6.1.4 Interpretation and Documentation

The ultrasound examination and the subsequent documentation of relevant findings of the visceral and retroperitoneal vessels depend on the clinical question to be answered. If an abdominal aortic aneurysm is diagnosed, the size is documented in the transverse plane; the report must also provide information on the localization and extent (infrarenal, relation to iliac arteries) as well as on the presence of thrombosis. Blood flow in the aorta should be documented by a longitudinally sampled Doppler waveform, though a color duplex scan may also be sufficient. In patients with suspected visceral artery stenosis, a Doppler spectrum is obtained from the origin of the respective artery, the preferred site of visceral stenosis, and the artery is scanned over a long stretch. The findings in patients evaluated for renal artery stenosis are documented by means of angle-corrected Doppler waveforms from the origins of both renal arteries. An angle-corrected waveform from the aorta is required as well. In fibromuscular dysplasia, either the findings in the middle thirds of both renal arteries are documented or Doppler waveforms from the origins and distal thirds (at the renal hilum) with comparison of resistance indices.

6.1.5 Clinical Role of Duplex Ultrasound

6.1.5.1 Aorta

6.1.5.1.1 Abdominal Aortic Aneurysm

Most ultrasound examinations of the retroperitoneal and intra-abdominal arteries are performed in patients with **suspected abdominal aortic aneurysm (AAA)**. Morphologically, an aneurysm is characterized by concentric or eccentric luminal dilatation. The vast majority of AAA are infrarenal (95%) and show variable degrees of thrombosis. In Europe, the underlying causes are as follows (in order of descending frequency):

- Atherosclerosis, 70–90%
- Idiopathic medial necrosis (Bollinger 1979), 8–10%
- Microbial infection including syphilis (which accounted for 20–30% of aneurysms in the 1960s), 4–5%
- Nonbacterial inflammatory aneurysms (arteritis), 3–5%
- Inflammation, 3–5%
- Congenital, 1–3%

Aneurysms predominantly occur in the elderly or in patients with multiple morbidity. They develop on the basis of rarefaction and fragmentation of the elastic membranes and atrophy of the muscular media of the vessel wall. Although the dilatative process primarily involves the media rather than the intimal and subintimal layers (the site of atherosclerotic lesions), aneurysms in the European population are typically associated with atherosclerosis and cigarette smoking. In other regions like Africa, nonbacterial inflammatory conditions such as arteritis or bacterial infections and their sequelae account for a much larger proportion of aneurysms (20–30%), with a greater number of younger persons being affected. The sonographic evaluation of the vessel wall can provide information on the underlying cause.

Ultrasound studies performed in the USA and Europe revealed a prevalence of 2.4% (n = 426) in the normal population aged 65–74 (>4 cm; Collin et al. 1988) and a prevalence of 4.9% (>3 cm) in an investigation of 1800 subjects over 50 years of age without concomitant vascular disease (Akkersdijk et al. 1991). The prevalence increases to 10–14% in individuals with peripheral arterial occlusive disease (PAOD) or hypertension (Galland et al. 1991; Twomey et al. 1984). Large multicenter studies confirm prevalences of 4–7% and also show that more than 90% of patients with aneurysms are smokers.

Because of the high prevalence of 4–7% in men over 65 (Scott et al. 1995; Ashton et al. 2002; Lindholt et al. 2005; Norman et al. 2004), several countries, including Germany, have installed screening programs for AAA. The results of a meta-analysis of 4 large multicenter studies including 125,000 men aged over 65 impressively confirm the clinical benefit and also the cost-effectiveness of screening based on simple B-mode ultrasound (measurement of infrarenal abdominal aortic diameter) (Lindholt and Norman 2008). In this meta-analysis, screening of the population at risk was found to significantly lower the rate of AAA rupture by 47%, aneurysm-related mortality by 7%, and emergency operations by 45%. On the other hand, there was a three-fold increase in elective operations for AAA, meaning that many patients were operated on for an AAA that never would have ruptured if left untreated.

The high prevalences of AAA quoted above mostly stem from studies conducted in the 1990s and around the turn of the millennium. Prevalences have since declined, mainly because fewer people are smoking. AAA is a disease of smokers, and there is a clear association with the amount and duration of smoking. A Swedish study conducted in 2009 reports a prevalence of 2.2% (Svensjö et al. 2011), and data from the Gloucestershire Aneurysm Screening Programme (GASP) show a decrease in the number of AAA (>3 cm; men >65 years) from 4.7% in 1990 to 1.1% in 2009 (Darwood et al. 2011). In view of these developments, we should reconsider the benefit of AAA screening programs, also in terms of cost effectiveness. According to Markow's simulation model, the threshold for cost-effectiveness of a screening program is 1% (Wanhainen et al. 2005).

Outside screening programs, most AAA are incidentally detected in patients undergoing an ultrasound examination for an unrelated problem (Allenberg et al. 1997). The therapeutic management of aortic aneurysms is guided by the **risk of rupture**, which increases with the diameter. When surgical repair is contemplated, the risk of rupture of the untreated AAA must be weighed against the risks of intraoperative and postoperative complications, which are considerable because aneurysms typically occur in older and multimorbid patients. The mortality risk is less than 5% in patients undergoing elective surgical resection and increases to more than 50–60% in emergency surgery for a ruptured aneurysm. Half of the patients with a ruptured AAA die before they reach the hospital.

Several follow-up studies of individuals with AAA (Limet et al. 1991; Nevitt et al. 1989; Zöllner et al. 1991) demonstrated a markedly **higher risk of rupture** for aneurysms greater than 5 cm, which is why a size of 5 cm evolved as the cutoff value for elective surgical resection (◘ Table 6.2a). Based on the UK Small Aneurysm Trial (1998), which compared the natural history and the risk of surgery, the cutoff diameter for surgical management was even elevated to 5.5 cm. Patients with an AAA smaller than 5.5 cm require close surveillance, and elective surgery is recommended if there is rapid growth of the aneurysm (>5 mm in 6 months), embolization to the periphery, pain, or the shape is very saccular. Other complications associated with AAA include compression of surrounding structures (veins, bowel) and fistulization.

Prevention of rupture is the guiding principle of management. Therefore, identification of factors contributing to the stabilization of an AAA is of crucial importance. Morphology seems to play a role (saccular aneurysms are more susceptible to rupture than spindle-shaped ones) as does thrombosis. Aneurysms with a thrombotic lining tend to grow more slowly, whereas growth appears to be accelerated by local pressure peaks associated with turbulent flow, which primarily occurs in saccular aneurysms.

Dissecting aneurysm (see ◘ Fig. 5.44 for aneurysm of the carotid artery) is caused by an intimal tear allowing blood to enter between the intima and media with formation of a false lumen along a segment of variable length where blood separates the intima from the media. The blood enters the false lumen at the upper point of entry and drains into the normal lumen at the distal end of the dissection (re-entry). Most aortic dissections originate in the thoracic aorta and from there may extend as far as the abdominal aorta. The distal extent serves to define different types of dissection, as in the De Bakey or Stanford classification. Transabdominal sonographic techniques are useful only for evaluating the abdominal aorta. Color duplex ultrasound is a valuable imaging modality, providing relevant information for therapeutic decision making including distal extent and involvement of visceral and renal arteries. The duplex examination will identify extension into aortic branches (renal and visceral arteries) or intermittent obstruction of the origins of these arteries by the intimal flap.

Hence, the ultrasound examination provides all the relevant information the surgeon needs **before open surgical aneurysm repair** with patch placement: site of the aneurysm (suprarenal/infrarenal abdominal aorta), involvement of common or internal iliac artery, aneurysm extent, and presence of atherosclerotic disease in the pelvic arteries and femoral bifurcation.

The **sonographic characterization of an AAA** also provides important clues for identifying aneurysms amenable to stenting rather than open surgery. In general, the following sonomorphologic features preclude an endovascular procedure (unless a Y-stent graft is used): a short and conical proximal aneurysm neck, proximal kink >60°, mural thrombosis at the renal artery origins, accessory lower pole renal arteries, severe kinking of an iliac artery, and aneurysm extension into the internal iliac artery.

Once the decision has been made to eliminate an AAA by endovascular aneurysm repair (EVAR), a CT scan is necessary to make the measurements required for selecting an adequate stent graft.

In the **postinterventional surveillance** of patients treated with a stent graft, color duplex imaging can contribute to the early identification of stent migration and endoleaks (types I, II, III) and thus help prevent complications. Contrast-enhanced ultrasound (CEUS) can improve endoleak detection.

◘ Table 6.2a Abdominal aortic aneurysm (AAA) size and estimated annual risk of rupture (Brewster et al. 2003)

AAA diameter (cm)	Annual rupture risk (%)
<3	0
3–3.9	0.4
4–4.9	1.1–2.0
5–5.9	3.3–9.4
6–6.9	9.5–15.9
7–7.9	24.0–36.0

6.1.5.1.2 Inflammatory and Atherosclerotic Conditions

Arteritis can also involve the aorta. Inflammation (e.g., giant cell arteritis, inflammatory aortic aneurysm) is suggested by thickening of the wall as opposed to thickening around the wall as is the case with retroperitoneal fibrosis (Ormond's disease). To make the distinction, the sonographer must carefully evaluate the proximal aortic branches and their origins as well as their relationship to the thickened area (see ◘ Figs. 6.38, 6.40 and 6.85 (Atlas)).

Autopsy studies show that **atherosclerosis**, which is well known to be a systemic disease, begins earlier in the abdominal aorta than in other arteries, with atherosclerotic lesions appearing in the aorta about 5–10 years earlier than in the carotid or coronary arteries.

This is why the **aortic arch** is increasingly the focus of the search for the **source of embolism** in patients with embolic cerebral infarction, after atherosclerotic lesions of the carotid system have been ruled out. However, transesophageal echocardiography (TEE) is needed to reliably identify and characterize aortic plaque as a potential source of embolism.

Stenosis of the abdominal aorta can also be evaluated by ultrasound as it will typically be found in the distal aorta and the aortic bifurcation. Bilateral intermittent claudication is the chief symptom as more severe ischemia is prevented by good collateral pathways. The rare condition of aortic thrombosis may originate from atherosclerotic plaques. Predisposing factors are clotting disorders, paraneoplasia, and oral contraceptives. Aortic thrombus does not cause occlusion, but rather grows into the lumen in a cone-shaped manner, typically first becoming clinically apparent when it causes embolism of a peripheral artery.

Leriche's syndrome is an occlusive disease of the aortic bifurcation with occlusion of both common iliac arteries and of the aorta up to the origin of the inferior mesenteric artery or even to the renal artery origins. In patients with this syndrome, blood to the legs is mainly supplied by collaterals arising from the mesenteric and epigastric arteries.

6.1.5.2 Visceral Arteries

Acute mesenteric ischemia is caused by inadequate blood flow through the mesenteric vessels and may ultimately result in bowel infarction. The most common cause is cardiac embolism. Other mechanisms include thrombosis of the mesenteric artery stem on the basis of pre-existing atherosclerotic stenosis, nonocclusive mesenteric ischemia, and severe acute venous thrombosis (e.g., acute occlusion of the superior mesenteric vein trunk).

Timely embolectomy or restoration of perfusion (within 8 h) is essential to prevent bowel infarction and resection of the involved segments. Patients who are operated on more than 12 h after symptom onset have a much poorer prognosis, facing resection of infarcted bowel segments, development of short bowel syndrome if extensive resection is required, and even death (▫ Table 6.2b). In early acute mesenteric ischemia, abdominal pain is the only symptom and laboratory parameters are normal (▫ Table 6.3). The clinical examination (no peritonism, no relevant tenderness) and B-mode ultrasound or X-ray provide no diagnostic clues either. A diagnostic test that can be used liberally in this situation is urgently needed. In a study of 57 patients presenting to a hospital with acute

▫ **Table 6.2b** Acute superior mesenteric artery occlusion. Mortality rates in relation to delay between onset of abdominal symptoms and surgery (From Walter et al. 1992)

Time from initial symptoms to surgery (h)	No.	Mortality
0–12	11	4 (36.3%)
12–24	16	10 (62.5%)
>24	19	18 (94.7%)
Total	46	32 (69.9%)

▫ **Table 6.3** Stages of acute mesenteric ischemia

Clinical and laboratory findings, diagnostic tests, treatment, prognosis	Initial stage: 1–6 h	Silent interval: 7–12 (24) h	Terminal stage: > (12) 24–48 h
Clinical presentation	Initial triad: 1. Severe abdominal pain without local or generalized signs of peritonitis, clinically normal abdomen 2. Signs of shock in about 20% of cases 3. Diarrhea (anoxic)	Receding pain Mild local changes, deteriorating general state, onset of intestinal paralysis	Paralytic ileus Peritonitis Protracted shock
Laboratory findings	⟶	Progressive leukocytosis Increase of serum lactate level Increasing CK and LDH levels Progressive acidosis	⟶
Plain radiography	Negative	Typically negative	Increased air content, fluid levels
B-mode ultrasound	Negative	Negative	Thickened bowel loops, air inclusions, (sub)total ileus of small intestine
Revascularization possible	+++	++	(+)
Bowel resection necessary	–	(+)	++
Prognosis	⟶	Deteriorating	⟶

mesenteric ischemia, only 32% were diagnosed correctly before surgery or death, and 81% died (Mamode et al. 1999). Little improvement has been achieved with overall mortality rates ranging from 60–90%. Only patients who receive adequate management within 8 (to 12) h of onset of ischemic symptoms have a significantly lower mortality rate below 30% (Endean et al. 2001; Lock 2001; Luther 2006; Kougias et al. 2007).

With its high sensitivity, **contrast-enhanced computed tomography** (CTA), especially multislice CT, is considered the method of first choice, while **digital subtraction angiography** (DSA) is used less and less frequently for diagnostic purposes alone. However, neither CTA nor DSA is readily and consistently available, particularly at night. Given this situation, it is surprising that so few published data are available on the role of color duplex ultrasound in the diagnosis of acute mesenteric ischemia. When performed with an adequate technique, color duplex allows good identification of proximal occlusion of the mesenteric artery trunk as well as peripheral occlusions during the initial stage, when insonation conditions are still adequate (i.e., during the first 8–12 h). Reliable identification of peripheral occlusions requires adequate adjustment of instrument settings and an understanding of indirect signs of downstream obstruction in Doppler waveforms obtained proximally. Color duplex ultrasound is noninvasive and well tolerable, making it an ideal imaging test for generous use in patients presenting with suspected mesenteric ischemia, who tend to be elderly and multimorbid.

Visceral artery aneurysm is uncommon but important to diagnose because of a high risk of rupture (in particular aneurysms of the splenic and hepatic arteries). Visceral aneurysm is often discovered incidentally in patients undergoing an ultrasound examination for evaluation of abdominal complaints. On color flow images, a visceral aneurysm is distinguished from other lesions, in particular pseudocysts of the pancreas, at first glance.

In patients with **clinical signs and symptoms of abdominal angina** (postprandial pain, weight loss), the sonographic duplex examination should include not only the superior mesenteric artery but also the celiac trunk and possibly the inferior mesenteric artery as well. There is good collateralization of mesenteric occlusion through the Riolan anastomosis from the inferior mesenteric artery as well as through the gastroduodenal artery, pancreaticoduodenal artery, and hepatic artery (celiac trunk) (◘ Fig. 6.23). This is why high-grade stenosis or occlusion of the superior mesenteric artery typically becomes clinically relevant only if there is concomitant stenosis or occlusion of a further visceral artery (celiac trunk or inferior mesenteric artery). Steno-occlusive lesions of these arteries are identified by spectral Doppler interrogation, which is mandatory for the differential diagnosis of abdominal pain and initiation of adequate treatment.

Stenosis of the celiac trunk is typically caused by atherosclerosis (at origin) and rarely by fibromuscular dysplasia. An important cause of stenosis due to **external compression** is the median arcuate ligament syndrome, or celiac artery compression syndrome. The significance of intermittent stenosis caused by the median arcuate ligament is still controversial. The most important criterion for ligamentous compression is the respiratory variation in the degree of stenosis. The accompanying pain is most likely due to mechanical irritation of the celiac plexus. A reduction in perfusion (see ◘ Figs. 6.19, 6.20, and 6.54 (Atlas)) resulting from intermittent compression seems unlikely as there is good collateralization of the visceral vessels. Intermittent compression may, however, damage the vessel wall, thus leading to secondary stenosis. This is confirmed by a study investigating the outcome of surgery, suggesting that a benefit can only be expected in patients with fixed celiac trunk stenosis (in both inspiration and expiration) and demonstration of a steal phenomenon by sonography and angiography (Walter et al. 1999). Surgery is indicated only in patients with epigastric pain and typical manifestations of abdominal angina such as postprandial symptoms and weight loss.

6.1.5.3 Renal Arteries

For adequate treatment of high blood pressure, it is necessary to differentiate essential hypertension from secondary hypertension and, among the patients with secondary hypertension, identify those with renovascular hypertension, which is amenable to causal treatment. The indications for an ultrasound examination of the renal arteries are:

- Workup of hypertension (atherosclerotic stenosis, fibromuscular dysplasia)
- Differentiation of <50% stenosis, higher-grade stenosis, and occlusion
- Follow-up after repair (operation, PTA with/without stenting)
- Suspected renal infarction
- Aortic aneurysm (spatial relationship to renal artery origins)
- Aortic dissection (possible involvement of renal arteries)
- Transplant kidney (anastomotic stenosis, rejection).

The average incidence of renovascular hypertension is 1–4% in unselected populations (van Bockel et al. 1989; Foster et al. 1973; Olbricht et al. 1991), but incidences as low as 0.18% and as high as 20% were also reported (Arlart and Ingrisch 1984; Tucker and Lebbarthe 1977). These discrepancies are due to the use of different screening methods and the investigation of different groups of normal subjects and patients (presence of vascular risk factors and concomitant diseases, specific patient subsets). Atherosclerotic stenosis virtually always occurs at the origins from the aorta or, very rarely, at the branchings into segmental arteries; it predominantly affects older men with other occlusive vascular conditions. In contrast, stenosis due to fibromuscular dysplasia nearly exclusively involves the middle thirds of the renal arteries and primarily occurs in young women (◘ Table 6.4). Hence, selective duplex imaging of the respective renal artery segments according to the suspected cause of stenosis can be performed.

In searching for renal artery stenosis (RAS) as a possible underlying mechanism of hypertension in older patients with atherosclerotic lesions, the examiner must therefore pay special attention to the origins of the renal arteries, where the stenosis is likely to be located in over 95% of this patient group. In younger patients, in whom a suspected stenosis may also be due to fibromuscular hyperplasia, the entire course of the renal arteries is carefully evaluated, in particular the middle third (◘ Table 6.4). Numerous studies have confirmed the validity of duplex sonography in identifying RAS (◘ Tables 6.5 and 6.6).

◘ **Table 6.4** Fibromuscular and atherosclerotic renal artery stenosis (RAS)

Parameter	Fibromuscular stenosis	Atherosclerotic stenosis
Proportion	<10%	>90%
Age	Typically <40 years	Typically >40 years
Sex	Predominantly women	Predominantly men
Preferred site	Typically middle and rarely distal third	Origin or proximal third
Poststenotic dilatation	Frequent	Rare
Repair method of choice	PTA (bypass)	PTA (reinsertion, bypass)

While angiography is the traditional method of diagnosing RAS, various alternative methods are available and there is an ongoing debate about their relative merits. The ACC/AHA 2005 Practice Guidelines for the Management of Patients with Peripheral Arterial Disease (Hirsch et al. 2006) favor duplex ultrasound imaging for diagnosing RAS, followed by computed tomography (in patients without renal insufficiency) and magnetic resonance imaging. Intra-arterial digital subtraction angiography (DSA), however, remains the gold standard. These guidelines do not recommend scintigraphic methods or laboratory tests (including captopril challenge test). Controversy also exists about the degree of stenosis (in terms of diameter reduction) above which RAS is able to induce hypertension and hence should be treated. As in other vascular territories, hemodynamic relevance (defined as >50% stenosis) does not automatically imply clinical relevance. Instead, clinical relevance of stenosis is defined by the diameter reduction that results in a relevant decrease in perfusion in the target organ. In the leg arteries, for instance, demand increases with activity, and hence a stenosis may cause problems only during activity but not at rest. For the carotid territory, a 60–70% diameter reduction is assumed to cause relevant perfusion reduction, and this threshold was also adopted for the renal arteries. However, simply applying these thresholds does not take into account that the renal arteries, unlike the extracranial carotid arteries, have no collaterals. Studies suggest that even stenosis causing only a 50% diameter reduction produces a marked increase in intra-arterial pressure gradients (Staub et al. 2007). In this study, the mean systolic pressure gradient

◘ **Table 6.5** Studies investigating the sensitivity and specificity of (color) duplex ultrasound in identifying hemodynamically significant renal artery stenosis (RAS >50%) using angiography as the gold standard (studies conducted before 1995)

Author	Total No. of renal arteries/No. of stenoses	Method/stenosis criteria	Sensitivity (%)	Specificity (%)	Reference angiography
Duplex imaging					
Avasthi et al. (1984)	52/26	PSV > 100 cm/s	89	73	IA DSA
Kohler and Strandness (1986)	43/–	RAR > 3.5	91	95	–
Ferretti et al. (1988)	104/27	PSV > 100 cm/s	100	92	Angio
Taylor et al. (1988)	58/14	RAR > 3.5	84	97	–
Strandness (1990)	58/14	RAR > 3.5	84	97	–
Hoffmann et al. (1991)	85/64	PSV > 180 cm/s	95	90	–
Schäberle (1989/1992)	91/44	PSV > 140 cm/s	86	83	IA DSA, Angio & X-ray densitometry
Color duplex imaging					
Breitenseher et al. (1992)	41/8	PSV > 120 cm/s	17	89	IA DSA
Karasch et al. (1993)	277/109	PSV > 180 cm/s	92.7	89.8	Angio, IA DSA, IV DSA
Spies et al. (1995)	268/42	–	93	92	IA DSA

PSV peak systolic velocity, *RAR* renal-aortic ratio, *IA DSA* intra-arterial digital subtraction angiography, *IV DSA* intravenous digital subtraction angiography, *Angio* cconventional angiography

Table 6.6 More recent studies investigating the accuracy of ultrasound in identifying hemodynamically relevant renal artery stenosis (RAS) using angiography as reference standard. Combination of different stenosis criteria (direct/indirect) for improving the diagnostic accuracy of ultrasound

Author	Number	Method/stenosis criteria	Sensitivity	Specificity	Reference method
Zeller et al. (2001)	69 (> 70% stenosis)	RAR > 3.5 ΔRI > 0.5 RAR > 3.5 and ΔRI > 0.05	100% 77.5% 76%	60% 99% 97%	Angiography Angiography Angiography
Krumme et al. (1996)	135 (> 50% stenosis)	PSV > 200 and ΔRI > 0.05	89%	92%	Angiography
Hong et al. (1999)	58 (60% stenosis)	PSV > 200 cm/s RAR > 3.5 AT >100 ms	91% 72% 50%	75% 92% 86%	Angiography Angiography
Conclusion: use of a combination of criteria is recommended					
Motew et al. (2000)	41 (>60% stenosis)	PSV > 180 cm/s AT >58 ms	94% 58%	88% 96%	Angiography Angiography
Conclusion: use of a combination of criteria is recommended					
Ripolles et al. (2001)	60 (>75% stenosis) Age < 50 Age > 50 Age < 50 Age > 50	AT >80 ms AT >80 ms AT >80 ms ΔRI > 0.05 ΔRI > 0.05	89% 100% 75% 90% 0%	99% 100% 97% 93% 100%	Angiography Angiography Angiography Angiography Angiography
Conclusion: ΔRI and AT are only reliable in patients younger than 50 years					
Radermacher et al. (1999)	226 (>50% stenosis)	PSV > 180 cm/s and hilar PSV < 25% of intrastenotic PSV AT > 70 ms	96%	98%	Angiography
Souza de Oliveira et al. (2000)	60 (>50% stenosis)	AT > 70 ms PSV > 150 cm/s	83.3%	89.3%	Angiography
Conkbayir et al. (2002)	50 (>60% stenosis)	PSV > 180 cm/s RAR > 3.0 AT >70 ms PSV > 180 cm/s or RAR >3.0 PSV > 180 cm/s or RAR > 3.0 or AT > 70 ms	89% 86% 48% 92% 87%	88% 97% 93% 88% 86%	Angiography Angiography Angiography Angiography Angiography
Conclusion: use of a combination of criteria is recommended					
Kawarada et al. (2006)	94 (>60% stenosis)	PSV > 219 cm/s	89%	89%	Angiography, pressure gradient across stenosis
Staub et al. (2007)	49 (>50% stenosis)	PSV > 200	92%	81%	Angiographic stenosis degree, intra-arterial measurement of pressure across stenosis
		RAR > 3.0 ΔRI > 0.05	83% 31%	91% 97%	Angiography Angiography
	49 (>70% stenosis)	PSV > 250 cm/s	89%	70%	Angiographic stenosis degree, intra-arterial measurement of pressure across stenosis
		RAR > 3.5 ΔRI > 0.05	84% 42	72% 91%	Angiography Angiography
Conclusion: PSV is recommended, may be combined with RAR (and ΔRI) to improve specificity					
Solar et al. (2011)	94 (>60% stenosis)	PSV > 180 cm/s	85%	84%	Angiography
AbuRahma et al. (2012)	313 (>60% stenosis)	PSV > 180 cm/s PSV > 285 cm/s RAR > 3.5 PSV > 180 cm/s and RAR > 3.5 PSV > 285 cm/s and RAR > 3.5	91% 67% 72% 73% 60%	41% 90% 81% 81% 94%	Angiography Angiography Angiography Angiography Angiography

AT acceleration time, *ΔRI* side-to-side difference in intrarenal resistive indices, *PSV* peak systolic velocity, *RAR* renal-aortic ratio

for angiographic stenosis of 50% was 24 mmHg. Other investigators found a significant upregulation of renin even for a 10% transstenotic pressure gradient (De Bruyne Manoharan et al. 2006; Hirsch et al. 2006).

Besides the need for a generally accepted threshold for clinically relevant RAS, the other issue to be resolved is the degree of stenosis above which an attempt at revascularization is justified (percutaneous transluminal angioplasty (PTA) with stenting/surgery). In the past, when surgery was the only treatment option, a higher cutoff was used because of the higher rate of morbidity compared with PTA. **Catheter dilatation with stenting** can be used more generously given the low complication rate and high success rate (internal quality assurance). It must be noted, however, that although studies show dilatation of RAS to be slightly superior to medical treatment in terms of lowering arterial blood pressure and improving renal function, there is no evidence-based proof for this superiority (Balk et al. 2006; Jaarsveld et al. 2003). The disagreement about the stenosis threshold that justifies interventional or surgical treatment is also at the root of the controversy regarding sonographic cutoff velocities and the diagnostic criteria to be used (direct or indirect): the largest group of authors advocate higher cutoff velocities, recommending PTA mainly for patients with higher-grade stenosis and severe renal dysfunction. Conversely, lower cutoff velocities are used by proponents of early PTA (typically to prevent fixed hypertension or parenchymal damage). The advocates of early PTA cannot make use of indirect sonographic criteria for diagnosis as these criteria yield reliable results only for higher-grade stenosis. Note also that PTA has no effect on essential hypertension in patients with secondary atherosclerotic wall lesions and RAS.

After RAS has been confirmed by duplex ultrasound, no further diagnostic tests are needed prior to angiography with simultaneous PTA. In patients having undergone PTA with or without stenting, ultrasound is also the follow-up method of choice for identifying residual or recurrent stenosis.

Color duplex ultrasound should be routinely used **after kidney transplant** and can help to prevent graft loss by timely detection of early postoperative vascular complications (Aschwanden et al. 2006; Urbancic and Buturovic-Ponikvar 2001). The sonographic parameters determined in this examination, in particular the resistance index (RI), also serve as baseline for subsequent follow-up examinations. In the further posttransplant course, a color duplex scan should be performed whenever a deterioration of graft function or an increase in arterial blood pressure is noted.

6.1.6 Measurement Parameters, Diagnostic Criteria, and Role of Ultrasound

6.1.6.1 Renal Arteries

A skilled examiner using a state-of-the-art high-end ultrasound machine should be able to identify and evaluate the renal arteries for stenosis in about 90% of cases. However, accessory renal arteries are more difficult to identify (Krumme et al. 1996). In the hands of an experienced examiner, sonographic evaluation of the renal arteries takes 10–20 min, depending on the acoustic window and clinical question to be answered (atherosclerotic stenosis: renal artery origins; fibromuscular dysplasia: middle thirds).

A wide range of different duplex scanning techniques and parameters have been proposed to differentiate normal findings and low-grade renal artery stenosis (RAS) from hemodynamically significant higher-grade stenosis. This situation shows that all methods have their specific limitations, which one tries to overcome by using different approaches. The fact that the poor visualization of the proximal and middle thirds of the renal arteries precludes velocity measurement for direct demonstration of stenosis has prompted some investigators (Bönhof et al. 1990; Schwerk et al. 1994) to measure and compare peripheral resistance indices in both renal arteries. This is done by spectral Doppler sampling in the distal thirds of the arteries from the flank approach (see ▸ Sect. 6.1.2.3).

In normal, unobstructed renal arteries, the **resistive index** (Pourcelot index, see ◘ Fig. 1.28) is roughly the same on both sides on condition that there is no unilateral renal parenchymal damage, which would lead to more pulsatile flow and thus affect the Pourcelot index as well. Distal to high-grade stenosis, flow is characterized by a delayed systolic upstroke and lower peak systolic velocity (PSV), while diastolic flow is increased, resulting in a lower Pourcelot index (◘ Fig. 6.8). A Pourcelot index <0.5 in the distal renal artery at the hilum suggests postocclusive changes due to upstream flow obstruction (◘ Fig. 6.6).

However, this method has poor sensitivity in patients with more pulsatile flow and higher Pourcelot indices resulting from a loss of vascular compliance due to atherosclerosis or medial sclerosis. In these patients, not even high-grade stenosis is associated with a Pourcelot index <0.5. On the other hand, unilateral reduction of the Pourcelot index of >0.05 (i.e., 10% decrease) compared with the contralateral side (◘ Fig. 6.67 (Atlas)) was found to have 82% sensitivity and 92% specificity for identifying >70% RAS using angiography as the gold standard (Schwerk et al. 1994). This method takes into account elasticity losses as well as systemic factors such as the effects of hypercirculation or hypertension, which may be a source of error in flow velocity measurements for stenosis quantification.

These indirect methods are limited by the fact that they will miss bilateral RAS. Moreover, the results are influenced by the presence of parenchymal damage, which affects the RI. Although renal damage with loss of parenchyma and renal atrophy can be identified by B-mode imaging and thus taken into account in the measurements, some uncertainty will remain. Parenchymal damage can also be caused by long-standing RAS. In these cases, a high resistance index is an indicator of parenchymal damage and can be used to identify those patients who will not benefit from renal artery recanalization due to the extent of kidney damage that has already occurred at the time of diagnosis. This is assumed to be the case if the ipsilateral intrarenal Pourcelot index is >0.8–0.85 (Radermacher et al. 2000).

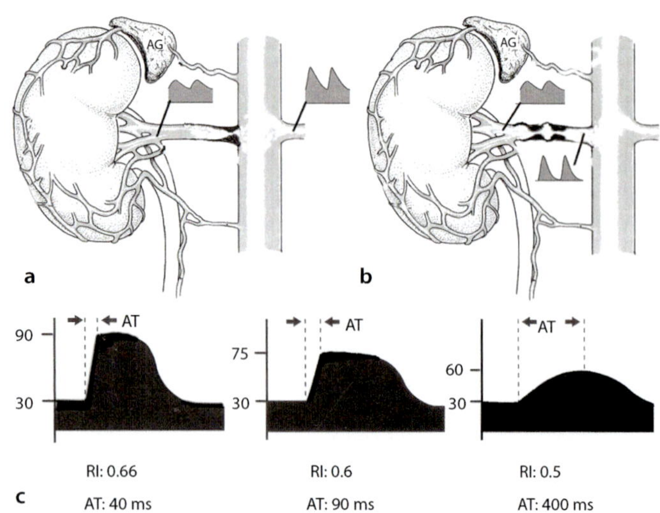

Fig. 6.8 a Atherosclerotic renal artery stenosis (at origin). Changes in postocclusive waveform: less pulsatile flow with delayed systolic upstroke, lower peak systolic velocity (PSV), and corresponding increase in diastolic flow. Lower resistance index (RI, Pourcelot index) as compared with nonstenosed, contralateral artery (see Figs. 6.6 and 6.68 (both Atlas)). **b** Fibromuscular dysplasia of renal artery. Prestenotic and poststenotic waveforms with changes resulting from stenosis in the middle third. Flow is more pulsatile upstream of the stenosis and becomes less pulsatile downstream with a markedly larger diastolic component and decreased RI (AG, adrenal gland). **c** Poststenotic renal artery Doppler waveforms obtained at renal hilum (evaluation for indirect stenosis criteria). Diagrams illustrating the changes seen with increasing stenosis severity (from left to right): normal to mild stenosis, moderate stenosis (60–70%), high-grade stenosis. The poststenotic decrease in pressure is associated with a decrease in peak systolic velocity (PSV), resulting in a lower RI (Pourcelot index). With increasing stenosis severity, the systolic upstroke (i.e., time to peak or acceleration time, AT) is delayed

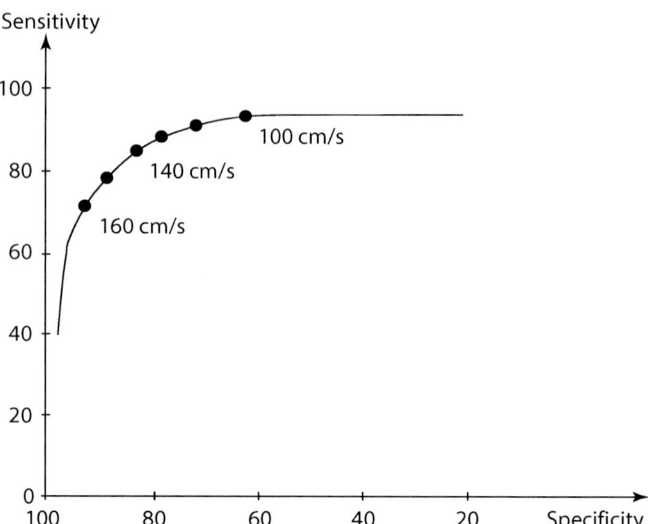

Fig. 6.9 Receiver-operating characteristic (ROC) curve for identifying the optimal peak systolic velocity (PSV) cutoff for differentiating a normal renal artery or low-grade stenosis from hemodynamically significant stenosis (>50%). A PSV threshold of 140 cm/s yields a sensitivity of 86% and a specificity of 83% compared with 75% and 93%, respectively, for a PSV of 160 cm/s (investigated in 170 renal arteries, including 44 with significant stenosis, and using X-ray densitometry as an additional reference method because reliable angiographic stenosis grading (in 2 planes) is generally not possible in the renal arteries) (Schäberle et al. 1992)

The resistance index can be regarded as a sensitive indicator of an early, relevant loss of kidney function. Especially in patients with signs of a hepatorenal syndrome, higher-grade liver cirrhosis is associated with vasoconstriction in the renal cortex, which is reflected in an increased RI. In these patients with advanced cirrhosis, the RI is increased before laboratory tests show any signs of impaired kidney function (Götzberger et al. 2008).

6.1.6.1.1 Role of Color Duplex Ultrasound in the Detection of Renal Artery Stenosis

Direct Criteria

As outlined above, various criteria have been proposed for detecting and grading renal artery stenosis (RAS), and the diagnostic accuracy reported for color duplex ultrasound (CDUS) depends on the criteria used. For peak systolic velocity (PSV), published sensitivities range from 71% to 98% with specificities of 62–98% compared with angiography as the gold standard. These ranges were obtained in studies defining hemodynamically relevant RAS as either >50% or >60% stenosis and using PSV cutoffs ranging from 100 to 220 cm/s (Tables 6.5 and 6.6). It is noteworthy that earlier investigators, using a combination of B-mode and Doppler ultrasound rather than CDUS, tended to identify lower PSV thresholds (<150 cm/s) (Avasthi et al. 1984; Schäberle 1989, 1992; Ferretti et al. 1988; Hansen et al. 1990) (Fig. 6.9, Table 6.5). Without the color mode for visualization of flowing blood (flow jet), however, PSV measurement is more prone to errors because angle correction is more difficult, especially in the more curved right renal artery (see Fig. 6.62d (Atlas)). Some studies conducted in the early 1990s (Berland et al. 1990; Breitenseher et al. 1992; Desberg et al. 1990) used PSVs of 100–120 cm/s to discriminate hemodynamically relevant RAS from moderate stenosis (based on PSV cutoffs used for grading internal carotid artery stenosis).

Later studies (especially after 1993; Table 6.6) using color duplex for placing the Doppler angle correction cursor mostly relied on higher PSV cutoffs on the order of 180–200 cm/s (Staub et al. 2007; Karasch et al. 1993; Motew et al. 2000; Conkbayir et al. 2003; Krumme et al. 1996; Solar et al. 2011). When cutoffs are defined using ROC curve analysis, the value identified to strike the best balance between sensitivity and specificity or positive predictive value (PPV) and negative predictive value (NPV) to some extent also reflects subjective bias and the specific situation for which the cutoff is defined. A more recent study (AbuRahma et al. 2012) found sensitivity, specificity, PPV, NPV, and overall accuracy (OA) to be 89, 54, 56, 88, and 68% for a PSV of 200 cm/s versus 67, 90, 81, 80, and 81% for a PSV of 285 cm/s. Based on their results, the authors proposed 285 cm/s as the ideal PSV cutoff for 60% RAS. Staub et al. (2007) reported a sensitivity, specificity, PPV, NPV, and accuracy of 96%, 69%, 81%, 93%, and 85% for a PSV of 180 cm/s; 92%, 81%, 87%, 88%, and 87% for a PSV of 200 cm/s; and 78%, 92%, 93%, 75%, and 84% for a PSV of 250 cm/s. Based on published data and clinical experience, the author considers **200 cm/s to be the best cutoff**. ROC curve analysis using angiography as the standard of reference will invariably yield lower sensitivity and higher specificity for higher PSV cutoffs and higher sensitivity with lower specificity for lower cutoffs.

Other factors contributing to the identification of **different PSV thresholds** in published studies are:

- the ultrasound technique used
- angle-correction errors (especially in the more curved right renal artery)
- the composition of the study population investigated (impact of greater rigidity of the vessel wall, chronic renal parenchymal damage, poorly controlled hypertension).

Published studies rarely discuss how the PSV is affected by systemtic factors such as blood pressure during the examination (a case in point is presented in ◘ Fig. 5.50 (Atlas)) and vessel wall rigidity.

Another issue that deserves more attention is how the results obtained for the method under investigation are degraded by **inherent limitations of the standard of reference**. As a rule, only oblique angiographic projections of the renal arteries are obtainable (while 2 projections are required for adequate stenosis grading). In most studies, sonographic PSV-based RAS grading is compared with anteroposterior angiograms. While angiography reportedly has good accuracy in the detection of RAS, interrater agreement regarding stenosis grading is poor (Van Jaarsveld et al. 1999). For this reason, radiodensitometry was used as an additional reference method in a study conducted by the author's group (Schäberle et al. 1992). In this study, a PSV cutoff of 140 cm was found to have 86% sensitivity and 83% specificity (◘ Fig. 6.9). Moreover, this study revealed good correlation (R = 0.84) in RAS grading before and after PTA between PSV-based sonographic grading and X-ray densitometry (see ◘ Figs. 6.66 (Atlas) and 6.14).

Discrepancies between angiographic and sonographic grading are especially large for **eccentric RAS**. The reason is that an eccentric plaque causing the same angiographic diameter reduction as a concentric plaque has a less severe hemodynamic effect (because the hemodynamic effect of a stenosis is based on the cross-sectional area reduction, which is 75% when caused by concentric plaque with 50% diameter reduction versus 50% when caused by eccentric plaque with the same diameter reduction). Duplex ultrasound evaluates the hemodynamic effect of a stenosis as a function of the cross-sectional area reduction. Therefore, the PSV measured in a concentric stenosis may be up to twice as high as the PSV in an eccentric stenosis with the same angiographic diameter reduction.

The other major direct parameter for predicting RAS is the **renal-aortic ratio (RAR)**. For identification of >60% RAS using an RAR **>3.5**, older studies reported 84–91% sensitivity and 95–97% specificity (Kohler et al. 1986; Taylor et al. 1988; Hawkins et al. 1989; Hansen et al. 1990). More recent studies found poorer diagnostic accuracies of 76–78% with sensitivities of 73–84% and specificities of 72–81% for this parameter (AbuRahma et al. 2012; Staub et al. 2007).

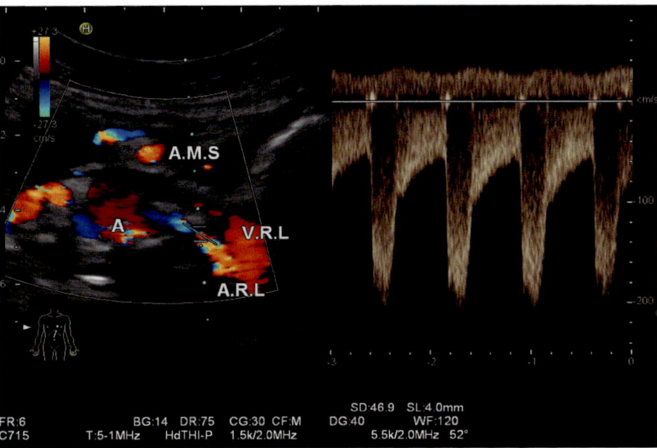

◘ **Fig. 6.10** Fibromuscular dysplasia causing 50–60% stenosis of the middle third of the renal artery (the preferred site of stenosis in patients with this condition). In this patient, renal artery stenosis (RAS) was graded based on the ratio of intrastenotic PSV to prestenotic PSV at the renal artery origin (continuity equation). The PSV ratio was 2.7 (from a PSV of 80 cm/s at the renal artery origin and an intrastenotic PSV of 220 cm/s)

Some investigators explored **end-diastolic velocity (EDV)** as a criterion for RAS. However, caution is in order because EDV strongly depends on the patient's heart rate and peripheral resistance and therefore becomes unreliable once renal parenchymal damage has occurred (which is associated with higher peripheral resistance and hence a decrease in EDV).

Studies specificially **validating the use of color duplex ultrasound (CDUS)** in patients with RAS due to **fibromuscular dysplasia** have not been conducted. The main challenge is overlying bowel gas, which may preclude adequate evaluation of the middle segment of the left renal artery. This diagnostic limitation can be overcome by comparing Doppler waveforms and resistive indices (RIs) from the origin of the renal artery and the hilum (◘ Fig. 6.8). In all patients with adequate evaluation of the mid-renal artery, calculation of the ratio of intrastenotic PSV and prestenotic PSV (in the proximal third of the artery) allows reliable stenosis grading according to the continuity equation (Schäberle 2015) (◘ Fig. 6.10). A ratio > 2 indicates >50% RAS and a ratio > 4 indicates >75% RAS (for concentric stenosis). As in the peripheral arteries, the PSV ratio is a more reliable parameter than absolute PSV.

▪ Indirect Criteria

Experience with waveform analysis in other vascular territories suggests that indirect stenosis criteria do not change appreciably unless **higher-grade stenosis** is present. Therefore, it is not surprising that a side-to-side difference in the resistive indice (ΔRI) of >0.05 (◘ Fig. 6.8c; ◘ Table 6.6) only has 31% sensitivity and 97% specificity (Staub et al. 2007) with a PPV of 93% and NPV of 50% for predicting 50% RAS versus 42% sensitivity and 91% specificity for predicting 70% stenosis (PPV of 69% and NPV of 77%). The poor sensitivity, even for >70% RAS, was confirmed by Zeller et al. (2001), who found 77%

sensitivity but 99% specificity, and by Ripolles et al. (2001), who reported only 50% sensitivity but 90% specificity (69% PPV, 92% NPV). Inerestingly, Ripolles et al. found the ΔRI >0.05 to yield adequate results in patients <50 years of age. In this age group, the parameter had 90% sensitivity and 99% sensitivity as opposed to 0% sensitivity and 100% specificity in patients >50 years. The poststenotic waveform strongly depends on vessel wall rigidity and renal parenchymal function. In elderly patients with atherosclerosis and parenchymal kidney damage, the typical poststenotic flow changes (markedly reduced PSV relative to EDV, delayed systolic upstroke) are less pronounced. Errors in interpreting ΔRI may also result in patients with asymmetrical parenchymal kidney damage.

Another indirect criterion is a delayed systolic rise (**prolonged acceleration time**) or a **reduced acceleration index** at the renal hilum (Kliewer et al. 1997; Stavros and Harshfield 1994; Postman et al. 1996; Nazzal et al. 1997; Patriquin et al. 1992). An acceleration time (AT) of >0.07 s is abnormal and indicates greater than 60% stenosis (Baxter et al. 1996; Kliewer et al. 1997; Stavros et al. 1992; Isaacson et al. 1995; Nazzal et al. 1997; Martin et al. 1991). However, recall that the indirect criteria are not helpful in identifying moderate stenosis (<70–80%) as the poststenotic blood flow abnormalities must reach a certain level before they are reliably reflected in changes in the indirect criteria that can be determined by sonographic evaluation at the renal hilum. This also holds true for AT, which shows poor sensitivity (on the order of 50%) but good specificity (around 95%) for <80 RAS (Conkbayir et al. 2003; Motew et al. 2000).

Many renal diseases and the renal damage they cause lead to an increase in the vascular RI; these include both acute and chronic conditions, glomerulonephritis, pyelonephritis, urinary tract obstruction, and steno-occlusive disease of the renal veins. AT is also affected by different factors such as arterial wall compliance and disturbed microcirculation in different conditions associated with renal parenchymal damage (in particular diabetic nephropathy).

Ipsilateral comparison of Pourcelot indices at the renal artery origin and at its distal end near the renal hilum is a useful criterion for identifying stenosis due to fibromuscular fibrosis if overlying bowel gas or obesity precludes adequate sonographic evaluation of the middle third of the artery. Obstruction by high-grade stenosis will lead to more pulsatile flow with a higher Pourcelot index upstream and a lower index downstream due to a decreased PSV and a corresponding increase in EDV (◘ Fig. 6.8a, b).

6.1.6.1.2 Therapy-Oriented Stenosis Grading

Although peak systolic velocity (PSV) with a cutoff of 180 cm/s (to 200 cm/s) is regarded as the most reliable parameter for detecting and grading renal artery stenosis (RAS), some investigators achieved inadequate sensitivities and specificities and therefore recommend various combinations of direct and indirect parameters (◘ Table 6.6). For the combination of PSV (>180 or 200 cm/s) and a renal-aortic ratio (RAR) of >3.5, three studies found sensitivities and specificities on the order of 90% (Staub et al. 2007; Conkbayir et al. 2003; Krumme et al. 1996).

AbuRahma et al. (2012) identified the combination of PSV >285 cm/s and RAR >3.5 to allow adequate RAS evaluation. This combination had only 60% sensitivity but 94% specificity using 60% angiographic stenosis for comparison. ROC curve analysis for a lower PSV of >180 cm/s in combination with the same RAR cutoff in this study by necessity resulted in a markedly better sensitivity of 73%, albeit at the cost of a lower specificity of 81% (◘ Table 6.6).

Determination of a combination of parameters is not feasible on a routine basis, which is why RAS grading in patients should primarily rely on PSV measurement. Additional parameters such as RAR or ΔRI can be determined in patients with inconclusive findings or in borderline cases. In patients with higher-grade RAS, color duplex ultrasound using PSV, or the other criteria discussed here, is superior to angiography.

The poststenotic pressure drop with decreased perfusion after higher-grade RAS simulates low systemic blood pressure, which is counterregulated by the renin-angiotensin system of the affected kidney. It was long assumed that this regulatory mechanism is not triggered unless severe RAS stenosis of at least 70% is present (corresponding to a PSV >280 cm/s). Hence, it was also assumed that only these higher-grade stenoses require treatment and need to be diagnosed reliably (Textor 1994; May et al. 1963; Muster et al. 1998; Guo and Fenster 1996). A stenosis of this magnitude can be diagnosed by additionally taking into account indirect criteria such as (audible) turbulence. For a therapy-oriented approach, the definition of a precise velocity cutoff for identifying stenosis with beginning hemodynamic effects (on the order of 50%) is less relevant, and the search for the best PSV cutoff becomes a purely academic pursuit.

Later studies including measurement of intra-arterial systolic pressure gradients suggest that renovascular hypertension can already be triggered by lower-grade stenosis (Gross et al. 2001; Staub et al. 2007). For a PSV of >200 cm/s (i.e., 50% angiographic stenosis), Staub et al. (2007) found a mean pressure gradient of >22 mmHg, which indicates significant stenosis with beginning upregulation of renin production (De Bruyne 2006). A limitation of these studies is that poststenotic pressure was measured with the transstenotic catheter in place (artificially contributing to luminal narrowing).

Strauss et al. (1993) found the intrastenotic pressure drop, validated by PSV measurement for iliac artery stenoses, to yield reliable results only when high-grade stenosis is present (simplified Bernoulli equation: pressure gradient $dP = 4 \times \text{intrastenotic } PSV^2$), for which the prestenotic PSV is considered negligible. When the stenosis is at the origin of the renal artery, the PSV measured in the aorta cannot be used as the prestenotic value. On the other hand, the poststenotic PSV occasionally used in the Bernoulli equation (Stock 2009) instead of the prestenotic PSV (dP = 4 × (intrastenotic PSV^2 − poststenotic PSV^2)) is inaccurate and neglects frictional and inertial losses across the stenosis.

The study of Staub et al. (2007) impressively illustrates the **problems encountered in defining cutoffs** for the major ultrasound-derived parameters of RAS (PSV, RAR, RI). A high sensitivity is achieved at the cost of specificity, and vice versa. For a therapy-oriented approach it thus follows that an ideal velocity cutoff for the renal arteries should detect all stenoses causing at least 70% diameter reduction, that is, it should have a high sensitivity combined with a high negative predictive value in order to reliably identify all patients for whom the majority of investigators advocate intervention (Zeller et al. 2003). In those cases where RAS can be treated by PTA with stenting, the diagnostic test should also reliably identify lower-grade stenosis (50%); the rationale here is that it has been shown that 50% stenosis is already associated with a poststenotic pressure drop and renin response. In these patients, PTA is an option if a benefit is expected based on the patient's clinical presentation and the effectiveness of other blood-pressure-lowering treatments. Hence, in this subset of patients, in whom PTA is contemplated as a realistic and beneficial treatment option, a lower PSV cutoff can be used even when it comes at the cost of a certain number of possibly unnecessary angiographies being performed, that is, in those patients who proceed to angiography with PTA (standby) based on the sonographic results (see graph in ◘ Fig. 6.9). However, note that in patients with borderline RAS, there are as yet no adequate evidence-based data available to prove any benefits of PTA over antihypertensive drug treatment (◘ Fig. 6.11). A high RI of >0.9 in the renal artery (◘ Fig. 6.11) indicates that parenchymal kidney damage has already occurred, and no blood-pressure-lowering effect can be expected from PTA (Radermacher et al. 2000); However, PTA may be indicated to maintain kidney function when there is very severe RAS.

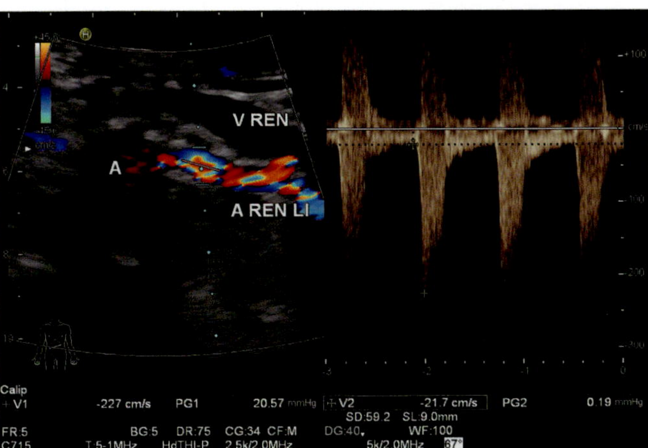

◘ **Fig. 6.11** Stenosis of the left renal artery with very turbulent flow and a peak systolic velocity (PSV) of 230 cm/s, corresponding to approx. 60% stenosis. Based on scientific data, this is a borderline finding with regard to whether or not PTA should be performed. The high resistive index (RI) of 0.9 indicates renal parenchymal damage. Therefore, no benefit in terms of blood pressure lowering is expected from interventional treatment of RAS in this patient

6.1.6.1.3 Contrast-Enhanced Ultrasound (CEUS)

Surprisingly good results were reported by the authors of a study investigating the clinical role of contrast-enhanced ultrasound (CEUS) in 120 patients with 38 stenotic renal arteries in comparison to color duplex ultrasound (CDUS) using angiography as the reference standard (Ciccone et al. 2011). This study reported a sensitivity, specificity, PPV, and diagnostic accuracy of 100% for CEUS compared with 84%, 0%, 80%, and 94% for CDUS. Claudon et al. (2000) described a 20% improvement in the detection of renal artery stenosis (RAS) by CEUS compared with CDUS (from 63.9% to 83.9%). In an earlier study, Missouris et al. (1996) found an increase in sensitivity from 85% to 94% and in specificity from 79% to 88% based on a 20 dB increase in Doppler intensity following administration of contrast microbubbles. Taken together, these study results indicate that CEUS can help resolve inconclusive CDUS findings in patients with suspected RAS.

CEUS is also highly sensitive in demonstrating active bleeding in patients with subcapsular renal hemorrhage and hematoma (posttraumatic or iatrogenic) (◘ Fig. 6.12).

6.1.6.1.4 Ultrasound Follow-Up After Renal Artery Stenting

Duplex ultrasound is the method of choice for the follow-up of patients after endovascular treatment of renal artery stenosis (RAS) (Schäberle 1993). In the postinterventional patient, the target site is known, and a spectral Doppler waveform enables good hemodynamic quantification of residual or recurrent RAS. Good visualization of the stent contributes to the good diagnostic performance of ultrasound in the identification of stent complications (◘ Figs. 6.13 and 6.14).

Data on recurrent RAS after stenting suggest that peak systolic velocity (PSV) and renal-aortic ratio (RAR) cutoffs defined for native arteries may overestimate in-stent restenosis (◘ Fig. 6.13) (Chi et al. 2009; Fleming et al. 2010). However, published reports present conflicting results. In the carotid territory, the need to use higher cutoffs for grading in-stent restenosis has been attributed to greater rigidity of the stented wall compared with native arteries and a narrower lumen of the stented segment. For >70% in-stent restenosis of the renal arteries, Chi et al. (2009) obtained optimal results using cutoffs of >395 cm/s for PSV and of >5.1 for RAR. Fleming et al. (2010) performed ROC curve estimates using PSV cutoffs of 180, 200, and 250 cm/s for identification of >60% in-stent RAS. They reported a sensitivity, specificity, PPV, and accuracy of 73%, 80%, 64%, and 77% for a PSV of 180 cm/s, 68%, 80%, 63%, and 76% for a

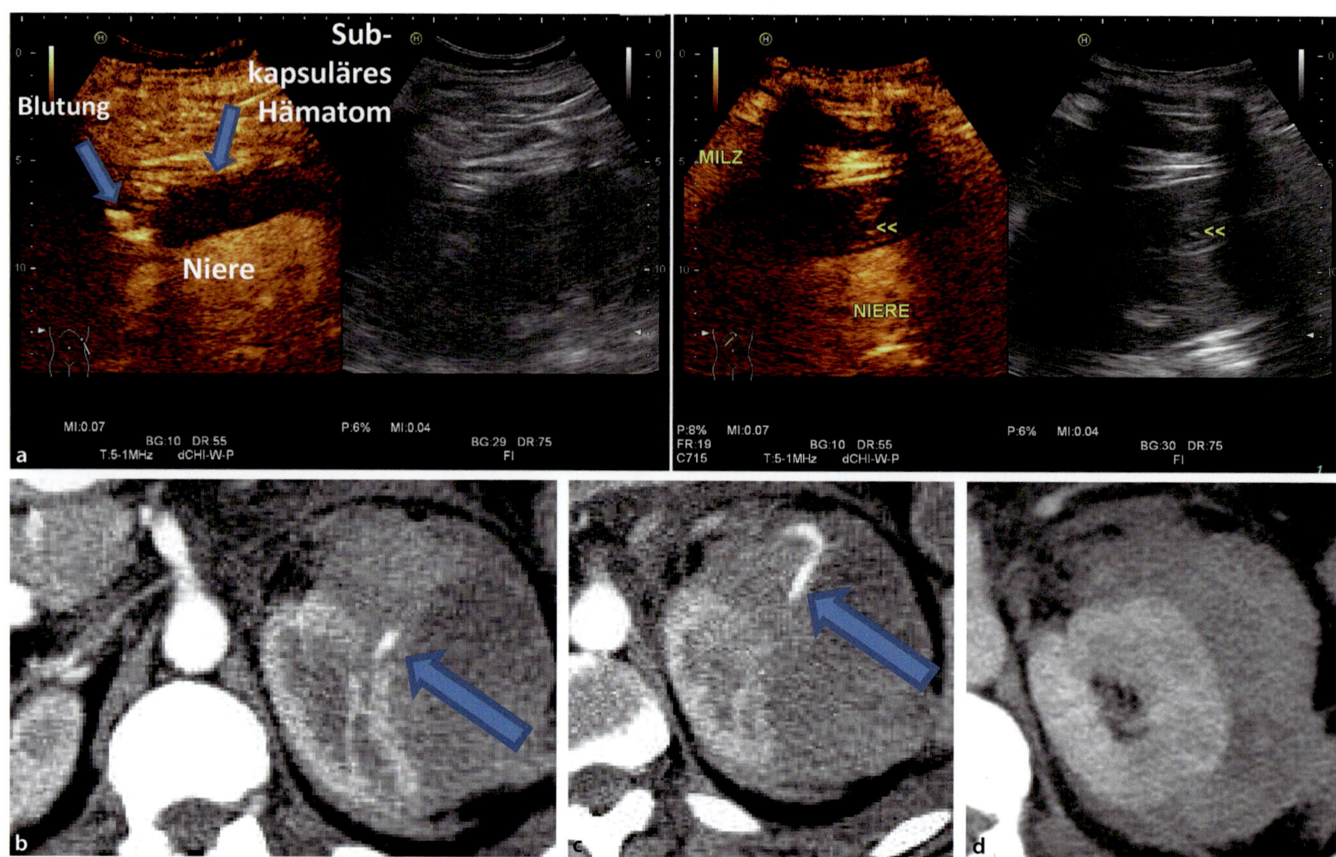

Fig. 6.12 **a** Iatrogenic renal injury (as a complication of abscess puncture in the paracolic gutter) with subcapsular renal hematoma and additional retroperitoneal hematoma. Contrast-enhanced ultrasound (CEUS) shows active bleeding from the puncture channel into the subcapsular hematoma (arrow); however, there is no diffuse bleeding into the surrounding tissue but to-and-fro flow at the site of the puncture channel. The bleeding stopped following thrombin injection treatment (for details of the method see ▶ Sect. 2.1.6.3). Directly after thrombin injection into the area of active bleeding (right CEUS image and corresponding gray-scale image), with the needle still in place (<<), bright spots are apparent lateral to the needle in the gray-scale image, indicating that the corresponding bright spots in the CEUS image are reflections of the injected thrombin and not due to the presence of microbubbles. The two images before (left) and after (right) thrombin injection show the same area; however, the left image was obtained from a more anterior approach (subcostal view) and the right image from a more posterior approach (intercostal view). **b**, **c**, **d** CT scans before thrombin treatment show bleeding from the puncture channel into the subcapsular renal hematoma during the arterial phase (**b** and **c**, arrow). The situation 7 days after ultrasound-guided thrombin injection is shown in **d** (compare **a**)

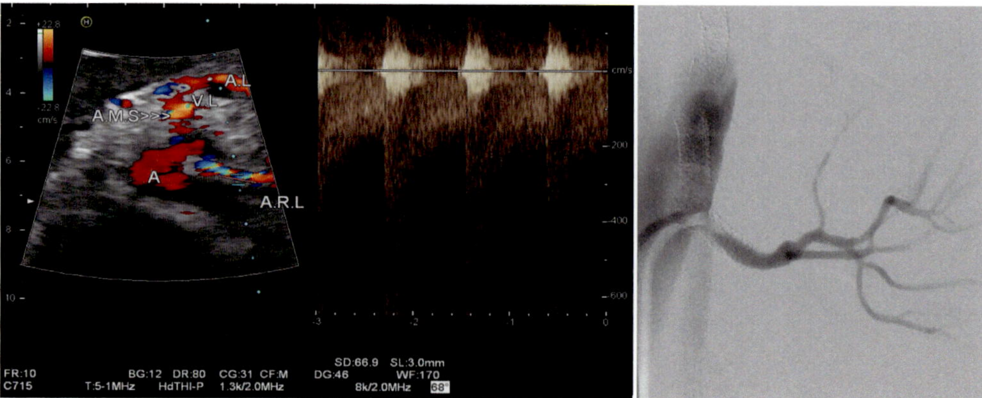

Fig. 6.13 **a** High-grade in-stent restenosis of the left renal artery with a peak systolic velocity (PSV) of 5.5 m/s and very turbulent flow (hyperechoic stent is seen extending into the aortic lumen). **b** Angiogram of the high-grade in-stent restenosis (proximal end of renal artery stent extends into the aorta). The patient has a second stent at the mesenteric artery origin (projected onto the aorta)

PSV of 200 cm/s, and 59%, 95%, 87%, and 83% for a PSV of 250 cm/s. Again, published ROC curve estimates suggest that there is no single cutoff for all situations. If the aim of sonographic evaluation is to identify all restenoses, a PSV cutoff of 180 cm/s yields the best results (highest sensitivity). However, if the aim is to identify the subset of patients with higher-grade stenosis who should have a reintervention, results are best when the PSV cutoff with the highest PPV and specificity is used (i.e., PSV of 250 cm according to the results of Fleming et al.).

Other investigators found similar velocity cutoffs for both stented and native arteries, for example a PSV of >200 cm/s and an RAR of >3.5 (Nolan et al. 2005) or a PSV >225 cm/s and a RAR >3.5 (Rocha-Singh et al. 2008). Napoli et al. even used lower cutoffs compared with the native renal arteries to improve the sensitivity and specificity for identifying in-stent RAS (PSV of 144 cm/s instead of 180 cm/s, RAR of 2.53 instead of 3.5). It may be speculated that, in this study, there was a larger proportion of patients with eccentric RAS (◘ Fig. 6.13). An eccentric stenosis with the same angiographic diameter reduction as a concentric stenosis causes a smaller cross-sectional area reduction and thus has a less severe hemodynamic effect, reflected in a smaller intrastenotic PSV increase (◘ Figs. 2.17 and 5.27).

The limitations resulting from the use of angiography as the gold standard in studies evaluating the diagnostic performance of ultrasound in native arteries also apply to studies investigating in-stent RAS, which are hampered by a number of additional factors. These additional limitations include small patient populations, a retrospective single-center design, selection bias (angiography only in patients with clinical and sonographic abnormalities), no information on insonation conditions (sonographic evaluability, angle correction errors), and failure to consider effects of systemic factors on hemodynamics. Some investigators are aware of these limitations and thus caution readers about generalizing their results (Chi et al. 2009; Fleming et al. 2010).

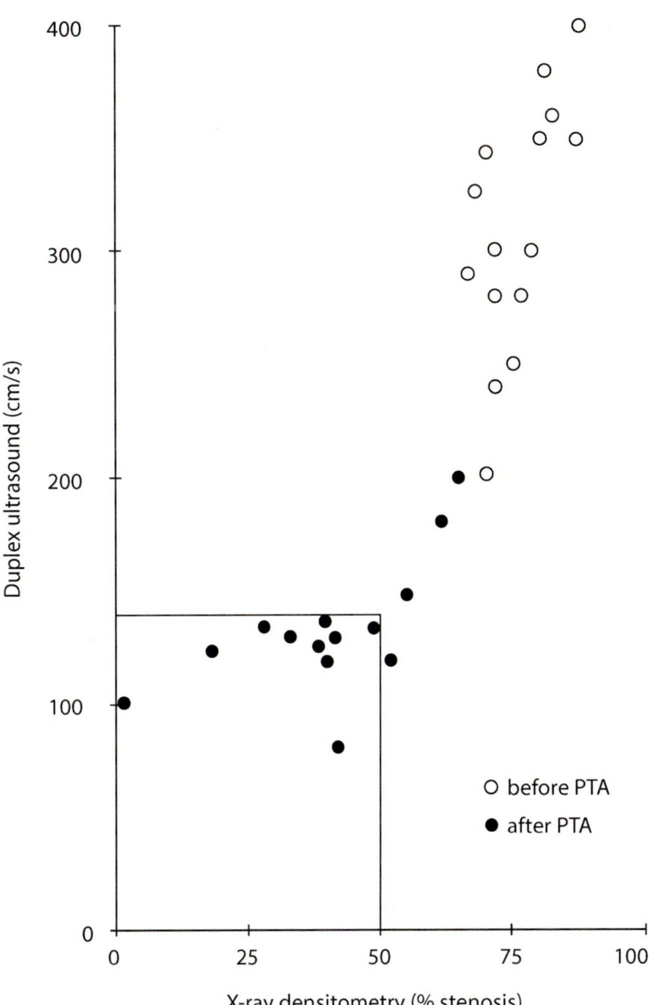

◘ **Fig. 6.14** Correlation of duplex ultrasonography and X-ray densitometry in 14 patients before and after percutaneous transluminal angioplasty (PTA) (R = 0.84). Hemodynamically significant stenosis is assumed at a peak systolic velocity (PSV) of >140 cm/s for duplex ultrasound and at >50% stenosis for X-ray densitometry (Schäberle et al. 1992)

6.1.6.1.5 Diagnostic Algorithm

Color duplex ultrasound (CDUS) is well suited as a first-line diagnostic test in patients with suspected renal artery stenosis (RAS). The most reliable parameter for identifying RAS is a peak systolic velocity (PSV) of >180 (to 200) cm/s. Inconsistenciens of published data on the best PSV cutoff reflect differences in study design and limitations of the standard of reference. In patients with inconclusive sonographic findings based on intrastenotic PSV, sensitivity and specificity can be improved by supplementary contrast-enhanced ultrasound (CEUS) or the additional use of indirect criteria (Schäberle 2015). If this extended sonographic approach still yields inconclusive findings or sonographic evaluation of the renal arteries is limited, magnetic resonance angiography (MRA) or computed tomography angiography (CTA) can be used for further diagnostic workup. Studies report sensitivities and specificities of 88–100% for MRA (Vasbinder et al. 2001) and 90–100% sensitivity and 92–98% specificity for CTA (Beregi et al. 1997; Kim et al. 1998; Wittenberg et al. 1999; Rountas et al. 2007). For CTA, the prospective multicenter Renal Artery Diagnostic Imaging Study in Hypertension (RADISH) reported a lower sensitivity of 64% and specificity of 92%.

Clinical experience can be at odds with the results obtained in trials with standardized study designs. As in other vascular territories, MRA tends to overestimate RAS severity by 26–32% (Glifeather et al. 1999; Krinsky et al. 1996; Steffens et al. 1997), and CT is limited in the identification of calcified plaque.

When the sonographic findings show borderline stenosis and a correct diagnosis is clinically warranted, angiography with PTA standby can be performed instead of supplementary CTA or MRA (◘ Fig. 6.15).

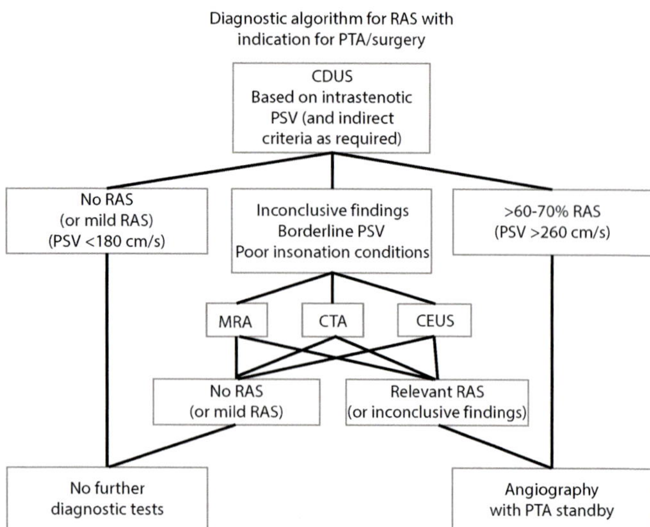

Fig. 6.15 Diagnostic algorithm for the sonographic workup of suspected renal artery stenosis (RAS) with indication for PTA/surgery. CDUS, color duplex ultrasound; CEUS, contrast-enhanced ultrasound; CTA, computed tomography angiography; MRA, magnetic resonance angiography; PSV, peak systolic velocity; PTA, percutaneous transluminal angioplasty

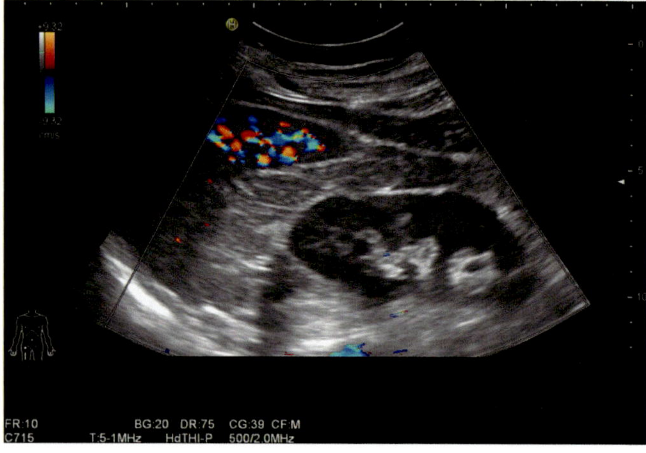

Fig. 6.16 Infarction of the left kidney. The color duplex image obtained with a lower PRF and higher receive gains shows no flow signals in the renal hilum or in the parenchymal region. True absence of flow in the kidney is confirmed by the fact that, with these instrument settings, flow signals are depicted from intraparenchymal vessels in the lower pole of the spleen

6.1.6.1.6 Renal Artery Occlusion

Renal artery occlusion may be suggested by poor visualization of the renal artery on gray-scale ultrasound and a very small kidney (<8–9 cm in length). Duplex imaging shows no flow at the renal artery origin or in the renal hilum and, at most, isolated intrarenal flow signals, indicating supply from capsular veins. Taken together, the results of several studies with small numbers of cases show an accuracy of 93% (Miralles et al. 1996; Hoffmann et al. 1991; Olin et al. 1995). For correct interpration of the sonographic findings, it is essential to use adequate settings including a low PRF and high enough gain (Fig. 6.16).

Renal artery occlusion may be missed if the acoustic window is poor or there is perfusion of the renal capsule and subcapsular parenchyma via collaterals, in particular from the retroperitoneum or the adrenal gland. However, in this situation, flow velocity is markedly reduced, and the flow profile shows characteristics of postocclusive flow as indirect signs. An additional contrast-enhanced ultrasound examination (CEUS) may be helpful and improve diagnostic accuracy (>95%), especially in patients with peripheral renal infarction or infarction due to occlusion of a segmental artery or lower pole artery.

6.1.6.1.7 Transplant Kidney

Two types of complications may occur after a kidney transplant: vascular complications and graft failure.

Vascular complications include:

- Postoperative occlusion of the anastomosed artery or vein in the early postoperative phase
- Transplant renal artery stenosis (TRAS) as a late complication (incidence of 2–25%)
- Aneurysm and arteriovenous fistula.

Anastomotic stenosis can occur during the first weeks after surgery or after many years. The connection of the transplant artery to the iliac artery (see Fig. 6.71 (Atlas)) and the more superficial localization of the transplant vessels facilitate evaluation by duplex ultrasound. Stenosis criteria are the same as for native kidneys, but indirect parameters should not be used. Instead, stenosis must be demonstrated directly on the basis of an increased blood flow velocity at the anastomosis or along the course of the transplant renal artery. An arteriovenous fistula mainly develops after needle biopsy and may resolve spontaneously. A persisting fistula is characterized by a mosaic of colors (due to vibration artifacts) and pulsatile flow in the draining vein (see Fig. 6.72 (Atlas) and ▶ Chap. 4).

Graft failure may occur immediately after transplantation (urine output less than 30 mL/h and progressive elevation of retention parameters). The most common cause is acute tubular necrosis. Perfusion is preserved while most patients have an excessively high resistive index (RI) of >0.9.

Secondary failure after primary graft function is chiefly caused by acute rejection, infection, or nephrotoxic drug effects. Function may be impaired by stenosis of the graft artery or of the ureter. In addition, late failure may be due to chronic rejection.

Acute rejection typically occurs within the first 3 months of transplantation and may be of vascular or interstitial origin. The vascular form of rejection with intimal and medial thickening, fibrinoid necrosis, and subsequent thrombus formation in the small vessels can be identified by an early acute RI increase in the renal artery. In the interstitial form with tubulitis and interstitial lymphocyte infiltration and interstitial edema,

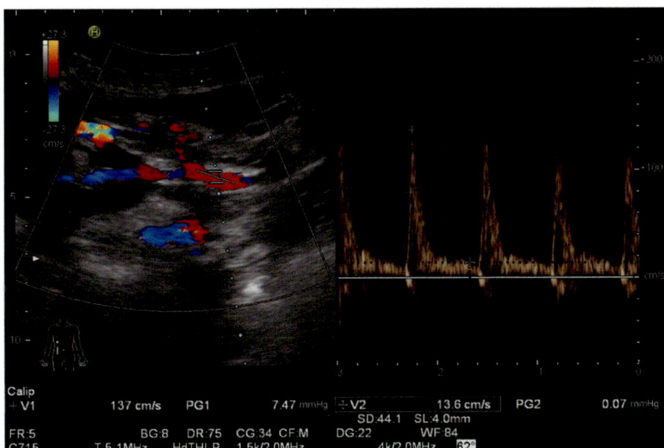

Fig. 6.17 Transplant kidney in subfascial location in the left true pelvis with rejection and a resistive index (RI) of 0.9, calculated from a peak systolic velocity (PSV) of 137 cm/s and an end-diastolic velocity (EDV) of 13 cm/s (RI = (PSV – EDV)/PSV). The sample volume is placed in the renal artery, and the transplant kidney is located to the left of it (with blood flow in segmental arteries). The iliac vessels are displayed posterior to the renal artery

there will be no significant increase in RI despite incipient dysfunction. In vascular rejection, the RI may increase 1–5 days before the diagnosis is suggested clinically; however, a reliable diagnosis of rejection in the case of an insidious increase in the RI can only be made on the basis of serial measurements, to then establish the indication for biopsy or treatment (Hollenbeck et al. 1994; Kubale 1987; Rigsby et al. 1987).

In the 1980s, the **resistive index (RI) of the transplant renal artery**, calculated as peak systolic velocity (PSV) minus end-diastolic velocity (EDV) divided by PSV (see Figs. 1.28 and 6.17), was overrated as a predictor of graft rejection. While certain forms of rejection are indeed associated with an increase in RI, it is not a sensitive marker and provides no clue as to the cause of a failing renal transplant (Tublin et al. 2003). However, another study found an RI of >0.8 to be a strong predictor of a poor prognosis (Radermacher et al. 2003). On the other hand, it is known that, in native arteries, atherosclerotic lesions or subclinical atherosclerosis (increase in intima-media thickness) can also lead to a higher RI, and such an increase in RI has been observed in transplant renal arteries as well.

The RI should be documented at each follow-up and a **change in RI** should prompt a search for the underlying cause, including vascular complications, which may be amenable to correction. Renal causes of an increased RI in patients with a kidney graft include acute and chronic rejection, acute tubular necrosis, renal vein thrombosis, pyelonephritis, and glomerulonephritis. Other causes are compression of the artery, urinary obstruction, and drug-induced dysfunction. A low heart rate can lead to an artificially high RI because the prolonged diastole results in a lower EDV.

Duplex ultrasound is well suited for identifying **vascular complications of the transplant renal vessels** as the underlying mechanism of transplant failure (Osman et al. 2003). The superficial location of a transplant kidney in the true pelvis often allows better sonographic evaluation with fewer artifacts compared to native kidneys. The only potential source of error in TRAS grading is inaccurate PSV measurement resulting from problems in Doppler angle correction in an arched transplant artery (see Fig. 1.23).

Renal vein thrombosis typically occurs in the first week after transplant and accounts for one third of all allograft losses in the early postoperative phase (Orlic et al. 2003; Giustacchini et al. 2002). The reported incidence is 1–3% (Aschwanden et al. 2006; Renoult et al. 2000). Sonographic findings in thrombosis of the transplant renal vein include dilatation and possibly a higher intraluminal echogenicity with absence of flow on color duplex imaging.

When venous drainage is obstructed, flow in the renal artery becomes more pulsatile with a decrease in the diastolic component or even diastolic backward flow (to-and-fro flow), similar to the flow profile in peripheral arteries (Aschwanden et al. 2006; Voiculescu et al. 2005). Prompt surgical thrombectomy is the only measure that can salvage the renal allograft in this situation. Thrombus may arise from renal vein stenosis, but the cause often remains unclear. Renal vein stenosis is suggested by an abrupt marked increase in venous flow velocity (three- to fourfold; Frauchiger et al. 1995; Baxter 2002); in the early postoperative phase, however, rather high flow velocities occur in the vein, particularly more centrally, where it crosses the iliac artery (Thalhammer et al. 2006).

Transplant renal artery stenosis (TRAS) becomes clinically apparent in deteriorating graft function and intractable arterial hypertension. TRAS can occur at the anastomosis, or it can be caused by kinking or atherosclerosis of the renal artery; the incidence is up to 10% (Baxter 2002; Bruno et al. 2004). In the color duplex examination, a stenosis along the course of the artery is revealed by an abrupt increase in flow velocity. The more common TRAS at the origin, or anastomosis with the iliac artery, is diagnosed by calculating a renoiliac ratio from PSV at the renal artery origin and PSV in the iliac artery. A PSV ratio > 2 is 80% sensitive and 100% specific for anastomotic stenosis (De Morais et al. 2003). The problem with using absolute PSV for grading TRAS is the same as in the native renal arteries. PSV cutoff values of 200–250 cm/s have been proposed in the literature, with sensitivities of 90–100% (De Morais et al. 2003; Baxter 2002; Patel et al. 2003).

Intra-arterial digital subtraction angiography (DSA) is the gold standard for **corroborating the diagnosis**, while magnetic resonance imaging is subject to artifacts and may lead to false-positive results or overestimate stenosis (Loubyre et al. 1996; Clerbaux et al. 2003).

Arteriovenous fistulas are iatrogenic complications with an incidence of 2–10% following biopsy (Furness et al. 2003; Merkus et al. 1993; Schwarz et al. 2005). If all patients

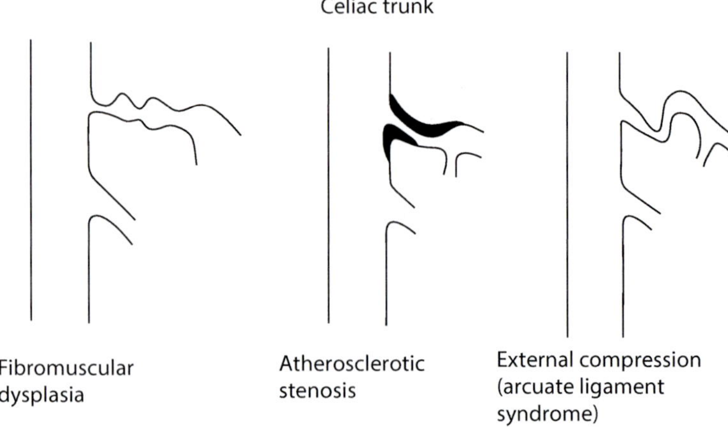

Fig. 6.18 Diagram of different types of celiac trunk stenosis and underlying pathologies (see Fig. 6.54 (Atlas))

were examined by color duplex after biopsy, the rate would probably be greater than 10%; however, 95% of all AV fistulas close spontaneously (Omoloja et al. 2002). As with all AV fistulas, the site is identified by a mosaic of colors due to perivascular tissue vibration. The higher flow volume results in an increase in EDV, and the RI is decreased due to direct drainage into the low-resistance venous system. Flow in the vein becomes more pulsatile and arterialized (see Fig. 6.72 (Atlas)).

6.1.6.2 Visceral Arteries

6.1.6.2.1 Celiac Trunk

Celiac Trunk Stenosis

Stenosis of the celiac trunk is rare and may be caused by atherosclerosis or fibromuscular dysplasia. The rare median arcuate ligament syndrome is caused by intermittent compression of the celiac trunk resulting from downward movement of the median arcuate ligament during expiration (Fig. 6.18). Atherosclerotic stenosis does not become clinically apparent unless several visceral arteries are obstructed.

In a study using a **peak systolic velocity (PSV) cutoff of 200 cm/s** for identifying angiographically proven celiac trunk stenosis greater 70%, duplex ultrasound had 87% sensitivity and 80% specificity (Moneta et al. 1993a, b, c). For 50% celiac trunk stenosis, Perko et al. (1997, 2001) found 94% sensitivity and specificity for a PSV cutoff of 200 cm/s. Note that these cutoffs yield valid results only in fasting patients with normal vascular anatomy.

Overall, published data and clinical experience suggest that a PSV of greater 220–250 cm/s (measured in fasting patients) reliably identifies hemodynamically relevant stenosis (>50%). However, it is likely that only higher-grade stenosis (>75%) with intrastenotic PSV of >280–300 cm/s becomes relevant in terms of compromising intestinal blood supply (see Fig. 6.22).

Celiac trunk occlusion (see Figs. 6.24 and 6.54 (Atlas)) can be bridged via collaterals coursing toward the splenic hilum or via the gastroduodenal artery. Depending on the collateral pathway, there will be retrograde flow in the splenic artery or hepatic artery. Blood flow velocity in the celiac territory is modulated by respiration and should therefore be measured at the resting end-expiratory position.

Median Arcuate Ligament Syndrome

Median arcuate ligament (MAL) syndrome or celiac artery compression syndrome (first operated on by Dunbar in 1965 and therefore also known as Dunbar's syndrome) is the intermittent compression of the celiac trunk near its origin (Fig. 6.19), and very rarely of the superior mesenteric artery.

It is controversial whether the nonspecific abdominal symptoms (upper abdominal pain, loss of appetite, vomiting) are due to hemodynamic disturbances or mechanical irritation of the celiac plexus (proven fibrosis). A primary vascular component appears unlikely given the rich collateral pathways (Fig. 6.54 (Atlas)).

Intermittent compression of the celiac trunk can damage the vessel wall and trigger deposition of thrombotic material, resulting in a so-called fixed stenosis and poststenotic dilatation, as in vascular compression syndromes of other body regions. Upper abdominal pain is most likely due to the pressure exerted by the arcuate ligament and diaphragmatic crura on the vegetative nerves encircling the celiac artery.

As with other compression syndromes that are confirmed by a function test, **duplex sonography** is the method of choice for diagnosing the median arcuate ligament syndrome. The examination is performed during both inspiration and expiration to confirm intermittent compression of the celiac trunk by the ligament. The intermittent constriction of the origin of the celiac trunk during expiratory downward movement of the diaphragm (Fig. 6.19) has a characteristic concave appearance on angiograms.

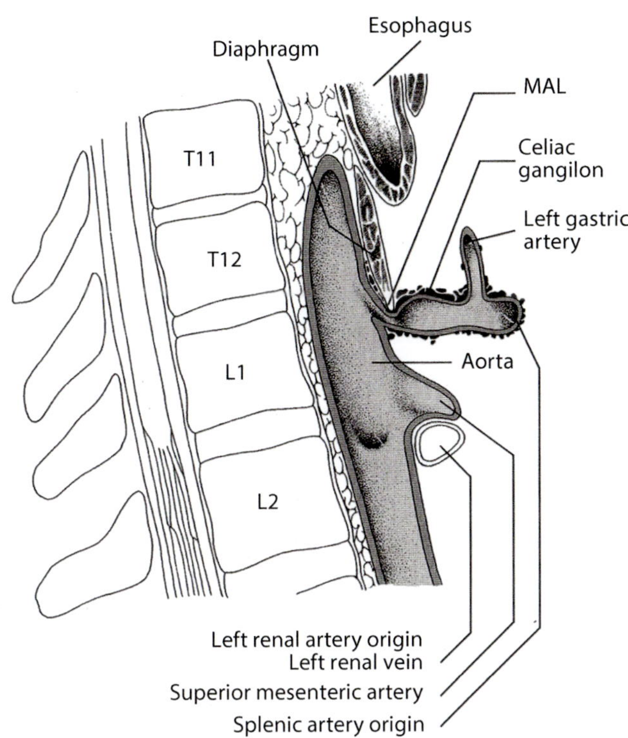

◘ **Fig. 6.19** Topographic relationships between the median arcuate ligament (MAL), aorta, celiac trunk, superior mesenteric artery, and celiac ganglion. Mechanism of compression of the proximal celiac trunk by the arcuate ligament (From Schwilden 1987)

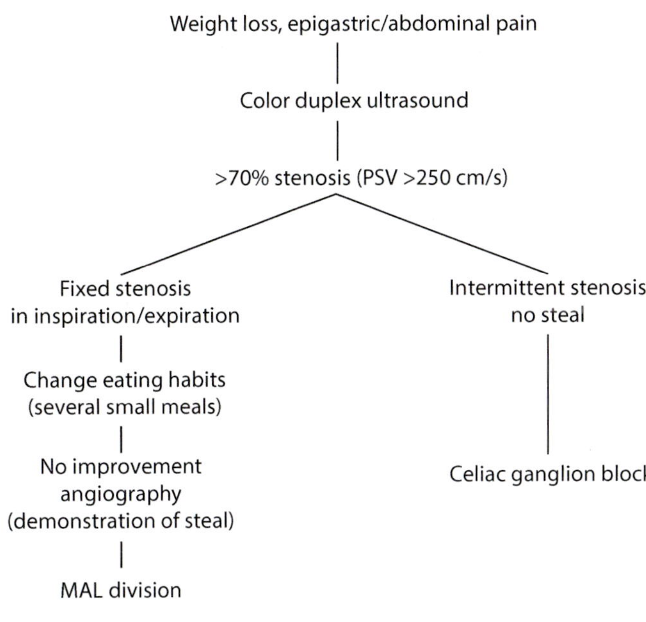

◘ **Fig. 6.20** Diagnostic and therapeutic decision algorithm in median arcuate ligament (MAL) syndrome

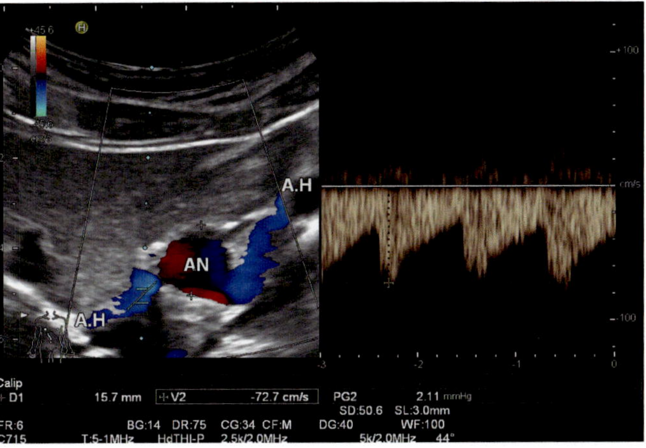

◘ **Fig. 6.21** Course of the hepatic artery in the hepatoduodenal ligament. There is a small aneurysm (AN) with turbulent flow (diameter of 16 mm)

Median arcuate ligament division is indicated if a fixed stenosis is present, identified by a PSV exceeding 280 cm/s during both inspiration and expiration. Surgery is promising and likely to eliminate the compression-related symptoms, especially in patients in whom a steal effect has been demonstrated by duplex ultrasound or by mesentericography and celiacography and in whom the clinical symptoms are due to this effect (abdominal angina with epigastric and postprandial pain and weight loss) and not to compression of the hypogastric plexus (pain).

Other possible causes such as atherosclerotic stenosis of the mesenteric arteries, tumor compression, or chronic pancreatitis must be ruled out (◘ Fig. 6.20).

6.1.6.2.2 Visceral Artery Aneurysm

Aneurysms of the visceral arteries are rare and most commonly affect the splenic artery (see ◘ Fig. 6.61 (Atlas)). A ruptured visceral artery aneurysm is a life-threatening emergency. The **risk of rupture** increases exponentially with the aneurysm diameter. Visceral aneurysm is congenital in rare cases. Other underlying mechanisms include atherosclerosis, trauma, mycosis, and inflammation. Up to 5–10% of patients with a many-year history of chronic pancreatitis develop a visceral artery aneurysm as a complication of this condition.

Visceral artery aneurysms are often detected incidentally and occasionally cause nonspecific symptoms with upper abdominal pain. They are conspicuous on B-mode scans as hypoechoic to anechoic round structures (see ◘ Fig. 6.27). Mural thrombosis is seen as echogenic layering. Aneurysms are **differentiated** from tumors or pseudocysts of the pancreas by the demonstration of flow in the color flow mode (◘ Fig. 6.21 and ◘ Fig. 6.61 (Atlas)). However, a large, mostly thrombosed aneurysm can be mistaken for a malignant tumor. A hepatic artery aneurysm requires precise preoperative localization, which determines the surgical approach (◘ Fig. 6.60 (Atlas)): an aneurysm of the common hepatic artery proximal to the origin of the gastroduodenal artery can be ligated without reconstruction because the liver will be supplied with blood via the gastroduodenal artery, while elimination of a more distal aneurysm (proper hepatic artery) additionally requires vascular reconstruction. Surgery can be planned on the basis of sonographic localization of the aneurysm and determination of its relationship to the origin of the gastroduodenal artery.

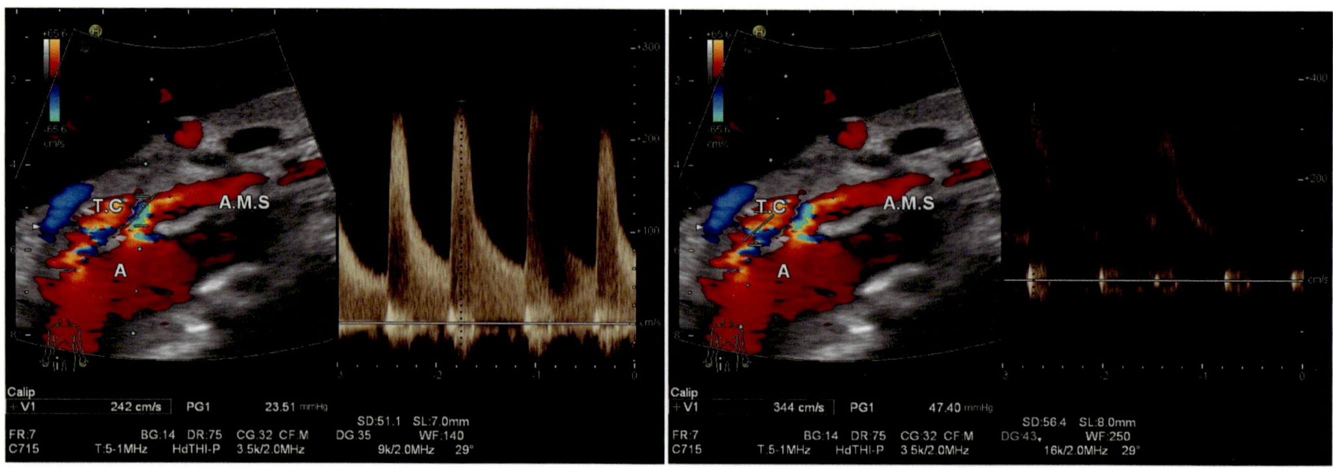

Fig. 6.22 Patient with approx. 50% stenosis of the superior mesenteric artery (A.M.S) with a peak systolic velocity (PSV) of 242 cm/s (left image and waveform) and >70% stenosis of the celiac trunk (T.C) with a PSV of 344 cm/s (right image and waveform). The high diastolic flow in this patient is due to a replaced right hepatic artery arising from the superior mesenteric artery (see Fig. 6.3b–d and Figs. 6.51 and 6.52 (both Atlas)). Note that enhanced flow may also be seen when the examination is performed after eating and that Doppler angle correction is difficult in the curved artery

6.1.6.2.3 Dissection

Dissections of the visceral arteries (see Fig. 6.88 (Atlas)), and of the renal arteries, occur either as extensions of aortic dissections (discussed in more detail in ► Sect. 6.1.6.3.6) or as iatrogenic complications of endovascular procedures (PTA). The severity depends on the dissection membrane, ranging from relatively asymptomatic cases to ischemic problems or even vascular occlusion. A dissection membrane extending from the aorta can be identified by color duplex ultrasound only if insonation conditions are very good. However, in most cases, there will be a characteristic abnormal flow signal due to the floating membrane in the bloodstream (see Fig. 6.88 (Atlas)) and the dissection-related flow obstruction (which may be static or dynamic).

6.1.6.2.4 Superior Mesenteric Artery

Hemodynamics and Measurement Technique

Because blood flow volumes and velocities in the mesenteric artery vary widely with demand, it is essential to examine patients in the fasting state in order to obtain standardized measurements and reliable results when applying velocity thresholds (Fig. 6.51 (Atlas)).

Mesenteric blood flow increases after eating (widening of the artery and increase in blood flow velocity) and is also affected by other physiologic and disease states as well as by pharmacologic agents. Decreases in blood flow velocity and volume are observed after physical exertion and under the influence of vasopressin. An increase in mesenteric peak systolic velocity (PSV) and blood flow volume can be observed after glucagon administration and in individuals with severe hyperthyroidism or during acute episodes of inflammatory bowel disease involving large segments of intestine (Derko 2001).

Quantification of mesenteric blood flow requires calculation of averaged flow velocity and precise measurement of the vessel diameter. Diameter measurements in the superior mesenteric artery by our group demonstrated variations of approx. 10% between systole and diastole with ensuing differences in the cross-sectional area of up to 35%. Therefore, accurate blood flow measurement makes it necessary to measure systolic and diastolic diameters separately and to calculate a mean vessel diameter according to the following formula, representing the two diameters according to their relative weight:

$$\text{Mean vessel diameter / radius}(R)$$
$$R = 1/3 \times \left(2 \times R_{\text{diastolic}} + R_{\text{systolic}}\right)$$

For vessels up to 12 mm in diameter, the diameter can be measured most reliably using the leading-edge method (see Fig. 1.28) and scanning with a low transmit power. This method results in slight overestimation of the diameter but, for diameters of up to 10 mm, the overestimation is smaller than the underestimation that would result from using the inner-wall-to-inner-wall method. Also, the method enables systematization of the measurement error, which is important for serial measurements.

Color duplex imaging facilitates the identification of the mesenteric and renal arteries. Once the target artery has been brought into view, a Doppler waveform is obtained for hemodynamic evaluation. Under good insonation conditions, color flow imaging will suggest a stenosis, but verification by spectral Doppler is necessary. Depending on the clinical question to be answered, spectral Doppler tracings should be sampled at the vessel origins, the preferred sites of atherosclerotic stenosis of the visceral arteries.

Atherosclerotic stenosis of visceral branches usually occurs at the origins from the aorta (Fig. 6.22). Involvement of the peripheral branches is only seen in diabetics with generalized medial sclerosis. If there is high-grade atherosclerotic stenosis of only one of the three visceral artery origins, compensatory dilatation of the preformed collateral pathways will ensure adequate perfusion in most cases.

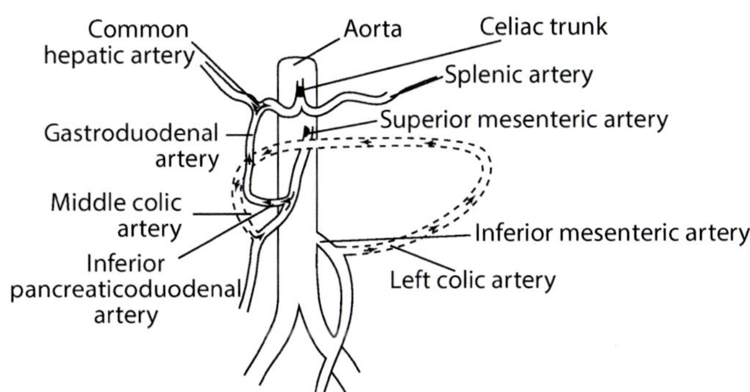

Fig. 6.23 Diagram of collateral pathways in occlusion of the celiac trunk and/or superior mesenteric artery: the Riolan anastomosis (dashed lines) between the superior mesenteric artery and the middle colic artery is the main collateral pathway in superior mesenteric artery occlusion. Collaterals between the celiac trunk and superior mesenteric artery include the pancreaticoduodenal artery and the gastroduodenal artery, which joins the hepatic artery

In general, **chronic intestinal ischemia** manifests as abdominal angina only if there is occlusion or stenosis of more than one visceral artery or in case of poor collateralization. The typical symptom is postprandial pain. Calcified plaques suggest a stenosis in the B-mode image, but definitive evidence is provided only by flow acceleration with turbulence or the absence of flow signals in case of occlusion.

Chronic mesenteric artery occlusion is due to atherosclerosis and is associated with extensive collateralization through the celiac trunk (primarily involving the pancreaticoduodenal artery) and the inferior mesenteric artery (Riolan anastomosis; Fig. 6.23). While the main collaterals (gastroduodenal, splenic, and inferior mesenteric arteries) are often detectable by ultrasound (Figs. 6.58b,c (Atlas) and 6.23), angiography provides a better overview and overall picture of collateral pathways. Specifically, the dilated gastroduodenal artery is visualized by duplex ultrasound at the pancreatic head. Ultrasound evaluation is facilitated by the fact that patients with chronic mesenteric ischemia tend to be thin because they suffer from abdominal angina (abdominal pain after eating). The superior mesenteric artery is filled distally and shows postocclusive flow with a delayed and reduced systolic rise and a decreased Pourcelot index (see Fig. 6.58 (Atlas)).

Color Duplex Ultrasound Grading of Mesenteric Artery Stenosis

Several studies, mostly in small series, report good results for color duplex ultrasound (CDUS) in the detection of hemodynamically relevant mesenteric artery stenosis in patients presenting with abdominal angina. While investigators consistently describe good sonographic evaluability of the mesenteric artery trunk and especially of the superior mesenteric artery origin, there is disagreement regarding the best velocity parameter (peak systolic velocity (PSV) versus end-diastolic velocity (EDV)) and optimal cutoff values (Table 6.7). Some authors advocate PSV as the most suitable parameters for mesenteric stenosis grading (Moneta et al. 1991; Bowersox et al. 1991; AbuRahma et al. 2012; Mitchell et al. 2009), while others opt for EDV (Zwolak 1999; Perko et al. 1997). PSV is well known to be influenced by a variety of factors including systolic blood pressure during the examination,

Table 6.7 Sensitivity, specificity, positive predictive value (PPV), negative predictive value (NPV), and overall accuracy (OA) of duplex ultrasound in the diagnosis of stenosis at the origin of the mesenteric artery. Results obtained with different cutoffs for peak systolic velocity (PSV), end-diastolic velocity (EDV), and PSV ratio. Cutoffs were identified using ROC curve analysis with angiography as the standard of reference

Parameter (study) (cutoff)	Sensitivity	Specificity	PPV	NPV	OA
PSV					
≥70% stenosis (Moneta 1993) (PSV ≥ 275 cm/s)	92%	59%	56%	93%	71%
≥50% stenosis (Bowersox 1991) (PSV ≥ 300 cm/s)	86%	89%	91%	83%	87%
>50% stenosis (Perko 1997) (PSV > 275 cm/s)	93%	80%			
>50% stenosis (AbuRahma 2012) (PSV > 295 cm/s)	87%	89%	90%	84%	88%
>70% stenosis (AbuRahma 2012) (PSV > 400 cm/s)	72%	93%	81%	85%	85%
EDV					
≥50% stenosis (Zwolak 1998) (EDV ≥ 45 cm/s)	79%	79%	84%	72%	79%
≥50% stenosis (Perko 2001) (EDV ≥ 70 cm/s)	47%	98%	97%	57%	68%
>50% stenosis (AbuRahma 2012) (EDV > 45 cm/s)	79%	79%	82%	69%	79%
>70% stenosis (AbuRahma 2012) (EDV > 70 cm/s)	65%	95%	86%	81%	84%
PSV ratio (superior mesenteric artery origin/aorta)					
>50% stenosis (AbuRahma 2012) (PSV ratio > 3.5)	69%	78%	79%	68%	73%
>70% stenosis (AbuRahma 2012) (PSV ratio > 4.5 cm/s)	67%	83%	65%	84%	78%

sympathetic tone, medications, and time since last meal. Even the respiratory phase appears to play a role, as some authors found a higher PSV during expiration (van Petersen et al. 2013; Seidl et al. 2010). This observation may be due to transient compression of the artery by the diaphragmatic crura (mild form of median arcuate ligament syndrome). A pitfall to be considered is that the proximal superior mesenteric artery segment may be more arched during expiration, leading to errors in setting the Doppler angle (see ◘ Fig. 6.55 (Atlas)).

To account for systemic factors affecting absolute PSV, some authors explored a PSV ratio calculated from intrastenotic PSV at the superior mesenteric artery origin and PSV in the aorta. However, AbuRahma et al. (2012) found poorer accuracies on the order of 70–80% using a PSV ratio >3.5 as a cutoff for identifying >50% stenosis and a ratio >4.5 for >70% stenosis compared with absolute PSV thresholds.

Another alternative velocity parameter, the EDV, also failed to improve accuracies (AbuRahma et al. 2012). EDV is influenced by even more additional factors than PSV (inflammatory bowel disease, heart rate). Anatomic variants also affect EDV. Of note, EDV is higher when the right hepatic artery arises from the superior mesenteric artery.

Errors in Doppler angle correction can cause errors in both PSV and EDV measurement. Aligning the angle correction cursor with the direction of blood flow is difficult when the proximal superior mesenteric artery takes an arched course. With downward movement of the diaphragm during inspiration, the bowel pulls down the mesenteric root, straightening the mesenteric artery and improving adjustment of the Doppler angle (see ◘ Fig. 6.55 (Atlas)).

The author's practical experience suggests that a PSV cutoff of 280 cm/s for >50% stenosis and of 350 cm/s for >70% provides adequate accuracies in the clinical setting. The relatively low sensitivity of 74% in conjunction with a high specificity of 93%, which AbuRaham et al. (2012) identified when using a PSV cutoff of 4 m/s for identifying 70% stenosis (◘ Table 6.7), indicates that this cutoff is slightly too high. It should also be noted that identification of 50% mesenteric stenosis is of little clinical relevance. Abdominal angina is caused by higher-grade stenosis, and because of good collateralization in this territory, steno-occlusive disease becomes relevant only when several arteries are affected (celiac trunk, inferior mesenteric artery). Finally, angiographic evaluation of the mesenteric artery origin in two planes is also technically challenging.

A stent alters hemodynamic parameters, and higher velocity thresholds should be used when evaluating **in-stent restenosis**. A stent reduces wall elasticity and the lumen of the artery, resulting in more pulsatile blood flow and a higher PSV. AbuRahma et al. (2012) propose a 20–30 cm/s higher velocity cutoff for stented mesenteric arteries, corresponding to a 10% higher PSV compared with stenosis in the native arteries (◘ Fig. 6.24a). Armstrong (2007) recommends angiography with reintervention in patients with an EDV of 50–70 cm/s or a poststenotic PSV <40 cm/s and an intrastenotic PSV >300 cm/s. This PSV appears rather low, and most asymptomatic patients with in-stent restenosis do not need a reintervention as long as intrastenotic PSV remains below 400 cm/s.

6.1.6.2.5 Acute Mesenteric Artery Occlusion

Acute mesenteric occlusion due to embolism is easily and reliably demonstrated by (color) duplex imaging as the absence of flow if the occlusion is located near the origin of the mesenteric artery from the aorta. Peripheral mesenteric artery occlusions, on the other hand, pose a diagnostic problem. If there is extensive infarction of the small intestine but the mesenteric artery trunk is patent, the embolus is typically lodged at the divisions into jejunal branches or further distally at the origins of the ileocolic and right colic arteries. If there are patent branches such as the middle colic artery or proximal segments of the jejunal branches, the trunk of the mesenteric artery is patent as well. The overall reduction in blood flow and peripheral dilatation in the territory of the patent branches, which provide collateral flow via the arcades, is reflected in the corresponding spectral Doppler waveforms (◘ Fig. 6.25; see ◘ Figs. 6.56 (Atlas) and 6.57 (Atlas)). Peak systolic velocity (PSV) is reduced, and the lower peripheral resistance results in a larger diastolic component and a lower Pourcelot index.

The waveform changes become more conspicuous with the number of occluded branches, which in turn increases the more proximal an embolus is located (see ◘ Fig. 6.57 (Atlas)). Consequently, these spectral Doppler changes in conjunction with the above-described decreases in the Pourcelot index and PSV should prompt a careful evaluation of the individual mesenteric branches distally in longitudinal and transverse planes using color duplex ultrasound to identify flow (◘ Fig. 6.26). The Doppler waveform changes are less marked when the mesenteric artery is occluded more distally (e.g., affecting only a few jejunal branches). However, the number of vessels involved has little clinical relevance and does not affect the patient's prognosis because the loss is compensated for by collateral flow through the patent branches and the arcades.

In the abdomen, **color duplex ultrasound** usually provides adequate resolution for evaluation of blood flow in the mesenteric artery trunk including its peripheral segment and the origins of the jejunal branches arising from it (◘ Figs. 6.26 and 6.57 (Atlas)). However, the sonographic detection of individual jejunal branch occlusions is of no therapeutic consequence. The foremost aim is the timely detection of mesenteric artery occlusion and surgical restoration of blood flow before ischemia causes extensive necrosis of the small bowel. For this, it is sufficient that the mesenteric artery trunk can be evaluated for flow from its origin to the umbilical level. When required, ultrasound of the mesenteric artery should include the origins of jejunal branches (◘ Fig. 6.26). Nonocclusive mesenteric ischemia (NOMI) is not detectable by duplex ultrasound; however, other imaging modalities such as CTA or angiography do not consistently detect NOMI either. NOMI often leads to necrosis and

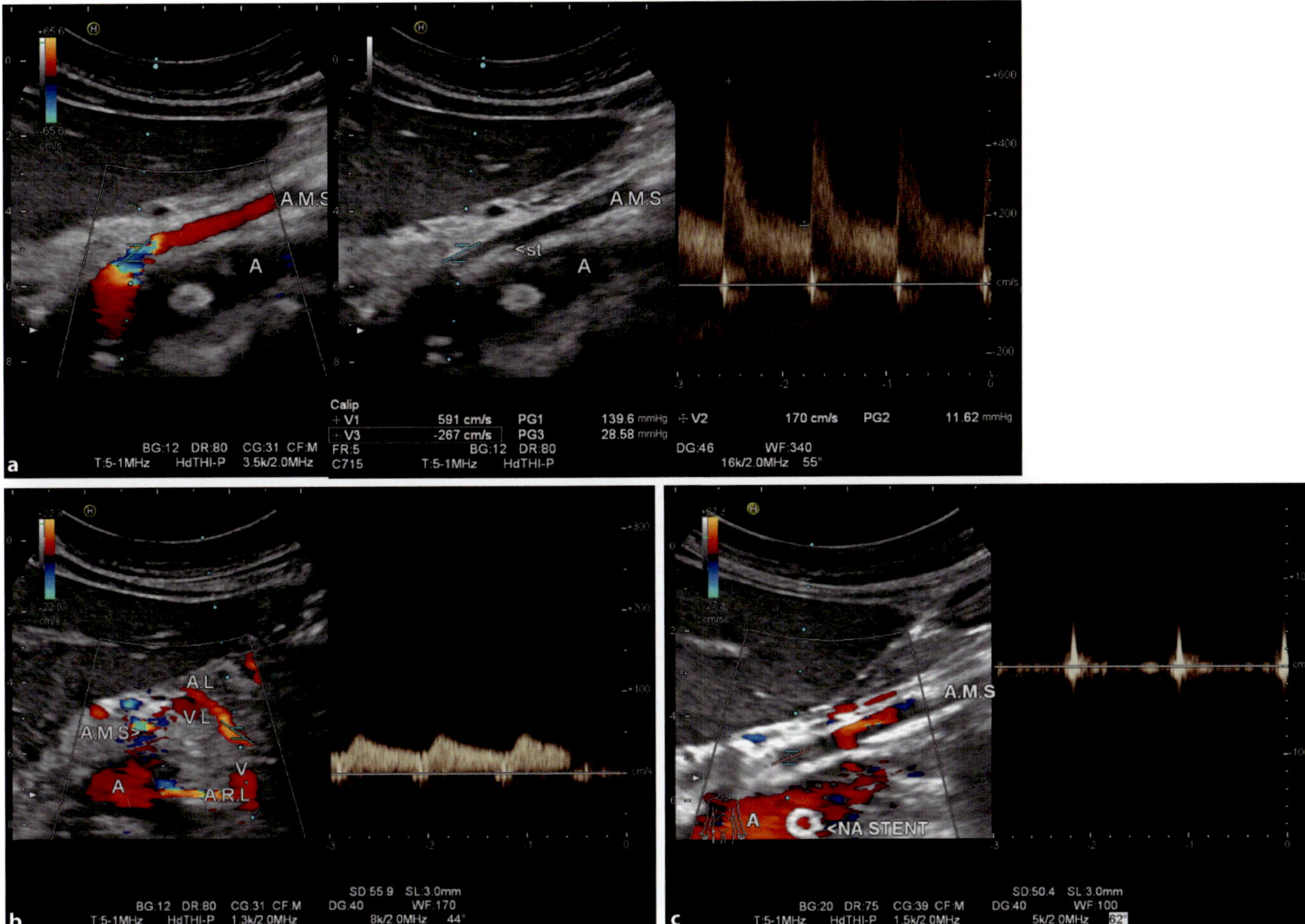

◻ **Fig. 6.24** **a** High-grade superior mesenteric artery in-stent restenosis with a peak systolic velocity (PSV) of 580 cm/s in a patient with a history of right-sided hemicolectomy for ischemic perforation (same patient as in ◻ Fig. 6.13). **b** There is concomitant celiac trunk occlusion, and the liver is supplied via the splenic artery, which shows reversed flow, i.e., flow toward the hepatic artery (red, toward transducer). The waveform from the splenic artery (A.L) shows little pulsatility. The splenic artery is supplied by small dilated arteries coursing from the pancreatic tail to the mesentery of the transverse colon. These arteries, in turn, are supplied by branches of the inferior mesenteric artery. The patient refused reintervention. **c** One year later, the patient presented with intestinal ischemia and occlusion of the stented superior mesenteric artery. The distal superior mesenteric artery is supplied via pancreaticoduodenal collaterals. The splenic artery (with regrograde flow) now supplies not only the liver but also the distal superior mesenteric artery (see ◻ Fig. 6.23). In conjunction with the patient's clinical presentation, these ultrasound findings prompted immediate endovascular reintervention

resection of affected bowel segments regardless of the time elapsed between symptom onset and surgery.

The **role of ultrasound** is confirmed by the author's experience in 101 consecutive patients seen from 1997 through 2004. These patients had a high clinical suspicion of mesenteric artery occlusion and a history of characteristic pain of less than 24-h duration. Suspected mesenteric artery occlusion was confirmed by duplex ultrasound using the above-described criteria in 19 patients (19%), who proceeded to surgical embolectomy based on the sonographic findings. The sonographic findings were confirmed intraoperatively. Nine of the patients operated on had occlusion of the peripheral mesenteric artery trunk only. Another four patients (4%) had NOMI due to obstruction of peripheral segments, which did not cause spectral waveform changes and was not detected by duplex ultrasound. In most of these cases, only a short intestinal segment had to be removed. In 62 patients (61%), ultrasound ruled out acute embolic mesenteric occlusion, and the findings were confirmed by the further clinical course or during surgery performed for other causes of acute abdomen. In 16 of the 101 patients (16%), angiography or CTA was performed because of poor insonation conditions or inconclusive spectral Doppler findings.

The results of Danse et al. (1996) confirm the ability of **Doppler sonography** to diagnose acute mesenteric artery occlusion. In this study of 770 patients with emergency admissions for acute abdominal pain, ultrasound correctly diagnosed superior mesenteric artery occlusion in 5 cases. The author of another, rather general overview (Cappell 1998) describes ultrasound as a nonstandard diagnostic test in acute mesenteric ischemia, though without providing sound scientific evidence for this conclusion.

B-mode imaging features can also provide clues in patients presenting with acute intestinal ischemia. Rapid development

6

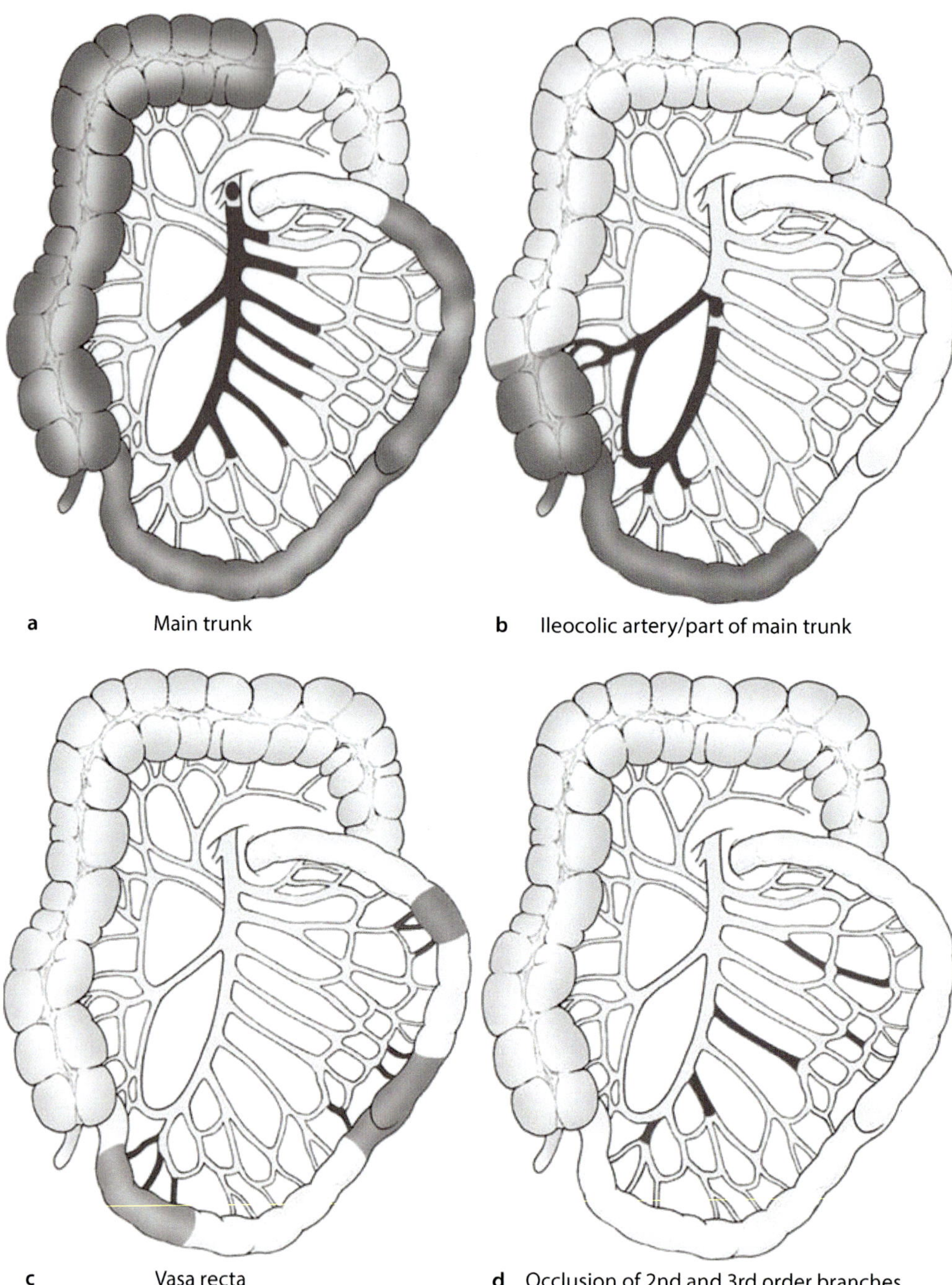

Fig. 6.25a–d Acute mesenteric artery occlusion. The extent of intestinal necrosis varies with the level of occlusion. Occlusion of individual jejunal branches only will not lead to acute intestinal ischemia as the arcades ensure collateral flow from patent jejunal branches (**d**). The vasa recta are involved in nonocclusive intestinal ischemia (**c**). Proximal occlusions in which the mesenteric trunk is still patent are associated with necrosis of long intestinal segments and have a poor prognosis. The Doppler waveform from the patent mesenteric artery shows abnormal changes (**a**, **b**). The remaining patent branches dilate to provide maximum blood supply via the arcades, resulting in less pulsatile, low-resistance flow. Nevertheless, overall flow through the patent mesenteric trunk is reduced (decreased PSV)

of intestinal wall edema is identified by the so-called bull's eye sign. The further course is characterized by intestinal wall necrosis and cessation of peristalsis along with further intestinal wall thickening and the appearance of free fluid around affected bowel loops. In the late phase, air bubbles appear in the intestinal wall and portal vein (Seitz and Rettenmaier 1994).

Ischemic bowel wall changes detected with B-mode ultrasound and unenhanced CT (Gebhardt et al. 1989; Danse et al. 1996, 2009) typically indicate irreversible damage, and no therapeutic measures can salvage the affected bowel segments. Nevertheless, color duplex ultrasound evaluation of intestinal wall thickening in acute abdomen may be helpful in that detection of flow signals near the wall rules out ischemia as the underlying cause.

When ultrasound identifies thickened bowel loops and ischemia is a possible differential diagnosis, a high-resolution ultrasound transducer can be used to search for flow signals in the bowel wall or in the adjacent mesentery (high gain without artifacts and low PRF). Flow detected by color duplex imaging should then be confirmed by obtaining a Doppler waveform from this area. Confirmation of flow rules out ischemia as the underlying cause, and a large diastolic flow component in the Doppler waveform points to an inflammatory cause (see Fig. 6.59 (Atlas)).

A **contrast-enhanced ultrasound (CEUS) examination** can also contribute useful information in patients with suspected mesenteric ischemia. Studies report sensitivities, specificities, PPV, and NPV of 94%, 100%, 100%, and 97%

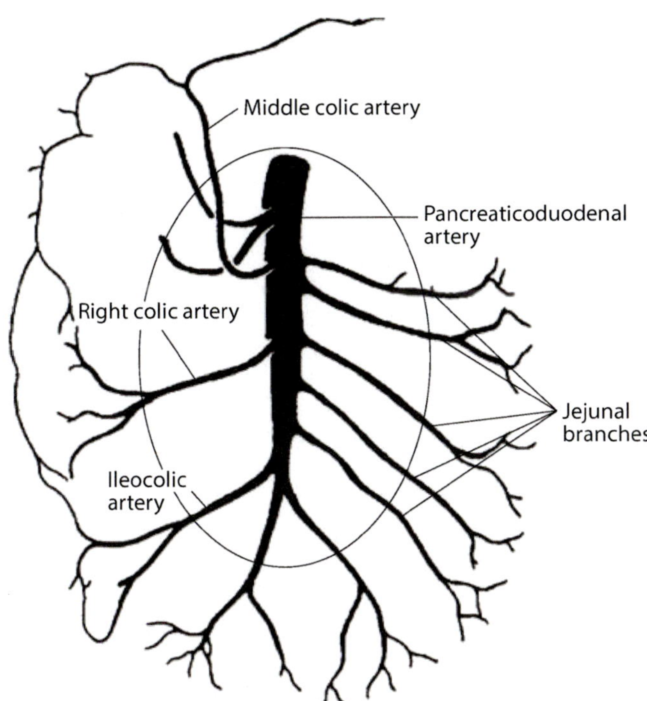

Fig. 6.26 Divisions of the superior mesenteric artery with side branches. Under good conditions, color duplex imaging visualizes the main trunk, the division into jejunal branches, the right colic artery, and ileocolic artery (visible area outlined) (According to Kubale 1994)

(Hamada et al. 2007) and of 85%, 100%, 100%, and 91% (Hata et al. 2005). However, in these studies, the authors did not investigate the mesenteric artery trunk but searched for enhancing flow (or absence of flowing blood) in the bowel wall of segments showing morphogic abnormalities on B-mode imaging (widening or wall thickening). CEUS is more time-consuming, and a literature search identified only one case report that describes the diagnosis of mesenteric artery trunk occlusion based on the use of ultrasound microbubbles (Giannetti et al. 2010).

It follows from the above that color duplex ultrasound is not the generally recommended first-line diagnostic imaging test, as it has several limitations including its examiner dependence, the reliance on good insonation conditions, and incomplete evaluability of the mesenteric territory. However, when performed by an experienced examiner with good methodological skills and use of adequate instruments settings, color duplex is a very time-efficient and accurate tool for identifying those forms of early acute mesenteric artery occlusion that are amenable to treatment in emergency patients. An ultrasound examination is routinely performed in patients presenting with abdominal pain, and supplementing this examination by a color duplex evaluation of the mesenteric artery trunk requires little extra time (<5 min). When color duplex yields a confident diagnosis, treatment can be initiated, while inconclusive findings need to be confirmed by CTA.

Insonation conditions are inadequate in the late phase of acute mesenteric artery occlusion, due to overlying air, pain, and poor patient compliance. At this stage, the indication for surgery is established on clinical grounds (but the prognosis is poor), and the sonographic findings are of little relevance. Conversely, in the earlier phase, when the clinical presentation alone would not necessarily justify emergency surgery (see Table 6.3), the insonation conditions in most patients allow adequate sonographic evaluation of the mesenteric artery trunk and its proximal divisions.

The resistive index (Pourcelot index) in the superior mesenteric artery is also decreased in patients with abdominal conditions associated with **peritonitis** or in patients with **septicemia**. However, in these patients, the RI is not required as a diagnostic marker, and the indication for surgery is established on clinical grounds or on the basis of additional diagnostic tests (B-mode ultrasound or other imaging modalities). The Doppler waveform in septicemia or peritonitis differs from that obtained in patients with distal mesenteric artery occlusion in that, while the diastolic component is increased, the PSV is still rather high and close to normal (while it is decreased in mesenteric artery occlusion).

Indirect sonographic criteria cannot be quantified and, if present, should prompt further diagnostic testing (angiography) or, if warranted in conjunction with the clinical presentation, laparotomy. Hypotension and tachycardia, as in septic shock, or generalized peritonitis also cause marked hemodynamic changes, resulting in abnormal Doppler waveforms. Thus, the spectral waveform from the mesenteric artery must always be interpreted in conjunction with the clinical presentation. However, the combination of a lower Pourcelot index with decreases in PSV and averaged blood flow velocities, demonstrated by spectral Doppler interrogation of the proximal superior mesenteric artery, always indicates peripheral occlusion of several mesenteric branches.

The **duplex ultrasound findings** in steno-occlusive disease of the superior mesenteric artery can be summarized as follows:

- **Stenosis:**
  - PSV >250–280 cm/s (fasting)
- **Proximal occlusion:**
  - Absence of flow signals at the origin of the superior mesenteric artery
- **Distal occlusion:**
  - Absence of flow in distal mesenteric artery trunk or occluded mesenteric branch (on condition that insonation conditions are adequate)
  - Indirect evidence from proximal Doppler interrogation:
    - Decrease in PSV when hemodynamically relevant flow obstruction is present distally
    - Reduced RI
    - Thump pattern immediately upstream of occlusion

The resistive index (RI), derived by spectral Doppler analysis, in the **superior mesenteric artery** is decreased or increased in the following physiologic and pathologic situations.

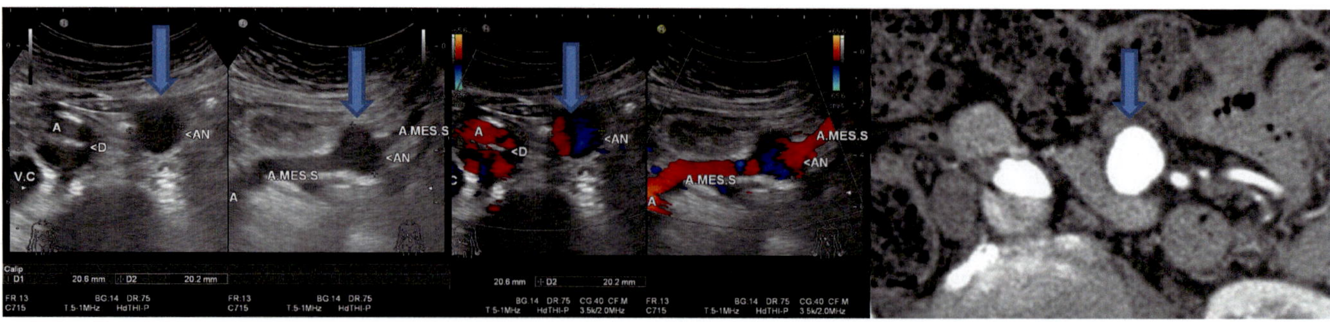

Fig. 6.27 Small aneurysm (<AN; arrow) with a diameter of 2.2 cm of the superior mesenteric artery (A.MES.S). The findings are presented in transverse and longitudinal views in the gray-scale mode on the left and in the color flow mode on the right. In addition, there is aortic dissection (A) with the dissection membrane (<D) visualized in the transverse gray-scale and color images. The corresponding axial abdominal CT image (rightmost) shows the mesenteric aneurysm (arrow) with a diameter of 2 cm and the aortic dissection with the dissection membrane to the left of the aneurysm

- **Lower RI** (Pourcelot index; Fig. 1.28c) with absolute or relative increase in diastolic flow component:
  - With increase in averaged flow velocity:
    - Postprandial
    - Medication-induced
    - Inflammatory
    - Tumor-related
    - Replaced hepatic artery (or the branch supplying the right liver) arising from the superior mesenteric artery (Fig. 6.3e)
  - With decrease in averaged flow velocity:
    - Distal mesenteric artery occlusion (widening of arteries recruited as collaterals)
- **Higher RI** with absolute or relative decrease in diastolic flow component:
  - Diabetes mellitus (medial sclerosis)
  - Acute severe mesenteric vein thrombosis.

In individuals with an abberrant hepatic artery arising from the superior mesenteric artery, the Doppler waveform obtained upstream of the origin will show a large diastolic component with a decrease in RI, because the flow pattern in this case is affected by the supply of a parenchymal organ. This must be borne in mind in interpreting the Doppler waveform (see Fig. 6.52 (Atlas)).

Nonocclusive intestinal ischemia (NOMI) has a poor prognosis and frequently occurs in patients with considerable comorbidity. The examiner must be aware of this condition as a **differential diagnosis of proximal mesenteric occlusion**. Circulatory insufficiency, sepsis, and diabetes mellitus play a role in the development of NOMI. Ultrasonography has no role in the diagnosis since only the smaller, distal mesenteric branches are affected, while the superior mesenteric artery and the proximal segments of the main branches are patent. The diagnosis is confirmed angiographically before therapy with intra-arterial vasodilators is initiated.

An increased pulsatility of the mesenteric artery may be due to reduced wall elasticity in diabetes mellitus or indicate disturbed peripheral venous drainage, as in extensive mesenteric vein thrombosis.

The **diagnostic value of color duplex ultrasound in evaluating infarction of the liver, spleen, or kidneys** due to acute peripheral artery occlusion depends on the insonation conditions. The extent of infarction varies with the site of occlusion and blood supply through collateral routes. B-mode ultrasound shows poorly delineated, inhomogeneous, and hypoechoic areas, but not earlier than 1–3 days after the acute event (Seitz and Rettenmaier 1994). There are some case reports describing the use of color duplex imaging in patients with renal or splenic infarction, but ultrasound is most beneficial in guiding interventional procedures such as abscess drainage in superinfection of necrotic areas.

Aneurysms of the visceral arteries are very uncommon but may present as emergencies when they rupture. They are typically detected incidentally in patients undergoing B-mode ultrasound for diagnostic workup of abdominal symptoms (which may be due to aneurysm-related pressure). They are differentiated from pseudocysts or other cystic tumorous lesions of the upper abdomen by their characteristic color duplex appearance. Locating the aneurysm to the splenic, superior mesenteric, or hepatic artery is important for planning the surgical procedure (see Fig. 6.61 (Atlas)). As with all other vascular territories, the diagnostic evaluation of aneurysms is the domain of color duplex ultrasound: the flexibility in choosing the orientation of the scan plane enables reliable diameter measurement, identification of thrombotic wall deposits, and assessment of the patent residual lumen.

Aneurysm of the superior mesenteric artery is rare (Fig. 6.27). Even less common are aneurysms of the gastroduodenal, pancreaticoduodenal, and inferior mesenteric arteries. They are typically mycotic aneurysms (staphylococci, salmonellae). Sonographically, they are located and measured as in other vascular territories. In planning the surgical procedure, it is crucial that their course and relationship to other vessels be determined exactly. Visceral aneurysms appear to be more common in patients with aberrant arteries.

6.1.6.3 Aorta

6.1.6.3.1 Aortic Stenosis and Thrombosis

Bilateral intermittent claudication may be caused by stenosis of the distal aorta. Therefore, the aorta should be evaluated if the Doppler waveform from the iliac artery shows poststenotic changes. High-grade stenosis of the abdominal aorta is indicated in the color duplex scan by a mosaic pattern resulting from perivascular vibration, as in an arteriovenous fistula. Severe atherosclerosis with calcified plaques impairs the detection of the stenosis jet in the duplex mode. On the other hand, extensive plaque with acoustic shadowing and poor delineation of the lumen in the B-mode scan often suggests high-grade stenosis of the aorta. The Doppler waveform sampled distal to the high-grade stenosis will show the typical postocclusive flow profile with a delayed systolic rise and large diastolic component.

Abdominal aortic stenosis occurs chiefly in the **distal infrarenal segment including the bifurcation**. In this setting, collateral supply with refilling of the iliac territory is mainly ensured by the inferior mesenteric artery, which will become dilated and show high peak systolic velocities (PSV) (often >200 cm/s) and end-diastolic velocities (EDV).

In acute occlusion of the distal aorta (Leriche's syndrome), the lumen is discriminated in the B-mode image by virtue of its being filled with hypoechoic material. If the occlusion is due to atherosclerosis, on the other hand, the aorta is difficult to differentiate from surrounding tissue. Flow is absent in both cases. In patients with poor visualization, chronic occlusion can be differentiated from high-grade stenosis by the absence of the mosaic pattern, caused by perivascular vibration, that is typical of stenosis.

Thrombosis of the aorta is visualized as a hypoechoic cone-like structure in the lumen. The tail of the thrombus is typically surrounded by flowing blood on all sides. Signs of luminal narrowing are seen on duplex scanning only when there is nearly complete occlusion. Most patients with aortic thrombosis present with embolism, often in both legs. Demonstration of flow around the hypoechoic thrombus on color flow images differentiates aortic thrombosis from an embolizing aneurysm (see ◘ Fig. 6.94 (Atlas)).

6.1.6.3.2 Abdominal Aortic Aneurysm

B-mode ultrasound (real-time gray-scale imaging) is the screening method of first choice for abdominal aortic aneurysm (AAA). The reported diagnostic accuracy approaches 100% (Beales et al. 2011; Hartshorne et al. 2011; Lindholt et al. 1999; Vidakovic et al. 2007; Mastracci and Cinà 2007; Thanos et al. 2008). To determine the true maximum diameter of the aneurysm, the largest transverse extension is identified to then rotate the transducer for measurement perpendicular to the vascular axis. Other important diagnostic features include the aneruysm shape, its topographic relationship to the renal artery origins, and possible iliac artery involvement. The therapeutically relevant **AAA features to be evaluated by color duplex** can be summarized as follows:

- Maximum AAA diameter (to establish surgical indication)
- Shape (saccular, spindle-shaped)
- Partial thrombosis
- Involvement of (common, internal) iliac arteries
- Infrarenal – suprarenal
- Other relevant features if endovascular repair is contemplated:
  - Distance from renal artery origins
  - Degree of angulation of elongated infrarenal aorta and possible iliac artery elongation
  - Conically shaped aneurysm neck

Color duplex ultrasound is only required to evaluate the patent lumen and differentiate it from mural thrombi and to obtain additional information in the differentiation of rare vascular conditions such as inflammatory AAA and aortitis (giant cell arteritis). However, the color flow information may facilitate evaluation of the topographic relationship to the renal artery origins and possible extension of a very long AAA aneurysm to the internal iliac artery origin.

Compared with angiography, which only depicts the residual lumen of an aneurysm, ultrasound provides much more detailed information regarding localization and extent as well as differentiation of thrombosed and patent portions. And the flexibility of ultrasound in selecting the scanning plane relative to the course of the abdominal aorta facilitates measurement of the **true aneurysm diameter**. Imaging modalities that use standardized axial sections may overestimate aneurysm size when the section in which the diameter is measured corresponds to an oblique (elliptical) plane through the aneurysm (◘ Fig. 6.30). This pitfall is attributable to concomitant elongation of the distal abdominal aorta, which is common in patients with atherosclerotic AAA (see ◘ Figs. 6.29 and 6.31).

AAA is a rare source of embolism. These aneurysms and aortic aneurysms with a very saccular shape require surgical management irrespective of their size. Saccular aneurysms tend to exhibit turbulent flow on color duplex imaging, while laminar flow is more likely in smaller, spindle-shaped aneurysms. The local pressure peaks occurring in turbulent flow are associated with more rapid growth and a higher risk of rupture. In the sonographic evaluation of patients with embolic occlusion of the leg arteries, thrombi in an aortic aneurysm should be ruled out as a source of embolism (see ◘ Fig. 6.74 (Atlas)).

In **inflammatory AAA**, concentric wall thickening is sonographically distinct from flowing blood in the patent lumen and, in patients with concomitant atherosclerotic lesions of the intima, also from thrombus in the aneurysm sac. In patients with inflammatory AAA, wall thickening tends to be confined to the aneurysmally dilated segment. Conversely, wall thickening in giant cell arteritis also involves the proximal abdominal aorta (and may be associated with concomitant aortic widening) (see ◘ Fig. 6.38).

6.1.6.3.3 Specific Aspects of the Ultrasound Examination in Abdominal Aortic Aneurysm

▪ Diameter Variation Through the Cardiac Cycle and Effect of Measurement Method

Exact sonographic measurement of the maximum diameter of the abdominal aorta is essential for identifying patients whose abdominal aortic aneurysm (AAA) should be operated on and for obtaining reliable serial measurements of AAA diameter in patients assigned to surveillance programs or undergoing follow-up after treatment. In addition, AAA

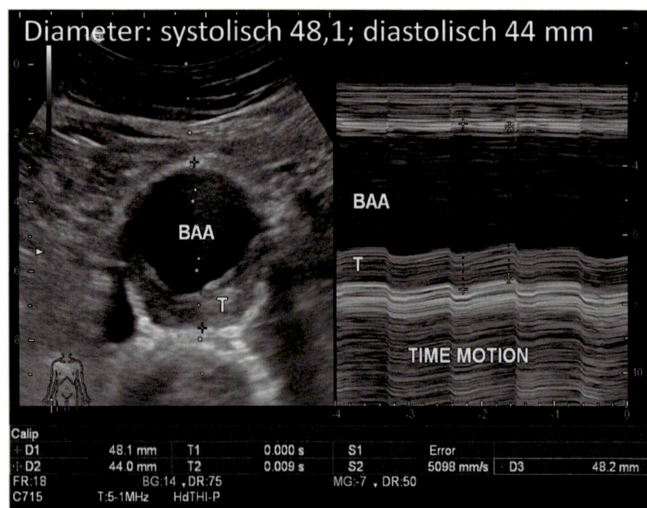

Fig. 6.28 Diameter variation of the abdominal aorta during the cardiac cycle in the time-motion mode. This mode systematically captures the full diameter range from 48 mm during systole to 44 m during diastole. In contrast, a single B-mode image (left) captures the diameter at a single point in time. In this example, the B-mode image incidentally shows the diameter during systole, which is 48 mm (measured using the leading-edge method)

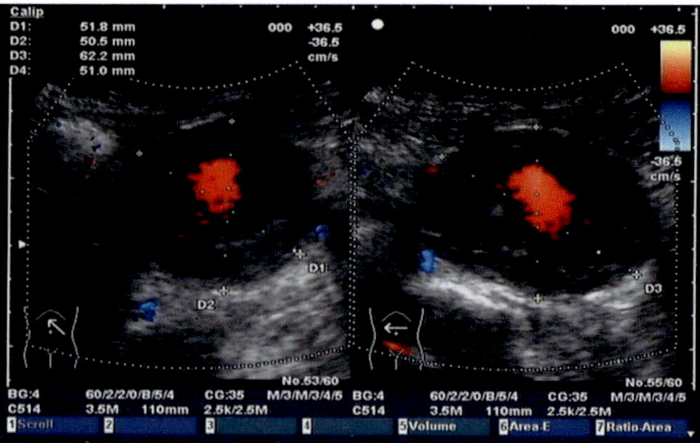

Fig. 6.29 Measurement of abdominal aortic aneurysm (AAA) diameter in a patient with elongation of the aorta and deviation to the left. Measurement in the transverse abdominal view (right image, see body marker) yields a diameter of 62.2 mm (D3). In contrast, measurement perpendicular to the longitudinal vessel axis after rotation of the transducer at the same level (left image) yields a diameter of 51.8 mm (D1). This is the orthogonal aneurysm diameter and reflects the true diameter. The anteroposterior (AP) diameter is the same in both views (50.5 mm (D2) and 51 mm (D4))

diameter is an important parameter in assessing the interobserver variability of ultrasound measurement and in comparing ultrasound with computed tomography (CT) or other imaging modalities. No standard exists for ultrasound- or CT-based aortic diameter measurement, and discrepancies resulting from the use of different methods are often ignored in the context of scientific investions (Long et al. 2012; Beales et al. 2011; Chiu et al. 2014).

There are several pitfalls the examiner should avoid. First, there is variation in the diameter of the normal aorta and of AAA during the cardiac cycle, resulting in a diameter difference of 1.5–4.3 mm from systole to diastole (Fig. 6.28) (Schäberle et al. 2014). In a small series of 30 patients with AAA analyzed by the author, the mean diameter variation through the cardiac cycle was 2.8 mm with diameters ranging from 3.6–7.6 cm. This issue is hardly ever addressed in sonographic studies (Grondal et al. 2012), and it simply cannot be considered due to inherent methodological limitations in static CT-based aortic diameter measurement (Chiu et al. 2014). Aortic diameter variation through the cardiac cycle explains some of the differences in serial measurements and in studies comparing different methods. ECG-gated ultrasound diameter measurement has been proposed to reduce variability and overcome this limitation (Bredahl et al. 2013); however, it is not feasible in clinical practice or in the setting of screening programs.

Another source of variability in sonographic aortic diameter measurement is whether the inner or outer wall reflection is used for measurement (see Fig. 1.28; Chiu et al. 2014). Investigators tend to uncriticially compare data from studies measuring the outer-to-outer-edge diameter (Ellis et al. 1991; Pleumeekers et al. 1998; Hartshorne et al. 2011) with results based on inner-to-inner-edge measurement (Lanne et al. 1997). While these sonographic methods were found to have good inter- and intraobserver agreement, the inner-edge method underestimated the diameter by an average of 4 mm compared with the outer-edge method (Chiu et al. 2014).

Measurement series in other vascular territories and in ultrasound phantoms show that the leading-edge method (see Figs. 1.28 and 6.28) yields the most reliable results because it avoids or systematizes errors resulting from blooming at interfaces between tissues with large differences in acoustic impedance such as the vessel wall (Schäberle 2009). With the leading-edge method, the vessel diameter is measured from the bright reflection of the outer wall close to the transducer to the inner wall reflection of the opposite wall (see Fig. 1.28).

Taken together, these limitations can result in a total variability in AAA diameter measurements of 5–6 mm. This variation is not harmful in initial screening but becomes relevant in patients with borderline AAA size and patients undergoing regular surveillance for AAA (where a size increase of 5 mm over 6 months is generally considered to be an indication for surgery). These issues are also relevant when AAA size is measured using CT and should be borne in mind when interpreting the results of studies comparing the diagnostic accuracy of ultrasound and CT.

Transducer Position and Multiplanar Reconstruction

The error resulting from measuring AAA diameter in the transverse abdominal view with oblique visualization of the aortic axis is more serious. When an AAA is present and increases in size, the aorta tends to become elongated and tortuous with lateral and sometimes anterior deviation. In this situation, measurement of the largest aortic diameter in the transverse upper abdominal view will overestimate AAA size. The same holds true for axial CT measurement. The elliptical slice of the aneurysm may overestimate its size by 1–2 cm compared with its true orthogonal diameter (Fig. 6.29). In

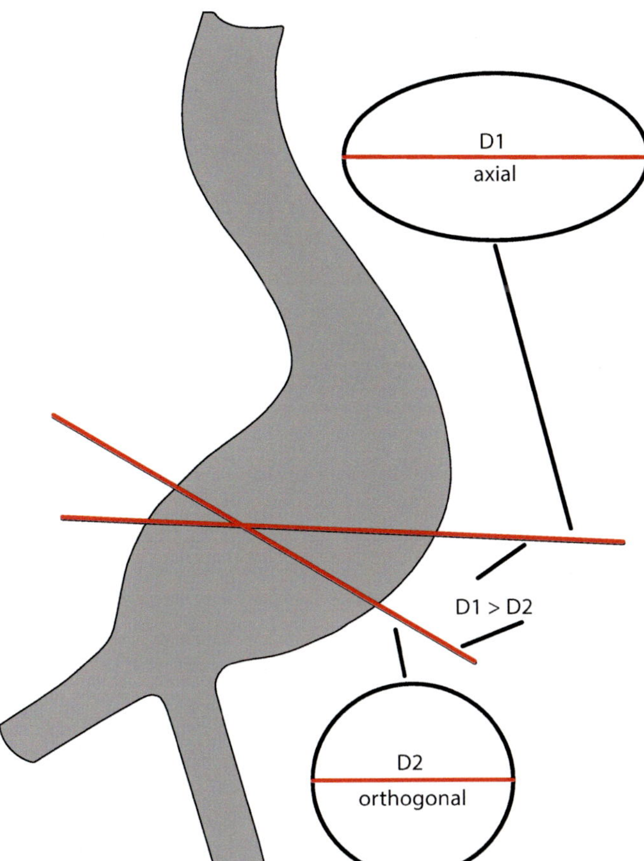

▣ **Fig. 6.30** Pitfall in measuring abdominal aortic aneurysm (AAA) diameter. Patients with an aortic aneurysm often have an elongated aorta with an outward curve to the left. When transverse images are obtained with the transducer in the normal abdominal position, this can lead to overestimation of the diameter because the aorta is being measured in an elliptical plane (D1). Overestimation of aneurysm size by measurement in the wrong scan plane can also lead to overestimation of the rupture risk. The correct diameter of the aneurysm is measured by rotating the transducer clockwise until a round image of the aorta comes into view (D2). With the transducer in this position, the true transverse diameter is measured orthogonally (perpendicular to the vessel axis)

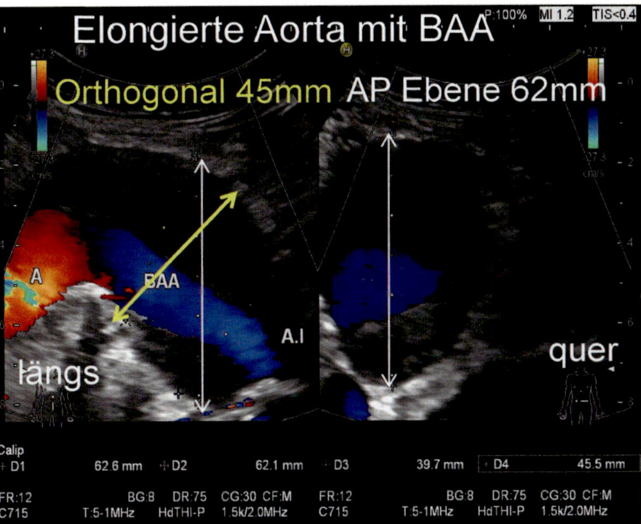

▣ **Fig. 6.31** Sources of variation in measuring the maximum abdominal aortic aneurysm (AAA) diameter in a patient with an elongated aorta and anterolateral deviation of its course. A maximum anteroposterior (AP) diameter of 62.6 mm (D1) is measured in the transverse abdominal view (right image), while the maximum orthogonal diameter measured perpendicular to the long axis of the aorta is 45.5 mm (left image). At the site of the AP diameter measurement in the transverse view, the orthogonal diameter is 39.7 mm (D3). The AP diameter is represented by the white line, the orthogonal diameter by the yellow line. The AP diameter measured in the right image corresponds to the CT-based diameter measurement in the axial plane (i.e., in the plane used for measuring AAA size when CT is performed without multiplanar reconstruction)

ultrasound, this error can be avoided by rotating the transducer from the transverse abdominal position until it is perpendicular to the long aortic axis (confirmed when the oval shape of the aorta becomes more rounded) (▣ Figs. 6.28, 6.29, and 6.30). When the elongated aorta deviates anteriorly, the diameter is best measured in the sagittal plane (▣ Fig. 6.31).

Without this **standardized approach**, it is not possible to take accurate and reproducible serial measurements of aortic diameter. This must be taken into account when interpreting discrepant results obtained with the same modality or with different modalities.

Studies show good intraobserver and interobserver agreement for sonographic measurement of the orthogonal AAA diameter, which is a prerequisite for obtaining meaningful results in serial measurements. Such a standardized approach is necessary to capture true size increases over time and avoid errors resulting from poor methodology (Sun 2006; AbuRahma 2006; Collins et al. 2007; Stavropoulos and Charagundla 2007).

Once again, adequate aortic diameter measurement requires clockwise rotation of the transducer from the position showing the largest aortic diameter to the view allowing diameter measurement perpendicular to the long aortic axis (change from elliptical to rounded shape of the aortic cross-section) (▣ Fig. 6.30).

In summary, the following procedure is recommended for the sonographic evaluation of the aorta and reliable AAA diameter measurement:

- Identify the aorta in the transverse plane and image its course from the suprarenal segment to the bifurcation
- Identify the renal artery origins and aortic bifurcation to determine AAA extent in relation to these structures
- Evaluate the entire aorta for possible elongation: may require transverse, oblique, or even longitudinal transducer positions
- Identify the widest (axial) aortic diameter
- From this position, rotate the transducer for measurement of AAA diameter perpendicular to the vascular axis (rounded rather than elliptical shape of the aortic cross-sectional area; may require a longitudinal view in some cases)
- Use the leading-edge method to measure AAA diameter
- Document findings and measurements

New techniques such as 3D ultrasound and ultrasound/CT image fusion have the potential to improve the accuracy of aneurysm size determination in the future, especially in serial examinations of patients with AAA (Bredahl et al. 2013; Pfister 2014).

6.1.6.3.4 Comparison of Ultrasound and Computed Tomography

No consistent picture emerges from studies comparing ultrasound and CT (Singh et al. 2004); discrepancies are often attributable to the study design (Beales et al. 2011). Investigators often fail to describe details of the ultrasound technique used to determine abdominal aortic aneurysm (AAA) size (e.g., transducer position, plane in which diameter is measured). In a study reviewing the methodology of maximum AAA diameter measurement (Long et al. 2012), only 40% of the studies included (n = 23) specified the plane of acquisition and 30% the caliper positions, and only 10% of the studies used the leading-edge method. Long et al. defined a quality score for the description of methodology in the studies reviewed and found a mean quality score of 2.5 (of a total of 4). Surprisingly, they found an even lower mean quality score of 1.6 for the description of methodology in guidelines for screening programs. Most of the guidelines they reviewed did not specify the axis of measurement or caliper positions (outer or inner diameter) (Long et al. 2012; Lederle et al. 1995), and these issues are rarely discussed (Moll et al. 2011). Overall, the review of Long et al. confirms that a range of different methods are in use for measuring AAA diameter.

Studies **comparing ultrasound and CT** show good agreement of the two modalities (correlation coefficient of 0.91) (Manning et al. 2009) with the majority of investigators concluding that ultrasound underestimates maximum aneurysm diameter compared with CT (mostly measured in AP plane) (Jaakkola et al. 1996, Sprouse et al. 2003, Manning et al. 2009, Long et al. 2012). Conversely, other authors point out that axial CT scans, without orthogonal reformation, often measure the diameter in oblique slices of the AAA, which tend to overestimate aneurysm diameter when there is relevant elongation of the aorta. This is clearly apparent from two studies performed by Sprouse et al. (2003 and 2004). In the earlier study, CT yielded larger diameters than ultrasound in 95% of cases. Specifically, AAA diameters by CT were 5.69 ± 0.89 cm versus 4.74 ± 0.91 cm by ultrasound (and the difference was significant, $p < 0.05$). In the later study, Sprouse et al. (2004) found good agreement between ultrasound and CT diameter measurements with a mean difference of only 0.8 mm when CT measurements were taken in reformatted slices allowing true orthogonal measurement. Comparison of axial and orthogonal AAA diameter measurements by CT revealed significantly larger mean diameters when measurements were taken in axial slices compared with orthogonal slices (58 mm versus 54.7 mm, $p < 0.05$). The overestimation of axially measured diameters increased with aortic angulation. These results clearly illustrate that selection of the correct slice for AAA diameter measurement affects ultrasound (◘ Figs. 6.29 and 6.30) and CT alike. Awareness of this pitfall is important both in clinical routine and in the setting of clinical studies (Long et al. 2012).

CT is generally considered the gold standard for measuring AAA diameter because it is not examiner-dependent and less susceptible to errors resulting from poor examination conditions. In view of the problems discussed here, there appears to be an urgent need to standardize measurements and ensure that we measure AAA diameter accurately and reproducibly in serial examinations. A consensus should specify how, where, and when to measure AAA diameter.

6.1.6.3.5 Abdominal Aortic Aneurysm Screening: Rupture Risk

Accurate and reproducible (orthogonal) measurement of aortic diameter is essential for preventing both excessive diagnostic testing (stressful for patients) and excessive treatment (surgical risk, complications, and postoperative morbidity) in screening and surveillance programs (◘ Figs. 6.36 and 6.37). Abdominal aortic aneurysm (AAA) is a non-malignant condition and it is therefore even more important not to put patients at risk through poor measurement methodology and operating on aneurysms that would never rupture during their lifetime. In addition, the low risk of rupture of <3–5%/year for AAA <5.5 cm must be weighed against the surgical risk and perioperative morbidity. Patients undergoing endovascular aneurysm repair (EVAR) also face several risks (endoleaks in up to 10% of cases, risk of stent graft limb occlusion of up to 5%) and require regular follow-up examinations with radiation and contrast medium exposure.

Clinically, AAA rupture is suggested by flank and back pain (occasionally abdominal pain), a palpable pulsating tumor, and shock. Gray-scale imaging depicts a hypoechoic structure of variable extent and comprising inhomogeneous or layered portions around the aorta in the retroperitoneum (◘ Fig. 6.75b (Atlas)). In patients with a contained aneuryms rupture, color duplex ultrasound demonstrates paravascular flow signals at the site of the leak. Leakage must be differentiated from other hypoechoic periaortic structures such as retroperitoneal fibrosis, horseshoe kidneys, or lymphoma, which may occur in conjunction with an aneurysm (see ► Sect. 6.1.6.3.8; ◘ Figs. 6.38, 6.39, and 6.40; ◘ Figs. 6.85, 6.86, and 6.87 (Atlas);). An examiner performing ultrasonography in emergency patients must pay special attention to such accompanying conditions as they have important implications.

If there is **perforation into the duodenum**, the intestine may appear fluid-filled. Fistula connections to the vena cava can be demonstrated by color duplex.

6.1.6.3.6 Aortic Dissection

Aortic dissection is only amenable to percutaneous ultrasound diagnosis if the intimal flap extends into the abdominal aorta. In the abdominal aorta, sonography is a valid method for assessing the extent of dissection, and spectral Doppler evaluation is helpful in identifying extension into arteries arising from the aorta or intermittent obstruction of blood flow at the origin of these arteries by the intimal flap moving synchronously with the heart (see ◘ Fig. 6.88 (Atlas)).

In a **dissecting aneurysm**, splitting of the arterial wall with tearing of the intima is suggested on gray-scale ultrasonography by the presence of a flap in the vessel lumen;

this flap can be identified by its hyperechoic reflection and typical undulating motion. Dissection is confirmed in the color mode by different flow velocities and directions in the true and false lumens (◘ Fig. 6.33). The power mode and contrast-enhanced ultrasound (CEUS) will help demonstrate slow flow in the false lumen and differentiate it from partial thrombosis. The color-coded flow directions contribute to the identification of the entry and re-entry sites. Knowledge of the relationships of the origins of the visceral and renal arteries to the true and false lumens determines the therapeutic management. As the dissected flap may extend into the groin, the iliac arteries must be included in the examination (see ◘ Figs. 6.88, 6.89, and 6.90 (Atlas)).

Spectral Doppler imaging at the sites of aortic branch origins for identifying **extension of the dissection into renal or visceral arteries** as well as intermittent occlusion or stenosis of a branch artery by the intimal flap (dynamic blood flow reduction) is important for the therapeutic approach. If there is extension into an aortic branch, the Doppler waveform will depict flow in the true and false lumens and may also contain signals produced by oscillation of the intimal flap. If there is narrowing or intermittent occlusion of a branch origin by the intimal flap, spectral Doppler will reveal signs of stenosis or systolic deceleration (decreased systolic velocity or even zero flow) (◘ Fig. 6.88 (Atlas)). Dissection with intermittent flow obstruction can lead to chronic ischemia and patients are at risk of acute ischemic events. Dynamic flow obstruction is difficult to detect with a morphologic imaging modality (CT, angiography) when the lumen is filled with contrast medium.

Conversely, with isolated dissection of the abdominal aorta, which is rare (Knabe et al. 2001), the proximal origin is typically not detectable by transcutaneous sonography (except with the transducer directed retrosternally from a jugular position). In these cases, transesophageal echocardiography (Link 1999), computed tomography, or magnetic resonance imaging is required for diagnosis. The diagnostic accuracies in aortic dissection are 70% for ultrasound (Nienaber et al. 1993), 98% for transesophageal echocardiography (Sommer et al. 1996), and 100% for MRI (Silverman 2000) and CT.

6.1.6.3.7 Follow-Up After Open Surgical and Endovascular Aneurysm Repair

▪ Diagnostic Algorithm

Follow-up (see ◘ Fig. 6.32) after open surgical repair of an abdominal aortic aneurysm (AAA) or patch angioplasty of aortic stenosis must ensure early identification of complications such as suture aneurysm, anastomotic stenosis, recurrent stenosis, or abscess.

Hypoechoic structures around a prosthesis, particularly at the sites of anastomosis, can be checked for the presence of flow using color duplex ultrasound to differentiate suture aneurysm from postoperative hematoma and abscess. Suture aneurysms are pseudoaneurysms and hence are characterized by to-and-fro flow (steam engine sound) in the Doppler waveform from the site of wall perforation (see ◘ Fig. 6.92 (Atlas)). An abscess suspected on clinical grounds can be confirmed by ultrasound-guided fine-needle aspiration biopsy.

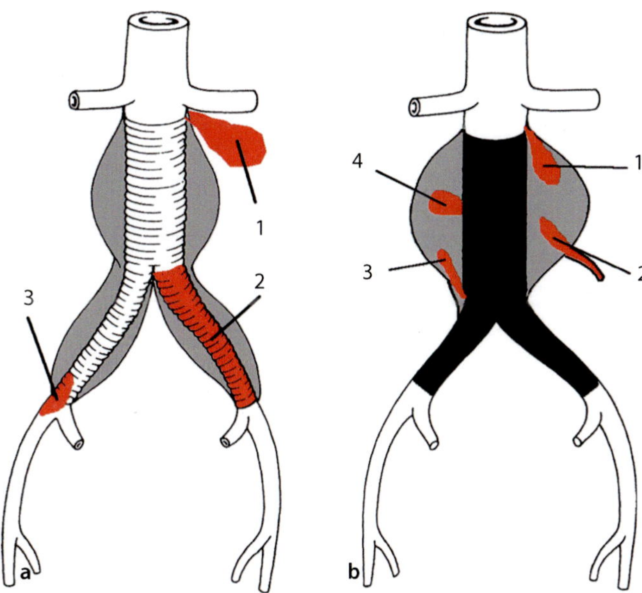

◘ **Fig. 6.32a, b** Complications of interventional and open surgical repair of abdominal aortic aneurysm (AAA). **a** Following surgical Y-prosthesis implantation: **1** suture aneurysm (typically at the upper anastomosis or, if the prosthesis extends into the femoral artery, at the lower anastomosis); **2** occlusion of an iliac limb; **3** anastomotic stenosis (distal anastomosis). **b** Types of endoleaks after endovascular aneurysm repair (EVAR): **1** type I endoleak, at the proximal or distal attachment site; **2** type II endoleak, from patent lumbar arteries; **3** type III endoleak, separation of modular components; **4** type IV endoleak, device failure (porosity)

After open surgical aneurysm repair, sonographic follow-up has sufficient validity to identify typical complications such as suture aneurysm (◘ Fig. 6.34), anastomotic stenosis, and iliac limb occlusion (in patients with a Y-stent graft).

The following **complications** of open surgical and endovascular AAA repair have therapeutic implications **and require special attention in sonographic follow-up**:

- After open surgical repair:
  - Recurrent aneurysm – suture aneurysm
  - Anastomotic stenosis/iliac limb occlusion
  - Abscess/infection
- After endovascular aneruysm repair (EVAR):
  - Endoleaks (types I, II, III)
  - Further sac growth
  - Stent graft migration/fracture (domain of conventional X-ray)
  - Iliac limb occlusion
  - Thrombotic deposits as a source of embolism or cause of luminal narrowing

After EVAR, patients should undergo imaging surveillance at 6-month intervals. AAA shrinkage indicates adequacy of the repair and rules out an endoleak (Giannoni et al. 1998; Thompson et al. 1998). Conversely, even a small further increase in aortic diameter (B-mode) points to a therapeutically relevant endoleak (with increasing pressure

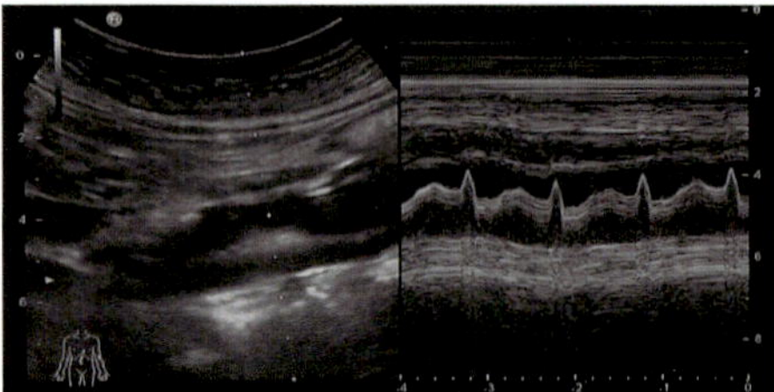

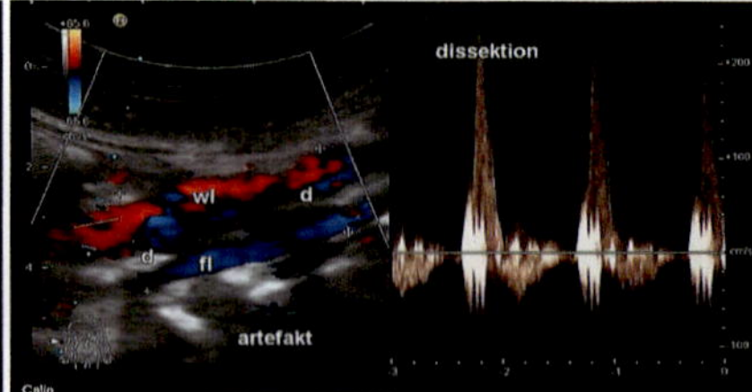

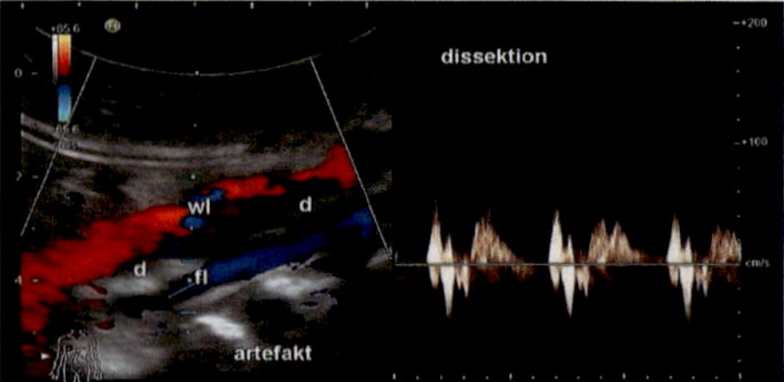

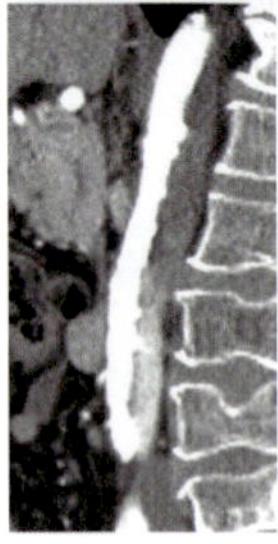

Fig. 6.33 Aortic dissection of longer duration with sclerotic thickening of the dissection membrane (same patient as in Fig. 6.27). In this patient, gray-scale imaging already shows the floating membrane (indicated by "d" in the color flow images) in the lumen and rules out intermittent obstruction of blood flow into arterial branches at their origins from the aorta. The waveforms shown along with the color flow images were obtained in the true lumen (wl) and false lumen (fl) (center and right, respectively). The bright artifact apparent in both waveforms in early systole is due to oscillation of the dissection membrane. The membrane is also apparent in the corresponding CTA scan

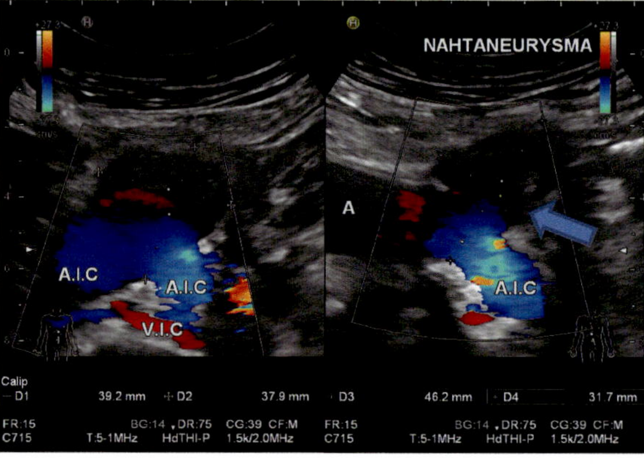

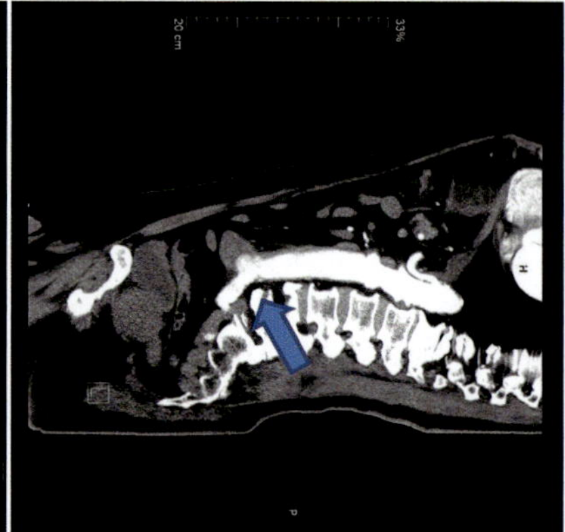

Fig. 6.34 Suture aneurysm after open surgical stent graft repair for abdominal aortic aneurysm (AAA). The arrow in the color flow images (transverse orientation on the left, longitudinal orientation on the right) indicates the site of leakage. The CT scan was obtained for stent graft sizing prior to interventional closure of the leak

in the aneurysm sac) and should prompt a careful search for the site of leakage using color duplex ultrasound (CDUS). If no endoleak is detected, the search should proceed using contrast-enhanced ultrasound (CEUS) or computed tomography angiography (CTA).

Serial ultrasound follow-up should be supplemented by an annual plain X-ray examination of the abdomen to rule out stent fracture, which can be identified sonographically only if an endoleak is presdent (type IV).

In summary, the following algorithm is proposed for the follow-up of patients after EVAR (in line with the general policy of stepwise diagnostic workup advocated throughout this book):

1. **B-mode ultrasound (follow-up at 6-month intervals):**
   - Development of AAA diameter over time
     - Diameter decreases → continue routine follow-up
     - Diameter remains constant or increases → search for endoleak, successively using CDUS, CEUS, and CTA (as required)
2. **CDUS** (PRF, gain): indicated if B-mode measurement shows constant or increasing sac diameter (orthogonal plane)
   - Type of endoleak
   - Types I and III: treatment
   - Type II (treatment required?):
     - Low-flow → follow-up (possibly at shorter intervals of 3 months)
     - High-flow → reintervention
3. **CEUS**: indicated if CDUS fails to identify an endoleak despite increasing AAA diameter
   - Same diagnostic accuracy as CTA
   - Superior in detecting small low-flow endoleaks (late retrograde blood flow into aneurysm sac via patent lumbar artery)
4. **CTA** (gold standard): indicated to search for suspected endoleak (B-mode findings) not detected by CDUS or CEUS

The basic idea of this stepwise approach is that the next test following in the recommended sequence of diagnostic procedures should only be performed if it is expected to provide therapeutically relevant information.

In addition, a systematic procedure is recommended to ensure reliable identification of endoleaks and other complications after EVAR (◘ Fig. 6.32):

- **Gray-scale examination** in transverse orientation to evaluate the upper stent end and its relationship to the renal artery origins.
- Gray-scale measurement of the largest orthogonal diameter of the residual aneurysm sac (see ◘ Figs. 6.77a and 6.82 (both Atlas)).
- **Transverse CDUS** (low pulse repetition frequency) of the aneurysm site and the stented segment from the renal artery origins to the bifurcation, focusing on the origins of the lumbar arteries and the inferior mesenteric artery (◘ Figs. 6.78 and 6.80 (both Atlas)).
- **Longitudinal CDUS** evaluation of the stent ends with spectral Doppler measurement to confirm patency, demonstrate stenosis, and identify type I endoleaks using an acute Doppler angle at the anchoring sites (◘ Fig. 6.79 (Atlas)).
- If CDUS reveals **flow in the aneurysm sac**, this must be confirmed by spectral Doppler interrogation. This is especially important in the early postinterventional phase before complete thrombosis of the aneurysm has occurred and movement of the stent can mimic flow signals (pseudoendoleak). Such pseudoendoleaks are differentiated from true endoleaks by the demonstration of to-and-fro flow in the spectral Doppler waveform (especially with the sample volume at the site of leakage, e.g., patent lumbar artery entering the aneurysm sac). This flow pattern is characteristic of endoleaks, which resemble pseudoaneurysms in terms of hemodynamics (see ◘ Fig. 6.80 (Atlas)). Mirror artifacts can be ruled out by insonation from different directions, supplemented by waveform information.
- Patients with **type II endoleaks** not requiring reintervention (patent lateral branches, lumbar arteries, inferior mesenteric artery) can be managed by shortening the follow-up interval (see ◘ Fig. 6.32). Higher-flow type I (failure of fixation) and type III endoleaks are reliably detected by ultrasound.

Whether the ultrasound examination allows adequate evaluation after AAA repair strongly depends on the individual acoustic window. Published data on the reliability of ultrasound are inconsistent, especially with regard to the identification of type II endoleaks (Ashoke et al. 2005; Sanford et al. 2006). Some authors showed CDUS to be sufficient to rule out endoleaks with reported sensitivities of 77–96% and specificities of 90–94% (D'Audiffret 2001; Golzarian et al. 2002; Sato et al. 1998; Sun 2006; AbuRahma 2006; Collins et al. 2007; Stavropoulos and Charagundla 2007); however, the patient populations investigated were small. The difficulty in detecting an endoleak is that it requires not only a good acoustic window and adequate machine settings (low pulse repetition frequency) but also great care in setting the Doppler angle correction cursor relative to the leak jet so as not to miss a type II endoleak. Moreover, motion and mirror artifacts in the excluded aneurysm sac can mimic flow in the color duplex examination, which must be differentiated from an endoleak by spectral Doppler interrogation (for technical details and optimization of settings see ► Sect. 6.1.2.1.2).

▪ Therapeutic Relevance of CDUS-derived Hemodynamic Information

Despite its inherent methodological limitations, color duplex ultrasound allows reliable evaluation for endoleaks after EVAR. Doppler waveforms contribute therapeutically relevant supplementary hemodynamic information not provided by CEUS or CTA (Schäberle et al. 2014).

The diagnostic questions to be answered by the sonographic examination of patients with a suspected endoleak can be summarized as follows:

- Is an endoleak present?
- If yes, which type (type I, II, III, or IV or a combined endoleak)?
- If a type II endoleak is present, is it fed by the inferior mesenteric artery or by a patent lumbar artery?
- How should the endoleak be managed?
  - Follow-up only
  - If treatment is required, how urgent is the reintervention?
    - elective
    - urgent
    - emergency intervention.

▪▪ Combined Endoleaks

Type I endoleaks develop in the early postinterventional period and tend to occur in conjunction with other endoleaks, commonly type II. A second endoleak can relieve the intrasac pressure buildup that would otherwise result from blood entering the sac through a type I endoelak. CDUS provides information on blood flow velocity and other flow characteristics at the entry point, which is relevant for estimating the acute risk of rupture associated with a type I endoleak. Like a pseudoaneurysm, a type I endoleak is characterized by to-and-fro flow with blood entering the sac during systole and leaving it during diastole. A monophasic waveform showing flow into the aneurysm sac but little or no backward flow indicates a high acute rupture risk or that the blood leaves the sac through a second, paradoxical endoleak, which may be termed an exoleak. Such a constellation is suggested by the demonstration of untypical orthograde flow in the lumbar artery or the inferior mesenteric artery draining the aneurysm through the endoleak (see ◘ Figs. 6.78 and 6.79 (both Atlas)). A Doppler waveform from the inferior mesenteric artery or origin of a patent lumbar artery provides the necessary hemodynamic information (flow character and direction) to fully capture the flow situation. This information is essential for estimating the risk of rupture and to plan an individual reintervention strategy.

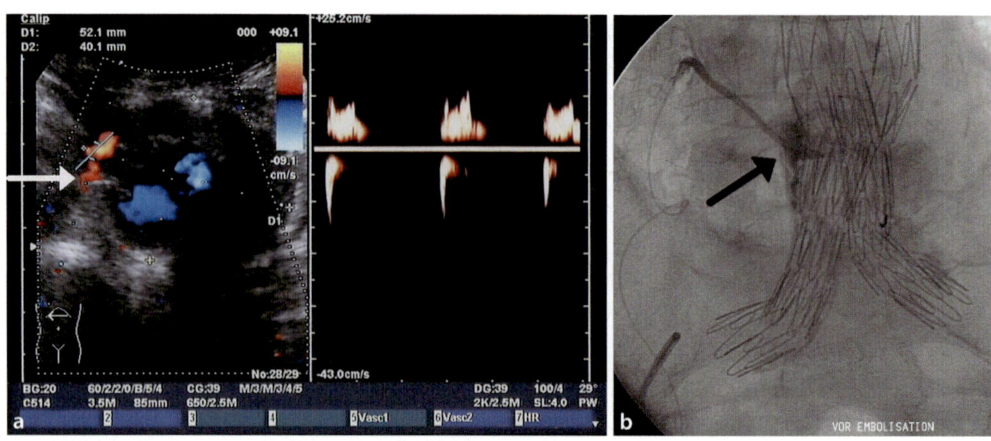

Fig. 6.35a, b Low-flow type II endoleak. **a** Flow in the former aneurysm sac fed by a patent right-sided lumbar artery (arrow) displayed in red (flow toward transducer) along with blue-coded flow in the stent graft (both iliac limbs). The waveform shows to-and-fro flow of very low frequency at the entry site, consistent with slow flow in the thin-caliber lumbar arteries and hence low flow volumes entering the aneurysm sac. These hemodynamic features suggest that there is no risk of rupture and that the endoleak is likely to close spontaneously. In addition, the anteroposterior aneurysm diameter has decreased from 5.7 to 5.1 cm. With this constellation of findings, no immediate reintervention is necessary. Instead, duplex ultrasound follow-up at 3-month intervals is indicated. **b** Angiogram with selective probing of the lumbar artery confirms a low-flow endoleak and blood flow in a small portion of the aneurysm sac. An endoleak with these features can be managed by watchful waiting. In this patient, coils were placed in the same angiography session

High-flow and Low-flow Type II Endoleaks

The Doppler waveform from the endoleak jet provides relevant information on **endoleak hemodynamics** (see Figs. 6.77, 6.78, 6.79, 6.80, and 6.81 (all Atlas)). A low-flow endoleak fed by a patent lumbar artery can be managed by watchful waiting as long as the aneurysm sac does not expand (see Figs. 6.81 and 6.82 (both Atlas). Because these type II endoleaks tend to close spontaneously, the risk of rupture is low (spontaneous thrombosis in up to 50% of type II endoleaks according to Carter et al. (2000)). However, validated criteria for the identification of low-flow endoleaks are not available for any imaging modality (Liewald et al. 2001; Parry et al. 2002; White et al. 2000). Time-intensity curves derived from CEUS allow quantitative analysis of endoleak flow dynamics. Again, validated data on the therapeutic relevance are not available. Methodologically, at least time-to-peak curves are required, while the sum of intensities alone is not sufficient.

Two **hemodynamic parameters** derived from **Doppler waveforms** obtained in the endoleak may be helpful in predicting the **risk of rupture**. On the one hand, the waveform shape provides information on resistance to blood flow. When a single endoleak is present, to-and-fro flow should predominate (due to the variation in pressure through the cardiac cycle, resulting in systolic flow into the aneurysm sac and diastolic flow back into the feeding artery). Consistent with this assumption, a higher spontaneous thrombosis rate was reported for endoleaks with bidirectional flow compared with endoleaks showing predominantly systolic inflow (similar to the flow profile of peripheral arteries) and little diastolic backward flow (Carter et al. 2000; Parent et al. 2002). Surprisingly, a more recent study identified bidirectional Doppler flow to be associated with a higher rate of sac growth (Beeman et al. 2010). This observation is counterintuitive because one would normally expect further aneurysm growth when inflow through an endoleak is higher than outflow (i.e., the waveform is monophasic), unless the blood leaves the sac via another route – an exoleak (see Fig. 6.79 (Atlas)). An aneurysm with blood entering the sac through one endoleak and leaving it through another is less likely to close spontaneously than a sac with bidirectional flow through a single endoleak. Correct placement of the sample volume for spectral Doppler interrogation is essential to capture blood flow directions at the endoleak site (patent lumbar artery or inferior mesenteric artery) (see Figs. 6.36 and 6.82 (Atlas)). Elsewhere in a perfused residual aneurysm sac, eddy flow with circulatory movement of blood (like in a pseudoaneurysm) may give rise to a monophasic waveform and misinterpretation of endoleak hemodynamics.

In addition, spectral Doppler can be used to measure flow velocity at the blood entry site (patent lumbar artery, inferior mesenteric artery) and thus estimate the flow volume. A high systolic velocity suggests a large endoleak volume or highly dynamic flow situation (Figs. 6.35, 6.36, 6.81 (Atlas), and 6.82 (Atlas)). A study investigating intrasac flow velocities proposed a Doppler cutoff >80 cm/s to identify endoleaks not expected to seal spontaneously (Arko 2003). In the author's experience, this cutoff is rather high and a cutoff on the order of 50–40 cm/s appears to better identify endoleaks requiring repair (Fig. 6.35b). However, Beeman et al. (2010) conclude that flow velocity in the aneurysm sac is not a relevant predictor of sac growth. Again, it is important to ensure that measurement is performed at the site of entry of a patent feeder into the aneurysm sac and with adequate Doppler angle correction (Fig. 6.36a). With a meticulous technique, the time-averaged velocity (intensity-weighted) during systolic inflow and diastolic outflow should be identical.

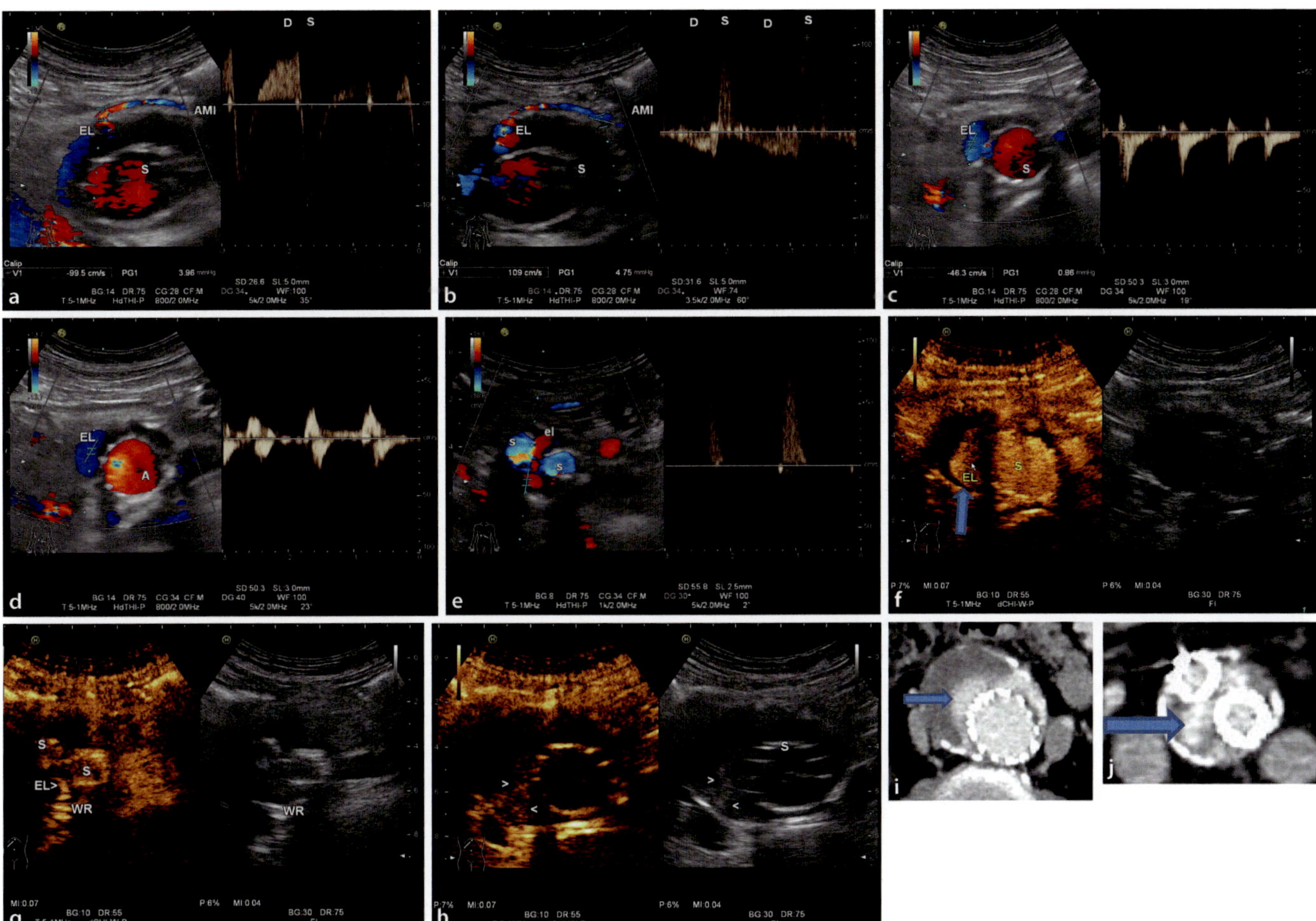

◻ Fig. 6.36a–j Sonographic endoleak characterization. **a** Endoleak in the upper portion of a stent graft following endovascular aneurysm repair (EVAR) for abdominal aortic aneurysm (AAA). There is blue-coded flow in the former aneurysm sac adjacent to red-coded flow in the stent graft (S). To determine whether a type I or type II endoleak is present, a Doppler waveform is obtained from the origin of the inferior mesenteric artery (AMI), which shows high-frequency bidirectional flow with flow into the aneurysm sac during systole (S) and a PSV of 100 cm. These findings are consistent with a high-flow endoleak. **b** To-and-fro flow with a PSV of 105 cm/s is confirmed along the course of the inferior mesenteric artery (AMI; systolic flow (S) toward the excluded aneurysm (toward transducer) and diastolic flow (D) away from transducer). While the waveform represents flow over time and thus captures its bidirectional nature, the color flow image selectively shows diastolic flow (blue-coded flow, away from transducer) and thus suggests orthograde flow. **c** Hemodynamic evaluation at an arbitrary site in the aneurysm rather than at the blood entry site is unsuitable for endoleak characterization. With the sample volume for spectral Doppler measurement placed away from the entry site (as done here for illustration), the PSV is 49 cm/s and flow is in one direction, which is usually due to circular flow in the sac. **d** Waveform from a site adjacent to the Doppler sampling site in **c**: PSV of only 25 cm/s but to-and-fro flow. **e** An additional endoleak is identified between the 2 iliac limbs of the stent graft, through which blood enters the inferior portion of the aneurysm sac (PSV of 1 m/s). Flow through this endoleak is unidirectional into the aneurysm sac with the blood taking a meandering course in the sac and leaving through the inferior mesenteric artery. **f** In the contrast-enhanced ultrasound (CEUS) examination, the large endoleak (EL) from the inferior mesenteric artery can only be suspected. **g** The second endoleak, fed by a patent lumbar artery between the iliac limbs, is visible in the same location as in the color flow image shown in **e**. This endoleak must be differentiated from the bright wall reflection (WR). **h** This CEUS image was obtained more inferiorly and is shown here to underline the importance of always interpreting contrast-enhanced images along with the corresponding unenhanced gray-scale images in order not to mistake bright spots for endoleaks. When such spots are present without and with contrast enhancement (indicated by arrowheads), they do not represent flow and hence do not suggest an endoleak. **i** The CTA examination in this patient demonstrates an endoleak with contrast medium extravasation (arrow) in the upper portion of the stent graft without allowing clear identification of the source of the endoleak. **j** Contrast medium extravasation into the aneurysm sac (arrow) is also seen more distally, and there appears to be a meandering communication between the upper and lower stent portion. The CTA appearance does not allow clear identification of the number of endoleaks present in this patient

To-and-fro flow is not physiologic and only occurs in endoleaks and pseudoaneurysms. A bidirectional waveform thus differentiates a true endoleak from mirror or pulsation artifacts.

Another sonographic parameter that can help the examiner in identifying patients requiring reintervention after EVAR is the (anteroposterior) aneurysm diameter in the time-motion mode. A pulsatile diameter variation of the aneurysm sac indicates an endoleak that should be treated (see ◻ Fig. 6.81 (Atlas)).

To the best of our knowledge, no published studies have investigated the possible diagnostic role of pulsation-related diameter variation of the residual aneurysm sac. In a small pilot study of 18 patients with type II endoleaks after EVAR conducted by the author, all 6 high-flow endoleaks showed a diameter variation of >2 mm through the cardiac cycle in the time-motion mode. Four of the 6 high-flow endoleaks led to sac growth within 6 months and were treated, while the other two showed a diameter increase >4 mm after another 3 months. Nine low-flow endoleaks showed no relevant pulsation (i.e., <2 mm variation through the cardiac cycle) and no sac growth over the next 6 months (measurement tolerance ±2 mm). Four of these 9 endoleaks closed spontaneously. However, 3 low-flow endoleaks showed relevant pulsation of 2–3 mm. Pulsation of the residual aneurysm sac is typically not observed when no endoleak is present.

The diagnostic and therapeutic relevance of sac pulsation in the time-motion mode might depend on the type of stent graft (structure of the prosthesis) used for EVAR. In this pilot study, all patients were treated with Endurant (Medtronic) or Zenith (Cook Medical) stent grafts.

▪▪ Preinterventional Identification of the Feeding Artery

When interventional closure of a type II endoleak is planned, it is helpful to know whether a patent lumbar artery or the inferior mesenteric artery is the culprit and whether it is a right-sided or left-sided lumbar artery. The side is difficult to identify using CEUS, and CTA at most provides some indirect clues. A Doppler waveform from the blood entry site with demonstration of **to-and-fro flow** allows identification of the side and also differentiation between an inferior mesenteric artery endoleak and a lumbar artery endoleak. A waveform showing unidirectional rather than bidirectional flow suggests that a second endoleak functioning as an exoleak is present and should be searched for (see ◘ Fig. 6.79 (Atlas)).

▪ Follow-Up of EVAR: CDUS Versus CEUS and CTA

While studies report adequate validity for **color duplex ultrasound (CDUS)** in identifying type II endoleaks that require intervention, contrast-enhanced ultrasound (CEUS) appears to be superior, especially in the detection of small endoleaks and in identifying endoleaks in patients with poor insonation conditions, and has even been reported to be comparable to computed tomography angiography (CTA) (Karthikesalingam et al. 2012). However, in all cases where CDUS identifies an endoleak that is confirmed by to-and-fro flow in the Doppler waveform, CEUS or CTA is not necessary before interventional endoleak closure (Carter et al. 2000; Chaer et al. 2009). Misinterpretation of mirror or pulsation artifacts in color flow imaging can be avoided by moving the transducer around to view the suspected endoleak from a different angle. Demonstration of to-and-fro flow confirms an endoleak, ruling out mirror or pulsation artifacts. When an endoleak has been identified by CTA or CEUS, CDUS can contribute therapeutically relevant information (see above). Spectral Doppler (possibly with echo enhancer) is also indispensable to identify steno-occlusive lesions at vessel origins in patients with a branched stent graft.

Studies consistently confirm that, with adequate insonation conditions, CDUS allows sufficient identification of **type I and III endoleaks** (◘ Figs. 6.78 and 6.79 (both Atlas)). These endoleaks, which may rupture, have higher flow velocities at the site of leakage and are detected with sensitivities and specificities of 95–100% (Karthikesalingam et al. 2012). Overall, most published data suggest that CDUS has adequate diagnostic accuracy for detection of type I and III endoleaks and identification of therapeutically relevant type II endoleaks after EVAR. An occasional patient requires supplementary CEUS or CTA to resolve inconclusive CDUS findings. While complications of CEUS are extremely rare, it must be borne in mind that it is an invasive examination and should only be performed by qualified examiners.

While a variety of diagnostic parameters exist, sac size remains the most important criterion in deciding about the **management of patients with type II endoleaks after EVAR** (surveillance versus intervention). Shrinkage of the residual aneurysm sac rules out a relevant endoleak, and the question regarding the best imaging modality becomes negligible. Conversely, when the sac expands, this points to a relevant endoleak, which must be identified using the full armentarium of imaging modalities. Since aneurysm diameter measurement is subject to some uncertainty, especially when insonation conditions are poor, an unchanged orthogonal diameter ± 0.5 cm should prompt a CDUS evaluation to rule out an endoleak. Patients with inconclusive CDUS findings should have a CEUS examination next. If the diagnosis still remains unclear, CTA is indicated.

Multiphase CTA is considered the gold standard for follow-up after EVAR. However, caution is required regarding the use of potentially nephrotoxic contrast agents in these patients, who are typically elderly and have multiple comorbidities including renal insufficiency. CDUS, which was initially used as an alternative to CTA in the follow-up of EVAR (◘ Figs. 6.35 and 6.36), shows discrepant results in terms of sensitivity and specificity compared with CTA. However, many investigators conclude CDUS follow-up to be sufficient or even equal to CTA, reporting sensitivities of 80–100% and specificities of 74–100% (Beeman et al. 2009; Chaer et al. 2009; Schmieder et al. 2009; Mirza et al. 2010; Sato et al. 1998; Wolf et al. 2000; Zannetti et al. 2000; Parent et al. 2002; McLafferty et al. 2002; Thompson et al. 1998; Fletcher et al. 2000). A review of the literature reports a mean sensitivity of 95% and mean specificity of 97% (McLafferty et al. 2002). Some investigators also point out advantages of CDUS over CTA such as the real-time evaluation of sac hemodynamics. This improves the detection of small lumbar artery endoleaks compared with CTA, which only displays the hemodynamic situation at individual points in time (e.g., venous phase). Other investigators reported inadequate diagnostic accuracy of CDUS for endoleak detection after EVAR (AbuRahma 2006; Schuster et al. 2009). A more recent meta-analysis including 25 studies with a total of 3975 paired scans found a pooled sensitivity of 0.74 and a pooled specificity of 0.96 for all types of endoleaks (predominantly type II endoleaks) compared with CTA (Karthikesalingam et al. 2012).

Several studies confirm that the sonographic detection and localization of endoleaks (especially of the more difficult to detect type II endoleaks) can be improved by the

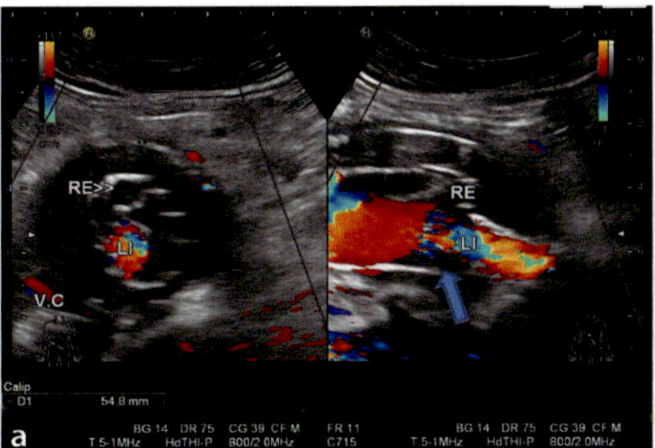

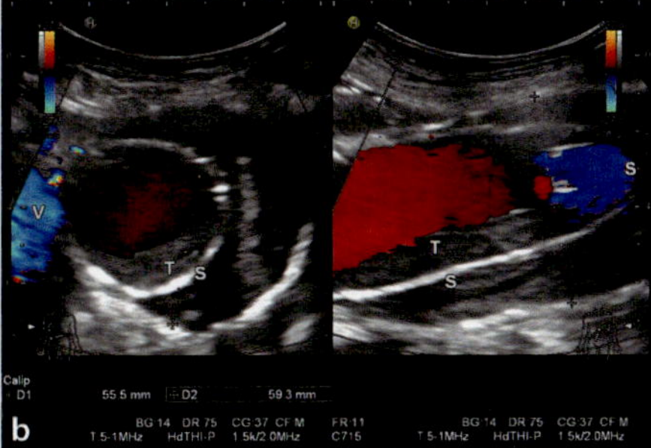

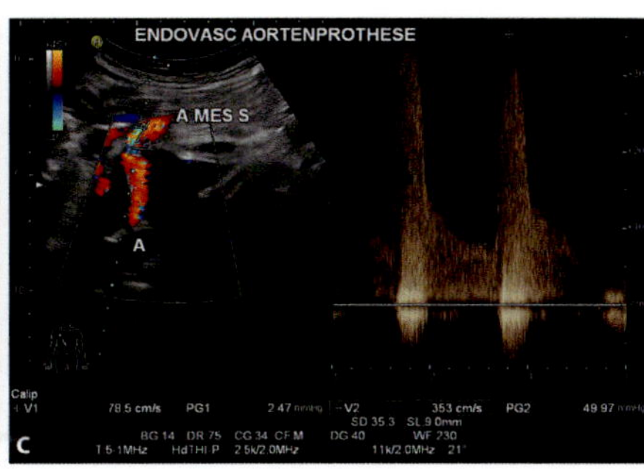

Fig. 6.37a–c Follow-up of a patient with a branched stent graft. **a** Ultrasound shows occlusion of the right iliac limb. The left iliac limb is patent but there is localized luminal narrowing (arrow) at its origin due to thrombus formation. **b** Thrombus formation (T) in the main stent graft body extending to the iliac limb origins (S). **c** Stenosis of the superior mesenteric artery (A.MES.S) at the end of the branched graft segment. The intrastenotic peak systolic velocity (PSV) is 350 cm/s (see sample volume) with a prestenotic PSV of 125 cm/s (not shown). The PSV ratio calculated from these velocities is 3, consistent with 60–70% stenosis. (The main stent graft body in the aorta (A) is patent; the absence of color flow signals is due to the obtuse angle of insonation and high PRF)

administration contrast microbubbles (Böhm et al. 2000; Henao et al. 2006; McWilliams et al. 2002; Bendick et al. 2003; Heilberger et al. 1997; Clevert et al. 2008; Sarlon et al. 2009; Giannoni et al. 2007).

CEUS in Endoleak Detection

Following injection of the microbubble contrast agent (for protocol details see ► Sect. 6.1.2.1.2), the examiner begins by searching for type I and III endoleaks at the stent graft ends (where the microbubbles arrive first). Type II endoleaks, which are fed by patent lumbar arteries or the inferior mesenteric artery, enhance later due to a longer transit time of the contrast microbubbles (and enhancement of these arteries may even persist into the venous phase). Following the search for endoleaks (for 2–3 min after microbubble administration), the next 2–5 min with persisting enhancement can be exploited to search for steno-occlusive lesions of the renal and mesenteric artery origins using color duplex utlrasound, which is especially important in patients with branched stent grafts.

In patients with an initially inconclusive contrast-enhanced scan, a second microbubble injection can be given to then focus on sites with suspicious or inconclusive findings after the first contrast bolus. If the results remain inconclusive, CTA should follow.

Published data consistently show CEUS to be comparable to CTA in detecting endoleaks and even superior in characterizing them (Iezzi et al. 2010; Pfister et al. 2009; Mirza et al. 2009). A meta-analysis of 11 studies with 981 paired scans comparing CEUS with CTA yielded a pooled sensitivity of 0.96 and a pooled specificity of 0.85 with follow-up and angiography often showing CEUS to be more accurate than CTA (Karthikesalingam et al. 2012). A small type II endoleak fed by retrograde flow in a patent lumbar artery enhances relatively late (longer transit time of microbubbles through long collateral pathways), and contrast medium extravasation may be missed, even during the venous phase of CT. The dynamic real-time CEUS examination (Fig. 6.36) is more flexible and thus better able to detect such late-enhancing endoleaks (Jung et al. 2008; Pfister et al. 2009).

In a study investigating contrast harmonic imaging (CHI) ultrasound (see ► Sect. 1.1.5) in 50 patients with suspected endoleaks following EVAR, CHI and CTA concordantly detected endoleaks in 30 cases and found no endoleak in 20 cases. In one patient, a combined type I/II endoleak was misclassified as type II. In another patient, a type II endoleak was initially only detected by CHI and later confirmed by follow-up CTA. Thus, CHI had 99% sensitivity, 93% specificity, 99% negative predictive value, and 95% positive predictive value. Time-intensity curve (TIC) analysis was used in this study to evaluate perfusion of the aneurysm (Pfister et al. 2009). Standardized signal analysis after echo enhancer administration can be used to compare enhancement in the stent graft and in the aneurysm sac; the intensity of enhancement varies with the amount of blood and can thus serve to quantify the endoleak, identifying at-risk aneurysms that warrant treatment.

Other Complications After EVAR

Ultrasound is clearly inferior to radiological imaging modalities in the detection of stent fracture and stent migration. Color duplex imaging will identify these complications only if they cause an endoleak (Fig. 6.84 (Atlas)). This is why surveillance programs for patients after EVAR should include an annual plain X-ray examination of the site of the former AAA.

Further complications after EVAR are occlusion of a stent graft limb with peripheral ischemia (Fig. 6.37a) and thrombus development in the main stent graft body, which may be a source of peripheral embolism (Fig. 6.37b), especially when the thrombus extends to the attachment site of a stent graft limb. Patients with a complex stent graft are additionally at risk of organic ischemia due to stenosis (Fig. 6.37c) or occlusion of the branched artery (renal artery, superior mesenteric artery).

6.1.6.3.8 Aortitis: Retroperitoneal Fibrosis – Inflammatory Abdominal Aortic Aneurysm

Inflammation of the aorta is rare compared with atherosclerosis. Aortitis may occur with or without dilatation and is complicated by obstruction, rupture and dissection. Underlying causes include endocarditis, local perivascular foci, and septicemia. The aorta is the most common site of bacterial infection. The differentiation of bacterial and nonbacterial aortitis can be difficult, dilatation is possible, and patients are at risk of aortic or aneurysm rupture (◘ Fig. 6.91 (Atlas)). Development of an eccentric or saccular aneurysm (mycotic aneurysm) is observed very early in the course of infection, and infectious aortitis is rarely detected before an aneurysm has formed (Narang and Rathlev 2007; Caspary 2016).

The aorta is involved in several large-artery vascular diseases including giant cell arteritis (◘ Fig 6.40b) and Takayasu's arteritis as well as Behçet's disease and Cogan's syndrome. Aortic involvement is typically asyomptomatic or presents with chest or back pain. Morphologic ultrasound findings include concentric wall thickening and sometimes dilatation of the aorta. Magnetic resonance angiography (MRA) and contrast-enhanced ultrasound (CEUS) may show increased aortic wall perfusion as a sign of local inflammation. The risk of aneurysm rupture or dissection is higher in patients with underlying vasculitis than in patients with atherosclerotic aneurysm.

Especially in Behçet's disease, dilatation is mostly eccentric, the increase in diameter can progress rapidly, and other complications such as concomitant superficial phlebitis or deep vein thrombosis may be present.

Occasionally, aortic inflammation is found in association with rheumatoid arthritis, systemic lupus erythematosus, sarcoidosis or inflammatory bowel diseases (Caspary 2016).

Isolated aortitis (possibly IgG4-related disease) is found in chronic periaortitis, retroperitoneal fibrosis (Ormond's disease), and in inflammatory aortic aneurysm. Inflammatory aortic aneurysm (◘ Fig. 6.39) may sometimes develop from degenerative aortic aneurysm in the presence of perivascular inflammation (Ketha et al. 2014) and after stent graft repair. In Ormond's disease (idiopathic in 70–80% of cases), inflammation extends beyond the periaortic area (◘ Fig 6.40a) and spreads within the retroperitoneal tissue.

Aortic wall thickening can be differentiated from perivascular, retroperitoneal conditions in the B-mode examination by assessing the course of arterial branches arising from the aorta. Retroperitoneal lymphomas are circumscribed round lesions but may become confluent. Retroperitoneal fibrosis is typically depicted as a more hypoechoic structure covering the aorta from anteriorly and involving the vena cava. It tapers off laterally and may also surround and compress the ureter.

Specifically, the course of the inferior mesenteric artery can help in differentiating wall thickening of the aorta and retroperitoneal fibrosis (◘ Figs. 6.38 and 6.40). In retroperitoneal fibrosis, the proximal inferior mesenteric artery is pushed against the aorta and thus courses between the aortic wall and the hypoechoic fibrosis for several centimeters before piercing through the hypoechoic fibrotic cap (see ◘ Fig. 6.85 (Atlas)). In inflammation of the aorta (e.g., giant cell arteritis), on the other hand, the inferior mesenteric artery pierces the hypoechoic layer around the patent lumen of the aorta directly at its origin to then descend into the left lower abdomen outside the hypoechoic thickening. Inflammatory wall

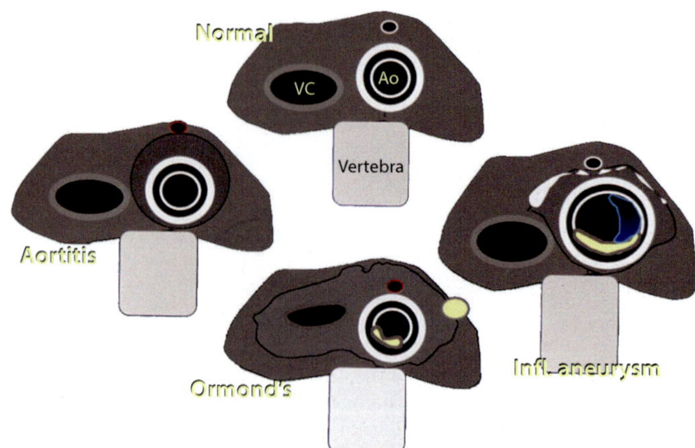

◘ **Fig. 6.38** Evaluation of the course of the proximal inferior mesenteric artery as it arises from the aorta for the differentiation of aortic wall thickening and retroperitoneal perivascular pathology (see ◘ Fig. 6.85 (Atlas)). The topmost diagram illustrates the normal anatomy of the aorta (Ao) and vena cava (VC). The diagram labeled "Aortitis" illustrates the situation in giant cell arteritis: the inferior mesenteric artery arises from the aorta and then courses outside the hypoechoic, concentrically thickened wall of the aorta. In this condition, the mesenteric artery takes the shortest path possible through the abnormal tissue (inflammatory aortic wall). The diagram labeled "Infl. aneurysm" illustrates the findings in inflammatory abdominal aortic aneurysm (AAA). In this condition, the inferior mesenteric artery also passes through the aneurysmatically dilated and thickened abdominal wall, taking the shortest path possible, to then descend toward the left lower abdomen outside the thickened structure. If atherosclerotic lesions are present, they can help in differentiating inflammatory wall thickening from thrombotic deposits in the aneurysm sac: atherosclerotic plaques make the intima appear bright, thus allowing differentiation of thrombotic deposits extending into the lumen from inflammatory wall thickening on the other side of the intima. The bottom diagram (labeled "Ormond's") illustrates the findings in retroperitoneal fibrosis. The proximal segment of the inferior mesenteric artery arising from the nonthickened aortic wall courses through the hypoechoic abnormal tissue before emerging out of it and passing to the left lower abdomen. In retroperitoneal fibrosis, the abnormal tissue pushes a longer proximal segment of the inferior mesenteric artery against the wall of the aorta. In patients with more advanced retroperitoneal fibrosis, which also encases the vena cava or even the ureter, the diagnosis and differentiation from other conditions are easier than in early disease with fibrotic tissue surrounding only the aorta. Therefore, the abnormal course of the proximal inferior mesenteric artery is the decisive criterion for making the differential diagnosis (Diagrams courtesy of K. Amendt)

thickening in aortitis and in inflammatory aortic aneurysm is circumferential and spares the vena cava (see ◘ Figs. 6.39 and 6.40). The flexible selection of scanning planes in the ultrasound examination facilitates determination of the relationships between the aorta, hypoechoic thickening, perivascular structures, and other vessels, thereby contributing to the differential diagnosis.

Thickening of the aortic wall due to vasculitis with aortic dilatation or inflammatory aortic aneurysm can be differentiated from intraluminal thrombi by its relationship to the intimal layer. While this is relevant for diameter measurement, differentiation is only possible when atherosclerotic plaque is present, which makes the intima appear brighter. The normal intima is not visible sonographically (◘ Figs. 6.38 and 6.39).

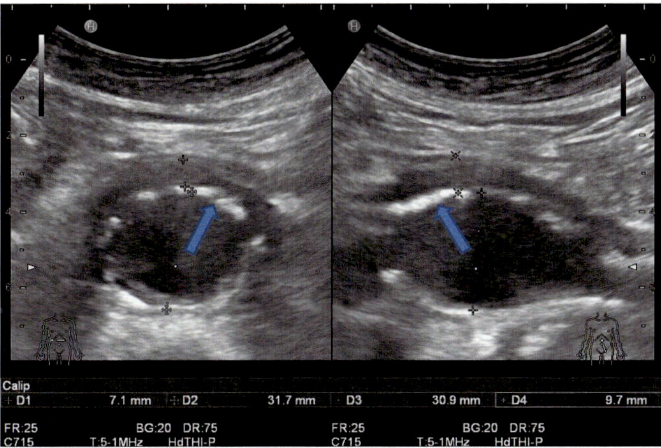

Fig. 6.39 Inflammatory abdominal aortic aneurysm (AAA). Transverse (left) and longitudinal (right) images show inflammatory wall thickening with a wall thickness of 9 mm. Here, the intima appears bright due to the presence of atherosclerotic plaque (arrow) and allows differentiation of vascular pathology on the luminal side from processes external to the intima. In this case, wall thickening involves the outer layers of the vessel wall. Thus, the relationship to the intima distinguishes inflammatory vessel wall thickening from thrombotic deposits, which would be seen to extend into the lumen from the inner side of the intima. The patent lumen is 31 mm in width

6.2 Visceral and Retroperitoneal Veins

6.2.1 Vascular Anatomy

6.2.1.1 Vena Cava

The inferior vena cava ascends parallel to the course of the aorta and to the right of the vertebral column. It is a capacitance vessel with an elliptical cross section and may vary in its anteroposterior diameter from 0.5 to 2.5 cm during the respiratory cycle. It is formed by the junction of the common iliac veins at the L4/L5 level slightly below the aortic bifurcation.

Variants and anomalies of the inferior vena cava are present in 1.5–4.0% of the population and are typically detected incidentally. They result from errors in the complex embryonic development with a disturbance in the transition from the symmetric venous system to the predominantly right-sided, asymmetric secondary system. The congenital anomalies were classified by Chuang et al. as early as 1974 (Table 6.8).

Vena cava anomalies typically involve the segment below the renal vein entries. Duplication (0.2–3%) and transposition (0.2–0.5%) are the most common anomalies. In both cases, the inferior vena cava, which runs to the left of the aorta,

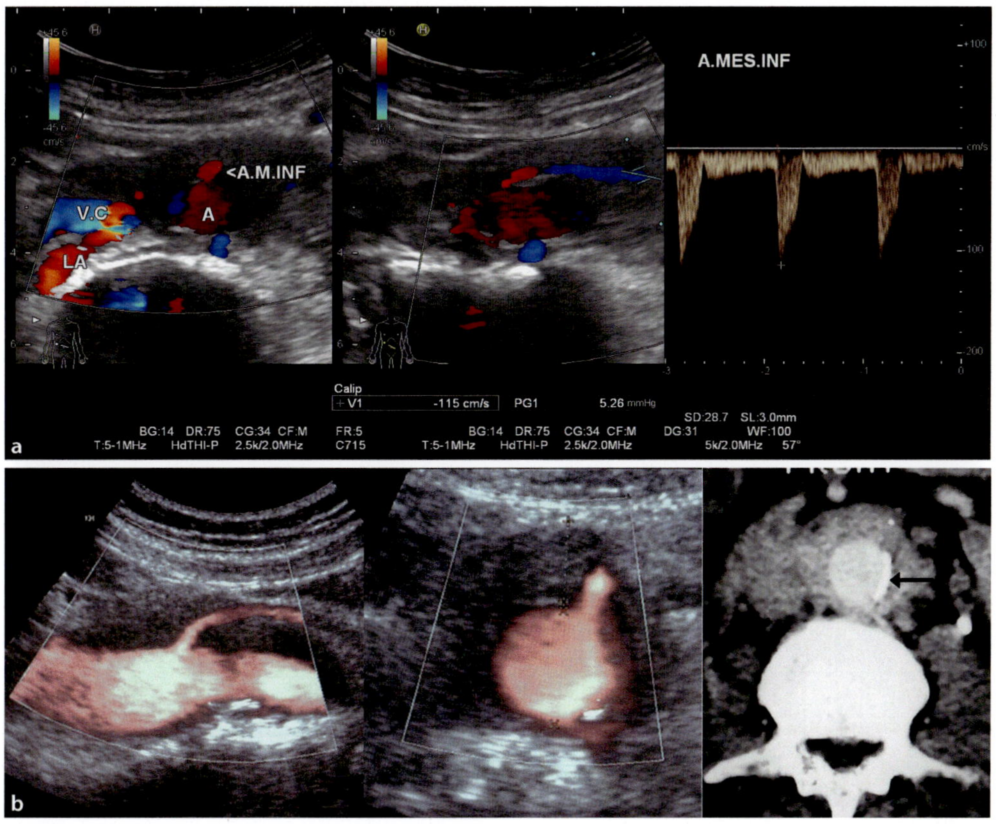

Fig. 6.40 **a** Retroperitoneal fibrosis (Ormond's disease) histologically proven by core biopsy. A thickened aortic wall as in vasculitis can be differentiated from retroperitoneal fibrosis by the course of the inferior mesenteric artery (<A.M.INF). The abnormal retroperitoneal tissue pushes the inferior mesenteric artery toward the aorta. The inferior mesenteric artery thus appears closer to the aortic lumen than in vasculitis. **b** Aortic wall thickening in giant cell arteritis (power mode images in longitudinal orientation on the left and transverse orientation on the right). The course of the inferior mesenteric artery at its origin confirms disease of the aortic wall as the artery pierces the thickened wall directly as it arises from the aorta rather than being pushed toward the aortic wall, as in fibrosis. The CT scan (rightmost image) shows circumferential wall thickening due to giant cell arteritis. Both ultrasound and CT additionally show plaque on the thickened wall in the lumen (Courtesy of K. Amendt)

6

Table 6.8 Classification of congenital anomalies of the inferior vena cava (According to Chuang et al. 1974)

Level	Segment	Description
I	Postrenal	
	Type A	Persistence of right posterior cardinal vein (retro- or circumaortic ureter)
	Type B	Persistence of right supracardinal vein (normal inferior vena cava)
	Type C	Persistence of left supracardinal vein (left-sided inferior vena cava)
	Type BC	Persistence of both supracardinal veins (duplicated inferior vena cava)
II	Renal	Persistence of renal venous ring (circumaortic ureter)
III	Prerenal or hepatic	Absence of hepatic segment (azygos or hemiazygos vein continuation)

crosses the aorta together with or as part of the left renal vein to then continue on its course on the right side of the aorta (see Fig. 6.42).

6.2.1.2 Renal Veins

The right renal vein courses anterior to the renal artery, and after 3–4 cm it empties into the vena cava at the level of the L1 vertebra. The left renal vein runs anterior and somewhat superior to the renal artery to then curve between the aorta and superior mesenteric artery and posteroinferior to the head of the pancreas on its way to the inferior vena cava. The left renal artery receives the ovarian or spermatic vein, which empty directly into the vena cava on the right (Fig. 6.1).

Variants include duplication of the renal veins and atypical terminations, for example, in the common iliac vein. Disturbed embryonic development may result in an atypical retroaortic course of the left renal vein.

6.2.1.3 Portal Venous System and Hepatic Veins

The portal vein is a thick trunk, normally 6–8 cm long, and has a transverse, anteroposterior elliptical diameter of 8–12 mm, rarely up to 16 mm, with wide physiologic variation. It passes through the hepatoduodenal ligament behind the proper hepatic artery and ascends to the porta hepatis, taking an oblique lateral course. Intrahepatically, it follows the branches of the hepatic artery and the bile ducts. The branching pattern of the portal vein provides the basis for the anatomic segmentation of the liver. The branches of the hepatic veins are intersegmental vessels.

The splenic vein passes behind the pancreas from the hilum of the spleen to the head of the pancreas, where it joins the superior mesenteric vein to form the portal vein (Fig. 6.41). The confluence of the two veins is situated to the left of and behind the pancreatic head, somewhat lateral and inferior to the origin of the mesenteric artery. The superior mesenteric vein courses to the right of the superior mesenteric artery and anterior to the aorta.

Blood is drained from the liver through the segmental branches into the three major veins, which empty directly into the inferior vena cava.

6.2.2 Examination Technique

6.2.2.1 Vena Cava

The aorta can serve as a landmark when examining the vena cava. When assessing the lower extremity vessels for thrombosis or when assessing patients with pulmonary embolism, the course of the vena cava is followed after evaluation of the pelvic and leg veins. Evaluation in the transverse plane is followed by longitudinal scanning for spectral Doppler

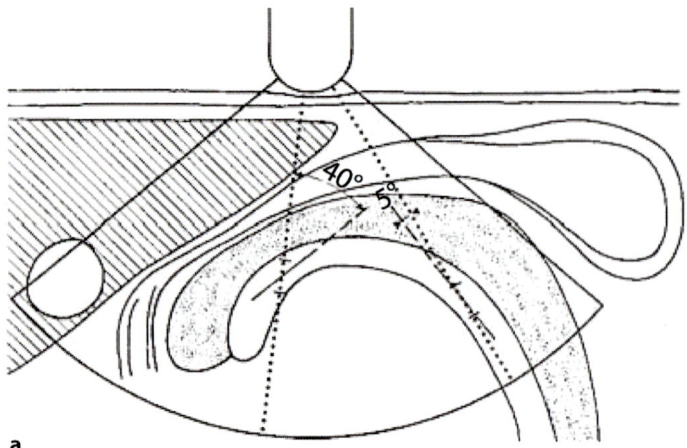

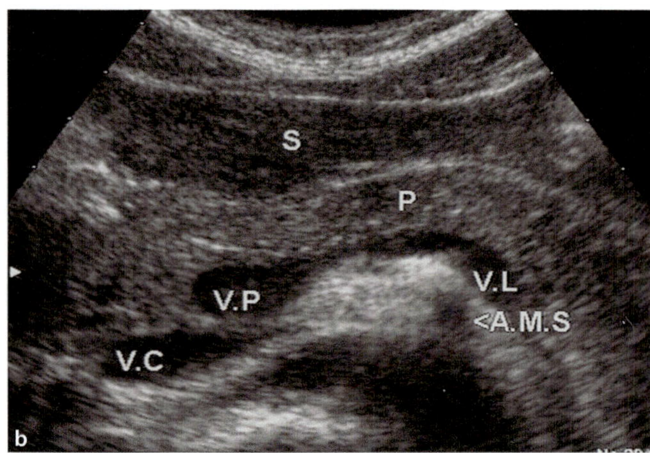

Fig. 6.41 **a** Transverse diagram showing the course of the splenic vein from right to left, where it joins the superior mesenteric vein to form the portal vein, below the head of the pancreas. **b** Course of the splenic vein (V.L), posterior to the pancreas (P) and anterior to the superior mesenteric artery (A.M.S), terminating in the portal vein (V.P)

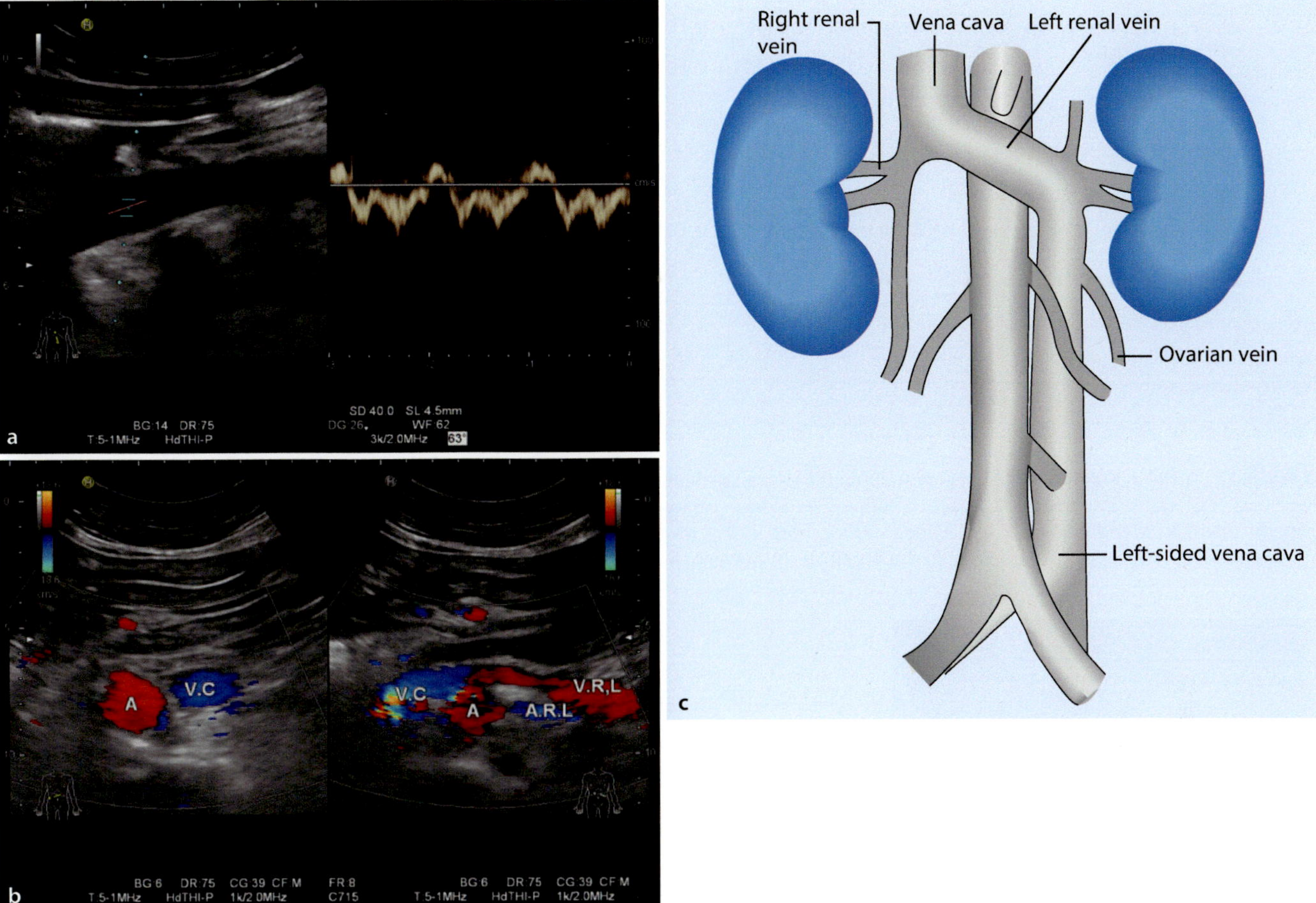

Fig. 6.42 **a** Cardiac modulation of the vena cava waveform (W-shaped). **b** Anatomic variant of the vena cava seen in transverse orientation on the left and longitudinal orientation on the right. The transverse image shows the infrarenal vena cava (V.C) to the left of the aorta (A). The transposed vena cava ascends to the left of the aorta, is joined by the left renal vein (V.R.L., longitudinal image), crosses the aorta, and then continues on its normal course, i.e., to the right of the aorta (A.R.L, left renal artery). **c** Diagram illustrating this anatomic variant: the transposed inferior vena cava ascends to the left of the aorta and, after receiving the left renal vein, crosses the aorta. The further ascent is orthotopic, i.e., to the right of the aorta

measurement. The confluence of the iliac veins at the level of the umbilicus can be identified using the aortic bifurcation at about the same level or slightly above for orientation.

In **pelvic vein thrombosis**, possible extension of the thrombus into the vena cava must be identified and the end of the thrombus evaluated for the presence of surrounding flow signals. The respiratory variation in vena cava diameter is determined in transverse or longitudinal images. Diameter variation is absent in thrombosis.

Compression ultrasound is unreliable in the abdomen (where compressibility is limited by anatomy), which is why (color) duplex ultrasound is necessary to exclude thrombosis. Only in slender patients is it possible to reliably compress the vena cava. The flow velocity determined from the Doppler waveform is likewise affected by respiratory phasicity and increasing cardiac pulsatility toward the heart (Fig. 6.42a). Below the kidneys, the liver can be used as an acoustic window with the portal vein being located anterior to the vena cava at the hilum of the liver.

The hepatic veins join the vena cava shortly before it passes through the diaphragm.

6.2.2.2 Renal Veins

The renal veins are scanned from the flank beginning at the renal hilum and following their course proximally (see Fig. 6.6). While the shorter right vein can be visualized from this position throughout its course to the inferior vena cava, the left vein (Fig. 6.43) must be scanned from a medial approach in transverse orientation to visualize the segment between the aorta and superior mesenteric artery and its termination.

The superior mesenteric artery can serve as a landmark to avoid confusion of the left renal vein with the slightly more anterocranial splenic vein. The left renal vein runs posterior to the superior mesenteric artery, that is, between the latter and the aorta; the splenic vein courses anterior to it and then crosses over the superior mesenteric artery to enter the portal vein.

When searching for **renal vein thrombosis** or intravascular tumor extension in the B-mode, the examiner must look for the absence of respiratory diameter fluctuations and the presence of echogenic intraluminal material dilating the vein. The absence of flow in the spectral Doppler recording is diagnostic of thrombosis.

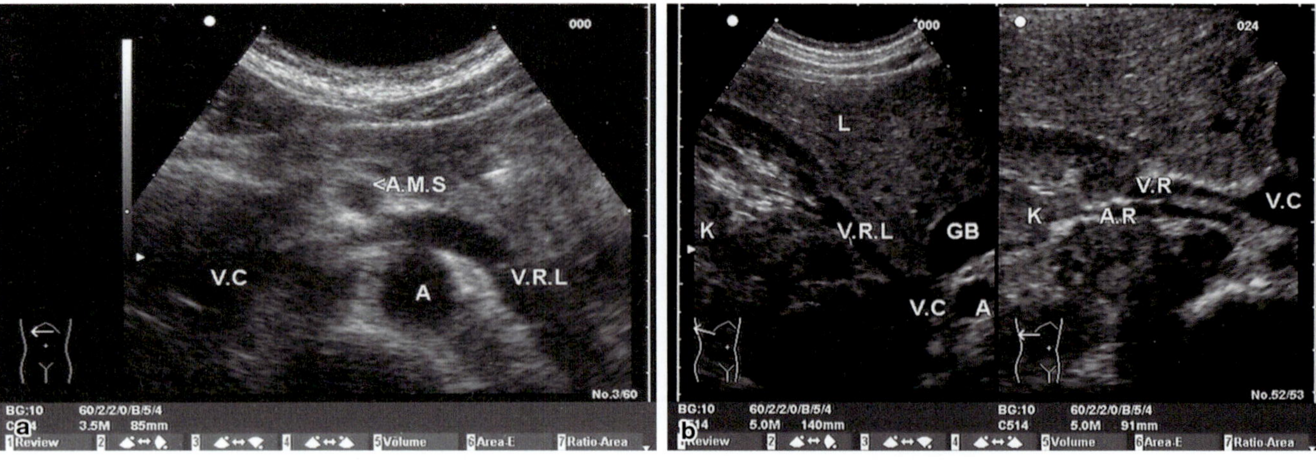

■ **Fig. 6.43** **a** The left renal vein (V.R.L) courses from the left renal hilum, between the aorta (A) and superior mesenteric artery (A.M.S), to the vena cava (V.C). Transverse epigastric image. **b** With the transducer on the right flank (left image), the right renal vein (V.R.) can easily be evaluated from the hilum (K) to the vena cava (V.C). With a slightly more medial transducer position (right image), the liver can be used as an acoustic window, and the renal vein can be seen deep to the liver (L) from the renal hilum (K) to the vena cava (V.C), coursing anterior to the renal artery (A.R.)

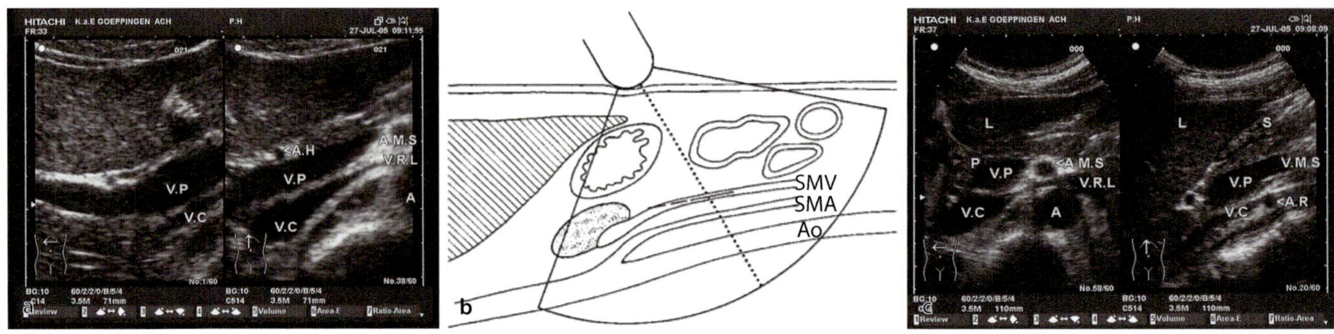

■ **Fig. 6.44** **a** In the subcostal oblique image (right upper abdomen), the portal vein formed by the confluence of the superior mesenteric and splenic veins posterior to the pancreatic head (right image) is seen anterior to the vena cava (V.C) on its course through the hepatoduodenal ligament to the liver hilum (left margin of left image). **b** Diagram of the course of the superior mesenteric vein (SMV; SMA, superior mesenteric artery; Ao, aorta). **c** The transverse upper abdominal image (left) shows the vena cava (V.C) to the left of the aorta (landmark); the portal vein (V.P) courses inside the hepatoduodenal ligament deep to the liver (L). The longitudinal image (right) shows the superior mesenteric vein (V.M.S.) coursing anterior to the vena cava (V.C, landmark) and terminating in the portal vein (V.P.) posterior to the pancreatic head

6.2.2.3 Portal Vein and Superior Mesenteric Vein

The course of the portal vein from below the pancreatic head to the liver hilum is most easily accessible from a subcostal approach in an oblique plane through the right upper abdomen (■ Fig. 6.44). If visualization is impaired by overlying bowel gas, the liver hilum can be identified and the portal vein followed distally from an intercostal position (right flank) using the liver as an acoustic window. Portal vein thrombosis is suggested by the presence of echogenic material in the lumen and absent respiratory diameter variation in the B-mode image, and is subsequently confirmed by (color) duplex imaging.

Suspected portal hypertension is easily demonstrated sonographically by the identification of portal vein collaterals. The evaluation for collateral circulation comprises the following steps:

- Flow in the portal vein: to-and-fro flow, retrograde flow, or reduced flow velocity (unreliable sign; augmentation maneuver may be necessary, which will elicit a less marked increase in flow).
- Flow direction in the splenic vein.
- Visualization of the falsiform ligament and reopening of the collapsed umbilical vein with hepatofugal flow (Cruveilhier–Baumgarten syndrome).
- Dilated left gastric vein (in longitudinal plane, arising from portal vein at the site of mesenteric vein termination).
- Varicose dilatation in the gallbladder wall.
- Identification of dilated gastroepiploic veins posterolateral to the left hepatic lobe and of splenorenal and splenogastric collaterals at the upper and lower poles of the kidney.

The **superior mesenteric vein** courses to the right of the superior mesenteric artery with a position to the left suggesting malrotation. The criteria for diagnosing thrombosis are the same as in the portal vein. If **mesenteric vein thrombosis** is suspected, the vein should be traced to the level of the jejunal branches, the ileocolic vein, and right colic vein. This is most easily accomplished in transverse orientation with slight angulation of the transducer in the color duplex mode.

6.2.3 Clinical Role of Duplex Ultrasound

6.2.3.1 Renal Veins

Acute renal vein thrombosis may be asymptomatic or present with pain and hematuria. The presentation depends on the extent of retroperitoneal collateralization, and based on this variability, it is assumed that renal vein thrombosis actually occurs more frequently than it is diagnosed. Thromboembolic complications are rare. Renal vein thrombosis can occur in patients with renal diseases such as nephrotic syndrome and glomerulonephritis, external compression of the renal vein by tumor or retroperitoneal lymphoma, and systemic conditions including clotting disorders and intra-abdominal inflammatory conditions such as acute pancreatitis or sepsis. The severity of renal impairment (from normal to acute renal failure) varies with the degree of thrombotic obstruction and the extent of retroperitoneal collateral flow (through capsular and suprarenal veins). This is why a duplex ultrasound examination of the renal vein is indicated not only in patients with clinical signs and symptoms but also in patients with a retroperitoneal tumor, so that prompt anticoagulation treatment can be initiated.

Renal vein evaluation is mandatory before surgery for a retroperitoneal tumor and especially before nephrectomy for renal cell carcinoma. The presence of tumor thrombus in the vein is especially important for the surgical approach in renal cell carcinoma; it has been shown that 20–40% of patients with a large renal tumor have tumor thrombus in the renal vein, among them 5–10% with extension of the thrombus into the vena cava (Goncharenko et al. 1979; Levine 1990).

6.2.3.2 Portal Venous System

In patients with chronic hepatic dysfunction, the examination focuses on **parenchymal damage**, ranging all the way to cirrhosis. It also includes damage of the vascular system, in particular portal hypertension, which typically develops secondary to cirrhosis. Portal hypertension can result from obstruction at different levels: sinusoidal obstruction (typical in cirrhosis); presinusoidal obstruction in schistosomiasis, Wilson's disease, and myeloproliferative diseases; prehaptic thrombosis or occlusion of the portal vein; postsinusoidal hepatic vein occlusion; compression of the vena cava; and severe right ventricular insufficiency.

In patients with **suspected cirrhosis**, evaluation of portal hypertension is important for the interpretation of the clinical findings and the patient's prognosis. Gray-scale ultrasound criteria are highly specific for liver cirrhosis, but sensitivity is very poor compared with liver biopsy and intraoperative findings. However, if portal hypertension is present and other underlying causes can be ruled out, then even with an inconclusive gray-scale examination, cirrhosis can be assumed. Criteria on gray-scale images include macroscopic and microscopic nodules, primarily identifiable as liver contour irregularities, and an increase in attenuation and echogenicity. Shrinkage of the right hepatic lobe with enlargement of the caudate lobe (caudate-to-right lobe ratio > 0.65) was found to be 90–100% specific for cirrhosis but with a poor sensitivity of only 43% (Harbin et al. 1980; Giorgio et al. 1986). Splenomegaly is common in portal hypertension but is also not very specific. Duplex imaging allows adequate evaluation of blood flow in the portal vein and in the splenic and mesenteric veins in 93–95% of patients (Patriquin et al. 1987; Yeh et al. 1996). The ultrasound criteria described below do not allow reliable exclusion of portal hypertension or cirrhosis.

6.2.4 Normal Findings

6.2.4.1 Vena Cava and Renal Veins

The normal vena cava has an average diameter of 1.5–3.0 cm with a maximum blood flow velocity of 40–100 cm/s. Intraindividually, the **diameter varies** from 0.5 to 2.5 cm **with respiration**. This variation is reflected in the Doppler waveform. Additional cardiac phasicity due to pressure changes in the right atrium results in an M-shaped flow profile. The first peak reflects the tricuspid valve movement during systole, followed by a decrease in flow velocity with increasing atrial filling and a second flow acceleration upon opening of the tricuspid valve, which produces the second peak. During atrial contraction, flow again becomes faster, sometimes with a short retrograde component.

The normal renal vein diameter is 4–10 mm with a maximum flow velocity of 20–40 cm/s. The **renal veins**, in particular the right one, also show **respiratory blood flow fluctuation**, which is reflected in the Doppler waveform by an increase in flow velocity during inspiration and a decrease during expiration. The left renal vein typically exhibits pulsatile variation due to brief compression of the vein during systole in the narrow passageway between the aorta and superior mesenteric artery. The left renal vein occasionally takes an atypical retroaortic course, and rarely multiple branches are present on the left (4% versus approx. 20% on the right). If the left renal vein is not depicted between the aorta and superior mesenteric artery, the examiner should look for it behind the aorta at about the level of the origin of the left renal artery.

The major branches of the hepatic venous system and the right renal vein have the same flow character as the vena cava (cardiac (atrial) pulsatility and respiratory phasicity).

6.2.4.2 Portal Venous System

The normal portal vein is depicted by gray-scale sonography with an anechoic, smoothly delineated lumen below the liver and shows less marked respiratory caliber variation than the vena cava (usually 8–13 mm, larger caliber during deep inspiration). The (color) duplex mode depicts flow toward the liver with respiratory variation. Maximum flow velocity (V_{max}) is 15–35 cm/s with a mean velocity (V_{mean}) of 10–25 cm/s (Seitz and Kubale 1988; Moriyasu et al. 1986;

Gaiani et al. 1989). Postprandially, flow velocity may exceed 35 cm/s. Altogether, flow velocities in the portal system are characterized by wide interindividual variation and also increase after a meal as in the mesenteric circulation (two- to threefold increase in flow volume in the superior mesenteric artery and vein). In fasting individuals, the normal superior mesenteric vein diameter is 4–12 mm with a maximum flow velocity of 10–45 cm/s, while the normal splenic vein diameter is 5–10 mm with a maximum flow velocity of 10–25 cm/s.

6.2.5 Documentation

Documentation of findings in the retroperitoneal veins as in the portal venous system depends on the clinical question to be answered. In addition to the B-mode findings and the Doppler waveform from the vein of interest, the perivenous findings should be documented as well. Specifically, vein compression and the extent of thrombotic changes must be recorded as well as collateral pathways in case of disturbed venous drainage, for example, retroperitoneal and splenorenal shunts in renal vein thrombosis and gastric or umbilical shunts in portal hypertension (liver cirrhosis, Cruveilhier–Baumgarten syndrome).

6.2.6 Abnormal Ultrasound Findings, Measurement Parameters, and Diagnostic Role

6.2.6.1 Vena Cava

The complex embryonic development of the venous system gives rise to numerous variants and malformations, all of which are rare. The vena cava can show the whole range of anomalies from aplasia to duplication (◻ Fig. 6.42).

Rare variants and atypical courses of the individual vessels are identified and differentiated from retroperitoneal lymph nodes in the color duplex mode (◻ Fig. 6.45). Compression of the vena cava is most commonly due to retroperitoneal lymph nodes or tumors, aortic aneurysm, or retroperitoneal fibrosis. Rare venous leiomyomas or leiomyosarcomas may also arise from the smooth muscle layer of the vena cava.

Since compression ultrasound is of limited use in demonstrating thrombosis of the retroperitoneal and visceral veins, duplex imaging and above all color-coded duplex imaging come in handy. However, there also exist B-mode criteria for thrombosis of the intra-abdominal or retroperitoneal veins.

Thrombus may be visualized directly as a hyperechoic structure. In addition, thrombosis is suggested if the respiratory caliber variation typical of the larger retroperitoneal veins, in particular the vena cava, is lost. This finding is unspecific, and dilatation of the vena cava with reduced or absent caliber fluctuation may also occur in right ventricular failure. Thrombosis should always be ruled out by color duplex imaging with a low pulse repetition frequency and high gain or by obtaining a Doppler waveform. Apart from thrombosis, venous drainage may be obstructed by tumor compression, tumor infiltration, or intravascular tumor growth (◻ Fig. 6.45).

The **clinical symptoms of thrombosis** depend on its site, temporal course, and collateralization. There is a risk of embolism, especially in pelvic vein and **vena cava thrombosis**. The latter is typically caused by an ascending thrombus from the pelvic and leg veins, less commonly by local obstruction (external tumor compression or infiltration), thrombus or **tumor extension** from the renal veins (renal cell carcinoma), or extension of hepatic vein thrombosis in Budd-Chiari syndrome.

Acute ascending thrombus is typically hypoechoic and may be difficult to identify on gray-scale ultrasound in obese patients. Over time, the thrombus undergoes hyalinization

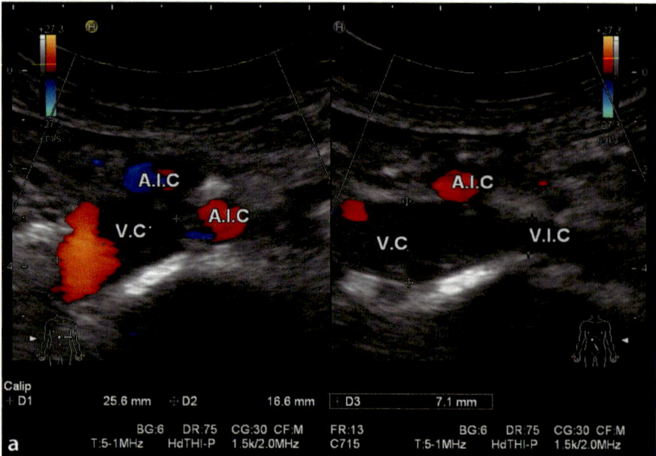

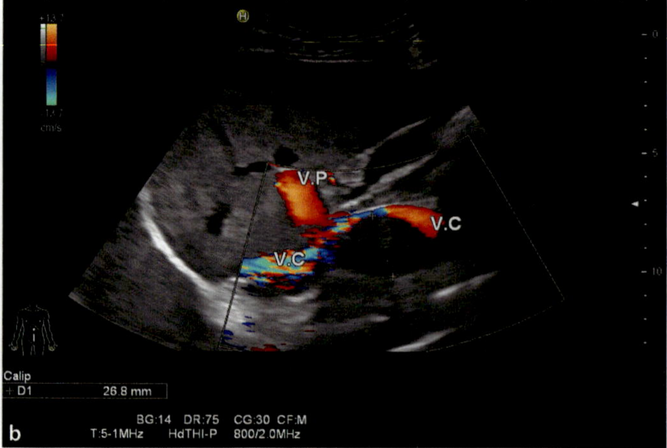

◻ **Fig. 6.45** **a** Transverse (left) and longitudinal image (right) of vena cava (V.C) thrombus due to ascending thrombosis from the common iliac artery (V.I.C). Vena cava thrombus must be differentiated from caval wall tumors and vena cava compression by outside structures. **b** Tumor of the vena cava wall (histologically diagnosed as leiomyoma) posterior to the liver hilum causes circumscribed luminal narrowing with aliasing (see ◻ Fig. 3.36). Sonomorphologically, a wall tumor cannot be differentiated from vena cava compression due to posteriorly located retroperitoneal tumors. Among the external tumors that can compress the vena cava, the relationship to the vena cava differentiates a retroperitoneal connective tissue tumor (sarcoma) from lymphoma, which is characterized by its paracaval or para-aortic position lateral or anterior to the vena cava

and becomes inhomogeneous. Thrombus organization with invasion of cells from the vessel wall and retraction of fibrin fibers results in increasing echogenicity and poorer delineation from the wall. Very old thrombi may undergo partial mural calcification.

Because a variety of **collateral pathways** exist, even occlusion of the vena cava may occasionally cause only a few clinical symptoms. Venous return occurs predominantly through the paravertebral plexus, the ascending lumbar and azygos venous systems, the superficial veins of the abdominal wall, and the portal collateral route. Color duplex scanning enables good evaluation of the collateral pathways in vena cava or pelvic vein thrombosis, though the findings have no clinical relevance in most cases.

Disturbed drainage of the pelvic and leg veins demonstrated by spectral Doppler (continuous flow without respiratory phasicity) may be due to central vena cava thrombosis caused by thrombus or tumor extension from the renal veins or compression of the vena cava by a retroperitoneal tumor or aortic aneurysm. Therefore, the examiner must carefully look for these possible causes. If the spectral waveform from the vena cava or pelvic veins shows pulsatile flow, a thorough search must be undertaken for an AV fistula, which may be caused by trauma, idiopathically, perforating aneurysm, or iatrogenically after surgery or puncture.

Tricuspid insufficiency or **right ventricular failure** affects caval blood flow, causing dilatation and changes in the Doppler waveform. Regurgitation into the right atrium in tricuspid insufficiency extends into the proximal vena cava, where it becomes apparent in the waveform by a reflux component during systole.

6.2.6.1.1 Membranous Vena Cava Obstruction

Congenital membranous structures can cause narrowing of the vena cava below the diaphragm (membranous stenosis) or at the termination of the left common iliac vein (venous spur). While often clinically asymptomatic, vena cava narrowing may give rise to descending thrombosis. In patients with good insonation conditions, color duplex imaging will demonstrate a slit-shaped stenosis with circumscribed flow acceleration. The fixed nature of the stenosis can be confirmed by a provocative test (Valsalva's maneuver with respiratory excursions).

6.2.6.2 Renal Veins

Just as in the inferior vena cava, thrombosis and central **tumor thrombus** of the renal veins can be identified sonographically in patients with adequate insonation conditions. Therefore, preoperative color duplex imaging of the renal veins is sufficient prior to tumor nephrectomy. Venography has a similar diagnostic yield only if it is performed as venacavography with compression or provocative maneuvers. For this reason, contrast-enhanced CT is the primary alternative imaging modality in the routine clinical setting.

The nephrotic syndrome associated with glomerulonephritis is the most common cause of **renal vein thrombosis**. Other factors promoting renal vein thrombosis include antithrombin III deficiency, sepsis, pregnancy, oral contraceptives, corticoid therapy, collagen diseases, and amyloidosis. Secondary renal vein thrombosis can be caused by obstruction due to retroperitoneal tumors, aortic aneurysm, or caval thrombosis as well as intravenous extension of renal tumors.

Unspecific features of renal vein thrombosis, detectable by gray-scale ultrasound, are enlargement of the kidney and reduced echogenicity of the renal parenchyma. In patients with an adequate acoustic window, the thrombus will be identified as a hypoechoic and partially inhomogeneous structure within the lumen of the dilated vein (▪ Fig. 6.106). Thrombosis is confirmed by the absence of flow in color duplex images or in the Doppler waveform. A partially occlusive thrombus may be seen as a defect in the color coding with a decrease or complete loss of cardiac pulsatility and respiratory phasicity of flow in the Doppler waveform. If there is good venous drainage through capsular veins and the suprarenal vein, venous flow may be detectable in the renal hilum even if there is complete occlusion of the renal vein.

An **indirect sign of acute renal vein thrombosis** is a marked reduction or even transient reversal of diastolic flow in the waveform from the renal artery. This is due to reflex vasoconstriction, and the flow pattern resembles that seen in rejection of a kidney transplant.

Apart from an increased peripheral resistance reflected in the waveform from the renal artery, acute renal vein thrombosis can also cause **kidney enlar**gement. The magnitude of these changes depends on the extent of collateral pathways of the thrombosed renal vein, which may involve splenorenal shunts or retroperitoneal routes such as venous connections to the adrenal gland. Recanalization after acute renal vein thrombosis is seen on color duplex as meander-like flow in an otherwise dilated and echogenic lumen.

Markedly **slower flow in the renal vein** with loss of cardiac pulsatility and respiratory phasicity is also seen in obstruction of the proximal inferior vena cava by a tumor or thrombosis or in right ventricular failure (acute: pulmonary embolism; chronic: tricuspid insufficiency).

Prior to tumor nephrectomy, sonographic evaluation of the renal veins is necessary to plan the extent of surgery according to the **stage of venous tumor extension**:

- **Stage I** is characterized by a button-like protrusion of tumor from the renal vein into the vena cava (see ▪ Fig. 6.107).
- In **stage II** the tumor extends farther into the vena cava but the upper margin is still below the level of the hepatic vein termination.
- In **stage III** the tumor extends to the level of the hepatic veins.
- In **stage IV** there is tumor extension into the atrium.

Adequate sonographic evaluation of venous thrombus or tumor thrombus is impaired by superimposed bowel gas and by flow phenomena, especially when examining obese patients, resulting in adequate duplex evaluation of the renal veins in only 50–80% cases (Schwerk et al. 1994; Didier et al. 1987; Dubbins 1986; London et al. 1989). When there is a

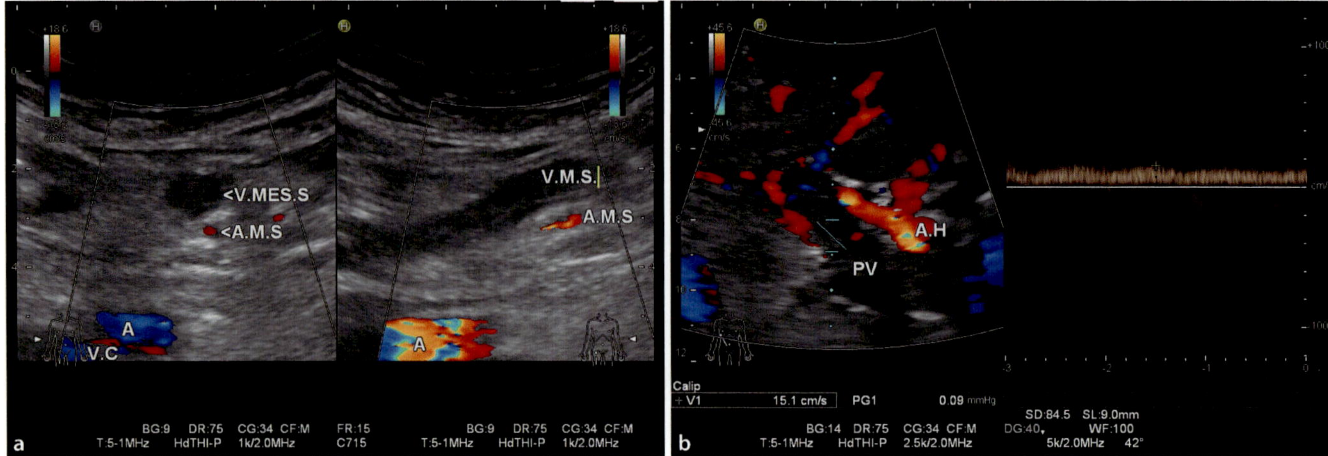

Fig. 6.46 **a** Occlusive thrombosis of the superior mesenteric vein (V.M.S): the lumen is dilated, slightly echogenic, and homogeneous. The vein can be identified adjacent to the superior mesenteric artery (A.M.S), which serves as a landmark. **b** Thrombosis of the portal vein (PV) with flow signals along the thrombus but no respiratory modulation (flow obstruction) and reduced flow velocity. There is flow displayed in red in the hepatic artery (A.H) and in venous collaterals in the liver hilum, particularly around the gallbladder

good acoustic window, ultrasound has 95–100% accuracy in detecting tumor thrombus. Because detailed evaluation of the renal veins by ultrasound is not always possible, **contrast-enhanced computed tomography and magnetic resonance imaging** are more accurate in preoperatively defining the extent of tumor thrombus in the renal vein and beyond and in planning the surgical resection. Given the importance of this information, these two imaging modalities should be used liberally as supplements to duplex ultrasound before surgery.

6.2.6.3 Superior Mesenteric Vein and Splenic Vein

Mesenteric vein thrombosis is a rare cause of intestinal necrosis. Therefore, duplex imaging performed to rule out mesenteric artery occlusion in patients presenting with the respective clinical symptoms should also include the mesenteric vein to exclude thrombosis there as well (Fig. 6.46). Edematous thickening of the intestinal walls is a conspicuous finding and will already be seen in the gray-scale image.

Causes of mesenteric vein thrombosis include hematologic diseases, clotting disorders, abscess or sepsis, and tumor occlusion. Apart from acute thrombosis presenting with acute symptoms of intestinal necrosis, there may be chronic thrombosis with unspecific findings such as fever, leukocytosis, or thrombocytosis.

An abnormal course of the superior mesenteric vein suggests **malrotation**, which is confirmed if the superior mesenteric vein lies to the left of the superior mesenteric artery. If the vein is anterior to the artery, malrotation is present in one third of the cases. These indirect signs of malrotation are easily detected by duplex ultrasound.

The **clinical severity of mesenteric vein thrombosis** depends on the extent and site of the thrombus (see Figs. 6.99 and 6.100 (both Atlas)) and collateralization. Partial thrombosis of the superior mesenteric vein, for instance, may be fairly asymptomatic and present with clinical signs of enteritis only. Conversely, patients with extensive central mesenteric vein thrombosis may present with an acute abdomen due to intestinal necrosis. Early diagnosis with initiation of anticoagulation therapy is essential for preventing progression. Therefore, the mesenteric vein should be included in the diagnostic workup of all patients with unspecific symptoms and intestinal wall thickening on B-mode images. The criteria for thrombosis of the superior mesenteric vein are the same as in other vascular territories: dilatation of the vein, absence of respiratory diameter variation, possibly depiction of the thrombus as an echogenic intraluminal structure on the B-mode image, and absence of flow signals or only residual flow signals near the wall surrounding a central thrombus on (color) duplex imaging (see Fig. 6.99 (Atlas)). Apart from intestinal wall thickening, another indirect sonographic sign, which can be seen in extensive mesenteric vein thrombosis, is an increase in pulsatility in the arterial waveform (see Fig. 6.100 (Atlas)) (Table 6.9).

Table 6.9 Mesenteric vein thrombosis

Criterion	Parameter
Risk factors	Portal hypertension Sepsis Diverticulitis Paraneoplastic syndrome Autoimmune disease Clotting disorder
Clinical presentation	From unspecific symptoms to acute abdomen (depending on the extent of collateralization)
Duplex ultrasound findings	Hyperechoic thrombus Dilated vein No intraluminal flow signals Diastolic flow in the superior mesenteric artery may be reduced Thickening of bowel loops in gray-scale image

The **left gastric vein** (coronary vein) and the **inferior mesenteric vein** play no role in routine clinical examinations of the abdomen; however, they can be recruited as collaterals in portal hypertension. If this is the case, the veins become enlarged, and sonographic demonstration of flow reversal is indicative of portal hypertension.

6.2.6.3.1 Splenic Vein Thrombosis

The splenic vein is part of the collateral pathway in portal hypertension and thus rarely thrombosed in these patients. More common causes of splenic vein thrombosis, besides systemic factors, include pancreatitis and pancreatic tumors. Clinical symptoms tend to be mild and the sonographic findings are the same as in other thrombosed veins. The thrombosed splenic vein is seen as a wormlike structure of low echogenicity posterior to the pancreas. Other findings include splenomegaly and absent or reduced flow (in partial thrombosis) on color duplex imaging.

Abnormalities of the splenic vein (such as thrombosis) are negligible, both clinically and in terms of their therapeutic consequences, because extensive collateral routes exist. However, the splenic vein should be included in the examination of patients with cirrhosis and portal hypertension, where it plays a role as a collateral.

6.2.6.4 Portal and Hepatic Veins

Atresia and hypoplasia of the portal vein are rare, as are anatomic variants and malformations. In individuals with a congenital extrahepatic portocaval shunt, portal venous blood from the mesentery and spleen drains directly into the inferior vena cava. As a result of this direct communication of the splenic and superior mesenteric veins with the vena cava (gray-scale scan), the cardiac pulsatility of venous return in the vena cava is transmitted to the mesenteric vein and reflected in the Doppler waveform from the latter.

Aneurysm of the portal vein is also rare and must be differentiated from pseudocysts of the pancreas, choledochal cysts, and liver cysts by the demonstration of flow in the color duplex mode.

6.2.6.4.1 Portal Vein Thrombosis

Portal vein thrombosis is diagnosed using the same sonomorphologic criteria as for other sites: dilatation of the lumen, absent respiratory diameter variation, and no flow signals or only residual flow signals around the thrombus on (color) duplex images.

Acute portal vein thrombus tends to be hypoechoic and is clearly delineated from perivascular structures, whereas older thrombi contain more inhomogeneous and hyperechoic portions and their contours become blurred, resulting in poorer sonographic discrimination of the thrombotic vein. The Doppler waveform sampled with an adequate angle will show absence of flow or flowing blood characterized by higher-frequency signals and loss of respiratory phasicity around a central thrombus.

Acute portal vein thrombosis (◘ Fig. 6.103 (Atlas)), like acute proximal mesenteric vein thrombosis, presents with acute symptoms. However, collateralization in portal vein thrombosis is more extensive if the superior mesenteric vein is not involved; the collateral vessels in this case include the splenic vein and gastric veins. The veins recruited as collaterals are expanded and can be detected by duplex ultrasound.

The causes of portal vein thrombosis include liver cirrhosis, paraneoplasia, clotting disorders, and sepsis. Other causes of thrombotic changes in the portal venous system are:

- Acute pancreatitis
- Chronic pancreatitis (may be associated with pseudocyst)
- Cancer (hepatocellular carcinoma, metastasis, pancreatic carcinoma)
- Idiopathic
- Abdominal infections
- Collagen diseases
- Myeloproliferative syndrome
- Trauma
- Status post splenectomy
- Pregnancy
- Medications
- Liver disease, cirrhosis, thrombocytosis
- Antiphospholipid antibody syndrome
- Deficiency of AT3, protein C, protein S.

Similar to portal hypertension in liver cirrhosis, acute portal vein thrombosis is associated with widening of the veins recruited as collaterals (splenic vein, esophagogastric vessels) and ascites. These features are detectable sonographically as secondary signs of portal vein thrombosis.

Ultrasound detects portal vein thrombosis with 89–100% sensitivity and 95–100% specificity, which is comparable to its accuracy in the detection of deep leg vein thrombosis (Zwiebel 2000). Very slow flow in severe portal hypertension with to-and-fro flow is difficult to detect sonographically and may pose a diagnostic problem.

As with older thrombosis in other territories, **chronic portal vein thrombosis** leads to shrinkage of the initially distended vessel, seen as an inhomogeneous, more hyperechoic thrombus within the lumen. In contradistinction to acute portal thrombosis, clinical signs and symptoms are relatively unspecific and mild, in particular when chronic portal thrombosis occurs secondary to liver cirrhosis.

The formation of collateral pathways in the liver hilum and partial recanalization of the thrombotic portal vein, so-called **cavernous transformation**, results in a worm-like meshwork of tortuous tubular structures, among which the former portal vein (with connective tissue structures) is at times difficult to identify by color duplex imaging. The sonographic appearance with meandering venous channels and a mosaic of colors, reflecting changing flow directions relative to the transducer, in and around the portal vein bed is pathognomonic (◘ Fig. 6.104 (Atlas)). However, despite recanalization in the form of cavernous transformation, many patients will have some kind of residual portal hypertension.

6.2.6.4.2 Portal Hypertension

Portal hypertension can be caused by obstruction of the portal venous system at different levels (◘ Fig. 6.47a) and is associated with complex circulatory changes. The pressure in the portal vein is typically 2–4 mmHg above that in the

6

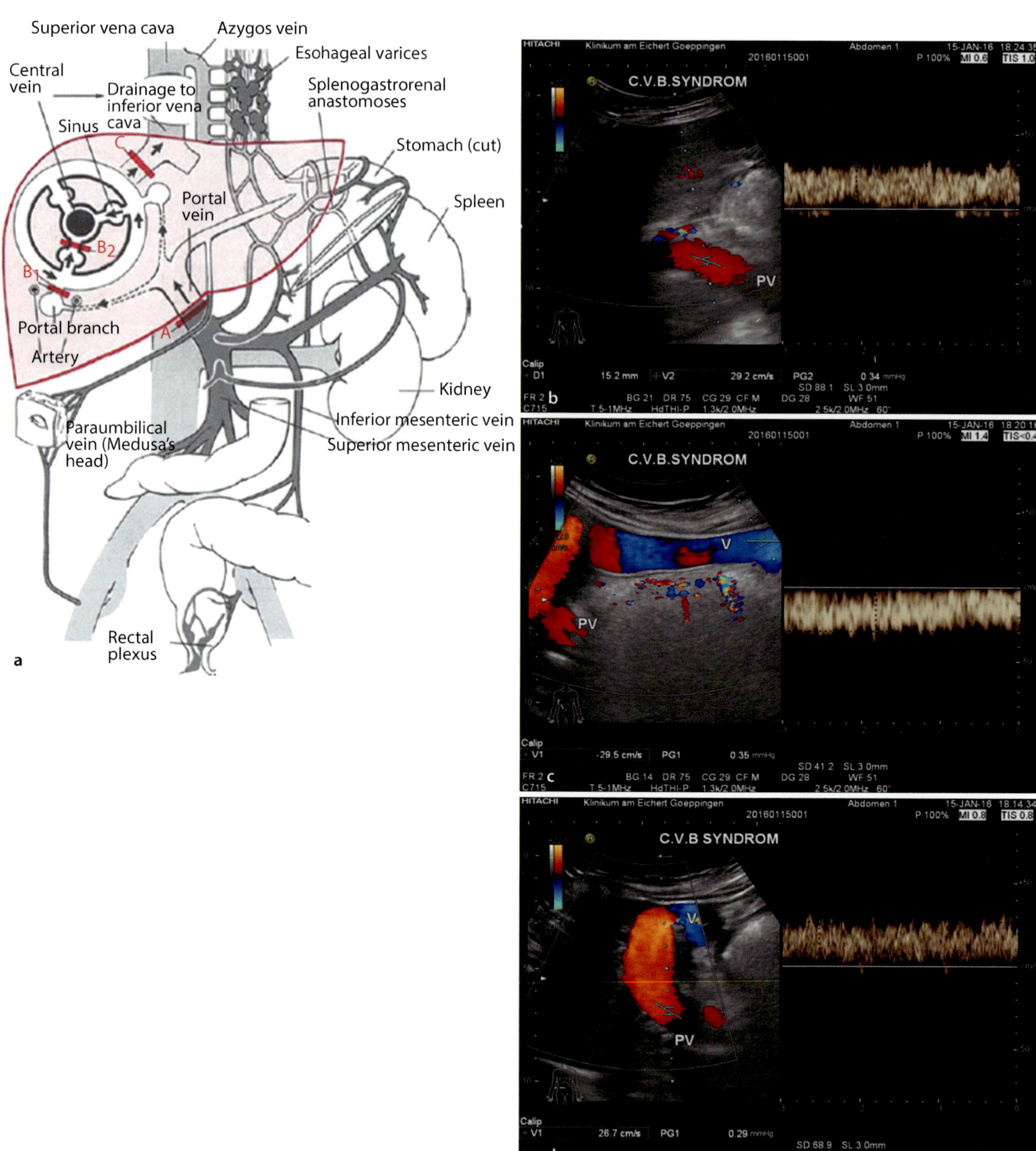

Fig. 6.47 **a** Portal venous system: Causes of portal hypertension and collateral circulation (From Droste 1989). Portal hypertension (>15 cm H2O in portal venous system) can be caused by: **A** Prehepatic obstruction: thrombosis of portal or splenic vein, tumor of adjacent organ (e.g., pancreas, stomach, duodenum, gallbladder). **B** Intrahepatic obstruction: **B1** Presinusoidal: schistosomiasis, Wilson's disease, myeloproliferative diseases (intrasinusoidal: chronic hepatitis, fatty liver); **B2** Postsinusoidal obstruction: liver cirrhosis (cause of portal hypertension in 90% of cases), cytostatics and other medications. **C** Posthepatic obstruction: hepatic vein occlusion (Budd-Chiari syndrome), compression of inferior vena cava, constrictive pericarditis. **b–d** Cruveilhier-Baumgarten syndrome (due to portal hypertension). **b** Portal hypertension in Child C cirrhosis with the portal vein dilated to 15 mm. There is continuous blood flow in the portal vein (loss of respiratory phasicity) with a maximum flow velocity of 29 cm/s (which is relatively high for portal hypertension; see collateral pathways in **a**). **c** The high flow velocity in the portal vein is due to supply from the widely patent umbilical vein (V) in Cruveilhier-Baumgarten syndrome. **d** The vein connecting the portal vein (PV) and patent umbilical vein (V) runs in the ligament. It is dilated and flow velocity is high (26 cm/s)

◘ Table 6.10 Ultrasound findings in portal hypertension	
Ultrasound technique	**Findings**
B-mode	Ascites, splenomegaly (sensitive but not very specific) Possibly cirrhotic changes of hepatic vessel architecture and parenchymal structure Signs of congestion of the gallbladder and stomach walls Dilated portal vein (rounded rather than oval cross section) Portocaval collaterals Portal vein thrombus (echogenic)
Duplex	Slower blood flow/reduced flow volume (highly sensitive) Hepatofugal blood flow (100% specificity) Loss of respiratory phasicity Reduced increase in flow velocity after a test meal Portosystemic collaterals (in 60–90%): left gastric vein, gastroesophageal varices, azygos vein, epigastric veins, paraumbilical veins (Cruveilhier-Baumgarten syndrome) Splenorenal shunts (100% specificity) Abnormal hepatic vein waveform (triphasic → monophasic) Additional parameters: – Increased resistance → reduced resistive index of hepatic artery – Increased damping index – Increased intrarenal resistive index >0.7 (highly specific for hepatorenal syndrome)
Color duplex	Portocaval collaterals Stagnating/reversed blood flow Portal vein thrombosis

inferior vena cava, and hypertension is defined as a pressure gradient of more than 11 mmHg that persists for an extended period.

Ultrasound Diagnosis

Duplex ultrasound performed for portal hypertension provides valid information on portal venous flow in 93–95% of patients (Patriquin et al. 1987; Yeh et al. 1996; Seitz and Kubale 1988). The **main criteria** are:

- Portal vein diameter measured by gray-scale ultrasound
- Hemodynamic information: flow direction, flow character, and blood flow velocity in the portal vein
- Identification of portocaval shunts/collateral pathways

The increased pressure in portal hypertension secondary to liver cirrhosis leads to widening of the portal vein (◘ Fig. 6.47b–d), its distal tributaries, and the veins recruited as collaterals (portocaval, gastroesophageal, splenorenal, umbilical), which may already be noted on B-mode ultrasound (◘ Table 6.10). Additionally, the normal respiratory diameter variation of the portal vein is lost (see ◘ Fig. 6.101 (Atlas)) or reduced (nicely seen in time-motion mode). A portal vein diameter of more than 13 mm indicates portal hypertension with a high sensitivity of 95–100% but a low specificity of only 45–50% (Bolondi et al. 1982), which is attributable to the wide variation in the normal portal vein diameter.

Dilatation and loss of respiratory diameter variation are observed not only in the portal vein but also in the mesenteric and splenic veins. An important supplementary sonographic criterion, also attributable to the increased intravascular pressure, is rounding of the normal oval cross section of these veins. Other supplementary findings include widening of the left gastric vein (diameter >4 mm) and high flow in the reopened umbilical vein (◘ Fig. 6.47).

The **spectral waveform in portal hypertension** is characterized by a reduced mean flow velocity and loss of respiratory phasicity (◘ Table 6.10; ◘ Figs. 6.97, 6.100, and 6.101 (Atlas)).

The main diagnostic role of color duplex ultrasonography is to follow up patients with portal hypertension and to timely identify complications such as thrombosis. Moreover, it provides useful diagnostic information in presinusoidal, extrahepatic portal hypertension. The most common causes are primary or secondary tumor thrombosis, inflammatory diseases like pancreatitis, and slow flow due to cirrhosis. The presentation of portal vein thrombosis varies with the temporal course and collateralization, ranging from unspecific abdominal symptoms to an acute abdomen in rare cases.

Depending on the severity of portal hypertension, spectral Doppler will demonstrate **antegrade flow with reduced velocity**, **to-and-fro flow**, or **flow reversal** when pressure exceeds 30 mmHg. Normal cardiac pulsatility of the liver veins is lost in cirrhosis.

The flow direction in the portal vein is determined not only by the severity of cirrhosis and the magnitude of intraportal blood pressure but also by the **direction of collateral drainage** (◘ Fig. 6.47a). Basically, portocaval collateral circulation may drain toward the center or toward the periphery and involves a variety of vessels:

1. **Shunts draining toward the center:**
   - Esophageal varices, gastric corpus and fundus varices (left gastric vein – azygos vein, short gastric veins – azygos vein)
   - Gastrosplenic shunts
   - Portorenal and splenorenal collaterals
   - Capsular veins of liver and spleen, diaphragmatic veins
2. **Shunts draining toward the periphery:**
   - Paraumbilical veins (Cruveilhier–Baumgarten syndrome)
   - Splenolumbar shunts
   - Mesenteric veins (superior and inferior mesenteric veins, ovarian vein, spermatic vein, rectal plexus)

The **demonstration of collateral pathways** is a highly sensitive direct sign of portal hypertension and is seen either as widening of the short gastric veins or left gastric vein with venous drainage to the esophageal plexus or as a patent umbilical vein (Cruveilhier–Baumgarten syndrome). Other collaterals including gastrorenal and splenorenal anastomoses and peripancreatic veins are less amenable to sonographic evaluation. When a systematic search is performed, 65–90% of the relevant portocaval collaterals can be identified by duplex imaging (Lafortune et al. 1987; Takayasu et al. 1984; Subramanyam et al. 1983).

The left gastric vein with a normal diameter of less than 4 mm is usually well visualized, making it of great diagnostic importance in duplex ultrasound. A diameter of over 7 mm and hepatofugal flow indicate portal hypertension (Lafortune et al. 1984; Morin et al. 1992). The demonstration of hepatofugal flow in the reopened umbilical vein, beginning in the round ligament, was found to have sensitivities and specificities of up to 100% (Gibson et al. 1989; Mostbeck et al. 1989). Occasionally, flow can be detected in the round ligament in individuals without portal hypertension; however, in these cases, blood flow velocity does not exceed 5 cm/s (Casarella 1995; Lafortune et al. 1984, 1987). It is also helpful to look for collaterals at the esophagogastric junction; these varices can be differentiated from enlarged lymph nodes by the demonstration of flow in the color duplex mode. Sonographic follow-up evaluation of the collateral pathways can also help in evaluating the outcome of treatment.

When the blood is chiefly drained through splenorenal or esophagogastric shunts and the pressure gradient is markedly increased, flow in the portal vein is backward (hepatofugal), while normal, hepatopetal flow may be preserved in patients with a patent umbilical vein (Cruveilhier–Baumgarten syndrome) (see collateral pathways in ◻ Fig. 6.47a). In these patients, there may even be retrograde flow in the right portal vein branch with normal flow direction in the left portal branch, which feeds the recanalized umbilical vein.

Venous blood flow is difficult to measure, mainly because the wide variation in vein diameter is difficult to quantify. This applies especially to the portal vein with its extreme variation in diameter between inspiration and expiration. Therefore, **mean blood flow velocity in the portal vein** is a more suitable quantitative parameter for discriminating between healthy individuals and patients with portal hypertension. Note, however, that mean flow velocity is influenced by the magnitude of collateralization and the veins recruited as collaterals. Most importantly, high flow in the patent and widened umbilical vein (Cruveilhier–Baumgarten syndrome) may mimic normal perfusion of the liver with a fairly normal flow velocity in the portal vein because the blood drains through the umbilical vein, circumventing the sinusoids (see ◻ Fig. 6.47).

Although the variable collateralization leads to a wide variation in mean portal flow velocities, both in intraindividual and interindividual comparison, significant differences are identified between healthy subjects and patients with portal hypertension when mean blood flow velocities (V_{mean}) determined in larger study populations are compared. Several such studies demonstrated a statistically significant decrease from 15 cm/s in healthy subjects to half that value in patients with cirrhosis (Seitz and Kubale 1988). Though maximum venous flow velocity is decreased to 7–15 cm/s (mean of 10 cm/s) in patients with cirrhosis, there is wide interindividual variation and overlap with the flow velocities in normal subjects, which may lead to misinterpretation in individual cases.

In summary, however, portal vein flow velocities allow the following conclusions to be drawn:

- Portal hypertension is unlikely if maximum flow velocity (V_{max}) in the portal vein is >30 cm/s
- Portal hypertension may be present if V_{max} is 10–30 cm/s
- Portal hypertension is likely if V_{max} is <10 cm/s.

Duplex imaging also allows evaluation of the decrease in portal blood flow in response to beta-blocker or somatostatin intake and of the increase after eating or after glucagon challenge. Cirrhotic patients show a less pronounced increase in portal blood flow velocity after a test meal.

Various tests were proposed to improve the differentiation of cirrhosis-induced portal hypertension from normal portal blood flow. Apart from the less marked increase in postprandial flow, drugs like beta-blockers or nifedipine also have a less pronounced effect on portal vein blood flow velocity in cirrhosis. Gaiani et al. (1989) compared 11 cirrhotic patients and healthy controls 60 min after a test meal and found a markedly lower increase in diameter of 3% in patients compared with 14% in controls, while the increase in flow velocity was 3.2% versus 24%. The flow volume after the test meal increased by only 8.5% in patients as opposed to 59% in controls. Such clearcut results were not always confirmed by other study groups.

Another parameter is the congestion index, which is the ratio between the cross-sectional area of the vein and blood flow velocity ($cm^2/cm/s = cm \times s$). The index is <0.07 cm $\times$ s in healthy individuals and increases to >0.1 cm $\times$ s in portal hypertension secondary to cirrhosis (Moriyasu et al. 1985; Siringo et al. 1994) (see ◻ Fig. 6.101 (Atlas)). Further studies are necessary to show whether glucagon-induced changes in portal venous flow can be used to estimate the hemodynamic reserve and whether measurement of portal flow velocity after propanolol administration, despite wide interindividual variation, may enable reliable identification of patients requiring treatment for portal hypertension.

Quantitative determination of blood flow is not necessary in the routine diagnostic workup of portal hypertension since there is no close correlation between portal blood flow and portal hypertension due to the highly variable and ramified collateral system.

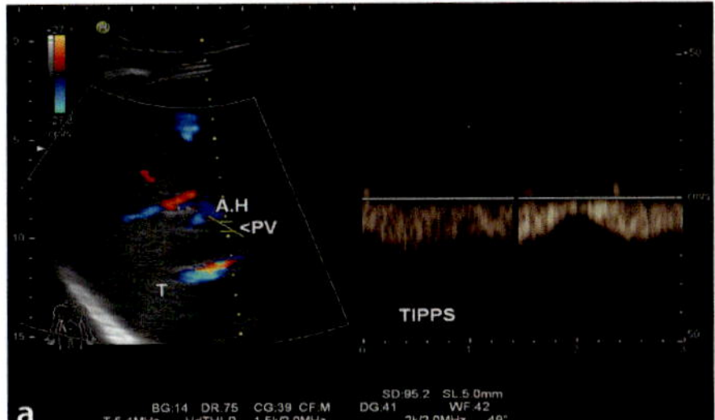

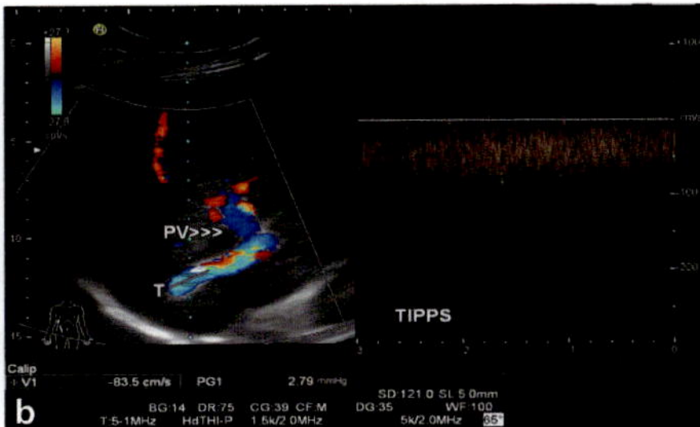

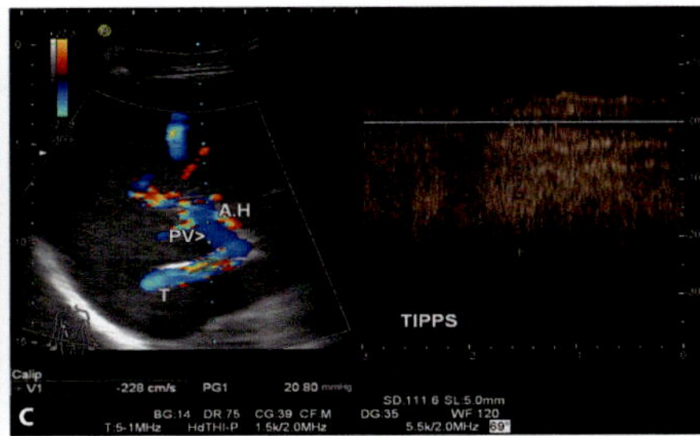

Fig. 6.48a–c Transjugular intrahepatic portosystemic stent shunt (TIPSS). **a** Color flow image showing reversed flow in the intrahepatic portal vein branch near the hilum after TIPPS. **b** The shunt is patent, flow direction is toward the heart (blue), and there is a normal flow velocity of 83 cm/s. **c** Nevertheless, continuous mapping of the shunt reveals a focal increase in flow velocity to 228 cm/s, which corresponds to 60% luminal narrowing (continuity equation, calculation of PSV ratio analogous to the method used for grading arterial stenosis)

The decreased portal blood flow in portal hypertension due to cirrhosis can lead to a compensatory increase in arterial perfusion, which is detectable sonographically. The higher perfusion can result in an enlargement of the cross-sectional areas of the hepatic arteries both within and outside the liver. Furthermore, progressive cirrhosis is associated with an increased resistance in the peripheral hepatic artery branches, resulting in a more pulsatile flow profile with increased resistive indices of 0.8 to 0.9.

Follow-Up After Treatment (TIPSS)

Endoscopic obliteration of esophageal varices and transjugular intrahepatic portosystemic stent shunt (TIPSS) procedures have led to a decrease in portocaval and splenorenal shunt operations. An important question to be answered before treatment is whether the portal, mesenteric, and splenic veins are patent. There is good evaluability of these veins by ultrasonography, which is why color duplex imaging has evolved into the method of choice. In the postoperative follow-up, ultrasound enables direct evaluation of shunt patency. The cardiac fluctuation of blood flow in the vena cava is transmitted to the anastomosed portal vein through the shunt.

When a distal splenorenal shunt (Warren shunt) is created, the relief of the portal vein leads to flow reversal in the splenic vein (hepatofugal flow). In the TIPSS procedure, a short circuit is established between the hepatic vein and portal vein under ultrasound guidance. Color duplex ultrasound can help in identifying a short puncture tract and is also useful for postinterventional surveillance of stent patency.

In-stent stenosis and shunt thrombosis are common, resulting in poor 1-year patency rates of 35–66% (Nazarian et al. 1994; Sterling and Darcy 1997; Kerlan et al. 1995). Patency can be improved by sonographic surveillance with timely revision. A sonographic examination should be performed within 24 h of stent placement to determine stent location and flow velocity and to confirm the technical success of the procedure, especially at the junctions between the stent ends and the native vein. Further examinations should follow at 3-month intervals with the following findings suggesting normalization and TIPSS adequacy (Fig. 6.48):

- Blood flow velocity in the shunt should be at least 50–60 cm/s (Chong et al. 1993; Foshager et al. 1995; Dodd et al. 1995; Feldstein et al. 1996). Normal peak shunt velocity ranges between 80 and 120 cm/s (Kanterman et al. 1997).
- Continuous color duplex imaging of the shunt (with an adequate pulse repetition frequency) should not reveal any mural thrombus: color-coded flow throughout the shunt lumen without gaps and without aliasing.
- Stent ends should extend just as far as necessary into the vena cava and portal vein.
- Doppler waveform should reveal largely continuous flow and at most slight cardiac pulsatility.
- Hepatopedal flow in the portal vein with a return to normal flow velocity.

Shunt stenosis is suggested by an abrupt doubling of shunt flow velocity (Fig. 6.48). A velocity of less than 50 cm/s within the shunt indicates inadequate shunt flow and should prompt a thorough search for shunt stenosis or other causes (Bodner et al. 2000; Murphy et al. 1998; Kanterman et al. 1997; Dodd et al. 1995). Stenosis is common at the stent ends but may occur anywhere along the course of the shunt. A drop in intrashunt blood flow also reduces flow velocity in the portal vein, and severe stenosis is associated with sonographic and clinical signs of portal hypertension.

When the **shunt is occluded**, there is no flow in color duplex imaging or in the Doppler waveform; the findings in the portal vein correspond to those of portal hypertension obtained before creation of the shunt.

6.2.6.4.3 Hepatic Veins

Like the vena cava, the hepatic veins are subject to both respiratory phasicity and **cardiac pulsatility**, giving rise to a triphasic waveform (Fig. 6.97 (Atlas)). Besides prandial fluctuations in blood flow volume, flow velocity varies with changing pressures in the chest cavity, right atrium, and abdomen. The triphasic, W-shaped waveform reflects the venous pressure variations during the cardiac cycle. The first velocity peak directed toward the vena cava occurs during systole and atrial filling. As the intra-atrial pressure increases, hepatofugal flow decreases in the hepatic veins and in the vena cava. Opening of the tricuspid valve leads to increased flow into the right ventricle and a second flow velocity peak in the hepatic veins and vena cava. During atrial contraction, there may be zero flow or retrograde, hepatopedal flow.

Another factor affecting the **Doppler waveform shape** of the hepatic veins is the **stiffness of the liver parenchyma**. As elasticity is lost and the parenchyma stiffens with progressive cirrhotic transformation, the waveform of the hepatic veins is increasingly flattened, changing from a triphasic to biphasic (loss of early diastolic backward flow) and, ultimately, monophasic appearance. In a population of 60 patients with portal hypertension confirmed by invasive measurement, 31.6% had a triphasic waveform, 46.7% a biphasic waveform, and 13% a monphasic waveform. In the healthy control group, 86.7% of subjects had a triphasic waveform, while 3% (1 subject) had a monophasic waveform and 10% a biphasic waveform (Hang et al. 2011).

The amount of flattening of the waveform correlates well with the severity of portal hypertension. Flattening of the waveform reflects increasing liver stiffness in progressive cirrhosis (see ◘ Fig. 6.97d,e (Atlas)). This is an important diagnostic criterion and also a prognostic factor (Bolondi et al. 1991; Ohta et al. 1994); for instance, a completely flat waveform from the the hepatic veins was reported to predict a life expectancy of less than 2 years. In a study of 52 patients with chronic hepatitis C, a markedly abnormal flow pattern in the hepatic veins was found to have a diagnostic accuracy of 77% and specificity of 78% for Child A cirrhosis (Colli et al. 1994).

Since blood flow in the hepatic veins is highly sensitive to parenchymal changes, which also occur in other liver conditions associated with severe fatty degeneration, flattening of the flow profile in the hepatic veins is not a specific indicator of cirrhosis. Moreover, there may be physiologic flattening of the waveform in advanced pregnancy.

Blood flow in the hepatic veins and the portal vein is also influenced by cardiac activity, and various cardiac diseases lead to a larger reflux component and increased pulsatility in these veins.

Budd–Chiari syndrome results from compromised hepatic venous outflow due to postsinusoidal obstruction. The obstruction may be caused by a mass (tumor, cyst, abscess), hepatic vein thrombosis, or a congenital anomaly with a connective tissue membrane in the termination of the middle and/or left hepatic veins. In acute hepatic vein thrombosis, color duplex ultrasound will show a dilated vein with intraluminal areas of higher echogenicity and absence of flow. In chronic thrombosis, there may be recanalization of an obstructed vein with sonographic identification of membranes and demonstration of venovenous and portosystemic shunts in the color duplex mode.

Duplex imaging is a valid modality for the routine diagnostic evaluation of portal hypertension including initial diagnosis, hemodynamic evaluation of the portal vein, and follow-up. Other imaging modalities are only needed to examine patients with poor insonation conditions (massive ascites, meteorism) and to answer specific diagnostic questions. The flexibility in choosing sonographic imaging planes enables hemodynamic assessment as well as precise determination of topographic relationships. This is an advantage of ultrasound over angiographic procedures as well as over magnetic resonance imaging, especially with regard to the determination of blood flow volumes and flow directions.

6.3 Atlas: Visceral and Retroperitoneal Vessels

◻ Table 6.11 lists the figures presented in the Atlas. The figures illustrate normal findings, methodology, and diseases of the visceral and retroperitoneal vessels.

◻ **Table 6.11** Visceral and Retroperitoneal Vessels – Figures

(continued)

Table 6.11 (continued)

Entity/Pathology	Figure
Abdominal aortic aneurysm with arterial embolism	Fig. 6.74 (Atlas), page 466
Abdominal aortic aneurysm	Fig. 6.75 (Atlas), page 466
Contained perforation of abdominal aortic aneurysm	Fig. 6.75 (Atlas), page 466
Abdominal aortic aneurysm due to nonatherosclerotic cause	Fig. 6.76 (Atlas), page 467
Follow-up after endovascular aneurysm repair (EVAR)	Fig. 6.77 (Atlas), page 467
Type Ib endoleak	Fig. 6.78 (Atlas), page 468
Type I endoleak after endovascular aneurysm repair (EVAR)	Fig. 6.79 (Atlas), page 469
Type II endoleak – high-flow	Fig. 6.80 (Atlas), page 469
Type II endoleak – when to treat	Fig. 6.81 (Atlas), page 470
Endoleak requiring repair – pulsation in time-mode mode	Fig. 6.81 (Atlas), page 470
Small type II endoleak	Fig. 6.81 (Atlas), page 470
Type II endoleak – high-flow versus low-flow (comparison with CT findings)	Fig. 6.82 (Atlas), page 471
Patent inferior mesenteric artery, not classified as a relevant endoleak	Fig. 6.82 (Atlas), page 471
Endoleak – stepwise diagnostic workup by CDUS, CEUS, CTA	Fig. 6.83 (Atlas), page 472
Type II endoleak missed by CDUS but detected with CEUS	Fig. 6.83 (Atlas), page 472
Stent graft rupture after EVAR	Fig. 6.84 (Atlas), page 473
Follow-up after EVAR – complication versus retroperitoneal fibrosis	Fig. 6.84 (Atlas), page 473
Retroperitoneal fibrosis – differential diagnosis: perforated abdominal aortic aneurysm	Fig. 6.85 (Atlas), page 474
Inflammatory abdominal aortic aneurysm	Fig. 6.86 (Atlas), page 474
Abdominal aortic aneurysm in a patient with horseshoe kidney	Fig. 6.87 (Atlas), page 475
Aortic dissection – dynamic versus static blood flow reduction	Fig. 6.88 (Atlas), page 475, 476
Infrarenal dissection	Fig. 6.89 (Atlas), page 476
Aortic dissection	Fig. 6.90 (Atlas), page 477
Aortic dissection after intervention	Fig. 6.90 (Atlas), page 477
Aortic perforation	Fig. 6.91 (Atlas), page 478
Differential diagnosis: aortic perforation – lumbar artery	Fig. 6.91 (Atlas), page 478
Mycotic aortic perforation	Fig. 6.91 (Atlas), page 478
Suture aneurysm after placement of a straight stent graft	Fig. 6.92 (Atlas), page 479
Suture aneurysm after placement of a straight stent graft	Fig. 6.93 (Atlas), page 479
Aortic thrombus (thrombolytic treatment) – aortic stenosis	Fig. 6.94 (Atlas), page 480, 481
Vena cava	Fig. 6.95 (Atlas), page 481
Situs inversus	Fig. 6.95 (Atlas), page 481
Right renal vein	Fig. 6.96 (Atlas), page 482
Left renal vein	Fig. 6.96 (Atlas), page 482

Table 6.11 (continued)

Entity/Pathology	Figure
Retroaortic left renal vein	Fig. 6.96 (Atlas), page 482
Normal and abnormal Doppler waveforms of hepatic veins	Fig. 6.97 (Atlas), page 482
Abnormal waveform of hepatic veins in liver cirrhosis	Fig. 6.97 (Atlas), apge 482
Waveform of hepatic vein in liver cirrhosis	Fig. 6.97 (Atlas), page 482
Portal vein and its tributaries	Fig. 6.98 (Atlas), page 482
Mesenteric vein thrombosis – surrounded by flowing blood	Fig. 6.99 (Atlas), page 483
Superior mesenteric vein thrombosis	Fig. 6.100 (Atlas), page 483, 484
Portal vein thrombosis	Fig. 6.100 (Atlas), page 483, 484
Portal hypertension	Fig. 6.101 (Atlas), page 484
Portal vein aneurysm	Fig. 6.102 (Atlas), page 484
Portal vein thrombosis	Fig. 6.103 (Atlas), page 485
Cavernous transformation of the portal vein	Fig. 6.104 (Atlas), page 485
Tumor compression	Fig. 6.105 (Atlas), page 485
Vena cava thrombosis	Fig. 6.106 (Atlas), page 486
Renal vein thrombus	Fig. 6.107 (Atlas), page 487
Tumor thrombus ascending in vena cava	Fig. 6.107 (Atlas), page 487
Varicose ovarian vein in nutcracker syndrome	Fig. 6.108 (Atlas), page 488
Vena cava umbrella	Fig. 6.109 (Atlas), page 489

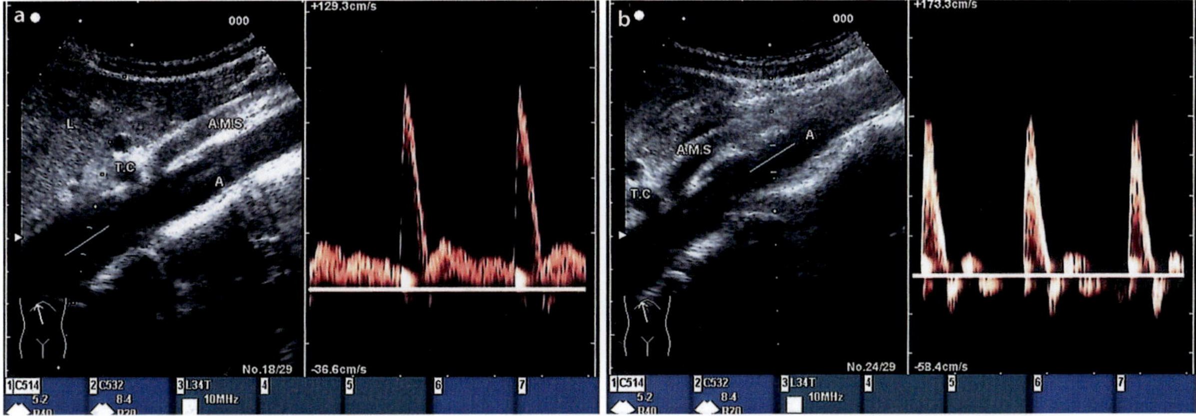

Fig. 6.49a, b (Atlas) Flow profile in the aorta.
a Proximal to the origins of the visceral arteries (T.C, celiac trunk; A.M.S., superior mesenteric artery), the flow profile in the abdominal aorta is predominantly determined by the supply to parenchymal organs: a dip in early diastole is followed by constant diastolic flow. Flow in the aorta is of a mixed type because it gives off arteries that supply parenchymal organs (monophasic flow profile – low peripheral resistance) and arteries that supply the extremities (triphasic profile – high peripheral resistance).
b Distal to the origins of the visceral and renal arteries, the aorta has a triphasic flow profile (supply to limbs)

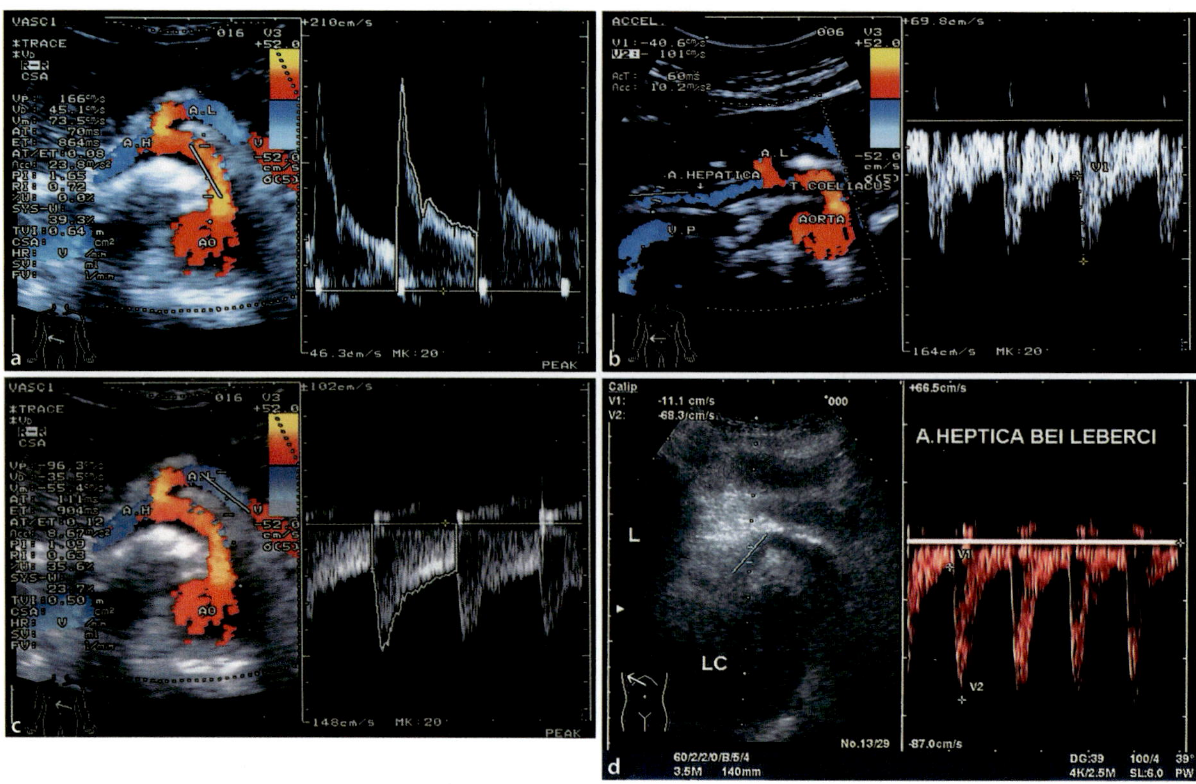

■ **Fig. 6.50a–d (Atlas) Celiac trunk.**

a Transverse view of the celiac trunk showing its origin from the abdominal aorta (AO) and division into the hepatic artery (A.H) and splenic artery (A.L). The bifurcation is said to resemble a palm leaf or gull's wings. Supplying parenchymal organs (spleen, liver), the celiac trunk, hepatic artery, and splenic artery show monophasic flow with a relatively large diastolic component, comparable to flow in the internal carotid artery. The aorta displayed in red gives off the celiac trunk anteriorly, likewise with flow depicted in red. The lighter color coding is not due to stenosis but to the angle of insonation. This is confirmed by the normal Doppler waveform with a peak systolic velocity (PSV) of 165 cm/s and an end-diastolic velocity (EDV) of 45 cm/s. Flow is synchronous with the cardiac cycle, exhibiting a low-frequency signal with a high amplitude due to wall motion in early systole.
b The hepatic artery courses to the liver hilum along the posterior aspect of the lower liver margin. The artery is coded in blue, indicating flow away from the transducer. The high diastolic flow is due to the low peripheral resistance of the liver. The splenic artery (A.L) first appears coursing in an anterior direction (toward transducer, coded red) and then turns posteriorly (blue) toward the splenic hilum.
c Splenic artery with typical Doppler waveform.
Hepatic artery in liver cirrhosis.
d Liver cirrhosis is associated with parenchymal transformation, resulting in an increase in flow resistance in the hepatic artery. This is reflected in an increased Pourcelot index, which correlates with the severity of parenchymal damage. In the case presented, the index is markedly increased to 0.83 (same patient as in ■ Fig. 6.101a–c (Atlas)). There is marked enlargement and hypoechogenicity of the caudate lobe (LC) as a sign of severe cirrhosis

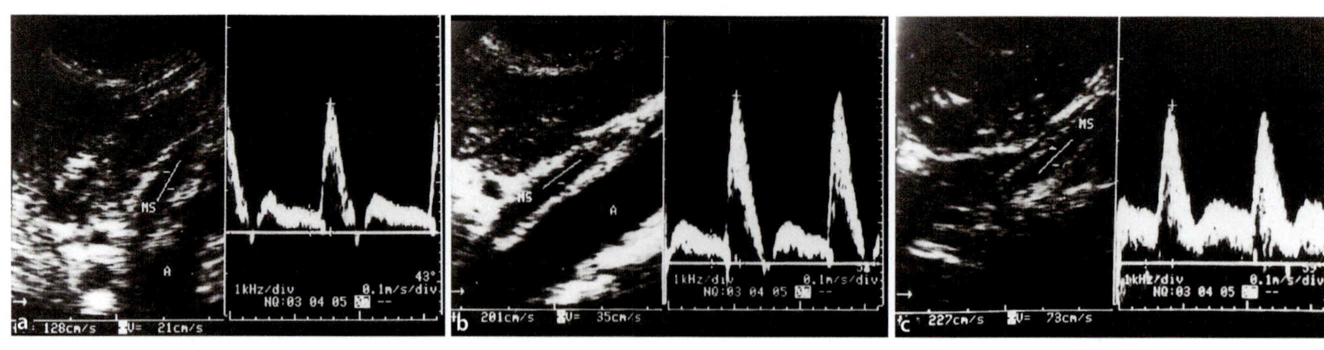

■ **Fig. 6.51a–c (Atlas) Mesenteric blood flow.**

a Superior mesenteric artery with typical Doppler waveform of the mixed type. The end-diastolic flow component is intermediate between that of a peripheral artery and that of an artery supplying a parenchymal organ. 24-year-old fasting subject: normal blood flow in the superior mesenteric artery shortly after its origin with a peak systolic velocity (PSV) of 128 cm/s, an end-diastolic velocity (EDV) of 21 cm/s, and pulsatile flow. The gray-scale image depicts the superior mesenteric artery (MS) arising from the aorta (A) at an acute angle.
b Same subject as in **a**. Following administration of 20 mg of nifedipine, PSV increases to 201 cm/s, EDV to 35 cm/s.
c Postprandial increase in mesenteric blood flow (PSV of 227 cm/s, EDV of 73 cm/s). Assuming a threshold of 200 cm/s for >50% stenosis, the increased flow velocity observed after nifedipine administration and after eating would indicate a 50–60% stenosis in a fasting patient

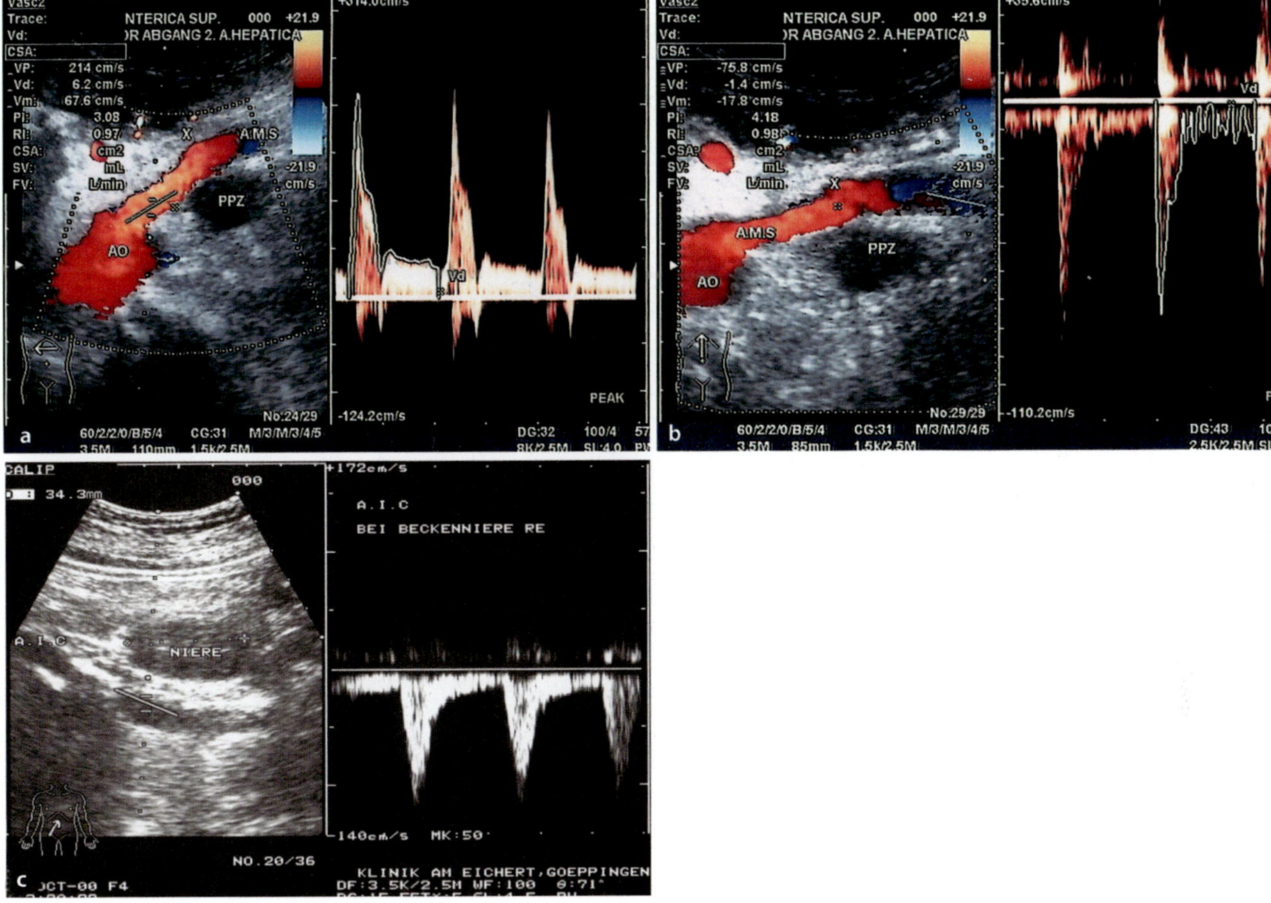

Fig. 6.52a–c (Atlas) Waveform patterns of anatomic variants.
a Flow in a vessel as reflected in the Doppler waveform is determined by the organs it supplies. If the hepatic artery arises from the superior mesenteric artery (see Fig. 6.3), peak systolic velocity (PSV) is high even in the absence of stenosis (fasting velocity of 214 cm/s in the case presented). The patient has chronic pancreatitis with a pancreatic pseudocyst (PPZ) between the aorta and the superior mesenteric artery. The cyst is hypoechoic in the B-mode image and can be differentiated from an aneurysm in the color duplex mode.
b Distal to the origin of the replaced hepatic artery (at the level of the pancreatic pseudocyst, where a second hepatic artery arises), the superior mesenteric artery shows flow with a smaller diastolic component and a reduced PSV. Proximal to the hepatic artery origin, flow is of the mixed type due to supply of two organs (liver and bowel). The examiner must be aware of these anatomic variants and their hemodynamic effects on Doppler waveforms obtained in this vascular territory.
c In individuals with pelvic kidneys, as shown here (or in a transplant kidney anastomosed to the iliac artery), the normal Doppler waveform of the iliac artery proximal to the renal artery origin is monophasic rather than triphasic. The image shows part of the pelvic kidney above the common iliac artery. The monophasic waveform is due to blood supply to both the peripheral arteries and the renal artery and does not suggest postocclusive flow despite the presence of plaque proximal to the sample volume. Distal to the renal artery origin, the external iliac artery exhibits triphasic flow

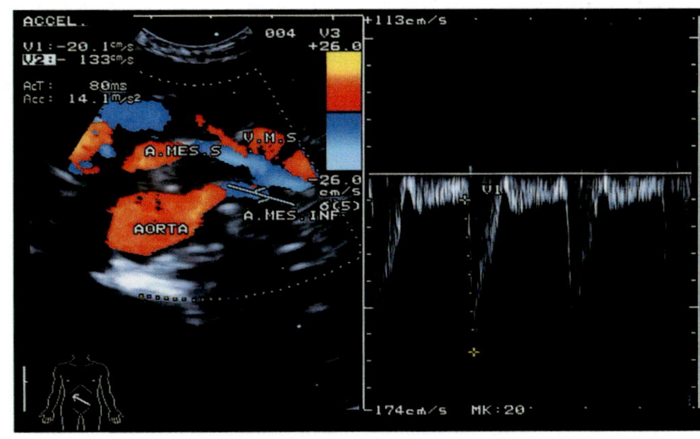

Fig. 6.53 (Atlas) Inferior mesenteric artery.
Origin of the inferior mesenteric artery from the aorta. The Doppler waveform resembles that of the superior mesenteric artery but may occasionally show a smaller diastolic flow component or even end-diastolic zero flow. Anteriorly, a jejunal branch is depicted (blue, away from transducer) distal to the division of the superior mesenteric artery. The superior mesenteric artery dividing into the ileocolic and right colic arteries is seen anterior to the aorta with flow in the same direction coded in red. Directly anterior to the origin of the jejunal artery (displayed in blue), the jejunal vein with flow in the opposite direction (red) courses parallel to the artery and empties into the superior mesenteric vein (V.M.S)

6

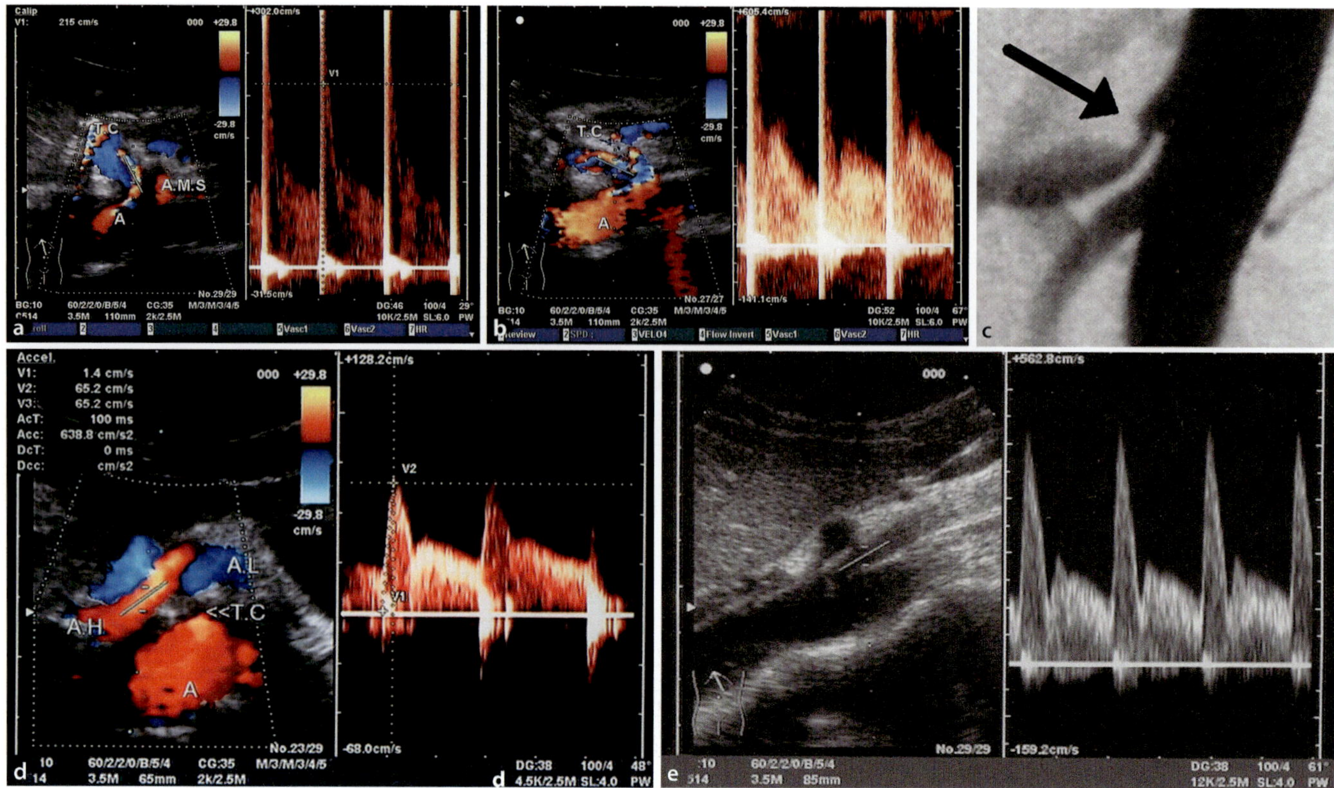

Fig. 6.54a–e (Atlas) Median arcuate ligament syndrome.
a, **b** There is aliasing at the origin of the celiac trunk (T.C) from the aorta (A), which is above the origin of the superior mesenteric artery (A.M.S). With the sample volume placed just anterior to the origin, the spectral Doppler measurement yields a peak systolic velocity (PSV) of 215 cm/s and an end-diastolic velocity (EDV) of 90 cm/s. Respiratory downward movement of the diaphragm displaces and compresses the celiac trunk, visible as a sharp bend in the proximal celiac segment in the color duplex image (in **b**). The corresponding spectral Doppler measurement (right) reveals a PSV of 6 m/s and EDV of 150 cm/s, consistent with marked compression of the celiac trunk. PSV is difficult to measure in the proximal portions of aortic branches because of superimposed high amplitudes from pulsatile wall motion in early diastole, which cannot be eliminated from the waveform by any wall filter.
c Angiogram confirming downward displacement and compression of the proximal celiac trunk by the median arcuate ligament.
Celiac trunk occlusion – changes in superior mesenteric artery waveform.
d Occlusion of the celiac trunk (T.C) is associated with retrograde blood flow in the hepatic artery (A.H) (red, flow toward transducer). The hepatic artery is refilled by the gastroduodenal artery and also supplies the splenic artery (A.L). The Doppler waveform is characteristic of an artery supplying a parenchymal organ and confirms retrograde flow in the hepatic artery. Blood flow direction in the splenic artery is normal.
e In occlusion of the celiac trunk, the liver and spleen are supplied by collaterals such as the pancreaticoduodenal and gastroduodenal arteries. The superior mesenteric artery (no stenosis) supplying these collaterals shows high blood flow velocity at its origin (average PSV of up to 4 m/s and EDV of 150 cm/s) with a flow profile similar to that of arteries supplying parenchymal organs. Chronic celiac trunk occlusion due to stenosis, as in this case, is associated with poststenotic dilatation (seen here above the superior mesenteric artery)

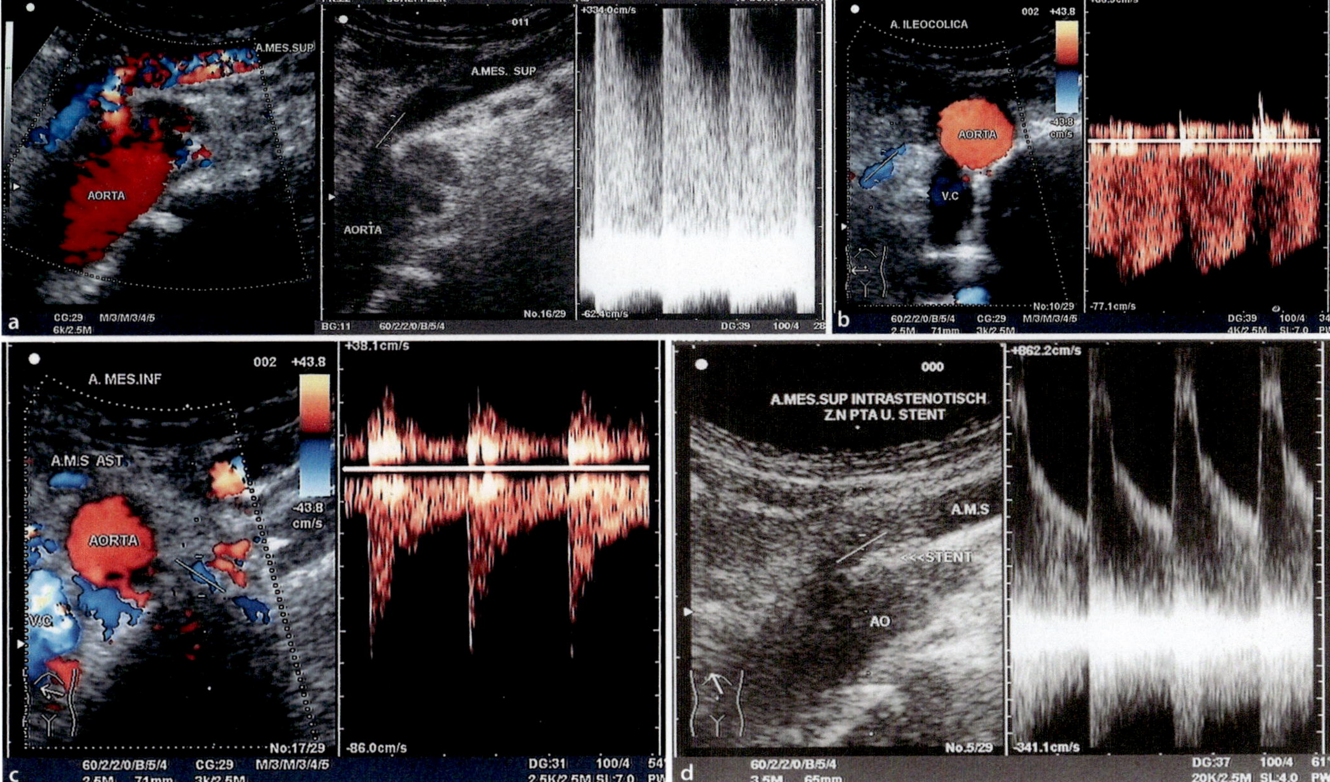

Fig. 6.55a–d (Atlas) High-grade mesenteric artery stenosis.
a Aliasing in the color mode suggests high-grade stenosis at the origin of the superior mesenteric artery. The scanning conditions are usually good in the very thin patients presenting with suspected abdominal angina, but the arched course of the superior mesenteric artery at its origin may impair adequate angulation of the Doppler beam (left image). In inspiration, this segment of the superior mesenteric artery is straightened, which facilitates adjustment of the angle correction cursor parallel to the vessel wall and reduces the angle setting error (compare gray-scale image and color duplex image).
b The Doppler waveform from the distal mesenteric branches (such as the ileocolic artery) shows the typical features of postocclusive flow with a markedly reduced pulsatility and an almost venous profile.
c The inferior mesenteric artery acts as a collateral via the Riolan anastomosis and hence shows an increased flow velocity, in particular in diastole.
d Sonographic follow-up after 2 months identifies the stent as a mesh-like structure in the wall area of the superior mesenteric artery. The Doppler waveform is characterized by a high-frequency signal with an angle-corrected PSV of over 8 m/s indicating high-grade restenosis

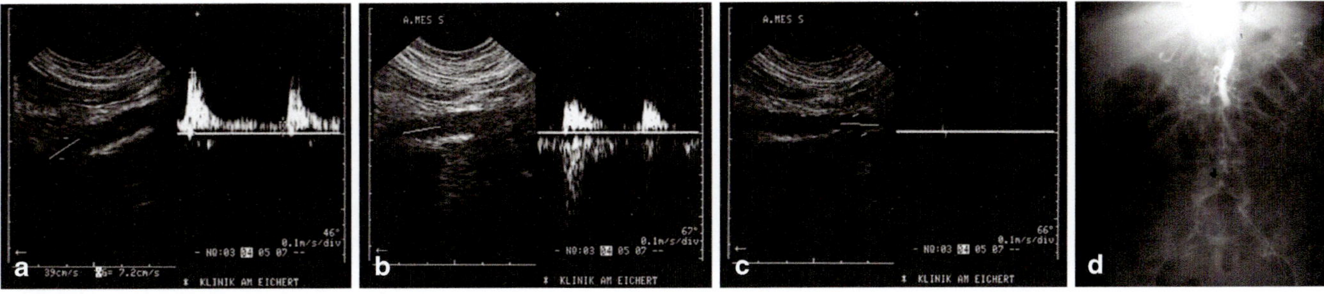

Fig. 6.56a–d (Atlas) Acute mesenteric artery occlusion.
a Patient presenting with acute abdomen. An abnormal Doppler waveform is obtained from the origin of the superior mesenteric artery with a decreased peak systolic velocity (PSV) of 39 cm/s. End-diastolic velocity (EDV) is 7.2 cm/s; the Pourcelot index is reduced.
b Continuous scanning of the superior mesenteric artery starting at its origin yields a flow profile more and more resembling a thump pattern with a decreasing flow velocity and absence of end-diastolic flow close to the occlusion. Flow in the mesenteric artery is toward the transducer and displayed above the baseline. The frequencies displayed below the baseline are from the middle colic artery, which arises near the sample volume.
c More distally, the superior mesenteric artery is occluded with zero flow in the Doppler waveform despite a high gain.
d Angiogram showing patency of the trunk of the superior mesenteric artery and occlusion distal to the origin of the middle colic artery

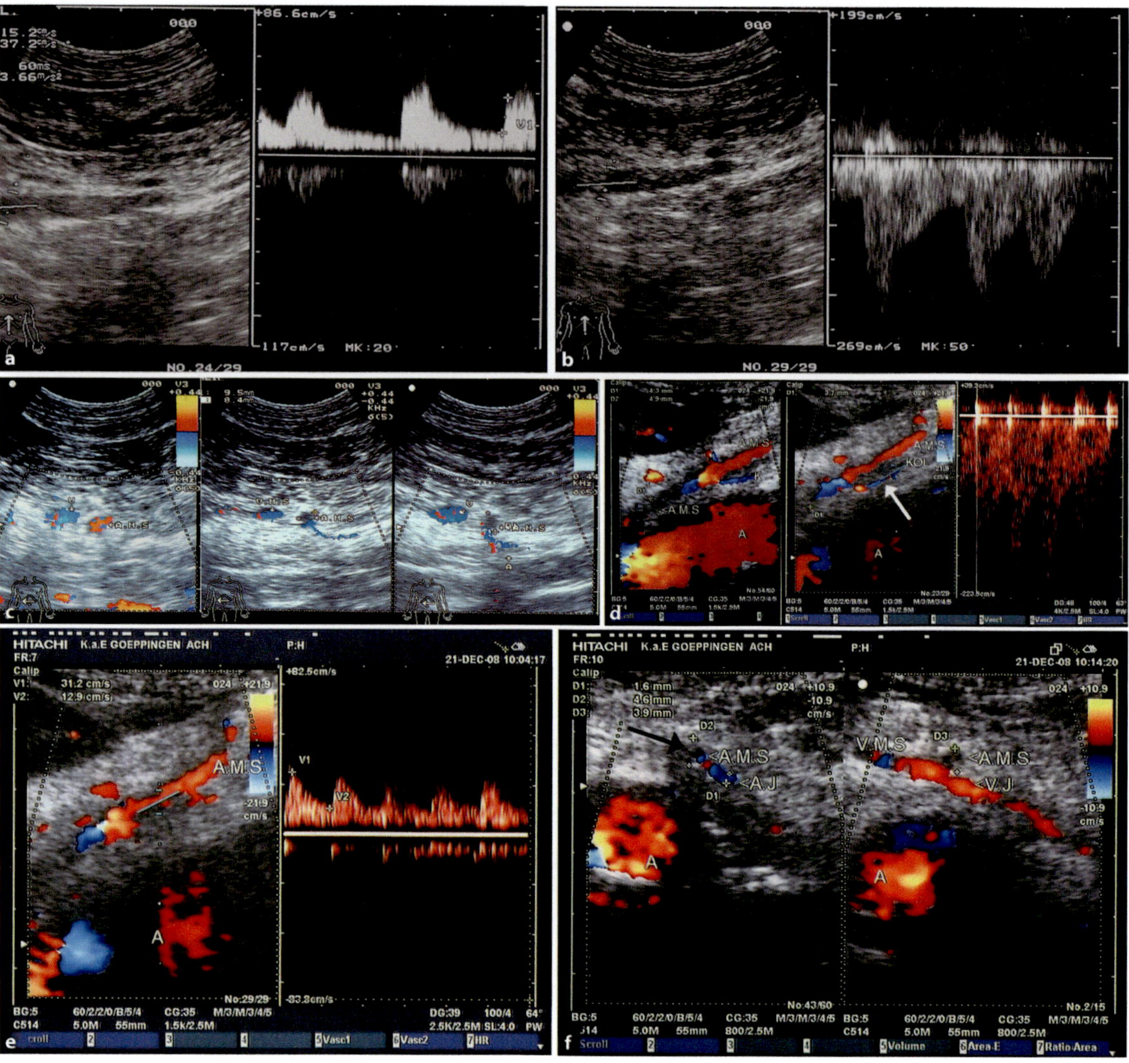

Fig. 6.57a–f (Atlas) Acute mesenteric artery occlusion.

a 42-year-old patient presenting with a 3-h history of severe abdominal pain, in part of a cramping nature. No abnormal laboratory values at this time (no leukocytosis, no acidosis, no elevated lactate level). The clinical examination reveals only mild tenderness, absence of peritonism, and diffuse abdominal pain. Normal B-mode ultrasound and radiologic examinations. No history of cardiac disease. Patient admitted to hospital in the evening with the tentative diagnosis of enteritis; analgesic therapy and follow-up contemplated. Additionally performed duplex ultrasound of the mesenteric arteries demonstrates an abnormal signal at the origin of the patent superior mesenteric artery. Peak systolic velocity (PSV) is markedly reduced to 37.2 cm/s with a relatively large diastolic component of 15.2 cm/s, resulting in an abnormal resistance index of 0.59.
b More distally, downstream of the origin of the middle colic artery, the Doppler waveform of the mesenteric artery shows a thump pattern.
c Color duplex imaging demonstrates a patent superior mesenteric artery to the level of the origins of the first jejunal branches. A proximal jejunal branch also shows color-coded flow signals. In the remainder of the superior mesenteric artery, neither color duplex nor spectral Doppler depicts flow signals. Emergency embolectomy with complete revascularization was performed without the necessity for bowel resection.
Mesenteric artery occlusion – acute versus chronic.
d A slim 82-year-old woman with a history of intermittent abdominal pain was hospitalized for severe abdominal pain. On admission, she had a regular heart rate of 95 beats/min but a history of embolectomy of the leg in the year before. The color duplex examination reveals occlusion of the proximal superior mesenteric artery segment from its origin to the level of the pancreaticoduodenal artery origin (K). The superior mesenteric artery (A.M.S) is refilled by the gastroduodenal artery (arising from the hepatic artery) and the pancreaticoduodenal artery (K). With the gastroduodenal artery acting as a collateral (KOL in the second image), flow in this artery is high and clearly visualized. The spectral Doppler recording with the sample volume in this artery reveals a PSV of 220 cm/s and an end-diastolic velocity (EDV) of 100 cm/s. These color duplex findings are consistent with chronic occlusion.
e With the sample volume placed in the superior mesenteric artery (A.M.S.), very low flow velocities of 31 cm/s during systole and 12 cm/s at end diastole are measured, suggesting poor collateralization or poor peripheral outflow.
f With the transducer in transverse orientation on the upper abdomen, the mesenteric artery trunk is examined in the color duplex mode with a low pulse repetition frequency, evaluating the jejunal origins for patency. Following the mesenteric artery downward, three jejunal branches are identified (A.J; left image) before the artery (A.M.S) first becomes partially occluded and then, more distally, completely occluded (no flow; right image). A jejunal vein branch (V.J) entering the mesenteric vein (V.M.S) is seen between the mesenteric artery anteriorly and the aorta (A) posteriorly. Taking these additional findings into account, the overall situation suggests acute embolic occlusion rather than chronic occlusion – despite the conclusion suggested by the findings described in **d**. Intraoperatively, a short embolic occlusion at the mesenteric artery origin from the aorta was seen and a second occlusion of the distal segment with some patent jejunal branches arising from the patent portion between these occlusions. The patent portion was supplied by the pancreaticoduodenal artery (as demonstrated by the sonographic examination)

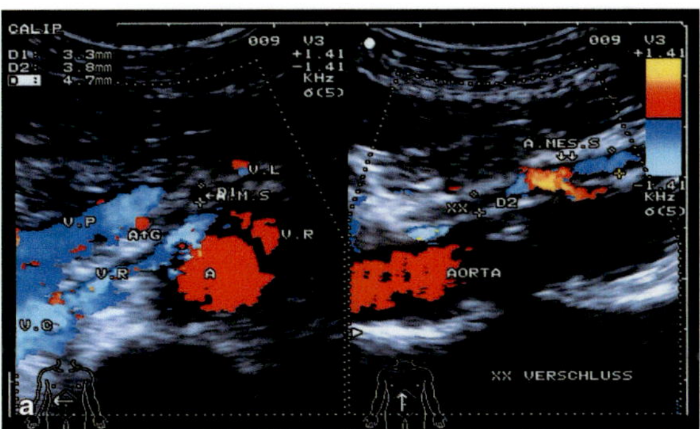

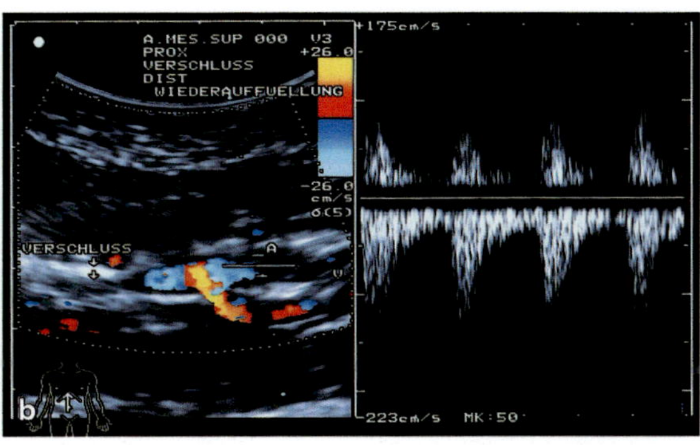

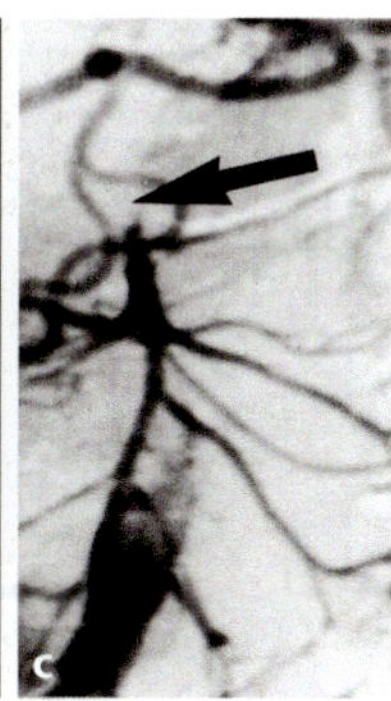

Fig. 6.58a–c (Atlas) Chronic mesenteric artery occlusion.
a 50-year-old patient with symptoms of abdominal angina caused by proximal occlusion of the superior mesenteric artery with refilling through the gastroduodenal and pancreaticoduodenal arteries about 4 cm distal to its origin, as demonstrated by color duplex ultrasound. Transverse image (left) depicting the renal vein (V.R) and superior mesenteric artery (A.M.S) anterior to the aorta (A). Color duplex fails to demonstrate flow in the occluded superior mesenteric artery (3.3 mm). More anteriorly, the splenic vein (V.L) is seen; the renal vein (V.R), including its termination in the vena cava (V.C), is depicted longitudinally (flow coded in blue), to the left of the aorta sectioned obliquely. Anteriorly, the portal vein (V.P) is shown with blue-coded flow. Between the renal and portal veins, the cross section of the red gastroduodenal artery is seen at its junction with the pancreaticoduodenal artery. It is depicted beneath the lower margin of the portal vein and marked (A↑G). In transverse orientation, this collateral pathway can be followed in its entire length including refilling of the superior mesenteric artery. The longitudinal image (right) depicts the superior mesenteric artery (A.MES.S) anterior to the obliquely sectioned aorta (red). Color signals are absent from the superior mesenteric artery segment in the left half of the image (XX), where it is merely seen as a hypoechoic, tubular structure. Along its course to the right of the image, it is refilled by the pancreaticoduodenal artery from posterolaterally (displayed in red, toward transducer). There is short backward flow in the unoccluded segment.
b The Doppler waveform shows rather high flow in the postocclusive segment of the superior mesenteric artery (flow toward the periphery coded in blue in the color duplex image) with a postprandial peak systolic velocity (PSV) of 120 cm/s and an end-diastolic velocity (EDV) of 30 cm/s, suggesting good collateral flow through the gastropancreaticoduodenal artery (coded red in the color image). Proximal to the entry of this collateral, the occluded segment of the superior mesenteric artery is depicted as a hypoechoic, tubular structure. Around the site of entry of the collateral, flow is highly turbulent. The postocclusive waveform shows a slightly delayed systolic rise, reduced pulsatility, and a larger end-diastolic component.
c Angiogram: Occlusion of the superior mesenteric artery at its origin (arrow) with refilling through the gastroduodenal and pancreaticoduodenal arteries. There is interference from the superimposed aorta at the lower margin. As a result of delayed contrast medium passage through the collateral pathways, the contrast medium has already disappeared from the aorta at the level of the celiac trunk and origin of the superior mesenteric artery by the time the refilled superior mesenteric artery becomes opacified

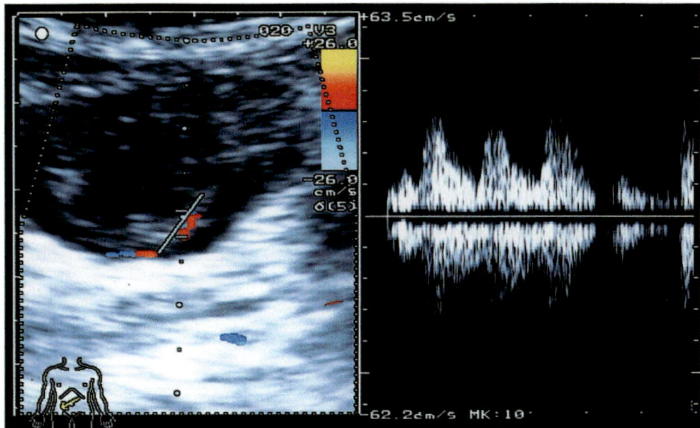

Fig. 6.59 (Atlas) Inflammatory bowel disease.
Acute abdomen with wall thickening of bowel loops on B-mode ultrasonography. The demonstration of flow in the bowel wall in the color duplex mode differentiates inflammatory thickening of the wall from thickening due to acute ischemia or mesenteric vein thrombosis, which exhibits the characteristic bull's eye sign. The inflammatory origin is also underlined by the large diastolic flow component in the Doppler waveform

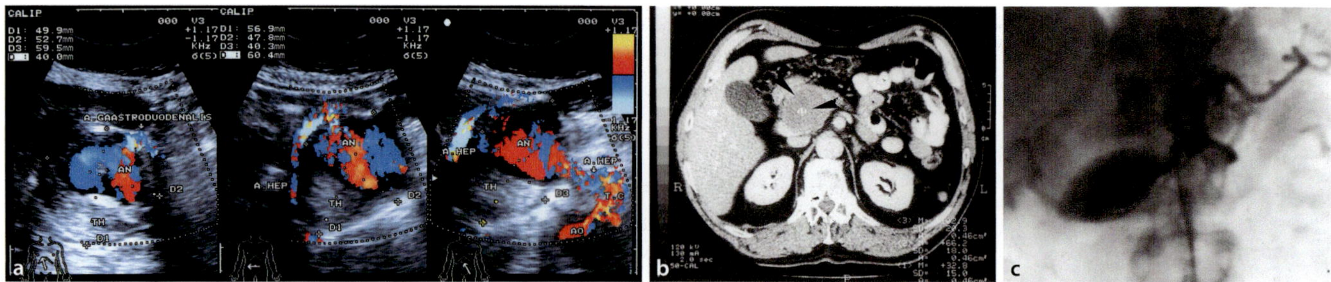

Fig. 6.60a–c (Atlas) Hepatic artery aneurysm.
a A structure of mixed echogenicity measuring 6 × 5 cm and showing flow signals in the color duplex mode is depicted in the portal hilum. Stagnation thrombus (TH) is seen in the posterior portion of the aneurysm. For the surgical procedure, it is important to precisely locate the vessels entering and arising from the aneurysm (AN), in particular the gastroduodenal artery, which is shown to arise from the anteroinferior aspect of the aneurysm (blue, left section). The middle section depicts the elongated proper hepatic artery (A.HEP) curving around the aneurysm. The right section shows the common hepatic artery (A.HEP) emptying into the aneurysm and arising from the celiac trunk (T.C) on the right side of the image. As the hepatic artery aneurysm also involves the gastroduodenal artery, reconstruction of the hepatic artery is necessary after resection of the aneurysm. If the aneurysm were localized proximal to the gastroduodenal artery, the latter would ensure arterial supply of the liver.
b Upper abdominal CT scan showing subhepatic mass (arrowhead): hepatic artery aneurysm with partial thrombosis (arrowhead).
c Angiogram depicting hepatic artery aneurysm (center)

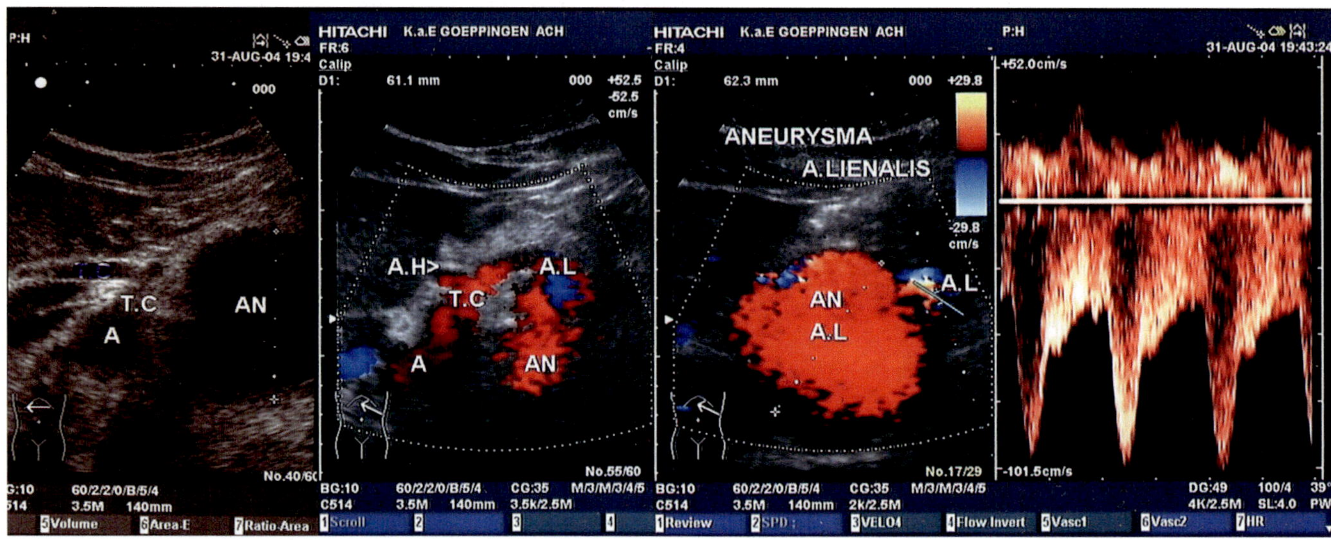

Fig. 6.61 (Atlas) Splenic artery aneurysm.
The B-mode image shows an anechoic cystic lesion in the omental bursa (leftmost). The diagnosis of an aneurysm is suggested by the color coding in the duplex mode (left center). The junction of the aneurysm with the vessel is seen upon rotation of the transducer; in this example the splenic artery (A.L) shortly after its origin from the celiac trunk (T.C; A = aorta, A.H = hepatic artery). Moving the transducer laterally to the left (right center), the distal splenic artery (A.L, with sample volume) can be traced along its course from the aneurysm (AN A.L) to the splenic hilum. The vascular relationships of the aneurysm are thus determined sonographically prior to surgery. The Doppler waveform (rightmost) shows the typical low-resistance flow of the splenic artery

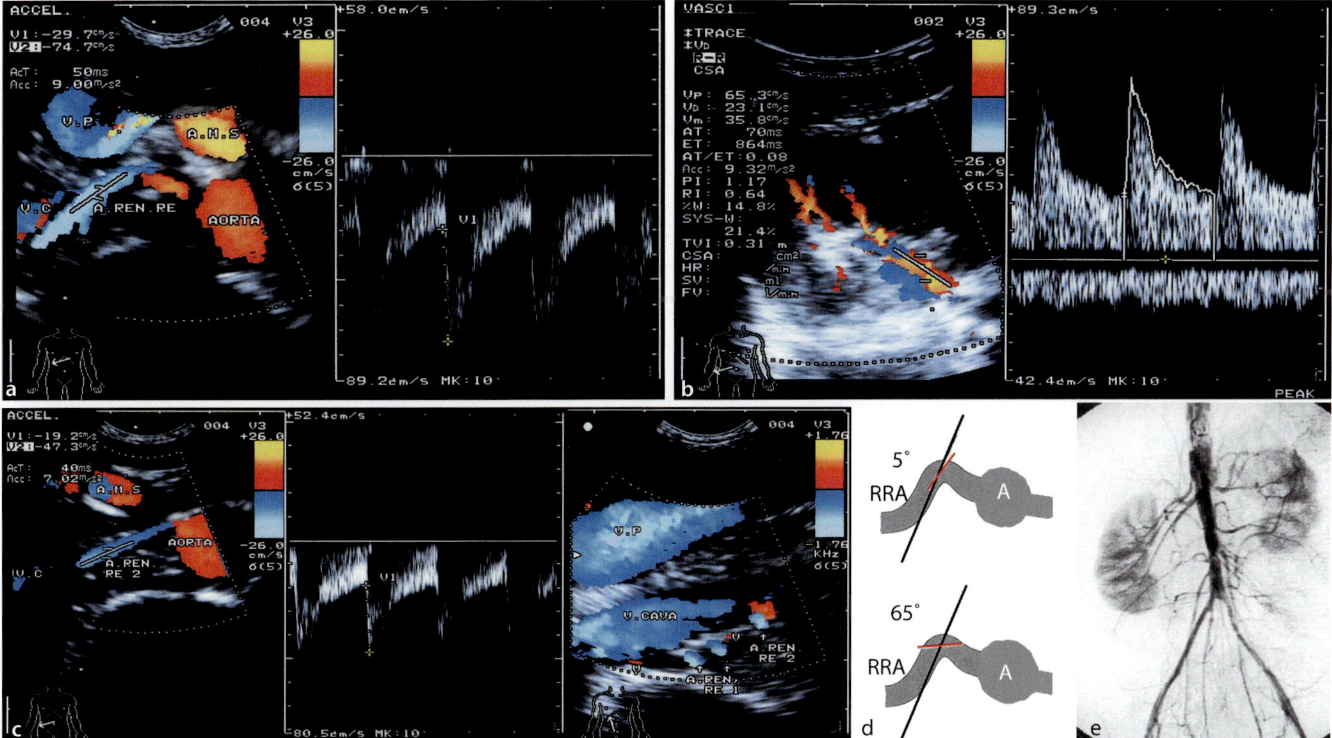

Fig. 6.62a–e (Atlas) Course of the renal arteries.

a Adequate diagnostic evaluation for renal artery stenosis (RAS) is crucially dependent on the meticulous visualization of the course of the renal artery. The transverse upper abdominal view on the left shows the right renal artery (A.REN.RE) following an arched course after arising from the aorta (proximal segment with flow in red toward transducer and distal segment with flow in blue away from transducer) below the vena cava (V.C). Anteriorly, the superior mesenteric artery (red, A.M.S) and portal vein (blue, V.P) are seen. A Pourcelot index of 0.6 is calculated for the origin of the renal artery from a peak systolic velocity (PSV) of 74.7 cm/s and an end-diastolic velocity (EDV) of 29.7 cm/s.

b Renal artery at the renal hilum imaged from the flank (in transverse orientation) with the beam striking the vessel at an adequate angle. The waveform and the Pourcelot index are the same at the hilum as at the origin, suggesting that no hemodynamically significant stenosis is present along the course of the renal artery between these two sampling sites.

c Since 25% of all kidneys are supplied by a paired renal artery and hypertension may be caused by stenosis at the origin of the second branch, the examiner must always look for a second renal artery branch by moving the transducer posteriorly in transverse orientation. Here, a second renal artery coded in blue arises from the aorta 1 cm from the origin of the first one. The characteristic renal artery waveform confirms the identity of the second artery. In longitudinal orientation (rightmost image), the renal arteries can be identified posterior to the vena cava with blood flow in the renal arteries and in the vena cava depicted in blue. Three renal artery branches with blood flow coded in blue are seen below the vena cava; this is due to early division of the inferior branch of the paired renal artery on this side.

d Diagram illustrating the difficulties in placing the angle correction cursor parallel to the direction of flow in a tortuous or curved renal artery segment, which is not uncommon at the origin of the right renal artery (RRA). These pitfalls must be borne in mind to ensure correct grading of atherosclerotic RAS, which tends to occur at the origin (see Fig. 1.23b).

e Angiogram: Two renal arteries arise from the aorta on the right with early division of the inferior branch

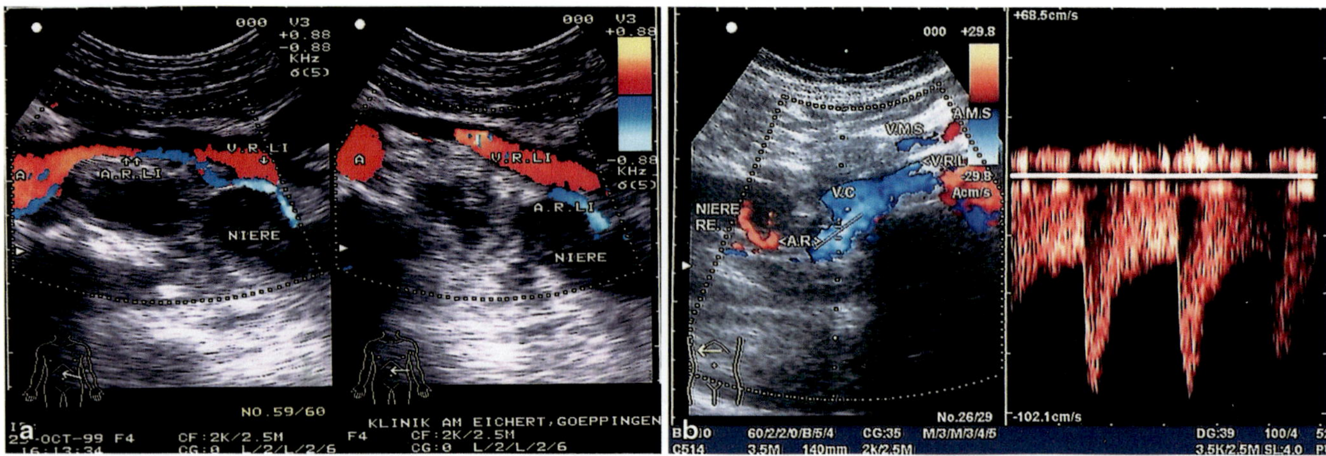

Fig. 6.63a, b (Atlas) **Sonoanatomy of the renal arteries.**

a The left renal artery usually has a length of 5–6 cm, from the aorta to the renal hilum. Scattering by bowel gas makes it difficult to scan the entire length of the left artery in a single plane. The left image depicts the renal artery with flow in red (toward transducer) at its origin and in blue at the renal hilum (away from transducer). The change in the color coding does not indicate an actual change in flow direction but only a change relative to the transducer. The right image depicts the left renal vein (flow in red, toward transducer) anterior to the artery along its course to the vena cava anterior to the aorta.

b The image shows the right renal artery undercrossing the vena cava. Its proximal and middle thirds are depicted with flow coded in blue (A.R). The vena cava (V.C, blue) is seen anterior to it and the aorta is sectioned transversely (A, red) at the right margin of the image. Anteriorly, the superior mesenteric artery (A.M.S) and vein (V.M.S) are seen. Between the aorta and the superior mesenteric artery, there is a short stretch of the left renal vein (V.R.L, blue). The distal third of the right renal artery is coded in red (flow toward transducer) at the renal hilum (NIERE RE). The Doppler waveform was obtained from the middle third (posterior to the vena cava), the preferred site of stenosis in fibromuscular dysplasia

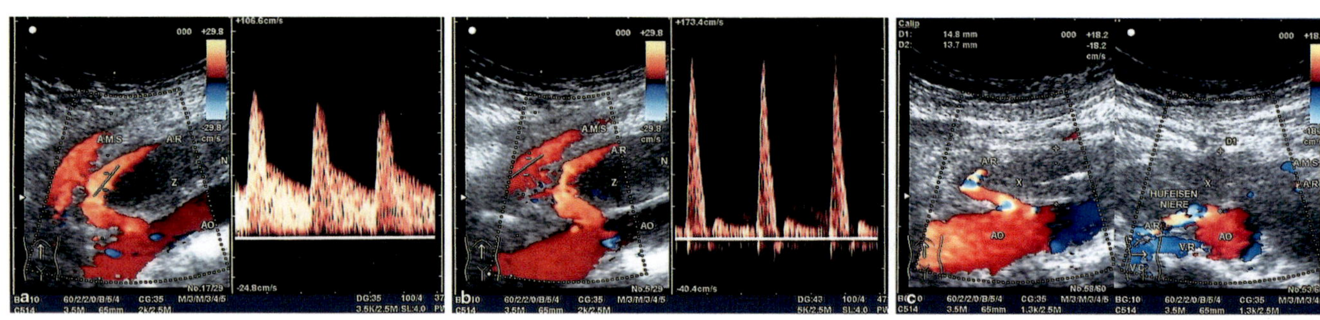

Fig. 6.64a–c (Atlas) **Horseshoe kidney.**

a Horseshoe kidneys have atypical arteries and veins. Besides additional lower pole vessels, a fifth renal artery supplying the renal bridge crossing over the aorta may be present as in the example shown. The young woman had an infected renal cyst (Z) in the preaortic bridge of the horseshoe kidney. Pus was drained from the cyst under ultrasound guidance. In inconclusive cases, the Doppler waveform can help to establish the identity of a vessel. Here, the inferior of the two vessels, coursing over the cyst (Z) and renal parenchyma, has the typical waveform of a renal artery and is thus identified as a supernumerary fifth renal artery (A.R).

b The artery coursing more superiorly (A.M.S) does not show the low-resistance flow typical of renal arteries but a mixed type characteristic of mesenteric arteries.

c Closer inspection of the vascular supply (transverse image on the right, longitudinal image on the left) shows the right lower polar artery (A.R) with flow in blue. This artery follows an atypical course, anterior to the vena cava on its way to the lower pole, after arising from the aorta (AO). A retroaortic renal vein with flow coded in blue (V.R) passes from the left lower pole into the vena cava (V.C). There is aliasing in the renal artery due to the low pulse repetition frequency used to detect slow venous (and arterial) flow. The longitudinal image on the left again shows the fifth renal artery (A.R) coursing to the renal parenchyma in front of the aorta (AO) after drainage of the infected cyst (site indicated by the X in the kidney)

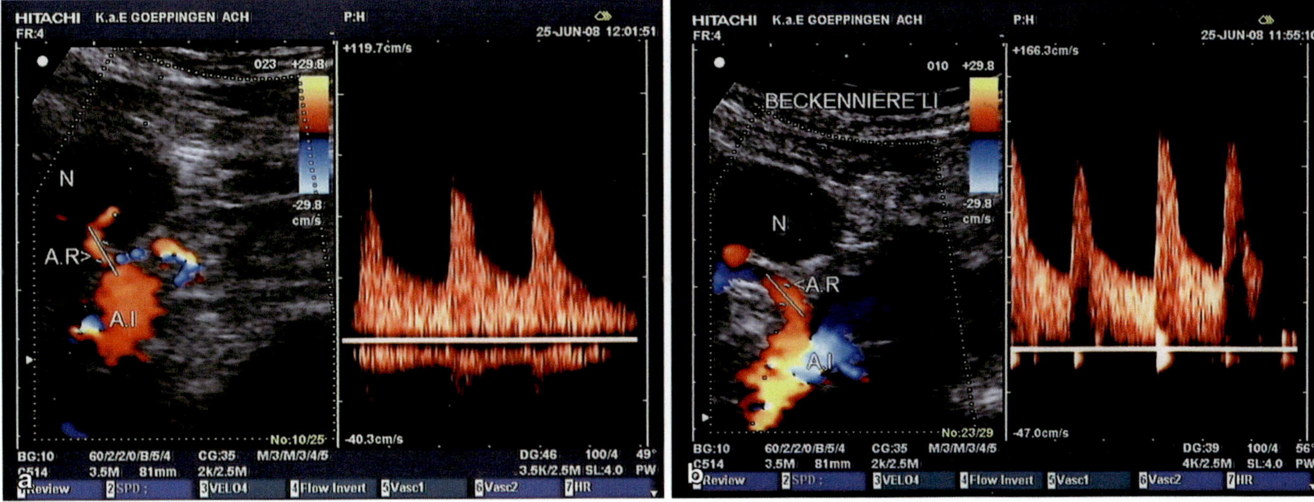

Fig. 6.65a, b (Atlas) Pelvic kidney.
If a kidney cannot be identified in its usual location in the flank, this should prompt a search for a pelvic kidney. The arterial supply of an ectopic pelvic kidney is highly variable with one or more renal arteries arising from the aorta or from the iliac artery. Also, the examiner must bear in mind that two polar arteries may be present and that stenosis in either of them can be the cause of hypertension. In the example, two polar arteries arising from the common iliac artery are identified; the two origins can be differentiated by moving and slightly rotating the transducer (lower pole artery in **a** and upper pole artery in **b**); stenosis in either artery is ruled out as flow velocity is below 120 cm/s. In patients with an ectopic kidney and aberrant arterial supply, renal hypertension can be caused by proximal common iliac artery stenosis

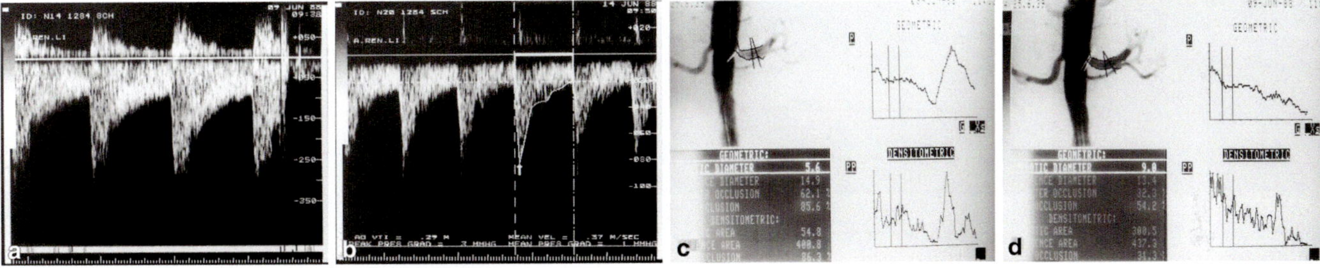

Fig. 6.66a–d (Atlas) Renal artery stenosis – PTA.
a Doppler waveform obtained in the presence of moderate to severe stenosis at the origin of the renal artery with marked turbulence and a peak systolic velocity (PSV) of 310 cm/s and end-diastolic velocity (EDV) of 100 cm/s.
b Doppler waveform from the same renal artery as in **a** after percutaneous transluminal angioplasty (PTA) shows return to normal flow velocity (PSV of 80 cm/s).
c X-ray densitometry (same patient as in **a**, before PTA): Measurement demonstrates a stenosis at the origin of the left renal artery with an area reduction of 86.3%.
d X-ray densitometry (same patient as before, after PTA; corresponding Doppler waveform in **b**): Residual stenosis with a 31.3% area reduction, which is hemodynamically nonsignificant. There is spectral broadening in the corresponding Doppler waveform but no accelerated flow

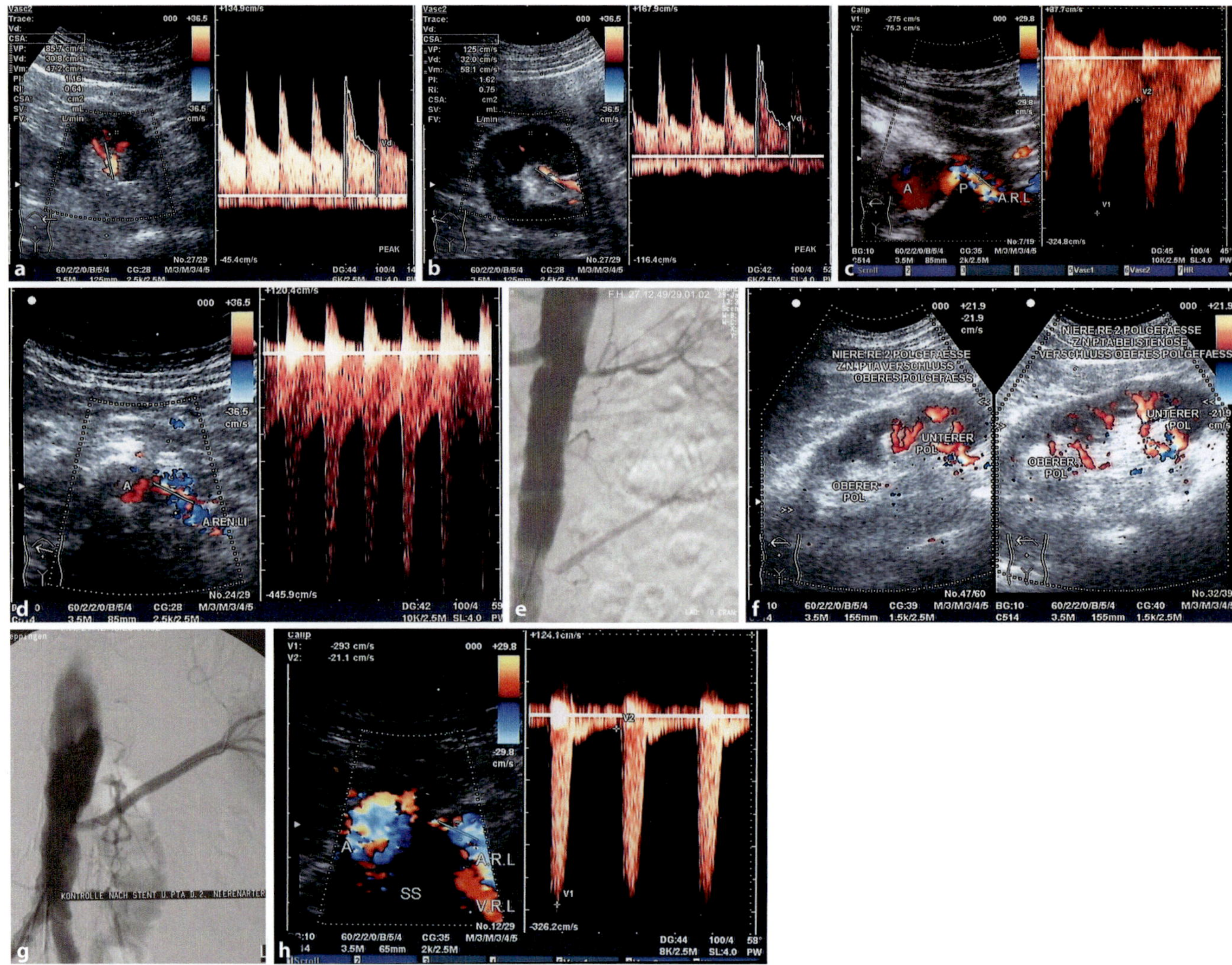

Fig. 6.67a–h (Atlas) Renal artery stenosis – indirect criteria.
The waveform from the renal hilum on the left yields a peak systolic velocity (PSV) of 85.7 cm/s and an end-diastolic velocity (EDV) of 47.2 cm/s, from which a resistance index (RI; Pourcelot index) of 0.64 is calculated.
b The corresponding values in the right renal artery are: PSV of 125 cm/s, EDV of 58.1 cm/s, and a resulting RI of 0.75. The 10% RI difference is consistent with the diagnosis of renal artery stenosis (RAS) and indicates postocclusive flow in the artery with the lower RI.
High-grade renal artery stenosis – PTA.
c Patient with two left renal arteries and a PSV of 275 cm/s in the upper pole artery, consistent with high-grade RAS caused by atherosclerotic plaque (P) at the origin of the artery. There is aliasing in the renal artery (A.R.L); the red flow signals anteriorly indicate the left renal vein (flow toward transducer).
d The Doppler waveform from the origin of the left renal artery confirms high-grade stenosis with a PSV over 4 m/s with the color flow image showing pronounced perivascular vibration (audible bruit on auscultation).
e Subsequent angiography with PTA confirms high-grade stenosis of both polar arteries on the left.
f Flank pain after PTA prompted a duplex ultrasound examination. In the lower pole of the kidney, both arterial and venous flow signals are obtained from the hilum to the periphery. The upper portion shows rarefied perfusion in the pole (capsular vessels) and no arterial flow at the hilum, consistent with occlusion of the upper pole artery after PTA.
g Angiogram confirms occlusion of the upper pole artery and normal flow in the lower pole artery.
Renal artery stenosis in diabetes mellitus – indication for PTA?
h High-grade stenosis of the left renal artery (A.R.L) with a PSV of 293 cm/s and an EDV of 21 cm/s, from which an RI of 0.9 is calculated. An RI of >0.8 indicates parenchymal damage and fixed hypertension, so that PTA is no longer a promising option. Stenotic plaque at the origin of the renal artery from the aorta (A) causes acoustic shadowing (SS). Retroaortic course of the left renal vein (V.R.L)

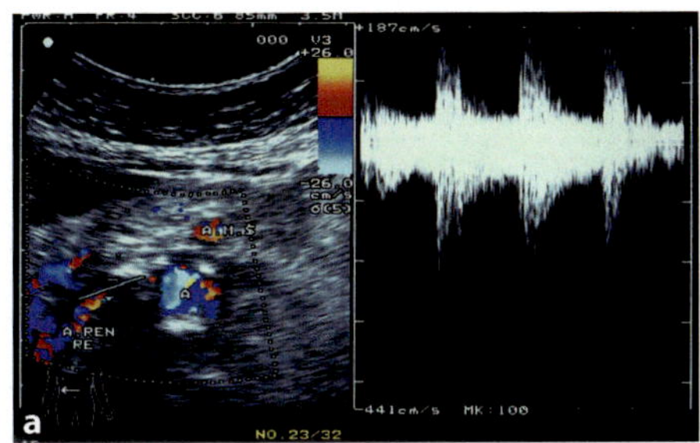

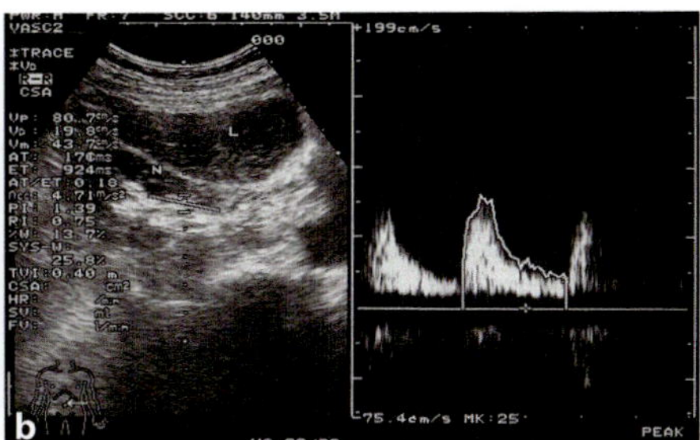

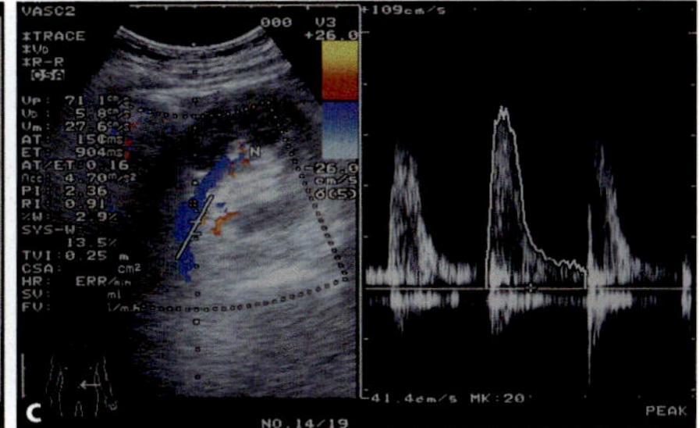

Fig. 6.68a–c (Atlas) Renal artery stenosis in diabetes mellitus – indirect criteria.
a In a patient with a long history of insulin-dependent diabetes mellitus and macro- and microangiopathy, the Doppler waveform obtained at the origin of the right renal artery shows turbulence and accelerated flow indicative of renal artery stenosis (RAS). Duplex imaging provides no adequate information for estimating the degree of stenosis due to plaque with acoustic shadowing at the origin. In interpreting the peak systolic velocity (PSV) of just over 2 m/s somewhat distal to the stenosis, one has to take into account possible hypertensive episodes during spectral Doppler sampling as well as the known higher pulsatility of blood flow with higher PSV in diabetics. In the case presented, for instance, the resistive index (Pourcelot index) is calculated from the Doppler spectra of both distal (hilar) renal artery segments for confirmation of the hemodynamic significance of the stenosis.
b The waveform from the right hilum yields a PSV of 80.7 cm/s and an end-diastolic velocity (EDV) of 19.8 cm/s with a Pourcelot index of 0.75. The gray-scale image depicts the liver (L) above the kidney.
c The waveform from the left hilum shows more pulsatile flow with a PSV of 71.1 cm/s and an EDV of 5.8 cm/s; the Pourcelot index is 0.91. Compared with the findings on the left side, the waveform of the right renal artery appears to be unusually normal, which is due to the fact that the effects of diabetes and stenosis cancel each other. The waveform from the left, which is too pulsatile for a renal artery, is attributable to medial sclerosis in long-standing diabetes mellitus and renal parenchymal damage. The much lower Pourcelot index of the right renal artery (over 10% in side-to-side comparison) is abnormal and indicates a hemodynamically significant proximal stenosis. This interpretation relies on the assumption that other factors explaining the difference such as asymmetric parenchymal kidney damage can be ruled out

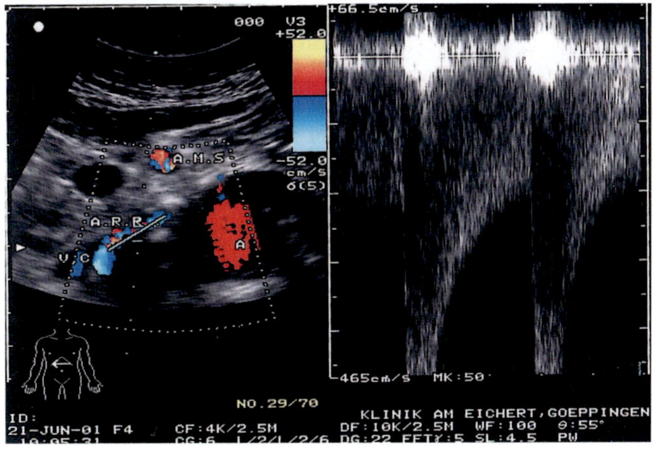

Fig. 6.69 (Atlas) Suprarenal aortic aneurysm with renal artery stenosis.
Sonographic evaluation of the renal artery is indicated to evaluate the relationship of its origin to an aortic aneurysm. The transverse upper abdominal view shows the right renal artery arising from an aortic aneurysm with partial thrombosis and a diameter of 4.5 cm at the level of the renal artery origin (hypoechoic, concentric thrombus also at the renal artery origin). In addition, there is high-grade renal artery stenosis with a peak systolic velocity (PSV) exceeding 5 m/s

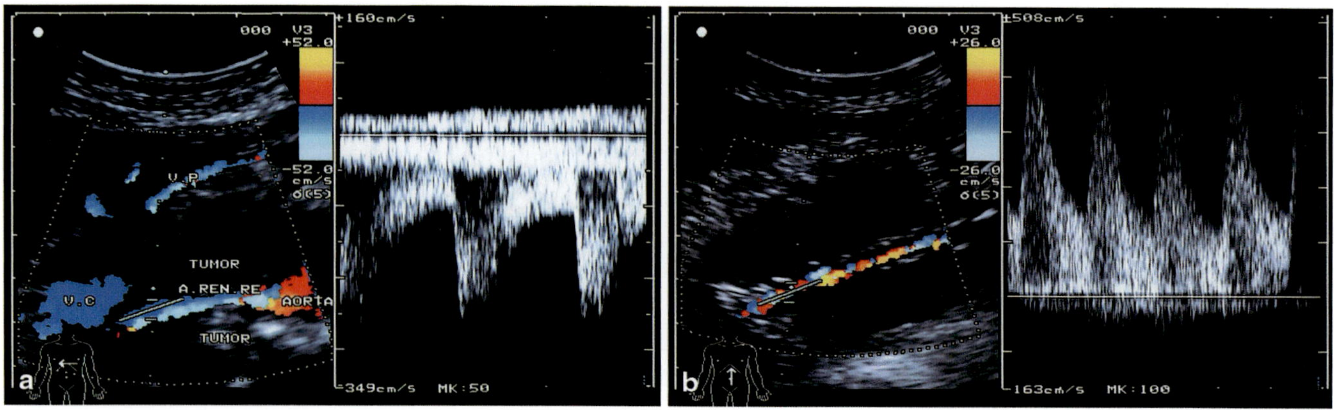

Fig. 6.70a, b (Atlas) Vessel compression by tumor.
a A leiomyosarcoma (confirmed by ultrasound-guided core biopsy) splays the vena cava (V.C) and aorta in the retroperitoneum. A long segment of the renal artery (A.REN.RE) running through the tumor is moderately constricted (Doppler-derived PSV of 250 cm/s). The vessels are located by color duplex imaging to avoid inadvertent vascular damage by subsequent ultrasound-guided core biopsy. Anteriorly, the portal vein (V.P) is also compressed by the tumor.
b The superior mesenteric artery encased by the tumor (sarcoma) at its root is also constricted along an extended segment (PSV of 450 cm/s)

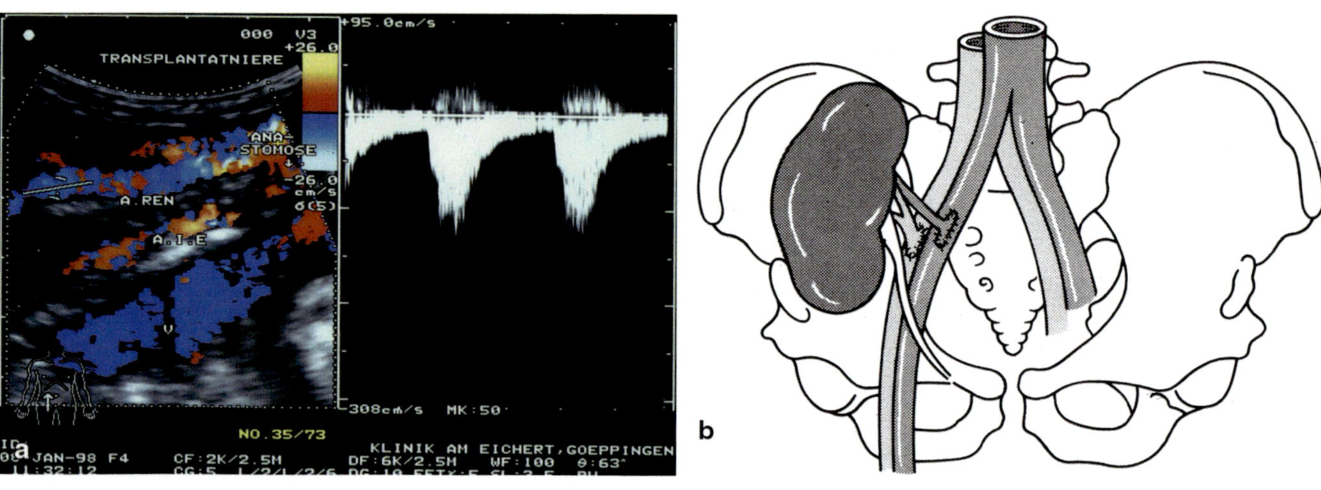

Fig. 6.71a, b (Atlas) Transplant kidney.
a Color duplex image depicting the artery of the transplant kidney, anastomosed to the iliac artery, with flow coded in blue (flow away from transducer), while the iliac artery is shown with flow in red (toward transducer). The Doppler waveform has a large diastolic component and the typical pattern of low-resistance flow indicating a functioning graft without rejection.
b Diagram of the connections of the renal transplant vessels to the iliac vessels

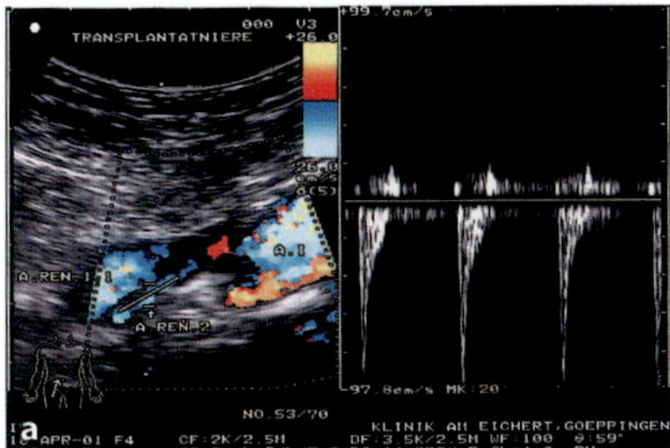

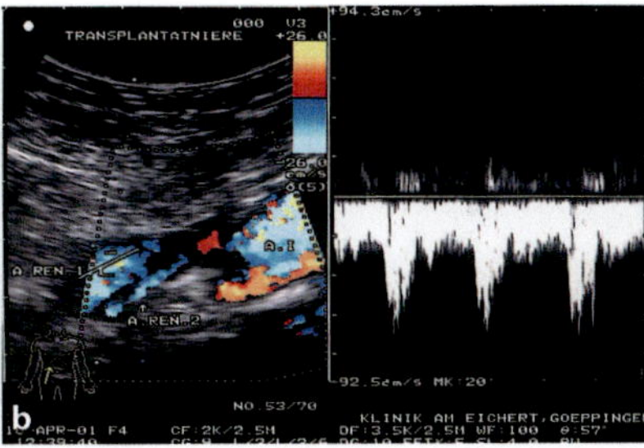

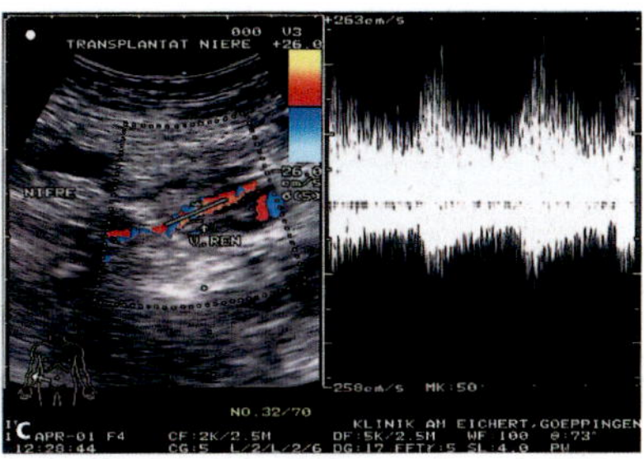

Fig. 6.72a–c (Atlas) Transplant kidney – rejection – fistula.
Analysis of the Doppler waveform from the renal artery is an integral component of the diagnostic evaluation of kidney graft function and rejection. The renal artery of a transplant kidney anastomosed to the iliac artery is often more easily accessible to sonographic evaluation than the native renal artery.
a The two renal arteries supplying the kidney are depicted at their origins from the iliac artery (A.I.). A highly pulsatile waveform comparable to that of an extremity artery is obtained from the origin of the second renal artery (A.REN.2). This flow profile indicates rejection.
b Surprisingly, the other transplant artery, inserted above the first one, has a monophasic waveform with the low-resistance flow typical of normal kidney function.
c The Doppler waveform of the renal vein (flow toward transducer in the direction of the iliac vein) depicts a pulsatile flow profile with marked turbulence, which is typical of venous flow downstream of an arteriovenous fistula. The patient had a history of repeated biopsy for suspected graft rejection, which led to the formation of a fistula and explains why the artery (A.REN.1) supplying the fistula shows low-resistance flow despite rejection (as documented in the second artery, labeled A.REN.2 in **a, b**)

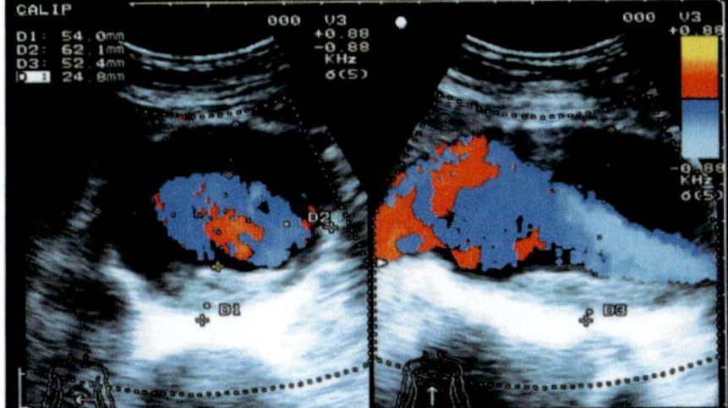

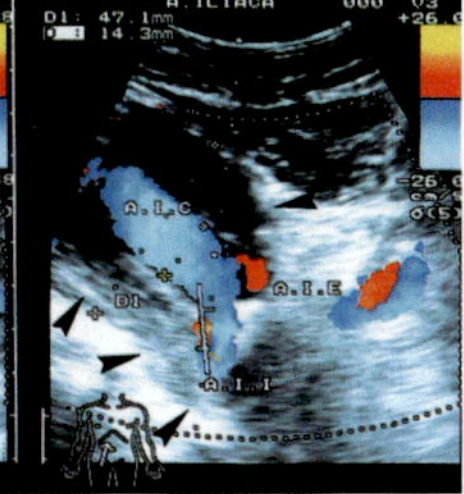

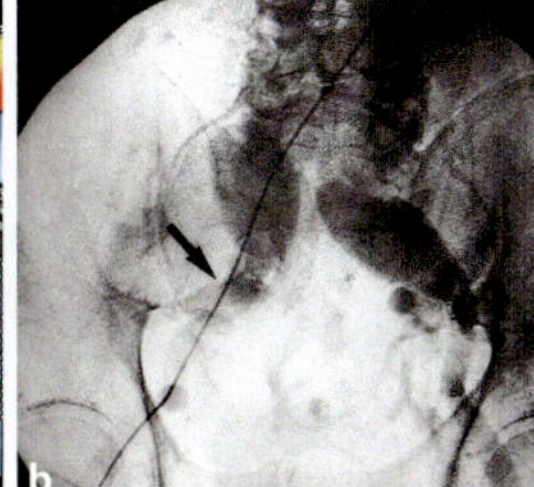

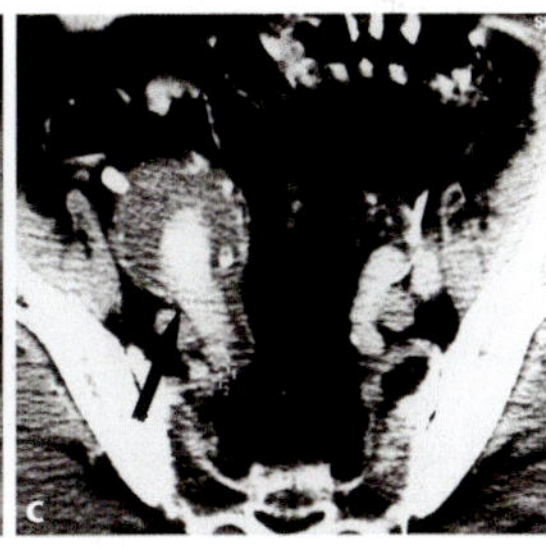

Fig. 6.73a–c (Atlas) Abdominal aortic and iliac artery aneurysm.
a Partially thrombosed infrarenal abdominal aortic aneurysm (AAA) shown in transverse orientation (left section) and longitudinally (middle section). Evaluation of the perfused lumen is improved in the color duplex mode. The total AAA diameter is 62 mm. The mural thrombosis lining the lumen appears hypoechoic around the patent lumen. The aneurysm (right section, arrowheads) involves the common iliac artery (A.I.C) and the proximal internal iliac artery (A.I.I). The elongated external iliac artery (A.I.E) leaves the scanning plane. At this level, the aneurysm has a total diameter of 47 mm with a patent lumen of 14 mm.
b Angiogram showing aneurysmal dilatation of the aorta and of the common iliac arteries. Due to mural thrombosis, the origin of the internal iliac artery on the right (arrow) seems not to be dilated.
c Contrast-enhanced CT: Aneurysm on the right (arrow) extending into the proximal internal iliac artery with mural thrombosis surrounding the perfused lumen. The internal iliac artery arises from the posterior aspect of the common iliac artery (see **a**)

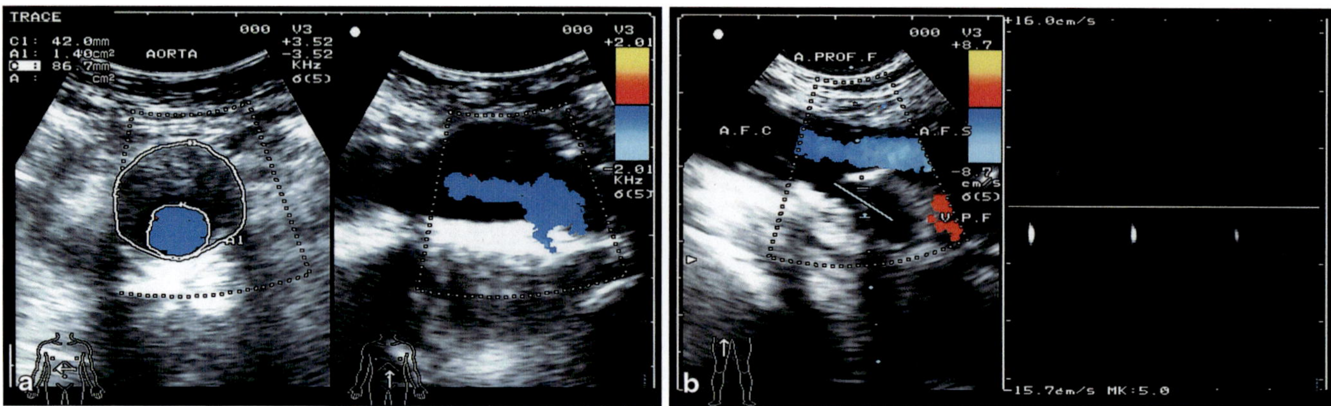

Fig. 6.74a, b (Atlas) Abdominal aortic aneurysm with arterial embolism.
a While the risk of rupture correlates with the diameter of the aneurysm, the risk of embolism associated with the presence of thrombosis in an aneurysm is independent of its size. The saccular aneurysm shown has a size of only 4 cm with mural thrombosis reducing the size of the lumen to that of the normal vessel, especially in the saccular portion; nevertheless, this aneurysm was the source of distal emboli (see **b**). This is an indication for surgery irrespective of aneurysm size. Angiography shows no abnormalities as the perfused lumen of the aneurysm corresponds to that of the normal width of the aorta. The white outline in the left image indicates the extent of the aneurysm; the longitudinal image on the right depicts the saccular anterior outpouching and the thrombotic lining.
b Isolated occlusion of the profunda femoris artery with a patent superficial femoral artery (A.F.S) and common femoral artery (A.F.C) is typically due to embolism rather than atherosclerosis. Neither color duplex nor the Doppler waveform demonstrates flow in the profunda femoris artery. The gray-scale mode shows not only a posterior plaque with acoustic shadowing but also hypoechoic thrombotic material extending from the profunda femoris artery (sample volume) into the bifurcation

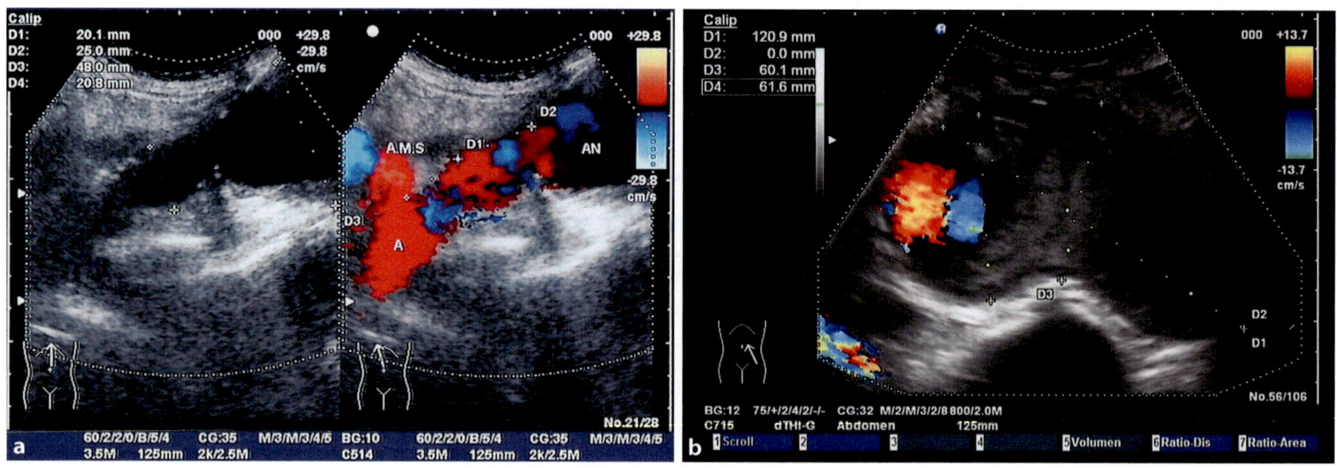

Fig. 6.75a, b (Atlas) Abdominal aortic aneurysm.
a The therapeutic management of an abdominal aortic aneurysm (AAA) is mainly dictated by its diameter, involvement of the iliac artery, presence of thrombosis, and infrarenal extent, including the distance to the renal artery origins, which is important when endovascular aneurysm repair (EVAR) is contemplated. Since the renal artery origins are best seen transversely, and the segment between the origins and the end of the aneurysm longitudinally, it is helpful to first identify the superior mesenteric artery in the longitudinal view and then use it as a guiding structure. The renal arteries arise 1–2 cm distal to the origin of the mesenteric artery. The segment between the end of the aneurysm and the superior mesenteric artery origin can thus be measured in longitudinal orientation. This value minus 2 cm is the distance between the renal artery origin and the aneurysm. This AAA cannot be eliminated by EVAR with a simple, nonbranched stent graft because thrombotic deposits in the aneurysm neck (posterior to the caliper in the left image) preclude firm proximal anchorage of the stent graft.
Contained perforation of abdominal aortic aneurysm.
b Infrarenal, partially thrombosed AAA measuring 6 cm (D3 + D4). The transverse lower abdominal scan reveals a contained perforation with complete thrombosis of the spilled blood at the time of the examination. The contour of the thrombosed aneurysm (arrow) is distinct from the clotted perivascular blood. The site of perforation is indicated by the contour disruption anterolaterally. The blood that escaped through the perforation into the psoas muscle has a total extent of 12 cm (D1). There are no flow signals at the site of perforation at the time of the examination

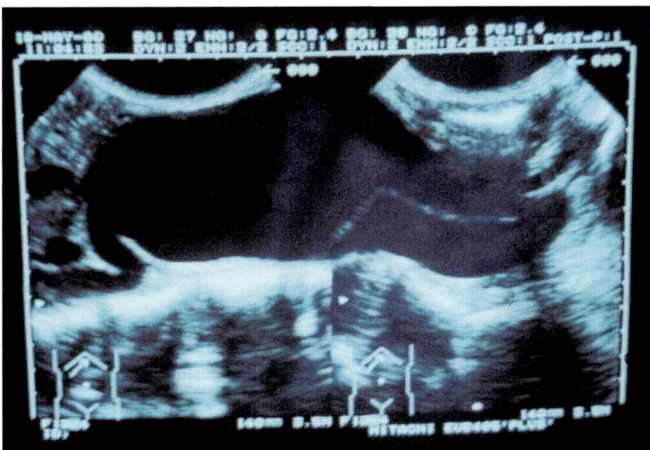

Fig. 6.76 (Atlas) Abdominal aortic aneurysm due to nonatherosclerotic cause.
Aneurysms of nonatherosclerotic or nonbacterial/noninfectious origin can grow to giant size before they rupture. In this young African woman (examined in Uganda) who presented with a tense abdomen, an aneurysm with a cross-sectional diameter of over 15 cm arising from the infrarenal aorta and extending to the iliac bifurcation on both sides filled most of the intra-abdominal cavity. The aneurysm is shown on a composite scan in longitudinal orientation. There is suprarenal kinking of the aorta, which thus extends from the vertebral column to the abdominal wall. The intestine is pushed to the side. Further down in the lower abdomen, with the transducer slightly rotated, the common iliac artery is shown to be aneurysmatically dilated to the level of the origin of the external iliac artery (normal lumen). Posterior to the common iliac artery, the common iliac vein is dilated due to congestion. There are no atherosclerotic lesions of the arterial wall. The patient has AIDS, making Cytomegalovirus infection (induced by immunodeficiency) the most likely cause of the aneurysm

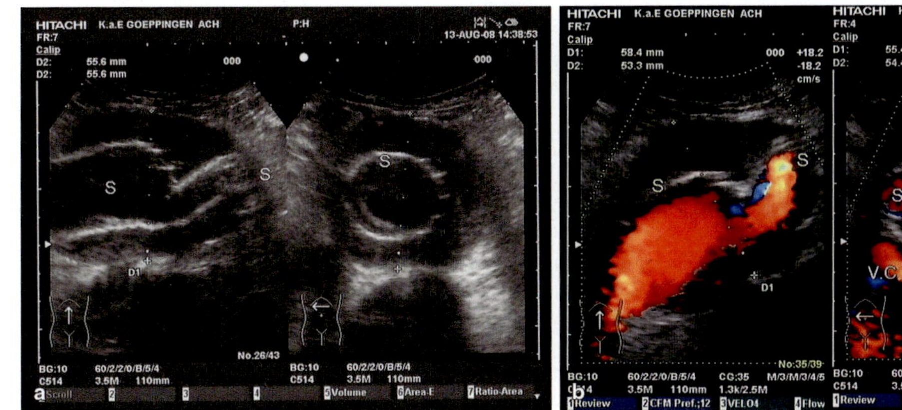

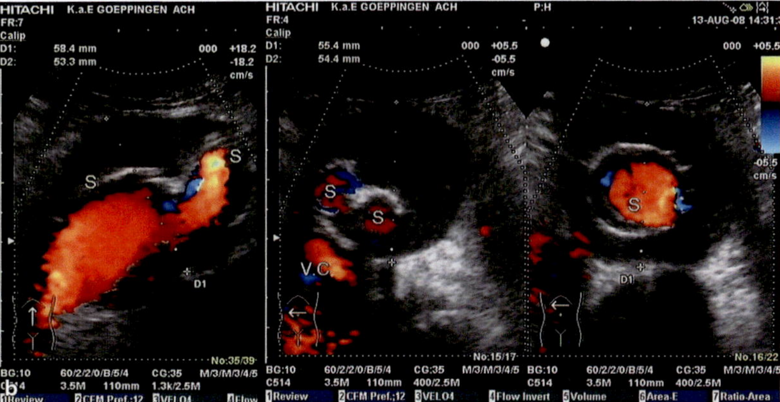

Fig. 6.77a, b (Atlas) Follow-up after endovascular aneurysm repair (EVAR).
a B-mode ultrasound follow-up after EVAR shows the stent graft (S) in the lumen of the abdominal aortic aneurysm (AAA) with properly connected left modular limb (longitudinal image on the left, transverse image on the right). The aneurysm diameter has decreased from 63 to 55 mm. Stent migration is difficult to identify by B-mode imaging.
b The aneurysm and stent graft are scrutinized carefully for endoleaks in longitudinal (leftmost section) and transverse orientation (middle and right sections) using color duplex imaging with a low pulse repetition frequency (in order not to miss low-flow endoleaks). In addition, the entire sac must be searched for flow from patent lumbar arteries (typically entering the aneurysm posterolaterally) or from a patent inferior mesenteric artery entering the sac anterolaterally (type II endoleak). The third step is to search for failure of the modular limb seal (type III endoleak) in longitudinal and transverse orientation. S indicates the two iliac limbs in longitudinal and transverse orientation (left and middle sections) and the main stent graft body in transverse orientation (right section). V.C, vena cava

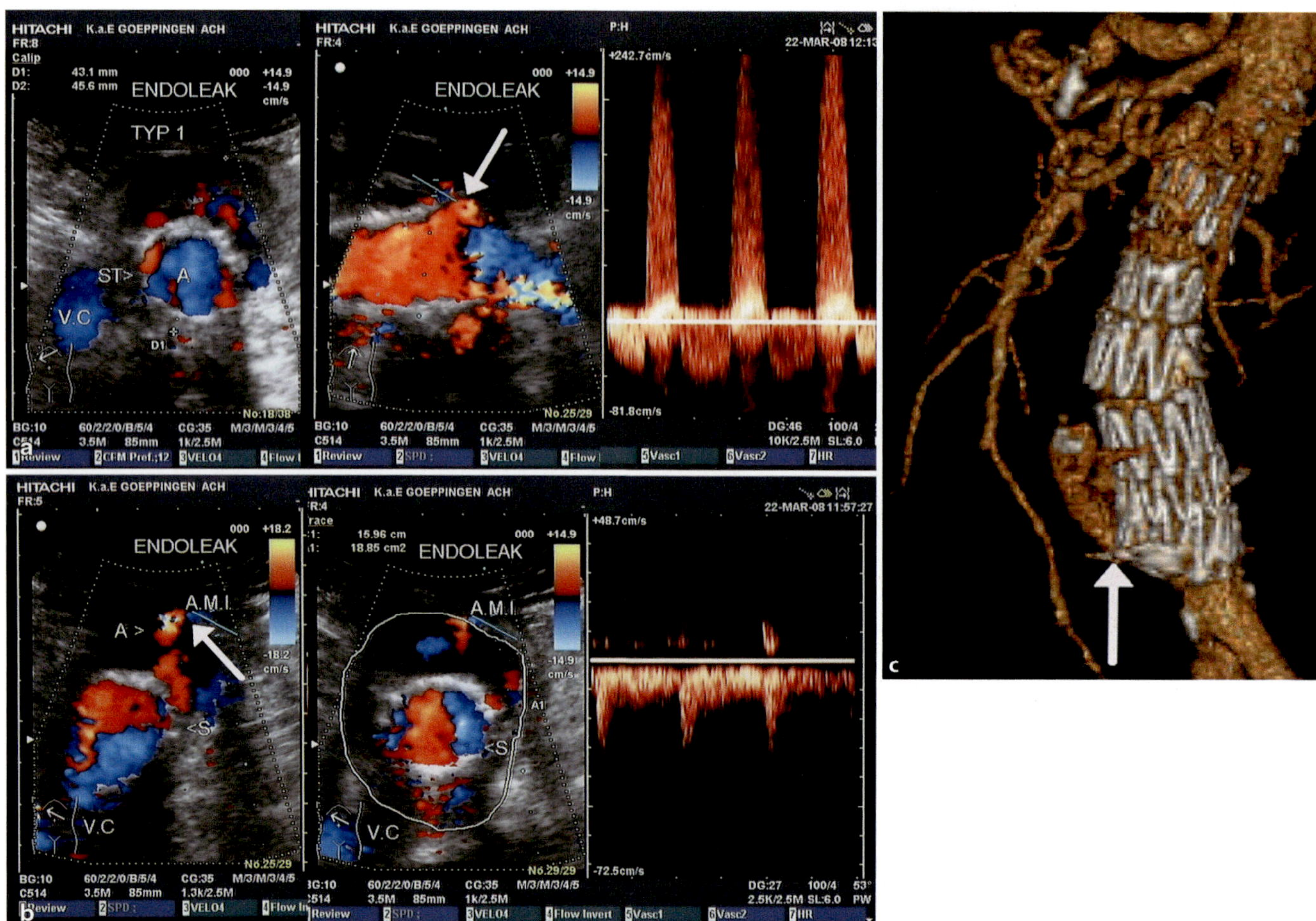

Fig. 6.78a–c (Atlas) Type Ib endoleak.

a Following implantation of a straight stent graft to isolate an infrarenal abdominal aortic aneurysm (AAA), there is flow in the distal aneurysm sac (V.C, vena cava; A, aorta; ST, stent). The middle section shows failure of the distal anastomotic seal at the level of the aortic bifurcation (type Ib endoleak, arrow). The Doppler waveform from this site shows high-frequency to-and-fro flow (with a PSV of 250 cm/s). Blood enters the aneurysm sac in systole and, in diastole, flows back into the distal aorta.

b Closer evaluation of flow within the aneurysm sac reveals that part of the blood flows along the stent graft toward the origin of the inferior mesenteric artery (coded in red, toward transducer). Directly at the origin of the inferior mesenteric artery (A.M.I), there is orthograde flow from the aneurysm (blue, away from transducer; below the baseline in the Doppler waveform). Flow at the origin of the inferior mesenteric artery is slow with a PSV of 30 cm/s. In the transverse image, the aneurysm sac is indicated by a white outline; the stent graft is visualized with color-coded flow, and bright echoes indicate the stent graft wall (S). The normal flow direction in the inferior mesenteric artery suggests that this is not a type II endoleak, but rather a type I endoleak with blood draining from the aneurysm sac through the inferior mesenteric artery. This example underscores the importance of evaluating blood flow directions for comprehensive evaluation after endovascular aneurysm repair (EVAR) and reliable identification of inflow and outflow. This information is important for correct interpretation of the situation and adequate management.

c 3D CT angiogram confirms the type I endoleak (arrow)

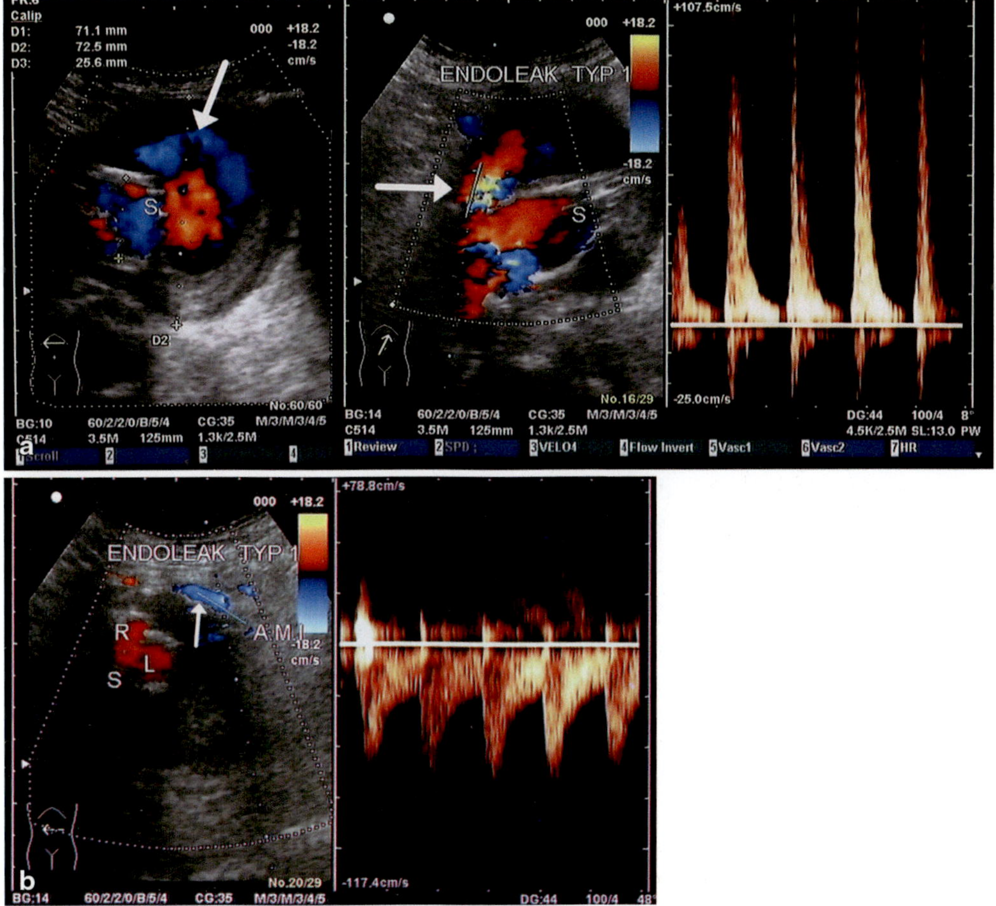

Fig. 6.79a, b (Atlas) Type I endoleak after endovascular aneurysm repair (EVAR).
a The color flow image shows flow within the stent graft (S) but also large color-coded areas indicating flow within the hypoechoic aneurysm sac. Blood enters the sac through a leak at the anastomotic seal below the renal artery origins (middle section), which is a type I endoleak (arrow). The Doppler waveform from the site of the leak shows high-frequency monophasic flow with a peak systolic velocity (PSV) of over 1 m/s. The to-and-fro flow characteristic of endoleaks and false aneurysms (identical hemodynamic situation) is absent here. Unidirectional flow into an aneurysm through an endoleak will lead to rupture within a short time if there is no adequate drainage, underscoring the importance of searching for an outflow in such situations.
b Here, blood leaves the aneurysm through the inferior mesenteric artery (A.M.I; coded in blue, away from transducer, indicated by arrow) visualized along the hypoechoic aneurysm sac with the stent graft (S) and the two iliac limbs (R and L). Farther to the left, the origin of the inferior mesenteric artery is seen with flow coded in red. The corresponding Doppler waveform from the inferior mesenteric artery reveals a rather large diastolic flow component

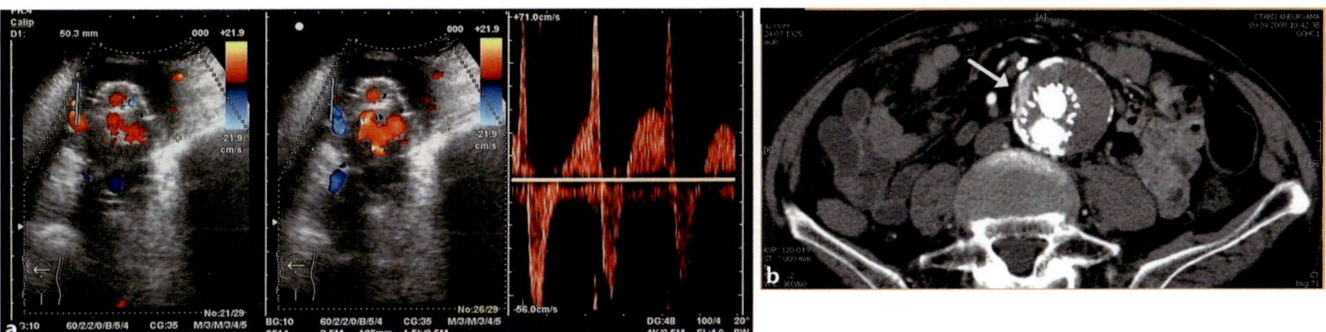

Fig. 6.80 a, b (Atlas) Type II endoleak – high-flow.
a When the color flow image shows flow in the residual sac following endovascular aneurysm repair (EVAR), true flow must be differentiated from artifacts (migration artifact, mirror artifact, and artifact from pulsatile stent graft movement in the thrombosed aneurysm sac, especially shortly after EVAR). Artifacts can be identified by insonation from different directions and spectral Doppler evaluation. Similar to false aneurysms in terms of hemodynamics, endoleak jets should exhibit to-and-fro flow from the lumbar artery perfusing the aneurysm sac (flow into the sac during systole and back into the lumbar artery during diastole).
b Contrast-enhanced CT scan demonstrates blood flow into the aneurysm sac from a lumbar artery (type II endoleak)

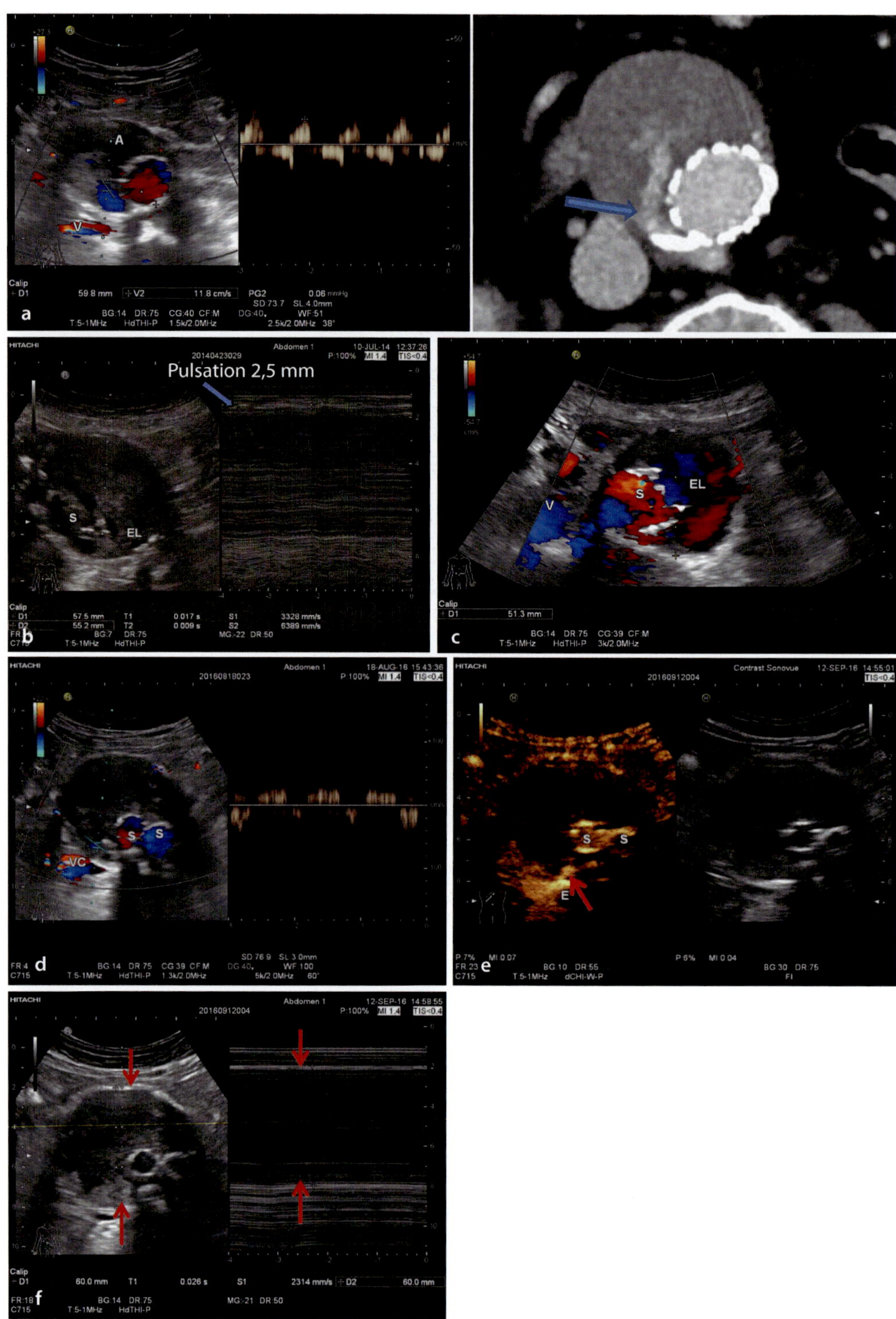

Fig. 6.81a–f (Atlas) Type II endoleak – when to treat.
a The example shows flow into the residual aneurysm sac from a lumbar artery on the right (coded in red, toward transducer); also visible is flow in both iliac limbs (blue). The waveform shows to-and-fro flow of very low frequency with a peak systolic velocity (PSV) <20 cm/s. The slow flow (measured at the site of entry of the feeding artery), combined with the small caliber of the feeding artery, means that the amount of blood entering the aneurysm is small. Such aneurysms often thrombose spontaneously, and there is no risk of rupture. They do not require treatment and can be managed by close monitoring (at 3-month intervals) to rule out further sac growth.
b, c Endoleak requiring repair – pulsation in time-mode mode.
b In the gray-scale image, inhomogeneous areas in the residual aneurysm sac already suggest an endoleak (EL) (S, stent). The diameter variation of 2.5 mm through the cardiac cycle (time-motion mode) indicates relevant blood flow into the residual sac. This endoleak requires repair.
c The color flow image confirms this diagnosis, showing blood flow in most of the residual aneurysm sac.
d–f Small type II endoleak.
Patient with a small type II endoleak fed by a patent posterolateral lumbar artery, which is identified by to-and-fro flow in the Doppler waveform (**d**) and by contrast-enhanced ultrasound (CEUS) (**e**). The absence of diameter variation of the residual aneurysm sac in the time-motion mode (**f**) indicates that there is no relevant pressure build-up in the aneurysm sac during systole

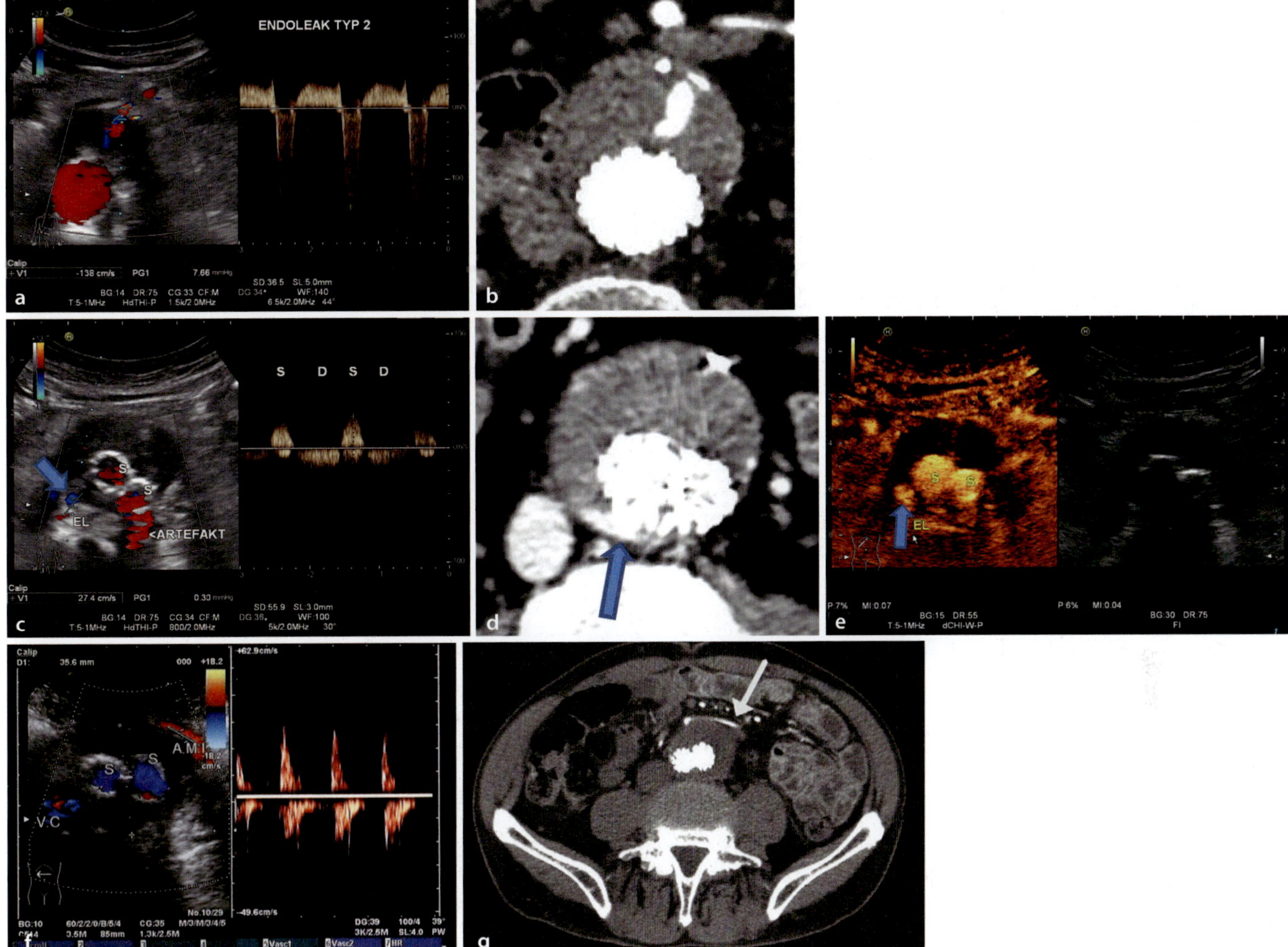

Fig. 6.82a–g (Atlas) Type II endoleak – high-flow versus low-flow (comparison with CT findings).
a Most endoleaks fed by an inferior mesenteric artery are high-flow endoleaks. In the case shown, peak systolic velocity (PSV) is 138 cm. Such high-flow endoleaks rarely close spontaneously, even if only a small portion of the excluded aneurysm sac shows flow signals.
b The CT angiogram confirms that flow is confined to a small portion of the aneurysm sac; however, flow into the sac is already seen during the arterial phase. Follow-up 3 months later confirmed a persistent high-flow endoleak (based on duplex ultrasound criteria) and an 8-mm increase in the diameter of the residual aneurysm sac (not shown). Endoleak embolization was performed.
c Follow-up 6 months later shows a new low-flow endoleak with a PSV of 27 cm/s (fed by a lumbar artery, flow coded in blue). The endoleak is located more peripherally, posterior to one of the iliac limbs. There is a mirror artifact with red-coded flow (same flow direction as within the stent graft). The waveform demonstrates to-and-fro flow with systolic inflow (S) and diastolic outflow (D), confirming the endoleak (as this is a flow pattern that does not occur physiologically). This small endoleak requires monitoring but no treatment.
d In the CT angiogram, the small endoleak cannot be identified with certainty. In addition, there is a small posterior plaque, which may be mistaken for an endoleak (in conjunction with the findings of contrast-enhanced ultrasound (CEUS)). Note that, in contrast-enhanced CTA, an endoleak fed by a patent lumbar artery may be opacified rather late, i.e., during the venous phase or even later (due to longer transit time of the contrast microbubbles through lumbar arteries). As a result, such endoleaks may even be missed by CTA.
e The type II endoleak identified by color duplex imaging in this patient and fed by a lumbar artery is more conspicuous in the CEUS examination (arrow) compared with CTA.
f,g Patent inferior mesenteric artery, not classified as a relevant endoleak.
f Sonographic mapping of an isolated aneurysm sac after EVAR for flow (using a low pulse repetition frequency) should also include a search for patent lumbar arteries supplying the sac or for a patent inferior mesenteric artery. Retrograde flow in the inferior mesenteric artery (A.M.I; red-coded flow toward transducer) is always suspicious for an endoleak even if no flow is detectable in the aneurysm sac. Here, the Doppler waveform demonstrates to-and-fro flow in the patent inferior mesenteric artery.
g CT angiogram confirms patency of the inferior mesenteric artery but without passage of contrast medium into the aneurysm sac, confirming the sonographic findings (this constellation of findings is very rare)

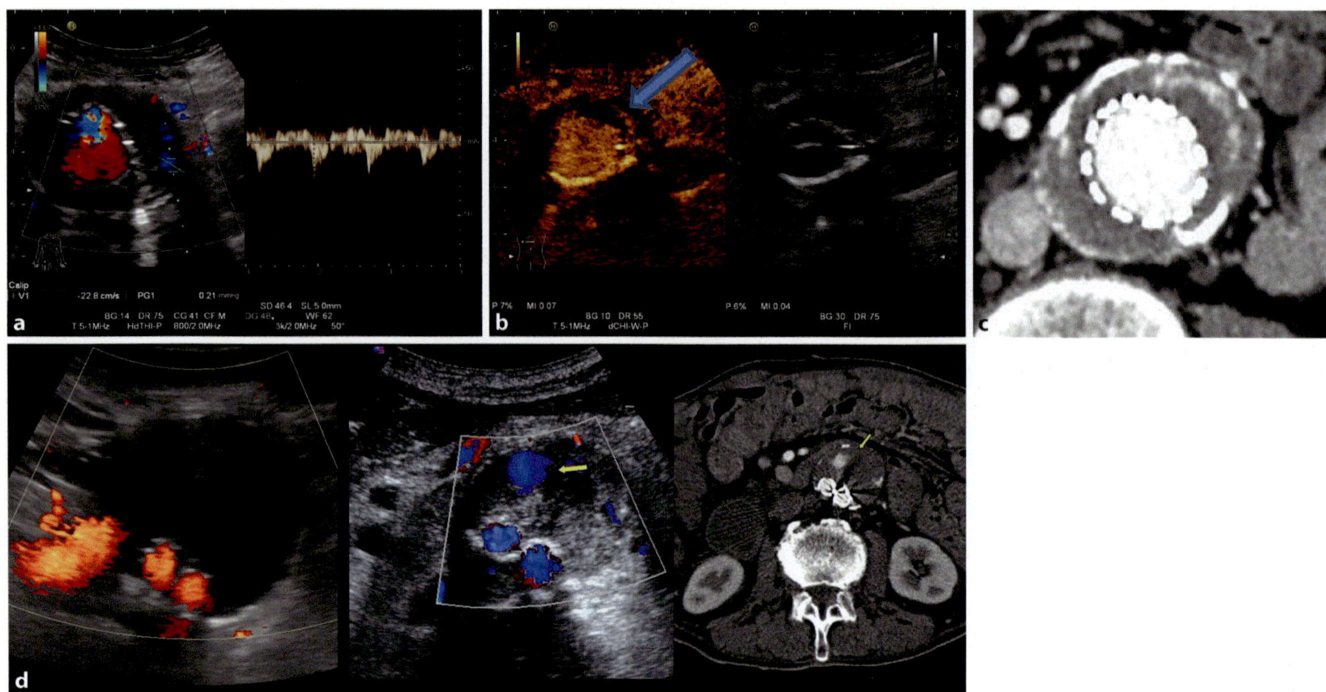

Fig. 6.83a–d (Atlas) Endoleak – stepwise diagnostic workup by CDUS, CEUS, CTA.
Stepwise diagnostic workup of a patient with unchanged diameter of abdominal aortic aneurysm (AAA) one year after endovascular aneurysm repair (EVAR): search for endoleak and evaluation of therapeutic relevance.
a Color duplex ultrasound (CDUS) identifies a small type II endoleak with to-and-fro flow.
b The endoleak is confirmed by contrast extravasation in the contrast-enhanced ultrasound (CEUS) examination.
c CT angiogram also shows contrast medium extravasation into the aneurysm sac.
Type II endoleak missed by CDUS but detected with CEUS.
d Color duplex examination (left image) following EVAR fails to identify an endoleak despite adequate settings. The two iliac limbs are depicted in the posterior portion of the aneurysm sac with the patent vena cava laterally (power mode display, which is less angle-dependent and improves the detection of slow-flowing blood; see Table 1.8). In the color duplex image obtained after contrast medium administration (middle), the signal enhancement reveals flow (arrow) in the aneurysm sac, consistent with a type II endoleak. The contrast-enhanced CT scan (right) confirms the endoleak (arrow) (Images courtesy of K. Pfister)

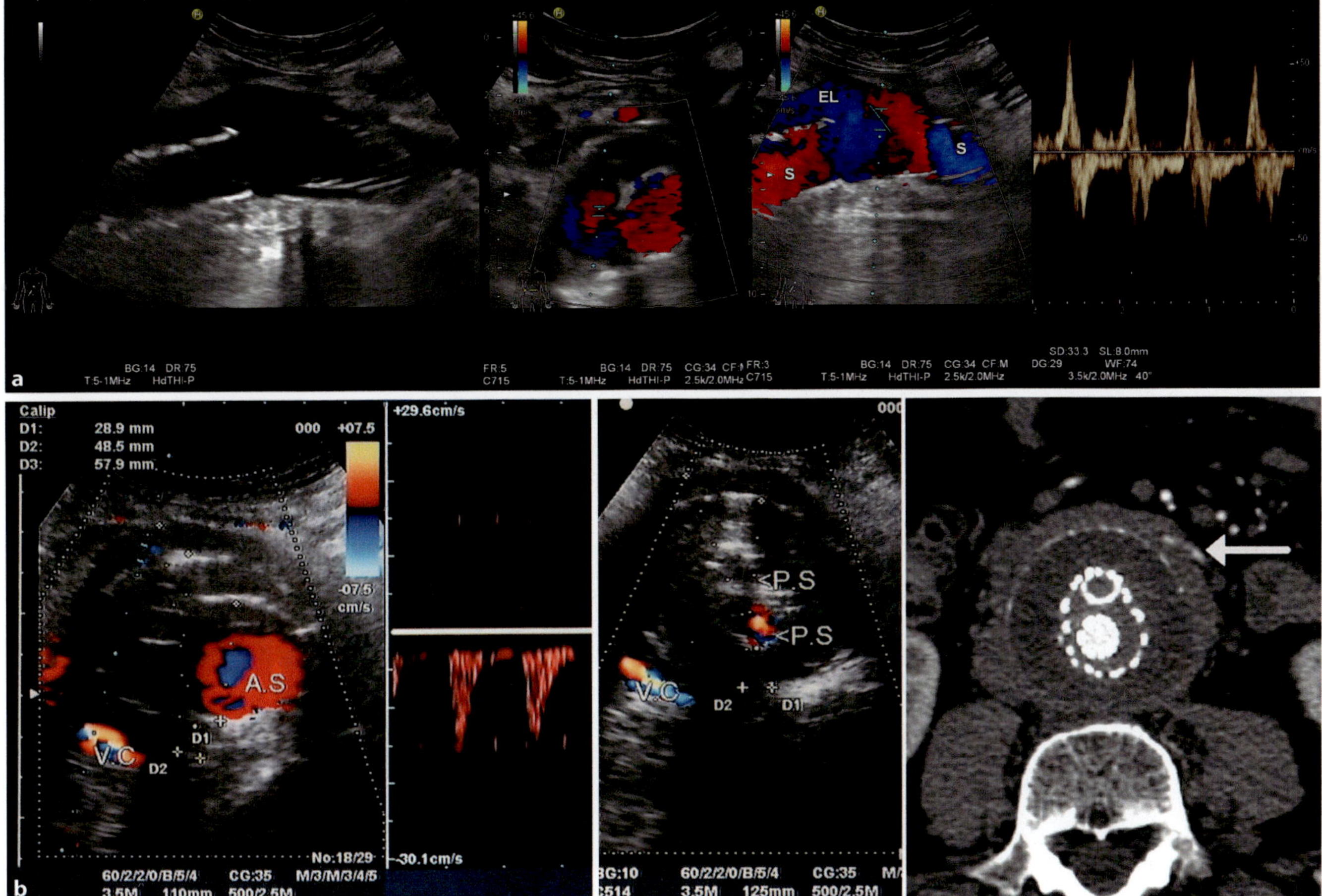

Fig. 6.84a, b (Atlas) Stent graft rupture after EVAR.
a The B-mode image already shows stent graft rupture; the color duplex images (transverse and longitudinal planes) confirm a type IV endoleak; and the waveform shows to-and-fro flow with a peak systolic velocity (PSV) of 60 cm/s.
Follow-up after EVAR – complication versus retroperitoneal fibrosis.
b Ultrasound follow-up 6 months after endovascular aneurysm repair (EVAR) identifies a margin of low echogenicity around the residual aneurysm sac. The residual diameter of the aneurysm sac in this plane (D2) is 48 mm (marked with calipers). The 1-cm margin around the stented aneurysm is most conspicuous anteriorly. Neither duplex ultrasound nor CT (rightmost image) demonstrates an endoleak. The Doppler waveform obtained from the area showing isolated color-coded flow signals within the hypoechoic margin (see sample volume) indicates normal intravascular blood flow and no to-and-fro flow (differential diagnosis: contained perforation). New-onset retroperitoneal fibrosis is suspected (differential diagnosis: perigraft reaction) and confirmed by ultrasound-guided biopsy. A.S = main stent graft body, V.C = vena cava.
The center right image (obtained at a slightly lower level) shows occlusion of the more anterior stent graft limb adjacent to the 1-cm hypoechoic margin surrounding the aneurysm sac (indicated by calipers); this is a complication occurring after EVAR. P.S = stent limb, V.C = vena cava.
The contrast-enhanced CT scan shows enhancing tissue around the aneurysm sac (interpreted to indicate inflammatory hyperemia). Retroperitoneal fibrosis also explains why shrinkage of the aneurysm sac after EVAR is minimal, even though neither contrast-enhanced CT nor color duplex imaging reveals an endoleak. Another CT finding consistent with retroperitoneal fibrosis is the demonstration of perfused arteries (arrow) coursing partially within the thickened margin and then being pushed back toward the aorta by perivascular fibrosis (see Figs. 6.37 and 6.85 (Atlas))

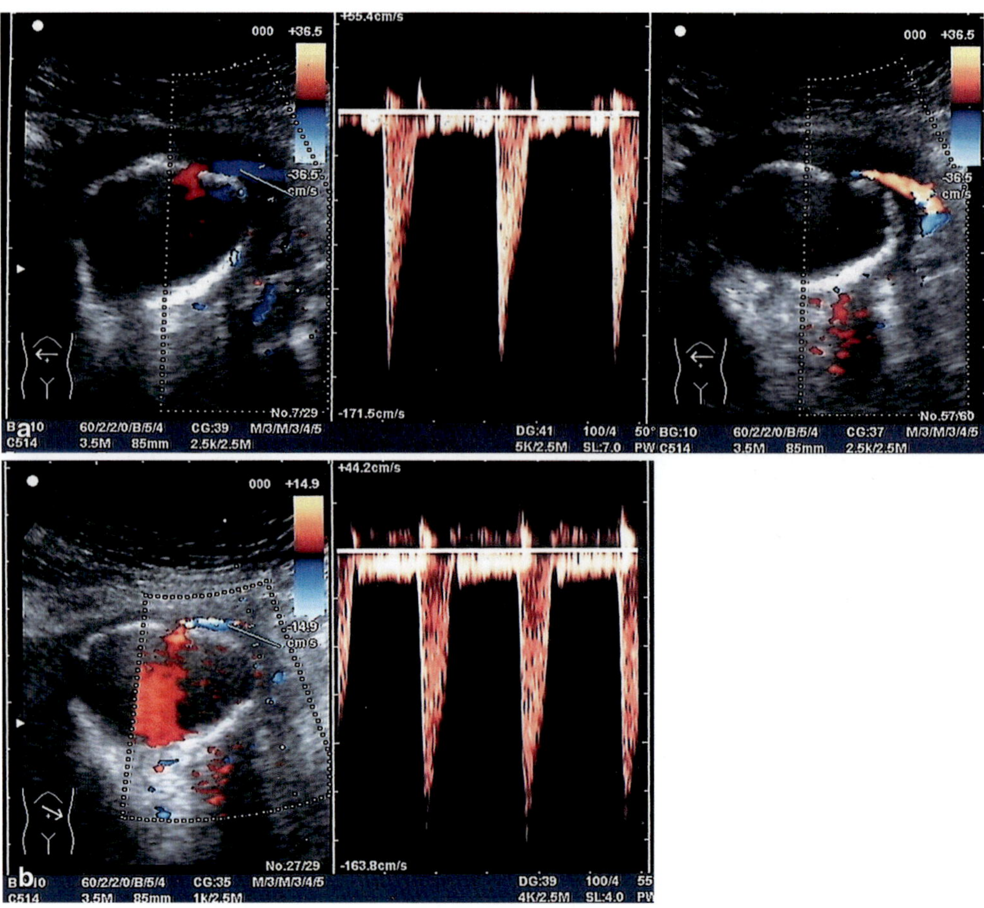

Fig. 6.85a, b (Atlas) Retroperitoneal fibrosis – differential diagnosis: perforated abdominal aortic aneurysm.
a Retroperitoneal fibrosis (Ormond's disease) may be visualized as a hypoechoic cap-like structure anterior to the aorta. This condition differs from aortitis and inflammatory aortic aneurysm in that the process also involves the vena cava, which is ensheathed by fibrotic tissue. The origin and proximal course of the inferior mesenteric artery are evaluated to establish the differential diagnosis. In the presence of retroperitoneal fibrosis, the mesenteric artery, after arising from the left lateral aspect of the aorta, is pushed against the aortic wall, where it runs for some centimeters before piercing through the hypoechoic fibrotic layer and continuing its intra-abdominal course in the mesentery. The image on the left depicts the inferior mesenteric artery arising from the aortic wall and the hypoechoic cap above. The image on the right obtained in slightly oblique orientation documents the course of the inferior mesenteric artery with flow displayed in blue (away from transducer). It is pushed against the aortic wall by the hypoechoic structure. The middle section shows the corresponding Doppler waveform.
b After a few months of cortisone treatment, the hypoechoic layers around the aorta and vena cava have markedly decreased in thickness, from 1 cm (see **a**) to 4 mm. However, the fibrotic tissue still pushes the inferior mesenteric artery against the aorta and its course remains unchanged. The Doppler waveform is from the inferior mesenteric artery

Fig. 6.86 (Atlas) Inflammatory abdominal aortic aneurysm. Transverse image (left) and longitudinal image (right) showing the typical appearance of an inflammatory abdominal aortic aneurysm (AAA). The aneurysm has a luminal diameter of 3.5 cm and exhibits atherosclerotic wall changes. The circumferential hypoechoic layer (1 cm) around the AAA confirms the inflammatory origin of the aneurysm. Furthermore, the presence of hyperechoic plaque allows identification of the intima and thus provides further evidence that the thickening is not due to thrombus (as it involves the arterial wall layer external to the intima; see Fig. 6.38)

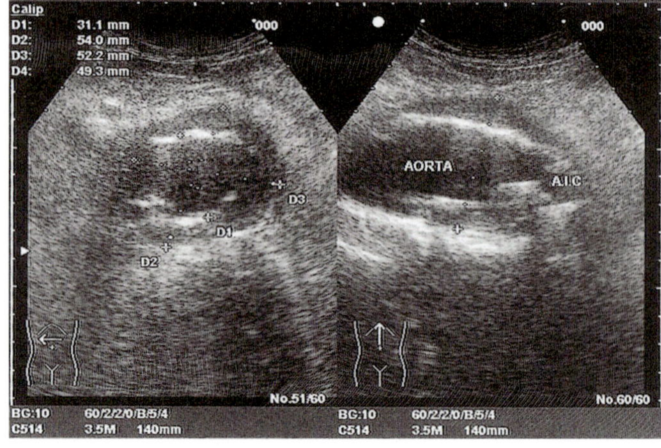

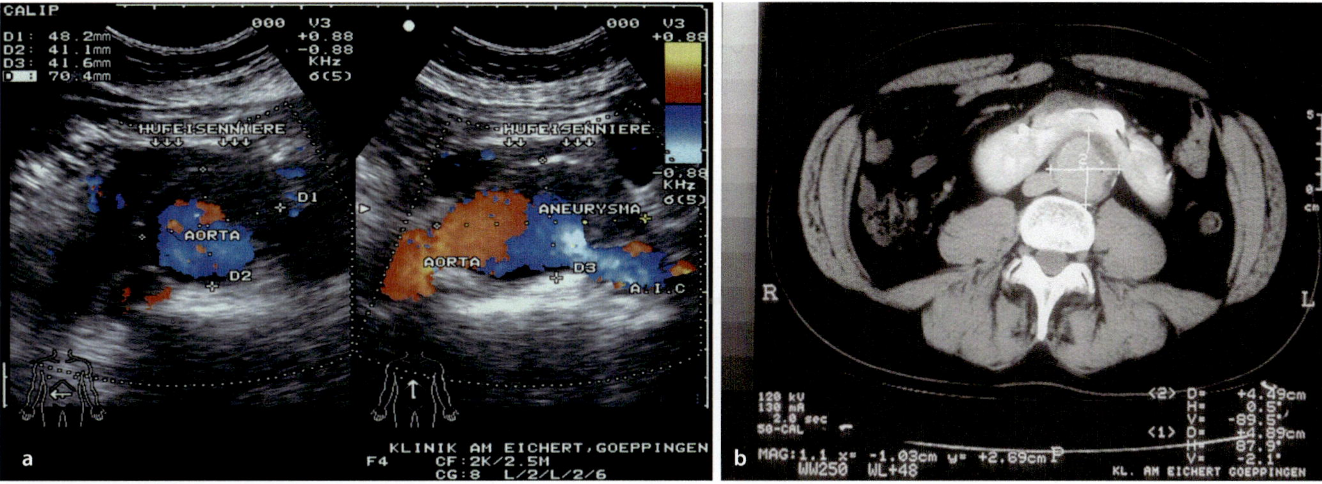

Fig. 6.87a, b (Atlas) Abdominal aortic aneurysm in a patient with horseshoe kidney.
a A horseshoe kidney is seen as a hypoechoic cap-like structure extending over the distal aorta. In the presence of a concomitant abdominal aortic aneurysm (AAA), as in this case, the abnormal kidney must be sonomorphologically differentiated from the aortic wall as well as from other retroperitoneal structures or contained aneurysm rupture.
b CT confirming AAA and horseshoe kidney

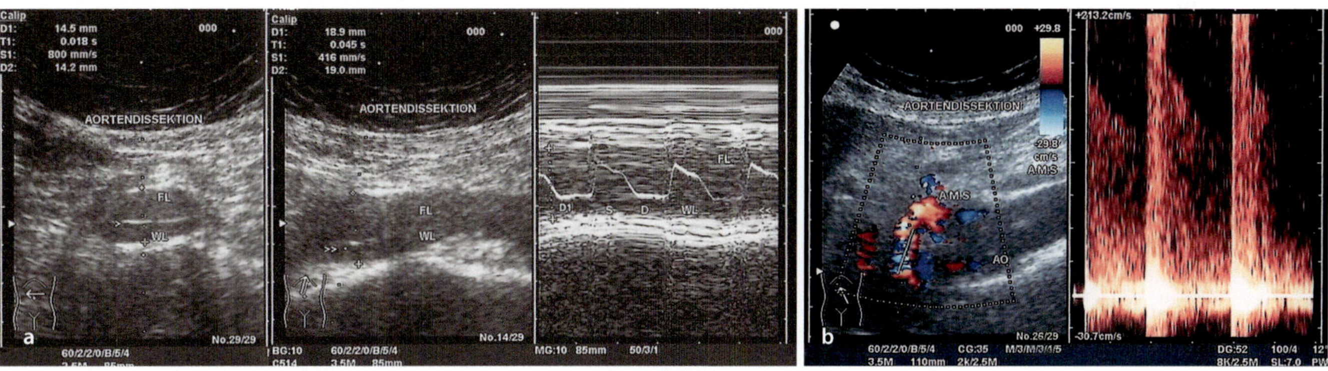

Fig. 6.88a–h (Atlas) Aortic dissection – dynamic versus static blood flow reduction.
a Aortic dissection can be demonstrated by B-mode ultrasound when the intimal flap is insonated at a right angle (transverse view on the left, longitudinal view in the middle). The time-motion mode on the right shows the systolic-diastolic flap movement in the lumen. Imaging at a perpendicular angle enables differentiation of the true (WL) and false lumen (FL). The false lumen is compressed as pressure increases during systole and expands again in diastole.
b The natural course and therapeutic measures in aortic dissection depend on the extent and involvement of aortic branches. Involvement of the superior mesenteric artery is associated with high-grade stenosis at the origin. Morphologically, the course of the intimal tear is difficult to identify. When the false lumen is located on the anterior side as in the case presented (see **a**), the superior mesenteric artery arises from the true lumen, and its origin is compressed by the false lumen or an intimal flap, resulting in flow obstruction with a typical stenotic waveform and a peak systolic velocity (PSV) of over 3 m/s (interpolated due to aliasing) (static flow reduction due to dissection membrane).
c Poststenotic Doppler waveform with the typical delay in systolic upstroke, turbulent flow, and a larger diastolic component. The color flow image shows the aorta (A) with the flap deep to the superior mesenteric artery.
d The Doppler waveform from the celiac trunk of the patient shows systolic deceleration with near-zero flow. This decrease in systolic flow velocity is due to intermittent obstruction of the celiac artery origin by the aortic intimal flap; normal orthograde flow during diastole occurs because of pressure reversal pushing the flap back into the lumen. This dangerous situation with imminent arterial occlusion cannot be adequately visualized by any of the merely morphologic imaging modalities and can only be identified on the basis of the hemodynamic information provided by spectral Doppler measurement (dynamic flow reduction due to dissection membrane).
e Diagram of type III aortic dissection according to De Bakey (examples in **b** and **c**). The mesenteric arteries arising from the true lumen are compressed by the false lumen or the intimal flap (From Heberer and van Dongen 1993).
f If dissection involves the origin of a renal artery, there may be superimposition of the Doppler frequency spectra from the true and false lumina or – depending on the re-entry site or the position of the sample volume in the dissected segment – to-and-fro flow as in the left renal artery shown.
g The waveform from a segmental artery in the left renal hilum demonstrates the typical postocclusive flow pattern with a reduced systolic upstroke and low PSV (25 cm/s) due to flow obstruction by the dissection.
h The right renal artery is not involved in the dissection and has a typical monophasic waveform with a PSV of 1 m/s. The further infrarenal course of the aortic dissection is shown in longitudinal (right center) and transverse planes (rightmost). The change in color coding may be due to the position of the re-entry site or physiologic flow reversal (early diastolic reflux)

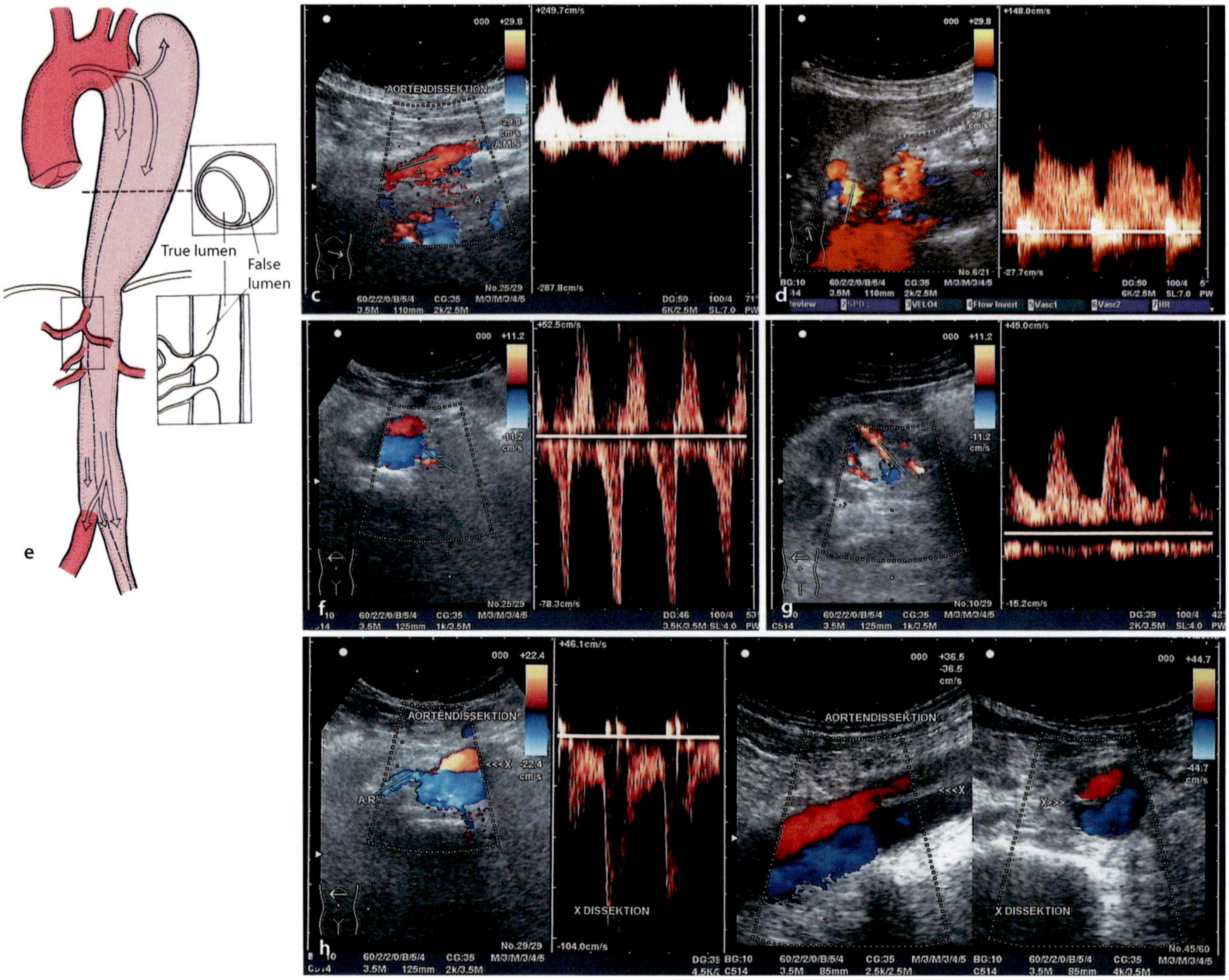

6

Fig. 6.88 (continued)

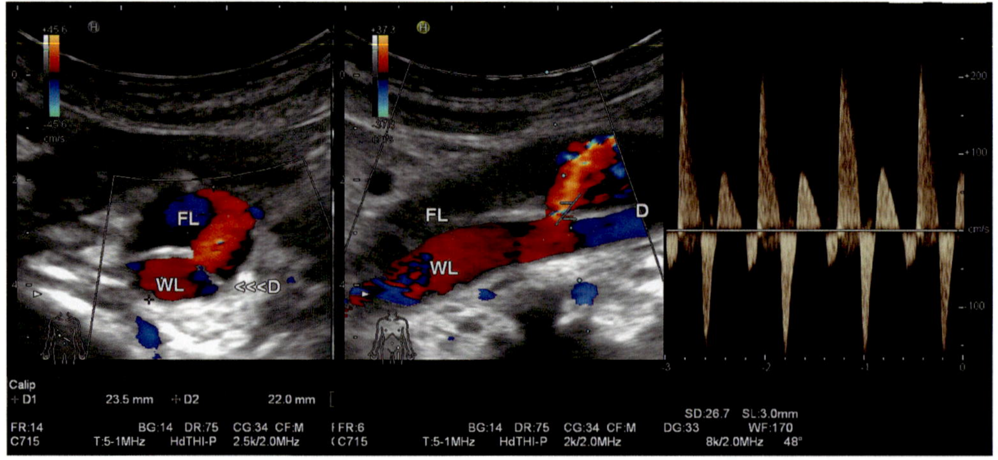

Fig. 6.89 (Atlas) Infrarenal dissection. Rare example of isolated infrarenal dissection with partial thrombosis. There is marked to-and-fro flow at the entry site (systolic inflow and diastolic outflow with additional forward and backward flow during diastole). A re-entry site is not identifiable. D indicates the dissection membrane; the true lumen (WL) is compressed; and the false lumen (FL) is partially thrombosed

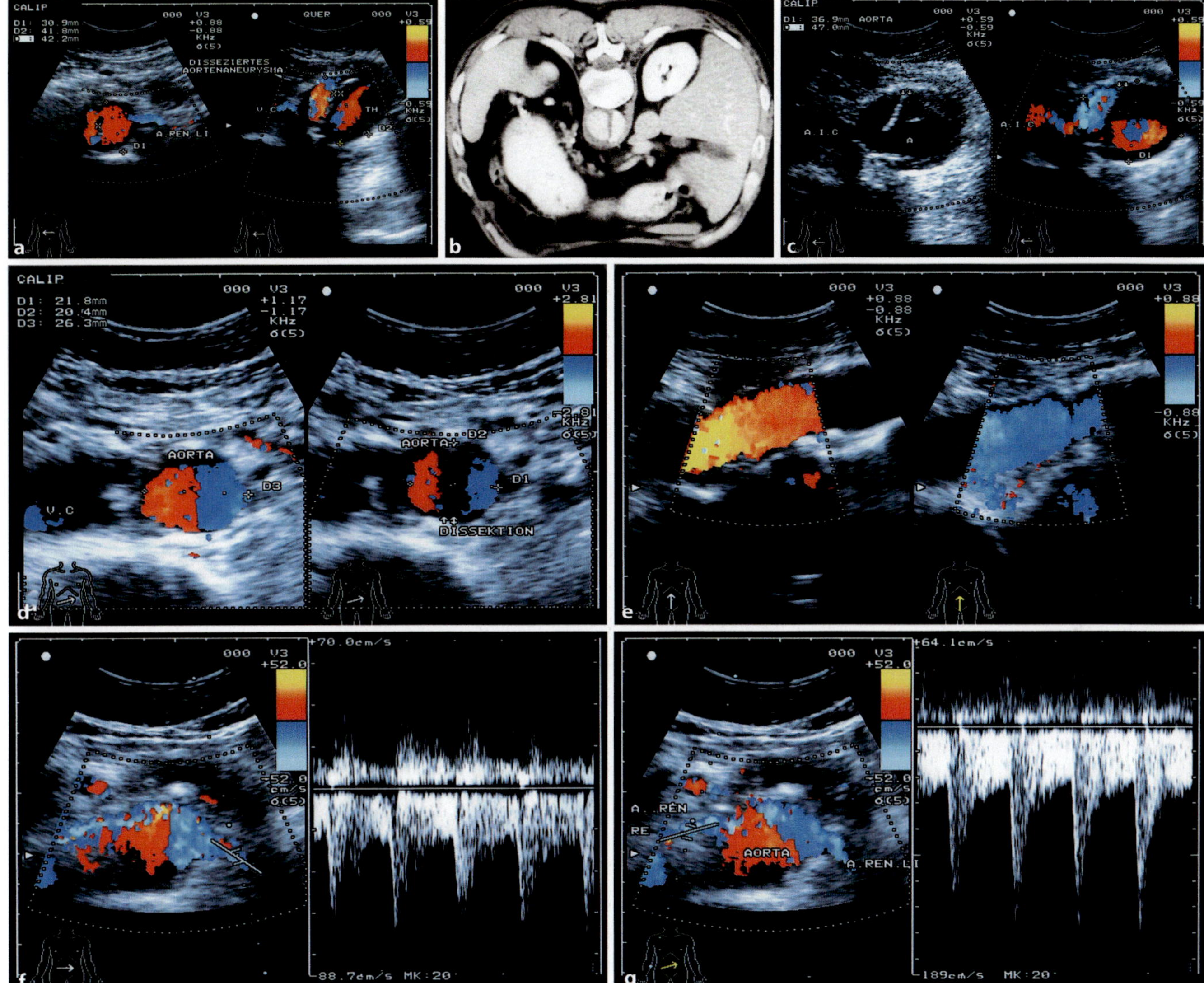

Fig. 6.90a–g (Atlas) Aortic dissection.

a Blood flow to the renal arteries is a crucial issue in the diagnostic evaluation of aortic dissection. At the level of the renal arteries (left image), both lumina of the dissected aorta exhibit antegrade flow, and the left renal artery (A.REN.LI) is displayed with blue-coded flow. The image on the right obtained 5 cm below clearly depicts the flap between the two lumina. The overall diameter is dilated to 42 mm due to aneurysmal changes.
b CT scan of dissected aortic aneurysm with visualization of the intimal flap.
c The second important diagnostic task in aortic dissection is to determine the relationship to the origins of the iliac arteries. Here, the dilated and dissected aorta with thrombotic wall deposits gives off the common iliac artery (A.I.C) on the right side, and the dissected aneurysm (A) extends into the left common iliac artery. The gray-scale image (left) depicts the flap and the thrombotic portion, while the color duplex image (right) shows the perfused lumina.

Aortic dissection after intervention.

d Aortic dissection as in the preceding example but with red-coded flow in the true lumen and blue-coded, retrograde flow in the false lumen. The image on the left fails to depict the intimal flap about 3 cm below the renal artery origins The image on the right demonstrates partial thrombosis of the false lumen just above the bifurcation. These findings reflect the status post surgery with closure of the thoracic entry.
e Following closure of the thoracic entry, the false lumen supplying the renal artery is filled retrogradely through the abdominal re-entry. The longitudinal image (right) demonstrates forward, red-coded flow in the true lumen and retrograde, blue flow in the false lumen (transducer moved to the left side).
f Patency of the false lumen is maintained through the outflow of blood into the left renal artery arising from it. The false lumen and the left renal artery are depicted with flow coded in blue. The Doppler waveform shows decreased flow with a peak systolic velocity (PSV) of 60 cm/s in the left renal artery compared to the contralateral side.
g The true lumen (red) gives off the blue-coded right renal artery, which arises from the posterior aspect and has a PSV of 165 cm/s and an end-diastolic velocity (EDV) of 45 cm/s

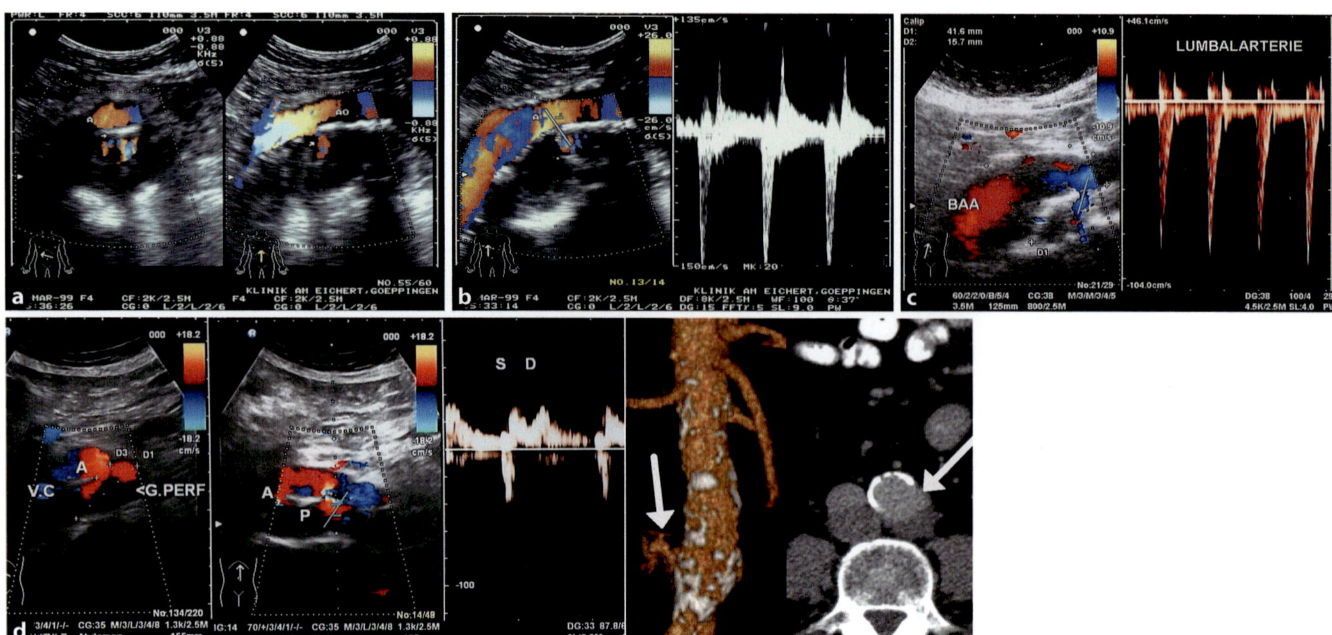

◻ Fig. 6.91a–d (Atlas) Aortic perforation.
a Diagnostic evaluation of suspected perforation in the abdomen and pelvis may be impaired by a poor insonation window or the occurrence of artifacts. Color duplex imaging is useful for demonstrating leakage, but the high susceptibility to artifacts in the abdomen makes it necessary to always confirm the color flow findings by spectral Doppler interrogation. In the example, color duplex imaging of a patient presenting with back pain identifies a leak in the posterior aortic wall with color-coded flow signals distal to it. Alternatively, these signals may represent mirror artifacts caused by the strong reflection of the aortic wall.
b The Doppler waveform (right) obtained from this area confirms the perforation by demonstrating to-and-fro flow (systolic influx with reflux throughout diastole), as it is also typical of pseudoaneurysm.
Differential diagnosis: aortic perforation – lumbar artery.
c Posteroinferior to a 41-mm infrarenal abdominal aortic aneurysm (BAA) a hypoechoic area is depicted adjacent to the aortic bifurcation (differential diagnosis: hematoma – retroperitoneal fibrosis – inflammatory vascular disease). As in **b** above, color flow imaging depicts blood flow signals coming out of the aorta (blue with sample volume) and passing the hypoechoic area. The Doppler waveform (right) shows the typical flow pattern of a lumbar artery, thus ruling out contained aortic perforation with typical to-and-fro flow.
Mycotic aortic perforation.
d The transverse and longitudinal color flow images show flow coded in red posterior to the aorta (P in the longitudinal image). Part of the escaped blood posterior to the aorta (A) is thrombosed and has low echogenicity. The Doppler waveform from the site of the leak (indicated by D3 in the transverse image) shows the characteristic to-and-fro flow of contained perforation (same as in pseudoaneurysm) with flow out of the artery in systole (S) and back into the artery in diastole (D). The longitudinal CT reconstruction of the aorta shows the site of perforation (arrow) in the distal aorta just above the bifurcation. The axial CT scan confirms the contained perforation (arrow) with perfused and thrombosed portions

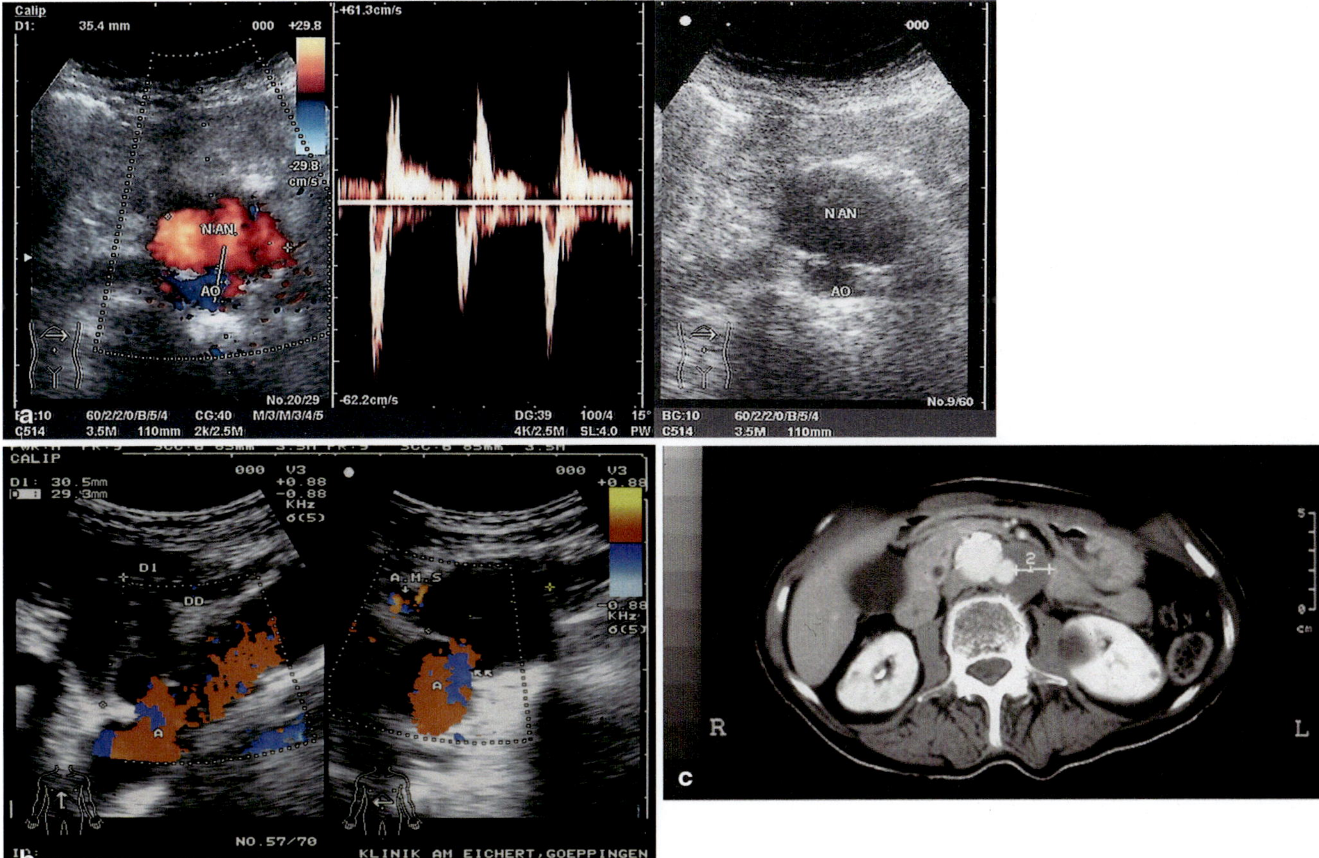

Fig. 6.92a–c (Atlas) Suture aneurysm after placement of a straight stent graft.
a Sonographic follow-up after aortic stent graft placement (e.g., for aneurysm) is indicated at 6-month intervals because an untreated suture aneurym, in particular at the superior anastomosis (N.AN), can lead to duodenal perforation, a potentially life-threatening complication. The anastomoses are evaluated in longitudinal and transverse planes for the presence of hypoechoic mushroom-like structures indicating a contained perforation or suture aneurysm. Color duplex imaging shows paravascular flow at the anastomosis, and the Doppler waveform from this site shows the flow profile characteristic of a pseudoaneurysm.
b With progressive thrombosis, the color-coded area becomes smaller and the aneurysm is more difficult to differentiate from other hypoechoic perivascular structures. In this setting, a suture aneurysm is suggested by a color-coded area extending beyond the wall directly next to the suture line (arrow).
c CT confirming the suture aneurysm with nearly complete thrombosis (2)

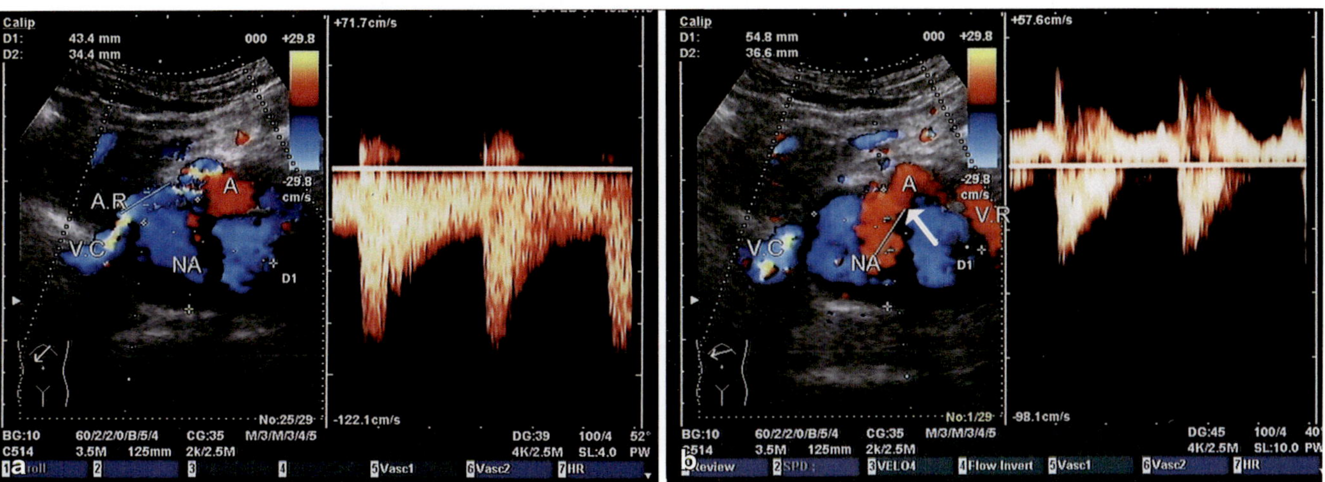

Fig. 6.93a, b (Atlas) Suture aneurysm after placement of a straight stent graft.
a Patient with suture aneurysm after implantation of a straight stent graft. The B-mode image shows a large hypoechoic area at the level of the renal artery origins with flow in the color duplex examination, consistent with a large retroperitoneal suture aneurysm. Doppler measurement in this area allows good differentiation of the suture aneurysm (NA) and renal artery (A.R).
b Unlike the waveform from the renal artery origin (A, see **a**), the Doppler waveform from the site of aortic leakage into the suture aneurysm (arrow) shows to-and-fro flow

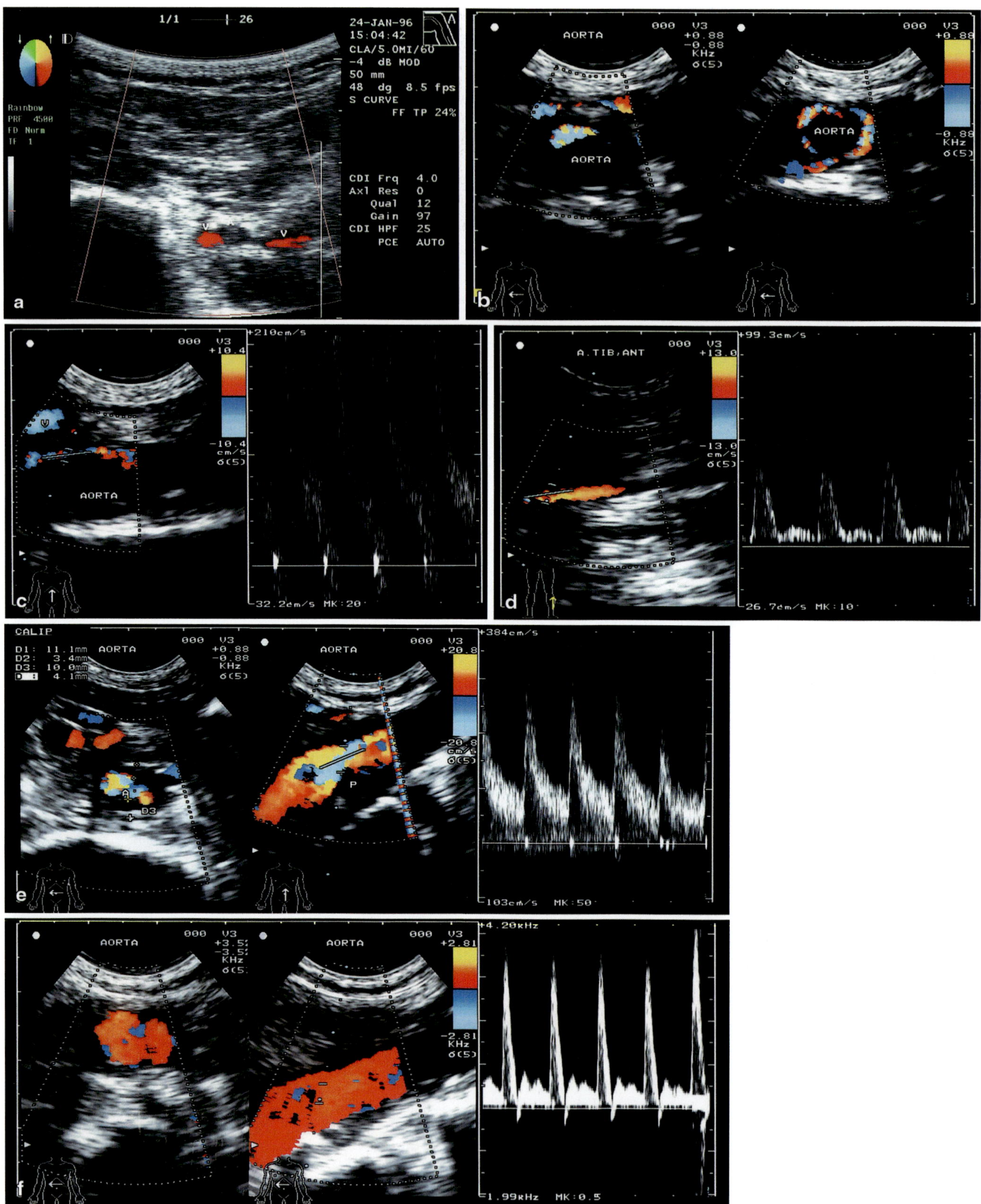
a
1/1 26
24-JAN-96
15:04:42
CLA/5.0MI/60
-4 dB MOD
50 mm
48 dg 8.5 fps
S CURVE
FF TP 24%
CDI Frq 4.0
Axl Res 0
Qual 12
Gain 97
CDI HPF 25
PCE AUTO
Rainbow
PRF 4500
V
b
AORTA
AORTA
AORTA
c
AORTA
+210cm/s
-32.2cm/s MK:20
d
A.TIB.ANT
+99.3cm/s
-26.7cm/s MK:10
e
CALIP
D1: 11.1mm
D2: 3.4mm
D3: 10.0mm
D3
AORTA
AORTA
P
+384cm/s
-103cm/s MK:50
f
AORTA
AORTA
+4.20kHz
1.99kHz MK:0.5

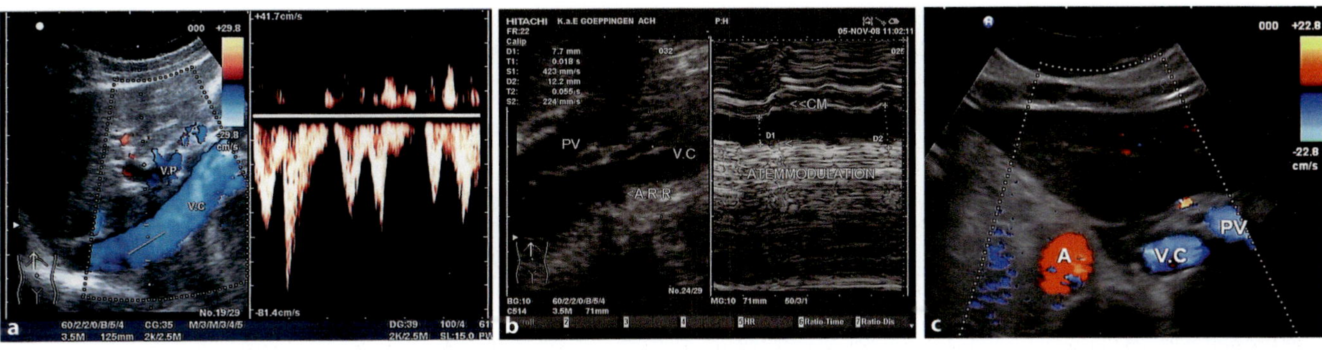

Fig. 6.95a–c (Atlas) Vena cava

a The cross-sectional area and flow velocity in the vena cava (V.C) vary with respiration. Blood flow is markedly faster during inspiration. In addition, blood flow is subject to cardiac (atrial) pulsatility. The Doppler waveform typically shows two peaks, one during systole and the other upon opening of the atrioventricular valves (W-shaped waveform). There is marked reduction, cessation, or even a short reversal of flow during atrial contraction.

b The usual oval cross section of the vena cava can show diameter variation due to changes in intravascular pressure during the respiratory cycle (W-shaped waveform); in addition, there may be variation due to cardiac pulsatility, indicated by "<<CM" in the time-motion display (right). **Situs inversus.**

c There are some extreme anatomic variants of the vena cava; these are rare and include absence, doubling with one vena cava on either side of the aorta, and a single vena cava to the left of the aorta as in the case shown (here, in accordance with ultrasound convention, the left-lying vena cava is displayed to the right of the aorta). In complete situs inversus, the liver is located in the left upper abdomen, and the portal vein (PV) also ascends toward the liver hilum on the left side

Fig. 6.94a–f (Atlas) Aortic thrombus (thrombolytic treatment) – aortic stenosis.

a 35-year-old woman presenting with very severe acute foot and calf pain due to bilateral occlusion of the below-knee arteries. For illustration, the occlusion of the anterior tibial artery is shown in transverse orientation. The artery blocked by a hypoechoic thromboembolus exhibits no flow, while there is flow coded in red in the paired anterior tibial vein (V) to the right and left of the artery. The acoustic shadow to the left of the tibial vein is caused by the fibula.

b In this case, embolic occlusion of the below-knee arteries is due to a thrombus in the distal aorta. The transverse image (left) depicts the thrombus 4 cm above the bifurcation. It is attached to the wall posteriorly with flow being confined to its anterior aspect (blue with aliasing). The right image depicts the hypoechoic thrombus in the aorta just above the bifurcation surrounded by flow with turbulent and high-frequency components on all sides.

c The longitudinal image shows the thrombus occupying most of the aortic lumen with some residual flow anteriorly. The Doppler waveform demonstrates marked flow acceleration with an end-diastolic velocity (EDV) of 50 cm/s and a peak systolic velocity (PSV) of 210 cm/s (aliasing); the waveform is monophasic. (Only the proximal segment of the aorta is depicted with color coding due to the small color box used.).

d On the basis of the duplex ultrasound findings obtained in this patient, angiography of the aorta was dispensed with because the manipulations might have triggered further distal embolism. Instead, bilateral intra-arterial thrombolytic treatment was initiated, which led to resolution of the thromboemboli in the below-knee arteries, as illustrated by the Doppler waveform from the recanalized anterior tibial artery. The waveform still shows abnormally increased diastolic flow, which is due to residual stenosis of the aorta and reactive hyperemia.

e Local thrombolytic treatment also had a systemic effect, resulting in dissolution of the thrombus in the aorta. The transverse image (left) and longitudinal image (right) still depict residual marginal thrombotic deposits. The color coding shows the patent lumen with aliasing (yellow – light blue) due to residual stenosis. The Doppler waveform indicates high-grade residual stenosis with a PSV of 300 cm/s and a monophasic flow profile.

f The patient refused further treatment. Follow-up 2 weeks later demonstrated autolysis of the residual thrombus in the distal aorta. The longitudinal image (middle section) shows hyperechoic posterior plaque and some residual, hypoechoic thrombotic deposits on the left wall with little luminal narrowing. Neither the Doppler waveform nor color duplex imaging demonstrates hemodynamically significant stenosis

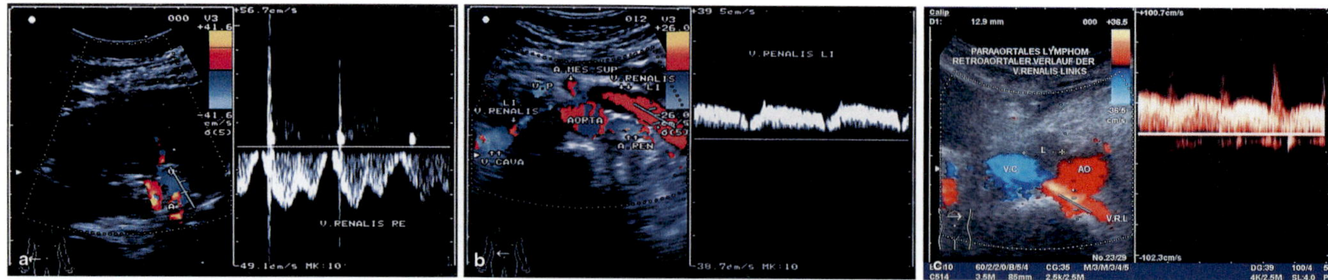

Fig. 6.96a–c (Atlas) Right renal vein.
a Cardiac pulsatility and respiratory phasicity of blood flow are transmitted as far as the right renal vein at the hilum (vein: blue, segmental artery: red).
Left renal vein.
b Cardiac pulsatility is typically lost in the left renal vein due to the narrow passage between the superior mesenteric artery and aorta. Instead, its flow variation is determined by the aortic pulse. Posterior to the red-coded renal vein, the renal artery is depicted in blue. The renal vein has a rather large caliber in front of the narrow passage and then continues as a relatively thin vessel (blue) to the vena cava.
Retroaortic left renal vein.
c If the left renal vein (V.R.L; red, flow toward transducer) is not identified between the aorta and superior mesenteric artery, the examiner must try and locate its entry into the vena cava (V.C) posterior to the aorta (AO). Identification of a retroaortic left renal vein is important prior to resection of an aortic aneurysm but is often an incidental finding, as in the case presented, where the atypical entry was identified in a patient in whom vascular sonography was performed prior to ultrasound-guided biopsy of a lymphoma (L)

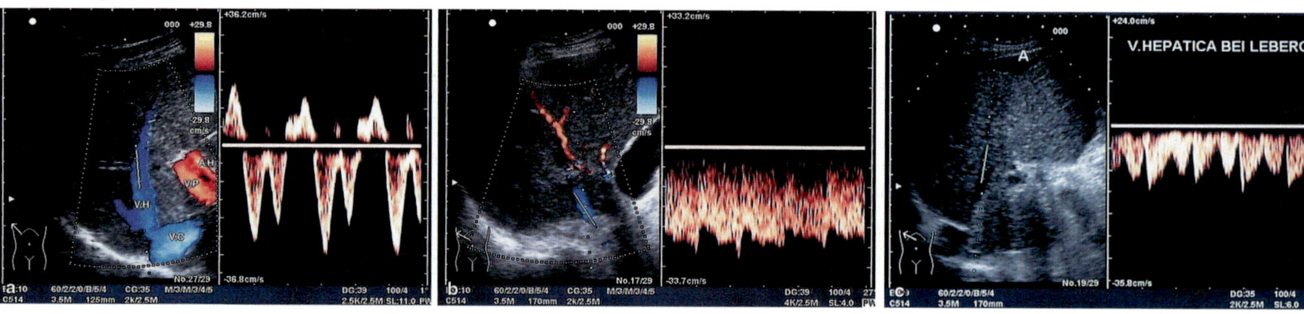

Fig. 6.97 (Atlas) Normal and abnormal Doppler waveforms of hepatic veins.
a W-shaped Doppler waveform with a first hepatofugal flow peak in systole, a second hepatofugal peak upon opening of the atrioventricular valves, and hepatopedal flow during atrial contraction. An abnormal waveform resembling a sinus wave with to-and-fro flow in the extreme case is seen in patients with right ventricular failure.
Abnormal waveform of hepatic veins in liver cirrhosis.
b The right hepatic vein in a patient with Child A liver cirrhosis scanned from the intercostal approach shows only residual cardiac pulsatility. The associated loss of parenchymal elasticity primarily prevents the decrease in flow velocity during atrial contraction, resulting in an increasingly band-like spectrum from the entry into the vena cava to peripheral branches (intermediate hepatic vein in blue, portal vein branch in red).
Waveform of hepatic vein in liver cirrhosis.
c Biphasic flow profile in the hepatic vein in a patient with liver cirrhosis (intercostal approach). Though the curve is flattened due to stiffening of the liver, some residual cardiac pulsatility is still present, and the curve is not as flat as in **b** (A, ascites) (same patient as in Fig. 6.101 (Atlas))

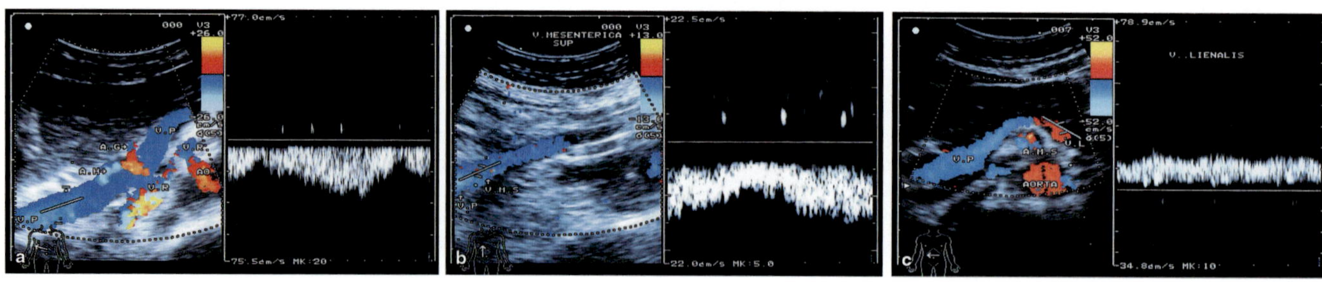

Fig. 6.98a–c (Atlas) Portal vein and its tributaries.
a The Doppler waveform from the portal vein is characterized by relatively wide variation in flow velocity, but flow is typically hepatocentral and slower during inspiration.
b The respiratory variation in blood flow velocity continues into the superior mesenteric vein, which is depicted to the right of the superior mesenteric artery.
c The splenic vein (V.L) is depicted at the lower edge of the pancreas with flow in red. It crosses over the root of the superior mesenteric artery (A.M.S) to enter (displayed in blue) the portal vein (V.P). The respiratory variation in flow velocity may continue into the splenic vein

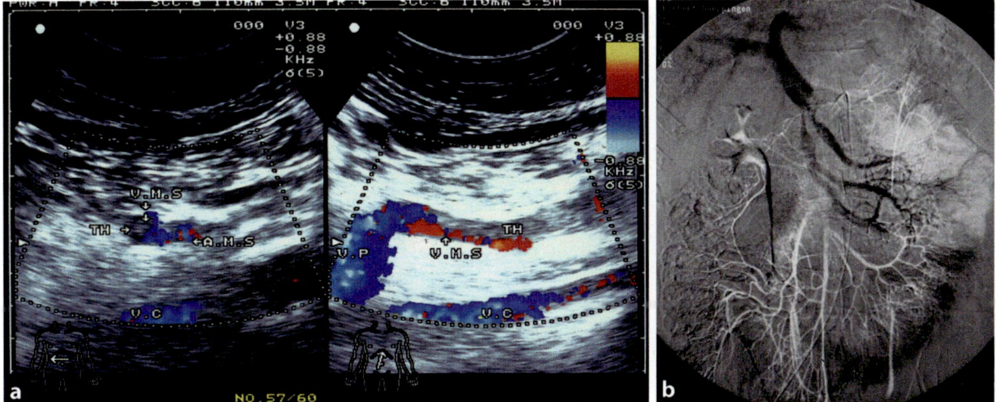

Fig. 6.99a, b (Atlas) Mesenteric vein thrombosis – surrounded by flowing blood.
a The extent of thrombosis and collateralization determine whether the clinical manifestation will be mild with flu-like symptoms or severe with an acute abdomen due to intestinal necrosis. A 38-year-old patient with diffuse abdominal pain was treated conservatively for several days. Sonography was performed to rule out appendicitis and pancreatitis. Closer evaluation of the superior mesenteric vein by color duplex imaging revealed thrombosis of individual jejunal vein branches with protrusion of a thrombus into the trunk of the superior mesenteric vein. Mural mesenteric vein thrombosis obstructs blood flow. Prompt initiation of full heparinization is necessary to prevent further appositional thrombus growth and intestinal necrosis.
b Digital subtraction angiogram confirms partial mesenteric vein thrombosis

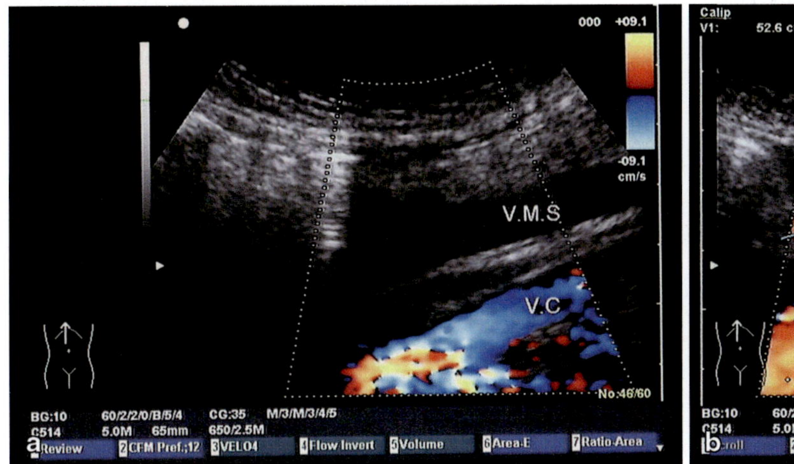

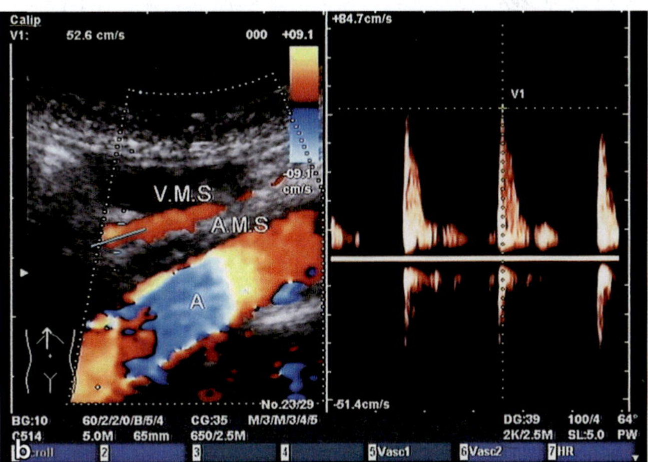

Fig. 6.100a–d (Atlas) Superior mesenteric vein thrombosis.
a Complete thrombosis of the superior mesenteric vein (V.M.S) is indicated by the absence of flow signals despite a low pulse repetition frequency (indicated by aliasing in the vena cava, V.C). The vena cava is depicted posterior to the superior mesenteric vein.
b The superior mesenteric artery (A.M.S, red) comes into view when the transducer is moved to the left side. There is aliasing in the aorta posteriorly (A). With this transducer position, the superior mesenteric artery appears deep to the confluence of the superior mesenteric vein (V.M.S) and the splenic vein. Occluding thrombosis of the superior mesenteric vein affects flow in the artery, giving rise to a preocclusive thump pattern. Peak systolic velocity (PSV) is markedly reduced (50 cm/s) and, along with the loss of diastolic flow, suggests high outflow resistance. Surprisingly, the 17-year-old woman had only mild diffuse abdominal pain (of the enteritic type) and mild meteorism, but no signs of peritonitis; there was mild leukocytosis without acidosis, and lactate levels were normal. The clinical symptoms persisted for 6 weeks before the diagnosis was made. Preexisting portal vein thrombosis in an abnormal vein with severe ectasia led to the formation of collateral pathways, mainly via the inferior mesenteric vein, which is why acute mesenteric vein thrombosis did not cause intestinal necrosis in this patient.
c, d Portal vein thrombosis.
c In portal vein thrombosis, there is a marked compensatory increase in blood flow in the hepatic artery with a peak systolic velocity (PSV) of approx. 2 m/s and an end-diastolic velocity (EDV) of 90 cm/s. The thrombosed portal vein (PV) is indicated by calipers.
d Good collateral drainage through small veins is confirmed by the depiction of flow in the hepatoduodenal ligament (continuous high-frequency flow with a velocity of 50 cm/s) and around the gallbladder

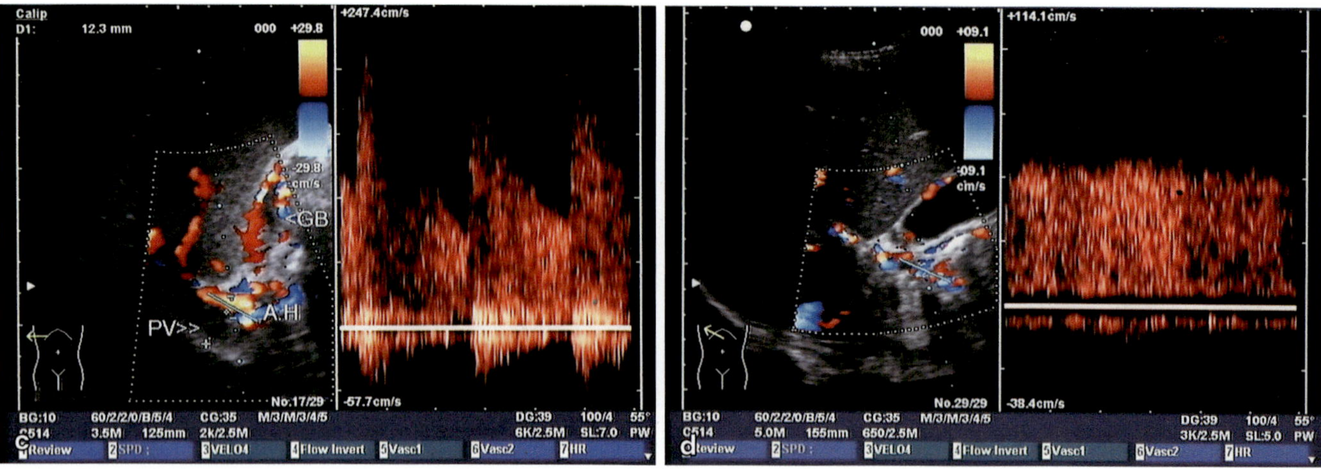

Fig. 6.100 (continued)

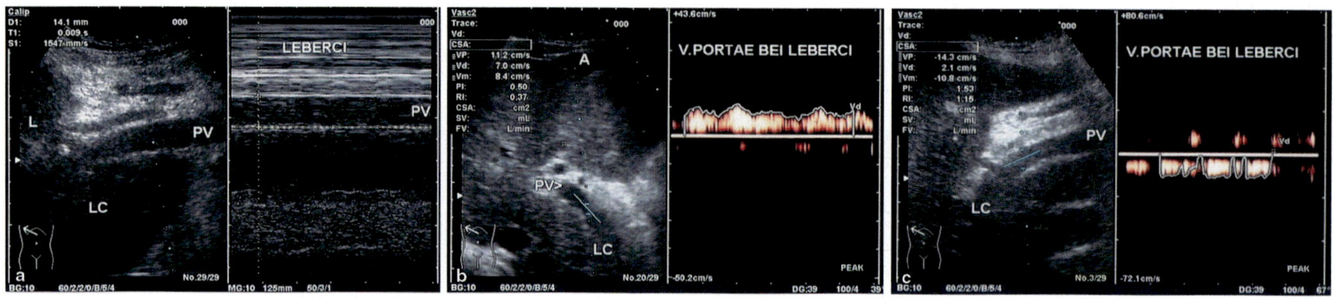

Fig. 6.101a–c (Atlas) Portal hypertension.
a Loss of respiratory diameter variation in gray-scale ultrasound is a sign of portal hypertension. In the example, the time-motion mode demonstrates a constant diameter of 14 mm of the portal vein (PV).
b The patient presented has portal hypertension and Child C liver cirrhosis. The peak flow velocity is markedly reduced to 11.2 cm/s with a mean flow velocity of 8.4 cm/s (intercostal transducer position). Other signs of liver cirrhosis depicted by ultrasound are perihepatic ascites (A) and the enlarged caudate lobe (LC). The congestion index is markedly increased to 0.2 cm × s.
c A reduced increase in postprandial flow velocity (mean flow velocity of 10.8 cm/s) is another sign of portal hypertension. With an unchanged diameter of 14 mm, postprandial flow velocity increases by only 20% (versus >60% in normal individuals). For didactic purposes, views of the portal vein from two transducer positions (**c**: subcostal; **b**: intercostal, from the flank) are shown with identical sample volumes in the vein. The intercostal approach permits smaller Doppler angles (38° versus 67° in the example), thus yielding more accurate flow velocity measurements. Serial examinations should be performed with identical transducer positions

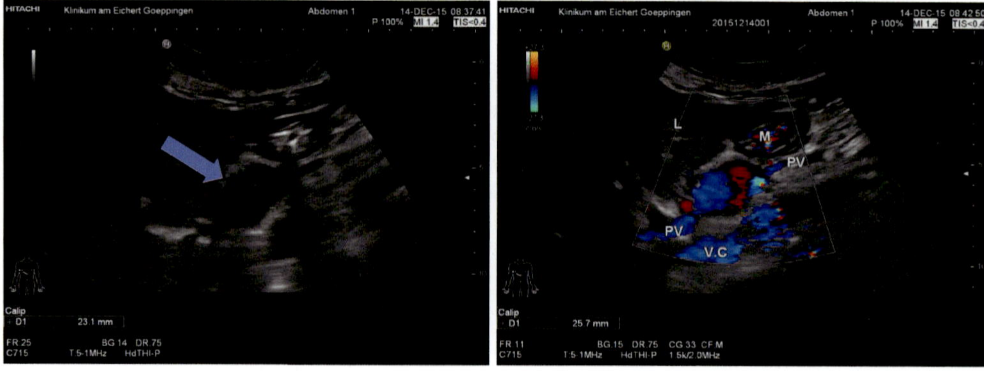

Fig. 6.102 (Atlas) Portal vein aneurysm.
Gray-scale image (left, arrow) and color duplex image (right) show a portal vein aneurysm measuring 25 mm in diameter; which is more than 4 times the normal portal vein (PV) diameter adjacent to the aneurysm (VC, vena cava; M, stomach; L, liver)

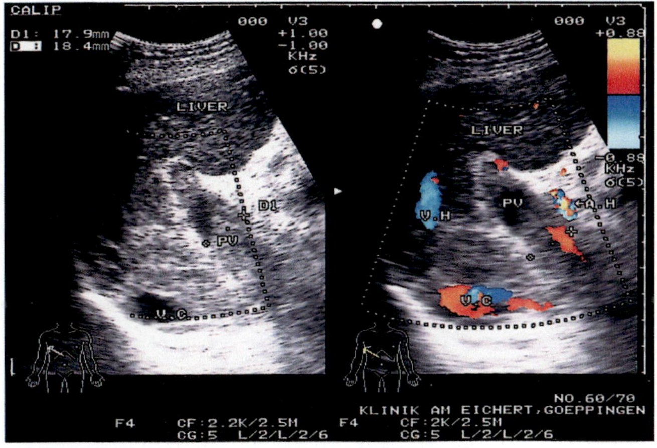

Fig. 6.103 (Atlas) Portal vein thrombosis.
Like thrombosis in other veins, portal vein thrombosis may already be suggested in the B-mode by a dilatation of the vessel and the presence of hyperechoic deposits in the lumen. Color duplex imaging from the intercostal approach using the liver as an acoustic window depicts flow signals (red, toward transducer). There is nearly complete thrombosis with residual flow close to the walls. The vena cava (V.C) is depicted posterior to the portal vein. There is aliasing in the hepatic artery (A.H) due to the low pulse repetition frequency (V.H, hepatic vein)

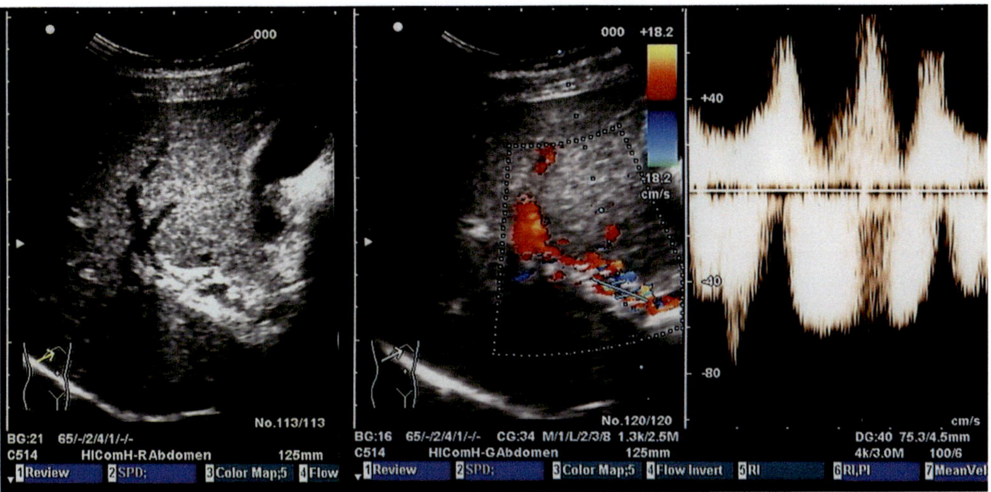

Fig. 6.104 (Atlas) Cavernous transformation of the portal vein.
Cavernous transformation is characterized by the failure to identify a normal-caliber portal vein in the liver hilum. Instead, there are numerous hyperechoic tubular structures with thickened walls occupying the portal vein bed, consistent with cavernous transformation secondary to portal vein thrombosis. The diagnosis is confirmed by the mosaic of colors seen in these channels in the color flow image. This color pattern does not indicate true flow reversal but only varying flow directions relative to the transducer in the tortuous venous channels.The Doppler waveform obtained from the transformed portal vein bed confirms blood flow toward and away from the transducer

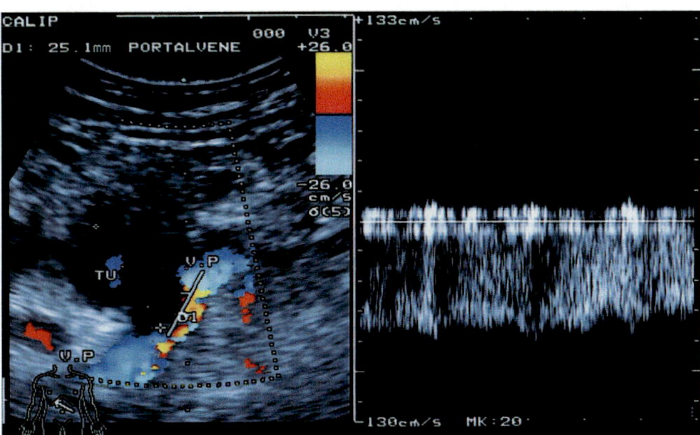

Fig. 6.105 (Atlas) Tumor compression.
Carcinoma of the pancreatic head with infiltration of the portal vein (V.P). The wall is poorly delineated and the lumen is compressed. Stenosis is suggested by aliasing in the color duplex image and in the Doppler waveform. There is an intratumoral vessel (TU) with flow coded in blue

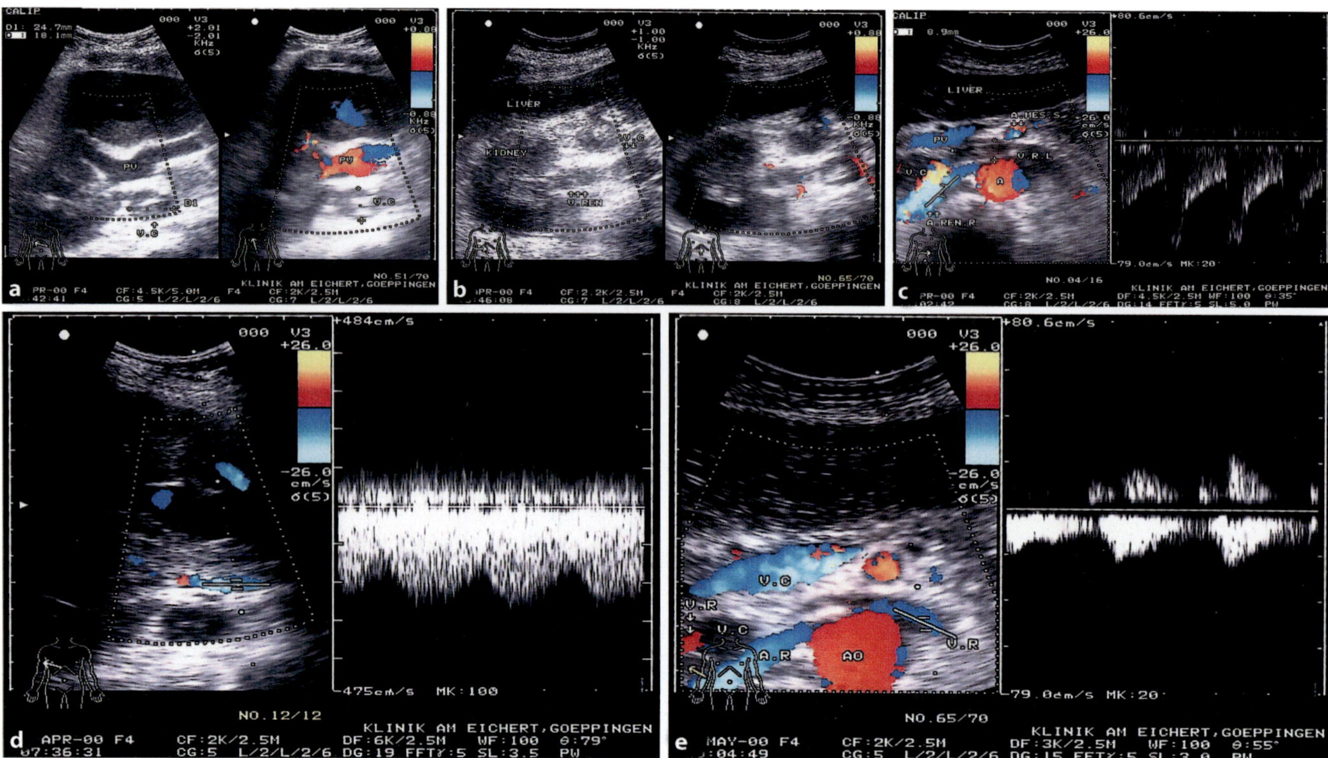

Fig. 6.106a–e (Atlas) Vena cava thrombosis.
Following laser-induced thermoablation of a large paracaval liver metastasis (presenting with right-sided upper abdominal pain), the patient developed subcapsular liver hemorrhage and complete thrombosis of the vena cava as a result of the local heat effect.
a B-mode image (left) and color duplex image (right) depicting the portal vein and vena cava (V.C) posterior to the liver hilum. The portal vein exhibits color-coded flow, while the vena cava (V.C) is depicted with hyperechoic internal echoes but without flow signals.
b The transverse view through the upper abdomen at a lower level shows residual flow near the walls displayed in red in the vena cava (right margin of right image) and no other flow signals. The images also depict the renal vein (V.REN) joining the vena cava. The flow signals next to the renal vein indicate venous return through retroperitoneal collaterals, chiefly the suprarenal vein.
c A tubular, hypoechoic structure without flow signals is depicted in the typical location of the left renal vein (V.R.L) between the superior mesenteric artery (A.MES.S) and the aorta (A), indicating thrombosis of this vein. The vein is markedly widened, and hyperechoic internal structures are depicted within the hypoechoic lumen. A vena cava thrombus next to the site of entry of the left renal vein is depicted with flow near the wall. Despite complete renal vein thrombosis, the right renal artery (A.REN.R) has a normal flow profile. This waveform and the uneventful clinical course (no increase in creatinine or urea despite complete bilateral renal vein thrombosis) confirm good collateral function of the sonographically depicted retroperitoneal veins, in particular the suprarenal vein and the capsular veins.
d Example of a retroperitoneal collateral vein with the typical venous flow signal depicted between the liver and the thrombosed vena cava (hypoechoic tubular structure posterior to the sample volume) in an oblique abdominal view.
e Color duplex examination 18 days later already demonstrates spontaneous recanalization of both renal veins with flow signals in the formerly completely thrombosed renal vein (V.R; see **c**) between the aorta and superior mesenteric artery; this finding is confirmed by the Doppler waveform. Blood flow is also demonstrated in the right renal vein (V.R/arrow), depicted in red near the left margin

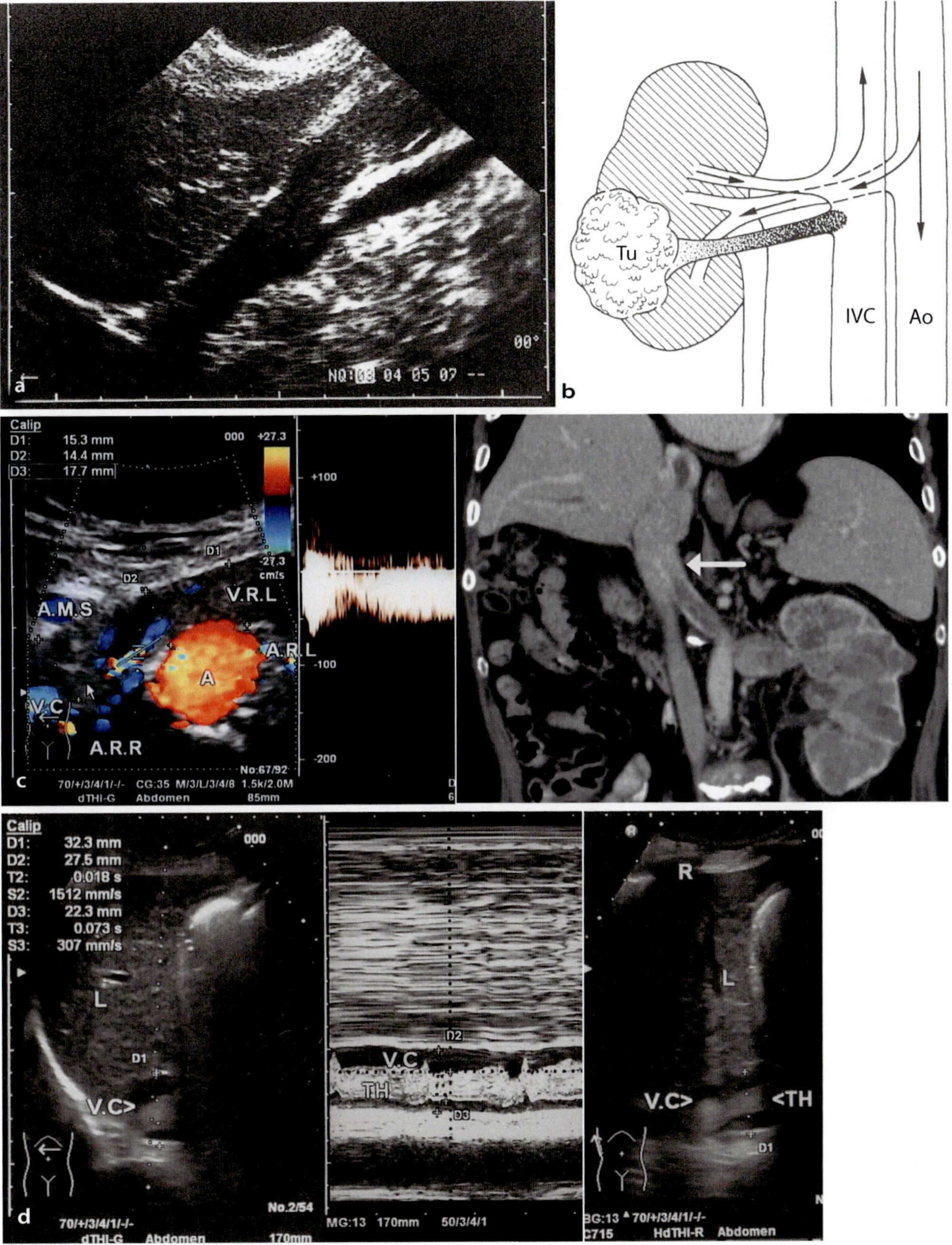

Fig. 6.107 (Atlas) Renal vein thrombus.
a The right renal vein coursing below the liver is occluded by a thrombus protruding into the vena cava (stage I, renal cell carcinoma).
b Diagram of renal vein thrombosis due to tumor. Two renal veins are present, and the drawing shows growth of a thrombus from a renal cell carcinoma (Tu) into the vena cava (IVC) through one of the veins.

Tumor thrombus ascending in vena cava

c Renal cell carcinoma of the left kidney with nearly complete occlusion of the left renal vein (V.R.L) by tumor thrombus. The sample volume is placed in the residual patent lumen next to the thrombus. The thrombus extends into the vena cava (V.C, indicated by arrow). (A.R.L = left renal artery, A.R.R = right renal artery, A.M.S. = superior mesenteric artery, A = aorta). The CT scan confirms the tumor thrombus in the left renal vein (arrow) with extension far into the vena cava (retrohepatic).
d Transverse and longitudinal images (from a lateral intercostal approach) showing floating tumor thrombus extending from the renal vein into the vena cava (with corresponding time-motion display). With this transducer position, the liver can be used as an acoustic window; however, there is acoustic shadowing from the ribs (R) (V.C = vena cava, TH = tumor thrombus, indicated by arrowhead; L = liver)

6

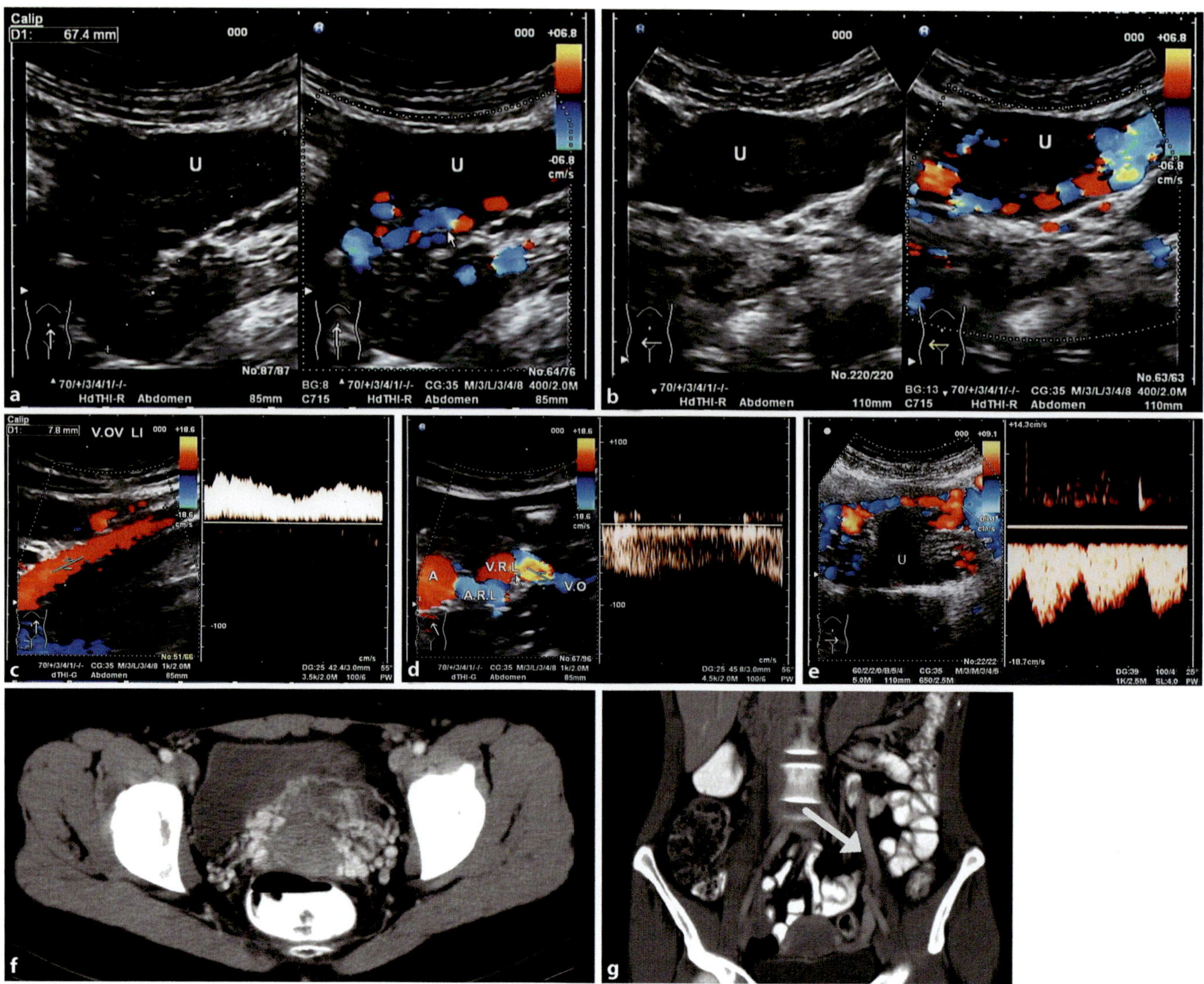

Fig. 6.108a–g (Atlas) Varicose ovarian vein in nutcracker syndrome.
a,b Patient with lower abdominal pain and a sensation of pressure increasing in the evening. The ultrasound examination (B-mode images on the left in **a** and **b**) reveals anechoic tubular structures surrounding the uterus, which correspond to a perfused varicose venous network that communicates with the ovarian vein in the color duplex mode (transverse images in **b** and longitudinal images in **a**). These changes are due to disturbed venous drainage in the left renal vein, which is entrapped between the superior mesenteric artery and the aorta (nutcracker syndrome). As a consequence, venous blood from the kidney drains into the left ovarian vein.
c There is high-frequency backward flow with little respiratory phasicity in the ovarian vein, which has a diameter of almost 10 mm (red, toward transducer).
d The ovarian vein (V.O, coded in blue) enters the left renal vein (V.R.L, red) anterior to the renal artery (A.R.L, blue). The Doppler waveform shows continuous retrograde high-frequency flow (toward the periphery) in the ovarian vein, while the blood flow direction in the renal vein proximal to the site of entry of the ovarian vein is normal. These flow directions reveal that the high retrograde flow in the dilated ovarian vein is responsible for the varicose degeneration of the periovarian and periuterine veins; laparoscopic ligation of the ovarian vein is indicated.
e Spectral Doppler imaging confirms venous flow in all dilated veins.
f Axial CT scan showing dilated varicose venous networks surrounding the uterus and ovary.
g CT scan showing the dilated ovarian vein between the left renal vein and the ovary but with no other anomalies. CT provides no hemodynamic information on blood flow in the dilated ovarian vein

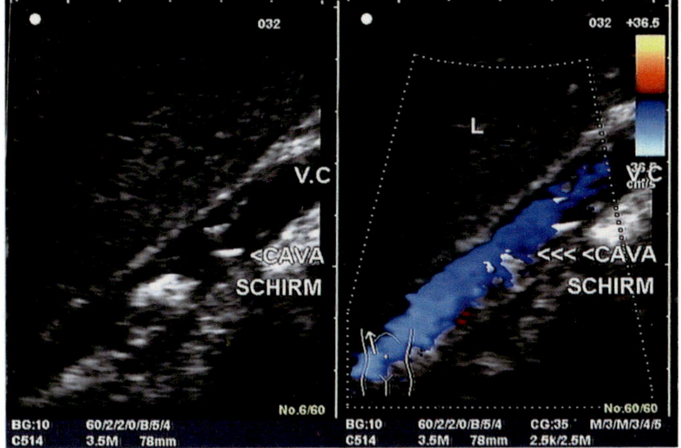

Fig. 6.109 (Atlas) **Vena cava umbrella.**
Color duplex ultrasound is ideal for confirming proper placement of a vena cava umbrella and patency of the vein

Penile and Scrotal Vessels

W. Schäberle, *Ultrasonography in Vascular Diagnosis*, https://doi.org/10.1007/978-3-319-64997-9_7

Erectile dysfunction is the lack of copulative power due to failure to initiate an erection or to maintain an erection. The causes of erectile dysfunction include psychologic, neurophysiologic, endocrinologic, and vasculogenic factors. The vascular mechanisms involved in the process of erection are an increased arterial inflow and reduced venous outflow. The incidence of erectile dysfunction due to vascular causes increases with age. About 10% of men suffer from erectile dysfunction.

7.1 Vascular Anatomy

7.1.1 Penile Vessels

The penis is supplied with blood by the internal pudendal artery, a branch of the internal iliac artery. The internal pudendal artery gives off scrotal branches and continues as the common penile artery, which divides into four terminal branches. These are the urethral or spongiosal artery, the dorsal penile artery (chiefly supplying the skin and glans penis), the bulbourethral artery, and the deep penile artery, which gives off branches to the corpora cavernosa (◘ Fig. 7.1). These branches course centrally in the cavernous bodies, which become rigid and enlarged when arterial inflow through these branches is increased. The other arteries play no relevant role in the erectile process.

Blood from the distal and middle portions of the corpora cavernosa is drained through the emissary and circumflex veins into the periprostatic plexus and from the proximal portion through the deep penile vein into the internal pudendal vein. The superficial dorsal vein of the penis drains primarily into the saphenofemoral junction through subcutaneous veins and the external pudendal veins. The blood from the deep penile vein flows out into the internal pudendal vein and the internal iliac vein (◘ Fig. 7.2).

In the flaccid state, the arterioles (helicine arteries) and the sinusoids in the cavernous spaces are contracted. There is only little blood flow due to high peripheral resistance. Conversely, the draining venules (emissary veins) are widely open; they drain the blood over a short stretch via the tunica albuginea into the circumflex vein and dorsal vein (◘ Fig. 7.3).

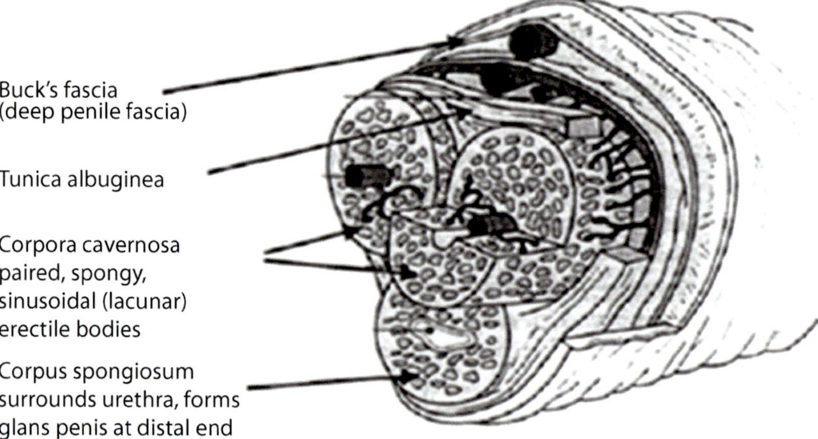

◘ Fig. 7.1 Anatomy of the erectile bodies of the penis

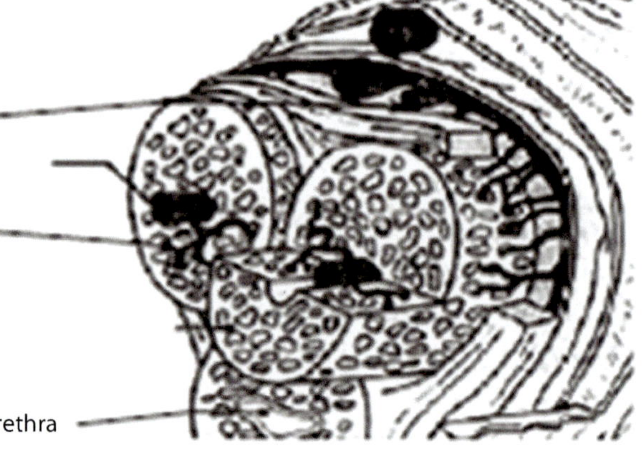

◘ Fig. 7.2 Arterial supply to the penis with arterial branches and venous drainage

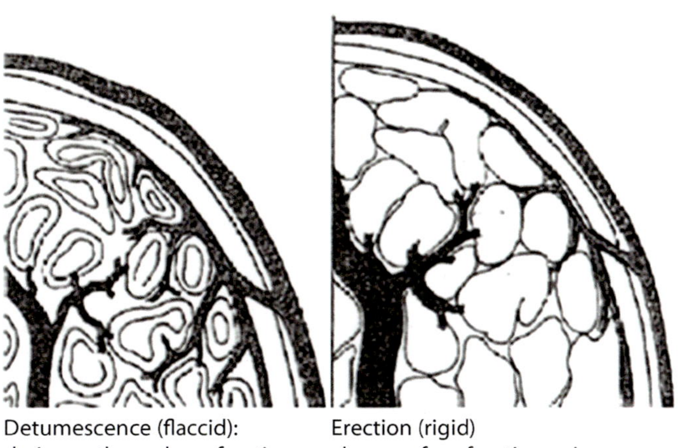

Fig. 7.3a, b Mechanism of penile erection. **a** In the flaccid state (detumescence), the helicine arteries and sinusoids are contracted, while the subtonic emissary veins are open. **b** The initial event in penile erection is relaxation of the smooth muscle of the helicine arteries, enabling increasing arterial inflow into the cavernous spaces. At the same time, venous outflow is increasingly blocked by compression of the emissary veins. Adequate closure of cavernosal outflow is crucial for maintaining an erection

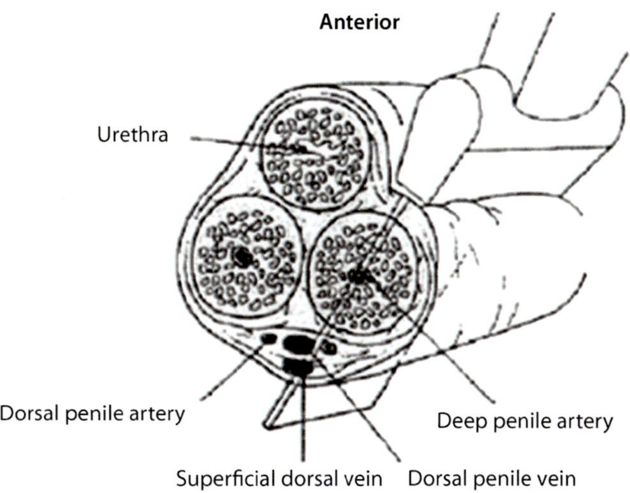

Fig. 7.4 Transducer position for evaluating arterial and venous perfusion. The penis rests on the patient's lower abdomen (as in erection)

7.1.2 Scrotal Vessels

The paired testicular artery arises from the abdominal aorta and courses from the retroperitoneum to the internal inguinal ring, from where it descends through the inguinal canal to the testis, surrounded by the veins of the pampiniform plexus and accompanied by the ductus deferens. The testicular veins drain the blood from the scrotum and testis via the pampiniform plexus. After having emerged from the internal inguinal ring, the right testicular vein courses to the inferior vena cava, the left testicular vein to the left renal vein.

7.2 Examination Technique

7.2.1 Erectile Dysfunction

7.2.1.1 Ultrasound Examination

The superficial course of the penile vessels enables their examination with a high-resolution, high-frequency transducer (7–10 MHz). The pulse repetition frequency and the wall filter should be set to detect slow flow.

With the patient in the supine position and the flaccid penis resting on the lower abdomen, the transducer is placed on the corpus carvernosum (anterior or posterior approach) near the base in transverse orientation (Fig. 7.4). In this position, the B-mode examination is performed with special attention given to the thickness of the tunica albuginea and the penile septum. The color mode is then switched on, and the deep penile artery is identified on both sides in transverse orientation with slight angulation of the transducer. The transducer is then rotated into the longitudinal plane for spectral Doppler interrogation of both arteries with calculation of angle-corrected flow velocities. To depict the slow flow velocities, a low pulse repetition frequency and wall filter are necessary, while the gain must be increased without allowing artifacts to occur (Table 7.1).

Table 7.1 Sonographic criteria

Technique	Criteria
B-mode image (longitudinal/ transverse)	Detumescence/erection Corpus cavernosum, homogeneous echotexture of normal tissue (scars) Atherosclerotic changes/plaques
Doppler	Waveform Peak systolic velocity (PSV) End-diastolic velocity (EDV) Resistive index (RI)
Course of erection	Changes in Doppler waveform (chiefly diastolic component) and RI during: detumescence – tumescence – erection – full erection
Pharmacologically induced erection	Intracavernous injection: 10 µg PGE1 or 30–60 mg papaverine Spectral Doppler recordings every 3–5 min Both deep penile arteries and deep dorsal vein Maximum tumescence after 8–20 min

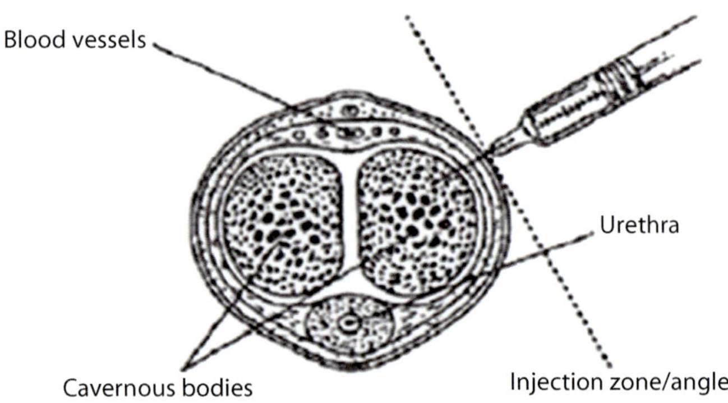

Fig. 7.5 Technique of intracavernous PGE1 or papaverine injection

7

Before scanning the penile vessels after **administration of a vasoactive agent**, written consent must be obtained from the patient after information about the examination and its possible side effects. For pharmacological induction of erection, prostaglandin (PGE1) or papaverine is injected into the left and right corpus cavernosum using a very fine needle (Fig. 7.5). To avoid side effects due to overdosage, the examination should be performed on 2 days with increasing dosages, beginning with 40 mg papaverine or 10 µg PGE1. If no adequate erection is achieved, 80 mg papaverine or 20 µg PGE1 should be injected into the right or left corpus cavernosum. Immediate outflow of the injected agent is prevented by short venous compression at the root of the penis. The erect penis is examined 4–5 min after injection by color duplex scanning in the same way as in the flaccid state. Following identification of the deep artery in transverse orientation, a spectral Doppler tracing is obtained from the proximal third of the artery near the base in longitudinal orientation with angle-corrected measurement of peak systolic (PSV) and end-diastolic flow velocities (EDV). Flow velocity measurement is repeated every 2–3 min until full erection is achieved. Finally, venous outflow in the deep femoral vein can be measured.

The pharmacologically induced erection should subside within 4–6 h. Immediate treatment is required in case of longer persistence or priapism, the most dreaded complication of PGE1 injection (Stief et al. 2000). This complication has an incidence of 1–4% and chiefly occurs if the dose is too high and in young patients with psychogenic erectile dysfunction (Wagner and Kaplan 1993). Treatment consists in injecting 5–10 mg Effortil in 5 ml saline solution with a thin needle. If there is progression to priapism, the intracavernous blood must be drained by aspiration.

7.2.2 Scrotal Vessels

The principal vessels involved in scrotal and testicular perfusion, the testicular artery and vein, course close to the surface in the inguinal canal and are thus accessible to duplex scanning with a high-resolution transducer. The spermatic artery passes through the abdominal wall together with the ductus deferens at the inner inguinal ring and can be traced sonographically in the B-mode in the inguinal canal, through which it descends to the scrotum as part of the spermatic cord. The testicular artery and vein are identified in the transverse plane in the color duplex mode to then obtain spectral Doppler tracings in longitudinal orientation. In addition, in patients evaluated for the presence of varicocele, the diameters of the veins are determined in longitudinal and transverse planes and the vessels are tracked downward (pampiniform plexus).

7.3 Normal Findings

7.3.1 Penile Vessels

B-mode images depict the corpus cavernosum as a roundish structure of a fairly homogeneous texture and low echogenicity that is surrounded by the more echogenic tunica albuginea. The septum separating the corpora is also echogenic.

In the flaccid state, the small-caliber deep artery of the penis may be difficult to identify in the B-mode. The Doppler spectrum recorded after identification of the artery in the color mode shows highly pulsatile flow due to high peripheral resistance. Intracavernous injection of PGE1 induces dilatation of the deep artery (seen in the B-mode) with an increase in systolic and diastolic flow velocities (Herbener et al. 1994; Mueller and Lue 1988; Quam et al. 1989). Normal arterial inflow results in a peak systolic velocity (PSV) of more than 30–35 cm/s 5–15 min after injection. The initially low peripheral resistance during the early phase of erection is associated with high end-diastolic velocity (EDV > 5–10 cm/s). The physiologic closure of venous outflow during erection leads to increased peripheral arterial resistance in the fully erect penis. This results in a marked decrease in end-diastolic flow, usually to zero (pulsatile flow), 5–25 min after injection. An EDV of 5 cm/s or above indicates venous insufficiency of the cavernous bodies.

Blood flow in the deep artery of the penis during tumescence is determined by arteriolar vasodilation and the changed pressure in the erectile tissue. Increasing filling of the cavernous spaces by inflowing blood results in a pressure increase in the corpora cavernosa as long as there is proper venous outflow closure. The ensuing increase in arterial flow resistance, in turn, leads to reduced diastolic flow (more pulsatile flow).

7.3.2 Scrotal Vessels

The testicular artery has a flow profile typical of a parenchyma-supplying vessel but with a rather small diastolic component. In a study of 30 men, a PSV of 14 cm/s (7.5–27.7 cm/s) and an EDV of 1.9 cm/s (0–4.7 cm/s) were found in the distal testicular artery. The resistance index (Pourcelot) was 0.84 (0.63–1; Middleton et al. 1989).

In the Valsalva test the testicular vein and pampiniform plexus veins exhibit zero flow after a brief reflux. Flow velocity varies with respiration; the normal diameter is less than 2–3 mm (Cvitanic et al. 1993).

7.4 Documentation

Transverse B-mode images of the penis depicting both cavernous bodies should be documented. The findings in the deep artery of the penis are documented together with the corresponding angle-corrected waveforms obtained in longitudinal orientation during penile flaccidity and in different phases of erection (at intervals of 2–3 min after PGE1 or papaverine injection). The waveforms should document the increase in PSV and EDV following injection as well as the subsequent decrease after full erection has been achieved.

The findings in the testicular artery are recorded at the level of the external inguinal ring in longitudinal orientation together with the waveform. In the same way, the findings in the pampiniform plexus veins are documented with the patient breathing spontaneously and while performing a Valsalva maneuver. The diameter of the veins is measured and recorded in the transverse plane.

7.5 Clinical Role of Duplex Ultrasound

7.5.1 Erectile Dysfunction

Accurate data on the **prevalence of erectile dysfunction** are difficult to obtain due to underreporting because of embarrassment or because the problem is not considered worthy of medical attention. It is well established that the incidence increases with age (Kinsey et al. 1948). Erectile problems are reported by 2% of men up to 40 years of age, 7% of men aged 41–50, 15% of men aged 51–60, and 75% of those over 70. In a population of 100 men (mean age, 37 years), 7% reported disturbed initiation of erection and another 9%, disturbed maintenance of erection (Frank et al. 1978). Until the end of the 1980s, it was assumed that erectile dysfunction was of psychogenic origin in 90% of cases (Borst 1987).

Various diagnostic modalities such as cavernosometry, cavernosography, CW Doppler, duplex ultrasound, and arteriography are available. They are used to measure intracavernosal pressure or perfusion parameters during erection or to detect arterial flow obstructions and demonstrate relevant organic abnormalities in 50–70% of men presenting with erectile dysfunction (Stief et al. 1988; Tamura et al. 1993; Whitehead et al. 1990). This leaves a percentage of only 30–50% with predominantly psychogenic dysfunction.

7.5.1.1 Pathophysiology of Erectile Dysfunction

Erectile dysfunction has organic, chiefly vasculogenic, causes in 50–70% of cases. Vascular causes can be arterial or venous.

- Arterial:
  - Stenosis, occlusion
  - Risk factors:
    - Atherosclerosis
    - Diabetes mellitus
    - Hypertension
    - Hypercholesterinemia
    - Smoking
- Venous:
  - Sinusoidal scar
  - Venous leakage
  - Peyronie's disease:
    - Plaques
    - Pain
    - Detumescence

Apart from vasculogenic causes, organic erectile dysfunction may be of neurogenic, endocrine, or drug-induced origin. Other causes include lesions of the cavernous bodies such as penile induration (Peyronie's disease). As with diabetes mellitus, vascular changes (macro- and microangiopathy) can aggravate a condition of primarily neurogenic origin (neuropathy of peripheral and autonomous nervous system). Vasculogenic erectile dysfunction may be caused by venous insufficiency of the corpora cavernosa with an incompetent veno-occlusive mechanism or by reduced arterial inflow due to stenosis or occlusion of the internal iliac artery or distal branches such as the pudendal artery.

Prior to any examination, a detailed history must be obtained to identify possible nonvascular causes of the patient's erectile problems. This includes information on medications taken by the patient as well as a sociopsychological interview pertaining to his social situation with special emphasis on the duration, severity, and character of the erectile dysfunction. Also important is a history of prior diseases and trauma including operations, especially of the true pelvis, in order to obtain clues as to whether the erectile dysfunction is primarily organic or psychogenic in nature. Information must also be obtained on vascular risk factors, and the subsequent clinical examination should be performed focusing on vascular disorders.

Identification of the underlying mechanism is of outmost importance for successful **treatment of erectile dysfunction**. In patients in whom a nonpsychogenic cause has been identified, therapeutic management is initiated according to the algorithm presented in ◘ Fig. 7.7 and on the basis of the history, clinical findings, and invasive and noninvasive diagnostic tests. The therapeutic measures may include pharmacologic treatment and, in case of vasculogenic erectile dysfunction, venous resection or arterial revascularization, depending on the duplex sonographic findings.

7.5.2 Acute Scrotum

In patients presenting with acute scrotum, testicular torsion and inflammatory conditions such as epididymitis must be differentiated, but this may be difficult on the basis of the clinical presentation and history alone. If either of these conditions is suspected, imminent loss of testicular function due to necrosis requires rapid intervention and may necessitate surgical exposure of the testis in inconclusive cases. Complete testicular torsion with arterial obstruction is distinguished from incomplete torsion. In the latter, only venous return is affected, but the testis is also at risk. A noninvasive duplex examination must therefore always include both arterial inflow and venous outflow.

7.5.3 Varicocele

Approx. 10–15% of sexually mature men suffer from varicocele, among them 5% with a severe form. Varicocele is a varicose condition of the veins of the pampiniform plexus that can be caused by valve incompetence of the spermatic vein. In addition, vascular anatomy also plays a role in the pathogenesis since the majority of varicoceles occur on the left side. While the right spermatic vein empties directly into the vena cava, the left vein joins the left renal vein. The higher hydrostatic pressure, compression by the inferior mesenteric artery, and an atypical course are among the factors that may explain why varicocele is more common on the left side. In a study of 45 patients with left-sided varicocele, 25% were found to have a retroaortic course of the renal vein, while a periaortic course was present in 31 cases (Justich 1982; impaired drainage through the renal vein).

It is likely that the pathologic constellation causing varicole is similar to that underlying the nutcracker syndrome in women (see ◘ Fig. 6.108 (Atlas)), namely marked compression of the left renal vein in the narrow anatomic passage between the aorta and superior mesenteric artery. This compression may not only obstruct drainage of the spermatic vein but can also lead to backward flow in the left renal vein (instead of forward flow into the vena cava) and a return of blood into the left spermatic vein via retroperitoneal collaterals, causing dilatation and valve incompetence of the spermatic vein with reversed flow into the periphery.

Although the exact mechanism of how a varicocele affects the spermiogram is not yet fully understood (hyperthermia, endocrine regulation, hypoxia/adrenal reflux), it is implicated as a cause of infertility as 30–50% of infertile men have a varicocele.

Surgery is indicated only in men with severe varicocele and manifest symptoms, unilateral testicular hypotrophy, or changes in the spermiogram with compromised spermiogenesis.

7.6 Abnormal Findings: Role of Duplex Ultrasound Parameters

7.6.1 Erectile Dysfunction

Characteristic ultrasound findings are obtained in arterial and venous erectile dysfunction:

- **Arterial erectile dysfunction:**
  - Arterial incompetence: PSV of <25 cm/s indicates severe arterial incompetence. Acceleration time is increased to over 120 ms. PSV of 25–30 cm/s indicates moderate arterial incompetence.
  - Note: Limited diagnostic accuracy in nervous patients and in psychogenic erectile dysfunction
- **Venous erectile dysfunction:**
  - Clinical presentation: poor rigidity despite normal arterial function
  - Duplex ultrasound:
    - Persistent diastolic flow >5 cm/s
    - Resistive index (RI) <1
    - Flow in deep dorsal vein
  - Note: Examination of venous competence only in patients with normal arterial function
  - Duplex scan provides only a preliminary diagnosis of venous incompetence, which needs to be confirmed by cavernosometry/cavernosography

B-mode sonography depicts **fibrosis** in the homogeneously hypoechoic corpus cavernosum as hyperechoic strands. Fibrosis and calcifications of the tunica albuginea (Peyronie's disease) are reliably identified by thickening and an increased echogenicity.

Extensive obstructive disease of the upstream arteries (both iliac arteries or pudendal artery) affect the flow character in the deep penile artery (postocclusive flow profile with decreased pulsatility) and thus suggest a **vasculogenic cause** of erectile dysfunction already in the flaccid state.

Injection of PGE1 or papaverine usually induces an increase in blood flow within 5–10 min (early tumescence phase) by lowering arterial resistance. As a result, PSV increases to more than 30–35 cm/s and EDV increases as well, while the Pourcelot index decreases. A pharmacologically induced PSV of less than 30 cm/s in the deep penile artery suggests inadequate arterial inflow. Studies demonstrated that a PSV below 25 cm/s after intracavernous injection was due to vascular obstruction, which was confirmed as the cause of erectile dysfunction in 88–100% of the patients by control angiography (Benson et al. 1993; Desai and Gilbert 1991; Quam et al. 1989). In another study of 42 patients with clinical signs of vasculogenic impotence, color duplex sonography was found to have 82% sensitivity and 88% specificity compared with selective penile DSA (Brandstetter et al. 1993). A delayed systolic upstroke in the Doppler waveform is another sign of proximal flow obstruction.

If arterial inflow appears normal, the failure to achieve or maintain an erection may be due to **dysfunction of the veno-occlusive mechanism**. As long as this mechanism is intact, the rise in intracavernous pressure leads to an increase in peripheral resistance with a decrease in the diastolic flow component. Conversely, if there is venous cavernous insufficiency, increased venous outflow results in persistent end-diastolic flow. An EDV of more than 5 cm/s indicates venous leakage with a sensitivity of over 90% (Quam et al. 1989). The magnitude of the EDV following maximum penile tumescence after intracavernous injection of a vasoactive agent correlates with venous outflow resistance and thus with the severity of venous leakage. Duplex sonography is a highly

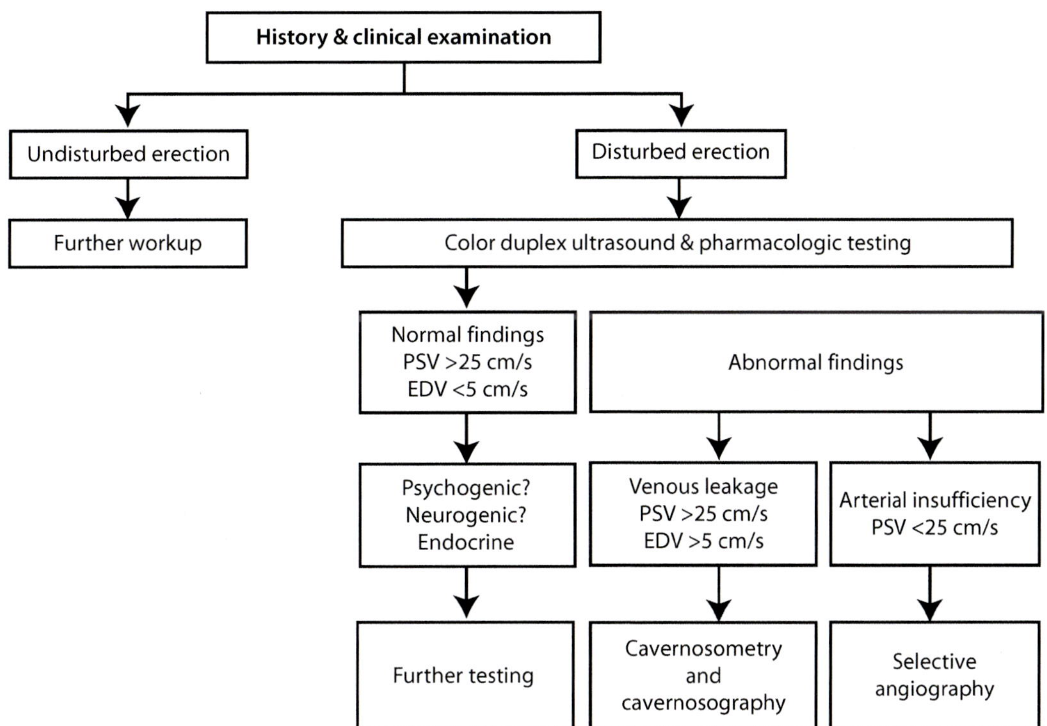

Fig. 7.6 Algorithm for the diagnostic management of patients with erectile dysfunction. Peak systolic velocity (PSV) and end-diastolic velocity (EDV) are measured by color duplex ultrasound

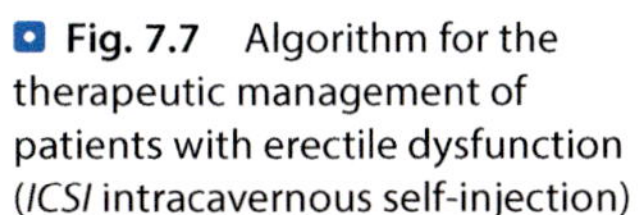
Fig. 7.7 Algorithm for the therapeutic management of patients with erectile dysfunction (*ICSI* intracavernous self-injection)

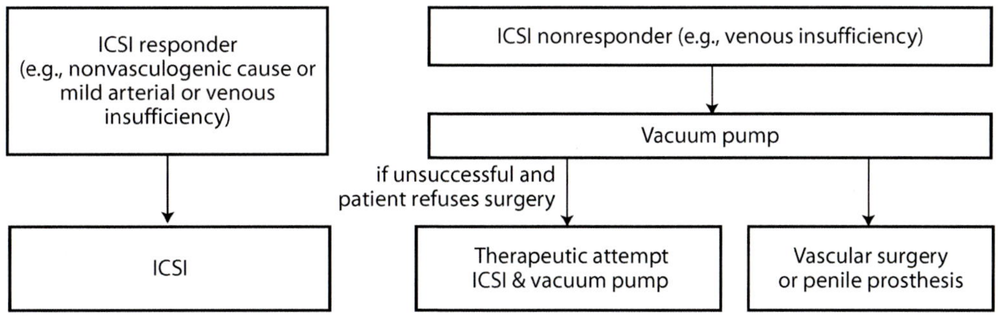

accurate tool for determining hemodynamic parameters during pharmacologically induced erection in the diagnostic evaluation and differentiation of vasculogenic causes of erectile dysfunction.

Based on the results of duplex imaging, further (invasive) diagnostic tests may be indicated; see algorithm for stepwise diagnostic workup in Fig. 7.6.

Treatment depends on whether initial intracavernous self-injection (ICSI) is successful or not (Fig. 7.7). Duplex measurements assist in choosing the most suitable therapy.

7.6.2 Acute Scrotum

In prepubertal boys, arterial flow is more difficult to detect due to the small testicular volume and slow blood flow; the scanner controls must be set to depict low frequency shifts, which means a low pulse repetition frequency and an adjusted gain. The normal testis appears uniform and is surrounded by a more echogenic capsule (tunica albuginea). Flow in the intratesticular segments of the testicular artery is monophasic with antegrade diastolic flow (low-resistance flow).

When Doppler measurement is performed between the external inguinal ring and the testis, care must be taken not to confuse the testicular artery with one of the supratesticular arteries, which supply the testicular coverings and cremaster and therefore lack a diastolic flow component (higher diastolic resistance).

In **testicular torsion**, the extent to which perfusion is compromised depends on the duration and severity. In incomplete torsion, the Doppler waveform is abnormal, but often shows some residual perfusion. In patients with suspected testicular torsion, spectral Doppler evaluation of the testicular artery is supplemented by color duplex imaging (low pulse repetition frequency) of the affected testis to evaluate arterial and venous flow. Spectral Doppler measurement of arterial and venous perfusion is necessary to rule out incomplete testicular torsion (acceleration time, flow velocity, side-to-side comparison).

Venous spectral Doppler measurement is necessary to confirm unimpaired venous drainage and **rule out incomplete testicular torsion** (which is characterized by unimpaired arterial inflow with impaired venous drainage).

In patients presenting with acute scrotum, duplex ultrasound has nearly 100% specificity for ruling out **acute ischemia** (Fitzgerald and Foley 1991). Several studies performed in small study populations found sensitivities of 86–100% and specificities of 100% in differentiating acute testicular or epididymal inflammation with hyperemia from testicular torsion with signs of acute ischemia (DeWire et al. 1992; Lerner et al. 1990; Middleton et al. 1990; Ralls et al. 1990). Inflammation is associated with low peripheral resistance, resulting in high diastolic flow. Conversely, testicular torsion is characterized by the absence of arterial flow in the twisted vessel segment and highly pulsatile flow without a diastolic flow component and a reduced PSV (compared to contralateral side) with a "knocking" waveform proximal to the lesion (in the inguinal ligament). Published studies rarely address the problem of incomplete testicular torsion with impaired venous drainage only. To exclude testicular damage resulting from venous compromise, the vein must be evaluated by color duplex imaging from the scrotal compartment to the level of the inguinal ligament. The normal waveform shows flow with respiratory phasicity.

Following spontaneous or manual **detorsion** after an ischemic interval, the compensatory increase in testicular perfusion can be detected by spectral Doppler measurement. Appendiceal torsion also presents with acute onset of pain; ultrasound demonstrates the twisted appendage as a mass adjacent to the echogenic testis or epididymis. Color duplex imaging demonstrates increased perfusion in adjacent testicular and epididymal tissue. Perfusion is also increased in epididymitis, and the increase can be demonstrated by a color duplex examination and comparison with the contralateral epididymis.

In a study of 31 patients, a cutoff value of 15 cm/s for PSV was found to have an accuracy of 90% for identifying **orchitis** and of 93% for **epididymitis** (Brown et al. 1995). Another parameter used was the ratio of PSVs on the affected side and the contralateral side, with a ratio of greater than 1.9 being defined as indicating epididymitis or orchitis.

Taken together, published studies suggest that ultrasound is a highly valid diagnostic modality for the evaluation of testicular and penile perfusion and detection of abnormalities. These reports, however, remain to be confirmed in larger patient populations. In unclear cases surgical exposure of the testis is still necessary.

7.6.3 Varicocele

Varicoceles are conspicuous as a convolution of veins in the scrotum (◘ Fig. 7.15 (Atlas)). Dilatation of the veins of the pampiniform plexus with a diameter of over 3 mm is considered abnormal. The Valsalva test performed in the standing patient will induce continuous backward flow in the abnormally dilatated veins, which can be demonstrated both by color duplex sonography and in the Doppler waveform (Fitzgerald and Foley 1991). In a study of 63 infertile men, color duplex was found to be highly accurate in the diagnosis of varicoceles with 97% sensitivity and 94% specificity compared to venography of the spermatic vein (Trum et al. 1996). However, the clinical significance of a sonographically diagnosed varicocele must not be overestimated. In an investigation of 26 fertile men, 42% were found to have dilatated pampiniform plexus veins with diameters of more than 2–3 mm and signs of reflux (Cvitanic et al. 1993). Sonographic criteria of varicocele are:

- Testicular size difference: >2 mL
- Plexus veins: >3 mm diameter
- (Color) duplex ultrasound: reflux during normal respiration in the standing patient

In addition, the termination of the spermatic vein and the course of the left renal vein should be imaged, including hemodynamic assessment (flow direction) of the proximal spermatic vein, to identify the underlying mechanism and assess the severity of outflow obstruction (▶ Sect. 7.5.3).

7.7 Atlas: Penile and Scrotal Vessels

◘ Table 7.2 lists the figures presented in the Atlas. The figures illustrate normal and abnormal findings in the ultrasound examination of the penile and scrotal vessels.

◘ **Table 7.2** Penile and scrotal vessels – figures

Entity/Pathology	Figure
Detumescence	◘ Fig. 7.8 (Atlas), page 500
Doppler waveform following prostaglandin injection	◘ Fig. 7.9 (Atlas), page 500
Doppler waveform – onset of erection	◘ Fig. 7.10 (Atlas), page 500
Doppler waveform – full erection	◘ Fig. 7.11 (Atlas), page 501
Doppler waveform – arterial insufficiency	◘ Fig. 7.12 (Atlas), page 501
Doppler waveform – venous leakage	◘ Fig. 7.13 (Atlas), page 501
Venous insufficiency of corpora cavernosa	◘ Fig. 7.14 (Atlas), page 502
Varicocele	◘ Fig. 7.15 (Atlas), page 502

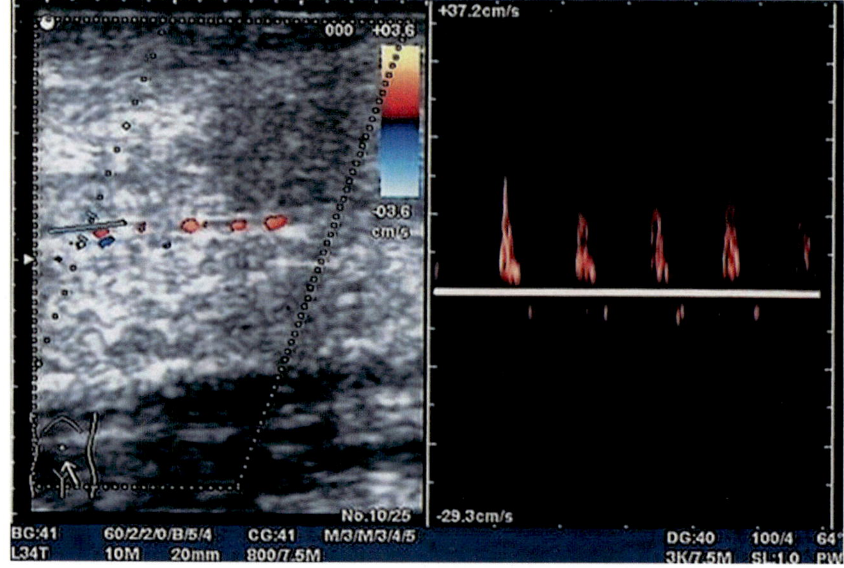

Fig. 7.8 (Atlas) Detumescence. In the flaccid state (detumescence), the deep artery of the penis demonstrates high-resistance flow with pulsatile systolic peaks but no significant diastolic flow

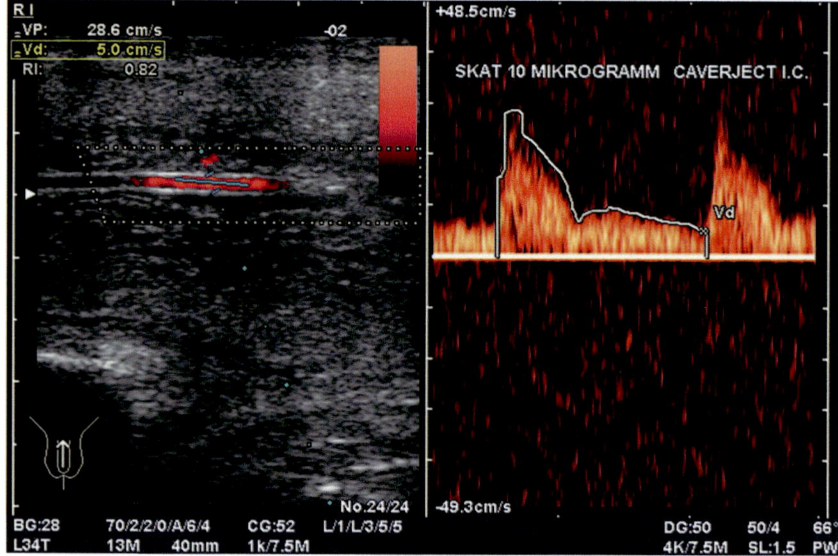

Fig. 7.9 (Atlas) Doppler waveform following prostaglandin injection. Markedly increased blood flow, especially in diastole, in the deep penile artery 10–15 min following injection of 10 µg PGE1 and relaxation of the smooth muscle of the sinusoids (low-resistance arterial inflow) (Courtesy of F. Trinkler)

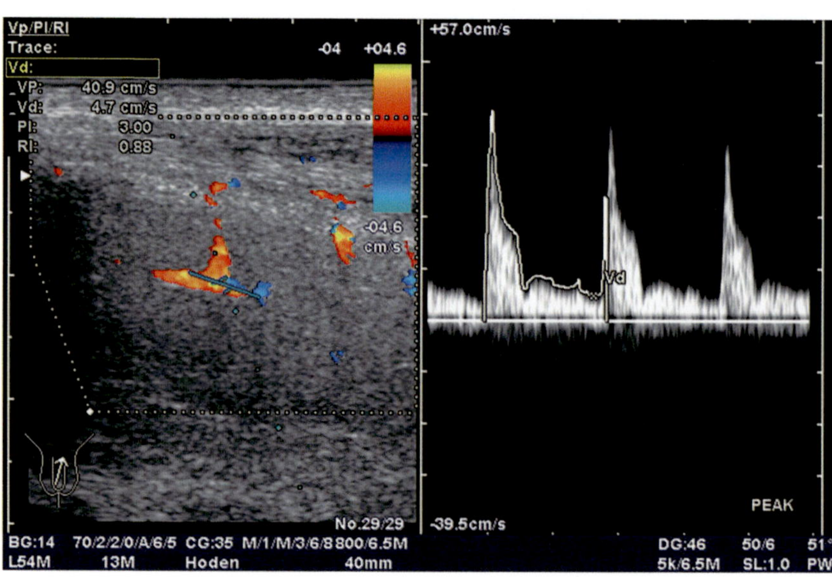

Fig. 7.10 (Atlas) Doppler waveform – onset of erection. With increasing erection brought on by continuous high arterial inflow, the sinusoids become filled, causing a build-up of counterpressure in the corpus cavernosum. As a result, peripheral resistance increases, and flow becomes more pulsatile. The diastolic flow component decreases and approaches zero in the further course. A peak systolic velocity (PSV) >30 cm/s indicates normal arterial blood supply. In the example, PSV is 40 cm/s (Courtesy of F. Trinkler)

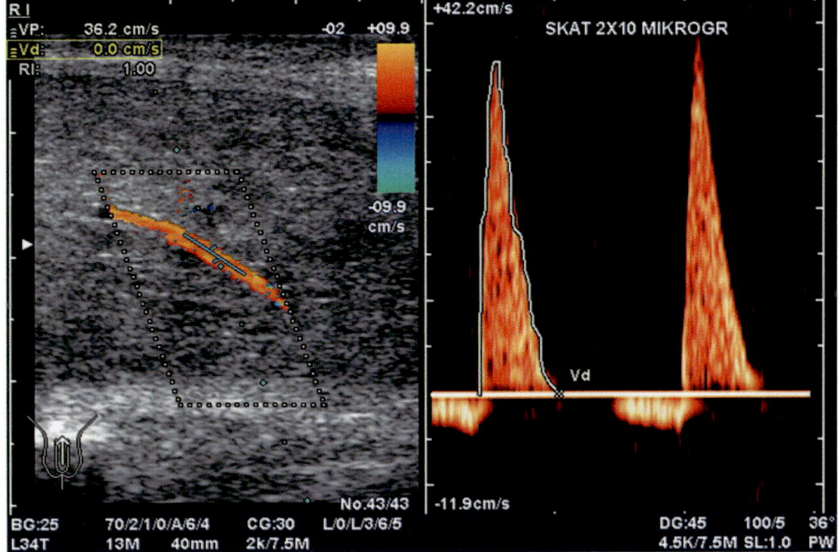

Fig. 7.11 (Atlas) Doppler waveform – full erection.
Flow decreases again due to the high intracavernous pressure in full erection with absence of flow or retrograde flow during diastole. This is associated with a decrease in PSV. No flow is detected in the deep vein of the penis (Courtesy of F. Trinkler)

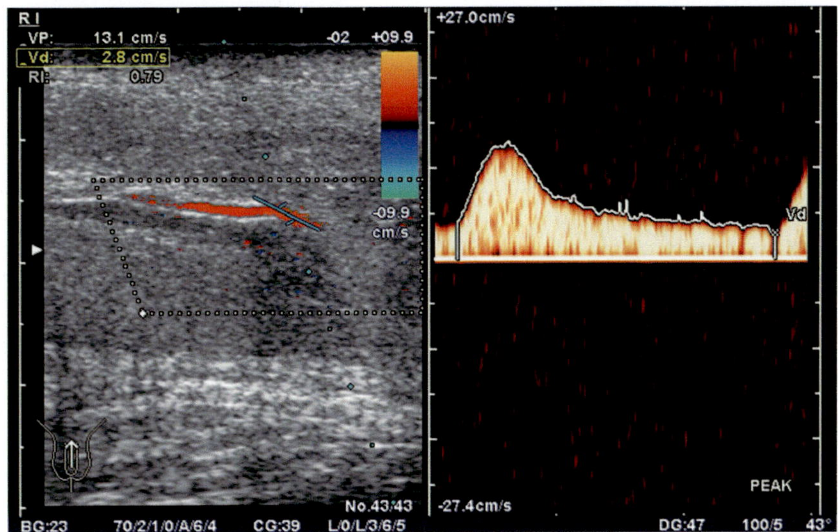

Fig. 7.12 (Atlas) Doppler waveform – arterial insufficiency.
Inadequate arterial inflow is characterized by a smaller increase in peak systolic velocity (PSV) in the deep penile artery. In severe insufficiency, PSV drops below 25 cm/s. In the case presented, intracavernous injection of 10 µg PGE1 does not induce erection, and there is no adequate increase in flow during systole after a reasonable delay (5–15 min). A PSV of only 12 cm/s, a delayed systolic upsurge (prolonged acceleration time), and a larger diastolic flow component are typical signs of postocclusive flow. Here, the postocclusive flow is caused by upstream atherosclerotic stenoses. Because of the patient's high-grade arterial insufficiency, it is not possible to reliably determine whether there is concomitant venous leakage

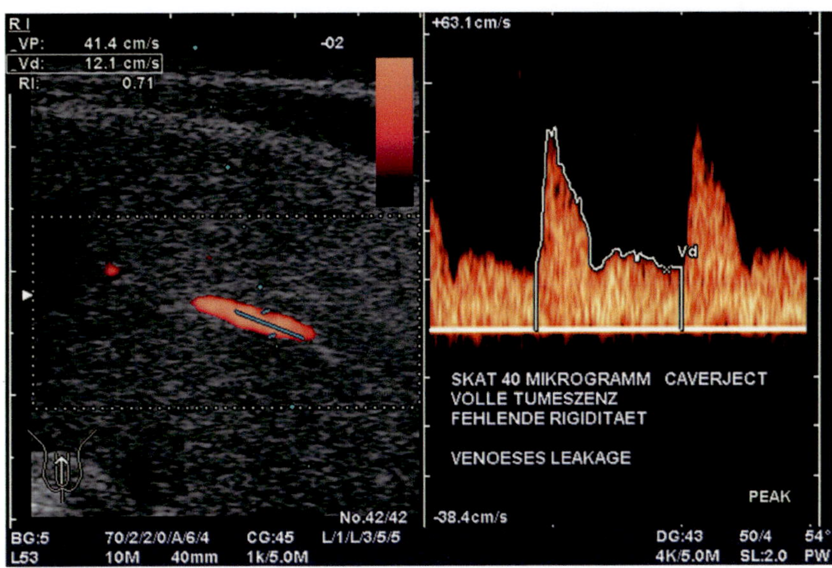

Fig. 7.13 (Atlas) Doppler waveform – venous leakage.
In patients with venous leakage, rigidity is inadequate although full tumescence is achieved. Following intracavernous PGE1 injection, the Doppler waveform from the deep penile artery demonstrates an adequate systolic increase with a PSV of 41 cm/s but no reduction during diastole. The high diastolic flow velocity indicates low peripheral resistance to venous outflow

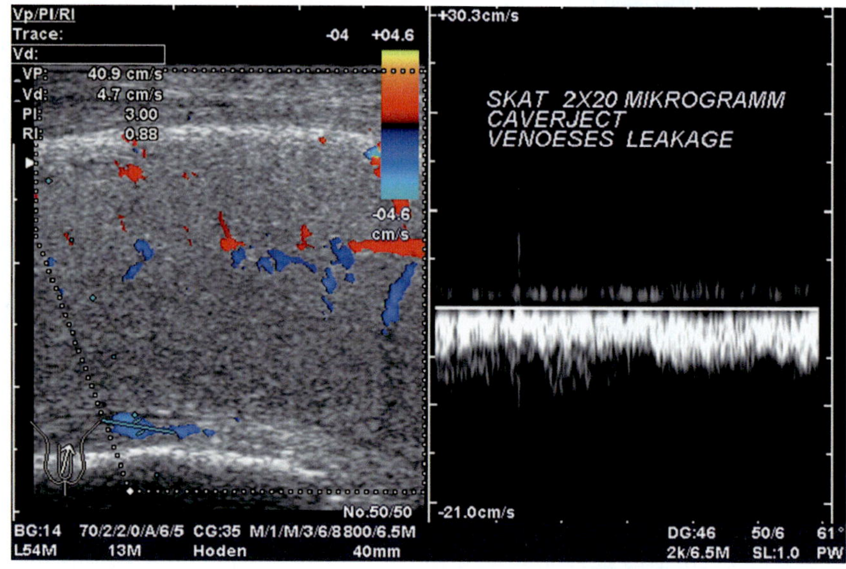

Fig. 7.14 (Atlas) Venous insufficiency of corpora cavernosa.
Under normal conditions, no venous flow signal is obtained from the deep dorsal vein in the phase of full tumescence. In the patient presented, venous leakage is suggested by the demonstration of venous flow with a velocity of 10–20 cm/s

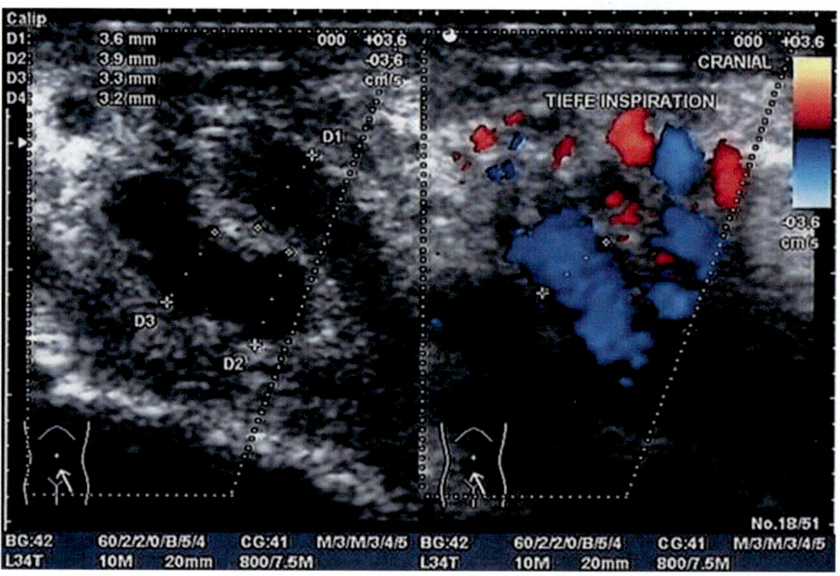

Fig. 7.15 (Atlas) Varicocele.
Varicocele is identified by duplex sonography as dilatation of the veins of the pampiniform plexus to over 3 mm (left image), along with backward flow toward the testes during deep inspiration or Valsalva's maneuver (color flow image on the right) (see Fig. 6.108 (Atlas))

Supplementary Information

W. Schäberle, *Ultrasonography in Vascular Diagnosis*, https://doi.org/10.1007/978-3-319-64997-9

References

Abou-Zamzam AM Jr, Moneta GL, Edwards JM, Yeager RA, Taylor LM Jr, Porter JM (2000) Is a single preoperative duplex scan sufficient for planning bilateral carotid endarterectomy? J Vasc Surg 31:282–288

AbuRahma AF (2006) Fate of endoleaks detected by CT angiography and missed by color duplex ultrasound in endovascular grafts for abdominal aortic aneurysms. J Endovasc Ther 13:490–495

AbuRahma AF, Robinson P, Decanio R (1989) Prospective clinicopathologic study of carotid intraplaque hemorrhage. Am Surg 55:169–173

AbuRahma AF, Richmond BK, Robinson PA et al (1995) Effect of contralateral severe stenosis or carotid occlusion on duplex criteria of ipsilateral stenoses: comparative study of various duplex parameters. J Vasc Surg 22:751–762

AbuRahma AF, Robinson PA, Killmer SM, Kioschos JM, Roberts MD (1996) A critical analysis of cerebral computed tomography scanning before elective carotid endarterectomy and its correlation to carotid stenosis. Surgery 119:248–251

AbuRahma AF, Kyer PD, Robinson PA, Hannay RS (1998) The correlation of ultrasonic carotid plaque morphology and carotid plaque hemorrhage: clinical implications. Surgery 124:721–728

AbuRahma AF, Robinson PA, Stickler DL et al (1998) Proposed new duplex classification for threshold stenoses used in various symptomatic and asymptomatic carotid endarterectomy trials. Ann Vasc Surg 12:349–358

AbuRahma AF, Burns W, Mullins DA (1999) Carotid artery dissection: a challenging diagnosis. W V Med J 95:17–19

AbuRahma AF, Covelli MA, Robinson PA, Holt SM (1999) The role of carotid duplex ultrasound in evaluating plaque morphology: potential use in selecting patients for carotid stenting. J Endovasc Surg 6:59–65

AbuRahma AF, Wulu JT Jr, Crotty B (2002) Carotid plaque ultrasonic heterogeneity and severity of stenosis. Stroke 33:1772–1775

AbuRahma AF, Abu-Halimah S, Bensenhaver J, Dean LS, Keiffer T, Emmett M et al (2008) Optimal carotid duplex velocity criteria for defining the severity of carotid in-stent restenosis. J Vasc Surg 48:589–594

AbuRahma AF, Welch CA, Mullins BB, Dyer B (2005) Computed tomography versus color duplex ultrasound for surveillance of abdominal aortic stent-grafts. J Endovasc Ther 12:568–573

AbuRahma AF, Mousa AY, Stone PA, Hass SM, Dean LS, Keiffer T (2012) Duplex velocity criteria for native celiac/superior mesenteric artery stenosis vs in-stent stenosis. J Vasc Surg 55:730–738

AbuRahma AF, Srivastava M, Stone PA, Mousa AY, Jain A, Dean LS, Keiffer T, Emmett M (2011) Critical appraisal of the Carotid Duplex Consensus criteria in the diagnosis of carotid artery stenosis. J Vasc Surg 53:53–60

AbuRahma AF, Srivastava M, Mousa AY (2012) Critical analysis of renal duplex ultrasound parameters in detecting significant renal artery stenosis. J Vasc Surg 56:1052–1060

AbuRahma AF, Stone PA, Srivastanva M et al (2012) Mesenteric/celiac duplex ultrasound interpretation criteria revisited. J Vasc Surg 55:428–436

ACAS (1995) Asymptomatic carotid atherosclerosis study. JAMA 273:1459–1461

Agrawal SK, Pinheiro L, Roubin GS et al (1992) Nonsurgical closure of femoral pseudoaneurysms complicating cardiac catheterization and percutaneous transluminal coronary angioplasty. J Am Coll Cardiol 20:610–615

Ahmad S, Blagg CR, Scribner BH (1998) Center and home chronic hemodialysis. In: Schrier RW, Gottschalk CW (eds) Diseases of the kidney, 4th edn, Little, Brown, pp 3281–3322

Aitken AGF, Godden DJ (1987) Real-time ultrasound diagnosis of deep venous thrombosis: a comparison with venography. Clin Radiol 38:309–313

Akbari CM, LoGerfo FW (1999) Diabetes and peripheral vascular disease. J Vasc Surg 30:373–384

Akkersdijk GJM, Puylaert JBCM, Vries A (1991) Abdominal aortic aneurysm as an incidental finding in abdominal ultrasonography. Br J Surg 78:1261–1263

Alanen A, Kormano M (1985) Correlation of the echogenicity and structure of clotted blood. J Ultrasound Med 4:421–425

Albrecht T, Urbank A, Mahler M et al (1998) Prolongation and optimization of Doppler enhancement with a microbubble US contrast agent by using continuous infusion: preliminary experience. Radiology 207:339–347

Albrecht T, Hoffmann CW, Schettler S et al (2000) B-mode enhancement at phase-inversion US with air-based microbubble contrast agent: initial experience in humans. Radiology 216:273–278

Albrechtson LL, Olson QCG (1976) Thrombotic side effects of lower limb phlebography. Lancet 1:723

Aldridge SC, Comerota AJ (1993) Popliteal venous aneurysm: report of two cases and review of the world literature. J Vasc Surg 18:708–715

Alexander JQ, Leos SM, Katz SG (2002) Is duplex ultrasonography an effective single modality for the preoperative evaluation of peripheral vascular disease? Am J Surg 68:1107–1110

Alexandrov AV, Bladin CF, Maggisano R, Norris JW (1993) Measuring carotid stenosis. Time for reappraisal. Stroke 24:1291–1296

Alexandrov AV, Brodie DS, McLean A et al (1997) Correlation of peak systolic velocity and angiographic measurement of carotid stenosis revisited. Stroke 28:339–342

Alexandrov AV, Vital D, Brodie DS, Hamilton Paul Grotta JC (1997) Grading carotid stenosis with ultrasound. Stroke 28:1208–1210

Allard L, Cloutier G, Durand L-G, Roederer GO, Langlois YE (1994) Limitation of ultrasonic duplex scanning for diagnosing lower limb arterial stenoses in the presence of adjacent segment disease. J Vasc Surg 19:650–657

Allenberg JR et al (1995) Endovascular reconstruction of infrarenal abdominal aortic aneurysm. Chirurg 66:870–877

Allenberg JR, Kallinowski F, Schumacher H (1997) Stand der Chirurgie des infrarenalen Aortenaneurysmas: Prävalenz und Versorgungssituation. Dt Ärztebl 94:A2830–A2834

Allon M, Robbin ML (2002) Increasing arteriovenous fistulas in hemodialysis patients: problems and solutions. Kidney Int 62:1109–1124

Alri M, Herba MJ, Reinhold C et al (1996) Accuracy of sonography in the evaluation of calf deep vein thrombosis in both postoperative surveillance and symptomatic patients. AJR 166:1361–1367

Alson MD, Lang EV, Kaufman JA (1997) Pedal arterial imaging. Vasc Interv Radiol 8:9–18

Aly S, Bishop CC (2000) An objective characterization of atherosclerotic lesion: an alternative method to identify unstable plaque. Stroke 31:1921–1924

Aly S, Jenskin MP, Zaidi FH, Coleridge Smith PD, Bishop CC (1998) Duplex scanning and effect of multisegmental arterial disease on its accuracy in lower limb arteries. Eur J Vasc Endovasc Surg 16:345–349

Aly S, Sommerville K, Adiseshiah M (1998) Comparison of duplex imaging and angiography in evaluation of lower limb arteries. Br J Surg 85:1099–1102

Amendt K (1998) Takayasu-Arteriitis. In: Amendt K, Diehm C (eds) Handbuch akrale Durchblutungsstörungen. Epidemiologie, Pathogenese, Diagnostik und Therapie. Barth, Heidelberg, pp 153–184

Anaya-Ayala JE, Pettigrew CD, Ismail N et al (2012) Management of dialysis access-associated "steal" syndrome with DRIL procedure: Challenges and clinical outcomes. J Vasc Access 13:299–304

Anderson IC, Baltaxe HA, Wolf GL (1979) Inability to show clot. One limitation of ultrasonography of the abdominal aorta. Radiology 132:693

Anjaria PD, Vaidya PN, Vahia VN et al (1973) Venous aneurysms. J Postgrad Med 20:142–144

Äppel RG, Bleyer AJ, Reavis S, Hansen KJ (1995) Renovascular disease in older patients beginning renal replacement therapy. Kidney Int 48:171–176

Appelman PT, de Jong TE, Lampman LE (1987) Deep venous thrombosis of the leg. Ultrasound findings. Radiology 163:743–746

Aprin H, Schwartz GB, Valderamma E (1987) Traumatic venous aneurysm. Clin Orthop 217:243–246

Araki CT, Back TL, Padberg FT, Thompson PN et al (1993) Refinements in the ultrasonic detection of popliteal vein reflux. J Vasc Surg 18:742–748

Arko FR (2003) Intrasac flow velocities predict sealing of type II endoleaks after endovascular abdominal aortic aneurysm repair. J Vasc Surg 37:8–15

Arlart IP, Ingrisch H (1984) Renovaskuläre Hypertonie. Radiologische Diagnostik und Therapie. Thieme, Stuttgart

Armstrong PA (2007) Visceral duplex scanning: evaluation before and after artery intervention for chronic mesenteric ischemia. Perspect Vasc Surg Endovasc Ther 19:386–392

Armstrong PA, Bandyk DF, Johnson BL et al (2007) Duplex scan surveillance after carotid angioplasty and stenting: A rational definition of stent stenosis. J Vasc Surg 46:460–465

Arning C (2001) Nonatherosclerotic disease of the cervical arteries: role of ultrasonography for diagnosis. Vasa 30:160–167

Arning C (2004) Die Karotidynie im Ultraschallbild: Mythos, Syndrom oder Krankheitsbild? Nervenarzt 75:1200–1203

Arning C (2005) Ultrasonographic criteria for diagnosing a dissection of the internal carotid artery. Ultraschall Med 26:24–28

Arning C, Grzyska U (2004) Color Doppler imaging of cervicocephalic fibromuscular dysplasia. Cardiovasc Ultrasound 2:7

Arning C, Oelze A, Lachenmayer L (1995) A rare cause of stroke: aortic dissection. Aktuell Neurol 22:189–192

Arning C, Hammer E, Kortmann H, Hahm H, Muller-Jensen A, Lachenmayer L (2003) Quantifizierung von A. carotis interna-Stenosen: Welche Ultraschallkriterien sind geeignet? Ultraschall Med 24:233–238

Arning C, von Reutern GM, Stiegler H, Gortler M (2010) Ultraschallkriterien zur Graduierung von Stenosen der A. carotis interna – Revision der DEGUM-Kriterien und Transfer in NASCET Stenosierungsgrade [Revision of DEGUM ultrasound criteria for grading internal carotid artery stenoses and transfer to NASCET measurement]. Ultraschall Med 31:251–257

Arning C, Görtler M, von Reuttern DM (2011) Carotisstenose: Definitionschaos wurde beseitigt. Dtsch Arztebl 108:A1794–A1795

Arnold JA, Modaresi KB, Thomas N, Taylor PR, Padayachee TS (1999) Carotid plaque characterization by duplex scanning: observer error may undermine current clinical trials. Stroke 30:61–65

Ascer E, Lorenso E, Pollina RM, Gennaro M (1995) Preliminary results of a nonoperative approach to saphenofemoral junction thrombophlebitis. J Vasc Surg 22:616–621

Ascer E, Pollina RM, Gennaro M, Lorensen E (1995) Noninvasive predictors of patency for infrapopliteal PTFE bypasses with combined arteriovenous fistula and vein interposition technique. Am J Surg 170:103–105

Ascer E, Mazzariol F, Hingorani A, Dalles-Cunba S, Gade P (1999) The use of duplex ultrasound arterial mapping as an alternative to conventional arteriography for primary and secondary infrapopliteal bypasses. Am J Surg 178:162–165

Ascher E, Hingorani A, Markevich N, Costa T, Kallakuri S, Khanimoy Y (2002) Lower extremety revascularization without preoperative contrast arteriography: experience with duplex ultrasound arterial mapping in 485 cases. Ann Vasc Surg 16:108–114

Ascher E, Hingorani A, Markevich N et al (2004) Role of duplex arteriography as the sole preoperative imaging modality prior to lower extremity revascularization surgery in diabetic and renal patients. Ann Vasc Surg 18:433–439

Aschulte-Altedorneburg G, Droste DW, Haas N (2000) Preoperative B-mode ultrasound plaque appearance compared with carotid endarterectomy specimen histology. Acta Neurol Scand 101:188–194

Aschwanden M, Hess P, Labs KH et al (2003) Dialysis access-associated steal syndrome: the intraoperative use of duplex ultrasound scan. J Vasc Surg 37:211–213

Aschwanden M, Thalhammer C, Schaub S, Wolff T, Steiger J, Jaeger KA (2006) Renal vein thrombosis after renal transplantation - early diagnosis by duplex sonography prevented fatal outcome. Nephrol Dial Transplant 21:825–826

Aschwanden M, Kesten F, Stern M et al (2010) Vascular involvement in patients with giant cell arteritis determined by duplex sonography of 2x11 arterial regions. Ann Rheum Dis 69:1356–1359

Aschwanden M, Daikeler T, Kersten F, Baldi T, Benz D, Tyndall A (2013) Temporal artery compression sign - a novel ultrasound finding for the diagnosis of giant cell arteritis. Ultraschall Med 34:47–50

Asciutto G, Mumme A, Marpe B, Hummel T, Geier B (2007) Different approaches in the treatment of cystic adventitial disease of the popliteal artery. Chir Ital 59:467–473

Ashoke R, Brown LC, Rodway A et al (2005) Color duplex ultrasonography is insensitive for the detection of endoleak after aortic endografting: a systematic review. J Endovasc Ther 12:297–305

Ashton HA, Buxton MJ, Day NE et al (2002) The Multicentre Aneurysm Screening Study (MASS) into the effect of abdominal aortic aneurysm screening on mortality in men: a randomised controlled trial. Lancet 360:1531–1539

Atri M, Herba MJ, Reinhold C, Leclerc J et al (1996) Accuracy of sonography in the evaluation of calf deep vein thrombosis in both postoperative surveillance and symptomatic patients. Am J Roentgenol 166:1361–1367

Aube C, Oberti F, Korali N et al (1999) Ultrasonographic diagnosis of hepatic fibrosis or cirrhosis. J Hepatol 30:472–478

Aune S, Pedersen OM, Trippestad A (1998) Surveillance of above-knee prosthetic femoropopliteal bypass. Eur J Vasc Endovasc Surg 16:509–512

Avasthi PS, Voyles WF, Greene ER (1984) Noninvasive diagnosis of renal artery stenosis by echo-Doppler velocimetry. Kidney Int 25:824–829

Avenarius JKA, Breek JC, Lampmann LEH et al (2002) The additional value of angiography after colour-coded duplex on decision making in patients with critical limb ischaemia. A prospective study. Eur J Vasc Endovasc Surg 23:393–397

AWMF-Leitlinien. Arteriitis cranialis. http://www.dgn.org/180.0.html

Baker WH, Stoney RJ (1972) Acquired popliteal entrapment syndrome. Arch Surg 105:780–781

Baker SR, Burnard KG, Sommerville KM, Thomas ML, Wilson NM (1993) Comparison of venous reflux assessed by duplex scanning and descending phlebography in chronic venous disease. Lancet 341:400–403

Bakken AM, Illig KA (2010) Long-term follow-up after endovascular aneurysm repair: is ultrasound alone enough? Perspect Vasc Surg Endovasc Ther 22:145–151

Bakker J, Beek FJ, Beutler JJ (1998) Renal artery stenosis and accessory renal arteries: accuracy of detection and visualization with gadolinium-enhanced breath-hold MR angiography. Radiology 207:497–504

Baldassarre D, Amato M, Bondioli A, Sirtori CR, Tremoli E (2000) Carotid artery intima-media thickness measured by ultrasonography in normal clinical practice correlates well with atherosclerosis risk factors. Stroke 31:2426–2430

Balk E, Raman G, Chung M et al (2006) Effectiveness of management strategies for renal artery stenosis: a systematic review. Ann Intern Med 145:901–912

Bandyk DF, Cato RF, Towne JB (1985) A low flow velocity predicts failure of femoropopliteal and femorotibial bypass grafts. Surgery 98:799–809

Bandyk DF, Scabrook GR, Moldenauer P et al (1988) Hemodynamics of vein graft stenoses. J Vasc Surg 8:688–695

Bandyk DF, Schmitt DD, Seabrook GR (1989) Monitoring functional patency of in situ saphenous vein bypasses: the impact of a surveillance protocol and elective revision. J Vasc Surg 9:286–296

Baril DT, Rhee RY, Kim J, Makaroun MS, Chaer RA, Marone LK (2009) Duplex criteria for determination of in-stent stenosis after angioplasty and stenting of superficial femoral artery. J Vasc Surg 49:133–139

Bärlin E, Schäberle W, Junge H, Seitz K, Rettenmaier G (1988) In-vitro-Untersuchung zur Meßgenauigkeit der mittleren Blutflußgeschwindigkeit bei Duplex-Geräten. Ultraschall Klin Prax 1(Suppl):69 (Abstr)

Barnes RW (1985) Doppler ultrasonic diagnosis of venous disease. In: Bernstein EF (ed) Noninvasive diagnostic techniques in vascular disease. Mosby, St. Louis, p 344

Barnes RW (1991) Noninvasive diagnostic assessment of peripheral vascular disease. Circulation 83(Suppl 2):120–127

Barnes RW, KK W, Hoak JC (1975) Fallibility of the clinical diagnosis of venous thrombosis. JAMA 234:605

Barnes RW, Nix ML, Barnes CL, Lavender RC et al (1989) Perioperative asymptomatic venous thrombosis: role of duplex scanning versus venography. J Vasc Surg 9:251–260

Barrelier MT (1993) Superficial venous thromboses of the legs. Phlebologie 46:633–639

Bartels E (1992) Farbkodierte Dopplersonographie der Vertebralarterien. Vergleich mit der konventionellen Duplexsonographie. Ultraschall Med 13:59–66

Bartels E, Flügel KA (1993) Advantages of color Doppler imaging for the evaluation of the vertebral arteries. J Neuroimaging 3: 229–233

Barwegen MGMH, van Dongen RJAM (1987) Neurovaskuläre Kompressionssyndrome an der oberen Thoraxapertur und ihre vaskulären Komplikationen. In: Heberer G, Van Dongen RJAM (Hrsg) Gefäßchirurgie. Springer, Berlin/Heidelberg/New York/Tokyo, pp S 571–S 584, Kirschnersche allgemeine und spezielle Operationslehre, Bd 11

Bassiouny HS, Sakaguchi Y, Mikucki SA et al (1977) Juxtalumenal location of plaque necrosis and neoformation in symptomatic carotid stenosis. J Vasc Surg 26:585–594

Baumgartner I, Maier SE, Koch M et al (1993) Magnetresonanzarteriographie, Duplexsonographie und konventionelle Arteriographie zur Beurteilung der peripheren arteriellen Verschlußkrankheit. Fortschr Röntgenstr 159:167–173

Baxter GM (2002) Imaging and renal transplantation. Imaging 14: 285–298

Baxter GM, McKechnie S, Duffy P (1990) Colour Doppler ultrasound in deep venous thrombosis: a comparison with venography. Clin Radiol 42:32–36

Baxter GM, Aitchison F, Sheppard D et al (1996) Colour Doppler ultrasound in renal artery stenosis: intrarenal waveform analysis. Br J Radiol 69:810–815

Bay WH, Henry ML, Lazarus JM et al (1998) Predicting hemodialysis access failure with color flow Doppler ultrasound. Am J Nephrol 18:296–304

Beach KW (1992) 1975–2000: a quarter century of ultrasound technology. Ultrasound Med Biol 18:377–388

Beales L, Wolstenhumlme S, Evans JA, West R, Scott DJ (2011) Reproducibility of ultrasound measurement of abdominal aorta. Br J Surg 98:1517–1525

Becker HM, Kortmann H (1987) Nahtaneurysmen. In: Heberer G, Van Dongen RJAM (Hrsg) Gefäßchirurgie. Springer, Berlin/Heidelberg/New York/Tokyo (Kirschnersche allgemeine und spezielle Operationslehre, Bd 11), pp 178–184

Becker D, Strobel D, Hahn EG (2000) Tissue harmonic imaging und contrast harmonic imaging. Verbesserung der Diagnose von Lebermetastasen. Internist 41:17–23

Beebe HG, Salles-Cunha SX, Scissons RP et al (1999) Carotid arterial ultrasound scan imaging: a direct approach to stenosis measurement. J Vasc Surg 29:838–844

Beeman BR, Doctor LM, Doerr K, McAfee-Bennett S, Dougherty MJ, Calligaro KD (2009) Duplex ultrasound imaging alone is sufficient for midterm endovascular aneurysm repair surveillance: a cost analysis study and prospective comparison with computed tomography scan. J Vasc Surg 50:1019–1024

Beeman BR, Murtha K, Doerr K et al (2010) Duplex ultrasound factors predicting persistent type II endoleak and increasing AAA sac diameter after EVAR. J Vasc Surg 52:1147–1152

Beil PRF, Brennan J (1991) Vein graft surveillance by duplex scanning and pressure measurement. In: Greenhalgh RM (ed) The maintenance of arterial reconstruction. Saunders WB, London, p 135

Belcaro G (1992) Evaluation of recurrent deep venous thrombosis using colour duplex scanning in comparison with venography. Vasa 21:22–26

Belcaro G, Nicolaides AN, Veller M (1995) Venous disorders. In: A manual of diagnosis and treatment. Saunders, London/Philadelphia/Toronto, p 99

Belkin M, Raftery KB, Mackey WC, McLaughlin RL, Umphrey SE, Kunkemueller A (1994) A prospective study of the determinants of vein graft flow velocity: implications for graft surveillance. J Vasc Surg 19:259–267

Bendick PJ et al (2003) Efficacy of ultrasound scan contrast agents in the noninvasive follow-up of aortic stent grafts. J Vasc Surg 37:381–385

Benninger DH, Baumgartner RW (2006) Ultrasound diagnosis of cervical artery dissection. Front Neurol Neurosci 21:70–84

Benninger DH, Georgiadis D, Gandjour J et al (2006) Accuracy of color duplex ultrasound diagnosis of spontaneous carotid dissection causing ischemia. Stroke 37:377–381

Benson CB, Aruny JE, Vickers MA (1993) Correlation of duplex sonography with arteriography in patients with erectile dysfunction. AJR Am J Roentgenol 160:71–73

Benvegna S, Cassina I, Giuntini G, Rusignuolo F, Talarico F, Florena M (1990) Atherothrombotic microembolism of the lower extremities (the blue toe syndrome) from atherosclerotic non-aneurysmal aortic plaques. J Cardiovasc Surg 31:87–91

Beregi JP, Louvegny S, Ceugnart L (1997) Helical x-ray computed tomography of renal arteries. Apropos of 300 patients. J Radiol 78:549–556

Bergamini TM, Tatum CM Jr, Marshall C, Hall-Disselkamp B, Richardson JD (1995) Effect of multilevel sequential stenosis on lower extremity arterial duplex scanning. Am J Surg 169:564–566

Bergqvist D, Bjorck M, Ljungman C (2006) Popliteal venous aneurysm – a systematic review. World J Surg 30:273–279

Berguer R, Hwang NHC (1974) Critical arterial stenosis:A theoretical and experimental solution. Ann Surg 180:39–50

Berland LL, Koslin DB, Routh WD, Keller FS (1990) Renal artery stenosis: prospective evaluation of diagnosis with color duplex US compared with angiography – work in progress. Radiology 174:421–423

Bernardi E, Prandoni P, Lensing AW et al (1998) D-dimer testing as an adjunct to ultrasonography in patients with clinically suspected deep vein thrombosis: prospective cohort study. The Multicentre Italian D-dimer Ultrasound Study Investigation Group. BMJ 317:1037–1040

Bernardi E, Camporese G, Büller H et al (2008) Serial 2-point ultrasonography plus D-dimer test vs whole-leg color-coded Doppler ultrasonography for diagnosing suspected symptomatic deep vein thrombosis. JAMA 300:1653–1659

Bettmann AM, Paulin S (1977) Leg phlebography: the incidence, nature and modifications of undesirable side effects. Radiol Diagn 122:101

Bettmann M, Salzman E, Rosenthal D et al (1980) Reduction of venous thrombosis complicating phlebography. AJR 134:1169–1172

Beven EG (1991) Thoracic outlet syndromes. In: Young JR, Graor RA, Olin JW, Bartholomew JR (eds) Peripheral vascular diseases. Mosby, St. Louis, pp 497–509

Biasi GM, Sampaolo A, Mingazzini P et al (1999) Computer analysis of ultrasonic plaque echolucency in identifying high risk carotid bifurcation lesions. Eur J Vasc Endovasc Surg 17:476–479

Biasi GM, Froio A, Diethrich EB et al (2004) Carotid plaque echolucency increases the risk of stroke in carotid stenting: the Imaging in Carotid Angioplasty and Risk of Stroke (ICAROS) study. Circulation 110:756–762

Bicknell CD, Cheshire NJ (2003) The relationship between carotid atherosclerotic plaque morphology and the embolic risk during endovascular therapy. Eur J Vasc Endovasc Surg 26:17–21

Biemans RGM (1987) Kompressionssyndrom der Arteria poplitea. In: Heberer G, Van Dongen RJAM (Hrsg) Gefäßchirurgie. Springer, Berlin/Heidelberg/New York/Tokyo, pp S593–S599, Kirschnersche allgemeine und spezielle Operationslehre, Bd 11

Biland L, Lemgo E, Widmer LK (1987) Zur Epidemiologie der venösen Thromboembolie. Internist 28:285

Blackshear WM, Phillips DJ, Chikos PM, Harley JD et al (1980) Carotid artery velocity patterns in normal and stenotic vessels. Stroke 11:67–71

Blätter W (1993) Komplikationen der Thrombophlebitis superficialis. Schweiz med Wschr 123:223–228

Blätter W, Bulling B, Hertel T, Rabe E (1996) Leitlinien zur Diagnostik und Therapie der Thrombophlebitis. Phlebologie 25:197–198

Blättler W, Linder C, Blättler IK et al (1996) Die ambulante Behandlung der akuten tiefen Beinvenenthrombose (TVT): eine randomisierte prospektive Studie. Schweiz Med Wochenschr 126(Suppl):74/I

Blättler W, Partsch H, Hertel T (1996) Leitlinien zur Diagnostik und Therapie der tiefen Bein- und Beckenvenenthrombose. Phlebologie 25:199–203

Bluth EL, Kay D, Merritt CRB et al (1986) Sonographic characterization of carotid plaque: detection of hemorrhage. AJR 146:1061–1065

Bluth EI, McVay LV, Merrit CRB, Sullivan MA (1988) The identification of ulcerative plaque with high resolution duplex sonographic carotid scanning. J Ultrasound Med 7:73–76

Bluth EL, Stavros AT, Marich KW, Wetzner SM, Aufrichtig D, Baker JD (1988) Carotid duplex sonography: a multicenter recommendation for standardized imaging and Doppler criteria. Radiographics 8:487–506

Bock RW, Gray-Weale AC, Mock PA et al (1993) The natural history of asymptomatic carotid artery disease. J Vasc Surg 17:160–171

Bodily K, Buttorff J, Nordesgaard A, Osborne R Jr (1996) Aortoiliac reconstruction without angiography. Am J Surg 171:505–507

Bodner G, Peer S, Fries D et al (2000) Color and pulsed Doppler ultrasound findings in normally functioning transjugular intrahepatic portosystemic shunts. Eur J Ultrasound 12:131–136

Böhm B, Heyne J, Seifert S, Rimpler H, Bartel M (2000) Der Wert der farbkodierten kontrastmittelgestützten Duplexsonographie bei der Erfassung von Endoleckagen nach Aortenstentimplantation im mittleren Nachuntersuchungszeitraum von 15 Monaten. Gefässchirurgie 5:225–231

Bollinger A (1979) Funktionelle Angiologie. Thieme, Stuttgart

Bollinger A, Franzeck UK (1982) Diagnose der tiefen Becken- und Beinvenenthrombose. Schweiz Med Wochenschr 112:550–556

Bolondi L, Gamrolfi L, Arienti V et al (1982) Ultrasonography in the diagnosis of portal hypertension: diminished response of portal vessels to respiration. Radiology 142:167–172

Bolondi L, Mazziotti A, Arienti V et al (1984) Ultrasonographic study of portal venous system in portal hypertension and after portosystemic shunt operations. Surgery 95:261–269

Bolondi L, Bassi SL, Gaiani S et al (1991) Liver cirrhosis: changes of Doppler waveform of hepatic veins. Radiology 178:513–516

Bolondi L, Gaiani S, Gebel M (1998) Portohepatic vascular pathology and liver disease: diagnosis and monitoring. Eur J Ultrasound 7(suppl 3):41–52

Bommer WJ, Miller L (1982) Real-time two dimensional color flow Doppler: enhanced Doppler flow imaging in the diagnosis of cardiovascular disease(abstr). Am J Cardiol 49:944

Bond MG, Wilmoth SK, Enevold GL et al (1989) Detection and monitoring of asymptomatic atherosclerosis in clinical trials. Am J Med 86:33–36

Bönhof J, Meairs SP, Wetzler H (1990) Duplex- und Farbdopplersonographische Kriterien von Nierenarterienstenosen. Ultraschall Klin Prax 5:187 (Abstr)

Bonnefous O, Pasque P (1986) Time domain formulation of pulse-Doppler ultrasound and blood velocity estimation by cross correlation. Academic. Ultrason Imaging 8:73–85

Bork-Wölwer L, Wuppermann TH (1991) Verbesserung der nichtinvasiven Diagnostik der V. saphena magna- und der Vena saphena parva-Insuffizienz durch die Duplex-Sonographie. Vasa 20:343–347

Börner N (1991) Diagnostische und prognostische Bedeutung der Echomorphologie tiefer Becken-Bein-Venenthrombosen. Habilitationsschrift Mainz

Börner N, Todt M, Schuter CJ, Meyer J (1987) Sonographie in der Diagnostik venöser Thromben. Klin Wochenschr 65(Suppl 9):37

Boström A, Ljungman C, Hellberg A et al (2002) Duplex scanning as the sole preoperative imaging method for infrainguinal arterial surgery. Eur J Vasc Endovasc Surg 23:140–145

Bots ML, de Jong PT, Hofmann A et al (1997) Left, right, near or far wall common carotid intima-media thickness measurements: associations with cardiovascular disease and lower extremity arterial atherosclerosis. J Clin Epidemiol 50:801–807

Bouchet C, Magne JL, Lacaze R, Lebrun D, Franco A (1986) L'anévrisme de la veine poplitée: une cause rare d'embolie pulmonaire à répétition. J Mal Vasc 11:190–193

Bouhoutsos J, Martin P (1974) Popliteal aneurysm, a review of 116 cases. Br J Surg 61:469–475

Bounameaux H (2002) Integrated diagnostic approach to suspected deep vein thrombosis and pulmonary embolism. Vasa 31:15–21

Bounameaux H, De Moerloose P, Reber G (1994) Plasma measurement of D-dimer as diagnostic aid in suspected venous thromboembolism: an overview. Thromb Haemost 71:1–6

Bowersox JC, Zwolak RM, Walsh DB et al (1991) Duplex ultrasonography in the diagnosis of celiac and mesenteric artery occlusive disease. Eur J Vasc Endovasc Surg 14:780–788

Brandl R, Orend KH, Becker HM (1993) Rekonstruktionsprinzipien bei peripherer arterieller Verschlußkrankheit der unteren Extremitäten. Dt Ärztebl 37:1616–1620

Brandstetter K, Schwarzer JU, Bautz W, Pickl U, Lenz M (1993) Vergleich der Farbduplexsonographie mit der selektiven penilen DSA bei der Abklärung der erektilen Dysfunktion. Fortschr Röntgenstr 158: 405–409

Braun B, Scheffler P, Kiehl R, Wenzel E (1986) A duplex system for evaluation of venous function. In: Maurer PC, Becker HM, Heidrich H, Hoffmann G, Kriessmann A, Müller-Wiefel H, Prätorius C (eds) What is new in angiology? Trends and controversies. Proceedings. Zuckschwerdt. Verlag, Munich

Braunwald E (1984) Heart disease. A textbook of cardiovascular medicine. WB Saunders, Philadelphia

Bredahl K, Eldrup N, Meyer C, Eiberg JE, Sillesen H (2013) Reproducibility of ECG-gated ultrasound diameter assessment of small abdominal aortic aneurysms. Eur J Vasc Endovasc Surg 45:235–240

Bredahl K, Taudorf M, Long A et al (2013) Three-dimensional ultrasound improves the accuracy of diameter measurement of the residual sac in EVAR patients. Eur J Vasc Endovasc Surg 46:525–532

Breitenseher M, Kainberger F, Hübsch P et al (1992) Screening von Nierenarterienstenosen. Fortschr Röntgenstr 156:228–231

Brescia MJ, Cimino JE, Appel K, Burwich BJ (1966) Chronic hemodialysis using venipuncture and a surgically created arteriovenous fistula. N Engl J Med 275:1089–1092

Brewster DC, Cronenwett JL, Hallet JW et al (2003) Guideline for the treatment of abdominal aortic aneurysms. Report of a subcommittee of the Joint Council of the American Association for Vascular Surgery and Society for Vascular Surgery. J Vasc Surg 37:1106–1117

Brittinger WD, Twittenhoff W-D, Walker G, Konrad N (1966) Revaskularisation des Dialyseshunts. Nieren- und Hochdruckkrankheiten 25:4–9

Brodmann M, Stark G, Pabst E, Seinost G et al (2001) Cystic adventitial degeneration of the popliteal artery – the diagnostic value of duplex sonography. Eur J Radiol 38:209–212

Brophy DP, Sheiman RG, Amatulle P, Akbari CM (2000) Iatrogenic femoral pseudoaneurysms: thrombin injection after failed US-guided compression. Radiology 214:278–282

Browman MW, Cooperberg PL, Harrison PB et al (1995) Duplex ultrasonography criteria for internal carotid stenosis of more than 70% diameter: angiographic correlation and receiver operating characteristic curve analysis. Can Assoc Radiol J 46:291–295

Brown JM, Hammers LW, Barton JW et al (1995) Quantitative Doppler assessment of acute scrotal inflammation. Radiology 197:427–431

Brunner U, Hauser M (1997) Hemodynamic assessment of venous aneurysm of lower leg and therapeutic consequences. Zentralbl Chir 122:809–812

Bruno S, Remuzzi G, Ruggenenti P (2004) Transplant renal artery stenosis. J Am Soc Nephrol 15:134–141

Bunk A, Buchcik R, Konopke R et al (2000) Farbdoppler, Power-Doppler, Echokontrastmittel. Verbesserung der perioperativen Diagnostik? Internist 41:29–36

Burckhardt CB (1993) Signalverarbeitung in Ultraschallabbildung, Doppler und Dopplerabbildung. Ultraschall Med 14:220–224

Burton BS, Syms MJ, Petermann GW et al (2000) MR imaging of patients with carotidynia. Am J Neuroradiol 21:766–769

Bushong SC, Archer BR (1991) Diagnostic ultrasound. Physics, biology and instrumentation. Mosby Year Book, St. Louis

Busuttil SJ, Franklin DP, Youkey JR et al (1996) Carotid duplex overestimation of stenosis due to severe contralateral disease. Am J Surg 172:144–148

Buth J, Disselhoff B, Sommeling C, Stam L (1991) Color-flow duplex criteria for grading stenosis in infrainguinal vein grafts. J Vasc Surg 14:716–726

Calligaro KD, Musser DJ, Chen AY et al (1996) Duplex ultrasonography to diagnose failing arterial prosthetic grafts. Surgery 120:455–459

Calligaro KD, Syrek JR, Dougherty MJ et al (1998) Selective use of duplex ultrasound to replace preoperative arteriography for failing arterial vein grafts. J Vasc Surg 27:89–95

Campbell WB, Milliar AW (1985) Cystic adventitial disease of the common femoral artery communicating with the hip joint. Br J Surg 72:537

Caplan LR (2008) Dissections of brain-supplying arteries. Nat Clin Pract Neurol 4:34–42

Cappell MS (1998) Intestinal (mesenteric) vasculopathy. I. Acute superior mesenteric arteriopathy and venopathy. Gastroenterol Clin N Am 27:783–825

Cardella JF, Young AT, Smith TP et al (1988) Lower extremity venous thrombosis. Comparison of venography, impedance plethysmography and intravenous manometry. Radiology 168:109

Carpenter JP, Holland GA, Baum RA, Owen RS, Carpenter JT, Cope C (1993) Magnetic resonance venography for the detection of deep venous thrombosis: comparison with contrast venography and duplex Doppler ultrasonography. J Vasc Surg 18:734–741

Carpenter JP, Lexa FJ, Davis JT (1995) Determination of sixty percent or greater carotid artery stenosis by duplex Doppler ultrasonography. J Vasc Surg 22:697–703

Carpenter JP, Lexa FJ, Davis JT (1996) Determination of duplex Doppler ultrasound criteria appropriate to the North American Symptomatic Carotid Endarterectomy Trial. Stroke 27:695–699

Carr S, Farb A, Pearce WH, Virmani R, Yao JST (1996) Atherosclerotic plaque rupture in symptomatic carotid artery stenosis. J Vasc Surg 23:755–766

Carter KA, Nelms CR, Bloch PHS et al (2000) Doppler waveform assessment of endoleak following endovascular repair of abdominal aortic aneurysm: predictors of endoleak thrombosis. J Vasc Technol 24:119–122

CASANOVA Study Group (1991) Carotid surgery versus medical therapy in asymptomatic carotid stenosis. Stroke 22:1229–1235

Casarella WJ (1995) Transjugular intrahepatic portosystemic shunt: a defining achievement in vascular and interventional radiology. Radiology 196:305

Caspary L (2016) Inflammatory diseases of the aorta. Vasa 45:17–29

Cassar K, Engeset J (2005) Cystic adventitial disease: a trap for the unwary. Eur J Vasc Endovasc Surg 29:93–96

Cave EM, Pugh ND, Wilson RJ et al (1995) Carotid artery duplex scanning: does plaque echogenicity correlate with patient symptoms? Eur J Vasc Endovasc Surg 10:77–81

Chaer RA, Gushchin A, Rhee R et al (2009) Duplex ultrasound as the sole long-term surveillance method post-endovascular aneurysm repair: a safe alternative for stable aneurysms. J Vasc Surg 49: 845–849

Chahlaoui J, Julien M, Nadeau P, Bruneau L, Roy P, Sylvestre J (1981) Popliteal venous aneurysm: a source of pulmonary embolism. AJR 136:415–416

Chahwan S, Miller MT, Pigott JP Whalen RC, Jones L, Comerota AJ (2007) Carotid arteria velocity characteristics after carotid artery angioplasty and stenting. J Vasc Surg 45:523–526

Chakfé N, Beaufigeau M, Geny B et al (1997) Extra-popliteal localization of adventitial cysts. Review of the literature. J Mal Vasc 22:79–85

Chalmers RTA, Hoballah JJ, Kresowik TF et al (1994) The impact of color duplex surveillance on the outcome of lower limb bypass with segments of arm veins. J Vasc Surg 19:279–288

Chang BB, Leather RP, Kaufman JL, Kupinski AM, Leopold PW, Shah DM (1990) Haemodynamic characteristics of failing infrainguinal in situ vein bypass. J Vasc Surg 12:596–600

Chang YJ, Lin SK, Ryo SJ, Wai YY (1995) Common carotid artery occlusion: evaluation with duplex sonography. Am J Neuroradiol 16:1099–1105

Charette S, Nehler MR, Whitehill TA et al (2001) Epithelioid hemangioendothelioma of the common femoral vein: Case report and review of the literature. J Vasc Surg 33:1100–1103

Chawla Y, Santa N, Dhiman RK et al (1998) Portal hemodynamics by duplex Doppler sonography in different grades of cirrhosis. Dig Dis Sci 43:354–357

Chengelis DL, Bendick PJ, Glover PJL, Brown OW, Ranaval TJ (1996) Prognosis of superficial venous thrombosis to deep vein thrombosis. J Vasc Surg 24:745–749

Chi YW, White CJ, Woods TC, Goldman CK (2007) Ultrasound velocity criteria for carotid in-stent restenosis. Catheter Cardiovasc Interv 69:349–354

Chi YW, White CJ, Thornton S, Milani RV (2009) Ultrasound velocity criteria for renal in-stent restenosis. J Vasc Surg 50:119–123

Chiche L, Barranger B, Cordoliani YS et al (1994) Two cases of cystic adventitial disease of the popliteal artery. Current diagnostic approach. J Mal Vasc 19:57–61

Chiu KW, Ling L, Tripathi V, Ahmed M, Shrivastava V (2014) Ultrasound measurement for abdominal aortic aneurysm screening: a direct comparison of the three leading methods. Eur J Vasc Endovasc Surg 47:367–373

Chong WK, Malisch TW, Mazer MJ et al (1993) Transjugular intrahepatic portosystemic shunts: US assessment with maximum flow velocity. Radiology 189:789–793

Choschzick M, Stosiek P, Hantschick M (1997) Cystic adventitial degeneration of the popliteal artery. Rare cause of intermittent claudication in middle-aged adults. Pathologe 18:467–473

Chuang VP, Mena CE, Hoskins PA (1974) Congenital anomalies of the inferior vena cava. Review of embryogenesis and presentation of a simplified classification. Br J Radiol 47:206–213

Ciccone MM, Cortese F, Fiorella A et al (2011) The clinical role of contrast-enhanced ultrasound in the evaluation of renal artery stenosis and diagnostic superiority as compared to traditional echo-color-Doppler flow imaging. Int Angiol 30:135–139

Ciulla MM, Paliotti R, Ferrero S, Vandone P, Magrini F, Zanchetti A (2002) Assessment of carotid plaque composition in hypertensive patients by ultrasonic tissue characterization: a validation study. J Hypertens 20:1589–1596

Clark TW, Cohen RA, Kwak A et al (2007) Salvage of nonmaturing native fistulas by using angioplasty. Radiology 242:286–292

Claudon M, Plouin PF, Baxter GM et al. for the Levovist Renal Artery Stenosis Study Group (2000) Renal arteries in patients at risk of renal arterial stenosis: multicenter evaluation of the echo-enhancer SHU 508 A at color and spectral Doppler US. Radiology 214:739–746

Claudon M, Cosgrove D, Albrecht T et al (2008) Guidelines and good clinical practice recommendations for contrast enhanced ultrasound (CEUS) – Update 2008. Ultraschall Med 29:28–44

Clevert DA, Johnson T, Michaely H (2006) High-grade stenoses of the internal carotid artery: comparison of high-resolution contrast enhanced 3D MRA, duplex sonography and power Doppler imaging. Eur J Radiol 60:379

Clevert DA, Minfaifar N, Weckbach S et al (2008) Color duplex ultrasound and contrast-enhanced ultrasound in comparison to MS-CT in the detection of endoleak following endovascular aneurysm repair. Clin Hemorheol Microcirc 39:121–132

Clevert DA, Jung EM, Reiser M, Rupp N Verbesserte diagnostische Sicherheit durch den Ultraschall B-Flow bei Gefäßdissektion. Institut für klinische Radiologie; München (DE); Radiologie; Passau (DE); Radiologie, München (DE)

Clevert DA, Sommer WH, Helck A, Reiser M (2011) Duplex and contrast enhanced ultrasound (CEUS) in evaluation of in-stent restenosis after carotid stenting. Hemorheal Microcirc 48:199–208

Clifford TA, Back T, Padberg FT, Thompson PN, Duran WN, Hobson RW (1993) Refinements in the ultrasonic detection of popliteal vein reflux. J Vasc Surg 18:742–748

Coelho JCU, Sigel B, Ryva JC, Machi J, Renigers SA (1982) B-mode sonography of blood clots. J Clin Ultrasound 10:323–327

Coffmann SW, Leon SM, Gupta SK (2000) Popliteal venous aneurysms: report of an unusual presentation and literature rview. Ann Vasc Surg 14:286–290

Cogo A, Lensing WA, Prandoni P, Hirsh J (1993) Distribution of thrombosis in patients with symptomatic deep vein thrombosis. Arch Intern Med 153:2777–2780

Cogo A, Lensing AWA, Koopman MMW et al (1998) Compression ultrasonography for diagnostic management of patients with clinically suspected deep vein thrombosis: a prospective cohort study. BMJ 316:17–20

Coleridge-Smith P, Labropoulos N, Partsch H, Myers K, Nicolaides A, Cavezzi A (2006) Duplex ultrasound investigation of the veins in chronic venous disease of the lower limbs–UIP consensus document. Part I. Basic principles. Eur J Vasc Endovasc Surg 31:83–92

Coley BD, Roberts AC, Fellmeth BD (1995) Postangiographic femoral artery pseudoaneurysms: further experience with US-guided compression repair. Radiology 194:307–311

Coli S, Magnoni M, Sangiorgi G et al (2008) Contrast-enhanced ultrasound imaging of intraplaque neovascularization in carotid arteries correlation with histology and plaque echogenicity. J Am Coll Cardiol 52:223–230

Colli A, Cocciolo M, Riva C et al (1994) Abnormalities of Doppler waveform of the hepatic veins in patients with chronic liver disease: correlation with histologic findings. AJR 162:833

Collin J, Auranja H, Sutton GLJ, Lindsell D, Oxford D (1988) Screening programme for abdominal aortic aneurysm in men aged 65 to 74 years. Lancet 2:613–615

Collins JT, Boros MJ, Combs K (2007) Ultrasound surveillance of endovascular aneurysm repair: a safe modality versus computed tomography. Ann Vasc Surg 21:671–675

Collins R, Burch J, Cranny G et al (2007) Duplex ultrasonography, magnetic resonance angiography, and computed tomography angiography for diagnosis and assessment of symptomatic lower limb peripheral arterial disease: systematic review. BMJ 334:1257

Colombier D, Elias A, Rousseau H, Otal P, Leger P, Joffre F (1997) Cystic adventitial disease: importance of computed tomography in the diagnostic and therapeutic management. J Mal Vasc 22:181–186

Comerota AJ, Katz ML (1990) The preoperative diagnosis of the ulcerated carotid atheroma. J Vasc Surg 11:505–510

Comerota AJ, Katz ML, Greenwald LL, Leefmans E, Czeredarczuk M, White JV (1990) Venous duplex imaging: should it replace hemodynamic tests for deep venous thrombosis? J Vasc Surg 11:53–59

Conkbayir I, Yucesoy C, Edguer T et al (2003) Doppler sonography in renal artery stenosis. An evaluation of intrarenal and extrarenal imaging parameters. Clin Imaging 27:256–260

Connell J (1978) Popliteal vein entrapment. Br J Surg 65:351

Cornus J, Pearson SD, Polak JF (1999) Deep venous thrombosis: complete lower extremity venous US examination in patients without known risk factors – outcome study. Radiology 211:637–641

Correas J-M, Hélénon O, Pourcelot L, Moreau J-F (1997) Ultrasound contrast agents. Acta Radiol 38(suppl 412):101–112

Corriere MA, Guzman RJ (2005) True and false aneurysms of the femoral artery. Semin Vasc Surg 18:216–223

Cosgrove D (1997) Echo enhancers and ultrasound imaging. Eur J Radiol 26:64–76

Cosgrove DO, Arger PH (1982) Intravenous echoes due to laminar flow – experimental observations. Am J Radiol 139:953–956

Cosgrove DO, Blomley MJK, Jayaram V et al (1998) Echo-enhancing (contrast) agents. Ultrasound Q 14:66–75

Cossman DV, Ellison JE, Wagner WH, Carroll RM et al (1989) Comparison of contrast angiography to arterial mapping with color-flow duplex imaging in the lower extremities. J Vasc Surg 10:522–529

Crawford ES, Hess KR (1989) Abdominal aortic surgery. N Engl J Med 321:1040–1042

Creutzig A, von der Lieth H, Majewski A, Caspary L, Oestmann J, Alexander K (1988) Vascular complications of the compression syndrome of the anterior thoracic aperture (thoracic outlet syndrome). Med Klin (Munich) 83:133–136

Cronan JJ (1993) Venous thromboembolic disease: the role of US. Radiology 186:619–630

Cronan JJ (1996) Deep venous thromosis: one leg or both legs? Radiology 200:323–324

Cronan JJ (1997) Controversies in venous ultrasound. Semin Ultrasound CT MR 18:33–38

Cronan J, Leen V (1989) Recurrent deep venous thrombosis: limitations of US. Radiology 170:739–742

Cronan JJ, Dorfman GS, Scola FH, Schepps B, Alexander J (1987) Deep venous thrombosis. US assessment using vein compression. Radiology 162:191–194

Cronan JJ, Dorfman GS, Gusmark J (1988) Lower-extremity deep venous thrombosis: further experience with and refinements of ultrasound assessment. Radiology 168:101

Cronan JJ, Froehlich J, Dorfman GS, Scola FH, Schepps B (1988) Serial compression ultrasonography in a patient population at high risk for deep vein thrombosis. Radiology 169(Suppl):321 (Abstr)

Cronenwett JL, Krupski WC, Rutherford RB (2000) Abdominal aortic and iliac aneurysms. In: Rutherford RB (ed) Vascular surgery, 5th edn. Saunders, Philadelphia, pp 1246–1280

Cvitanic OA, Cronan JJ, Sigman M, Landau ST (1993) Varicoceles: postoperative prevalence – a prospective study with color Doppler US. Radiology 187:711–714

Czerny M, Trubel W, Claeys L et al (1997) Acute mesenteric ischemia. Zentralbl Chir 122:538–544

D'Audiffret A (2001) Follow-up evaluation of endoluminally treated abdominal aortic aneurysms with duplex ultrasonography: validation with computed tomography. J Vasc Surg 33:42–50

Daher A, Jones V, da Silva AF (2001) The role of popliteal vein incompetence in the diagnosis of saphenous-popliteal reflux using continuous wave Doppler. Eur J Vasc Endovasc Surg 21:350–352

Dahl JR, Freed TA, Burke MF (1976) Popliteal vein aneurysm with recurrent pulmonary thromboemboli. JAMA 236:2531–2532

Danse EM, Van Beers BE, Goffette P, Dardenne AN, Latterre PF, Pringot J (1996) Acute intestinal ischemia due to occlusion of superior mesenteric artery: detection with Doppler sonography. J Ultrasound Med 15:323–326

Danse EM, Kartheuser A, Paterson HM et al (2009) Color Doppler sonography of small bowel changes. J Belg Radiol 92:202–206

Darwood R, Earnshaw JJ, Turton G, Shaw E, Whyman M, Poskitt K et al (2012) Twenty-year review of abdominal aortic aneurysm screening in men in the county of Gloucestershire, United Kingdom. J Vasc Surg 56:8–14

Dasbach G, Schmitz I, Niehoff L, Edelmann M, Müller K-M (1998) Arteriosklerose der Karotisregion. Gefässchirurgie 3:151–157

Dauzat MM, Laroche J-R, Charras CC, Blin B, Domingo-Faye MM (1986) Real-time B-mode ultrasonography for better specificity in the noninvasive diagnosis of deep vein thrombosis. J Ultrasound Med 5:625–631

Davidson JT, Callis JT (1993) Arterial reconstruction of vessels in the foot and ankle. Ann Surg 217:699–708

Davies KN, Humphrey PR (1993) Complications of cerebral angiography in patients with symptomatic carotid territory ischaemia screened by carotid ultrasound. J Neurol Neurosurg Psychiatry 56:967–972

Davies AH, Hawdon AJ, Sydes MR, Thompson SG (2005) Is duplex surveillance of value after leg vein bypass grafting? Principal results of the Vein Graft Surveillance Randomised Trial (VGST). Circulation 112:1985–1991

Davis SM, Donnan GA (2003) Is carotid angiography necessary? Editors disagree. Stroke 34:1819

Dawson DL (1996) Noninvasive assessment of renal artery stenosis. Semin Vasc Surg 9:172–181

De Bakey ME, Henly WS, Cooley DA et al (1965) Surgical management of dissecting aneurysms of the aorta. J Thorac Cardiovasc Surg 49:130–148

De Bray JM, Glatt B (1994) Quantification of atheromatous stenosis in the extracranial internal carotid artery. Cerebrovasc Dis 5:414–426

De Bray JM, Baud JM, Dauzat M on behalf of the Consensus Conference (1997) Consensus concerning the morphology and the risk of carotid plaques. Cerebrovasc Dis 7:289–296

De Bruyne Manoharan G, Pijls NHJ et al (2006) Assessment of renal artery stenosis severity by pressure gradient measurement. J Am Coll Cardiol 48:1851–1855

De Haan MW, Kroon AA, Flobbe K (2002) Renovascular disease in patients with hypertension: detection with duplex ultrasound. J Hum Hypertens 16:501–507

De Morais RH, Muglia VF, Mamere VF et al (2003) Duplex Doppler sonography of transplant renal artery stenosis. J Clin Ultrasound 31:135–141

De Morais Filho D, Miranda F, Del Carmen Janeiro Peres M et al (2004) Segmental waveform analysis in diagnosis of peripheral arterial occlusive diseases. Ann Vasc Surg 18:714–724

De Smet AA, Kitslaar PJ (1990) A duplex criterion for aorto-iliac stenosis. Eur J Vasc Surg 4:275–278

De Smet AA, Emers EJ, Kitslaar PJ (1996) Duplex velocity characteristics of aortoiliac stenosis. J Vasc Surg 23:628–636

De Valois JC, van Schaik CC, Verzijlbergen F, van Ramshorst B, Eikelboom BC, Meuwissen OJAT (1990) Contrast venography: from gold standard to "golden backup" in clinically suspected deep vein thrombosis. Eur J Radiol 11:131–137

DEGUM, Arbeitskreis Gefäßdiagnostik (1986) Richtlinien für die Durchführung dopplersonographischer Untersuchungen der Becken- und Beinvenen. Deutsche Ges Angiologie, Mitt 3. Demeter, Gräfelfing

Delcker A, Diener HC (1992) Die verschiedenen Ultraschallmethoden zur Untersuchung der A. vertebralis: Eine vergleichende Wertung. Ultraschall Med 13:213–220

Delin A, Johansson G, Silfverswärd C (1990) Vascular tumors in occlusive disease of the iliac-femoral vessels. Eur J Vasc Surg 4:539–542

Denzel C, Balzer K, Muller KM, Fellner F, Fellner C, Lang W (2003) Relative value of normalized sonographic in vitro analysis of arteriosclerotic plaques of internal carotid artery. Stroke 34:1901–1906

Denzel C, Fellner F, Wutke R, Bazler K, Muller KM, Lang W (2003) Ultrasonographic analysis of arteriosclerotic plaques in the internal carotid artery. Eur J Ultrasound 16:161–167

Denzel C, Balzer K, Merhof D, Lang W et al (2009) 3D cross sectional view to investigate the morphology of internal carotid artery plaques. Is 3D ultrasound superior to 2D ultrasound? Ultraschall Med 29: 291–296

Derkx FH, Schalekamp MA (1994) Renal artery stenosis and hypertension. Lancet 344:237–239

Desai KM, Gilbert HG (1991) Noninvasive investigation of penile artery function. In: Kirby RS, Carson CC, Webster GD (eds) Impotence: diagnosis and management of male erectile dysfunction. Butterworth-Heinemann, Oxford, pp 81–91

Desberg AL, Paushter DM, Lammert GK et al (1990) Renal artery stenosis: evaluation with color Doppler flow imaging. Radiology 177:749–753

Deutsch AL, Hyde J, Miller SM, Diamond CG, Schanche AF (1985) Cystic adventitial degeneration of the popliteal artery: CT demonstration and directed percutaneous therapy. AJR 145:117–118

DeWire DM, Begun FP, Lawson RK, Fitzgerald S, Foley WD (1992) Color Doppler ultrasonography in the evaluation of the acute scrotum. J Urol 147:89–91

Diamaria G, Zittoun R, Reynes M (1981) Anévrisme veineux poplité révélé par une embolie pulmonaire. Ann Cardiol Angeiol 30: 337–338

Diehm C (1998) Buerger Syndrom (Thrombangiitis obliterans). In: Handbuch akrale Durchblutungsstörungen. Epidemiologie, Pathogenese, Diagnostik und Therapie. Barth, Heidelberg, pp 185–203

Dietrich CF, Averkiou MA, Correas JM (2012) An EFSUMB introduction into Dynamic Contrast-Enhanced Ultrasound (DCE-US) for quantification of tumour perfusion. Ultraschall Med 33:344–351

Dion JE, Gates PC, Fox AJ, Barnett HJM, Blom RJ (1987) Clinical events following neuroangiography: a prospective study. Stroke 18:997–1004

Disselhof B, Buth J, Jakimowicz J (1989) Early detection of stenosis of femoro-distal grafts. A surveillance study using colour-duplex scanning. Eur J Vasc Surg 3:43–48

Diwan A, Sarkar R, Stanly JC (2000) Incidence of femoral and popliteal artery aneurysms in patients with abdominal aortic aneurysms. J Vasc Surg 31:863–869

Dix FP, McDonald M, Obomighie J et al (2006) Cystic adventitial disease of the femoral vein presenting as deep vein thrombosis: a case report and review of the literature. J Vasc Surg 44:871–874

Do DD, Zehender T, Mahler F (1993) Farbkodierte Duplexsonographie bei iatrogenen Aneurysmata spuria in der Leiste. Dtsch Med Wochenschr 118:656–660

Do DD, Braunschweig M, Baumgartner I, Furrer M, Mahler F (1997) Adventitial cystic disease of the popliteal artery: percutaneous US-guided aspiration. Radiology 203:743–746

Dodd GD III, Zajko AB, Orons PD et al (1995) Detection of transjugular intrahepatic portosystemic shunt dysfunction: value of duplex Doppler sonography. Am J Roentgenol 164:1119–1124

Doelman C, Duijm LE, Liem YS et al (2005) Stenosis detection in failing hemodialysis access fistulas and grafts: comparison of color Doppler ultrasonography, contrast-enhanced magnetic resonance angiography and digital subtraction angiography. J Vasc Surg 42:739–746

Donald IP, Edwards RD (1982) Fatal outcome from popliteal venous aneurysm associated with pulmonary embolism. Br J Radiol 55:930–931

Dorweiler B, Neufang A, Kreitner KF et al (2002) Magnetic resonance angiography unmasks reliable target vessels for pedal bypass grafting in patients with diabetes mellitus. J Vasc Surg 35:766–772

Dougherty MJ, Calligaro KD, DeLaurentis DA (1998) The natural history of "failing" arterial grafts in a duplex surveillance protocol. Ann Vasc Surg 12:255–259

Droste, v. Planta (1989) Memorix, 2. korrigierte Auflage: VCH Verlagsgesellschaft, Weinheim (Bundesrepublik Deutschland)

Droste DW, Karl M, Bohle RM, Kaps M (1997) Comparison of ultrasonic and histopathological features of carotid artery stenosis. Neurol Res 19:380–384

Dubbins PA (1986) Renal artery stenosis: duplex Doppler evaluation. Br J Radiol 59:225–229

Duerschmied D, Rossknecht A, Olsson L et al (2005) Contrast ultrasound perfusion imaging of lower extremities in peripheral arterial disease – a novel diagnostic method. Ultraschall Med 26:S39

Dunant JH, Eugenidis N (1973) Cystic degeneration of the popliteal artery. Vasa 2:156–159

Dyet JF, Nicholson AA, Eitles OF (2000) Vascular imaging and Intervention in peripheral arteries in the diabetic patient. Diabetes Metab Res Rev 16(Suppl 1):16–22

Dzsinich C, Gloviczki P, Van Heerden J et al (1992) Primary venous leiomyosarcoma: a rare but lethal disease. J Vasc Surg 15:592–603

Ebrahim S, Papacosta O, Whincup P et al (1999) Carotid plaque, intima media thickness, cardiovascular risk factors, and prevalent cardiovascular disease in men and women: The British Regional Heart Study. Stroke 30:841–850

Eckstein HH, Winter R, Eichbaum M et al (2001) Grading of internal carotid artery stenosis: validation of Doppler/duplex ultrasound criteria and angiography against endarterectomy specimen. Eur Vasc Endovasc Surg 21:301–310

ECST Collaborative Group (1996) Endarterectomy for moderate symptomatic carotid stenosis: interim results from the MRC European Carotid Surgery Trial. Lancet 347:1591–1593

ECST European Carotid Surgery Trialists Collaborative Group (1991) MRC European Carotid Surgery Trial: interim results for symptomatic patients with severe (70–90%) or with mild (0–29%) carotid stenosis. Lancet 337:1235–1243

Edmondson HT, Crowe JA (1972) Popliteal artery and venous entrapment. Am Surg 38:657–659

Edwards JM, Coldwell DM, Goldman ML, Strandness DE Jr (1991) The role of duplex scanning in the selection of patients for transluminal angioplasty. J Vasc Surg 13:69–74

Edwards JM, Moneta GL, Papanicolaou G et al (1995) Prospective validation of a new duplex ultrasound criteria for 70%–99% internal carotid stenosis. JEMU 16:3–7

Effeney DJ, Fiedmann MB, Gooding GAW (1984) Iliofemoral venous thrombosis: real-time ultrasound diagnosis, normal criteria, and clinical application. Radiology 150:787–792

Egbring J, Görg C (2007) Die asymptomatische Lungenembolie: Sollte jeder Patient mtit tiefer Beinvenenthrombose am Thorax geschallt werden? Ultraschall Med 28:375–379

Eiberg JP, Jensen F, Gronvall Rasmussen JB, Schroeder TV (2001) Screening for aortoiliac lesions by visual interpretation of the common femoral Doppler waveform. Eur J Vasc Endovasc Surg 22:331–336

Eiberg JP, Madycki G, Hansen MA, Christiansen S, Gronvall Rasmussen JB, Schroeder TV (2002) Ultrasound imaging of infrainguinal arterial disease has a high interobserver agreement. Eur J Vasc Endovasc Surg 24:293–299

Eichlisberger R, Jäger K (1989) Beeinflussung der venösen Hämodynamik durch Venenpharmaka. Nachweis mittels Duplexsonographie. Was gibt es Neues in der Phlebologie (Kurzfassung)

El-Barghouty N, Geroulkas G, Nicolaides A, Androulakis A, Bahal V (1995) Computer-assisted carotid plaque characterization. Eur J Vasc Endovasc Surg 9:389–393

El-Barghouty N, Nicolaides A, Bahal V, Geroulakos G, Androulakis A (1996) The identification of the high risk carotid plaque. Eur J Vasc Endovasc Surg 11:470–478

El-Barghouty NM, Levine T, Ladva S, Flanagan A, Nicolaides A (1996) Histological verification of computerised carotid plaque characterisation. Eur J Vasc Endovasc Surg 11:414–416

Elgersma OE, van Leersum M, Buijs PC et al (1998) Changes over time in optimal duplex threshold for the identification of patients eligible for carotid endarterectomy. Stroke 29:2352–2356

Elhammady MS, Baskaya MK, Sonmez OF et al (2007) Persistent primitive hypoglossal artery with retrograde flow from the vertebrobasilar system: a case report. Neurosurg Rev 30:345–349

Elias A, Le Croff G, Bouvier JL, Benichou A, Serradimigni A (1987) Value of real-time B-mode ultrasound imaging in the diagnosis of deep vein thrombosis of the lower limbs. Int Angiol 6:175–182

Elias A, Mallard L, Elias M et al (2003) A single complete ultrasound investigation of the venous network for the diagnostic management of patients with a clinically suspected first episode of deep venous thrombosis of the lower limbs. Thromb Haemost 89:221–227

Eliasziw M, Rankin RN, Fox AJ, Hynes RB, Barnett HJ (1995) Accuracy and prognostic consequences of ultrasonography in identifying severe carotid artery stenosis. North American Symptomatic Carotid Endarterectomy Trial (NASCET) Group. Stroke 26:1747–1752

Elkind MS, Cheng J, Boden-Albala B, Paik MC, Sacco RL (2001) Elevated white blood cell count and carotid plaque thickness: Northern Manhattan Stroke Study. Stroke 32:842–849

Ellis M, Powell JT, Greenhalg RM (1991) Limitations of ultrasonography in surveillance of small abdominal aortic aneurysms. Br J Surg 78:614–616

Elsman BH, Legemate DA, van der Heijden FA, de Vos HJ, Mali WP, Eikelboom BC (1995) Impact of ultrasonographic duplex scanning on therapeutic decision making in lower-limb arterial disease. Br J Surg 82:630–633

Elsman BH, Legemate DA, van der Heyden FW et al (1996) The use of color-coded duplex scanning in the selection of patients with lower extremity arterial disease for percutaneous transluminal angioplasty: a prospective study. Cardiovasc Intervent Radiol 19:313–316

Elsman BH, Legemate DA, de Vos HJ, Mali WP, Eikelboom BC (1997) Hyperaemic colour duplex scanning for the detection of aortoiliac stenoses. A comparative study with intra-arterial pressure measurement. Eur J Vasc Endovasc Surg 14:462–467

Elster EA, Hewlett S, DeRienzo DP, Donovan S, Georgia J, Yavorski CC (2002) Adventitial cystic disease of the axillary artery. Ann Vasc Surg 16:134–137

Endean ED, Barnes SL, Kwolek CJ et al (2001) Surgical management of thrombotic acute intestinal ischemia. Ann Surg 233:801–808

Engberding R (1990) Untersuchungstechniken in der Echokardiographie. Springer, Berlin/Heidelberg/New York, pp S183–S193

Enzinger F, Weiss S (1993) Hemangioendothelioma: vascular tumor of intermediate malignancy. In: Enzinger F, Weiss S (eds) Soft tissue tumors. C.V. Mosby, St Louis, pp 627–640

Erickson SJ, Mewissen MW, Foley WD et al (1989) Stenosis of the internal carotid artery: assessment using color imaging compared with angiography. Am J Roentgenol 152:1299–1305

European Carotid Plaque Study Group (1995) Carotid artery plaque composition - relationship to clinical presentation and ultrasound B-mode imaging. Eur J Vasc Endovasc Surg 10:23–30

Evers EJ, Wuppermann T (1995) Ultraschalldiagnostik bei postthrombotischem Syndrom. Eine vergleichende Untersuchung mittels Farbduplex, CW-Doppler, und B-Bildsonographie. Ultraschall Med 16:259–263

Evers EJ, Wuppermann T (1997) Die Charakterisierung des postthrombotischen Refluxes mittels farbkodierter Duplexsonographie. Vasa 26:190–193

Evers EJ, Wuppermann T (1997) Langzeitverlaufbeobachtung der venösen Hämodynamik bei postthrombotischem Syndrom mittels Farbdopplersonographie. Ultraschall 18(S1):54

Eyding J, Geier B, Staub D (2011) Current strategies and possible perspectives of ultrasonic risk stratification of ischemic stroke in internal carotid artery disease. Ultraschall Med 32:267–273

Faggioli GL, Pini R, Mauro R et al (2011) Identification of carotid 'vulnerable plaque' by contrast-enhanced ultrasonography: correlation with plaque histology, symptoms and cerebral computed tomography. Eur J Vasc Endovasc Surg 41:238–248

Falk E (1992) Why do plaques rupture? Circulation 86:III-30–III-42

Falk RL, Smith DF (1987) Thrombosis of upper extremity thoracic inlet veins: diagnosis with duplex Doppler sonography. Am J Radiol 149:677–682

Falls G, Eslami MH (2010) Recurrence of a popliteal venous aneurysm. J Vasc Surg 51:458–459

Faught WE, Mattos MA, van Bemmelen PS et al (1994) Color-flow duplex scanning of carotid arteries: new velocity criteria based on receiver operator characteristic analysis for threshold stenoses used in the symptomatic and asymptomatic carotid trials. J Vasc Surg 19:818–828

Favaretto E, Pili C, Amato A et al (2007) Analysis of agreement between duplex ultrsound scanning and arteriography in patients with lower limb artery disease. J Cardivasc Med 8:337–341

Fay JJ (1985) Anévrisme veineux poplité. Thèse Médicine, n° 78 Lille

Federman J, Anderson ST, Rosengarten DS, Pitt A (1977) Pulmonary embolism secondary to anomalies of deep venous system of the leg. Br Heart J 39:547–552

Feigenbaum H (ed) (1986) Echocardiography. Lea & Febiger, Philadelphia, pp 1–49

Feinstein SB, Cheirif J, ten Cate FJ et al (1990) Safety and efficacy of a new transpulmonary ultrasound contrast agent: initial multicenter clinical results. J Am Coll Cardiol 16:316–324

Feldstein VA, Patel MD, LaBerge JM (1996) Transjugular intrahepatic portosystemic shunts: accuracy of Doppler US in determination of patency and detection of stenoses. Radiology 201:141–147

Fell G, Phillips DJ, Chikos PM, Harley JD, Thiele BL, Strandness DE (1981) Ultrasonic duplex scanning for disease of the carotid artery. Circulation 64:1191–1195

Fellmeth BD, Roberts AC, Bookstein JJ et al (1991) Post-angiographic femoral artery injuries: nonsurgical repair with US-guided compression. Radiology 178:671–675

Fellner F, Janka R, Fellner C et al (1999) Post occlusion visualization of peripheral arteries with "floating table" MR angiography. Magn Reson Imaging 17:1235–1237

Ferrer EJM, Samso J, Serrando R et al (2000) Use of ultrasound in the diagnosis of carotid artery occlusion. J Vasc Surg 31:736–741

Ferretti G, Salomone A, Castagno PL (1988) Renovascular hypertension: a non-invasive duplex scanning screening. Int Angiol 7:219–223

Fillinger MF, Baker RJ Jr, Zwolak RM et al (1996) Carotid duplex criteria for 60% or greater angiographic stenosis: variation according to equipment. J Vasc Surg 24:856–864

Finkenzeller T, Tacke J, Clevert DA et al (2008) Quantification of extracranial ICA stenoses with vessel ultrasound by CCDS and B-flow in comparison to 64-slice multidector CTA, contrast-enhanced MRA and DSA. Ultraschall Med 29:294–301

Finlay DE, Longley DG, Foshager MC, Letourneau JG (1993) Duplex and color Doppler sonography of hemodialysis arteriovenous fistulas and grafts. Radiographics 13:983–989

Fisher AJ, Paulson EK, Kliewer MA et al (1998) Doppler sonography of the portal vein and hepatic artery: measurement of a prandial effect in healthy subjects. Radiology 207:711–715

Fitzgerald SW, Foley WD (1991) Genitourinary system. In: Lanzer P, Yoganathan AP (eds) Vascular imaging by color Doppler and magnetic resonance. Springer, Berlin

Fitzgerald SW, Erickson S, DeWire DM et al (1992) Color Doppler sonography in the evaluation of the adult acute scrotum. J Ultrasound Med 11:543–548

Flanigan DP, Burnham SJ, Goodreau JJ et al (1979) Summary of cases of adventitial cystic disease of the popliteal artery. Ann Surg 189: 165–175

Flanigan DP, Ballard JL, Robinson D et al (2008) Duplex ultrasound of the superficial femoral artery is a better screening tool than ankle-brachial index to identify at risk patients with lower extremity atherosclerosis. J Vasc Surg 47:789–792

Fleming SH, Ross PD, Timothy EC (2010) Accuracy of duplex sonography scans after renal artery stenting. J Vasc Surg 52:953–958

Fletcher JP, Kershaw LZ, Barker DS (1990) Ultrasound diagnosis of lower limb deep venous thrombosis. Med J Aust 153:453–455

Fletcher J, Saker K, Baptiste P et al (2000) Colour Doppler diagnosis of perigraft flow following endovascular repair of abdominal aortic aneurysm. Int Angiol 19:326–330

Flückiger F, Steiner H, Rabl H, Waltner F (1991) Zystische Adventitia-Degeneration der Arteria poplitea: Sonographische Sicherung der Diagnose. Ultraschall Med 12:84–87

Fobbe F (1993) Periphere Venen. In: Wolf KJ, Fobbe F (eds) Farbkodierte Duplexsonographie. Thieme, Stuttgart/New York, pp 114–129

Fobbe F, Wolf K-J (1988) Erste klinische Erfahrungen mit der Angiodynographie. Fortschr Röntgenstr 148:259–264

Fobbe F, Koennecke H-C, El Bedewi M, Heidt P, Boese-Landgraf J, Wolf K-J (1989) Diagnostik der tiefen Beinvenenthrombose mit farbkodierter Duplexsonographie. Fortschr Röntgenstr 151:569

Fobbe F, Ruhnke-Trautmann M, van Gemmeren D, Hartmann CA, Kania U, Wolf K-J (1991) Altersbestimmung venöser Thromben im Ultraschall. Fortschr Röntgenstr 155:344–348

Foley WD (1991) Color Doppler flow imaging. Andover Medical Publishers, Boston

Foley WD, Middleton WD, Lawson TL, Erickson S, Quiroz FA, Macrander S (1989) Color Doppler ultrasound imaging of lower-extremity venous disease. AJR Am J Roentgenol 152:371–376

Föllinger O (1982) Laplace- and Fourier-transformation. AEG-Telefunken, Berlin

Fontcuberta J, Flores A, Langsfeld M et al (2005) Screening algorithm for aortoiliac occlusive disease using duplex ultrasonography-acquired velocity spectra from the distal external iliac artery. Vascular 13:164–172

Foo FJ, Hammond CJ, Goldstone AR et al (2011) Agreement between computed tomograpghy and ultrasound on abdominal aortic aneurysms and implications on clinical decisions. Eur J Vasc Endovasc Surg 42:608–614

Forsberg F, Liu J-B, Burns PN, Merton DA, Goldberg BB (1994) Artifacts in ultrasonic contrast agent studies. J Ultrasound Med 13:357–365

Forster S, Embree PM, O'Brien WD (1990) Flow velocity profile via time-domain correlation: error analysis and computer simulation. IEEE Trans Ultrason Ferroelectr Freq Control 37:164–175

Foshager MC, Ferral H, Nazarian GK et al (1995) Duplex sonography after transjugular intrahepatic portosystemic shunts (TIPS): normal hemodynamic findings and efficacy in predicting shunt patency and stenosis. Am J Roentgenol 165:1–7

Foster JH, Dean RH, Pinkterton JA, Rhamy RK (1973) Ten years experience with the surgical management of renovascular hypertension. Ann Surg 177:755–760

Fox R, Kahn M, Adler J et al (1985) Adventitial cystic disease of the popliteal artery: Failure of percutaneous transluminal angioplasty as a therapeutic modality. J Vasc Surg 2:165–175

Franco G, Nguyen Khac G (1997) Anévrisme veineux de la fosse poplitee: exploration ultrasonographique. Phlebologie 50:31–35

Francois GF, Jausseran JM, Giuly J (1988) Anévrisme veineux poplité. Presse Méd 17:755

Frank E, Anderson C, Rubinstein D (1978) Frequency of sexual dysfunction in "normal" couples. N Engl J Med 299:111–115

Fraser JD, Anderson DR (1999) Deep venous thrombosis: recent advances and optimal investigation with US. Radiology 211:9–24

Frauchiger B, Holtz D, Eichlisberger R, Jäger KA (1995) Duplexsonographie zur Abklärung der renovaskulären Hypertonie und bei Durchblutungsstörungen der Transplantatniere. In: Jäger KA, Eichlisberger R (eds) Sono-Kurs – Ein konzentrierter Refresherkurs über die gesamte Ultraschalldiagnostik. Karger, Basel, pp 114–127

Frauchiger B, Schmid HP, Roedel C, Moosmann P, Staub D (2001) Comparison of carotid arterial resistive indices with intima-media thickness as sonographic markers of atherosclerosis. Stroke 32:836–841

Frederick MG, Hertzberg BS, Kliewer MA et al (1996) Can the US examination for lower extremity deep venous thrombosis be abbreviated? A prospective study of 755 examinations. Radiology 199:45–47

Frimann-Dahl J (1935) Postoperative Röntgenuntersuchungen. Acta Chir Scand 76(Suppl):36

Frühwald F, Blackwell DE (1992) Atlas der farbkodierten Dopplersonographie. Springer, Wien/New York, p 101

Fukudome Y, Abe I, Onaka U et al (1998) Regression of carotid wall thickening after corticosteroid therapy in Takayasu's arteritis evaluated by B-mode ultrasonography: report of 2 cases. J Rheumatol 25:2029–2032

Furness PN, Philpott CM, Chorbadijan MT et al (2003) Protocol biopsy of the stable renal transplant: a multicenter study of methods and complication rates. Transplantation 76:969–973

Fürst G, Kuhn FP, Trappe RP, Modder U (1990) Diagnostik der tiefen Beinvenenthrombose. Farb-Doppler-Sonographie versus Phlebographie. Fortschr Geb Röntgenstr Neuen Bildgeb Verfahr 152:151–158

Fürst G, Saleh A, Wenserski F et al (1999) Reliability and validity of noninvasive imaging of internal carotid artery pseudo-occlusion. Stroke 30:1450–1455

Gabrielli R, Vitale S, Constanzo A, Carra A (2010) Our experience of popliteal vein aneurysm. Interact Cardiovasc Thorac Surg 11:835–837

Gaiani S, Bolondi L, Li Bassi S et al (1989) Effect of meal on portal hemodynamics in healthy humans and in patients with chronic liver disease. Hepatology 9:815–819

Gaitini D (1990) Late changes in veins after deep venous thrombosis: ultrasonic findings. Fortschr Röntgenstr 153:68–72

Gaitini D, Kaftori JK, Pery M, Weich YL, Markel A (1988) High-resolution real-time ultrasonography in the diagnosis of deep vein thrombosis. Fortschr Roentgenstr 149:26

Galen SR, Gambino RS (1975) Beyond normality. The predictive value and efficiency of medical diagnoses. Wiley, New York, pp 10–14

Gallacher JJ, Hageman JH (1985) Popliteal vein aneurysm causing pulmonary embolus. Arch Surg 120:1173–1175

Galland RB, Simmons MJ, Torrie EPH (1991) Prevalence of abdominal aortic aneurysm in patients with peripheral vascular disease. Br J Surg 78:1259–1260

Garovic VD, Textor SC (2005) Renovascular hypertension and ischemic nephropathy. Circulation 112:1362–1374

Gartenschlager M, Klose KJ, Schmidt JA (1996) Diagnose flottierender venöser Thromben mittels Phlebo-Spiral-CT. Fortschr Geb Röntgenstr Neuen Bildgeb Verfahr 164:376–361

Garth KE, Carroll BA, Sommer FG, Oppenheimer DA (1983) Duplex ultrasound scanning of the carotid arteries with velocity spectrum analysis. Radiology 147:823–827

Gebhardt J et al (1989) Sonographische Akutdiagnostik der Darmischämie. Ultraschall 10:158–163

Geelkerken RH, Delahunt TA, Schultze Kool LJ et al (1996) Pitfalls in the diagnosis of origin stenosis of die coeliac and superior mesenteric arteries with transabdominal color duplex examination. Ultrasound Med Biol 22:695–700

Geiger A, Hammel D, Scheld HH, Böcker W (1991) Fallbericht: Ungewöhnlich großer Tumor eines Glomus caroticum. Angio 13:279–283

Gentile AT, Mills JL, Gooden MA et al (1997) Identification of predictors of lower extremity vein graft stenosis. Am J Surg 174:218–221

Gerlach HE, Schellong SM, Hach-Wunderle V et al (2009) Non-implementation of guideline recommendations for diagnosis of deep venous thrombosis in Germany. J Thromb Haemost 7:491

Geroulakos G, Ramaswami G, Nicolaides A et al (1993) Characterization of symptomatic and asymptomatic carotid plaques using high-resolution real-time ultrasonography. Br J Surg 80:1274–1277

Geroulakos G, Domjan J, Nicolaides A, Stevens J et al (1994) Ultrasonic carotid artery plaque structure and risk of cerebral infarction on computed tomography. J Vasc Surg 20:263–266

Gerson L, Martin H (1981) Ectasie veineuse d'origine traumatique. Angiologie 33:275–278

Giannetti A, Biscontri M, Randisi P, Cortese B, Minacci C, Stumpo M (2010) Contrast-enhanced sonography in the diagnosis of acute mesenteric ischemia: Case Report. J Clin Ultrasound 38:156–160

Giannoni MF, Bilotta F, Fiorani L, Fiorani P (1998) Regarding "Reduction in aortic aneurysm size: early results after endovascular graft replacement". Letter. J Vasc Surg 27:981

Giannoni MF, Fanelli F, citone M, Cristina Acconcia M, Speziale F, Gossetti B (2007) Contrast ultrasound imaging: the best method to detect type II endoleak during endovascular aneurysm repair follow-up. Interact Cardiovasc Thorac Surg 6:359–362

Gibson NS, Schellong SM, Kheir DY et al (2009) Safety and sensitivity of two ultrasound strategies in patients with clinically suspected deep venous thrombosis: a prospective managemend study. J Thromb Haemost 7:2035–2041

Gillespie DL, Villavicencio JL, Gallagher C et al (1997) Presentation and management of venous aneurysms. J Vasc Surg 26:845–852

Giorgio A, Amoroso P, Lettieri G et al (1986) Cirrhosis: value of caudate to right lobe ratio in diagnosis with US. Radiology 161:443–445

Giustacchini P, Pisanti F, Citterio F et al (2002) Renal vein thrombosis after renal transplantation: an important cause of graft loss. Transplant Proc 34:2126–2127

Giyanani VL, Krebs CA, Nall LA, Eisenberg RL, Parvey HR (1989) Diagnosis of abdominal aortic dissection by image-directed Doppler sonography. J Clin Ultrasound 17:445–448

Glickerman DJ, Obregon RG, Schmiedl UP et al (1996) Cardiac-gated MR angiography of the entire lower extremity: a prospective comparison with conventional angiography. AJR 167:445–451

Glifeather M, Yoon HC, Siegelman ES (1999) Renal artery stenosis: evaluation with conventional angiography versus gadolinium-enhanced MR angiography. Radiology 210:367–372

Golledge J, Beattie DK, Greenhalg RM, Davies AH (1996) Have the results of infrainguinal bypass improved with the widespread utilisation of postoperative surveillance? Eur J Vasc Endovasc Surg 11:388–392

Golledge J, Iannos J, Walsh JA, Burnett JR, Foreman RK (2001) Critical assessment of the outcome of infrainguinal vein bypass. Ann Surg 234:697–701

Golzarian J et al (2002) Evaluation of abdominal aortic aneurysm after endoluminal treatment: comparison of color Doppler sonography and biphasic helical CT. AJR Am J Roentgenol 178:623–628

Gonçalves I, Moses J, Pedro LM et al (2003) Echolucency of carotid plaques correlates with plaque cellularity. Eur J Vasc Endovasc Surg 26:32–38

Gonçalves I, Lindholm MW, Pedro LM et al (2004) Elastin and calcium rather than collagen or lipid content are associated with echogenicity of human carotid plaques. Stroke 35:2795–2800

Gooding GAW, Perez S, Rapp JH, Drupski WC (1991) Lower-extremity vascular grafts placed for peripheral vascular disease. Prospective evaluation with duplex Doppler sonography. Radiology 180: 379–386

Goodman LR, Lipchick RJ (1996) Diagnosis of acute pulmonary embolism: time for a new approach. Radiology 199:25–27

Gorenstein A, Katz S, Schiller M (1987) Congenital aneurysms of the deep veins of the lower extremities. J Vasc Surg 5:765–768

Görtler M, Niethammer R, Widder B (1994) Differentiating subtotal carotid artery stenoses from occlusions by colour-coded duplex sonography. J Neurol 241:301–305

Gottlieb RH, Voci S, Syed L et al (2003) Randomized prospective study comparing routine versus selective use of sonography of the complete calf in patients with suspected deep venous thrombosis. AJR 180:241–245

Götzberger M, Kaiser C, Landauer N, Dieterle C, Heldwein W, Schiemann U (2008) Intrarenal resistance index for the assessment of early renal function impairment in patients with liver cirrhosis. Eur J Med Res 13:383–387

Gramiak R, Shah PM (1968) Echocardiography of the aortic root. Investig Radiol 3:356–366

Grant EG, Perrella RR (1990) Wishing won't make it so: duplex Doppler sonography in die evaluation of renal transplant dysfunction. AJR 155:538–539

Grant EG, Duerinckx AJ, El Saden S et al (1999) Doppler sonographic parameters for the detection of carotid stenosis. Am J Roentgenol 172:1123–1129

Grant EG, Duerinckx AJ, El Saden SM et al (2000) Ability to use duplex US to quantify internal carotid stenoses: fact or fiction? Radiology 214:247–252

Grant EG, Benson CB, Moneta GL et al (2003) Carotid artery stenosis: gray-scale and Doppler US diagnosis – Society of Radiologists in Ultrasound Consensus Conference. Radiology 229:340–346

Grassbaugh JA, Nelson PR, Rzucidlo EM, Schermerhorn ML, Fillinger MF, Powell RJ et al (2003) Blinded comparison of preoperative duplex ultrasound and contrast arteriography for planning revascularisation at the level of the tibia. J Vasc Surg 37:1186–1190

Grassi CJ, Polak JF (1990) Axillary and subclavian venous thrombosis: follow-up evaluation with color Doppler flow US and venography. Radiology 175:651–654

Gray-Weale AC, Graham JC, Burnett JR et al (1988) Carotid artery atheroma: comparison of preoperative B-mode ultrasound appearance with carotid endarterectomy specimen. J Cardiovasc Surg 29:115–123

Gray-Weale AC, Graham JC, Burnett JR et al (1988) Comparison of preoperative B-mode ultrasound appearance with carotid endarterectomy specimen pathology. J Cardiovasc Surg 29:676–681

Green RM, McNamara J, Ouriel K, DeWeese JA (1990) Comparison of infrainguinal graft surveillance techniques. J Vasc Surg 11: 207–214

Greenwood LH, Yrizarry JM, Hallett JW (1982) Peripheral venous aneurysms with recurrent pulmonary embolism: report of a case and review of the literature. Cardiovasc Intervent Radiol 5:43–45

Greiner L (2005) Quantifizierung des Nichtquantifizierbaren oder: Maß und Zahl sind Schall und Rauch. Ultraschall Med 26:183–184

Griewig B, Morganstern C, Driesner F et al (1996) Cerebrovascular disease assessed by color flow and power Doppler ultrasonography. Comparison with digital subtraction angiography in internal carotid artery stenosis. Stroke 27:95–100

Grigg MJ, Nicolaides AN, Wolfe JHN (1988) Detection and grading of femorodistal vein graft stenoses: duplex velocity measurements compared with angiography. J Vasc Surg 8:661

Grigg MJ, Wolfe JHN, Tovar A, Nicolaides AN (1988) The reliability of duplex derived haemodynamic measurements in the assessment of femoro-distal grafts. Eur J Vasc Surg 2:177–181

Grogan J, Castilla M, Lozanski L et al (2005) Frequency of critical stenosis in primary arteriovenous fistulae before hemodialysis access: should duplex ultrasound surveillance be the standard of care? J Vasc Surg 41:1000–1006

Grogan JK, Shaalan WE, Cheng H (2005) B-mode ultrasonographic characterization of carotid atherosclerotic plaques in symptomatic and asymptomatic patients. J Vasc Surg 42:435–441

Grøndal N, Bramsen MB, Thomsen MD, Rasmussen CB, Lindholdt JS (2012) The cardiac cycle is a major contributor to variability in size measurements of abdominal aortic aneurysms by ultrasound. Eur J Vasc Endovasc Surg 43:30–33

Grønholdt ML, Nordestgaard BG, Nielsen TG, Sillesen H (1996) Echolucent carotid artery plaques are associated with elevated levels of fasting and postprandial triglyceride-rich lipoproteins. Stroke 27:2166–2172

Gronholdt ML, Wiebe BM, Laursen H (1997) Lipid-rich carotid artery plaques appear echolucent on ultrasound B-mode images and may be associated with intraplaque haemorrhage. Eur J Vasc Endovasc Surg 14:439–445

Grønholdt ML, Nordestgaard BG, Wiebe BM, Wilhjelm JE, Sillesen H (1998) Echo-lucency of computerized ultrasound images of carotid atherosclerotic plaques are associated with increased levels of triglyceride-rich lipoproteins as well as increased plaque lipid content. Circulation 97:34–40

Grønholdt ML, Nordestgaard BG, Schroeder TV, Vorstrup S, Sillesen H (2001) Ultrasonic echolucent carotid plaques predict future strokes. Circulation 104:68–73

Gronholdt ML, Nordestgaard BG, Bentzon J (2002) Macrophages are associated with lipid-rich carotid artery plaques, echolucency on B-mode imaging, and elevated plasma lipid levels. J Vasc Surg 35:137–145

Gross CM, Kramer J, Weingartner O et al (2001) Determination of renal arterial stenosis severity: comparison of pressure gradient and vessel diameter. Radiology 220:751–756

Grosser S, Kreymann G, Guthoff A et al (1990) Farbkodierte Duplexsonographie bei Phlebothrombosen. Dtsch Med Wochenschr 115:1939–1944

Grosser S, Kreymann G, Kühns A (1991) Duplex-sonographisch quantifiziertes Shuntvolumen und dessen klinische Relevanz. Angio Arch 22:74–77

Gruss JD, Geissler C (1997) Aneurysms of the subclavian artery in thoracic outlet syndrome. Zentralbl Chir 122:730–734

Gubler FM, Laan R, van der Veen F (1996) The value of palpation, varicoscreen contact thermography and colour Doppler ultrasound in the diagnosis of varicocele. Hum Reprod 11:1232–1235

Guo Z, Fenster A (1996) Three-dimensional power Doppler imaging: A phantom study to quantify vessel stenosis. Ultrasound Med Biol 22:1059–1069

Haas SB, Tribus CB, Insall JN, Becker MW, Windsor RE (1992) The significance of calf thrombi after total knee arthroplasty. J Bone Joint Surg Br 74:799–802

Haaverstadt R, Fougner R, Myhre HO (1995) Venous haemodynamics and the occurrence of leg oedema in patients with popliteal aneurysm. Eur J Vasc Endovasc Surg 9:204–210

Haaverstadt R, Johnsen H, Saether OD, Myhre HO (1995) Lymph drainage and the development of post-reconstructive leg oedema is not influenced by the type of inguinal incision. A prospective randomised study in patients undergoing femoropopliteal bypass surgery. Euro Vasc Endovasc Surg 10:316–322

Habscheid W (1988) Einsatz der Real-Time-Sonographie zur Diagnostik der tiefen Beinvenenthrombose auf einer internistischen Intensivstation. Intensivmed Notfallmed 25:326

Habscheid W (1998) Stellenwert der Duplexsonographie in der Beinvenendiagnostik. DMW 132:1185–1190

Habscheid W (2006) Sonographie der Beinvenenthrombose. Ultraschall Med 27:512–532

Habscheid W, Landwehr P (1990) Diagnostik der akuten tiefen Beinvenenthrombose mit der Kompressionssonographie. Ultraschall Med 11:268–273

Habscheid W, Wilhelm T (1988) Diagnostik der tiefen Beinvenenthrombose durch Real-time-Sonographie. Dtsch Med Wochenschr 113:586–591

Habscheid W, Becker W, Höhmann M (1989) Diagnostik der tiefen Beinvenenthrombose. Dtsch Med Wochenschr 114:837

Habscheid W, Höhmann M, Klein S (1990) Kompressionssonographie als Verfahren zur Diagnose der akuten tiefen Beinvenenthrombose. Med Klin 85:6–12

Hach W (1981) Spezielle Diagnostik der primären Varikose. Demeter, Gräfelfing

Hach W, Hach-Wunderle V (1994) Die Rezirkulationskreise der primären Varikose. Springer, Berlin/Heidelberg

Hach W, Hach-Wunderle V (1996) Phlebographie der Bein- und Beckenvenen. Schnetztor, Konstanz, pp 89–120

Hach W, Hach-Wunderle V (1998) Diagnostik der tiefen Bein- und Beckenthrombosen durch Phlebographie und Duplex-Sonographie. Hämostaselogie 18:11–17

Hach W, Girth E, Lechner W (1977) Einteilung der Stammvarikose der V. saphena magna in 4 Stadien. Phlebol Proktol 6:116–123

Hach-Wunderle V, Blätter W, Gerlach H, Konstantinides St, Noppenney T, Pillny M, Riess H, Schellong S, Stiegler H, Wildberger JE (2010) Diagnostik und Therapie der Venenthrombose und der Lungenembolie. Interdisziplinäre S2 Leitlinie. VASA (Suppl) S78/2010. www.awmf.org/uploads/tx_szleitlinien/065-002_S2_Diagnostik_und_Therapie_der Venenthrombose_und_der_Lungenembolie_06_2010_2_pdf

Haerten R (1998) Power-Doppler-Verfahren. In: Bogdahn U, Becker G, Schlachetzki F (eds) Echosignalverstärker und transkranielle Farbduplex-Sonographie. Blackwell Wissenschafts-Verlag, Berlin/Wien, pp 93–99

Haerten R, Kim J (1993) Verfahren der Farbdoppler-Sonographie – Ein Methodenvergleich. Ultraschall Med 14:225–230

Haimov H, Giron F, Jacobsen JH (1979) The expanded polytetrafluoroethylene graft. Three years` experience with 362 grafts. Arch Surg 114:673–677

Haire WD, Lynch TG, Lund GB, Lieberman RP, Edney JA (1991) Limitations of magnetic resonance imaging and ultrasound-directed (duplex) scanning in the diagnosis of subclavian vein thrombosis. J Vasc Surg 13:391–397

Hallam MJ, Reid JM, Cooperberg PL (1989) Color-flow Doppler and conventional duplex scanning of the carotid bifurcation: prospective double-blind correlative study. Am J Roentgenol 152:1101–1105

Halliday A, Harrison M, Hayter E (2010) 10-year stroke prevention after successful carotid endarterectomy for asymptomatic stenosis (ACST-1): a multicentre randomised trial. Lancet 376:1074–1084

Hamada T, Yamauchi M, Hashimoto Y, Nakai K, Suenaga K (2007) Prospective evaluation of contrast-enhanced ultrasonography with advanced dynamic flow for the diagnosis of intestinal ischemia. Br J Radiol 80:603–608

Hamann H, Cyba-Altunbay S, Schäfer H, Vollmar JF (1986) Asymptomatic carotid artery stenosis. Surgery versus medical treatment (Casanova Study). In: Maurer PC, Becker HM, Heidrich H, Hoffmann G, Kriessmann A, Müller-Wiefel H (eds) What is new in angiology? Zuckschwerdt, München, p 305

Hamulyak K, Lensing AWA, van der Meer J, Smid WM, van Ooy A, Hoek JA (1995) Subcutaneous low molecular-weight heparin or oral anticoagulants for the prevention of deep-vein thrombosis in elective hip and knee replacement? Thromb Haemost 76:1428–1431

Handa N, Matsumoto M, Maeda H, Hougaku H, Kamada T (1995) Ischemic stroke events and carotid atherosclerosis. Results of the Osaka Follow-up Study for Ultrasonograhic Assessment of Carotid Atherosclerois (the OSACA Study). Stroke 26:1781–1786

Hankey GJ, Warlow CP, Sellar RJ (1990) Cerebral angiographic risk in mild cerebrovascular disease. Stroke 21:209–222

Hansen LG, Boris P (1986) Aneurysma der Vena femoralis und poplitea. Radiologe 26:210

Hansen KJ, Tribble RW, Reavis SW (1990) Renal duplex sonography: evaluation of clinical utility. J Vasc Surg 12:227–236

Harbin WP, Robert NH, Ferrucci JT (1980) Diagnosis of cirrhosis based on regional changes in hepatic morphology. Radiology 135:273–283

Harloff A, Strecker C, Reinhard M et al (2006) Combined measurement of carotid stiffness and intima-media thickness improves prediction of complex aortic plaques in patients with ischemic stroke. Stroke 37:2708–2712

Harnoss B-M, Keller F, Häring R, Distler A, Maurer PC (Hrsg) (1991) Der Dialyseshunt als chirurgische und nephrologische Aufgabe. Angio Archiv 22

Harns PL, de Cossart L, Moody P, Douglas H (1988) How can we detect and manage fibrous strictures within new grafts? Are these more problematical with reversed than in situ bypass? In: Greenhalgh RM (ed) Limb salvage and amputation for vascular disease. Saunder WB, London, p 221

Harolds JA, Friedman MH (1977) Venous aneurysms. South Med J 70:719–721

Harrer JU, Sasse A, Klötzsch C (2006) Intimal flap in a conmon carotid artery in a patient with Marfan's syndrome. Ultraschall Med 27: 487–488

Harris E, Taylor L, Porter J (1989) Epithelioid hemangioendothelioma of external iliac vein: a primary vascular tumor presenting as traumatic venous obstruction. J Vasc Surg 10:697–699

Hartshorne TC, CN MC, Earnshaw JJ, Morris J, Nasim A (2011) Ultrasound measurement of aortic diameter in a national screening programme. Eur J Vasc Endovasc Surg 42:195–199

Hassen S, Barrellier MT, Seinturier C, Bosson JL, Genty C, Long A, Pernod G (2011) High percentage of non-diagnostic compression ultrasonography results and the diagnosis of ipsilateral recurrent proximal deep vein thrombosis. J Thromb Haemost 9:414–416

Hata J, Kamada T, Haruma K, Kusunoki H (2005) Evaluation of bowel ischemia with contrast-enhanced US: initial experience. Radiology 236:712–715

Hatle L, Angelson B (1985) Doppler ultrasound in cardiology. Lea & Febiger, Philadelphia, pp 22–26

Hatsukami TS, Prornozich JF, Zierler RE et al (1992) Color Doppler imaging of infrainguinal arterial occlusive disease. J Vasc Surg 16: 527–533

Hauser M, Brunner U (1994) Neue pathophysiologische und funktionelle Gesichtspunkte zur Insuffizienz der Vena saphena parva. Vasa 22:338–341

Hawkins PG, McKnoulty LM, Gordon RD (1989) Noninvasive renal artery duplex ultrasound and computerized nuclear renography to screen for and follow progress in renal artery stenosis. J Hypertens 7(Suppl):184–185

Heberer G, Van Dongen RJAM (eds) (1993) Gefäßchirurgie. Springer, Berlin/Heidelberg/New York/Tokyo. Kirschnersche allgemeine und spezielle Operationslehre, Bd 11

Hecking C, Aschwanden M, Dickenmann M et al (2006) Efficient haemodialysis despite complete central venous thrombosis. Vasa 35:243–244

Hedblad B, Wikstrand J, Janzon L et al (2001) Low-dose metroprolol CR/XL and fluvastatin slow progression of carotid intima-media thickness: main results from the Beta-Blocker Cholesterol-Lowering Asymptomatic Plaque Study (BCAPS). Circulation 103:1721–1726

Heilberger P et al (1997) Postoperative color flow duplex scanning in aortic endografting. J Endovasc Surg 4:262

Heine GH, Gerhart MK, Girndt M et al (2006) Intrarenale Widerstandsindices und Subklinische Artherosklerose als Prognosemarker bei nierentransplantierten Menschen. Ultraschall Med 27:S62

Heinrich U (1993) In-vitro-Untersuchungen an Gefäßstenosen mit der farbkodierten Duplexsonographie unter besonderer Berücksichtigung der Stenosegradbestimmung. Universität Würzburg, Med Diss

Hellings WE, Peeters W, Moll FL et al (2010) Composition of carotid atherosclerotic plaque is associated with cardiovascular outcome: a prognostic study. Circulation 121:1941–1950

Henao EA, Hodge MD, Felkai DD et al (2006) Contrast-enhanced duplex surveillance after endovascular abdominal aortic aneurysm repair: improved efficacy using a continuous infusion technique. J Vasc Surg 43:259–264

Henderson RD, Steinman DA, Eliasziw M, Barnett HJ (2000) Effect of contralateral carotid artery stenosis on carotid ultrasound velocity measurements. Stroke 31:2636–2640

Hendrickx PH, Roth U, Brassel F et al (1990) Phantomuntersuchungen zur Wertigkeit der farbkodierten Doppler-Sonographie bei der arteriellen Verschlußkrankheit der unteren Extremitäten. Fortschr Röntgenstr 152:1–5

Hendrickx PH, Roth U, von der Lieth H (1991) Wertigkeit der Angiodynographie zur Verlaufskontrolle chirurgischer Gefäßprothesen. Ultraschall Med 12:188–192

Hennerici M, Meairs S (2000) Imaging arterial wall disease. Cerebrovasc Dis 10(Suppl 5):9–20

Hennerici M, Neuerburg-Heusler D (1988) Gefäßdiagnostik mit Ultraschall. Thieme, Stuttgart

Hennerici M, Steinke W, Rautenberg W (1989) High-resistance Doppler flow pattern in extracranial carotid dissection. Arch Neurol 46: 670–672

Henricksen JH, Moller S, Schifter S et al (1999) Increased arterial compliance in decompensated cirrhosis. J Hepatol 31:712–718

Herbener TE, Seftel AD, Nehra A, Goldstein I (1994) Penile ultrasound. Semin Urol 12:320–332

Hermus L, Tielliu IF, Wallis de Vries BM, van den Dungen JJ, Zeebregts CJ (2010) Imaging the vulnerable carotid artery plaque. Acta Chir Belg 110:159–164

Hermus L, van Dam GM, Zeebregts CJ (2010) Advanced carotid plaques imaging. Eur J Vasc Endovasc Surg 39:125–133

Herzog P, Anastasiu M, Wollbrink W, Herrmann W, Holtermüller K-H (1991) Real-time Sonographie bei tiefer Becken- und Beinvenenthrombose. Med Klinik 86:132–137

Hill SL, Donato AT (1994) Ability of the carotid duplex scan to predict stenosis, symptoms and plaque structure. Surgery 116:914–920

Hirsch AT, Haskal ZJ, Hertzer NR et al (2006) ACC/AHA 2005 practice guidelines for the management of patients with peripheral arterial disease (lower extremities, renal, mesenteric, and abdominal aortic): a collaborative report from the American Association for Vascular Surgery/Society for Vascular Surgery, Society for Cardiovascular Angiography and Interventions, Society for Vascular Medicine and Biology, Society of Interventional Radiology, and the ACC/AHA Task Force on Practice Guidelines (Writing Committee to Develop Guidelines for the Management of Patients With Peripheral Arterial Disease). Circulation 113:e463–e654

Hirschl M, Bernt R (1990) Normalwerte, Reproduzierbarkeit und Aussagekraft duplexsonographischer Kriterien in der Venenfunktionsdiagnostik. Ultraschall. Klin Prax 5:81–84

Hoballah JJ, Nazzal MM, Ryan SM et al (1997) Is color duplex surveillance of infrainguinal polyetrafluoroethylene grafts worthwhile? Am J Surg 174:131–135

Hoffmann U, Edwards JM, Carter S et al (1991) Role of duplex scanning for the detection of atherosclerotic renal artery disease. Kidney Int 39:1232–1239

Hofmann W, Forstner R, Sattlegger P, Ugurluoglu A, Magometschnigg H (2001) Die bildgebende Diagnostik pedaler Anschlussgefäße, Gefäßchirurgie. Springer, Originalarbeit 6:98–102

Hofmann WJ, Walter J, Ugurluoglu A, Czerny M, Forstner R, Magometschnigg H (2004) Preoperative high-frequency duplex scanning of potential pedal target vessels. J Vasc Surg 39:169–175

Hollenbeck M, Hilbert N, Meusel F, Grabensee B (1994) Increasing sensitivity and specificity of Doppler sonographic detection of renal

transplant rejection with serial investigation technique. Clin Investig 72:609–615
Hollerweger A, Macheiner P, Rettenbacher T, Gritzmann N (2000) Sonographische Diagnose von Muskelvenenthrombosen des Unterschenkels und deren Bedeutung als Emboliequelle. Ultraschall Med 21:66–72
Homma S, Ishii T, Tsugane S, Hirose N (1997) Different effects of hypertension and hypercholesterolemia on the natural history of aortic atherosclerosis by the stage of intimal lesion. Atherosclerosis 125:85–95
Homma S, Hirose N, Inagaki T, Suzuki M, Wakida Y (1999) Lifestyle, familial history and social background of Japanese centenarians. In: Tauchi H, Sato T, Watanabe T (eds) Japanese centenarians – medical research for the final stages of human aging. Editorial and Publishing Office of Japanese Centenarians, Aichi, pp 20–35
Homma S, Hirose N, Ishida H, Ishii T, Araki G (2001) Carotid plaque and intima-media thickness assessed by B-mode sonography in subjects ranging from young adults to centenarians. Stroke 32:830–835
Honda O, Sugiyama S, Kugiyama K et al (2004) Echolucent carotid plaques predict future coronary events in patients with coronary artery disease. J Am Coll Cardiol 43:1177–1184
Hong JS, Lee KB, Kim DK, Kim DI (2007) Cystic adventitial disease of the popliteal artery: report of a case. Surg Today 37:719–722
Hood DB, Mattos MA, Mansour A et al (1996) Prospective evaluation of new duplex criteria to identify 70% internal carotid artery stenosis. J Vasc Surg 23:254–261
Hoogi A, Adam D, Hoffman A (2011) Carotid plaque vulnerability: quantification of neovascularization on contrast-enhanced ultrasound with histopathologic correlation. AJR Am J Roentgenol 96:431–436
Horrow MM, Stassi J, Shurman A, Brody JD, Kirby CL, Rosenberg HK (2000) The limitations of carotid sonography: interpretive and technology-related errors. Am J Roentgenol 174:189–194
Hua HT, Hood DB, Jensen CC et al (2000) The use of color flow duplex scanning to detect significant renal artery stenosis. Ann Vasc Surg 14:118–124
Huber TS, Ozaki CK, Flynn TC et al (2002) Prospective validation of an algorithm to maximize native arteriovenous fistulae for chronic hemodialysis access. J Vasc Surg 36:452–459
Hull R, Hirsh J, Sackett D et al (1981) Clinical validity of a negative venogram in patients with clinically suspected venous thrombosis. Circulation 64:622–625
Hull R, Raskop G, Leclerc J, Jay R, Hirsh J (1984) The diagnosis of clinically suspected venous thrombosis. Clin Chest Med 5:439–456
Hunink MG, Polak JF, Barlan MM, O'Leary DH (1993) Detection and quantification of carotid artery stenosis: efficacy of various Doppler velocity parameters. AJR Am J Roentgenol 160:619–625
Hust MH, Schuler A (1992) Farb-Doppler-gesteuerte Kompressionstherapie eines großen Aneurysma spurium der Arteria femoralis nach Linksherzkatheterisierung. Dtsch Med Wochenschr 117:1675–1678
Hust MH, Schuler A, Claußnitzer R, Wild K, Metzler B (1993) Farbdopplergesteuerte Kompressionstherapie. Dtsch Ärztebl 90:B2536–B2541
Huston J, James E, Brown RD Jr et al (2000) Redefined duplex ultrasonographic criteria for the diagnosis of carotid artery stenosis. Mayo Clin Proc 75:1133–1140
Iacob M, Ifrim S, Tanasescu C et al (2005) Duplex ultrasound evaluation of patients with carotid stenosis treated with stent implantation. Ultraschall Med 26:S104
Idu MM, Buth J, Hop WC, Cuypers P, van de Pavoordt ED, Tordoir JM (1998) Vein graft surveillance: is graft revision without angiography justified and what criteria should be used? J Vasc Surg 27:399–411. Discussion 412–413
Idu MM, Buth J, Hop WC, Cuypers P, van dc Pavoordt ED, Tordoir JM (1999) Factors influencing the development of vein-graft stenosis and their significance for clinical management. Eur J Vasc Endovasc Surg 17:15–21
Iezzi R, Basilico R, Giancristofaro D, Pascali D, Cotroneo AR, Storto ML (2009) Contrast-enhanced ultrasound versus color duplex ultrasound imaging in the follow-up of patients after endovascular abdominal aortic aneurysm repair. J Vasc Surg 49:552–560
Ihlberg L, Luther M, Tierala E, Lepäntalo M (1998) The utility of duplex scanning in infrainguinal vein graft surveillance: results from a randomised controlled study. Eur J Vasc Endovasc Surg 16:19–27
Ihnat DM, Mills JL, Dawson DL et al (1999) The correlation of early flow disturbances with the development of infrainguinal graft stenosis: a 10-year study of 341 autogenous vein grafts. J Vasc Surg 30:8–15
Ikeda M, Fujimori Y, Tankawa H, Iwata H (1984) Compression syndrome of the popliteal vein and artery caused by popliteal cyst. Angiology 35:245–251
Insua JA, Young JR, Humphries AW (1970) Popliteal artery entrapment syndrome. Arch Surg 101:771–775
Irninger W (1963) Histologische Altersbestimmung von Thrombosen und Embolien. Virchows Archiv Path Anat 336:220–237
Isaacson JA, Neumyer MM (1995) Direct and indirect renal arterial duplex and Doppler colour flow evaluations. J Vasc Technol 193:309–316
Isaacson JA, Zierler RE, Spittell PC, Strandness DE (1995) Noninvasive screening for renal artery stenosis: comparison of renal artery and renal hilar duplex scanning. J Vasc Technol 19:105–110
Ishikawa K (1987) Cystic adventitial disease of the popliteal artery and of other stem vessels in the extremities. Jpn J Surg 17:221–229
Iwai T, Sato S, Yamada T et al (1987) Popliteal vein entrapment caused by the third head of the gastrocnemius muscle. Br J Surg 74:1006–1008
Jaakkola P, Hippeläinen M, Farin P, Rytkönen H, Kainulainen S, Paranen K (1996) Interobserver variability in measuring the dimensions of the abdominal aorta: comparison of ultrasound and computed tomography. Eur J Vasc Endovasc Surg 12:230–237
Jaarsveld BC, Krijnen P, Pieterman H et al (2003) The effect of balloon angioplasty on hypertension in atherosclerotic renal-artery stenosis. N Engl J Med 342:1007–1014
Jack CR, Sharma R, Vemuri RB (1984) Popliteal venous aneurysm as a source of pulmonary emboli in a male. Angiology 35:55–57
Jacob A, Stock KW, Proske M, Steinbrich W (1996) Lower extremity angiography: improved image quality and outflow vessel detection with bilaterally antegrade selective digital subtraction angiography. A blinded prospective intraindividual comparison with aortic flush digital subtraction angiography. Investig Radiol 31:184–193
Jacobs NM, Grant EG, Schellinger D et al (1985) Duplex carotid sonography: criteria for stenosis, accuracy, and pitfalls. Radiology 154: 385–391
Jäger K (1987) Apparative Untersuchungen zur Diagnose der tiefen Venenthrombose. Internist 28:299–307
Jäger K (1989) Neuere diagnostische Methoden zur nichtinvasiven Lokalisation und hämodynamischen Beurteilung arterieller Obstruktionen. Internist 30:397–405
Jäger K, Bollinger A (1986) Blood flow velocity and diameter of the popliteal vein. Phlebology 85:260–263
Jäger K, Martin PDL, HC RL, Roederer GO, Langlois YE, Strandness DE (1985a) Noninvasive mapping of lower limb arterial lesions. Ultrasound Med Biol 11:515–521
Jäger K, Ricketts HJ, Strandness DE (1985b) Duplex scanning for the evaluation of lower limb arterial disease. In: Bernstein EF (ed) Noninvasive diagnostic techniques in vascular disease. Mosby, St. Louis
Jäger K, Bollinger A, Siegenthaler W (1986a) Duplex-Sonographie in der Gefäßdiagnostik. Dtsch Med Wochenschr 111:1608–1613
Jäger K, Bollinger A, Valli C, Ammann R (1986b) Measurement of mesenteric blood flow by duplex scanning. J Vasc Surg 3:462–469
Jäger K, Seifert H, Bollinger A (1989) M-mode echovenography. A new technique for the evaluation of venous wall and venous valve motion. Cardiovasc Res 23:25–30
Jäger K, Eichlisberger R, Frauchiger B (1993) Stellenwert der bildgebenden Sonographie für die Diagnostik der Venenthrombose. Haemostaseologie 13:116–124
Jahromi AS, Ciná CS, Liu Y, Clase CM (2005) Sensitivity and specificity of color duplex ultrasound measurement in the estimation of internal carotid artery stenosis: A systematic review and meta-analysis. J Vasc Surg 41:962–972
Janzarik WG, Ringleb PA, Reinhard M et al (2007) Recurrent carotid artery vasospasms. Report of 2 cases. Stroke 37:2170–2173

Jennersjo CM, Fragerberg ICH, Karlander SG et al (2005) Normal D-dimer concentration is a common finding in symptomatic outpatients with distal vein thrombosis. Blood Coagul Fibrinolysis 16:517–523

Jiang S, Stewart G, Barnes E et al (2013) Effect of vascular access surveillance program on service provision and access thrombosis. Semin Dial 26:361–365

Johnson BF, Manzo RA, Bergelin RO, Strandness DE (1995) Relationship between changes in the deep venous system and the development of the postthrombotic syndrome after an acute episode of lower limb deep vein thrombosis: a one- to six-year follow-up. J Vasc Surg 21:307–313

Johnson SA, Stevens SM, Woller SC et al (2010) Risk of deep vein thrombosis following a single negative whole-leg compression ultrasonography. A systematic review and meta-analysis. JAMA 303:438–445

Johnston KW, Rutherford RB, Tilson MD et al (1991) Suggested standards for reporting on arterial aneurysms. Ad Hoc Committee on Reporting Standards, Society for Vascular Surgery and North American Chapter, International Society for Cardiovascular Surgery. J Vasc Surg 13:452–458

Johnston DC, Chapman KM, Goldstein LB (2001) Low rate of complications of cerebral angiography in routine clinical practice. Neurology 57:2012–2014

Jongbloets LM, Lensing AW, Koopman MM, Buller HR, Cate JW (1994) Limitations of compression ultrasound for the detection of symptomless postoperative deep vein thrombosis. Lancet 343:114–144

Jorgensen JO, Hanel KC, Morgan AM, Hunt JM (1993) The incidence of deep venous thrombosis in patients with superficial thrombophlebitis of the lower limbs. J Vasc Surg 18:70–73

Juenemann KP, Persson-Juenenemann C, Alken P (1990) Pathophysiology of erectile dysfunction. Semin Urol 8:80

Jung M (1990) Diagnosis of deep leg vein thrombosis: can we dispense with phlebography? Vasa 30(Suppl):30–33

Jung EM, Kubale R, Clevert DA et al (2007) B-flow and B-flow with 3D and SRI postprocessing before intervention and monitoring after stenting of the internal carotid artery. Clin Hemorheol Microcirc 36:35–46

Jung EM, Kubale R, Ritter G et al (2007) Diagnostics and characterisation of preocclusive stenoses and occlusions of the internal carotid artery with B-flow. Eur Radiol 17:439–447

Justich E (1982) The compression syndrome of the left renal vein. Rofo 136:404–412

Jutley RS, Cadle I, Cross KS (2001) Preoperative assessment of primary varicose veins: a duplex study of venous incompetence. Eur J Vasc Endovasc Surg 21:370–373

Kagawa R, Moritake K, Shima T, Okada Y (1996) Validity of B-mode ultrasonographic findings in patients undergoing carotid endarterectomy in comparison with angiographic and clinicopatholgic features. Stroke 27:700–705

Kakkar VV (1972) The diagnosis of deep vein thrombosis using the 125I-fibrinogen test. Arch Surg 104:152–159

Kakkar VV, Howe CT, Flanc C et al (1969) Natural history of postoperative deep venous thrombosis. Lancet 2:230–232

Kakkos SK, Stevens JM, Nicolaides AN et al (2007) Texture analysis of ultrasonic images of symptomatic carotid plaques can identify those plaques associated with ipsilateral embolic brain infarction. Eur J Vasc Endovasc Surg 33:422–429

Kallmayer M, Tsantilas P, Zieger C, Ahmed A, Söllner H, Zimmermann A, Eckstein H (2014) Ultrasound surveillance after CAS and CEA: What's the evidence? J Cardiovasc Surg 55:33–41

Kanazawa R, Ishihara S, Okawara M et al (2008) A successful treatment with carotid artery stenting for a symptomatic internal carotid artery severe stenosis with ipsilateral persistent primitive hypoglossal artery: case report and review of the literature. Minim Invasive Neurosurg 51:298–302

Kanterman RY, Vesely TM, Pilgram TK et al (1995) Dialysis access graft: anatomic location of venous stenosis and result of angioplasty. Radiology 195:135–139

Kanterman RY, Darcy MD, Middleton WD et al (1997) Doppler sonography findings associated with transjugular intrahepatic portosystemic shunt malfunction. Am J Roentgenol 168:467–472

Kaps M, Seidel G (1999) Echokontrastverstärkung in der neurologischen Ultraschalldiagnostik. Dt Ärztebl 96:A 276–A 280

Karacagil S, Almgren B, Bergström R, Bowald S, Eriksson I (1989) Postoperative predictive value of a new method of intraoperative angiographic runoff assessment in femoropopliteal bypass grafting. J Vasc Surg 10:400–407

Karacagil S, Löfberg AM, Almgren B et al (1994) Duplex ultrasound scanning for diagnosis of aortoiliac and femoropopliteal arterial disease. Vasa 23:325–329

Karacagil S, Löfberg AM, Granbo A, Lörelius LE, Bergqvist D (1996) Value of duplex scanning in evaluation of crural and foot arteries in limbs with severe lower limb ischaemia – a prospective comparison with angiography. Eur J Vasc Endovasc Surg 12:300–303

Karasch T, Rieser R, Grün B et al (1993) Bestimmung der Verschlusslänge in Extremitätenarterien. Farbduplexsonographie versus Angiographie. Ultraschall Med 14:247–254

Karasch T, Strauss AL, Grün B et al (1993) Farbcodierte Duplexsonographie in der Diagnostik von Nierenarterienstenosen. Dtsch Med Wochenschr 118:1429–1436

Karasch T, Strauss AL, Worringer M, Neuerburg-Heusler D, Roth FJ, Rieger H (1993c) Vergleich der Farbduplexsonographie mit verschiedenen angiographischen Verfahren in der Diagnostik arteriosklerotischer Nierenarterienstenosen und -verschlüsse. Ultraschall Klin Prax 8:180

Karasch T, Neuerburg-Heusler D, Strauss A, Rieger H (1994) Farbduplexsonographische Kriterien zur Diagnose arteriosklerotischer Nierenarterienstenosen und -verschlüsse. In: Keller E, Krumme B (Hrsg) Farbkodierte Duplexsonographie in der Nephrologie. Springer, Berlin/Heidelberg/New York/Tokyo

Kardoulas DG, Kastamouris AN, Gallis PT (1996) Ultrasonographic and histologic characteristics of symptom-free and symptomatic carotid plaque. Cardiovasc Surg 4:580–590

Karthikesalingam A, Al-Jundi W, Jackson D et al (2012) Systematic review and meta-analysis of duplex ultrasonography, contrast-enhanced ultrasonography or computed tomography for surveillance after endovascular aneurysm repair. Br J Surg 99:1514–1523

Kasai C, Namekawa K, Koyano R, Omoto R (1985) Real-time two-dimensional blood flow imaging using an autocorrelation technique. IEEE Trans Son Ultrason 32:458–463

Kathrein H (1991) Duplexsonographie von Dialyseshunts. Springer, Berlin/Heidelberg/New York/Tokyo

Kathrein H, König P, Dittrich P, Judmeier G (1988) Nichtinvasisve Beurteilung von Cimino-Brescia-Fisteln und PTFE-Shunts mit der Duplexsonographie. Vasa 26(Suppl):39–41

Katsamouris AN, Giannoukas AD, Tsetis D et al (2001) Can ultrasound replace arteriography in the management of chronic arterial occlusive disease of the lower limp? Eur J Vasc Endovasc Surg 21:155–159

Katz ML, Johnson M, Pomajzl MJ et al (1983) The sensitivity of real time B-mode carotid imaging in detection of ulcerated plaque. Bruit 8:13–16

Kawarada O, Yokoi Y, Takemoto K, Morioka N, Nakata S, Shiotani S (2006) The performance of renal duplex ultrasonography for the detection of hemodynamically significant renal artery stenosis. Catheter Cardiovasc Interv 68:311–318

Kearon C, Julian JA, Newnan TE, Ginsberg JS (1998) Noninvasive diagnosis of deep vein thrombosis. McMaster Diagnostic Imaging Practice Guidelines Initiative. Ann Intern Med 128:663–677

Keleinouridis V, Eckstein MR, Dembner AG, Waitman AG, Athanasoulis CA (1985) The normal leg venogram: significance in suspected vein thrombosis. Int Angiol 4:369–371

Keller F, Loewe HJ, Bauknecht KJ, Schwarz A, Offermann G (1988) Kumulative Funktionsraten von orthotopen Dialysefisteln und Interponaten. Dtsch Med Wschr 113:332–336

Keller F, Harnoss B-M, Czerlinsky H (1991) Umfrageergebnisse zur Technik der Ciminofistel. Angio. Archiv 22:7–9

Keo HH, Baumgartner I, Schmidli J, Do DD (2007) Sustained remission 11 years after percutaneous ultrasound guided aspiration for cystic adventitial degeneration in the popliteal artery. J Endovasc Ther 14:364–365

Kerlan RK Jr, LaBerge JM, Gordon RL, Ring EJ (1995) Transjugular intrahepatic portosystemic shunts: current status. Am J Roentgenol 164:1059–1066

Kerr TM, Canley JJ, Johnson JR et al (1990) Analysis of 1084 consecutive lower extremities involved with acute venous thrombosis diagnosed by dublex scanning. Surgery 108:520–527

Kerr TM, Lutter KS, Moeller DM et al (1990) Upper extremity venous thrombosis diagnosed by dublex scanning. Am J Surg 160:202–206

Kessler C, von Maravic M, Bruckmann H, Kompf D (1995) Ultrasound for the assessment of the embolic risk of carotid plaques. Acta Neurol Scand 92:231–234

Ketha SS, Pipitone N, Salvarani C (2014) Inflammatory abdominal aortic aneurysm: a case report and review of the literature. Vasc Endovasc Surg 48:65–69

Khan S, Khan M, Bradley B et al (2011) Utility of duplex ultrasound in detecting and grading de novo femoropopliteal lesions. J Vasc Surg 54:1067–1073

Khaw KT (1997) Does carotid duplex imaging render angiography redundant before carotid endarterectomy? Br J Radiol 70:235–238

Khoury M (2004) Failed angioplasty of a popliteal artery stenosis secondary to cystic adventitial disease. Vasc Endovasc Surg 38:277–280

Kiews P-W (1991) Color velocity imaging – Ein Vergleich der Verfahren zur farbkodierten Sonographie. Roentgenstrahlen (Philips Medizin Systeme) 65:1–6

Kiews P-W (1993) Physik und Technik der farbkodierten Duplexsonographie (FKDS). In: Wolf KJ, Fobbe F (eds) Farbkodierte Duplexsonographie. Thieme, Stuttgart/New York, pp 248–295

Killewich LA, Bedford GR, Beach KW, Strandness DE Jr (1989) Diagnosis of deep venous thrombosis. A prospective study comparing duplex scanning to contrast venography. Circulation 79:810–814

Killewich LA, Fisher C, Bartlett ST (1990) Surveillance of in situ infrainguinal bypass grafts: conventional vs color flow duplex ultrasonography. J Cardiovasc Surg 31:662

Killewich LA, Nunnelee JD, Auer AI (1993) Value of lower extremity venous duplex examination in the diagnosis of pulmonary embolism. J Vasc Surg 17:934–1030

Killewich LA, Bedford GR, Beach KW, Standness DE (1998) Spontaneous lysis of deep venous thrombi: rate and outcome. J Vasc Surg 9:89–97

Kim TS, Chung JW, Park JH (1998) Renal artery evaluation: comparison of spiral CT angiography to intra-arterial DSA. J Vasc Interv Radiol 9:553–559

Kim ES, Sun Z, Kapadia S et al (2012) Characteristics of duplex sonographic parameters over time after successful carotid artery stenting. J Ultrasound Med 31:1169–1174

Kimura K, Yasaka M, Moriyasu H, Tsuchiya T, Yamaguchi T (1994) Ultrasonographic evaluation of vertebral artery to detect vertebrobasilar axis occlusion. Stroke 25:1006–1009

Kinney EV, Bandyk DF, Mewissen MW et al (1991) Monitoring functional patency of percutaneous transluminal angioplasty. Arch Surg 126:743–747

Kirsch JD, Wagner LR, James EM et al (1994) Carotid artery occlusion: positive predictive value of duplex sonography compared with angiography. J Vasc Surg 19:642–649

Kitamura A, Iso H, Imano H et al (2004) Carotid intima-media thickness and plaque characteristics as a risk factor for stroke in Japanese elderly men. Stroke 35:2788–2794

Klein-Weigel P, Fish J, Fraedrich G (2015) Strategien für die präinterventionelle Bildgebung bei peripherer arterieller Verschlusskrankheit. Gefässchirurgie 20:441–447

Kliewer MA, Tupler RH, Hertzberg BS et al (1994) Doppler evaluation of renal artery stenosis: interobserver agreement in the interpretation of waveform morphology. Am J Roentgenol 162:1371–1376

Kliewer MA, Herzberg BS, Keogan MT et al (1997) Early systole in the healthy kidney: variability of Doppler US waveform parameters. Radiology 205:109–113

Koelemay MJ, den Hartog D, Prins MH, Kromhout JG, Legemate DA, Jacobs MJ (1996) Diagnosis of arterial disease of the lower extremities with duplex ultrasonographie. Br J Surg 83:404–409

Koelemay MJ, Legemate DA, van Gurp J, Ponson AE, Reekers JA, Jacobs MJ (1997) Colour duplex scanning and pulse-generated run-off for assessment of popliteal and cruropedal arteries before peripheral bypass surgery. Br J Surg 84:1115–1119

Koelemay MJW, Legemate DA, van Gurp JA, de Vos H, Balm R, Jacobs MJHM (2001) Interobserver variation of colour duplex scanning of the popliteal, tibial and pedal arteries. Eur J Vasc Endovasc Surg 21:160–164

Koelemay MJ, Lijmer JG, Stoker J, Legemate DA, Bossuyt PM (2001) Magnetic resonance angiography for the evaluation of lower extremity arterial disease: a meta-analysis. JAMA 285:1338–1345

Koennecke HC, Fobbe F, Hamed MM, Wolf KJ (1989) Diagnostik arterieller Gefäßerkrankungen der unteren Extremitäten mit der farbkodierten Duplexsonographie. Fortschr Röntgenstr 151:42–46

Kohler TR (1990) Doppler evaluation of lower limb vessels. Clin Diagn Ultrasound 26:139–148

Kohler TR, Strandness DE Jr (1986) Noninvasive testing for the evaluation of chronic venous disease. World J Surg 106:903–910

Kohler TR, Zierler RE, Martin RL (1986) Noninvasive diagnosis of renal artery stenosis by ultrasonic duplex scanning. J Vasc Surg 4: 450–456

Kohler TR, Nance DR, Cramer MM et al (1987) Duplex scanning for diagnosis of aortoiliac and femoropopliteal disease: a prospective study. Circulation 76:1074–1080

Koksoy C, Kuzu A, Kutlay J, Erden I, Ozcan H, Ergin K (1995) The diagnostic value of colour Doppler ultrasound in central venous catheter related thrombosis. Clin Radiol 50:687

Kono Y, Pinell SP, Sirlin CB (2004) Carotid arteries: contrast-enhanced US angiography – preliminary clinical experience. Radiology 230: 561–568

Koopman MMW, Prandoni P, Piovella F et al (1996) Treatment of venous thrombosis with intravenous unfractionated heparin administered in the hospital as compared with subcutaneous low-molecular-weight heparin administered at home. N Engl J Med 334:677–681

Koppenhagen K, Fobbe F (1993) Diagnostik der tiefen Beinvenenthrombose. Hamostaseologie 13(Suppl):12–14

Korten E, Toonder IM, Schrama YC et al (2007) Dialysis fistulae patency and preoperative diameter ultrasound measurement. Eur J Vasc Endovasc Surg 33:467–471

Kougias P, Lau D, El Sayes HF et al (2007) Determinants of mortality and treatment outcome following surgical interventions for acute mesenteric ischemia. J Vasc Surg 46:467–474

Krause U, Kock HJ, Kröger K, Albrecht K, Rudofsky G (1998) Prevention of deep venous thrombosis associated with superficial thrombophlebitis of the leg by early saphenous vein ligation. Vasa 27:34–38

Kreitner KF, Kalden P, Neufang A et al (2000) Diabetes and peripheral arterial occlusive disease: prospective comparison of contrast enhanced three-dimensional MR angiography with conventional digital subtraction angiography. Am J Roentgenol 174:171–179

Kremkau FW (1990) Doppler Ultrasound: Principles and Instruments. Saunders, Philadelphia

Kriessmann A, Bollinger A (Hrsg) (1978) Ultraschall-Doppler-Diagnostik in der Angiologie. Thieme, Stuttgart

Kriessmann A, Bollinger A, Keller H (Hrsg) (1982) Praxis der Doppler-Sonographie. Thieme, Stuttgart

Krings W, Adolph J, Diederich S, Urhahne S, Vassallo P, Peters PE (1990) Diagnostik der tiefen Becken- und Beinvenenthrombose mit hochauflösender real-time und CW-Doppler-Sonographie. Radiologe 30:525–531

Krinsky G, Rofsky N, Giangola G (1996) Gadolinium-enhanced three-dimensional MR angiography of acquired arch vessel disease. AJR Am J Roentgenol 167:981–987

Krishnabhakdi S, Espinola-Klein C, Kurz G, Neufang A, Schmidt W, Oelert H (2001) Sonographisches Venenmapping – Stellenwert in der distalen Bypasschirurgie. Ultraschall Med 22(Suppl):60

Kroegel C (2003) Advances in the diagnosis and treatment of pulmonary embolism. Pulmonary embolism – how can you mend a broken clot? Respiration 70:4–6

Kroegel C, Reissig A (2003) Principle mechanisms underlying venous thromboembolism: epidemiology, risk factors, pathophysiology and pathogenesis. Respiration 70:7–30

Krumme B, Lehnert T, Wollschläger H, Keller E (1995) Möglichkeiten und Grenzen der farbduplexgesteuerten Kompressionstherapie von punktionsbedingten Gefäßläsionen in der Leiste. Fortschr Röntgenstr 163:158–162

Krumme B, Blum U, Schwertfeger E et al (1996) Diagnosis of renovascular disease by intra- and extrarenal Doppler scanning. Kidney Int 50:1288–1292

Krysiewicz S, Mellinger BC (1989) The role of imaging in the diagnostic evaluation of impotence. Am J Roentgenol 153:1133–1139

Kubale R (1987) Renovaskuläre Erkrankungen. In: Seitz K, Kubale R. Duplex Sonographie der abdominellen und retroperitonealen Gefäße. VCH, Weinheim

Kubale R (1993) Abdominelle Venen, portalvenöses System und Leber. In: Wolf K-J, Fobbe F (Hrsg) Farbkodierte Duplexsonographie. Thieme, Stuttgart, pp 158–184

Kubale R (1994) Abdominelle und retroperitoneale Gefäße. In: Rettenmaier G, Seitz KH (Hrsg) Sonographische Differentialdiagnostik. Chapman & Hall, Weinheim, pp 865

Kudlicka J, Kavan J, Tuka V et al (2012) More precise diagnosis of access stenosis: ultrasonography versus angiography. J Vasc Access 13:310–314

Kutzner H, Schneider-Stock R (2009) Vaskuläre Tumoren (Kap. 18). In: Klöppel G et al (eds) Pathologie, 3rd edn. Springer, Heidelberg/ Berlin, p 543

Kuzniec S, Kauffman P, Molnar LJ et al (1998) Diagnosis of limb and neck arterial trauma using duplex ultrasonography. Cardiovasc Surg 6:358–366

Kwon BJ, Jung C, Sheen SH (2007) CT angiography of stented carotid arteries: comparison with Doppler ultrasonography. J Endovasc Ther 14:489–497

Labropoulos N, Volteas SK, Giannoukas AD, Toulpoupakis E, Delis K, Nicolaides AN (1996) Asymptomatic popliteal vein aneurysms. Vasc Surg 6:453–458

Labropoulos N, Leon LR Jr, Gonzalez-Fajardo JA et al (2007) Nonatherosclerotic pathology of the neck vessels: prevalence and flow patterns. Vasc Endovasc Surg 41:417–427

Labs K-H (1991) Die Aussagekraft der Dopplerspektralanalyse für die praktische Diagnostik. Vasa 32(Suppl):72–84

Ladleif M, Langholz J, Heidrich H, Blank B (1998) Wertigkeit der farbkodierten Duplexsonographie bei der Diagnostik von Fingerarterienverschlüssen. Vasa 52(Suppl):44

Lafortune M, Marleau D, Breton G et al (1984) Portal venous system measurements in portal hypertension. Radiology 151:27–30

Lafortune M, Patriquin H, Pomier G et al (1987) Hemodynamic changes in portal circulation after portosystemic shunts: use of duplex sonography in 43 patients. Am J Roentgenol 149:701–706

Lagerstedt CL, Olsson CC, Fagher BO, Öqvist BW, Albrechtsson U (1985) Need for long-term anticoagulant treatment in symptomatic calf-vein thrombosis. Lancet 2:515–518

Lal BK, Hobson RW, Goldstein J, Chakhtoura EY, Duran WN (2004) Carotid artery stenting: is there a need to revise ultrasound velocity criteria? J Vasc Surg 39:58–66

Lal BK, Hobson RW, Hameed M et al (2006) Noninvasive identification of the unstable carotid plaque. Ann Vasc Surg 20:167–174

Lal BK, Hobson RW II, Tofighi B, Kapadia I, Cuadra S, Jamil Z (2008) Duplex ultrasound velocity criteria for the stented carotid artery. J Vasc Surg 47:63–73

Landry GJ, Moneta GL, Taylor LM et al (1999) Duplex scanning alone is not sufficient imaging before secondary procedures after lower extremity reversed vein bypass graft. J Vasc Surg 29:270–280

Landwehr P, Lackner K (1990) Farbkodierte Duplexsonographie vor und nach PTA der Arterien der unteren Extremität. Fortschr Röntgenstr 152:35–41

Landwehr P, Tschammler A, Höhmann M (1990) Gefäßdiagnostik mit der farbkodierten Duplexsonographie. Dtsch Med Wochenschr 115:343–351

Lang W (2002) Arterielle Gefäßdiagnostik beim diabetischen Fußsyndrom. Gefässchirurgie 7:122–127

Lange P, Houe T, Helgstrand UJV (2001) The efficacy of ultrasound-guided compression of iatrogenic femoral pseudo-aneurysms. Eur J Vasc Endovasc Surg 21:248–250

Lange SF, Trampisch HJ, Pittrow D et al. for the getABI Study Group (2007) Profound influence of different methods for determination of the ankle brachial index on the prevalence estimate of peripheral arterial disease. BMC Public Health 7:147

Langerstedt CL, Olsson CG, Fagher BO et al (1985) Need for long-term anticoagulant treatment in symptomatic calf vein thrombosis. Lancet 2:515–518

Langholz JP (1997) Ultrasound contrast agents in peripheral vascular disease. In: Nanda NC, Schlief R, Goldberg BB (eds) Advances in echo imaging using contrast enhancement, 2nd edn. Kluwer, Dordrecht, pp 543–560

Langholz J (1998) Investigation of peripheral arterial disease: the expanding role of echo-enhanced color flow Doppler and duplex sonography. Eur J Ultrasound 7(Suppl 3):53–61

Langholz J, Heidrich H (1991) Sonographische Diagnose der tiefen Becken–/Beinvenenthrombose: Ist die farbkodierte Duplexsonographie "überflüssig"? Ultraschall Med 12:176–181

Langholz J, Schlief R, Heidrich H (1992) Verbesserung der farbcodierten Duplexsonographie durch Kontrastmittelgabe bei schwer untersuchbaren Regionen der peripher-arteriellen Becken-Bein-Strombahn. Ultaschall Med 13:234–238

Langholz J, Maul R, Heidrich H (1994) Was ist eine "hypoplastische" A. vertebralis? Überlegungen auf der Basis duplexsonographischer Untersuchungen. Vasa 43(Suppl):50 (Abstr)

Langholz J, Ladleif M, Blank B, Heidrich H, Behrendt C (1997) Colour coded duplex sonography in ischemic finger artery disease - a comparison with hand arteriography. Vasa 26:85–90

Langsfeld M, Hershey FB, Thorpe L et al (1987) Duplex B-mode imaging for the diagnosis of deep venous thrombosis. Arch Surg 122: 587–591

Langsfeld M, Gray-Weale AC, Lusby RJ (1989) The role of plaque morphology and diameter reduction in the development of new symptoms in asymptomatic carotid arteries. J Vasc Surg 9:548–557

Länne T, Sandgren T, Mangell P, Sonesson B, Hansen F (1997) Improved reliability of ultrasonic surveillance of abdominal aortic aneurysms. Eur J Vasc Endovasc Surg 13:149–153

Länne T, Solvig J, Eriksson A, Olofsson PA, Marsal K, Hansen F (1997) Time domain ultrasonography – a reliable method of percutaneous volume flow measurement in large arteries. Clin Physiol 17: 371–382

Lanzer P, Yoganathan AP (1991) Vascular imaging by color Doppler and magnetic resonance. Springer, Berlin/Heidelberg/New York/Tokyo

Larch E (1993) Farbcodierte Duplexsonographie zur Beurteilung der Unterschenkelarterien bei peripherer arterieller Verschlußkrankheit. Vasa 41(Suppl):14

Larch E, Minar E, Ahmadi R et al (1997) Value of color duplex sonography for evaluation of tibioperoneal arteries in patients with femoropopliteal obstruction: a prospective comparison with anterograde intra-arterial digital subtraction angiography. J Vasc Surg 25:629–636

Laub G (1999) Principles of contrast-enhanced MR angiography. Basic and clinical applications. Magn Reson Imaging Clin N Am 7: 783–795

Lausen M, Jensen R, Wille-Jorgensen P et al (1995) Colour Doppler flow imaging ultrasonography versus venography as screening method for asymptomatic postoperative deep venous thrombosis. Eur J Radiol 20:200–204

Lederle FA, Wilson SE, Johnson GR et al (1995) For the Abdominal Aortic Aneurysm Detection and Management Veterans Administration Cooperativ Study Group. Variability in measure of abdominal aortic aneurysms. J Vasc Surg 21:945–952

Lee HM, Wang Y, Sostman HD et al (1998) Distal lower extremity arteries: evaluation with two-dimensional MR digital subtraction angiography. Radiology 207:505–512

Lee VS, Hertzberg BS, Workman MJ, Smith TP et al (2000) Variability of Doppler US measurements along the common carotid artery: effects on estimates of internal carotid arterial stenoses in patients with angiographically proved disease. Radiology 214:387–392

Legemate DA, Teeuwen C, Hoemeveld H, Ackerstaff RG, Eickelboom BC (1991a) Spectral analysis criteria in duplex scanning of aortoiliac and femoropoliteal arterial disease. Ultrasound Med Biol 17: 769–776

Legemate DA, Teeuwen C, Hoeneveld H, Eikelboom BC (1991b) Value of duplex scanning compared with angiography and pressure measurement in the assessment of aortoiliac arterial lesions. Br J Surg 78:1003–1008

Leiner T, de Haan MW, Nelemans PJ et al (2005) Contemporary imaging techniques for the diagnosis of renal artery stenosis. Eur Radiol 15:2219–2229

Lensing AWA, Prandoni P, Brandjes D et al (1989) Detection of deep vein thrombosis by real-time B-mode ultrasonography. New Engl J Med 320:342–345

Lensing AWA, Prandoni P, Brandjes D et al (1989) Detection of deep-vein thrombosis by real-time B-mode ultrasonography. New Engl J Med 320:392–398

Lensing AWA, Doris CI, McGrath FP et al (1997) A comparison of compression ultrasound with color Doppler ultrasound for the diagnosis of symptomless postoperative deep vein thrombosis. Arch Intern Med 157:765–768

Lepore T, Savran J, van de Water J, Harrower H, Yablonski M (1978) Screening for lower extremity deep venous thrombosis. Am J Surg 135:529–534

Lerner RM, Medorach RA, Hulbert WC, Rabinowitz R (1990) Color Doppler US in the evaluation of acute scrotal disease. Radiology 176:355–358

Leu HJ (1973) Histologische Altersbestimmung von arteriellen und venösen Thromben und Embolie. Vasa 2:265–273

Leu HJ, Bollinger A, Pouliadis G, Brunner U, Soyka P (1977) Pathologie, Klinik, Radiologie und Chirurgie der zystischen Adventitia-Degeneration peripherer Blutgefäße. Vasa 6:94–99

Leung A, Hampson SJ, Singh MP et al (1983) Ultrasonic diagnosis of bilateral congenital internal jugular venous aneurysms. Br J Radiol 56:588–591

Lev M, Saphir O (1952) Endophlebohypertrophy and phlebosclerosis: II. The external and common iliac veins. Am J Pathol 28(3):401–411

Levien LJ, Benn CA (1998) Adventitial cystic disease: a unifying hypthesis. J Vasc Surg 28:193–205

Levine M, Gent M, Hirsh J et al (1996) A comparison of low-molecular-weight heparin administered primarily at home with unfractionated heparin administered in the hospital for proximal deep vein thrombosis. N Engl J Med 334:677–681

Levy MM, Baum RA, Carpenter JP (1998) Endovascular surgery solely based on noninvasive preprocedural imaging. J Vasc Surg 28: 995–1003

Lewis SC, Wardlaw JM (2002) Which Doppler velocity is best for assessing suitability for carotid endarterectomy? Eur J Ultrasound 15:9–20

Lewis BD, James EM, Charboneau JW et al (1989) Current applications of color Doppler imaging in the abdomen and extremities. Radiographics 9:599–631

Lewis BD, James EM, Welch TJ, Joyce JW, Hallett JW, Weaver AL (1994) Diagnosis of acute deep venous thrombosis of the lower extremities: prospective evaluation of colour Doppler flow imaging versus venography. Radiology 192:651–655

Li R, Cai J, Tegeler C et al (1996) Reproducibility of extracranial carotid atherosclerotic lesions assessed by B-mode ultrasound: the ARIC Study. Ultrasound Med Biol 22:791–799

Liapis CD, Gugulakis A, Misiakos E, Verkokos C, Dousaitou B, Sechas M (1994) Surgical treatment of extracranial carotid aneurysms. Int Angiol 13:290–295

Liapis CD, Kakisis JD, Kostakis AG (2001) Carotid stenosis: factors affecting symptomatology. Stroke 32:2782–2786

Libby P (2002) The fire within. Sci Am 286:46–55

Liewald F et al (2001) Influence of treatment of type II leaks on the aneurysm surface area. Eur J Vasc Endovasc Surg 21:339–343

Ligush J, Reavis SW, Preisser JS, Hansen KJ (1998) Duplex ultrasound scanning defines operative strategies for patients with limb-threatening ischemia. J Vasc Surg 28:482–491

Limberg B (1991) Duplexsonographische Diagnose der portalen Hypertension bei Leberzirrhose. Einfluss einer standardisierten Testmahlzeit auf die portale Hämodynamik. Dtsch Med Wochenschr 116:1384–1387

Limet R, Sakalihassan N, Albert A (1991) Determination of the expansion rate and incidence of rupture of abdominal aortic aneurysms. J Vasc Surg 14:540–548

Lindholt JS, Norman P (2008) Screening for abdominal aortic aneurysm reduces overall mortality in men. A meta-analysis of the mid- and long-term effects of screening for abdominal sortic aneurysms. Eur J Vasc Endovasc Surg 36:167–171

Lindholt JS, Vammen S, Juul S, Henneberg EW, Fasting H (1999) The validity of ultrasonographic scanning as screening method for abdominal aortic aneurysm. Eur J Vasc Endovasc Surg 17:472–475

Lindholt JS, Juul S, Fasting H, Henneberg EW (2005) Screening for abdominal aortic aneurysm: single centre randomised controlled trial. BMJ 330:750–753

Lindholt JS, Sorensen J, Sogaard R, Henneberg EW (2010) Long-term benefit and cost-effectivness analysis of screening for abdominal aortic aneurysms from a randomized controlled trial. Br J Surg 97:826–834

Lindholt JS, Søgaard R, Laustsen J (2012) Prognosis of ruptured abdominal aortic aneurysms in Demark form 1994-2008. Clin Epidemiol 4:111–113

Lindquist R (1977) Ultrasound as a complementary diagnostic method in deep vein thrombosis of the leg. Acta Med Scand 201:435

Lippert H, Pabst R (1985) Arterial variations in man. Bergmann, Munich

Lock G (2001) Acute intestinal ischemia. Best Pract Res Clin Gastroenterol 15:83–88

Lockhart ME, Robbin ML (2001) Hemodialysis access ultrasound. Ultrasound Q 17:157–167

Lockhart ME, Robbin MI, Allon M (2004) Preoperative sonographic radial artery evaluation and correlation with subsequent radiocephalic fistula outcome. J Ultrasound Med 23:161–168

Lohr JM, Kerr TM, Lutter KS, Cranley RD (1991) Lower extremity calf thrombosis: to treat or not to treat? J Vasc Surg 14:618–623

London GM, Safar ME (1989) Abnormalities of intrarenal hemodynamics in essential and renovascular hypertension in man. Presse Med 18:1459–1460

London GM, Safar ME (1989) Renal hemodynamics in patients with sustained essential hypertension and in patients with unilateral stenosis of the renal artery. Am J Hypertens 2:244–252

Londrey GL, Hodgson KJ, Spadone DP, Ramsey DE, Barkmeier LD, Summer DS (1990) Initial experience with colour-flow duplex scanning of infrainguinal bypass grafts. J Vasc Surg 12:284–290

Long A, Rouet L, Lindholdt JS, Allaire E (2012) Measuring the maximum diameter of native abdominal aortic aneurysms: review and critical analysis. Eur J Vasc Endovasc Surg 43:515–521

Longo JM, Bilbao JI, Rousseau HP et al (1992) Color Doppler guidance in transjugular placement of intrahepatic portosystemic shunts. Radiology 184:281–283

Lopez JA, Espeland MA, Jarow JP (1992) Interpretation and quantification of penile blood flow studies using duplex ultrasonography. J Urol 146:1271

Lossef FV, Rajan S, Calcagno D, Jelinger E, Patt R, Barth KH (1992) Spontaneous rupture of an adventitial cyst of the popliteal artery: confirmation with MR imaging. J Vasc Interv Radiol 3:95–97

Lovelace TD, Moneta GL, Abou-Zamzam AM Jr et al (2001) Optimizing duplex follow-up in patients with an asymptomatic internal carotid artery stenosis of less than 60%. J Vasc Surg 33:56–61

Lovett JK, Gallagher PJ, Hands LJ, Walton J, Rothwell PM (2004) Histological correlates of carotid plaque surface morphology on lumen contrast imaging. Circulation 110:2190–2197

Lovett JK, Redgrave JN, Rothwell PM (2005) A critical appraisal of the performance, reporting and interpretation of studies comparing carotid plaque imaging with histology. Stroke 36:1091–1097

Lowery AJ, Hynes N, Manning BJ, Mahendran M, Tawfik S, Sultan S (2007) A prospective feasibility study of duplex ultrasound arterial mapping, digital-subtraction angiography and magnetic resonance angiography in management of critical lower limb ischemia by endovascular revascularization. Ann Vasc Surg 21:443–451

Ludwig M (1991) Quantitative Flußmessungen an Venen. Ultraschall-dreiländertreffen, Lausanne

Ludwig M, Stumpe KO (1994) Karotisultraschall in der Früherkennung der Atherosklerose. Dtsch Ärztebl 91:745–746

Ludwig D, Schwarting K, Korbel CM, Bruning A, Schiefer B, Stange EF (1998) The postprandial portal flow is related to the severity of portal hypertension and liver cirrhosis. J Hepatol 28:631–638

Ludwig M, Mv P-K, Stumpe KO (2003) Intima media thickness of the carotid arteries: early pointer to arteriosclerosis and therapeutic endpoint. Ultraschall Med 24:162–174

Lue TF (1991) Physiology of penile erection. In: Jonas U, Thon WF, Stief CG (eds) Erectile dysfunction. Springer, Berlin/Heidelberg/New York, pp 44–65

Lujan S, Criado E, Puras E, Izquierdo LM (2002) Duplex scanning or arteriography for preoperative planning of lower limb revascularisation. Eur J Vasc Endovasc Surg 24:31–36

Lundell A, Lindblad B, Bergqvist D, Hansen F (1995) Femoropopliteal-crural graft patency is improved by an intensive surveillance program: a prospective randomized study. J Vasc Surg 21:26–34

Lundin P, Svensson A, Henriksen E et al (2000) Imaging of aortoiliac arterial disease. Duplex ultrasound and MR angiography versus digital subtraction angiography. Acta Radiol 41:125–132

Lusby RJ (1993) Plaque characterisation: does it identify high risk groups? In: Bernstein EF, Callow AD, Nicolaides AN, Shifrin EG (eds) Cerebral revascularisation. Med-Orion, London/Los Angeles/Nicosia, pp 93–107

Luska G, Risch U, Pellengahr M, von Boetticher H (1990) Farbcodierte dopplersonographische Untersuchungen zur Morphologie und Hämodynamik der Arterien des Beckens und der Beine bei gesunden Probanden. Fortschr Röntgenstr 153:246–251

Luther B (2006) Akute viszerale Ischämie. Gefässchirurgie 11:167–172

Luther B (Hrsg) (2014) Techniken der offenen Gefäßchirurgie. Springer Verlag, Berlin/Heidelberg

Lutter KS, Kerr TM, Roedersheimer LR, Lohr JM, Sampson MSG, Cranley JJ (1991) Superficial thrombophlebitis diagnosed by duplex scanning. Surgery 110:42–46

MacMathuna P, Vlavianos P, Westaby D, Williams R (1992) Pathophysiology of portal hypertension. Dig Dis 10(Suppl 1):3–15

Maged IM, Kron IL, Hagspiel KD (2009) Recurrent cystic adventitial disease of the popliteal artery: Successful treatment with percutaneous transluminal angioplasty. J Vasc Endovasc Surg 43:399–402

Magnusson MB, Nelzen O, Risberg B, Sivertsson R (2001) A colour doppler ultrasound study of venous reflux in patients with chronic leg ulcers. Eur J Vasc Endovasc Surg 21:353–360

Makris SA, Karkos CD, Awad S, London NJ (2006) An "all-comers" venous duplex scan policy for patients with lower limb varicose veins attending a one-stop vascular clinic: is it justified? Eur J Vasc Endovasc Surg 32:718–724

Maleti O, Lugli M, Collura M (1997) Anévrysmes veineaux poplités: exppérience personelle. Phlebologie 50:53–59

Mamode N, Pickford I, Leiberman P (1999) Failure to improve outcome in acute mesenteric ischemia: Seven-year review. Eur J Surg 165:203–208

Mannami T, Baba S, Ogata J (2000) Potential of carotid enlargement as a useful indicator affected by high blood pressure in a large general population of a Japanese city: the Suita study. Stroke 31:2958–2965

Manning BJ, Kristmundsson T, Sonesson B, Resch T (2009a) Abdominal aortic aneurysm diameter: a comparison of ultrasound measurements with those from standard and three-dimensional computed tomography reconstracions. J Vasc Surg 50:263–268

Manning BJ, O'Neill SM, Haider SN et al (2009b) Duplex ultrasound in aneurysm surveillance following endovascular aneurysm repair: a comparison with computed tomography aortography. J Vasc Surg 49:60–65

Manthey J, Munderloh KH, Mautner JP, Köhl M, Fröhlich G (1994) Popliteal venous aneurysm with pulmonary and paradoxical embolization. Vasa 23:264–267

Marin J, Gosselin J, Khayat A (1978) A propos d'un cas d'anévrisme de la veine poplitée avec embolie pulmonaire. Phlebologie 31: 433–438

Markel A, Manzo RA, Bergelin RO, Strandness DE (1992a) Valvular reflux after deep vein thrombosis: incidence and time of occurrence. J Vasc Surg 15:377–384

Markel A, Monzo R, Bergelin RO, Strandness DE (1992b) Pattern and distribution of thrombi in acute venous thrombosis. Arch Surg 127:305–309

Marshall M (1990a) Die Duplex-Sonographie bei phlebologischen Fragestellungen in Praxis und Klinik. Ultraschall. Klin Prax 5:51–56

Marshall M (1990b) Sklerosierungsreaktion großer Varizen im hochauflösenden Ultraschallbild. Phlebol Proktol 19:205–214

Martin RL, Nanra RS, Wlodarczyk J et al (1991) Renal hilar Doppler analysis in the detection of renal artery stenosis. J Vasc Technol 15:173–180

Mastracci TM, Cinà CS (2007) Screening for abdominal aortic aneurysm in Canada: review and position statement of the Canadian Society for Vascular Surgery. J Vasc Surg 45:1268–1276

Mathiesen EB, Bonaa KH, Joakimsen O (2001) Echolucent plaques are associated with high risk of ischemic cerebrovascular events in carotid stenosis: the Tromso Study. Circulation 103:2171–2175

Mathis G (2009) Two silver standards in the imaging of pulmonary embolism. Ultraschall Med 30:497–498

Mathis G, Bitschnau R, Gehmacher O et al (1999) Chest ultrasound in diagnosis of pulmonary embolism in comparison to helical CT. Ultraschall Med 20:54–59

Mathis G, Blank W, Reißig A et al (2005) Thoracic ultrasound for diagnosing pulmonary embolism. A prospective multicenter study of 352 patients. Chest 128:1531–1538

Matsagas MI, Vasdekis SN, Gugulakis AG et al (2000) Computer-assisted ultrasonographic analysis of carotid plaques in relation to cerebrovascular symptoms, cerebral infarction, and histology. Ann Vasc Surg 14:130–137

Mattos MA, Londrey GL, Leutz DW et al (1992) Color-flow duplex scanning for the surveillance and diagnosis of acute deep venous thrombosis. J Vasc Surg 15:366–376

Mattos MA, van Bemmelen PS, Barkmeier ID et al (1993) Routine surveillance after carotid endarterectomy: does it affect clinical management? J Vasc Surg 17:819–830

May R, Mignon G (1976) Spindelförmiges Aneurysma der Vena fibularis. Fortschr Röntgenstr 25:563–564

May R, Nissl R (1968) Aneurysma der Vena poplitea. Fortschr Röntgenstr 108:402–403

May R, Nissl R (1973) Die Phlebographie der unteren Extremität. Thieme, Stuttgart/New York

May AG, Deweese JA, CG ROB (1963) Hemodynamic effects of arterial stenosis. Surgery 53:513–524

Mazzariol F, Ascher E, Salles-Cunha S, Grade P, Hingorani A (1999) Values and limitations of duplex ultrasonography as the sole imaging method of preoperative evaluation for popliteal and infrapopliteal bypasses. Ann Vasc Surg 13:1–10

Mazzariol F, Hingorani A, Gunduz Y, Yorkovich W, Salles-Cunha S (2000) Lower-extremity revascularisation without preoperative contrast arteriography in 185 cases: lessons learned with duplex ultrasound arterial mapping. Eur J Vasc Endovasc Surg 19:509–515

McDevitt DT, Lohr JM, Martin KD, Welling RE, Sampson MG (1993) Bilateral popliteal vein aneurysms. Ann Vasc Surg 7:282–286

McLachan MSF, Thomson JG, Taylor DW, Kelly ME, Sackett DL (1979) Observer variation in the interpretation of lower limb venograms. Am. J Radiol 132:227–229

McLafferty RB, McCrary BS, Mattos MA et al (2002) The use of color-flow duplex scan for the detection of endoleaks. J Vasc Surg 36:100–104

McWilliams RG et al (2002) Detection of endoleak with enhanced ultrasound imaging: comparison with biphasic computed tomography. J Endovasc Ther 9:170–179

Meairs S, Hennerici M (1999) Four-dimensional ultrasonographic characterization of plaque surface motion in patients with symptomatic and asymptomatic carotid artery stenosis. Stroke 30:1807–1813

Meerbaum S (1997) Microbubble fluid dynamics of echocontrast. In: Nanda NC, Schlief R, Goldberg BB (eds) Advances in echo imaging using contrast enhancement, 2nd edn. Kluwer, Dordrecht, pp 11–38

Mehta M, Paty PS, Roddy SP (2011) Treatment options for delayed AAA rupture following endovascular repair. J Vasc Surg 53:14–20

Meissner MH, Caps MT, Zierler BK, Bergelin RO, Manzo RA, Strandness DE (2000) Deep venous thrombosis and superficial venous reflux. J Vasc Surg 32:48–56

Melany ML, Grant EG, Farooki S et al (1999) Effect of US contrast agents on spectral velocities: in vivo evaluation. Radiology 211:427–431

Meltzer RS, Tickner EG, Sahines TP, Popp RL (1980) The source of ultrasound contrast effect. J Clin Ultrasound 8:121–127

Mendes RR, Farber MA, Marston WA et al (2002) Prediction of wrist arteriovenous fistula maturation with preoperative vein mapping with ultrasonography. J Vasc Surg 36:460–463

Mercer KG, Scott DJA, Turton EPL, Berridge DC, Weston MJ (1999) Can intra-operative flow measurements identify grafts for intensive duplex surveillance? St James University Hospital NHS Trust, Leeds

Merkus JW, Zeebregts CJ, Hoitsman AJ et al (1993) High incidence of arteriovenous fistula after biopsy of kidney allografts. Br J Surg 80:310–312

Merritt CRB, Bluth EI (1992) Ultrasound identification of plaque composition. In: Labs KH et al (eds) Diagnostic vascular ultrasound. Arnold, London, pp 213–223

Metz V, Braunsteiner A, Grabenwöger F et al (1988) Farbcodierte Doppler-Sonographie der Becken-Bein-Arterien: Überprüfung der Wertigkeit der Methode im Vergleich zur Angiographie. Fortschr Röntgenstr 149:314–316

Metz V, Dock W, Grabenwöger F et al (1992) Wertigkeit unterschiedlicher klinischer und bildgebender Verfahren für die postoperative Verlaufskontrolle extraanatomischer Bypasses. Fortschr Röntgenstr 154:172–175

Mewissen MW, Kinney EV, Bandyk DF et al (1992) The role of duplex scanning versus angiography in predicting outcome after balloon angioplasty in the femoropopliteal artery. J Vasc Surg 15:860–864

Meyer P, Strobel M (2008) Intima-Media-Dicke-Messung. Medizinische Verlagsgesellschaft, Berlin, pp 9–21

Meyer P, Rudofsky G, Nobbe N (1986) Das Histogramm des Okklusionsmaterials – ein neuer Prognoseparameter der thrombolytischen Therapie bei tiefer Beinvenenthrombose. In: Hansmann M, Koischwitz D, Lutz H, Trier HG (eds) Ultraschalldiagnostik 86. Springer, Berlin/Heidelberg/New York/Tokyo, p 138

Meyer JL, Khalil RM, Obuchowski NA, Baus LK (1997) Common carotid artery: variability of Doppler US velocity measurements. Radiology 204:339–341

Michaels JA, Galland RB (1993) Management of asymptomatic popliteal aneurysms: the use of a Markovic decision tree to determine the criteria for a conservative approach. Eur J Vasc Surg 7:136–143

Mickley V (2006) Central vein obstruction in vascular access. Eur J Vasc Endovasc Surg 32:439–444

Middleton WD, Melson GL (1989) Testicular ischemia: color Doppler sonographic findings in five patients. AJR Am J Roentgenol 152:1237–1239

Middleton WD, Foley WD, Lawson TL (1988) Color flow Doppler imaging of carotid artery abnormalities. Am J Roentgenol 150:419–425

Middleton WD, Kellman GM, Melson GL, Madrazo BL (1989a) Postbiopsy renal transplant arteriovenous fistulas: color Doppler US characteristics. Radiology 171:253–257

Middleton WD, Thorne DA, Melson GL (1989b) Color Doppler ultrasound of the normal testis. AJR Am J Roentgenol 152:293–297

Middleton WD, Siegel BA, Melson GL, Yates CK, Andriole GL (1990) Acute scrotal disorders: prospective comparison of color Doppler US and testicular scintigraphy. Radiology 177:177–181

Miller N, Satin R, Tousignant L, Sheiner NM (1996) A prospective study comparing duplex scan and venography for diagnosis of lower-extremity deep vein thrombosis. Cardiovasc Surg 4:505–508

Millner R (Hrsg) (1987) Ultraschalltechnik. Physik, Weinheim, pp 41–46

Mills JL Sr (2001) Infrainguinal vein graft surveillance: how and when. Semin Vasc Surg 14:169–176

Mills JL, Harris EJ, Taylor LM, Beckett WC (1990) The importance of routine surveillance of distal bypass grafts with duplex scanning: a study of 379 reversed vein grafts. J Vasc Surg 12:379–386

Mills JL, Fujitani RM, Taylor SM (1993) The characteristics and anatomic distribution of lesions that cause reversed vein graft failure: a five-year prospective study. J Vasc Surg 17:195–206

Mills JL, Bandyk DF, Gathan V, Esses GE (1995) The origin of infrainguinal vein graft stenosis: a prospective study based on duplex surveillance. J Vasc Surg 21:16–22

Mills JL Sr, Wixon CL, James DC, Devine J, Westerband A, Hughes JD (2001) The natural history of intermediate and critical vein graft stenosis: recommendations for continued surveillance or repair. J Vasc Surg 33:273–278

Miralles M, Cairols M, Cotillas J et al (1996) Value of Doppler parameters in the diagnosis of renal artery stenosis. J Vasc Surg 23:428–435

Mirza TA, Karthikesalingam A, Jackson D et al (2010) Duplex ultrasound and contrast-enhanced ultrasound versus computed tomography for the detection of endoleak after EVAR: systematic review and bivariate meta-analysis. Eur J Vasc Endovasc Surg 39:418–428

Missouris CG, Allen CM, Balen FG, Buckham T, Lees WR, MacGregor GA (1996) Non-invasive screening for renal artery stenosis with ultrasound contrast enhancement. J Hypertens 14:519–524

Mitchell DG (1990) Color Doppler imaging: principles, limitations and artifacts. Radiology 177:1–10

Mitchell EL, Chang EY, Landry GJ et al (2009) Duplex criteria for native superior mesenteric artery stenosis overestimate stenosis in stented superior mesenteric arteries. J Vasc Surg 50:335–340

Mödder U (1992) Farbcodierte Duplexsonographie (Angiodynographie). Fortschr Röntgenstr 157:204–209

Mofidi R, Kelman J, Berrry O, Bennett S, Murie JA, Dawson AR (2007) Significance of the early postoperative duplex result in infrainguinal vein bypass surveillance. Eur J Vasc Endovasc Surg 34:327–332

Mofidi R, Pandanaboyana S, Flett MM, Nagy J, Griffiths GD, Stonebridge PA; East of Scotland Vascular Network (2009) The value of vein graft surveillance in bypasses performed with small-diameter vein grafts. Ann Vasc Surg 23:17–23

Mohan CR, Hoballah JJ, Schueppert MT et al (1995) Should all in situ saphenous vein bypasses undergo permanent duplex surveillance? Arch Surg 130:483–487

Mohan IV, Laheij RJF, Harris PL (2001) Risk factors for endoleak and the evidence for stent-graft oversizing in patients undergoing endovascular aneurysm repair. Eur J Vasc Endovasc Surg 21:344–349

Moll R, Habscheid W, Landwehr P (1991) Häufigkeit des Aneurysma spurium der Arteria femoralis nach Herzkatheteruntersuchung und PTA. Fortschr Röntgenstr 154:23–27

Moll FL, Powell JT, Fraedrich G et al (2011) Management of abdominal aortic aneurysms. Clinical practice guidelines of the European Society of Vascular Surgery. Eur J Vasc Endovasc Surg 41:51–58

Moneta GL, Taylor DC, Helton WS, Mulholland MW, Strandness DE (1988) Duplex ultrasound measurement of postprandial intestinal blood flow: effect of meal composition. Gastroenterology 95: 1294–1301

Moneta GL, Yeager RA, Dalman R et al (1991) Duplex ultrasound criteria for the diagnosis of splanchnic artery stenosis or occlusion. J Vasc Surg 14:511–520

Moneta GL, Yeager RA, Antonovic R et al (1992) Accuracy of lower extremity arterial duplex mapping. J Vasc Surg 15:275–284

Moneta GL, Yeager RA, Antonovic R et al (1992) Accuracy of lower extremity arterial duplex mapping. J Vasc Surg 17:511–520

Moneta GL, Edwards JM, Chitwood RW et al (1993) Correlation of North American Symptomatic Carotid Endarterectomy Trial (NASCET): Angiographic definition of 70% to 99% internal carotid artery stenosis with duplex scanning. J Vasc Surg 17:152–157. Discussion 157–159

Moneta GL, Lee RW, Yeager RA et al (1993) Mesenteric duplex scanning: a blinded prospective study. J Vasc Surg 17:79–86

Moneta GL, Yeager RA, Lee RW, Porter JM (1993c) Noninvasive localisation of arterial occlusive disease: a comparison of segmental Doppler pressures and arterial duplex mapping. J Vasc Surg 17:578–582

Moneta GL, Edwards JM, Papanicolaou G et al (1995) Screening for asymptomatic internal carotid artery stenosis: duplex criteria for discriminating 60% to 99% stenosis. J Vasc Surg 21:989–994

Monreal M, Montserrat E, Salvador R et al (1989) Real-time ultrasound for diagnosis of symptomatic venous thrombosis and for screening of patients at risk. Correlation with ascending conventional venography. Angiology 39:527

Montefusco von Kleist CM, Bakal C, Sprayregen S, Rhodes BA, Veith FJ (1993) Comparison of duplex ultrasonography and ascending contrast venography in the diagnosis of venous thrombosis. Angiology 44:169–175

Monzer MAY, Wiese JA, Shamma AR (1987) The to-and-fro-sign: duplex Doppler evidence of femoral artery pseudoaneurysm. Am J Roentgenol 150:632–634

Moore WS (2003) For severe carotid stenosis found on ultrasound, further arterial evaluation is unnecessary. Stroke 34:1816–1817

Moreau P, Albat B, Thévenet A (1994) Surgical treatment of extracranial internal carotid artery aneurysm. Ann Vasc Surg 8:409–416

Morin C, Lafortune M, Pomier G et al (1992) Patent paraumbilical vein: anatomic and hemodynamic variants and their clinical importance. Radiology 185:253–256

Moriyasu F, Nishida O, Ban N et al (1986) "Congestion index" of the portal vein. Am J Roentgenol 146:735–739

Moriyasu F, Ban N, Nishida O et al (1986) Clinical application of an ultrasonic duplex system in the quantitative measurement of portal blood flow. J Clin Ultrasound 14:579–588

Moriyasu F, Ban N, Nishida O et al (1986) Portal hemodynamics in patients with hepatocellular carcinoma. Radiology 161:707–711

Moser KM, LeMoine JR (1981) Is embolic risk conditioned by location of deep venous thrombosis? Ann Intern Med 94:439–444

Mosso M, Jung HH, Baumgartner RW (2007) Recurrent spontaneous vasospasm of cervical carotid ophthalmic and retinal arteries causing repeated retinal infarcts: a case report. Cerebrovasc Dis 24:381–384

Motew SJ, Cherr GS, Craven TE (2000) Renal duplex sonography: main renal artery versus hilar anaylsis. J Vasc Surg 32:462–471

Moucka J, Jäger K (1990) Rationelle Abklärung bei peripherer arterieller Verschlußkrankheit. Schweiz Rundsch Med Prax 79:1553–1559

Mueller SC, Lue TF (1988) Evaluation of vasculogenic impotence. Urol Clin North Am 15:65–76

Muhm M, Polterauer P, Gstottner W, Temmel A et al (1997) Diagnostic and therapeutic approaches to carotid body tumors: review of 24 patients. Arch Surg 132:279–284

Müller-Schwefe CH, von Klinggräf G, Riepe G, Schröder A (1991) Das inflammatorische Bauchaortenaneurysma. Ultraschall Med 12: 158–163

Müller-Wiefel H (1974) Untersuchungen zur Hämodynamik in den Venen der unteren Extremität. In: Physiologische, phathophysiologische und klinische Aspekte. Schattauer, Stuttgart

Mulligan SA, Matsuda T, Tanzer P et al (1991) Peripheral arterial occlusive disease: prospective comparison of MR angiography and color duplex US with conventional angiography. Radiology 178:695–700

Multicentre Aneurysm Screening Study Group (2002) Multicentre aneurysm screening study (MASS): cost effectiveness analysis of screening for abdominal aortic aneurysms based on four year results from randomised controlled trial. BMJ 325:1135. and Lancet 360: 1531–1539

Munda R, First MR, Alexander JW, Linnemann CC, Fidler JP, Kittur D (1983) Polytetrafluoroethylene graft survival in hemodialysis. J Am Med Assoc 249:219–222

Murphy TP, Cronan JJ (1990) Evolution of deep venous thrombosis: a prospective evaluation with US. Radiology 177:543–548

Murphy TP, Beechman RP, Kim HM et al (1998) Long-term follow-up after TIPS: use of Doppler velocity criteria for detecting elevation of portosystemic gradient. J Vasc Interv Radiol 9:275–281

Muster BR, Williams DM, Prince MR (1998) In vitro model of arterial stenosis: correlation of MR signal dephasing and trans-stenotic pressure gradients. Magn Reson Imaging 16:301–310

Naidich JB, Feinberg AW, Karp-Harmann H, Ka Tyma CG, Stein HL (1988) Contrast venography. Reassessment of its role. Radiology 168:97

Naidich JB, Torre JR, Pellerito JS et al (1996) Suspected deep venous thrombosis: is US of both legs necessary? Radiology 200:429–431

Naim C, Douziech M, Therasse E et al (2014) Vulnerable atherosclerotic carotid plaque evaluation by ultrasound, computed tomography angiography, and magnetic resonance imaging: an overview. Can Assoc Radiol J 65:275–286

Nanto M, Takado M, Mohbuchi H et al (2012) Rare variant of a persistent primitive hypoglossal artery arising from the external carotid artery. Neurol Med Chir 52:513–515

Napoli V, Pinto S, Bargellini I, Vignali C, Cioni R, Petruzzi P (2002) Duplex ultrasonographic study of the renal arteries before and after renal artery stenting. Eur Radiol 12:796–803

Narang AT, Rathlev NK (2007) Non-aneurysmal infectious aortitis: a case report. J Emerg Med 32:359–563

NASCET – North American Symptomatic Carotid Endarterectomy Trial Collaborators (1991) Beneficial effect of carotid endarterectomy in symptomatic patients with high-grade carotid stenosis. N Engl J Med 325:445–453

National Kidney Foundation (2006) KDOQI Clinical Practice Guidelines and Clinical Practice Recommendations for 2006 Updates: Hemodialysis Adequacy, Peritoneal Dialysis Adequacy and Vascular Access. Am J Kidney Dis 48(suppl 1):S1–S322

Nazarian GK, Gerral H, Castańeda-Zúńiga WR et al (1994) Development of stenoses in transjugular intrahepatic portosystemic shunts. Radiology 192:231–234

Nazzal MM, Hoballah JJ, Miller EV et al (1997) Renal hilar Doppler analysis is of value in the management of patients with renovascular disease. Am J Surg 174:164–168

Nchimi A, Biquet JF, Brisbois D et al (2003) Duplex ultrasound as first-line screening test for patients suspected of renal artery stenosis: prospective evaluation in high-risk group. Eur Radiol 13: 1413–1419

Neale ML, Chambers JL, Kelly AT et al (1994) Reappraisal of duplex criteria to assess significant carotid stenosis with special reference to reports from the North American Symptomatic Carotid Endarterectomy Trial and the European Carotid Surgery Trial. J Vasc Surg 20:642–649

Nederkoorn PJ, Brown MM (2009) Optimal cut-off criteria for duplex ultrasound for the diagnosis of restenosis in stented carotid arteries: review and protocol for a diagnostic study. BMC Neurol 22:36

Neglen P, Raju S (1992) A comparison between descending phlebography and duplex Doppler investigation in the evaluation of reflux in chronic venous insufficiency: a challenge to phlebography as the gold standard. J Vasc Surg 16:687–693

Nelemans PJ, Leiner T, de Vet HC, van Engelshoven JM (2000) Peripheral arterial disease: meta-analysis of the diagnostic performance of MR angiography. Radiology 217:105–114

Neuerburg J, Vorwerk D, Günther RW, Keulers P (1991) Intravascular ultrasound for support in percutaneous interventional treatment. Vasa 33(Suppl):298–299

Neuerburg-Heusler D (1984) Dopplersonographische Diagnostik der extrakraniellen Verschlußkrankheit. Vasa 12(Suppl):59–70

Neuerburg-Heusler D, Hennerici M (1995) Gefäßdiagnostik mit Ultraschall. In: Doppler und farbcodierte Duplexsonographie. Thieme, Stuttgart

Neuerburg-Heusler D, Karasch TH (1991) Farbkodierte Duplex-Sonographie – Erweiterung der gefäßdiagnostischen Möglichkeiten? In: Maurer PC, Dörrler J, von Sommogy ST (Hrsg) Gefäßchirurgie im Fortschritt. Thieme, Stuttgart

Neville RF, Abularrage CJ, White PW et al (2004) Venous hypertension associated with arteriovenous hemodialysis access. Semin Vasc Surg 17:50–56

Nevitt MP, Ballard DJ, Hallett JW Jr (1989) Prognosis of abdominal aortic aneurysms. A population-based study. N Engl J Med 321:1009–1014

Nichols WN, O'Rourke MF (eds) (1990) McDonald's blood flow in arteries. Theoretical, experimental and clinical principles, 3rd edn. Edward Arnold, London, pp 54–76

Nicolaides AN (1995) Asymptomatic carotid stenosis and risk of stroke: identification of a high risk group (ACSRS): a natural history study. Int Angiol 14:21–23

Nielsen TG, von Jessen F, Sillesen H (1993) Doppler spectral characteristics of infrainguinal vein bypasses. Eur J Vasc Surg 7:610–615

Nielsen TG, Sillesn H, Schroeder TV (1995) Simple hyperaemia test as a screening method in a postoperative surveillance of infrainguinal in situ vein bypasses. Eur J Vasc Endovasc Surg 10:298–303

Nolan BW, Schermerhorn ML, Powell RJ, Rowell E (2005) Restenosis in gold-coated renal artery stents. J Vasc Surg 42:40–46

Noon GP, Jose LZ, Graig M et al (1984) Popliteal vein pseudoaneurysm: a case report. Surgery 96:942–945

Noppeney T, Noppeney J, Winkler M (2007) Das venöse Poplitealaneurysma. Gefässchirurgie 12:187–190

Norgren L, Hiatt WR, Dormandy JA, Nehler MR, Harris KA, Fowkes FGR (2007) Inter-Society Consensus for the Management of Peripheral Arterial Disease (TASC II). Eur J Vasc Endovasc Surg 33:S1–S75

Norman PE, Jamrozik K, Lawrence-Brown MM, Le MT, Spencer CA, Tuohy RJ et al (2004) Population based randomised controlled trial on impact of screening on mortality from abdominal aortic aneurysm. BMJ 329:1259–1264

Norris CS, Greenfield LJ, Hermann JB (1985) Free-floating iliofemoral thrombus. Arch Surg 120:806–808

Numata K, Tanaka K, Kiba T et al (1999) Hepatic artery resistance after mixed-meal ingestion in healthy subjects and patients with chronic liver disease. J Clin Ultrasound 27:239–248

O'Donnell TF Jr, Erdoes L, Mackey WC et al (1985) Correlation of B-mode ultrasound imaging and arteriography with the pathologic findings of carotid endarterectomy. Arch Surg 120:443–449

O'Leary DH, Holen J, Ricotta JJ et al (1987) Carotid bifurcation disease: prediction of ulceration with B-mode ultrasound. Radiology 162:523–525

O'Leary D, Glagov S, Zarins C, Giddens D (1991) Carotid artery disease. In: Rifkin MD, Charboneau JW, Laing FC (eds) Ultrasound 1991: Special Course Syllabus, 77th Scientific Assembly and Annual Meeting. RSNA, Oak Park, pp 189–200

O'Leary DH, Polak JF, Kronmal RA, Manolio TA, Burke GL, Wolfson SK Jr (1999) Carotid-artery intima and media thickness as a risk factor for myocardial infaction and stroke in older adults. Cardiovascular Health Study Collaborative Research Group. N Engl J Med 340:14–22

Oates CP, Pickard RS, Powell PH, Murthy LNS, Whittingham TAW (1995) The use of duplex ultrasound in the assessment of arterial supply to the penis in vasculogenic impotence. J Urol 153:354–357

Ohta M, Hashizume M, Tomikawa M et al (1994) Analysis of hepatic vein waveform by Doppler ultrasonography in 100 patients with portal hypertension. AJG 89:170–175

Olbricht CJ, Wanke B, Haubitz M, Koch KM (1991) Captopril spürt Stenosen der Nierenarterien auf. Med Trib 16:27

Older RA, Gizienski TA, Wilkowski MJ et al (1998) Hemodialysis access stenosis: early detection with color Doppler US. Radiology 207: 161–164

Olin JW (2002) Atherosclerotic renal artery disease. Cardiol Clin 20: 547–562

Olin JW, Piedmonte MR, Young JR (1995) The utility of duplex ultrasound scanning of renal arteries for diagnosing significant renal artery stenosis. Ann Intern Med 122:833–838

Olojugba DH, McCarthy MJ, Naylor AR, Bell PR, London NJ (1998) At what peak velocity ratio should duplex detected infrainguinal vein graft stenoses be revised? Eur J Vasc Endovasc Surg 15:258–260

Omoloja AA, Racadio JM, McEnery PT (2002) Post-biopsy renal arteriovenous fistula. Pediatr Transplant 6:82–85

Orlic P, Vukas D, Drescik I et al (2003) Vascular complications after 725 kidney transplantations during 3 decades. Transplant Proc 35:1381–1384

Ortiz MW, Lopera JE, Gimenez CR et al (2006) Bilateral cystic adventitial disease of the popliteal artery: A case report. Cardiovasc Intervent Radiol 29:306–310

Ortmann J, Widmer MK, Gretener S et al (2009) Cystic adventitial degeneration: ectopic ganglia from adjacent joint capsules. Vasa 38:374–377

Osman Y, Shokeir A, Ali-El-Dein B et al (2003) Vascular complications after live donor renal transplantation: study of risk factors and effects on graft and patient survival. J Urol 169:859–862

Ota H, Takase K, Rikimaru H et al (2005) Quantitative vascular measurements in arterial occlusive disease. Radiographics 25:1141–1158

Owen WJ, Mc Coll I (1980) Venous aneurysm of the axilla simulating a soft tissue tumour. Br J Surg 67:577–578

Owen RS, Carpenter JP, Baum RA, Perloff U, Cope C (1992) Magnetic resonance imaging of angiographically occult runoff vessels in peripheral arterial occlusive disease. N Engl J Med 326:1577–1581

Pages S et al (2001) Comparison of color duplex ultrasound and computed tomography scan for surveillance after aortic endografting. Ann Vasc Surg 15:155–162

Painter TA, Hertzer NR, Beven EG, O'Hara PJ (1985) Extracranial carotid aneurysms: report of six cases and review of the literature. J Vasc Surg 2:312–318

Palareti G, Cosmi B, Lessiani G et al (2010) Evolution of untreated calf deep-vein thrombosis in high risk symptomatic outpatients: the blind, prospective CALTHRO study. Thromb Haemost 104:1063–1070

Pan LG, Forster HV, Ohtake PJ, Lowry TF, Korducki MJ, Forster AL (1985) Effect of carotid chemoreceptor denervation on breathing during ventrolateral medullary cooling in goats. J Appl Physiol 79: 1120–1128

Pan XM, Saloner D, Reilly LM et al (1995) Assessment of carotid artery stenosis by ultrasonography, conventional angiography, and magnetic resonance angiography: correlation with ex vivo measurement of plaque stenosis. J Vasc Surg 21:82–88

Papanicolaou G, Beach KW, Zierler RE, Strandness DE (1995) The relationship between arm-ankle pressure difference and peak systolic velocity in patients with stenotic lower extremity vein grafts. Ann Vasc Surg 9:554–560

Parent FN et al (2002) The incidence and natural history of type I and II endoleak: a 5-year follow-up assessment with color duplex ultrasound scan. J Vasc Surg 35:595–597

Parent NF, Meier GH, Godxiachvili V et al (2002) The incidence and natural history of type I and II endoleak. A 5 year follow-up assessment with color duplex ultrasound scan. J Vasc Surg 35:474–481

Park AE, McCarthy WJ, Pearce WH, Matsumura JS, Yao JST (1998) Carotid plaque morphology correlates with presenting symptomatology. J Vasc Surg 27:872–879

Park SH, Chung JW, Lee JW, Han MH, Park JH (2001) Carotid artery involvement in Takayasu's ateritis: evaluation of the activity by ultrasonography. J Ultrasound Med 20:371–378

Parks A (1961) Intraneural ganglion of the lateral popliteal nerve. J Bone Joint Surg 43B:784

Parmar J, Aslam M, Standfield N (2007) Pre-operative radial arterial diameter predicts early failure of arteriovenous fistula (AVF) for haemodialysis. Eur J Vasc Endovasc Surg 33:113–115

Parry DJ et al (2002) Type II endoleaks: predictable, preventable, and sometimes treatable? J Vasc Surg 36:105–110

Partsch H (1976) "A-sounds" or "S-sounds" for Doppler ultrasonic evaluation of pelvic vein thrombosis. Vasa 5:16–19

Partsch H (1996) Diagnose und Therapie der tiefen Beinvenenthrombose. Vasa 46(Suppl):5–53

Partsch H, Lofferer O (1972) Die Doppler-Detektoruntersuchung als Suchtest und Verlaufskontrolle von Bein-Beckenvenenthrombosen. Wien Klin Wochenschr 84:760–763

Partsch H, Mostbeck A (1979) Die Früherkennung der tiefen Unterschenkelvenenthrombophlebitis. Vasa 8:237–246

Partsch H, Oburger K, Mostbeck A et al (1992) Frequency of pulmonary embolism in ambulant patients with pelvic vein thrombosis: a prospective study. J Vasc Surg 16:715–722

Pascarella L, Al-Tuwaijri M, Bergan JJ, Mekenas LM (2005) Lower extremity superficial venous aneurysms. Ann Vasc Surg 19:69–73

Passman MA, Moneta GL, Nehler MR, Taylor LM et al (1995) Do normal early color-flow duplex surveillance examination results of infrainguinal vein grafts preclude the need for late graft revision? J Vasc Surg 22:476–484

Patel KR, Semel L, Oauss RH (1988) Extended reconstruction rate for limb salvage with intraoperative prereconstruction angiography. J Vasc Surg 7:531–537

Patel MR, Kuntz KM, Klufsa RA (1995) Preoperative assessment of the carotid bifurcation. Can magnetic resonance angiography and duplex ultrasonography replace contrast arteriography? Stroke 26:1753–1758

Patel SG, Colli DA, Wardlaw JM (2002) Outcome, observer reliability and patient preferences if CTA, MRA or Doppler ultrasound were used, individually or together, instead of digital subtraction angiography before carotid endarterectomy. J Neurol Neurosurg Psychiatry 73:21–28

Patel U, Khaw KK, Hughes NC (2003) Doppler ultrasound for detection of renal transplant artery stenosis - threshold peak systolic velocity needs to be higher in a low-risk or surveillance population. Clin Radiol 58:772–777

Patriquin H, LaFortune M, Burns PN, Dauzat M (1987) Duplex Doppler examination in portal hypertension: technique and anatomy. Am J Roentgenol 149:71–76

Patriquin HB, LaFortune M, Jéquier J-C et al (1992) Stenosis of the renal artery: assessment of slowed systole in the downstream circulation with Doppler sonography. Radiology 184:470–485

Paty PS, Kaufman JL, Koslow AR, Chang BB, Leather RP, Shah DM (1992) Adventitial cystic disease of the femoral vein: a case report and review of the literature. J Vasc Surg 15:214–217

Paulson WD, Moist L, Lok CE (2013) Vascular access surveillance: Case study of a false paradigm. Semin Dial 26:281–286

Pavela J, Ahanchi S, Steerman SN, Higgins JA, Panneton JM (2014) Grayscale median analysis of primary stenosis and restenosis after carotid endarterectomy. J Vasc Surg 59:978–982

Pedersen OM, Aslaksen A, Vik-Mo H, Bassoe AM (1991) Compression ultrasonography in hospitalized patients with suspected deep venous thrombosis. Arch Intern Med 151:2217–2220

Pedro LM, Pedro MM, Gonçalves I et al (2000) Computer-assisted carotid plaque analysis: characteristics of plaques associated with cerebrovascular symptoms and cerebral infarction. Eur J Vasc Endovasc Surg 19:118–123

Pedro LM, Fernandes e Fernandes J, Pedro MM (2002) Ultrasonographic risk score of carotid plaques. Eur J Vasc Endovasc Surg 24:492–498

Pennestri F, Loperfido SMP et al (1984) Assessment of tricuspid regurgitation by pulsed Doppler ultrasonography of the hepatic veins. J Cardiol 54:363–368

Perkins JM, Galland RB, Simmons MJ, Magee TR (2000) Carotid duplex imaging: variation and validation. Br J Surg 87:320–322

Perko MJ (2001) Duplex ultrasound for assessment of superior mesenteric artery blood flow. Eur J Vasc Endovasc Surg 21:106–117

Perko MJ, Just S, Schroeder TV (1997) Importance of diastolic velocities in the detection of celiac and mesenteric artery diesease by duplex ultrasound. Eur J Vasc Endovasc Surg 26:288–293

Perlin SJ (1992) Pulmonary embolism during compression US of the lower extremity. Radiology 184:165–166

Perrier A, Bounameaux H (2001) Cost-effective diagnosis of deep vein thrombosis and pulmonary embolism. Thromb Haemost 86: 475–487

Perrier A, Desmarais S, Miron MJ et al (1999) Noninvasive diagnosis of venous thromboembolism in outpatients. Lancet 353:190–195

Persson BG, Donner M, Peterson B, Eklof B, Wintzell K (1980) Aneurysm of the popliteal vein as a cause of pulmonary embolism. Acta Med Scand 208:407–410

Persson AV, Jones C, Zide R, Er J (1989) Use of the triplex scanner in diagnosis of deep venous thrombosis. Arch Surg 124:593

Peterson BG, Longo M, Kibbe MR, Matsumura JS, Blackburn D, Astleford P, Eskandari MK (2005) Duplex ultrasound remains a reliable test even after carotid stenting. Ann Vasc Surg 19:793–797

Petrick J (1996) Spektralanalyse von Ultraschall-Doppler-Signalen mit und ohne Ultraschallkontrastmittel an Modellen von Blutgefäßen. PhD Thesis, Berlin 1995. Köster, Berlin

Petrick J, Schlief R, Zomack M, Langholz J, Urbank A (1992) Pulsatiles Strömungsmodell mit elastischen Gefäßen für duplexsonographische Untersuchungen. Ultraschall Med 13:277–282

Petros JA, Andriole GL, Middleton WD, Picus DA (1991) Correlation of testicular color Doppler ultrasonography, physical examination and venography in the detection of left varicoceles in men with infertility. J Urol 145:785–788

Pezzullo JA, Perkins AB, Cronan JJ (1996) Symptomatic deep vein thrombosis: diagnosis with limited compression US. Radiology 198: 67–70

Pfeil W, Jacksch R, Kotzerke M, Störk T, Selbach J. Behandlung von Pseudoaneurysmen der Femoralarterie mit Thrombininjektion – Das deutsche Multicenter-Register. Cardioangiologisches Centrum Bethanien, Frankfurt/M (DE); St. Vincenzkrankenhaus Essen (DE); Hegau Klinikum; Singen (DE); Karl Olga Krankenhaus; Stuttgart (DE); Caritas Krankenhaus; Bad Mergentheim (DE)

Pfister K et al (2009) Detection and characterization of endoleaks following endovascular treatment of abdominal aortic aneurysms using Contrast Harmonic Imaging (CHI) with quantitative perfusion analysis (TCI) compared to CT angiography (CTA). Ultraschall Med. in press

Pfister K, Krammer S, Janotta M et al (2010) Welche Nachkontrolle ist bei endovaskulärer Versorgung von abdominellen Aortenaneurysmen empfehlenswert? Zentralbl Chir 135:409–415

Pietura R, Janczarek M, Zaluska W et al (2005) Colour Doppler ultrasound assessment of well-functioning mature arteriovenous fistulas for haemodialysis access. Eur J Radiol 55:113–119

Piovella F, Crippa L, Barone M, Viganò D'Angelo S, Serafini S, Galli L, Beltrametti C, D'Angelo A (2002) Normalization rates of compression ultrasonography in patients with a first episode of deep vein thrombosis of the lower limbs: association with recurrence and new thrombosis. Haematologica 87:515–522

Planken RN, Keuter XH, Kessels AG et al (2006) Forearm cephalic vein cross-sectional area changes at incremental congestion pressures: towards a standardized and reproducible vein mapping protocol. J Vasc Surg 44:353–358

Pleumeekers HJ, Hoes AW, Mulder PG et al (1998) Differences in observer variability of ultrasound measurements of the proximal and distal abdominal aorta. J Med Screen 5:104–108

Ploenes C, Strauss A (1999) Die Wertigkeit der Farbduplexsonographie in der Diagnose von Nierenarterienstenosen und -verschlüssen. Vasa 55:47

Podhaisky H, Hänsgen K, Seifert H, Taute BM (1996) Parameter und Einflußfaktoren der sonographischen Untersuchung des peripheren arteriellen Gefäßsystems. Herz/Kreisl 28:129–133

Polak JF (1992) Peripheral vascular sonography: a practical guide. Williams & Wilkins, Baltimore

Polak JF, Cutter SS, O'Leary DH (1988) Doppler color flow imaging of the calf veins. Description of method and preliminary results. Radiology 169(Suppl):318 (Abstr)

Polak JF, Culter S, O'Leary D (1989) Deep veins of the calf: assessment with color Doppler flow imaging. Radiology 171:481–485

Polak JF, Dobkin GR, O'Leary DH, Wang A-M, Cutler SS (1989) Internal carotid artery stenosis: accuracy and reproducibility of color-Doppler-assisted duplex imaging. Radiology 173:793–798

Polak JF, Donaldson MC, Dobkin GR et al (1990) Early detection of saphenous vein arterial bypass graft stenosis by color-assisted duplex sonography: a prospective study. AJR 154:857–861

Polak JF, Karmel MI, Mannick JA, O'Leary DH, Donaldson MC, Whittemore AD (1990) Determination of the extent of lower-extremity peripheral arterial disease with color-assistend duplex sonography: comparison with angiography. AJR 155:1085–1089

Polak JF, Magruder CD, Whittemore AD et al (1990) Pulsatile masses surrounding vascular prostheses: real-time US color flow imaging. Radiology 170:363–366

Polak JF, Mitchell MI, Mannick JA, O'Leary DH, Donaldson MC, Whittemore AD (1990) Determination of the extent of lower-extremity peripheral arterial disease with color-assisted duplex sonography. Am J Roentgenol 155:1085–1089

Polak KF, Karmel MI, Meyerowitz JA (1991) Accuracy of color Doppler flow mapping for evaluation of the severity of femoropopliteal arterial disease, a prospective study. J Vasc Interv Radiol 2: 471–476

Polak JF, Bajakian RL, O'Leary DH, Anderson MR, Donaldson MC, Jolesz FA (1992) Detection of internal carotid artery stenosis: comparison of MR angiography, color Doppler sonography, and arteriography. Radiology 182:35–40

Polak JF, O'Leary DH, Kronmal RA et al (1993) Sonographic evaluation of carotid artery atherosclerosis in elderly: relationship of disease severity to stroke and TIA. Radiology 188:363–370

Polak JF, Shemanski L, O'Leary DH, Lefkowitz D et al (1998) Hypoechoic plaque at US of the carotid artery: an independent risk factor for incident stroke in adults aged 65 years or older. Radiology 208: 649–654

Poli A, Tremoli E, Colombo A et al (1988) Ultrasonographic measurement of the common carotid arterial wall thickness in hypercholesterolemic patients. Atherosclerosis 70:253–261

Pomposelli FB Jr, Marcaccio EJ, Gibbons GW et al (1995) Dorsalis pedis arterial bypass: durable limb salvage for foot ischemia in patients with diabetes mellitus. J Vasc Surg 21:375–384

Porst H (1987) Erektile Impotenz. Enke, Stuttgart, pp S73–S77

Porter TR (1998) Transient response imaging. In: Bogdahn U, Becker G, Schlachetzki F (eds) Echosignalverstärker und transkranielle Farbduplex-Sonographie. Blackwell, Berlin Wien, pp 192–203

Postman CT, Bijlstra PJ, Rosenbusch G, Thien T (1996) Pattern recognition of loss of early systolic peak by Doppler ultrasound has a low sensitivity for the detection of renal artery stenosis. J Hum Hypertens 10:181–184

Prabhakaran S, Rundek T, Ramas R et al (2006) Carotid plaque surface irregularity predicts ischemic stroke: the Northern Manhattan Study. Stroke 37:2696–2701

Prandoni P (1993) Symptomatic deep vein thrombosis and the incidence of postthrombotic syndrome. Int Union of Angiology, Beaune, Oct. 6

Prandoni P, Kahn SR (2009) Post-thrombotic syndrome: prevalence, prognostication and need for progress. Br J Haematol 145:286–295

Prandoni P, Cogo A, Bernardi E, Villalta S et al (1993) A simple ultrasound approach for detection of recurrent proximal vein thrombosis. Circulation 88:1730–1735

Prandoni P, Polistena P, Bernardi E et al (1997) Upper-extremity deep vein thrombosis: risk factors, diagnosis and complications. Arch Intern Med 157:357–362

Prandoni P, Lensing AW, Prins MH et al (2002b) Residual venous thrombosis as a predictive factor for recurrent venous thromboembolism. Ann Intern Med 137:955–960

Prandoni P, Lensing AW, Bernardi E, Villalta S, Bagatella P, Girolami A (2002a) The diagnostic value of compression ultrasonography in patients with suspected recurrent deep vein thrombosis. Thromb Haemost 88:402–406

Prandoni P, Prins MH, Lensing AW et al. AESOPUS Investigators (2009) Residual thrombosis on ultrasonography to guide the duration of anticoagulation in patients with deep venous thrombosis: a randomized trial. Ann Intern Med 150:577–585

Pross C, Shortsleeve CM, Baker JD et al (2001) Carotid endarterectomy with normal findings from a completion study: is there need for early duplex scan? J Vasc Surg 33:963–967

Prountjos P, Bastounis E, Hadjinikolaou L, Felekuras E, Balas P (1991) Superficial venous thrombosis of the lower extremities co-existing with deep venous thrombosis. A phlebographic study on 57 cases. Int Angiol 10:63–65

Pursell R, Torrie P, Gibson M, Galland B (2004) Spontaneous and permanent resolution of cystic adventitial disease of the popliteal artery. J R Soc Med 97:77–78

Quam JP, King BF, James EM et al (1989) Duplex and color Doppler sonographic evaluation of vasculogenic impotence. AJR Am J Roentgenol 153:1141–1147

Quandalle P, Sandement A, Chambon JP, Wurtz A (1989) L'anévrisme des veines profondes des membres inférieurs. J Chir 126:586–590

Quéré I, Leizorovicz A, Galanaud JP et al (2012) Superficial venous thrombosis and compression ultrasound imaging. J Vasc Surg 56:1032–1038

Radermacher J, Chavan A, Bleck J et al (2000) Use of Doppler ultrasonography to predict the outcome of therapy for renal-artery stenosis. N Engl J Med 334:410–417

Radermacher J, Chavan A, Schäffer J et al (2000) Detection of significant renal artery stenosis with color Doppler sonography: combining extrarenal and intrarenal approaches to minimize technical failure. Clin Nephrol 53:333–343

Radermacher J, Mengel M, Ellis S et al (2003) The renal arterial resistance index and renal allograft survival. N Engl J Med 349:115–124

Ragavendra BN, St H, Hilton S, Subramanyam BR, Rosen RJ, Lam SL (1986) Deep venous thrombosis: detection by probe compression of veins. J Ultrasound Med 5:89–95

Raghavendra BN, Rosen J, Lam S, Riles T, Horii SC (1984) Deep venous thrombosis. Detection by high-resolution real-time ultrasonography. Radiology 152:789

Rai S, Davies RS, Vohra RK (2008) Failure of endovascular stenting for popliteal cystic disease. Ann Vasc Surg 23:410.el–5

Rajfer J, Rosciszweski A, Mehringer M (1988) Prevalence of corporeal venous leakage in impotent men. J Urol 140:69

Ralls PW, Jensen MC, Lee KP, Mayekawa DS, Johnson MB, Halls JM (1990) Color Doppler sonography in acute epididymitis and orchitis. J Clin Ultrasound 18:383–386

Ranke C, Trappe JH (1997) Blood flow velocity measurements for carotid stenosis estimation: interobserver variation and interequipment variability. Vasa 26:210–214

Ranke C, Hendrickx PH, Brasel F et al (1990) Duplexsonographie: Genauigkeit, Reproduzierbarkeit und Fehlermöglichkeiten. Dtsch Med Wochenschr 115:528–533

Ranke C, Creutzig A, Alexander K (1992) Duplex scanning of the peripheral arteries: correlation of the peak velocity ratio with angiographic diameter reduction. Ultrasound Med Biol 18:433–440

Ranke C, Rieder M, Creutzig A, Alexander K (1995) A nomogram of duplex ultrasound quantification of peripheral arterial stenoses. Studies of the cardiovascular model and in angiography patients. Med Klin(Munich) 90:72–77

Ranke C, Creutzig A, Becker H, Trappe HJ (1999) Standardization of carotid ultrasound: a hemodynamic method to normalize for interindividual and interequipment variability. Stroke 30:402–406

Rao AB, Koeller KK, Adair CF (1999) Paragangliomas of the head and neck: Radiologic-pathologic correlation. Radiographics 19: 1605–1632

Ratiff DA, Gallagher PJ, Hames TK et al (1985) Characterization of carotid artery disease: comparison of duplex scanning with histology. Ultrasound Med Biol 11:835–840

Redekop G, Marotta T, Weill A (2001) Treatment of traumatic aneurysms and arteriovenous fistulas of the skull base by using endovascular stents. J Neurosurg 95:412–419

Redgrave JN, Gallagher P, Lovett JK (2008) Critical cap thickness and rupture in symptomatic carotid plaques; the Oxford Plaque Study. Stroke 39:1722–1729

Reid JA, Wolsley C, Lau LL et al (2005) The effect of pravastatin on intima media thickness of the carotid artery in patients with nomal cholesterol. Eur J Vasc Endovasc Surg 30:464–468

Reilly LM (1990) Carotid intraplaque hemorrhage: noninvasive detection and clinical significance. In: Bernstein EF (ed) Noninvasive diagnostic techniques in vascular disease. Mosby, St Louis, pp 99–107

Reilly LM (1993) Importance of carotid plaque morphology. In: Bernstein EF (ed) Vascular diagnosis, 4th edn. Mosby Year Book, St. Louis, pp 333–340

Reilly LM, Lusby RJ, Hughes L et al (1983) Carotid plaque histology using real-time ultrasonography: clinical and therapeutic implications. Am J Surg 146:188–193

Reiter M, Horvat R, Puchner S et al (2007) Plaque imaging of the internal carotid artery – correlation of B-flow imaging with histopathology. AJNR Am J Neuroradiol 28:122–126

Reiter M, Effenberg I, Sabeti S (2008) Increasing carotid plaque echolucency is predictive of cardiovascular events in high-risk patients. Radiology 248:1050–1055

Reix T, Sevestre H, Sevestre-Petri M et al (1998) Primary malignant tumors of the venous system in the lower extremities. Ann Vasc Surg 12:589–596

Reuther GR, Wanjura D, Bauer H (1989) Acute renal vein thrombosis in renal allografts: detection with duplex Doppler US. Radiology 170:557–558

Rich NM (1982) Popliteal entrapment and adventitial cystic disease. Surg Clin North Am 62:449–465

Rich NM, Hughes CW (1967) Popliteal artery and vein entrapment. Am J Surg 113:696–698

Rich NM, Collins GJ, Mc Donald PT, Kozloff L, Clagett GP, Collins JT (1979) Popliteal vascular entrapment. Arch Surg 114:1377–1384

Richter G, Böhm S, Görg DH, Schwerk WB (1992) Verlaufsbeobachtungen zur Echogenität venöser Gerinnungsthromben. Ultraschall Klin Prax 7:69–73

Richtlinien für die Durchführung Doppler- und duplexsonographischer Untersuchungen peripherer Arterien und Venen, extrakranieller hirnversorgender Halsarterien und intrakranieller Arterien des Arbeitskreises Gefäßdiagnostik der DEGUM (1991) Mitteil Angiol 1:10–17

Ricotta JJ (1990) Plaque characterization by B-mode scan. Surg Clin North Am 70:191–199

Rieger H (1985) Durchblutungsstörungen. Adam Pharma Verlag GmbH, Essen

Rieger H, Schoop W (eds) (1998) Klinische Angiologie. Springer, Berlin/Heidelberg/New York, pp 627–666

Riehl J, Clasen W, Schmidt H, Kierdorf H, Sieberth HG (1989) Altersabhängige Veränderungen der renalen Hämodynamik: Untersuchungen mittels Duplex-Sonographie. Ultraschall Klin Prax 1(Suppl):129

Righini M, Paris S, Le Gal G, Laroche JP, Perrier A, Bounameaux H (2006) Clinical relevance of distal deep vein thrombosis. Review of literature data. Thromb Haemost 95:56–64

Rigsby C, Burns PN, Weltin GG, Chen B, Bia M, Taylor KJW (1987) Doppler signal quantitation in renal allografts: comparison in normal and rejecting transplants with pathologic correlation. Radiology 162:39–42

Ripolles T, Aliaga R, Morote V et al (2001) Utility of intrarenal Doppler ultrasound in the diagnosis of renal artery stenosis. Eur J Radiol 40:54–63

Riviere J, Soury P, Poli P, Peillon C, Watelet J, Testart J (1994) Importance of complementary peroperative examinations in the treatment of adventitial cystic degeneration of the popliteal artery. J Mal Vasc 19:251–252

Robbin ML, Oser RF, Allon M et al (1998) Hemodialysis access graft stenosis: US detection. Radiology 208:655–661

Robbin ML, Chamberlain NE, Lockhart ME et al (2002) Hemodialysis arteriovenous fistula maturity: US evaluation. Radiology 225:59–64

Robinson WP, Belkin M (2009) Acute limb ischemia due to popliteal artery aneurysm: a continuing surgical challenge. Semin Vasc Surg 22:17–24

Rocha-Singh K, Jaff MR, Lynne Kelly E (2008) RENAISSANCE Trial Investigators. Renal artery stenting with noninvasive duplex ultrasound follow-up: 3-year results from the RENAISSANCE renal stent trial. Catheter Cardiovasc Interv 72:853–862

Rofsky NM, Adelman MA (2000) MR angiography in the evaluation of atherosclerotic peripheral vascular disease. Radiology 214:325–338

Rollins DL, Semrow CM, Friedell ML, Buchbinder D (1987) Use of ultrasonic venography in the evaluation of venous valve function. Am J Surg 154:189–191

Roobottom CA, Dubbins PA (1995) Significant disease of the celiac and superior mesenteric arteries in asymptomatic patients: predictive value of Doppler sonography. AJR 161:985–988

Roobottorn CA, Hunter JD, Weston MJ, Dubbins PA (1995) Hepatic venous Doppler waveforms: changes in pregnancies. J Clin Ultrasound 23:477–482

Rooijens PP, TordoirJH ST et al (2004) Radiocephalic wrist arteriovenous fistula for hemodialysis: meta-analysis indicates a high primary failure rate. Eur J Vasc Endovasc Surg 28:583–589

Rose SC, Zwiebel WJ, Nelson BD et al (1990) Symptomatic lower extremity deep venous thrombosis: accuracy, limitations and role of color duplex flow imaging in diagnosis. Radiology 175:639–644

Rose SC, Zwiebel WJ, Miller FJ (1994) Distribution of acute lower extremity deep venous thrombosis in symptomatic and asymptomatic patients: imaging implications. J Ultrasound Med 13:243–250

Rosen MP, Sheiman RG, Weintraub J, McArdle C (1996) Compression sonography in patients with indeterminate or low-probability lung scans: lack of usefulness in the absence of both symptoms of deep vein thrombosis and thromboembolic risk factor. AJR 166:285–289

Rosfors S, Eriksson M, Hoglund N, Johansson G (1993) Duplex ultrasound in patients with suspected aorto-iliac occlusive disease. Eur J Vasc Surg 7:513–517

Rosner NM, Doris PE (1988) Diagnosis of femoropopliteal venous thrombosis: comparison of duplex sonography and plethysmography. Am J Roentgenol 150:623–627

Ross B, Sherriff L, Walton L (1984) Diagnosis of deep-vein thrombosis: comparison of clinical evaluation, ultrasound, plathysmography, and venoscan with X-ray venogram. Lancet 2:716–719

Ross GJ, Violi L, Barber LW et al (1988) Popliteal venous aneurysm. Radiology 168:721–722

Rosvall M, Janzon L, Berglund G, Engstrom G, Hedblad B (2005) Incident coronary events and case fatality in relation to common carotid intima-media thickness. J Intern Med 257:430–437

Roth SM, Back MR, Bandyk DF et al (1999) A rational algorithm for duplex scan surveillance after carotid endarterectomy. J Vasc Surg 31:838–839

Rothwell PM (2003) For severe carotid stenosis found on ultrasound, further arterial evaluation prior to carotid endarterectomy is unnecessary: the argument against. Stroke 34:1817–1819

Rothwell PM, Warlow CP (1999) Prediction of benefit from carotid endarterectomy in individual patients: a risk-modelling study. European Carotid Surgery Trialists' Collaborative Group. Lancet 353:2105–2110

Rothwell PM, Gibson RJ, Slattery J et al (1994) Equivalence of measurements of carotid stenosis: a comparison of three methods on 1001 angiograms. Stroke 25:2435–2439

Rothwell PM, Gibson R, Warlow CP (2000) Interrelation between plaque surface morphology and degree of stenosis on carotid angiograms and the risk of ischemic stroke in patients with symptomatic carotid stenosis. On behalf of the European Carotid Surgery Trialists Collaborative Group. Stroke 31:615–621

Rothwell PM, Warlow CP, on behalf of the European Carotid surgery Trialists' Collaborative Group (2000) Low risk of ischemic stroke in patients with reduced internal carotid artery lumen diameter distal to severe symptomatic carotid stenosis: cerebral protection due to low poststenotic flow? Stroke 31:622–630

Rotter W (1981) Gefäßveränderungen bei frischer und älterer Thrombose. In: Vinazzer H (ed) Thrombose und Embolie. Anästhesie Intensivmed 134: 171–177

Rountas C, Vlychou M, Vassiou K (2007) Imaging modalities for renal artery stenosis in suspected renovascular hypertension: prospective intraindividual comparison of color Doppler US, CT angiography, GD-enhanced MR angiography and digital subtraction angiography. Ren Fall 29:295–302

Roy-Chaudhury P, Kelly BS, Miller MA et al (2001) Venous neointimal hyperplasia in polytetraflouroethylene dialysis grafts. Kidney Int 59:2325–2334

Rubin JM, Bude RO, Carson PL et al (1994) Power Doppler US: a potentially useful alternative to mean frequency-based color Doppler US. Radiology 190:853–856

Rubin BG, Beak BI, Reilly JM (1995) Fusiform aneurysms of the popliteal vein. In: The American venous forum 7th annual meeting, 1995 Feb. 23–25, Fort Lauderdale. Abstract Book p 39

Rutherford RB, Flanigan DP, Gupta SK, Johnston KW, Karmody A, Whittemore AD (1986) Suggested standards for reports dealing with lower extremity ischemia. J Vasc Surg 4:80–94

Rutherford RB, Baker D, Ernst C et al (1997) Recommended standards for reports dealing with lower extremity ischaemia: revised version. J Vasc Surg 26:517–538

Saal JG, Dürk H (1994) Rationale Labordiagnostik in klinischer Immunologie und Rheumatologie. Internist 35:633–639

Saba L, Caddeo G, Sanfilippo R (2007) CT and ultrasound in the study of ulcerated carotid plaque compared with surgical results: potentialities and advantages of multidetector row CT angiography. AJNR Am J Neuroradiol 28:1061–1066

Sabba C, Ferraioli G, Genecin P et al (1991) Evaluation of postprandial hyperemia in superior mesenteric artery and portal vein in healthy and cirrhotic humans: an operator-blind echo-Doppler study. Hepatology 13:114–118

Sacks D, Robinson ML, Marinelli DL, Perlmutter GS (1990) Evaluation of the peripheral arteries with duplex after angioplasty. Radiology 176:39–44

Safian RD, Textor SC (2001) Renal-artery stenosis. N Engl J Med 344: 431–442

Sakaguchi M, Kitagawa K, Nagai Y et al (2003) Equivalence of plaque score and intima-media thickness of carotid ultrasonography for predicting severe coronary artery lesion. Ultrasound Med Biol 29:367–371

Sandler DA, Duncan JS, Ward P et al (1984) Diagnosis of deep veinthrombosis. Comparison of clinical evaluation, ultrasound, plethysmography and venoscan with x-ray venogram. Lancet 2:716

Sandok BA (1983) Fibromuscular dysplasia of the internal carotid artery. Neurol Clin 1:17–26

Sanford RM, Bown MJ, Fishwick G et al (2006) Duplex ultrasound scanning is reliable in the detection of endoleak following endovascular aneurysm repair. Eur J Vasc Encovasc Surg 32:537–541

Sarap MD, Wheeler WE (1988) Venous aneurysms. J Vasc Surg 8:182–183

Sarkar R, Ro KM, Obrand DI, Ahn SS (1998) Lower extremity vascular reconstruction and endovascular surgery without preoperative angiography. Am J Surg 176:203–207

Sarlon G, Lapierre F, Sarlon E, Bartoli MA, Magnan PE, Branchereau A (2009) Endovascular aneurysm repair follow-up by unenhanced and contrast-enhanced duplex ultrasound. J Mal Vasc 34:121–132

Sato DT et al (1998) Endoleak after aortic stent graft repair: diagnosis by color duplex ultrasound scan versus computed tomography scan. J Vasc Surg 28:657–663

Scali ST, Chang CK, Raghinaru D et al (2013) Prediction of graft patency and mortality after distal revascularization and interval ligation for hemodialysis access-related hand ischemia. J Vasc Surg 57:451–458

Scarpato R, Gembarowicz R, Farber S et al (1981) Intraoperative prereconstruction arteriography. Arch Surg 116:1053–1055

Schäberle W (1992) Diagnosis of venous aneurysm by ultrasound examination. In: Eurodop 92. Br Med Ultrasound Soc, London, p 157 (Abstr)

Schäberle W (1993) Ultraschall in der Venendiagnostik. Springer, Heidelberg

Schäberle W (2011) Ultrasonography in Vascular Diagnosis. Springer Verlag, Heidelberg

Schäberle W (2014) Technische Diagnostik. In: Nüllen et al. Venöse Thrombembolien. Springer Verlag, Heidelberg

Schäberle W, Eisele R (1990) Duplexsonographische Kriterien eines distalen Mesenterialarterienverschlusses. Ultraschall Klin Prax Suppl 5:197

Schäberle W, Eisele R (1991) Das sonographische Bild einer zystischen Adventitiadegeneration. Vasa 33:207–208

Schäberle W, Eisele R (1991) Duplexsonographie versus Phlebographie in der Diagnostik der tiefen Beinvenenthrombose. Phlebologie 5:45

Schäberle W, Eisele R (1992) Duplexsonographische Diagnostik der Fossa poplitea zur Differenzierung seltener arterieller und venöser Gefäßerkrankungen. Ultraschall. Klin Prax 7:148

Schäberle W, Eisele R (1996) Die sonographische Diagnostik, Verlaufsform und Therapie der cystischen Adventitiadegeneration. Ultraschall Med 17:131–137

Schäberle W, Eisele R (1996) Ultrasound diagnosis, follow-up and therapy of cystic degeneration of the adventitia. 2 case reports and review of the literature. Ultraschall Med 17:131–137

Schäberle W, Eisele R (2001) Das venöse Aneurysma tiefer Beinvenen – Wertigkeit der Duplexsonographie in Operationsindikation und Therapieplanung. Ultraschall Med 22(Suppl):60–61

Schäberle W, Leyerer L (2013) Sonographischer Stenosegrad ist nicht gleich sonographischer Stenosegrad ist nicht gleich angiographischer Stenosegrad. Messmethodische Aspekte und Fehlerquelle der hämodynamischen und der morphologischen Graduierung femoropoplitealer Stenosen. Gefässchirurgie 18: 292–297

Schäberle W, Leyerer L (2013) Venenaneurysma – Therapieentscheidung duch sonographische Diagnostik der Hämodynamik. Gefässchirurgie 18:659–664

Schäberle W, Leyerer L (2014) Structured, time-efficient and therapy-oriented ultrasonography diagnostics for dialysis shunt problems. Gefässchirurgie 19:471–480

Schäberle W, Neuerburg Heusler D (1989) Wertigkeit der Duplexsonographie in der Diagnostik der Nierenarterienstenose. Klin Wochenschr 67(Suppl XVI):177

Schäberle W, Seitz K (1988) Meßmethodische Probleme der Durchmesser- und Querschnittsbestimmung für die duplexsonographische Stromzeitvolumenmesseung. Ultraschall Klin Prax Suppl 1:68

Schäberle W, Seitz K (1991) Duplexsonographische Blutflußmessung in der Arteria mesenterica superior. Ultraschall Med 12:277–282

Schäberle W, Bärlin E, Seitz K (1988) Meßmethodische Probleme zur Durchmesser- bzw. Querschnittsbestimmung für die duplexsonographische Stromzeitvolumenmessung. Ultraschall Klin Prax Suppl 1: 68 (Abstr)

Schäberle W, Schock D, Eisele R (1992) Der isolierte Poplitealarterienverschluß: Wertigkeit der Duplexsonographie in Differential-diagnose und Therapieplanung. Vasa 35(Suppl):69–70

Schäberle W, Strauss A, Neuerburg-Heusler D, Roth FJ (1992) Wertigkeit der Duplexsonographie in der Diagnostik der Nierenarterienstenose und ihre Eignung in der Verlaufskontrolle nach Angioplastie (PTA). Ultraschall Med 13:271–276

Schäberle W, Ulrich C, Meyer H, Eisele R (1995) Großes Aneurysma spurium in der A. poplitea nach arthroskopischer Meniskektomie. Arthroskopie 8:41–43

Schäberle W, Leyerer L, Pfister K (2012) Sportabitur trotz Gefäßverschluss. Gefässchirurgie 17:775–778

Schäberle W, Leyerer L, Kabiri R, Richter P (2013) Zystische Adventitiadegeneration. Sonographische Diagnostik und Therapieoptionen. Gefässchirurgie 18:572–577

Schäberle W, Rupp-Heim G, Leyerer L et al (2013) Thrombuszapfen oder Venenwandtumor. Differenzialdiagnose in der Bildgebung und Literaturübersicht epitheloides Hämangioendotheliom. Gefässchirurgie 18:216–221

Schäberle W, Rupp-Heim G, Leyerer L (2013) Duplexsonographische Diagnostik von Beckenarterienstenosen Stenosegraduierung und zeiteffizientes Vorgehen durch Spektralanalyse. Gefässchirurgie 18:44–51

Schäberle W, Rupp-Heim G, Leyerer L (2013) Persistierende primitive Hypoglossusarterie (PPHA). Gut kollateralisierter A.-carotis-interna-Verschluss. Gefässchirurgie 18:131–138

Schäberle W, Rupp-Heim G, Leyerer L (2013) Sonographische Verlaufskontrolle nach Karotisstentimplantation (CAS): Graduierung von Rezidivstenosen und Stentdislokation. Gefässchirurgie 18:394–399

Schäberle W, Leyerer L, Giebeler C et al (2014) Color duplex sonography in chronic and acute ischemia of the mesenteric artery. Is color duplex sonography relevant for diagnostics? Gefässchirurgie 19:247–256

Schäberle W, Rupp-Heim G, Leyerer L (2014) Is color duplex ultrasonography still important compared to contrast-enhanced sonography in endoleak diagnostics after EVAR. Gefässchirurgie 19:147–152

Schäberle W, Leyerer L, Schierling W, Pfister K (2015) Ultrasound diagnostics of the abdominal aorta. Gefässchirurgie 20:22–27

Schäberle W, Leyerer L, Schierling W, Pfister K (2015) Ultrasound diagnostic of renal artery stenosis. Stenosis criteria, CEUS and recurrent in-stent stenosis. Gefässchirurgie 20:102–111

Scharnke W, Claußnitzer R, Wild K, Schuler A (1995) Aneurysma der V. poplitea als Ursache von Lungenembolien. Diagnose mittels FDS. Ultraschall Med 16:114

Schatz IJ, Fine G (1962) Venous aneurysms. N Engl J Med 266:1310–1312

Schellong S (1993) Vaskulitiden. In: Alexander K (Hrsg) Gefäßkrankheiten. Urban & Schwarzenberg, München/Wien/Baltimore

Schellong MS, Schwarz T, Halbritter K et al (2003) Complete compression ultrasonography of the leg veins as a single test for the diagnosis of deep vein thrombosis. Thromb Haemost 89:228–234

Schenk EA, Bond MG, Aretz TH et al (1988) Multicenter validation study of real-time ultrasonography, arteriography, and pathology: pathologic evaluation of carotid endarterectomy specimens. Stroke 19:289–296

Schiff MJ, Feinberg W, Naidisch JB (1987) Noninvasive venous examinations as a screening test for pulmonary embolism. Arch Intern Med 147:505

Schild H, Berg S, Weber W, Schmied W, Steegmuller KW (1992) The venous aneurysm. Aktuelle Radiol 2:75–80

Schindler JM, Kaiser M, Gerber A, Vuilliomenet A, Popovic A, Bertel O (1990) Colour coded duplex sonography in suspected deep vein thrombosis of the leg. BMJ 301:1369–1370

Schlager O, Francesconi M, Haumer M et al (2007) Duplex sonography versus angiography for assessment of femoropopliteal arterial disease in a "real-world" setting. J Endovasc Ther 14:452–459

Schmidberger H, Hackl A, Ludwig G (1979) Aneurysma der Vena poplitea. Fortschr Röntgenstr 131:553–554

Schmidt WA (2006) Takayasu and temporal arteritis. Front Neurol Neurosci 21:96–104

Schmidt WA, Blockmans D (2005) Use of ultrasonography and positron emission tomography in the diagnosis and assessment of large-vessel vasculitis. Curr Opin Rheumatol 17:9–15

Schmidt WA, Gromnica-Ihle E (2002) Incidence of temporal arteritis in patients with polymyalgia rheumatica: a prospective study using color Doppler ultrasonography of the temporal arteries. Rheumatology (Oxford) 41:46–52

Schmidt JA, Bierbrauer A, Wichert P (1993) Vaskulitiden großer Arterien. Internist 34:615–621

Schmidt WA, Kraft HE, Vorpahl K, Völker L, Gromnica-Ihle EJ (1997) Color duplex ultrasonography in the diagnosis of temporal arteritis. N Engl J Med 337:1336–1342

Schmidt W, Seifert A, Gromnica-Ihle E, Krause A, Natusch A (2008) Ultrasound of proximal upper extremity arteries to increase the diagnostic yield in large-vessel giant cell arteritis. Rheumatology 47:96–101

Schmieder GC, Stout CL, Stokes GK, Parent FN, Panneton JM (2009) Endoleak after endovascular aneurysm repair: duplex ultrasound imaging is better than computed tomography at determining the need for intervention. J Vasc Surg 50:1012–1018

Schminke U, Motsch L, Hilker L, Kessler C (2000) Three-dimensional ultrasound observation of carotid artery plaque ulceration. Stroke 31:1651–1655

Schmitt HE (1974) Möglichkeiten und Grenzen der antegraden Phlebographie. Vasa 3:440–445

Schmitt HE (1977) Aszendierende Phlebographie bei tiefer Beinvenenthrombose. Huber, Bern

Schneider PA, Ogawa DY (1998) Is routine preoperative aortoiliac arteriography necessary in the treatment of lower extremity ischemia? J Vasc Surg 28:28–36

Schneider JR, Walsh DB, McDaniel MD, Zwolak RM, Besso SR, Cronenwett JL (1993) Pedal bypass versus tibial bypass with autogenous vein: a comparison of outcome and hemodynamic results. J Vasc Surg 17:1029–1038

Schneider PA, Ogawa DY, Rush MP (1999) Lower extremity revascularization without contrast arteriography: a prospective study of operation based upon duplex mapping. Cardiovasc Surg 7:699–703

Schöllhorn J (1985) Cystic adventitial degeneration as a cause of dynamic stenosis of the popliteal artery: a case report. Angiology 36:809–814

Scholz H (1998) Der adäquate Gefäßzugang für die Hämodialyse. Bard, Impra, München

Schönhofer B, Bechthold H, Renner R, Bundschu HD (1991) Asymptomatische Lungenembolie bei Varikophlebitis der V. saphena magna: Sonographische Dokumentation von Wachstum und Ablösung eines Appositionsthrombus. Phlebologie 20:48

Schönhofer B, Bechthold H, Renner R et al (1992) Sonographische Befunde bei Varikophlebitis der Vena saphena magna. Dtsch Med Wochenschr 117:51–55

Schönhofer B, Bundschu HD, Wolf K, Grehn S (1992) Farbkodierte Duplexsonographie im Vergleich zur Phlebographie bei tiefer Bein- und Beckenvenenthrombose. Med Klin 87:172–178

Schoop W (1988) Praktische Angiologie. Thieme, Stuttgart/New York, p 127

Schopohl J, Haen E, Ullrich T, Gärtner R (2000) Sildenafil (Viagra). Dt Ärztebl 97: A-311–A-315

Schraverus P, Dulieu J, Milleux P, Coulier B (1997) Cystic adventitial disease of the popliteal vein: report of a case. Acta Chir Belg 97:90–92

Schröder JO, Euler HH (1993) Systemischer Lupus erythematodes. Internist 34:351–361

Schröder A, Peters A, Riepe G et al (2001) Vascular tumors simulating occlusive disease. Vasa 30:62–66

Schroeder WB, Bealer JF (1992) Venous duplex ultrasonography causing acute pulmonary embolism: a brief report. J Vasc Surg 15: 1082–1083

Schuler A, Wild K, Hofstätter F, Claussnitzer R, Blank W, Braun B (1993) Seltene Aneurysmalokalisationen – Farbdopplersonographische (FDS) Diagnostik. Ultraschall. Klin Prax 8:201

Schuler A, Claußnitzer R, Dinkelacker S, Blank B, Braun B (1995) Farbdopplersonographie bei ascendierenden Thrombophlebitiden der unteren Extremität. Ultraschall Med 16:76

Schulte-Altedorneburg G, Droste DW, Haas N et al (2000) Preoperative B-mode ultrasound plaque appearance compared with carotid endarterectomy specimen histology. Acta Neurol Scand 101:188–194

Schürmann R, Balzer TH, Schlief R (1992) Diagnostisches Potenzial von Ultraschall-Kontrastmitteln in der Gefäßdiagnostik. Ultraschall Med 13:234–238

Schwartz RA, Kerns DB, Mitchell DG (1991) Color Doppler ultrasound imaging in iatrogenic arterial injuries. Am J Surg 162:4–8

Schwarz A, Gwinner W, Hiss M et al (2005) Safety and adequacy of renal transplant protocol biopsies. Am J Transplant 5:1992–1996

Schweizer J, Oehmichen F, Brandt HG, Altman E (1993) Farbkodierte Duplexsonographie und kontrastmittelverstärkte Duplexsonographie bei tiefer Beinvenenthrombose. Vasa 22:22–25

Schwerk WB, Restrepo IK, Stellwaag M et al (1994) Renal artery stenosis: grading with image-directed Doppler US. Evaluation of renal resistive index. Radiology 190:785–790

Scoble JE (1996) The epidemiology and clinical manifestations of atherosclerotic renal disease. In: Novick A, Scoble J, Hamilton G (eds) Renal vascular disease. WB Saunders, London/Philadelphia/Toronto, pp 303–314

Scott RA, Wilson NM, Ashton HA, Kay DN (1995) Influence of screening on the incidence of ruptured abdominal aortic aneurysm: 5-year results of a randomized controlled study. Br J Surg 82:1066–1070

Sebatai MM, Tegos TJ, Nicolaides AN (2000) Hemispheric symptoms and carotid plaque echomorphology. J Vasc Surg 31:39–49

Sebenik M, Ricci A, DiPasquale B et al (2005) Undifferentiated intimal sarcoma of large systemic blood vessels. Am J Surg Pathol 29: 1184–1192

Seidel G, Cangür H, Meyer-Wiethe K et al (2006) On the ability of ultrasound parametric perfusion imaging to predict the area of infarction in acute ischemic stroke. Ultraschall Med 27:543–548

Seidl H, Tuerck J, Schepp W, Schneider R (2010) Splanchnic arterial blood flow is significantly influenced by breathing – assessment by duplex-Doppler ultrasound. Ultrasound in Med. Biol 36:1677–1681

Seino Y, Fujimori H, Shimai S et al (1994) Popliteal venous aneurysm with pulmonary embolism. Intern Med 33:779–782

Seitz K, Kubale R (1988) Duplexsonographie der abdominellen und retroperitonealen Gefäße. Weinheim, VCH

Sensier Y, Hartshorne T, Thrush A et al (1996) The effect of adjacent segment disease on the accuracy of colour duplex scanning for the diagnosis of lower limb arterial disease. Eur J Vasc Endovasc Surg 12:238–242

Sensier Y, Bell PR, London NJ (1998) The ability of qualitative assessment of the common femoral Doppler waveform to screen for significant aortoiliac disease. Eur J Vasc Endovasc Surg 15:357–364

Sensier Y, Fishwick G, Owen R, Pemberton M, Bell PR, London NJ (1998) A comparison between color duplex ultrasonography and arteriography for imaging infrapopliteal lesions. Eur J Vasc Endovasc Surg 15:44–50

Sensier Y, Thrust A, Loftus I et al (2000) A comparison of colour duplex ultrasonography, papaverin testing and common femoral Doppler waveform analysis for assessment of the aortoiliac arteries. Eur J Vasc Endovasc Surg 20:29–35

Sessa C, Nicolini P, Perrin M et al (2000) Management of symptomatic and asymptomatic popliteal venous aneurysm: a retrospective analysis of 25 patients and review of the literature. J Vasc Surg 32:902–912

Setacci F, Sirignano P, de Donato G, Chisci E, Palasciano G, Setacci C (2008) Adventitial cystic disease of the popliteal artery: experience of a single vascular and endovascular center. J Cardiovasc Surg 49:235–239

Sevestre MA, Labarere J, Casez P et al (2009) Accuracy of complete compression ultrasound in ruling out suspected deep venous thrombosis in the ambulatory setting. A prospective cohort study. Thromb Haemost 102:166–172

Shaalan WE, French-Sherry E, Castilla M, Lozanski L, Bassiouny HS (2003) Reliability of common femoral artery hemodynamics in assessing the severity of aortoiliac inflow disease. J Vasc Surg 37:960–969

Shah F, Balan P, Weinberg M et al (2007) Contrast-enhanced ultrasound imaging of atherosclerotic carotid plaque neovascularization: a new surrogate marker of atherosclerosis? Vasc Med 12:291–297

Shalhoub J, Monaco C, Owen DR (2011) Late-phase contrast-enhanced ultrasound reflects biological features of instability in human carotid atherosclerosis. Stroke 42:3634–3636

Shawn H, Fleming MD, Ross P et al (2010) Accuracy of duplex sonography scans after renal artery stenting. J Vasc Surg 52:953–958

Sheiman RG, McArdle CR (1995) Bilateral lower extremity US in the patient with unilateral symptoms of deep venous thrombosis: assessment of need. Radiology 194:171–173

Sheiman RG, McArdle CR (1999) Clinically suspected pulmonary embolism: use of bilateral lower extremity US as the initial examination – a prospective study. Radiology 212:75–78

Sheiman RG, Weintraub JL, McArdle CR (1995) Bilateral lower extremity US in the patient with bilateral symptoms of deep venous thrombosis: assessment of need. Radiology 196:379–381

Shetty AN, Bis KG, Kirsch M (2000) Contrast-enhanced breath-hold three-dimensional magnetic resonance angiography in the evaluation of renal arteries: optimization of technique and pitfalls. J Magn Reson Imaging 12:912–923

Shrikhande GV, Graham AR, Aparajita R et al (2011) Determining criteria for predicting stenosis with ultrasound duplex after endovascular intervention in infrainguinal lesions. Ann Vasc Surg 25:454–460

Sidhu PS, Allan PL, Cattin F et al (2006) Diagnostic efficacy of SonoVue, a second generation contrast agent, in the assessment of extracranial carotid or peripheral arteries using colour and spectral Doppler ultrasound: a multicentre study. Br J Radiol 79:44–51

Sieunarine K, Lawrence-Brown MM, Kelsey P (1991) Adventitial cystic disease of the popliteal artery: early recurrence after CT guided percutaneous aspiration. J Cardiovasc Surg 32:702–704

Silva MB Jr, Hobson RW, Pappas PJ et al (1998) A strategy for increasing use of autogenous hemodialysis access procedures: impact of preoperative noninvasive evaluation. J Vasc Surg 27:302–307

Silverstein MD, Heit JA, Mohr DN, Petterson TM, O'Fallon WM, Melton LJ (1998) Trends in the incidence of deep vein thrombosis and pulmonary embolism. Arch Intern Med 158:585–593

Silvestri M, Villain P, Boursier JL, Elias A (1987) L'anévrisme veineux poplité: une cause rare d'embolie pulmonaire. Presse Méd 16:2127

Singh K, Jacobsen BK, Solberg S, Kumar S, Arnesen E (2004) The difference between ultrasound and computed tomography (CT) measurements of aortic diameter increases with aortic diameter: analysis of axial images of abdominal aortic and common iliac artery diameter in normal and aneurismal aortas. The Tromsø Study, 1994-1995. Eur J Vasc Endovasc Surg 28:158–167

Siragusa S, Malato A, Anastasio R et al (2008) Residual vein thrombosis to establish duration of anticoagulation after a first episode of deep vein thrombosis: the Duration of Anticoagulation based on Compression Ultrasonography (DACUS) study. Blood 112:511–515

Siragusa S, Malato A, Saccullo G, Iorio A, Di Ianni M, Caracciolo C, Coco LL, Raso S, Santoro M, Guarneri FP, Tuttolomondo A, Pinto A, Pepe I, Casuccio A, Abbadessa V, Licata G, Battista Rini G, Mariani G, Di Fede G (2011) Residual vein thrombosis for assessing duration of anticoagulation after unprovoked deep vein trhombosis of the lower limbs: the extended DACUS study. Am J Hematol 86:914–917

Siringo S, Bolondi L, Gaiani S et al (1994) The relationship of endoscopy, portal Doppler US flowmetry, and clinical and biochemical tests in cirrhosis. J Hepatol 20:11

Sitzer M, Müller W, Rademacher J (1990) Color-flow Doppler-assisted duplex imaging fails to detect ulceration in high-grade internal carotid artery stenosis. J Vasc Surg 23:461–465

Sitzer M, Fürst G, Fischer H, Siebler M et al (1993) Between-method correlation in quantifying internal carotid stenosis. Stroke 24:1513–1518

Sitzer M, Muller W, Siebler M, Hort W et al (1995) Plaque ulceration and lumen thrombus are the main sources of cerebral microemboli in high-grade internal carotid stenosis. Stroke 26:1231–1233

Sitzer M, Wolfram M, Jörg R et al (1996) Color flow Doppler-assisted duplex imaging fails to detect ulceration in high-grade internal carotid artery Stenosis. J Vasc Surg 24:461–465

Skillman JJ, Kent KC, Porter DH, Kim D (1990) Simultaneous occurrence of superficial and deep thrombophlebitis in the lower extremity. J Vasc Surg 11:818–824

Smets D, Debing E, De Raeve H, Van den Brande P (1997) Venous aneurysm four years after greater saphenous vein stripping. Acta Chir Belg 97:194–195

Smith JC, Watkins GE, Smith D et al (2012) Accuracy of digital subtraction angiography, computed tomography angiography, and magnetic resonance angiography in grading of carotid artery stenosis in comparison with actual measurement in an in vitro model. Ann Vasc Surg 26:338–343

Solar M, Zizka J, Krajina A et al (2011) Comparison of duplex ultrasonography and magnetic resonance imaging in the detection of significant renal artery stenosis. Acta Med (Hradec Kralove) 54:9–12

Soulez G, Therasse E, Robillard P et al (1999) The value of internal carotid systolic velocity ratio for assessing carotid artery stenosis with Doppler sonography. Am J Roentgenol 172:207–212

Souza de Oliveira IR, Widmann A, Molnar LJ et al (2002) Colour Doppler ultrasound: a new index improves the diagnosis of renal artery stenosis. Ultrasound Med Biol 36:41–47

Sperschneider H, Stein G (1996) Update Nephrologie – Teil III. Nierenarterienstenose Rationelle Diagnostik. Med Klin 91:517–520

Spies KP, Fobbe F, El-Bedewi M, Wolf KJ, Distler A, Schulte KL (1995) Color-coded duplex sonography for noninvasive diagnosis and grading of renal artery stenosis. Am J Hypertens 8:1222–1231

Spronk S, den Hoed PT, de Jonge LC et al (2005) Value of the duplex waveform at the common femoral artery for diagnosing obstructive aortoiliac disease. J Vasc Surg 42:236–242

Sprouse LR, Meier GH, Lesar CJ, DeMasi RJ, Parent FN, Gayle RG (2003) A comparison of abdominal aortic aneurysm diameter measurements obtained by ultrasound and computerized tomography: is there a difference? J Vasc Surg 38:466–471

Sprouse LR, Meier GH, Parent FN, DeMasi RJ, Glickman MH, Barber GA (2004) Is ultrasound more accurate than axial computed tomography for determination of maximal abdominal aortic aneurysm diameter? Eur J Vasc Endovasc Surg 28:28–35

Stammler F, Ysermann M, Mohr W, Kuhn C, Goethe S (2000) Value of color-coded duplex ultrasound in patients with polymyalgia rheumatica without signs of temporal arteritis. Dtsch Med Wochenschr 125:1250–1256

Stanziale SF, Wholey MH, Boules TN, Selzer F, Makaroun MS (2005) Determining in-stent stenosis of carotid arteries by duplex ultrasound criteria. J Endovasc Ther 12:346–353

Staub D (2015) Atherosclerotic plaque neovascularization and inflammation – is there a link? Vasa 44:163–165

Staub D, Canevascini R, Huegli R et al (2007) Best duplex-sonographic criteria for the assessment of renal artery stenosis – correlation with intra-arterial pressure gradient. Ultraschall Med 28:45–51

Staub D, Schinkel AF, Coll B (2010) Contrast-enhanced ultrasound imaging of the vasa vasorum: from early atherosclerosis to the identification of unstable plaques. JACC Cardiovasc Imaging 3:761–771

Staub D, Partovi S, Schinkel AFL et al (2011) Correlation of carotid artery atherosclerotic lesion echogenicity and severity at standard US with intraplaque neovascularization detected at contrast-enhanced US. Radiology 258:618–626

Staub D, Partovi S, Imfeld S et al (2013) Novel applications of contrast-enhanced ultrasound imaging in vascular medicine. Vasa 42:17–31

Stavropoulos SW, Charagundla SR (2007) Imaging techniques for detection and management of endoleaks after endovascular aortic aneurysm repair. Radiology 243:641–655

Stavros T, Harshfield D (1994) Renal Doppler, renal artery stenosis, and renovascular hypertension: direct and indirect duplex sonographic abnormalities in patients with renal artery stenosis. Ultrasound Q 12:217–263

Stavros AT, Parker SH, Yakes WF et al (1992) Segmental stenosis of the renal artery: pattern recognition of tardus and parvus abnormalities with duplex sonography. Radiology 184:487–492

Steckmeier B, Spengel FA, Küffer G et al (1989) Richtlinien zur Diagnostik und Therapie des Kompressionssyndroms der A. poplitea. Angio 11:105–113

Steffens JC, Link J, Graessnerr J (1997) Contrast-enhanced, K-space-centered, breath-hold MR angiography of renal arteries and the abdominal aorta. J Magn Reson Imaging 7:617–622

Stein PD, Hull RD, Saltzman HA, Pineo G (1993) Strategy for diagnosis of patients with suspected acute pulmonary embolism. Chest 103:1553–1559

Steinke W, Kloetzsch C, Hennerici M (1990) Carotid artery disease assessed by color Doppler flow imaging: correlation with standard Doppler sonography and angiography. Am J Roentgenol 154:1061–1068

Steinke W, Els T, Hennerici M (1992) Comparison of flow disturbances in small carotid atheroma using a multi-gate pulsed Doppler system and Doppler color flow imaging. Ultrasound Med Biol 18:11–18

Steinke W, Hennerici M, Rautenberg W, Mohr JP (1992) Symptomatic and asymptomatic high-grade carotid stenoses in Doppler color-flow imaging. Neurology 42:131–138

Steinmetz E, Rubin BG, Sanchez LA et al (2004) Type II endoleak after endovascular abdominal aortic aneurysm repair: a conservative approach with selective intervention is safe and cost-effective. J Vasc Surg 39:306–313

Steinweder C, Schutzenberger W, Fellner F (2009) 64-Detector CT angiography in renal artery stent evaluation: prospective comparison with selective catheter angiography. Radiology 252:299–305

Sterling KM, Darcy MD (1997) Stenosis of transjugular intrahepatic portosystemic shunts: presentation and management. Am J Roentgenol 168:239–244

Sterpetti AV, Schultz RD, Feldhaus RJ et al (1988) Ultrasonographic features of carotid plaque and the risk of subsequent neurologic deficits. Surgery 104:652–660

Sterpetti AV, Hunter WJ, Schultz RD (1991) Importance of ulceration of carotid plaque in determining symptoms of cerebral ischemia. J Cardiovasc Surg 32:154–158

Stevens SM, Elliott CG, Chan KJ, Egger MJ, Ahmed KM (2004) Withholding anticoagulation after negative result on duplex ultrasonography for suspected symptomatic deep venous thrombosis. Ann Intern Med 140:985–991

Stevenson SM, Woller SC, Graves KK et al (2013) Withholding anticoagulation following a single negative whole-leg ultrasound in patients at high pretest probability for deep vein thrombosis. Clin Appl Thromb Hemost 19:79–85

Stewart MT, Moritz MW, Smith RB (1986) The natural history of carotid dysplasia. J Vasc Surg 3:305–310

Stief CG, Wetterauer U (1988) Erectile responses to intracavernous papaverine and phentolamine: comparison of single and combined delivery. J Urol 140:1415–1416

Stief CG, Bähren W, Gall H, Scherb W (1988) Functional evaluation of penile hemodynamics. J Urol 139:734–737

Stief CG, Truss MC, Becker AJ, Kuczyk M, Jonas U (2000) Pharmakologische Therapiemöglichkeiten der Erektionsstörung. Dt Ärztebl 97:A-457–A-460

Stiegler H, Weichhain B, Chatzopulos D, Mathies R, Standl R, Mehnert H (1991) Untersuchungen zur Häufigkeit und Symptomatologie der Lungenembolie in Abhängigkeit von der Lokalisation der tiefen Beinvenenthrombose. Vasa 20:119–124

Stiegler H, Rotter G, Standl R et al (1993) Wertigkeit der Duplexsonographie in der Diagnose insuffizienter Vv. perforantes (Abstract). Vasa 41(suppl):15

Stiegler H, Rotter G, Standel R et al (1994) Wertigkeit der Farbduplexsonographie in der Diagnose insuffizienter Vv. perforantes. Vasa 23:109–114

Stierli P, Aeberhard P, Livers M (1992) The role of colour flow duplex screening in infrainguinal vein grafts. Eur J Vasc Surg 6: 293–298

Stock KF (2009) Ultraschalldiagnostik der Nierengefäße und der Transplantatniere. Radiologe 49:1040–1047

Strandness DE (1977) Thrombosis detection by ultrasound, plethysmography, and phlebography. Semin Nucl Med 7:213–218

Strandness DE (1990) Duplex scanning in diagnosis of renovascular hypertension. Surg Clin North Am 70:109–117

Strauch BS, O'Conell RS, Geoly KL et al (1992) Forecasting thrombosis of vascular access with Doppler color flow imaging. Am J Kidney Dis 19:554–557

Strauss AL (2001) Farbduplexsonographie der Arterien und Venen. Springer, Berlin/Heidelberg/New York

Strauss A (2002) Duplexsonographie der Arterien und Venen. Radiologe 42:235–248

Strauss AL, Beller KD (1996) Duplexsonographie mit Echokontrastmittel. Ultraschall Med 17:260–265

Strauss AL, Beller KD (1997) Arterial parameters under echo contrast enhancement. Eur J Ultrasound 5:31–38

Strauss AL, Schäberle W, Rieger H, Neuerburg-Heusler D, Roth F-J, Schoop W (1989) Duplexsonographische Untersuchungen der A. profunda femoris. Z Kardiol 78:567–572

Strauss AL, Scheffler A, Rieger H (1990) Dopplersonographische Bestimmung des Druckabfalls über peripheren Modell-arterienstenosen. Vasa 19:207–211

Strauss AL, Schäberle W, Rieger H, Roth FJ (1991) Use of duplex scan in the diagnosis of arteria profunda femoris stenosis. J Vasc Surg 13:698–704

Strauss AL, Roth FJ, Rieger H (1991) Duplexsonographische Bestimmung des Druckabfalls über Iliakaarterienstenosen. Med Klin 86:498–502

Strauss AL, Roth F-J, Rieger H (1993) Noninvasive assessment of pressure gradients across iliac artery stenoses: duplex and catheter correlative study. J Ultrasound Med 12:17–22

Strauss AL, Weber G, Karasch T et al (1995) Quantifizierung hämodynamisch wirksamer Arterienstenosen mit Farbduplexsonographie. In: Ludwig M et al (eds) Doppler–/Duplex-Sonographie in der Intensivmedizin. Bonn, Kagerer Kommunikation, p 18

Strauss AL, Ludwig M, Stein HJ et al. für den Arbeitskreis Gefäßdiagnostik der Deutschen Gesellschaft für Ultraschall in der Medizin (DEGUM), Sektion Ultraschall der Deutschen Gesellschaft für Angiologie (DGA) und Kassenärztliche Vereinigung Koblenz (1999) Empfehlungen zur Qualitätssicherung in der Ultraschalldiagnostik der Gefäße (1996) Vasa 28:135–139

Streifler JY, Benavente OR, Fox AJ, for the NASCET Group (1991) The accuracy of angiographic detection of carotid plaque ulceration. Results from the NASCET. Stroke 22:149

Stritecky-Kähler T (1994) Chirurgie der Krampfadern/Tomas Stritecky-Kähler. Thieme, Stuttgart/New York

Strotham G, Blebea J, Fowl RJ, Rosenthal GR (1995) Contralateral duplex scanning for deep venous thrombosis is unnecessary in patients with symptoms. J Vasc Surg 22:543–547

Sturzenegger M, Mattle HP, Rivoir A, Baumgartner RW (1995) Ultrasound findings in carotid artery dissection: analysis of 43 patients. Neurology 45:691–698

Subramaniam RM, Heath R, Chou T, Cox K, Davis G, Swarbrick M (2005) Deep venous thrombosis: withholding anticoagulation therapy after negative complete lower limb US findings. Radiology 237:348–352

Subramanyam BR, Balthazar EJ, Madamba MR et al (1983) Sonography of porto-systemic collaterals in portal hypertension. Radiology 146:161–166

Sullivan DE, Peter DJ, Cranley JJ (1984) Real-time B-mode venous ultrasound. J Vasc Surg 1:465

Sumner OS, Lamberth A (1979) Reliability of Doppler ultrasound in the diagnosis of acute venous thrombosis both above and below the knee. Am J Surg 138:205

Sun Z (2006) Diagnostic value of color duplex ultrasonography in the follow-up of endovascular repair of abdominal aortic aneurysm. J Vasc Interv Radiol 17:759–764

Sun Y, Cheng-Huai L, Chien-Jung L et al (2002) Carotid atherosclerosis, intima media thickness and risk factors – an analysis of 1781 asymptomatic subjects in Taiwan. Atherosclerosis 164:89–94

Sutton-Tyrrell K, Wolfson SK, Thompson T, Kelsoey SF (1992) Measurement variability in duplex scan assessment of carotid atherosclerosis. Stroke 23:215–220

Svensjö S, Björck M, Gürtelschmid M, Gidlund K, Hellberg A, Wanhainen A (2011) Low prevalence of abdominal aortic aneurysm among 65-year-old Swedish men indicates a change in the epidemiology of the disease. Circulation 124:1118–1123

Sys J, Michielsen J, Bleyn J (1997) Adventitial disease of the popliteal artery in a triathlete: A case report. Am J Sports Med 25:854–857

Sztajzel R (2005) Ultrasonographic assessment of the morphological characteristics of the carotid plaque. Swiss Med Wkly 135:635–643

Sztajzel R, Momjian-Mayor I, Comelli M et al (2006) Correlation of cerebrovascular symptoms and microembolic signals with the stratified gray-scale median analysis and color mapping of the carotid plaque. Stroke 37:824–829

Takayasu K, Moriyama N, Shima Y et al (1984) Sonographic detection of large spontaneous spleno-renal shunts and its clinical significance. Br J Radiol 57:565–570

Takiuchi S, Rakugi H, Honda K (2000) Quantitativ ultrasonic tissue characterization can identify high-risk atherosclerotic alteration in human carotid arteries. Circulation 102:766–770

Talbot SR (1982) Use of real-time imaging in identifying deep venous obstruction: a preliminary report. Bruit 6:41–42

Tamura M, Iriguchi H, Miyamoto T et al (1993) Postoperative results of ligation of crura penis for impotence with corporal venoocclusive insufficiency. Nippon Hinokika Gakkai Zasshi 84:473–478

Tamura M, Iriguchi H, Miyamoto T et al (1993) Transition of diagnosis and treatment for impotence. Nippon Hinyokika Gakkai Zasshi 84:1397–1403

Tan M, Velthuis SI, Westerbeek RE, van Rooden CJ, van der Meer FJM, Huisman MV (2010) High percentage of non-diagnostic compression ultrasonography results and the diagnosis of ipsilateral recurrent proximal deep vein thrombosis. J Thromb Haemost 8: 848–850

Tan M, Mol GC, van Rooden CJ, Klok FA, Westerbeek RE, Iglesias Del Sol A, van de Ree MA, de Roos A, Huisman MV (2014) Magnetic resonance direct thrombus imaging differentiates acute recurrent ispilateral deep vein thrombosis from residual thrombosis. Blood 124:623–627

Taniguchi N, Itoh K, Honda M et al (1997) Comparative ultrasonographic and angiographic study of carotid arterial lesions in Takayasu's arteritis. Angiology 48:9–20

Tartarini G, Bertoli D, Baglini R, Balbarini A, Mariani M (1988) Diagnosis of aortic dissection by color-coded Doppler. J Nucl Med 32:127–130

Taylor DC, Kettler MD, Moneta GL et al (1988) Duplex ultrasound in the diagnosis of renal artery stenosis: a prospective evaluation. J Vasc Surg 7:363–369

Taylor PR, Wolfe JHN, Tyrrell MR, Mansfield AO, Nicolaides AN, Houston RE (1990) Graft stenosis: justification for 1-year surveillance. Br J Surg 77:1125–1128

Taylor PR, Tyrell MR, Crofton M et al (1992) Colour flow imaging in the detection of femoro-distal graft and native artery stenosis: improved criteria. Eur J Vasc Surg 6:232–236

Taylor KJW, Burns PN, Wells PNT (1995) Clinical applications of Doppler ultrasound. Raven, New York, pp 1–33

Tegos TJ, Sabetai MM, Nicolaides AN, Pare G, Elatrozy TS, Dhanjil S (2000a) Comparability of the ultrasonic tissue characteristics of carotid plaques. J Ultrasound Med 14:399–407

Tegos TJ, Sohail M, Sabetai MM et al (2000b) Echomorphologic and histopathologic characteristics of unstable carotid plaques. AJNR Am J Neuroradiol 21:1937–1944

Tegos TJ, Stavropulos P, Sabetai MM (2001) Determinants of carotic plaque instability: echoicity versus heterogenity. Eur J Vasc Endovasc Surg 22:22–30

Teichgräber U, Gebel M, Benter T, Manns MP (1997) Duplexsonographische Charakterisierung des Lebervenenflusses bei Gesunden. Ultraschall Med 18:267–271

Tellis VA, Kohlberg WI, Bhat DJ, Driscoll B, Veith FJ (1979) Expanded polytetrafluoroethylene graft fistula for chronic hemodialysis. Ann Surg 189:101–105

Telman G, Kouperberg E, Sprecher E et al (2006) Duplex ultrasound verified by angiography in patients with primary and restenosis of internal carotid artery. Ann Vasc Surg 20:478–481

Ten Cate-Hoek AJ, Ten Cate H, Tordoir J et al (2010) Individually tailored duration of elastic compression therapy in relation to incidence of the postthrombotic syndrome. J Vasc Surg 52:132–138

Ten Kate GL, Sijbrands EJ et al (2010) Noninvasive imaging of the Vulnerable Atherosclerotic Plaque. Curr Probl Cardiol 25:556–591

Tessler FN, Gehring BJ, Gomes AS et al (1991) Diagnosis of portal vein thrombosis: value of color Doppler imaging. Am J Roentgenol 157:293–296

Textor SC (1994) Renovascular hypertension. Endocrinol Metab Clin N Am 23:235–253

Thalhammer C, Aschwander M, Mayr M et al (2006) Duplex sonography after living donor kidney transplantation: new insights in the early postoperativ phase. Ultraschall Med 27:141–145

Thanos J, Rebeira M, Shragge BW, Urbach D (2008) Vascular ultrasound screening for asymptomatic abdominal arotic aneurysm. Health Policy 4:75–83

Theodotou BC, Whaley R, Mahaley MS (1987) Complications following transfemoral cerebral angiography for cerebral ischemia: report of 159 angiograms and correlation with surgical risk. Surg Neurol 28:90–92

Thetter O (1987) Das Kompressionssyndrom des Arcus tendineus M. solei. In: Heberer G, Van Dongen RJAM (Hrsg) Gefäßchirurgie. Springer, Berlin/Heidelberg/New York, pp 600–602, Kirschnersche allgemeine und spezielle Operationslehre, Bd 11

Thiele BL, Strandness DE Jr (1983) Accuracy of angiographic quantification of peripheral atherosclerosis. Prog Cardiovasc Dis 26:223–236

Thiele BL, Bandyk DF, Zierler RE, Strandness DE Jr (1983) A systematic approach to the assessment of aortoiliacal disease. Arch Surg 118:477–481

Thomas ML, Mc Donald LM (1978) Complications of ascending phlebography of the leg. Br Med J 2:317

Thomas CHR, Röder H-U, Möser GH (1989) Diagnostische Wertigkeit der Angiodynographie bei pulsierenden Raumforderungen. Fortschr Röntgenstr 150:454–457

Thomas PR, Shaw JC, Asthon HA, Kay DN, Scott RA (1994) Accuracy of ultrasound in a screening programme for abdominal aortic aneurysms. J Med Screen 1:3–6

Thompson MM, Boyle JR, Hartshorn T et al (1998) Comparison of computed tomography and duplex imaging in assessing aortic morphology following endovascular aneurysm repair. Br J Surg 85:346–350

Tian J, Hu S, Sun Y et al (2013) Vasa vasorum and plaque progression, and responses to atorvastatin in a rabbit model of artheriosclerosis: contrast-enhanced ultrasound imaging and intravascular ultrasound study. Tian. Heart 99:48–54

Tinder TN, Bandyk DF (2009) Detection of imminent vein graft occlusion: what is the optimal surveillance program? Semin Vasc Surg 22:252–260

Tinder CN, Chavanpun JP, Bandyk DF et al (2008) Efficacy of duplex ultrasound surveillance after infrainguinal vein bypass may be enhanced by identification of characteristics predictive of graft stenosis development. J Vasc Surg 48:623–628

Tonelli M, James M, Wiebe N et al (2008) Ultrasound monitoring to detect access stenosis in hemodialysis patients: a systematic review. Am J Kidney Dis 61:630–640

Tordoir JHM, De Bruin HG, Hoeneveld H, Eikelboom BC, Kitslaar PJ (1989) Duplex ultrasound scanning in the assessment of arteriovenous fistulas created for hemodialysis access: comparison with digital subtraction angiography. J Vasc Surg 10:122–128

Tordoir J, Canaud B, Haage P et al (2007) EBPG on vascular access. Nephrol Dial Transplant 22:ii88–ii117

Toursarkissian B, Allen BT, Petrinec D (1997) Spontaneous closure of selected iatrogenic pseudoaneurysms and arteriovenous fistulae. J Vasc Surg 25:803–808

Tranquet T, Bescos JM, Reparaz B (1989) Noninvasive methods in the diagnosis of isolated superior mesenteric vein thrombosis: US and CT. Gastrointest Radiol 14:321–325

Tratting S, Hübsch P, Schuster H, Pötzleitner D (1990) Color-coded Doppler imaging of normal vertebral arteries. Stroke 21:1222–1225

Tratting S, Hübsch P, Schwaighofer B, Karnel F, Eilenberger M (1991) Vaskuläre Raumforderungen der Arteria carotis – Nachweis mit der farbkodierten Dopplersonographie. Ultraschall Med 12:70–73

Tratting S, Schwaighofer B, Hübsch P, Schwarz M, Kainberger F (1991) Color-coded Doppler sonography of vertebral arteries. J Ultrasound Med 10:221–226

Tratting S, Hübsch P, Frühwald F (1992) Farbkodierte Dopplersonographie der Vertebralarterien. In: Frühwald F, Blackwell DE (Hrsg) Atlas der farbkodierten Doppersonographie. Gefäße und Weichteile des Halses und der oberen Extremität. Springer, Wien/New York, p 138

Tratting S, Plötzleitner D, Hübsch P, Kaha K, Matula CH, Magometschnigg H (1992) Nicht-invasive Verlaufskontrolle mittels farbkodierter Doppler-Sonographie nach operativen Eingriffen an den extrakraniellen hirnversorgenden Arterien. Fortschr Röntgenstr 156: 224–227

Treiman GS, Lawrence PF, Bhirangi K, Gazak CE (1999) Effect of outflow level and maximum graft diameter on velocity parameters of reversed vein grafts. J Vasc Surg 30:16–25

Trickett JP, Scott RA, Tilney HS (2002) Screening and management of asymptomatic popliteal aneurysms. J Med Screen 9:92–93

Trum JW, Gubler FM, Laan R, van der Veen F (1996) The value of palpation, varicoscreen contact thermography and color Doppler ultrasound in the diagnosis of varicocele. Hum Reprod 11:1232–1235

Tsang WY, Chan JK (1993) The family of epithelioid vascular tumors. Histol Histopathol 8:187–212

Tsilimparis N, Hanack U, Yousefi S, Alevizakos P, Rückert RI (2007) Cystic adventitial disease of the popliteal artery: an argument of the developmental theory. J Vasc Surg 45:1249–1252

Tsolakis IA, Walvatne CS, Caldwell MD (1998) Cystic adventitial disease of the popliteal artery: diagnosis and treatment. EJVES 13: 188–194

Tucker RM, Lebbarthe DR (1977) Frequency of surgical treatment for hypertension in adults in the Mayo Clinic from 1973–1975. Mayo Clin Proc 52:542–555

Tucker RM, Strog CG, Brennan LA, Sheps SG (1978) Renovascular hypertension: relationship of surgical curability to renin-angiotensin activity. Mayo Clin Proc 53:373–377

Turmel-Rodrigues L, Pengloan J, Baudin S et al (2000) Treatment of stenosis and thrombosis in haemodialysis fistulas and grafts by interventional radiology. Nephrol Dial Transplant 15:2029–2036

Turmel-Rodrigues L, Mouton A, Birmele B et al (2001) Salvage of immature forearm fistulas for haemodialysis by interventional radiology. Nephrol Dial Transplant 16:2365–2371

Turton EP, Scott DJ, Richards SP et al (1999) Duplex-derived evidence of reflux after varicose vein surgery: neoreflux or neovascularisation? Eur J Vasc Endovasc Surg 17:230–233

Twomey A, Twomey EM, Wilinks RA (1984) Unrecognized aneurysm disease in male hypertensive patients. Br J Surg 71:307–308

Ubbink DT, Legemate DA, Llull JB (2002) Color-flow duplex scanning of the leg arteries by use of a new echo-enhancing agent. J Vasc Surg 35:392–396

Uematsu M, Okada M (1999) Primary venous aneurysms: case reports. Angiology 50:239–244

UK Small Aneurysm Trial Participants (1998) Mortality results for randomised controlled trial of early elective surgery or ultrasonographic surveillance for small abdominal aortic aneurysms. Lancet 352:1649–1660

Umemura A, Yamada K (2000) B-mode flow imaging of the carotid artery. Stroke 32:2055–2057

Umscheid T et al (2001) Nachuntersuchungen bei Patienten nach endovaskulärer Aortenprothesen-Durchführung, Anforderungen und Probleme. Gefässchirurgie 6:185–193

Urbancic A, Buturović-Ponikvar J (2001) Emergency intra- and perioperative doppler after kidney transplantation – a guide for immediate surgical intervention. Transplant Proc 33:3320–3321

Uthoff H, Staub D, Meyerhans A et al (2008) Intima media thickness and carotid resistive index: progression over 6 years and predictive value for cardiovascular events. Ultraschall Med 29:604–610

Uthoff H, Schwob A, Staub D et al (2010) Thrombophlebitis – what else? Ultraschall Med 31:335–338

Vachharajani TJ (2012) Diagnosis of arteriovenous fistula dysfunction. Semin Dial 25:445–450

Valentine RJ (2003) Asymptomatic internal carotid artery aneurysm. J Vasc Surg 37:210

Valji K, Bookstein JJ (1993) Diagnosis of arteriogenic impotence: efficacy of duplex sonography as a screening tool. Am J Roentgenol 160:65–69

Valois de JC, van Schaik CC, Verzijlbergen F et al (1990) Contrast venography: from gold standard to "golden backup" in clinically suspected deep vein thrombosis. Eur J Radiol 11:131–137

Van Bemmelen PS, Bedford G, Beach K, Strandness DE (1989) Quantitative segmental evaluation of venous valvular reflux with duplex ultrasound scanning. J Vasc Surg 10:425–431

Van Bockel JH, van Schilfgaarde R, Van Brummelen P, Terpsta JL (1989) Renovascular hypertension. Surg Gynecol Obstet 169:467–478

Van Damme H, Demoulin JC, Zicot M, Creemers E, Trotteur G, Limet R (1992) Pathological aspects of carotid plaques. J Cardiovasc Surg 33:46–53

Van Damme H, Sakalihasan N, Limet R (1999) Fibromuscular dysplasia of the internal carotid artery: personal experience with 13 cases and literature review. Acta Chir Belg 99:163–168

Van der Hulst VP, van Baalen J, Kool LS et al (1996) Renal artery stenosis: endovascular flow wire study for validation of Doppler US. Radiology 200:165–168

Van der Velde EF, Toll DB, Ten Cate-Hoek AJ et al (2011) Comparing the diagnostic performance of 2 clinical decision rules to rule out deep vein thrombosis in primary care patients. Ann Fam Med 9:31–36

Van der Zaag ES, Legemate DA, Nguyen T, Balm R, Jacobs MJ (1998) Aortoiliac reconstructive surgery based upon the results of duplex scanning. Eur J Vasc Endovasc Surg 16:383–389

Van Gemmeren D, Fobbe F, Ruhnke-Trautmann M (1991) Diagnostik tiefer Beinvenenthrombosen mit der farbkodierten Duplexsonographie und sonographische Altersbestimmung der Thrombose. Z Kardiol 80:523–528

Van Jaarsveld BC, Pieterman H, van Dijk LC et al (1999) Inter-observer variability in the angiographic assessment of renal artery stenosis. DRASTIC study group. Dutch Renal Artery Stenosis Intervention Cooperative. J Hypertens 17(12 Pt 1):1731–1736

Van Petersen AS, Meerwaldt R, Kolkman JJ et al (2013) The influence of respiration on criteria for transabdominal duplex examination of the splanchnic arteries in patients with suspected chronic splanchnic ischemia. J Vasc Surg 57:1603–1611

Van Ramshorst B, Legemate DA, Verzijlbergen JF et al (1991) Duplex scanning in the diagnosis of acute deep vein thrombosis of the lower extremity. Eur J Vasc Surg 5:255–260

Van Ramshorst B, van Bemmelen PS, Hoeneveld H, Eikelboom BC (1994) The development of valvular incompetence after deep vein thrombosis: a follow-up study with duplex scanning. J Vasc Surg 20:1059–1066

Vandendriessche M, Thiery L (1986) Aneurisma van de vena poplitea. Acta Chir Belg 86:37–40

Vasbinder GB, Nelemans PJ, Kessels AG (2001) Diagnostic tests for renal artery stenosis in patients suspected of having renovascular hypertension: a meta-analysis. Ann Intern Med 135:401–411

Vasbinder GB, Nelemans PJ, Kessels AG (2004) Renal Artery Diagnostic Imaging Study in Hypertension (RADISH) Study Group. Accuracy of computed tomographic angiography and magnetic resonance angiography for diagnosing renal artery stenosis. Ann Intern Med 141:674–682

Vascular Access 2006 Work Group (2006) Clinical practice guidelines for vascular access. Am J Kidney Dis 48:S176–S247

Vasdekis SN, Clarke GH, Hobbs JT, Nicolaides AN (1989) Evaluation of non-invasive and invasive methods in the assessment of short saphenous termination. Br J Surg 76:929–932

Vasdekis SN, Clarke GH, Nikolaides A (1989) Quantification of venous reflux by means of duplex scanning. J Vasc Surg 10:670–677

Vasovic L, Milenkovic Z, Jovanovic I et al (2008) Hypoglossal artery: A review of normal and pathological features. Neurosurg Rev 31:385–396

Vavuranakis M, Sigala F, Vrachatis DA et al (2013) Quantitativ analysis of carotid plaque vasa vasorum by CEUS and correlation with histology after endarterectomy. Vasa 42:184–195

Vermeulen EGJ, Umans U, Rijbroek A, Rauwerda JA (2000) Percutaneous duplex-guided thrombin injection for treatment of iatrogenic femoral artery pseudoaneurysms. Eur J Vasc Endovasc Surg 20:302–304

Vicente DC, Kazmers A (1999) Acute mesenteric ischemia. Curr Opin Cardiol 14:453–458

Vidakovic R, Feringa HH, Kuiper RJ et al (2007) Comparison with computed tomography of two ultrasound devices for diagnosis of abdominal aortic aneurysm. Am J Cardiol 100:1786–1791

Visser K, Idu MM, Buth J, Engel GL, Hunink MG (2001) Duplex scan surveillance during the first year after infrainguinal autologous vein bypass grafting surgery: costs and clinical outcomes compared with other surveillance programs. J Vasc Surg 33:123–130

Vitovec J (1976) Aneurysma venae poplitae. Cesk Radiol 30:328–340

Vogel P, Laing FD, jr JRB, Wing VW (1987) Deep venous thrombosis of the lower extremity: US evaluation. Radiology 163:747–751

Voiculescu A, Hollenbeck M, Müller B et al (2005) Reversed diastolic flow after renal transplantation. A sign for a poor prognosis. Ultraschall Med 26:S73

Vollmar J (1982) Rekonstruktive Chirurgie der Arterien. Thieme, Stuttgart, pp 137–202

Von Behren P (1998) Harmonic imaging. In: Bogdahn U, Becker G, Schlachetzki F (eds) Echosignalverstärker und transkranielle Farbduplex-Sonographie. Blackwell Wiss.-Verlag, Berlin/Wien, pp 183–191

Vosshenrich R, Kopka L, Castillo E, Bottcher U, Graessner J, Grabbe E (1998) Electrocardiograph-triggered two-dimensional time-of-flight versus optimized contrast-enhanced three-dimensional MR angiography of the peripheral arteries. Magn Reson Imaging 16:887–892

Wagner G, Kaplan HS (1993) The new injection treatment for impotence. Brunner/Mazel, New York, pp 85–93

Waibel P, Fahrländer J, Ludin H (1966) Die chirurgische Behandlung der Angina abdominalis. Bedeutung der Diagnose in der Prophylaxe des arteriellen Mesenterialinfarktes. Schweiz med Wschr 96:10

Wain RA, Berdejo GL, Delvalle WN et al (1999) Can duplex scan arterial mapping replace contrast arteriography as the test of choice before infrainguinal revascularization? J Vasc Surg 29:100–107

Wallner B, Kratzsch G, Friedrich JM, Roth J (1989) Die intraarterielle DSA der Handarterien in der Diagnostik entzündlicher Bindegewebserkrankungen. RöFo 151:565–568

Walter P, Lindemann W, Koch P, Feifel G (1992) Der akute Mesenterialinfarkt. Klinikarzt 21:457–463

Walter P, Kubale R, Gross G, Beraneck E (1999) Das Kompressionssyndrom des Truncus coeliacus. Gefässchirurgie 4:28–33

Wang H, Spinner RJ, Amrami KK (2007) Adventitial cyst of the radial artery with a wrist joint connection. J Hand Surg 32:126–130

Wanhainen A, Berqvist D, Björck M (2002) Measuring the abdominal aorta with ultrasonography and computed tomography – difference and variability. Eur J Vasc Endovasc Surg 24:428–434

Wanhainen A, Lundkvist J, Bergqvist D, Björck M (2005) Cost-effectiveness of different screening strategies for abdominal aortic aneurysm. J Vasc Surg 41:741–751

Ward B, Baker AC, Humphrey VF (1997) Nonlinear propagation applied to the improvement of resolution in diagnostic medical ultrasound. J Acoust Soc Am 101:143–154

Wardlaw JM, Chappell FM, Best JJK, Wartolowska K, Berry E, on behalf of the NHS Research and Development Health Technology Assessment Carotid Stenosis Imaging Group (2006) Non-invasive imaging compared with intra-arterial angiography in the diagnosis of symptomatic carotid stenosis: a meta-analysis. Lancet 367:1503–1512

Watanabe F, Yoshida T, Akizuki M, Mukai M (1993) Development of multiple subcutaneous nodules in a patient with rheumatic arthritis during methotrexate therapy. Ryumachi 33:74–79

Waugh J, Sacharias N (1992) Arteriographic complications in the DSA era. Radiology 182:243–246

Webber GW, Jang J, Gustavson S (2007) Contemporary management of postcatheterization pseudoaneurysms. Circulation 115:2666–2674

Weber J, May R (1990) Funktionelle Phlebologie. Thieme, Stuttgart

Weber G, Strauss AL, Rieger H, Scheffler A, Eisenhoffer J (1992) Validation of Doppler measurement of pressure gradients across peripheral model arterial stenosis. J Vasc Surg 16:10–16

Wein AJ, van Arsdalen K, Hanno PM, Levin RM (1991) Anatomy of male sexual function. In: Jonas U, Thon WF, Stief CG (eds) Erectile dysfunction. Springer, Berlin/Heidelberg/New York, pp 3–15

Weingarten MS, Branas CC, Czeredarzuk M, Schmidt JD, Wolferth CC (1993) Distribution and quantification of venous reflux in lower extremity chronic venous stasis disease with duplex scanning. J Vasc Surg 18:753–759

Weinmann S, Sandbichler P, Flora G (1986) Aneurysma der Vena poplitea als Quelle der Lungenembolie. Langenbecks Arch Chir 367:107–112

Weinmann EE, Chayen D, Kobzantzev ZV, Zaretsky M, Bass A (2002) Treatment of postcatheterisation false aneurysms: ultrasound-guided compression vs ultrasound-guided thrombin injection. Eur J Vasc Endovasc Surg 23:68–72

Weiss S, Enzinger F (1982) Epitheloid hemangioendothelioma: A vascular tumor often mistaken for a carcinoma. Cancer 50:970–981

Welch HJ, Young CM, Semegran AB, Iafrati MD, Mackey WC, O'Donnell TF (1996) Duplex assessment of venous reflux and chronic venous insufficiency: The significance of deep venous reflux. J Vasc Surg 24:755–762

Welger D, Müller JH (1988) Assoziierte thrombotische Prozesse des oberflächlichen, perforierenden und intramuskulären Venensystems bei Patienten mit akuter Phlebothrombose der unteren Extremitäten. Z Ges Inn Med Grenzgeb 43:15–18

Wells DH (1992) Physical and technical aspects of colour flow ultrasound. In: Labs KH et al (eds) Diagnostic vascular ultrasound. Arnold, London, pp 145–152

Wells PS, Lensing AWA, Davidson BL, Prins MH, Hirsh J (1995) Accuracy of ultrasound for the diagnosis of deep venous thrombosis in asymptomatic patients after orthopedic surgery. Ann Intern Med 122:47–53

Wells PS, Hirsh J, Anderson DR, Lensing AW, Foster G et al (1995) Accuracy of clinical assessment of deep vein thrombosis. Lancet 345:1326–1330

Wells PS, Anderson DR, Bormanis J et al (1997) Value of assessment of pretest probability of deep-vein thrombosis in clinical management. Lancet 350:1795–1798

Wells PS, Anderson DR, Rodger M et al (2003) Evaluation of D-dimer in the diagnosis of suspect deep-vein thrombosis. N Engl J Med 349:1227–1235

Wermke W, Gassmann B (1998) Tumordiagnostik der Leber mit Echosignalverstärker. Springer

Weskot H, Özden N, Von Leitner E (2005) Stellenwert der kontrastverstärkten Sonograpie der ambulanten Diagnostik: Zuverlässigkeit und Ökonomie. Ultraschall Med 26:S73

Wesley S, Moore MD (2003) For severe carotid stenosis found on ultrasound, further arterial evaluation is unnecessary. Stroke 34:1816–1817

Westerband A, Mils JK, Kistler S, Berman SS, Hunter GC, Marek JM (1997) Prospective validation of threshold criteria for intervention in infrainguinal vein undergoing duplex surveillance. Ann Vasc Surg 11:44–48

Westerbeek RE, Van Rooden CJ, Tan M, Van Gils AP, Kok S, De Bats MJ, De Roos A, Huisman MV (2008) Magnetic resonance direct thrombus imaging of the evolution of acute deep vein thrombosis of the leg. J Thromb Haemost 6:1087–1092

Wheeler AHB (1985) Diagnosis of deep vein thrombosis. Am J Surg 150:7–14

Whelan TJ (1984) Popliteal artery entrapment. In: Rutherford RB (ed) Vascular surgery. Saunders, Philadelphia

White RH (2012) Identifying risk factors for venous thromboembolism. Circulation 125:2051–2053

White GH et al (2000) How should endotension be defined? History of a concept and evolution of a new term. J Endovasc Ther 7:435–438

Whitehead ED, Klyde BJ, Zussman S, Salkin P (1990) Diagnostic evaluation of impotence. Postgrad Med 88:123–26, 129–136

Whyman MR, Hoskins PR, Leng GC et al (1993) Accuracy and reproducibility of duplex ultrasound imaging in a phantom model of femoral artery stenosis. J Vasc Surg 17:524–530

Whyman MR, Ruckley CV, Fowkes FG (1993) A prospective study of the natural history of femoropopliteal artery stenosis using duplex ultrasound. Eur J Vasc Surg 7:444–447

Widder B (1999) Doppler- und Duplexsonographie der hirnversorgenden Arterien. Springer, Berlin/Heidelberg/New York/Tokyo

Widder B, Görtler M (2004) Doppler- und Duplexsonographie der hinversorgenden Arterien. Springer, Heidelberg

Widder B, von Reutern GM, Neuerburg-Heusler D (1986) Morphologische und dopplersonographische Kriterien zur Bestimmung von Stenosierungsgraden an der A. carotis interna. Ultraschall Med 7:70–75

Widder B, Berger G, Bressmer H et al (1988) Reproduzierbarkeit sonographischer Kriterien zur morphologischen Beurteilung von Karotisstenosen. Ultraschall Klin Prax 5(Suppl 1)

Widder B, Arnolds B, Drews S (1990) Terminologie der Ultraschallgefäßdiagnostik. Ultraschall Med 11:214–218

Widder B, Berger G, Hackspacher J et al (1990) Reproduzierbarkeit sonographischer Kriterien zur Charakterisierung von Karotisstenosen. Ultraschall Med 11:56–61

Widder B, Paulat K, Hackspacher J et al (1990) Morphological characterization of carotid artery stenosis by ultrasound duplex scanning. Ultrasound Med Biol 16:349–354

Widder B, Kleiser B, Hackspacher J, Reuchlin G, Dürr A (1992) Sonomorphological prediction of progressive carotid artery stenoses. In: Oka M et al (eds) Recent advances in neurosonology. Elsevier, Amsterdam, pp 425–429

Widmann MD, Sumpio BE (1992) Persistent hypoglossal artery: an anomaly leading to false-positive carotid duplex sonography. Ann Vasc Surg 6:176–178

Wijeyaratne SM, Jarvis S, Stead LA et al (2003) A new method for characterizing carotid plaque: multiple cross-sectional view echomorphology. J Vasc Surg 37:778–784

Wilbur AC, Spigos DG (1986) Adventitial cyst of the popliteal artery: CT-guided percutaneous aspiration. J Comput Assist Tomogr 10: 161–163

Wilkinson R (1996) Epidemiology and clinical manifestation. In: Novick A, Scoble J, Hamilton G (eds) Renal vascular disease. Saunders, London/Philadelphia/Toronto, pp 171–184

Willoteaux S, Faivre-Pierret M, Moranne O (2006) Fibromuscular dysplasia of the main renal arteries: comparison of contrast-enhanced MR angiography with digital subtraction angiography. Radiology 241:922–929

Wilson YG, Davies AH, Currie IC, Morgan M, McGrath C, Baird RN (1996) Vein graft stenosis: incidence and intervention. Eur J Vasc Endovasc Surg 11:164–169

Wittenberg G, Schindler T, Tschammler A, Kenn W, Hahn D (1998) Wertigkeit der farbkodierten Duplexsonographie bei der Beurteilung von Armgefäßen -Arterien und Hämodialyseshunt. Ultraschall Med 19:22–27

Wittenberg G, Kenn W, Tschammler A (1999) Spiral CT angiography. Eur Radiol 9:546–551

Wixon CL, Mills JL, Westerband A, Hughes JD, Ihnat DM (2000) An economic appraisal of lower extremity bypass graft maintenance. J Vasc Surg 32:1–12

Wolf KJ, Fobbe F (1993) Farbkodierte Duplexsonographie. Thieme, Stuttgart

Wolf Y et al (2000) Duplex ultrasound scanning versus computed tomographic angiography for postoperative evaluation of endovascular abdominal aortic aneurysm repair. J Vasc Surg 32:1142–1148

Wölfle KD, Neudert S, Mayer B, Storm G, Bruijnen H, Loeprecht H (1992) Duplexsonographische Überwachung von infrainguinalen arteriellen Rekonstruktionen: Kann dadurch ein drohender Bypassverschluss erkannt werden? Zentrbl Chir 117:540–546

Wölfle KD, Bruijnen H, Mayer B, Loeprecht H (1994) Verlaufskontrolle infrainguinaler Bypassoperationen: Bedeutung von systolischer Spitzengeschwindigkeit und Arm-Knöchel-Index für die Bewertung femorodistaler Rekonstruktionen. Vasa 23:349–356

Wölfle KD, Bruijnen H, Limmer S, Loeprecht H (1999) Autologe Distal-origin-Bypasses zur Überbrückung infrapoplitealer Verschlussprozesse bei Diabetikern mit kritischer Fußischämie. Gefässchirurgie 4:220–228

Wolverson MK, Bashiti HM, Peterson GJ (1983) Ultrasonic tissue characterization of atheromatous plaques using a high resolution real time scanner. Ultrasound Med Biol 6:669–709

Wong JK, Duncan JL, Nichols DM (2003) Whole-leg duplex mapping for varicose veins: observations on patterns of reflux in recurrent and primary legs, with clinical correlation. Eur J Vasc Endovasc Surg 25:267–275

Wong TH, Tay KH, Sebastian MG, Tan SG (2013) Duplex ultrasonography arteriography as first-line investigation for peripheral vascular disease. Singap Med J 54:271–274

Woodcock JP, Fitzgerald DE, Labs KH et al (1992) Consensus on problem areas in diagnostic vascular ultrasound. In: Labs KH et al (eds) Diagnostic vascular ultrasound. Arnold, London, pp 321–325

Woods VL, Zvaifler NJ (1985) Pathogenesis of systemic lupus erythematosus. In: Kelly WN, Harris ED, Ruddy SR, Siedge CB (eds) Textbook of rheumatology, 3rd edn. Saunders, Philadelphia/London/Toronto, pp 1077–1100

Wuppermann T (1986) Varizen, Ulcus cruris und Thrombose. Springer, Berlin/Heidelberg/New York/Tokyo

Wuppermann T, Exler U, Mellmann J, Kestilä M (1981) Noninvasive quantitative measurement of regurgitation insufficiency of the superior saphenous vein by Doppler-ultrasound: a comparison with clinical examination and phlebography. Vasa 10:24–27

Wuppermann T, Knospe E, Reiss HD, Mellmann J (1981) Diagnostik insuffizienter Venae perforantes: Trefferquoten verschiedener Untersuchungsmethoden bei der primären Varikosis. In: May R, Partsch H, Staubesand J (eds) Venae perforantes. Urban & Schwarzenberg, Munich

Xiong L, Deng YB, Zhu Y (2009) Correlation of carotid plaque neovascularization detected by using contrast-enhanced US with clinical symptoms. Radiology 251:583–589

Yan F, Li X, Jin Q (2012) Ultrasonic imaging of endothelial CD81 expression using CD81-targeted contrast agents in in vitro and in vivo studies. Ultrasound Med Biol 38:670–680

Yao JST, Van Bellen B, Flinn WR, Bergan JJ (1982) Aneurysms of the venous system. In: Bergan JJ, Yao JST (eds) Aneurysms, diagnosis and treatment. Grune & Stratton, New York, pp 515–529

Yao JST, Flinn WR, McCarty WJ, Bergan JJ (1986) The role of noninvasive testing in the evaluation of chronic venous problems. World J Surg 10:911–918

Yeh H-C, Stancato-Pasik A, Ramos R, Rabinowitz JG (1996) Paraumbilical venous collateral circulations: colour Doppler ultrasound features. J Clin Ultrasound 24:359–366

Yilmaz E, Ilgit E, Taner D (1995) Primitive persistent carotid-basilar and carotid vertebral anastomosis. A report of seven cases and a review of the literature. Cin Anat 8:36–43

Yuasa H, Mitake S, Oguri T et al (2005) A case of transient blindness due to severe stenosis of the internal carotid artery with persistent primitive hypoglossal artery (PPHA). Rinsho Shinkeigaku 45:579–582

Yurcel EK, Fisher JS, Egglin TK, Geller SC, Waltman AC (1991) Isolated calf venous thrombosis: diagnosis with compression ultrasound. Radiology 179:443–446

Yurdakul M, Tola M, Cumhur T (2006) B-flow imaging for assessment of 70% to 99% internal carotid artery stenosis based on residual lumen diameter. J Ultrasound Med 25:211–215

Zachrisson BE, Norback B (1974) Phlebographic diagnosis of a soleus vein aneurysm. Vasa 3:308

Zannetti S, De Rango P, Parente B et al (2000) Role of duplex scan in endoleak detection after endoluminal abdominal aortic aneurysm repair. Eur J Vasc Endovasc Surg 19:531–535

Zanow J, Petzold K, Petzold M et al (2006) Flow reduction in high-flow arteriovenous access using intraoperative flow monitoring. J Vasc Surg 44:1273–1278

Zarins CK, Giddens DP, Bharadvaj BK (1983) Carotid bifurcation atherosclerosis; quantitative correlation of plaque localization with flow velocity profiles and wall shear stress. Circ Res 53:502–514

Zeller T, Frank U, Späth M (2001) Farbduplexsonographische Darstellbarkeit von Nierenarterien und Erkennung hämodynamisch relevanter Nierenarterienstenosen. Ultraschall Med 22:116–121

Zeller T, Frank U, Müller C et al (2003) Predictors of improved renal function after percutaneous stent-supported angioplasty of severe atherosclerotic ostial renal artery stenosis. Circulation 108: 2244–2249

Zhang Z, Berg M, Ikonen A (2005) Carotid stenosis degree in CT angiography: assessment based on luminal area versus luminal diameter measurements. Eur Radiol 15:2359–2365

Zhang WW, Harris LM, Dryjski ML (2006) Should conventional angiography be the gold standard for carotid stenosis? J Endovasc Ther 13:723–728

Zhou W, Felkai DD, Evans M, McCoy SA, Lin PH, Kougias P et al (2008) Ultrasound criteria for severe in-stent restenosis following carotid artery stenting. J Vasc Surg 47:74–80

Zierler RE (1999) Vascular surgery without arteriography: use of duplex ultrasound. Cardiovasc Surg 7:74–82

Zierler RE (2001) Is duplex scanning the best screening test for renal artery stenosis? Semin Vasc Surg 14:177–185

Zöllner N, Zoller WG, Spengel FA, Weigold B, Schewe CK (1991) The spontaneous course of small abdominal aortic aneurysms. Aneurysmal growth rates and life expectancy. Klin Wochenschr 69: 633–639

Zuber M, Koch B, Gause A, Pfreundschuh M (1996) Diagnose- und Klassifikationskriterien in der Rheumatologie: Kollagenosen. Dtsch Med Wochenschr 121:913–919

Zwiebel WJ (1987) Spectrum analysis in carotid Doppler sonography. Ultrasound Med Biol 13:625–636

Zwiebel WJ (1997) Doppler parameters for carotid stenosis. Semin Ultrasound CT MR 18:66

Zwiebel WJ (2000) Vascular disorders of the liver. In: Zwiebel WJ (ed) Introduction to vascular ultrasonography. Saunders, Philadelphia/London/Toronto, pp 431–454

Zwolak RM (1999) Can duplex ultrasound replace arteriography in screening for mesenteric ischemia. Semin Vasc Surg 12:252–260

Zwolak RM (2000) Arterial duplex scanning. In: Rutherford RB (ed) Vascular surgery, 5th edn. Saunders, Philadelphia/London/Sydney, pp 192–214

Zwolak RM, Fillinger MF, Walsh DB et al (1998) Mesenteric and celiac duplex scanning: a validity study. J Vasc Surg 27:1078–1108

Subject Index

A

B

C

D

E

F

G

H

I

R

S

T

Z

Printed by Printforce, the Netherlands